D1209266

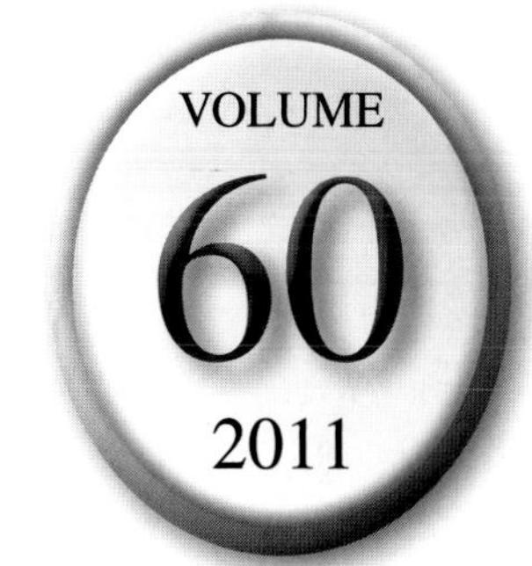

Instructional Course Lectures

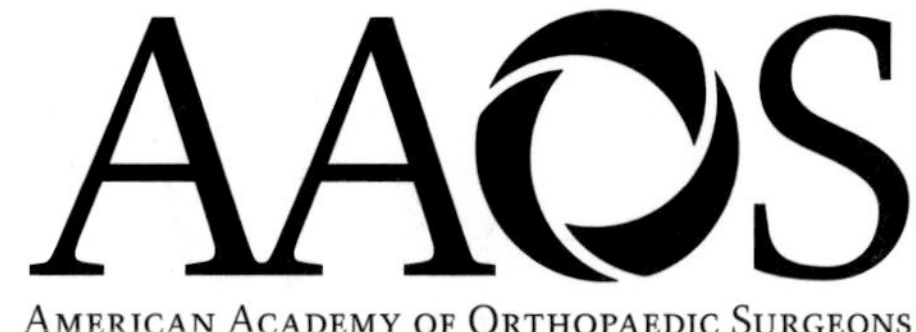

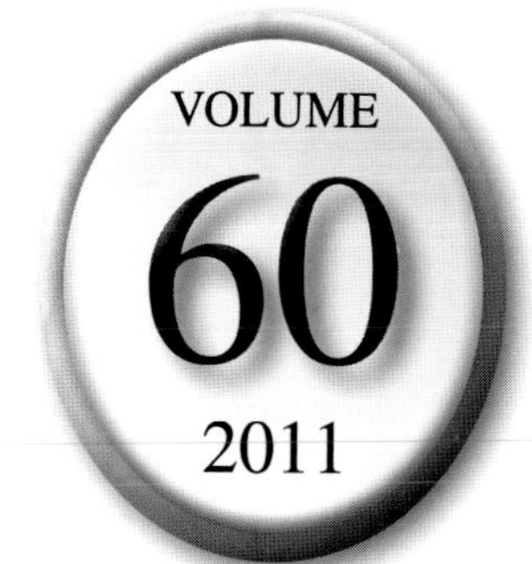

Instructional Course Lectures

Edited by

Kenneth A. Egol, MD
Professor of Orthopaedic Surgery
Department of Orthopaedic Surgery
New York University School of Medicine
New York University Hospital for Joint Diseases
New York, New York

Paul Tornetta III, MD
Professor and Residency Program Director
Department of Orthopaedic Surgery
Boston University School of Medicine
Director of Orthopaedic Trauma
Boston Medical Center
Boston, Massachusetts

Published 2011 by the
American Academy
of Orthopaedic Surgeons
6300 North River Road
Rosemont, IL 60018

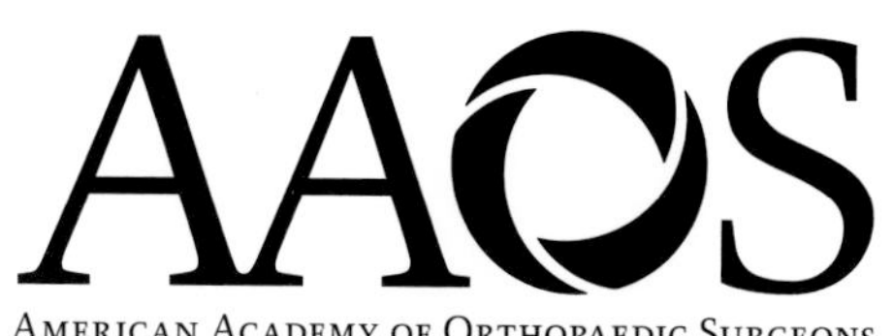

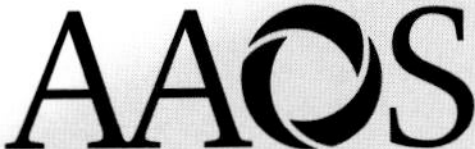

American Academy of Orthopaedic Surgeons

Staff

Mark W. Wieting, *Chief Education Officer*

Marilyn L. Fox, PhD, *Director, Department of Publications*

Lisa Claxton Moore, *Managing Editor*

Kathleen A. Anderson, *Senior Editor*

Mary Steermann Bishop, *Senior Manager, Production and Archives*

Courtney Astle, *Assistant Production Manager*

Susan Morritz Baim, *Production Coordinator*

Suzanne O'Reilly, *Graphic Designer*

Anne Raci, *Database Coordinator*

Karen Danca, *Permissions Coordinator*

Abram Fassler, *Production Database Associate*

Charlie Baldwin, *Page Production Assistant*

Hollie Benedik, *Page Production Assistant*

Michelle Bruno, *Publications Assistant*

Instructional Course Lectures Volume 60
American Academy of Orthopaedic Surgeons

The material presented in the *Instructional Course Lectures 60* has been made available by the American Academy of Orthopaedic Surgeons for educational purposes only. This material is not intended to present the only, or necessarily best, methods or procedures for the medical situations discussed, but rather is intended to represent an approach, view, statement, or opinion of the author(s) or producer(s), which may be helpful to others who face similar situations.

Some drugs or medical devices demonstrated in Academy courses or described in Academy print or electronic publications have not been cleared by the Food and Drug Administration (FDA) or have been cleared for specific uses only. The FDA has stated that it is the responsibility of the physician to determine the FDA clearance status of each drug or device he or she wishes to use in clinical practice.

Furthermore, any statements about commercial products are solely the opinion(s) of the author(s) and do not represent an Academy endorsement or evaluation of these products. These statements may not be used in advertising or for any commercial purpose.

First Edition

ISBN 978-0-89203-744-5

Printed in the USA

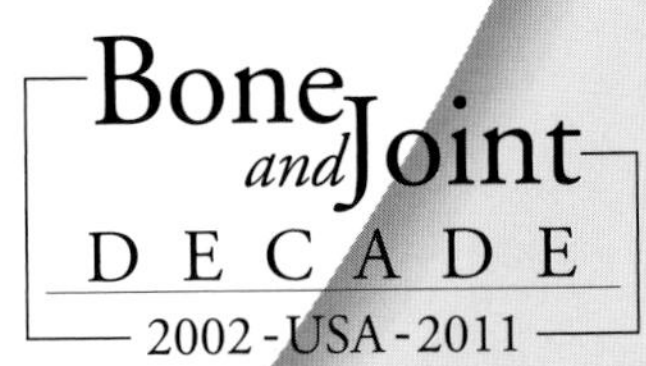

Contributors

Christopher S. Ahmad, MD
Associate Professor, Department of Orthopaedic Surgery, Columbia University, New York, New York

D. Greg Anderson, MD
Associate Professor, Department of Orthopaedic Surgery, Thomas Jefferson University, Philadelphia, Pennsylvania

April D. Armstrong, MD
Associate Professor, Department of Orthopaedics and Rehabilitation, Penn State Milton S. Hershey Medical Center, Hershey, Pennsylvania

Kyriacos Athanasiou, PhD, PE
Professor and Chair, Department of Biomedical Engineering, University of California, Davis, Davis, California

George S. Athwal, MD, FRCSC
Assistant Professor, Hand and Upper Limb Center, University of Western Ontario, London, Ontario, Canada

Sue D. Barber-Westin, BS
Director of Clinical and Applied Research, Cincinnati SportsMedicine Research and Education Foundation, Cincinnati, Ohio

Joseph U. Barker, MD
Sports Medicine Fellow, Department of Orthopaedics, Rush University Medical Center, Chicago, Illinois

Keith R. Berend, MD
Associate, Joint Implant Surgeons, Clinical Associate Professor, Department of Orthopedics, The Ohio State University, New Albany, Ohio

Christopher T. Born, MD, FACS
Director of Orthopaedic Trauma and Professor of Orthopaedic Surgery, Department of Orthopaedics, Rhode Island Hospital, Alpert Medical School of Brown University, Providence, Rhode Island

Michael J. Bosse, MD
Department of Orthopaedic Surgery, Carolina Medical Center, Charlotte, North Carolina

Joel L. Boyd, MD
Department of Orthopedics, Tria Orthopedic Center, Bloomington, Minnesota

Thomas D. Brown, PhD
Richard and Janice Johnston Chair of Orthopaedic Biomechanics, Department of Orthopaedics and Rehabilitation, University of Iowa, Iowa City, Iowa

Matthew L. Busam, MD
Associate Director, Cincinnati SportsMedicine and Orthopaedic Center, Cincinnati, Ohio

Ryan Carr, MD
Resident, Department of Orthopaedics, University of Illinois, Chicago, Illinois

Charles Carroll IV, MD
Associate Professor of Clinical Orthopaedic Surgery, Illinois Hand Center, Northwestern Orthopaedic Institute, Feinberg School of Medicine, Northwestern University, Chicago, Illinois

Robert M. Cercek, MD
Orthopaedic Surgeon, The CORE Institute, Phoenix, Arizona

Justin W. Chandler, MD
Shoulder and Elbow Fellow, Department of Orthopaedic Surgery, Rothman Institute at Jefferson, Philadelphia, Pennsylvania

Ryan C. Chen, MD
Orthopaedic Surgeon, Resurgens Orthopaedics, Marietta, Georgia

J.F. Myles Clough, MD, DPhil, FRCSC
Clinical Instructor, Department of Orthopaedic Surgery, University of British Columbia, Vancouver, British Columbia, Canada

Terry A. Clyburn, MD
Clinical Associate Professor, Baylor College of Medicine, University of Texas, Houston, Texas

Brian J. Cole, MD, MBA
Orthopaedic Surgeon, Department of Orthopaedics, Midwest Orthopaedics at Rush, Chicago, Illinois

Peter A. Cole, MD
Professor, Department of Orthopaedic Surgery, University of Minnesota, Chief of Orthopaedic Surgery, Regions Hospital, St. Paul, Minnesota

Clifford W. Colwell Jr, MD
Medical Director, Shiley Center for Orthopaedic Research and Education, Scripps Clinic, Department of Clinical Research Services, Scripps Health, La Jolla, California

John E. Conway, MD
Texas Health Resources, Fort Worth, Texas

Craig J. Della Valle, MD
Associate Professor and Adult Reconstruction Fellowship Director, Department of Orthopaedic Surgery, Rush University Medical Center, Chicago, Illinois

Demetris Delos, MD
Orthopaedic Resident, Department of Orthopaedics, Hospital for Special Surgery, New York, New York

David M. Dines, MD
Assistant Attending Orthopaedic Surgeon, Department of Sports Medicine and Shoulder Service, Hospital for Special Surgery, New York, New York

Joshua S. Dines, MD
Assistant Attending Orthopaedic Surgeon, Department of Sports Medicine and Shoulder Service, Hospital for Special Surgery, New York, New York

Douglas R. Dirschl, MD
Professor and Chairman, Department of Orthopaedics, University of North Carolina School of Medicine, Chapel Hill, North Carolina

Kenneth A. Egol, MD
Professor of Orthopaedic Surgery, Department of Orthopaedic Surgery, New York University School of Medicine, New York University Hospital for Joint Diseases, New York, New York

Neal S. ElAttrache, MD
Director of Sports Medicine Fellowship, Kerlan-Jobe Orthopaedic Clinic, Los Angeles, California

J. Kent Ellington, MD
Foot and Ankle Fellow, Institute for Foot and Ankle Reconstruction, Mercy Medical Center, Baltimore, Maryland

James C. Esch, MD
Voluntary Assistant Clinical Professor, Department of Orthopaedics, University of California School of Medicine, San Diego, Orthopaedic Specialists of North County, Oceanside, California

Richard P. Evans, MD
Chief of Adult Reconstruction, Department of Orthopedic Surgery, University of Arkansas for Medical Science, Little Rock, Arkansas

Gregory C. Fanelli, MD
Department of Orthopaedic Surgery, Geisinger Orthopaedics, Danville, Pennsylvania

Jack Farr, MD
Director, Cartilage Restoration Center, OrthoIndy, Indianapolis, Indiana

Rachel M. Frank, BS
Feinberg School of Medicine, Northwestern University, Chicago, Illinois

Richard J. Friedman, MD, FRCSC
Clinical Professor of Orthopaedic Surgery, Medical University of South Carolina, Charleston, South Carolina

John P. Fulkerson, MD
Clinical Professor of Orthopedic Surgery, University of Connecticut, Orthopedic Associates of Hartford, Farmington, Connecticut

Leesa M. Galatz, MD
Associate Professor, Shoulder and Elbow Service, Department of Orthopaedic Surgery, Washington University School of Medicine, St. Louis, Missouri

Marc T. Galloway, MD
Associate Director, Cincinnati SportsMedicine and Orthopaedic Center, Cincinnati, Ohio

Michael J. Gardner, MD
Assistant Professor, Department of Orthopaedic Surgery, Washington University School of Medicine, St. Louis, Missouri

Trevor R. Gaskill, MD
Resident, Division of Orthopaedic Surgery, Duke University Hospital, Durham, North Carolina

Charles L. Getz, MD
Assistant Professor, Department of Orthopaedic Surgery, Thomas Jefferson Medical School, Rothman Institute, Philadelphia, Pennsylvania

Scott D. Gillogly, MD
Atlanta Sports Medicine and Orthopaedic Center, Atlanta, Georgia

Andrew H. Glassman, MD
Staff Surgeon, Department of Orthopaedic Surgery, Grant Medical Center, Columbus, Ohio

S. Raymond Golish, MD, PhD
Clinical Instructor, Department of Orthopaedic Surgery, Stanford University, Palo Alto, California

Andreas H. Gomoll, MD
Assistant Professor of Orthopaedic Surgery, Harvard Medical School, Cartilage Repair Center, Brigham and Women's Hospital, Boston, Massachusetts

Mark H. Gonzalez, MD, MEng
Professor and Head, Department of Orthopedic Surgery, University of Illinois at Chicago, Chicago, Illinois

John T. Gorczyca, MD
Professor of Orthopaedic Surgery, Department of Orthopaedic Surgery, University of Rochester Medical Center, Rochester, New York

David J. Hak, MD, MBA
Associate Professor, Department of Orthopaedic Surgery, University of Colorado, Denver Health Medical Center Denver, Colorado

Edward J. Harvey, MD, FRCSC
Chief of Orthopaedic Trauma, Department of Orthopaedic Surgery, McGill University, Montreal, Quebec, Canada

Andrew Haskell, MD
Department of Orthopedic Surgery, Palo Alto Medical Foundation, Palo Alto, California

Roman A. Hayda, MD
Co-Director of Orthopaedic Trauma, Associate Professor of Orthopaedic Surgery, Department of Orthopaedics, Rhode Island Hospital, Alpert Medical School of Brown University, Providence, Rhode Island

Martin J. Herman, MD
Associate Professor of Orthopedic Surgery and Pediatrics, Drexel University College of Medicine, St. Christopher's Hospital for Children, Philadelphia, Pennsylvania

Kristin Hitchcock, MSI
Medical Research Librarian, Department of Research and Scientific Affairs, American Academy of Orthopaedic Surgeons, Rosemont, Illinois

David J. Jacofsky, MD
Chairman, The CORE Institute, Phoenix, Arizona

Kyle J. Jeray, MD
Program Director, Department of Orthopaedic Surgery, Associate Professor of Clinical Orthopaedic Surgery, University of South Carolina School of Medicine, Greenville Hospital System, Greenville, South Carolina

Jay D. Keener, MD
Department of Orthopaedic Surgery, Washington University, St. Louis, Missouri

John D. Kelly, MD
Associate Professor, Department of Orthopaedics, University of Pennsylvania, Philadelphia, Pennsylvania

James S. Kercher, MD
Fellow, Division of Sports Medicine, Rush University Medical Center, Chicago, Illinois

Michael W. Kessler, MD, MPH
Department of Orthopaedic Surgery, Long Island Jewish Medical Center, New Hyde Park, New York

Choll W. Kim, MD, PhD
Executive Director, Society for Minimally Invasive Spine Surgery, Spine Institute of San Diego, Center for Minimally Invasive Spine Surgery at Alvarado Hospital, San Diego, California

Graham J.W. King, MD, FRCSC
Professor, Department of Surgery, University of Western Ontario, London, Ontario, Canada

Paul F. Lachiewicz, MD
Consulting Professor, Department of Orthopaedic Surgery, Duke University Medical Center and the Durham Veterans Administration Medical Center, Durham, North Carolina

Bruce A. Levy, MD
Assistant Professor, Department of Orthopaedic Surgery, Mayo Clinic, Rochester, Minnesota

Jason S. Lin, MD
Foot and Ankle Fellow, The Institute for Foot and Ankle Reconstruction, Mercy Medical Center, Baltimore, Maryland

Peter B. MacDonald, MD, FRCS
Section of Orthopedics, University of Manitoba, Winnipeg, Manitoba, Canada

Robert G. Marx, MD, FRCSC
Professor of Orthopedic Surgery and Public Health, Sports Medicine and Shoulder Service, Hospital for Special Surgery, New York, New York

Frederick A. Matsen III, MD
Professor, Department of Orthopaedics and Sports Medicine, University of Washington Medical Center, Seattle, Washington

James McCarthy, MD
Associate Professor, Department of Orthopedics and Rehabilitation, University of Wisconsin Hospital and Clinics, Madison, Wisconsin

Charles T. Mehlman, DO, MPH
Associate Professor of Pediatrics, Department of Pediatric Orthopaedic Surgery, Cincinnati Children's Hospital Medical Center, Cincinnati, Ohio

R. Michael Meneghini, MD
Director, Center for Joint Preservation and Replacement, New England Musculoskeletal Institute, Department of Orthopaedic Surgery, University of Connecticut Health Center, Farmington, Connecticut

William M. Mihalko, MD, PhD
Associate Professor, Campbell Clinic, Department of Orthopaedics, Chief Science Officer, InMotion Orthopaedic Research Center, Memphis, Tennessee

Tom Minas, MD
Director, Cartilage Repair Center, Brigham and Women's Hospital, Department of Orthopedics, Associate Professor, Harvard Medical School, Boston, Massachusetts

Keith O. Monchik, MD
Clinical Instructor of Orthopaedics, Department of Orthopaedic Surgery, Alpert Medical School of Brown University, Rhode Island Hospital, Providence, Rhode Island

Claude T. Moorman III, MD
Director of Sports Medicine, Division of Orthopaedic Surgery, Duke University Hospital, Durham, North Carolina

Bernard F. Morrey, MD
Consultant and Professor of Orthopedic Surgery, Department of Orthopedic Surgery, Mayo Clinic, Rochester, Minnesota

Michael J. Morris, MD
Joint Implant Surgeons, New Albany, Ohio

Calin S. Moucha, MD
Department of Orthopaedic Surgery, Mount Sinai School of Medicine, New York, New York

Anand M. Murthi, MD
Associate Professor and Chief, Shoulder and Elbow Service, Department of Orthopaedics, University of Maryland School of Medicine, Baltimore, Maryland

Mark S. Myerson, MD
Director, The Institute for Foot and Ankle Reconstruction, Mercy Medical Center, Baltimore, Maryland

Roman M. Natoli, MD, PhD
Resident, Department of Orthopaedic Surgery and Rehabilitation, Loyola University, Chicago, Illinois

David L. Nelson, MD
Private Practice, San Francisco, California

Frank R. Noyes, MD
Chairman and CEO, Cincinnati SportsMedicine and Orthopaedic Center, President and Medical Director, Cincinnati SportsMedicine Research and Education Foundation, Clinical Professor (Volunteer), Department of Orthopaedic Surgery, University of Cincinnati College of Medicine, Cincinnati, Ohio

Steven A. Olson, MD, FACS
Professor and Chief of Orthopaedic Trauma, Department of Orthopaedic Surgery, Duke University, Durham, North Carolina

Shital N. Parikh, MD
Assistant Professor, Division of Orthopaedic Surgery, Cincinnati Children's Hospital Medical Center, Cincinnati, Ohio

Javad Parvizi, MD, FRCS
Professor, Department of Orthopaedic Surgery, Thomas Jefferson University, Rothman Institute, Philadelphia, Pennsylvania

Deepan Patel, MD
Orthopaedic Surgery Resident, Department of Orthopaedic Surgery, New York University Hospital for Joint Diseases, New York, New York

Frank M. Phillips, MD
Professor of Orthopaedic Surgery, Rush University Medical Center, Chicago, Illinois

Peter D. Pizzutillo, MD
Director of Pediatric Orthopaedic Surgery, St. Christopher's Hospital for Children, Philadelphia, Pennsylvania

Andrew N. Pollak, MD
Associate Professor and Head, Division of Orthopaedic Traumatology, University of Maryland School of Medicine, Baltimore, Maryland

Laura Prokuski, MD
Sonoran Orthopedic Trauma Surgeons, Scottsdale, Arizona

CDR Matthew T. Provencher, MD, MC, USN
Associate Professor of Orthopaedic Surgery, Uniformed Services University of the Health Sciences, Director of Orthopaedic Sports Surgery, Naval Medical Center, San Diego, California

Kevin J. Pugh, MD
Director of Limb Reconstruction, Department of Orthopaedic Trauma and Reconstructive Surgery, Grand Medical Center, Columbus, Ohio

Matthew L. Ramsey, MD
Associate Professor of Orthopedic Surgery, Shoulder and Elbow Service, Rothman Institute, Thomas Jefferson University, Philadelphia, Pennsylvania

David Ring, MD, PhD
Orthopaedic Hand and Upper Extremity Service, Massachusetts General Hospital, Boston, Massachusetts

Craig S. Roberts, MD, MBA
Professor and Residency Program Director, Department of Orthopaedic Surgery, University of Louisville, Louisville, Kentucky

Scott A. Rodeo, MD
Co-Chief of Sports Medicine and Shoulder Service, Attending Orthopaedic Surgeon, Hospital for Special Surgery, New York, New York

Anthony A. Romeo, MD
Professor, Department of Orthopaedic Surgery, Rush University Medical Center, Chicago, Illinois

Joaquin Sanchez-Sotelo, MD, PhD
Consultant and Associate Professor, Department of Orthopedic Surgery, Mayo Clinic, Rochester, Minnesota

Susan A. Scherl, MD
Associate Professor of Pediatric Orthopaedics, Department of Orthopaedics, The University of Nebraska, Omaha, Nebraska

Nicholas A. Sgaglione, MD
Department of Orthopaedic Surgery, Long Island Jewish Medical Center, New Hyde Park, New York

Anup Shah, MD
Shoulder Fellow, Harvard Shoulder Service, Massachusetts General Hospital, Boston, Massachusetts

Peter F. Sharkey, MD
Professor of Orthopaedic Surgery, Jefferson Medical College, Rothman Institute, Philadelphia, Pennsylvania

Krzysztof Siemionow, MD
Spine Fellow, Department of Orthopedics, Rush University Medical Center, Chicago, Illinois

Rafael J. Sierra, MD
Assistant Professor and Consultant, Department of Orthopedic Surgery, Mayo Clinic, Rochester, Minnesota

Scott M. Sporer, MD
Assistant Professor, Department of Orthopaedic Surgery, Rush University Medical Center, Chicago, Illinois

James P. Stannard, MD
Chairman and J. Vernon Luck Distinguished Professor, Department of Orthopaedic Surgery, University of Missouri Health Care, Columbia, Missouri

Scott P. Steinmann, MD
Professor of Orthopedic Surgery, Mayo Clinic College of Medicine, Rochester, Minnesota

Eric J. Strauss, MD
Sports Medicine Fellow, Department of Orthopaedic Surgery, Rush University Medical Center, Chicago, Illinois

Michael J. Stuart, MD
Professor and Vice-Chairman, Department of Orthopedics, Mayo Clinic, Rochester, Minnesota

Nirmal C. Tejwani, MD
Associate Professor of Orthopaedics, Department of Orthopaedics, New York University Hospital for Joint Diseases, Chief of Orthopaedic Trauma, Bellevue Hospital, New York, New York

Ryan M. Tibbetts, MD
Clinical Instructor, Rockwood Shoulder and Elbow Fellowship, Department of Orthopedic Surgery, University of Texas Health Science Center, San Antonio, Texas

Dominick A. Tuason, MD
Resident, Department of Orthopaedic Surgery, University of Pittsburgh Medical Center, Pittsburgh, Pennsylvania

Mark A. Vitale, MD, MPH
Resident, Department of Orthopaedic Surgery, Columbia University, New York, New York

James E. Voos, MD
Fellow, Sports Medicine and Shoulder Service, Hospital for Special Surgery, New York, New York

Sharon Walton, MD
Orthopedic Resident, Department of Orthopedic Surgery, University of Illinois at Chicago, Chicago, Illinois

Jon J.P. Warner, MD
Chief, Harvard Shoulder Service, Department of Orthopaedic Surgery, Massachusetts General Hospital, Boston, Massachusetts

Lawrence X. Webb, MD
Professor of Orthopaedics, Mercer University School of Medicine, Medical Center of Central Georgia, Macon, Georgia

David S. Wellman, MD
Resident, Department of Orthopaedic Surgery, Northwestern University Feinberg School of Medicine, Chicago, Illinois

Lawrence Wells, MD
Assistant Professor, Department of Orthopaedic Surgery, Children's Hospital of Philadelphia, Philadelphia, Pennsylvania

Daniel B. Whelan, MD, FRCSC
Assistant Professor, Department of Surgery, University of Toronto, St. Michael's Hospital, Toronto, Ontario, Canada

Gerald R. Williams Jr, MD
Professor of Orthopaedic Surgery, Director, Shoulder and Elbow Center, Jefferson Medical College, Rothman Institute, Philadelphia, Pennsylvania

R. Baxter Willis, MD, FRCSC
Professor of Surgery, University of Ottawa, Department of Surgery, Division of Orthopaedic Surgery, Children's Hospital of Eastern Ontario, Ottawa, Ontario, Canada

Michael A. Wirth, MD
Professor and Charles A. Rockwood Jr Chair of Orthopaedic Surgery, University of Texas Health Science Center, San Antonio, Texas

Jennifer Moriatis Wolf, MD
Associate Professor of Orthopaedic Surgery, Department of Orthopaedics, University of Colorado, Denver, Colorado

Philip R. Wolinsky, MD, FACS
Professor, Vice Chair, Chief of Orthopaedic Trauma Surgery, Department of Orthopaedic Surgery, University of California, Davis, Sacramento, California

Dane K. Wukich, MD
Associate Professor of Orthopaedic Surgery, University of Pittsburgh School of Medicine, Pittsburgh, Pennsylvania

Preface

Sir William Osler once said, "to study disease without books is to sail an unchartered sea, while to study books without patients is not to go to sea at all." The goal of *Instructional Course Lectures, Volume 60* is to help orthopaedic surgeons chart a course of effective treatment within the field of orthopaedic disease. This ICL volume is meant to aid the practicing orthopaedic surgeon in his or her commitment to lifelong learning. These 49 chapters were selected from more than 200 outstanding courses offered at the 2010 Annual Meeting of the American Academy of Orthopaedic Surgeons. The chapters present the latest and most cutting-edge concepts and treatments available to physicians who treat musculoskeletal conditions.

I would like to thank each and every one of the 129 authors who took time out of their busy practices to aid in the education of their colleagues, both at the Annual Meeting and in this volume. The efforts put forth to produce such high quality manuscripts in a very short amount of time and adhere to some very tight deadlines demonstrate a dedication to the AAOS mission of providing continuing education for orthopaedic surgeons. The information provided by the authors will be of great use to the profession for years to come.

Volume 60 was made possible because of the dedicated Academy staff, including Marilyn L. Fox, PhD, director of the AAOS publications department; Lisa Claxton Moore, managing editor for the ICL series; and especially Kathleen A. Anderson, senior editor for this volume. The video for the accompanying DVD, which enhances the educational content of this ICL volume, was organized and edited by Reid L. Stanton, the manager of electronic media programs, and his staff.

It has been my honor to serve as Chair of the AAOS 2010 Instructional Courses Committee and as the editor of ICL 60. I am grateful to Dr. Joseph D. Zuckerman, the immediate Past President of the AAOS, who trained and mentored me as a resident and then welcomed me back as a member of the staff at the New York University Hospital for Joint Diseases. His unwavering support and loyalty over the past 17 years have afforded me numerous opportunities that have enriched my life and career as a physician within the field of orthopaedic surgery.

I would like to acknowledge the fine work of my colleagues on the Instructional Courses Committee over the past 3 years, including Mary I. O'Connor, MD; Mark W. Pagnano, MD; Frederick M. Azar, MD; Paul J. Duwelius, MD; Paul Tornetta III, MD; James D. Heckman, MD; and Dempsey S. Springfield, MD. Special thanks to Paul Tornetta for serving as my assistant editor for this volume and sharing in the peer review process. Special thanks also go to Drs. Springfield, Heckman, and Vernon Tolo, MD for selecting the instructional course lectures for presentation in *The Journal of Bone and Joint Surgery*. I would be remiss if I did not thank Kathie Niesen for the support and guidance given to me as a member and as the Chair of the AAOS Instructional Courses Committee.

Finally, I would like to dedicate this volume to my family—my wife, Lori, and my children, Alex, Jonathan, and Gabby—for understanding the time this project took and for their support for everything I do in the field of orthopaedic surgery.

Kenneth A. Egol, MD
New York, New York

Table of Contents

Section 1: Trauma

Section 2: Shoulder

Section 3: Elbow

Section 4: Adult Reconstruction: Hip and Knee

Section 5: Foot and Ankle

Section 6: Spine

Section 7: Pediatrics

Section 8: Sports Medicine

Section 9: Orthopaedic Medicine

Section 10: The Practice of Orthopaedics

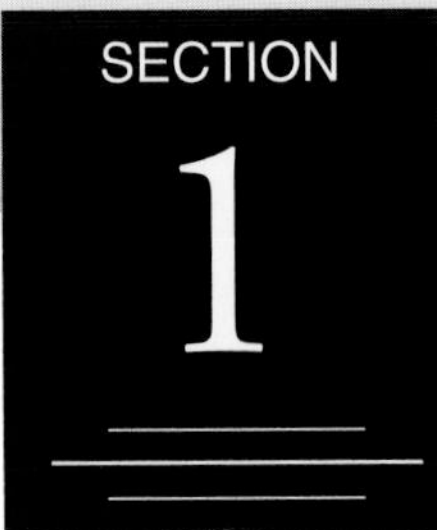

Trauma

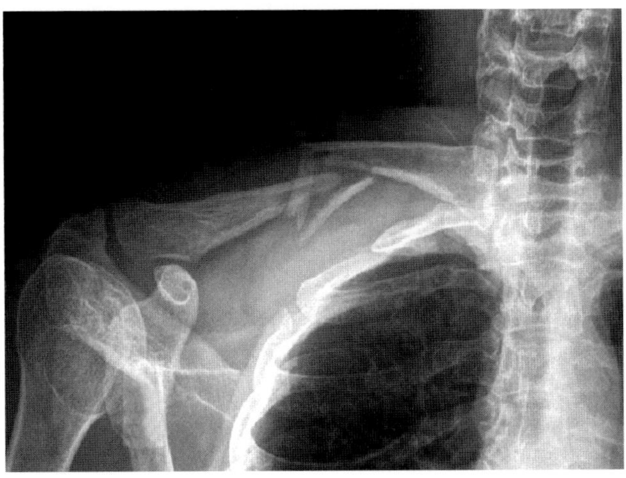

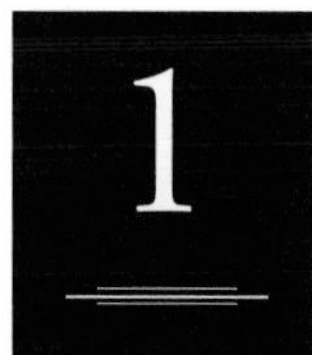

Essentials of Disaster Management: The Role of the Orthopaedic Surgeon

Christopher T. Born, MD, FACS
Keith O. Monchik, MD
Roman A. Hayda, MD
Michael J. Bosse, MD
Andrew N. Pollak, MD

Abstract

Disaster preparedness and management education is essential for allowing orthopaedic surgeons to play a valuable, constructive role in responding to disasters. The National Incident Management System, as part of the National Response Framework, provides coordination between all levels of government and uses the Incident Command System as its unified command structure. An "all-hazards" approach to disasters, whether natural, man-made, intentional, or unintentional, is fundamental to disaster planning. To respond to any disaster, command and control must be established, and emergency management must be integrated with public health and medical care. In the face of increasing acts of terrorism, an understanding of blast injury pathophysiology allows for improved diagnostic and treatment strategies. A practical understanding of potential biologic, chemical, and nuclear agents and their attendant clinical symptoms is also prerequisite. Credentialing and coordination between designated organizations and the federal government are essential to allow civilian orthopaedic surgeons to access systems capable of disaster response.

Instr Course Lect 2011;60:3-14.

The ability to respond to large-scale disasters is recognized as an increasingly important obligation of physicians and surgeons. This has been underscored within the United States by events such as the terrorist attack on September 11, 2001, large-scale wildfires in California, and Hurricane Katrina. The 2004 tsunami in Indonesia resulted in at least 230,000 deaths. The January 2010 earthquake in Haiti resulted in as many fatalities as the Indonesian tsunami and caused a massive number of musculoskeletal injuries in the survivors. All these events presented enormous challenges with respect to the response organizations. It is clear from lessons learned that the keys to response are preparation, plan-

Dr. Born or an immediate family member serves as a board member, owner, officer, or committee member of the American College of Surgeons, the Orthopaedic Trauma Association, the American Academy of Orthopaedic Surgeons, and the Foundation for Orthopaedic Trauma; serves as a paid consultant to or is an employee of Stryker and Illuminoss; has received research or institutional support from Stryker; and owns stock or stock options in BioIntraface and Illuminoss. Dr. Monchik or an immediate family member serves as a paid consultant to or is an employee of Mitek and has received research or institutional support from Stryker. Dr. Hayda or an immediate family member is a member of a speakers' bureau or has made paid presentations on behalf of AONA and serves as an unpaid consultant to BioIntraface. Dr. Pollak or an immediate family member serves as a board member, owner, officer, or committee member of the Orthopaedic Trauma Institute and the National Trauma Institute; has received royalties from Extraortho; is a member of a speakers' bureau or has made paid presentations on behalf of KCI and Smith & Nephew; serves as a paid consultant to or is an employee of Extraortho and Smith & Nephew; and has received research or institutional support from Stryker and Smith & Nephew. Neither Dr. Bosse nor any immediate family member has received anything of value from or owns stock in a commercial company or institution related directly or indirectly to the subject of this chapter.

Portions of this chapter adapted from Born CT, Monchik KO: Disaster and mass casualty preparedness, in Schmidt AH, Teague DC, eds: Orthopaedic Knowledge Update: Trauma 4. *Rosemont, IL, American Academy of Orthopaedic Surgeons, 2010, pp 95-106.*

Table 1
Emergency Support Function (ESF) Annexes

ESF #1 Transportation
ESF #2 Communications
ESF #3 Public works and engineering
ESF #4 Firefighting
ESF #5 Emergency management
ESF #6 Mass care, emergency assistance, housing, and human services
ESF #7 Logistics management and resource support
ESF #8 Public health and medical services
ESF #9 Search and rescue
ESF #10 Oil and hazardous materials response
ESF #11 Agriculture and natural resources
ESF #12 Energy
ESF #13 Public safety and security
ESF #14 Long-term community recovery
ESF #15 External affairs

ning, risk analysis, training, and a system of coordinated incident management that has the ability to expand or contract to meet the needs of any given event—a unified, all-hazards response plan. Events themselves may be vastly different (for example, man-made versus geophysical disasters). Preparation should begin with a hazard vulnerability analysis (HVA). Drills and rehearsals are an important part of preparation. Certain medical principles come into play as part of a disaster response plan and include the concepts of search and rescue, triage, surge capacity, and resupply. During a situation in which resources may be limited, a paradigm shift may need to occur, whereby medical care may be withheld from more severely injured patients to provide for the larger population of victims. Industrial accidents and terrorism have added to the complexity of disaster response, making a fundamental knowledge of hazardous materials management and the pathophysiology of blast injury a requisite part of response preparation.

Structure of Government Response to Disaster

The National Incident Management System (NIMS) was established as a result of the 2001 terrorist attack on the World Trade Center in New York City. President George W. Bush issued Homeland Security Presidential Directive V, which called for the development of NIMS. The purpose of NIMS was to improve the coordination of incident response between all levels of government, the private sector, and nongovernment organizations. NIMS defines how the nation responds in a unified and coordinated manner through an all-hazards planning approach. The response is flexible and scalable because response assets can be deployed to address small or large incidents caused by any type of event. Most events are managed on a local basis; however, as events increase in size, duration, or the number of victims, the involvement of state, national, or even international assets can be increased. Therefore, NIMS governs how the nation responds in a unified and coordinated manner to small, contained incidents, such as the collapse of an interstate highway bridge, to large, open, catastrophic events, such as a hurricane or an earthquake.

NIMS is part of the larger National Response Framework (NRF) that describes in a core document the overall national response precepts, including response actions and organizations, roles and responsibilities, and planning requirements.[1] There are several associated subdocuments (annexes) that identify assets or groups of assets that may be needed to meet specific situations. The Emergency Support Function annexes enumerate the 15 most commonly used federal resources that might be required to respond to an incident (such as transportation, communications, or medical response)[2] (**Table 1**). Other support annexes and incident annexes outline assistive administrative platforms (such as financial management or volunteer and private sector coordination), as well as broad incident categories (such as nuclear/radiologic, biologic, or mass evacuation). NIMS response elements can be implemented at any level and at any time; these elements help to improve coordination among all response partners and ensure that they use standard command and management structures. The NRF defines the key response partners and their interrelationships at local, state, federal, and tribal levels. Incident responses are tiered and scalable depending on the scope and nature of the event. Coordination between states may need to take place through mutual aid and assistance agreements, such as the Emergency Management Assistance Compact, by which a state can request and receive assistance from other member states. At the federal level, the president ultimately commands the federal response effort, which is coordinated by the secretary of the US Department of Homeland Security with the assistance of a regional administrator of the Federal Emergency Management Agency. In circumstances in which a state's emergency plan has been activated, the governor of a particular state can request federal assistance through 1 of the 10 regional administrators of the Federal Emergency Management Agency. A significant delay in carrying out this important step by the governor of Louisiana during Hurricane Katrina in 2005 contributed to the overall delay in response to the disaster.

The key organizational component of the NRF is the Incident Command System (ICS) (**Figure 1**). The ICS is the standard for emergency manage-

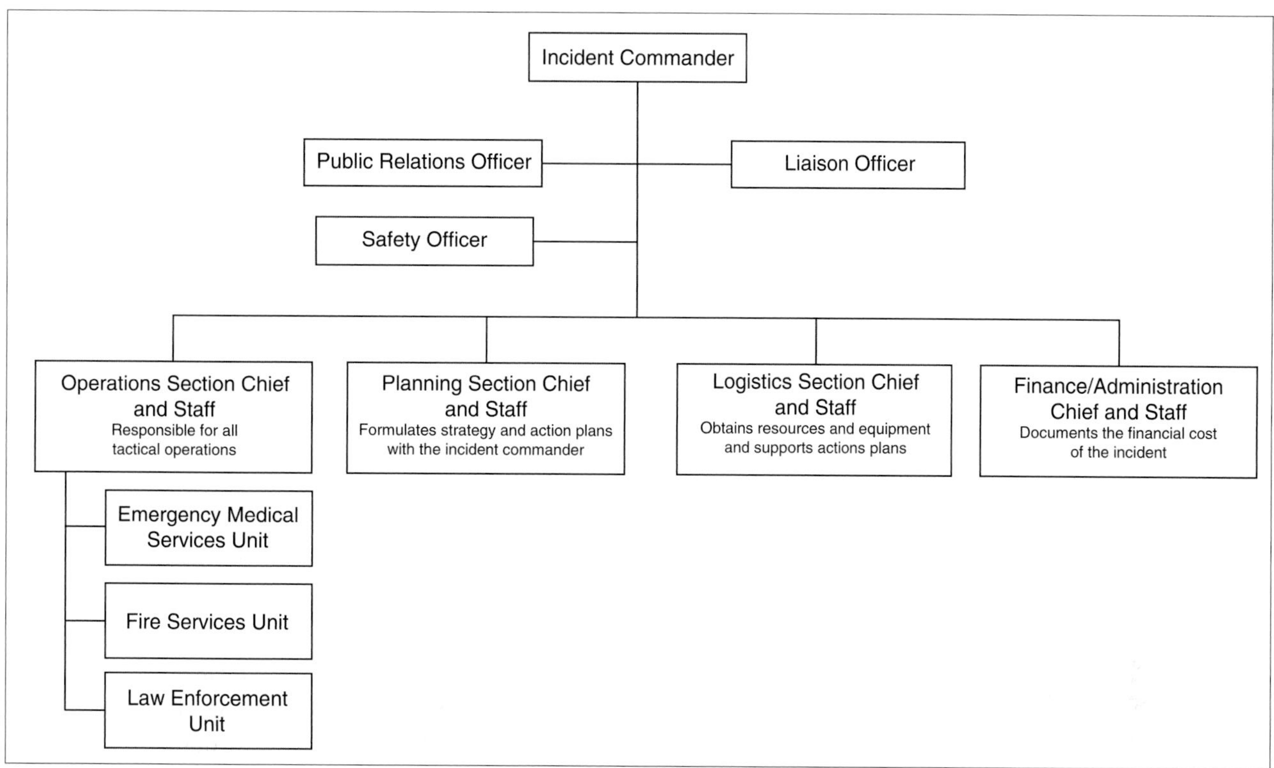

Figure 1 The organizational structure of the ICS shows the relationship between the command staff, the general staff, and the section chiefs. The modular structure allows for the ICS to be expanded or contracted according to the changing needs of a disaster situation. Additional units are added as needed under each of the section chiefs. (Adapted from the FEMA National Incident Management System at http://www.fema.gov/emergency/nrf/. Accessed March 30, 2010.)

ment across the country, and adoption of this system is a prerequisite for receiving federal emergency preparedness funding. The local emergency operations center (EOC) coordinates information resources and provides support to the incident commander at the event scene. A unified command structure is a hallmark of the ICS, which incorporates five management functions. The size of each component can expand or contract depending on the scope and requirements of the incident. The incident commander is the person in overall charge of the incident response. The incident commander is supported by a command staff consisting of a public information officer, a safety officer, and a liaison officer. The public information officer interfaces with the public and the media and is generally charged with disseminating timely and accurate information. Rumor and hearsay will have a negative effect on the public's response to an event. The safety officer is charged with ensuring the overall safety and security of the responders and victims. The liaison officer is in charge of gathering information about support agencies. The incident commander, public information officer, safety officer, and liaison officer constitute the command staff for the organization. The general staff consists of four sections: operations, planning, logistics, and finance/administration.[1]

The operations section performs all of the tactical efforts needed to manage an event, including medical care, search and rescue, hazardous waste removal, and power restoration. The planning, logistics, and finance/administration sections provide the support functions necessary for the operations section to carry out the physical aspects of the response, all under the direction of the incident commander and the command staff.

Disaster Definitions and Classifications

Disasters can be categorized as natural or man-made. Natural events include geophysical disasters, such as a hurricane or an earthquake, and man-made disasters include both intentional and unintentional events. The 1995 destruction of the Murrah Federal Building in Oklahoma City was an intentional event. An industrial accident or a disaster caused by a technologic failure would be considered an unintentional event (for example, a refinery explosion or the accidental release of a virus from a research laboratory). Disasters can be geographically confined or can expand across an entire region. They may be time limited or open.

The January 2010 earthquake that devastated Haiti was initially a time-limited event that was relatively geographically confined to the region along the Enriquillo-Plaintain Garden fault line that passes just south of Port-au-Prince, Haiti.[3] The devastation to the nation's capital and the governmental health care, communications, transportation, and cultural infrastructure, coupled with the vast number of deaths and injuries, transformed this disaster into an ongoing event that required international intervention for many months.

The type of injuries and the number of casualties generated are important considerations for any disaster response effort. These factors will define the types of resources that will be needed and how and where resources will be deployed. A level I response requires the use of local resources only, whereas a level II response necessitates the activation of regional resources. Level III responses require national or even international assistance.

The past 20 years have seen a significant increase in acts of terrorism. In 2005 there were 758 terrorist events in 45 countries, more than half of which were bombings. These acts resulted in more than 3,000 deaths and 8,000 injuries, including 400 first responders. In the United States alone, the Federal Bureau of Investigation has reported 324 confirmed terrorist bombings between 1980 and 2001. Threats from classic chemical, ordnance, biologic, and radiologic weapons of mass destruction remain a serious cause for concern. Bombs are the most common weapon used by terrorist organizations because they are inexpensive, easy to make and transport, and readily achieve the terrorist's aim of maximum casualty generation and lethality.[4] Chemical, biologic, and radiologic/nuclear devices require relatively greater levels of scientific and engineering sophistication and are generally related to nation-states rather than individual terrorist groups.

Mass casualty events are distinguished from routine patient care by the relationship between total casualty needs and available local resources. A true mass casualty event is quite different from the routine care of patients on a busy Saturday night in the emergency department. A multiple casualty event is characterized by strained resources over a limited period of time, whereas a mass casualty event is characterized by a need for casualty care that far exceeds the available resources.

Planning

Although disasters can be random and unpredictable, there is a widespread misconception that planning and preparation cannot take into account the entire spectrum of possible events. Most types of disasters have predictable common patterns and elements that allow analysis and comparison and provide experience-based knowledge that can prove helpful in dealing with future events. Preparation and planning based on prior experiences can enable successful disaster management and response. The integration of many stakeholders, including hospitals; local, regional, and state agencies; nongovernmental organizations; volunteer organizations; and the federal government must also be taken into consideration.

The planning process is performed using an all-hazards approach by which all potential threats are considered and a single overall response structure is developed. This means that there is one plan but the plan is modular, flexible, and scalable and can be appropriately modified to manage a specific event by drawing on various response assets as needed. Having one overarching plan is more effective and efficient than having several plans for many different types of situations. It is important that any response plan incorporate lessons learned from past experience, define the roles and responsibilities of participants, be continuously updated, and avoid complacency.[5] Training and rehearsal are critical; failure to practice exercise response components can be a key barrier to a successful response outcome. Disincentives to the planning process include financial, time, and manpower investments necessary for adequate disaster preparation rehearsal.

Effective health care preparation and response to disasters has three fundamental components: competency, capability, and capacity. The keys to implementation are the coordinated efforts among the public health sector, emergency management agencies, and the health care delivery system. Although the health care delivery system is most commonly associated with medical response, this would be incomplete without public health and emergency management integration. Such interfaces promote a competent and capable response with the capacity to provide care appropriate to the event.

The response should not start with the detection of an event but rather with advanced risk identification, planning, and mitigation of possible threats (for example, container screening at a seaport). Mitigation reduces the possibility that these identifiable hazards will occur, and preparation lessens the impact of such events when they do occur. A response must be in place for disasters that involve all types of mechanisms and hazards, recognizing elements common to all disaster types (for example, meeting the basic needs of large numbers of victims) and unique facets of particular hazards. A building collapse will generate fundamentally different response needs than an influenza pandemic. The response plan should have the flexibility and adaptability required to successfully meet the unique demands of different situations. A HVA can be used to determine many of the credible threats to a community or region. A port city that is a terminal for an oil refinery will have different planning issues and needs from a farming community in a tornado-prone area. All-hazards planning can consider in advance many of the potential threats that are unique to a community. The HVA identifies these potential risks and assigns an estimate of the likelihood of occurrence to each risk.[6] These prioritized risks are then matched to an assessment of preparedness, and targets for improvement are identified. Disaster plans ultimately should be developed around the HVA.

Prehospital Management

For most disasters, the initial response begins at the scene. There are four primary phases to scene response, starting with chaos and moving through reorganization, site clearing, and recovery. The chaos typically lasts 10 to 20 minutes and is characterized by widespread confusion at the scene. Panic is evident by those at "ground zero" of the event. During this period, there is no medical command. Walking wounded and bystanders may act as initial rescuers. Casualties are most vulnerable during this phase, and the longer it lasts—determined by the rapidity and effectiveness of the scene response—the more lives may be lost. Essential to order is the establishment of command and control, which occurs when someone takes charge and effectively becomes the incident commander at the scene. Initially this can be any qualified citizen who can see the big picture and has the ability to organize those around him or her. Frequently, this role will then be assumed by the first senior emergency medical services responder at the scene and ultimately by the incident commander designated by the local disaster plan. It is critical, early in the event, to have a strong authority to establish leadership. Reorganization then begins to establish control to overcome the chaos. The scene incident commander is responsible for establishing a scene command post that centralizes responder leadership across police, fire, and emergency medical services. This joint command across all disciplines assures that all operational activities are initiated.

The scene command post should be set up near the scene, not at the scene, in a safe location. The scene incident commander must have direct communication with the overall incident commander, who is usually located at a remote EOC. During the World Trade Center attack in lower Manhattan on September 11, the scene command post was set up inside the north tower of the center—with disastrous consequences. Following the Oklahoma City bombing, the scene command post had to be relocated three times in the first few hours as scene hazards became evident and rumors of additional bombs could not be discounted. Local authorities may choose to open an EOC that is remote from the scene, which serves as the central incident command post with a designated incident commander who is responsible for overall coordination of the response. The EOC is responsible for initiating additional general public safety measures, such as curfew, quarantine, and large-scale evacuation. The EOC also notifies state and federal authorities of the event and response, which may lead to requests for state and federal assistance.

The first priority of the scene incident commander is to rapidly assess the scene and report critical information to local authorities, including existing and potential hazards, an estimate of the dead and injured, and the immediate resource needs. As reorganization progresses, responders become more organized and coordinated. Safety during the reorganization phase is paramount. Disaster scenes are inherently dangerous because of unstable structures as well as compromised power and gas lines. Panicked survivors or gangs trying to take advantage of an unstable civil situation can be a serious threat to rescuers.

Disaster scenes also have the potential for the discharge of a variety of biohazardous contaminants. Dust has short-term (eye, nose, throat, and lung irritation) and long-term (chronic pulmonary disease) consequences. There is a potential for toxic exposures to asbestos (from pulverized insulation), silica (from pulverized concrete), and chemicals of combustion. Infectious exposures exist from human blood and tissue (hepatitis and human immunodeficiency viruses). The area may have been deliberately contaminated by radioactive, chemical, or biologic agents. Specialized equipment may be needed to detect contamination and toxins. Temperatures at the scene can vary at the extremes, leading to dehydration, heat exhaustion, and hypothermia, depending on the setting. Establishing a safe environment at the scene is the first priority in the prehospital response. Protection not only involves avoiding hazards but also anticipating otherwise unavoidable hazards by using the appropriate level of personal protective equipment, which can be cumbersome and confining and lead to physical stress, discomfort, and dehydration.[7]

A "second hit" is a significant incident that occurs sometime after the primary event that causes further injuries at the scene. This can be intentional, such as a second terrorist bomb planted to kill and injure first responders. Nonintentional second hits would include explosions from gas leaks or other combustible materials or a delayed structural collapse as occurred at the World Trade Center. The consequences of second hits can be profound. The number of casualties increases, adding to the mass casualty burden. The rescue effort becomes compromised because responders are now casualties. Confusion and fear at the scene increases.

Responder safety must come first if casualties are to have their best chance of survival. Scene security starts with local police and may require help from state and federal law enforcement as the event unfolds. The National Guard is an asset of state governments and an important resource for security. The disaster scene may be a crime scene, so it is important to work with law enforcement to preserve forensic evidence.

The only triage at the scene is the determination of who is alive and who is dead. Site clearing is the phase during which casualties who are alive are quickly identified and moved to a casualty collection point close to, but not at, the disaster site. This differs from search and rescue in which teams work with dogs and other detection equipment to find and extricate trapped casualties. Search and rescue teams have special technical skills, which are practiced together and often. The survival of these casualties is related to the time of extrication, with the probability of survival decreasing considerably after 24 hours. Search and rescue is hazardous for rescuers. Seventy percent of fatalities in confined space rescue are the rescuers themselves.

The site of the casualty collection point should be safe from hazards at the scene, and should be located upwind and uphill from the contaminated environment. The site should be easily visible to casualties, so that the walking wounded can find the site. The site also should have convenient routes for entry and exit for both ground and air evacuation. Casualties should receive only the most minimal interventions at the scene (for example, stopping obvious bleeding). Once rescued and determined to be alive, these individuals are transported to casualty collection points away from the scene for triage and brief life-saving care before being sent to hospitals. At the casualty collection point, triage is performed to identify the critically injured among the victim population.[5] The triage decision triggers life-saving interventions involving airway, release of tension pneumothorax, and hemorrhage control. Evacuation occurs from this point by ground and air transport. The most critically injured are evacuated first. Typically, patients will gravitate to the hospital nearest the event scene. A coordinated distribution of casualties to outlying or specialty hospitals is desirable to avoid any one facility from being overwhelmed while others remain unused. Such a systematic effort requires good planning and early incident command leadership. There are technical considerations for the distribution of patients to hospitals, including the distance/time between the casualty collection point and various facilities. Bad weather can effectively eliminate air transport, and roads may be impassable. The basic principles of decontamination apply to transport of the injured. Casualties taken from the scene should be presumed contaminated until proven otherwise.

After the living casualties have been rescued and moved away from the scene, recovery efforts begin. The shift from rescue to recovery can take an emotional toll on responders and the community. Remains require identification and tracking. After the Haiti earthquake, public health considerations required that bodies be buried in mass graves, so identification was not always possible.

Communication is perhaps the most common pitfall in disaster response. Without it, the entire response will lack cohesiveness. Communication is initially threatened by a loss of infrastructure and power. The remaining operable systems become overwhelmed. Poor planning also increases the risk of communications failure by not recognizing in advance incompatible systems across responders and facilities. A lack of redundancy and contingency systems (satellite phones, walkie-talkies, ham radios, broadcast media, independent power sources) and using discipline-specific jargon are additional sources of communication problems that are avoidable with advanced planning.

Hospital Response

As an event develops, chaos can move into the hospital, transforming it into a secondary disaster scene.[8] In the hospital, a chaotic situation may result from the unexpected appearance of casualties. This chaos is prevented by early institution of the hospital disaster plan. To switch to a disaster plan, a hospital system needs to be prepared through planning to address several elements for an effective response.[9]

The hospital incident command system is an extension of the general incident command management system and should be implemented early. The hospital is integrated into the system-wide response and transforms its organization from its day-to-day structure into one more capable of meeting the requirements for disaster response. The hospital incident command system defines clear lines of authority and reporting and gives staff clear instruction and direction for accountability (**Figure 2**). This system uses the same framework for all events yet (like the incident command system) allows flexibility and adaptability for event specifics. Its common lan-

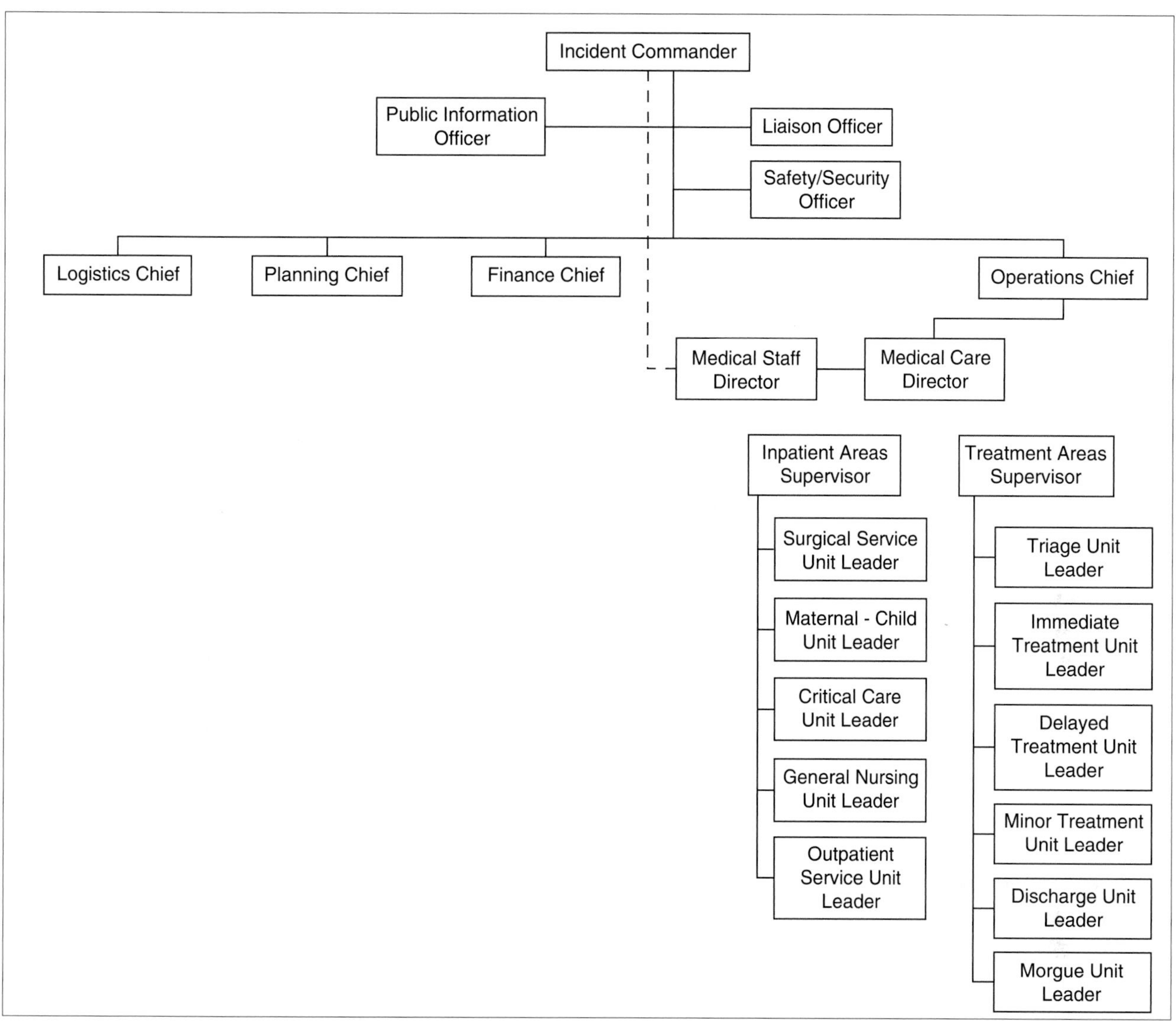

Figure 2 The organizational structure of the hospital incident command system follows the same basic structure and terminology as the incident command system. The hospital incident command system varies from the incident command system in that the units under the four section chiefs are created for the specific needs of the hospital setting. (Adapted from the FEMA National Incident Management System at http://www.fema.gov/emergency/nrf/. Accessed March 30, 2010.)

guage facilitates a cohesive response.

An emergency operations plan and the hospital command center (the hospital EOC) should be activated. Using identification vests serves as a visual cue for staff and prehospital responders to know who is responsible for performing specific activities in this new structure. Working communication devices, such as walkie-talkies and cell phones, are essential for connecting the organization internally and externally. A well-developed hospital incident command system prevents unnecessary communications and keeps networks functional.[10] Job action sheets are checklists to ensure that needed actions occur relative to specific roles. There is one job action sheet for each functional position in the hospital incident command system. These sheets are maintained for easy access and distribution by the incident commander and general staff. They define the purpose of the position, communication and reporting links, and critical action considerations. Job action sheets are an integral component of a hospital's disaster plan and should be reviewed at each training exercise.

Security is responsible for maintaining a safe environment within the hospital. Facility and perimeter lockdown should be implemented. All staff must remain vigilant to the possibility of a second hit at the hospital. Controlling hospital access means allowing designated staff and casualties into the casualty evaluation lane and keeping mass providers, spontaneous unaffiliated volunteers, media, families, and worried bystanders out (this is easier said than done and may involve techniques in crowd and riot control). Designating a place for these groups to gather under staff supervision is key to preventing confusion. Other safety measures include decontamination external to the facility, using personal protective equipment, and a functional personnel and vehicle identification system.

The units under the medical care branch collectively provide assessment and care for the critically injured, noncritically injured, and psychiatric casualties. Clinical support services, including radiology and laboratory units, should be minimized for initial casualty care. Triage is designed to direct the critically injured into the hospital. Minimal acceptable care is the standard of care in mass casualty incidents because this level of care promotes the greatest good for the greatest number of injured victims. Formal radiologic imaging and laboratory testing should be minimized during the acute casualty influx, with reassessment after the casualty influx subsides. Focused assessment with sonography and a handheld blood analyzer can be swift adjuncts for the initial casualty evaluation. One model of medical response involves small teams grouped per stretcher. The team then stays with the casualty for all casualty acute care needs. This enhances the operational span of control and casualty tracking while reducing the risk of missed injuries. Rarely is there an adequate supply of these teams, so "overtriage" can rapidly deplete this resource. A typical medical response team may include a surgeon, an anesthesiologist, two nurses, and a respiratory technician. Additional assets may include residents, medical and nursing students, and prescreened volunteers.

Casualty flow must be unidirectional in the forward direction, otherwise congestion in acute care areas will quickly develop. Casualty areas must be designated with assigned triage officers and care teams. Triage officers reassess casualties for any change in status that would indicate a change in priority. Outpatient areas with the walking wounded will likely have the highest number of casualties and must be staffed to prevent these patients from seeking care in other parts of the hospital. A secondary triage area or staging unit facilitates the forward flow of casualties and disposition within the hospital. Those casualties awaiting disposition after leaving the emergency department for radiologic evaluation should not return to the emergency department; new casualties will have replaced them. Patient tracking and good clinical documentation enhances the continuity of care, reduces redundant care in a situation of scarce resources, and is essential for outcomes analyses. Key elements include the triage level, primary survey findings, and identified injuries with interventions. It is best to adapt familiar forms, rather than introduce entirely new forms. If used, electronic medical records may enhance this process, but users must be familiar with the technology in advance rather than learning on the job.

Hospital incident command system logistics involve supply and resupply, facilities management, and support of responding personnel. One common problem is that hospitals in a region are often dependent on the same suppliers for equipment and services. In normal daily functioning this is fine, but in the disaster setting, a bottleneck will occur when each facility calls for urgent resupply at the same time.[10] Within the hospital, space for workers must be expanded, and shift adjustments may be necessary to prevent fatigue. The basics of daily living, such as sleep, food, and reassurance that child, family, and pet care are being provided, are critical considerations because these will become competing priorities in the minds of responder staff. The hospital also requires external linkage with responders in the field, local authorities, public health officials, state and federal officials, the media, and the families of casualty victims. Pre-event tested internal and external communication networks provide the system for sharing critical information, intelligence, and continuous situation updates, all using common language. Multilayered technology with redundancy is the most effective means to keep these systems working.

The incident command system planning section provides situation updates; screens and tracks volunteers and their assignments; assists with demobilization after the event, which includes critical incident stress management; and facilitates conduct of the hospital after action review.

A hospital's incident action plan (disaster plan) needs to build in surge capacity and surge capability needs. Surge capacity is the ability to accommodate an increased casualty load without compromising standards of care. Once this capacity is exceeded, the level of care drops precipitously as the critical casualty load increases. To address surge capacity, hospitals will discharge noncritical patients and place a hold on any nonessential surgery. New space is created (for example, the postanesthesia care unit can become an intensive care unit, and the cafeteria a care area for the walking wounded or a family holding area). Alternate sites may be considered and contracted in advance. Surge capability is defined as the ability to provide specialty expertise, such as burn, geriatric,

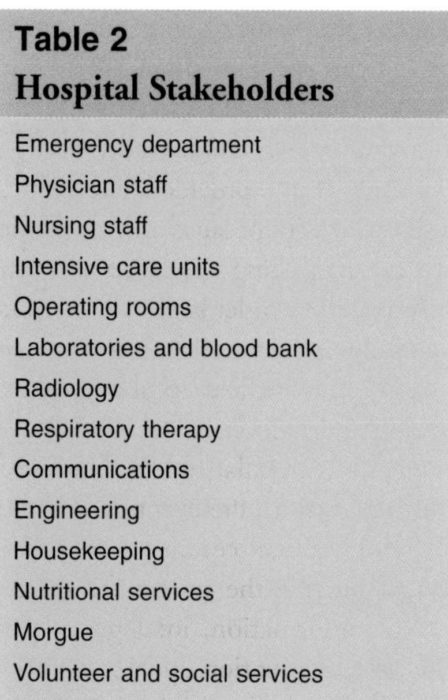

Table 2 Hospital Stakeholders
Emergency department
Physician staff
Nursing staff
Intensive care units
Operating rooms
Laboratories and blood bank
Radiology
Respiratory therapy
Communications
Engineering
Housekeeping
Nutritional services
Morgue
Volunteer and social services
Security
Administration

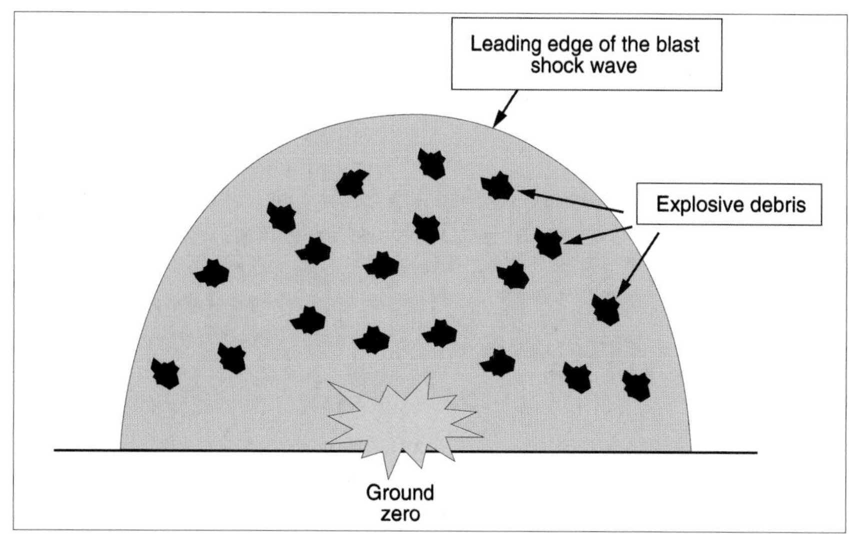

Figure 3 After the blast event, the area of blast overpressure rapidly expands but decays in strength. Air is highly compressed at the leading edge of the blast shock wave. Primary blast injuries occurs proximate to ground zero, whereas secondary, tertiary, and quaternary injuries can extend far beyond the area of the primary blast.

and pediatric care; intensive care unit/ventilator capability; dialysis; and neurosurgical services.

Barriers to a successful hospital response include a "business as usual but just busier" mind-set. This is a recipe for chaos at the hospital. Using exclusive, nonincident command system language and terminology in the plan and planning that neglects input from all stakeholders within the hospital system will present an additional pitfall to an organized response (**Table 2**). Inadequate staff education and training and nonsubstantive "check-the-box" drills designed to meet regulatory requirements are also problematic. Just because a hospital may not be a trauma center does not mean it will not receive casualties. Experience has shown that casualties in need of care view all hospitals as equivalent, regardless of trauma center status.

Blast Injury and Chemical, Ordnance, Biologic, and Radiologic Weaponry

Concern over the use of weapons of mass destruction has increased as the incidences of terrorism increase. As a result, part of disaster management response must include some level of education on the pathophysiology of weaponry. It is also important to remember that catastrophic events involving chemical, ordnance, biologic, and radiologic elements can occur outside the context of terrorism. Industrial accidents have killed or injured thousands of people at one time, and response preparation must include these nonmilitary elements.

Blast physics is described as the rapid transformation of a liquid or a solid into a gas that takes place over milliseconds and causes a rapid spike in the local air pressure. This very high, overpressure wave moves outward from the explosion source at hypersonic speeds (**Figure 3**). Blast injuries are frequently categorized as primary, secondary, tertiary, and quaternary.[11] This pressure front is the source of primary blast injuries. It moves through the victim's body in the form of shock, stress, and shear waves that cause implosion, spalling, and acceleration-deceleration injury to tissue and organs. Severe internal damage can sometimes cause death in the absence of obvious external damage. The destructive magnitude of the blast has several determinants, including the amount and nature of the explosive material used, the distance from the blast epicenter, and the environment in which the blast occurs. Explosives are categorized as either low- or high-energy depending on the rapidity and completeness of the reaction (**Table 3**). C-4 plastic explosives and nitroglycerin are considerably more powerful than gunpowder or a gasoline-fueled Molotov cocktail. Ammonium nitrate is a high-energy explosive that is commonly used by terrorists because it is inexpensive and the components are readily available. Blast waves can be reflected off solid objects, thereby increasing their magnitude; a blast in a confined space, such as a bus or a building, is predictably more lethal. Positive pressure blast waves are propa-

Table 3
Explosive Types

High-Energy Explosives	Low-Energy Explosives
Trinitrotoluene (TNT)	Pipe bombs
C-4	Gunpowder
Semtex	Pure petroleum-based bombs
Nitroglycerine	Molotov cocktail
Dynamite	
Ammonium nitrate fuel oil	

gated farther and faster under water. In the air, as the blast wave moves away from the source, its strength deteriorates approximately as the inverse cube of the distance.

Primary blast injury has its most significant effect at air-fluid interfaces (such as the bowel or tympanic membrane), as well as at the alveolar-capillary interface. Vascular disruption and hemorrhage can cause blast lung and bowel infarction. Those exposed to significant blast overpressure should be monitored for at least 24 hours because visceral injury may not be immediately identifiable. Blast lung can present with symptoms similar to acute respiratory distress syndrome. Traumatic amputation can occur in those in proximity to the blast and may sometimes be used as a marker for triage management following a bombing.

Secondary blast injuries caused by missiles composed of either bomb fragments or projectiles that have been imbedded within the device are designed to increase wounding. In addition, local materials loosened by the blast, such as glass and pieces of building materials, can also become airborne as secondary fragmentation. Careful examination of the victim for small puncture wounds, which may be caused by these forms of shrapnel, can be misleading regarding the size, amount, and position of embedded fragments; the liberal use of radiographs is recommended as part of the evaluation process.

Tertiary blast injury stems from the victim being thrown by the blast, resulting in potentially significant blunt head and musculoskeletal injuries. Quaternary blast injury arises from building collapse, thermal injuries from the blast itself, and secondary fires, as well as smoke and dust inhalation. Building collapse after a bombing can be particularly vexing because extrication prolongs the victim's time to treatment for crush and other musculoskeletal injuries.[12]

Chemical weapons are generally classified into five different physiologic agent categories that include nerve, blood, pulmonary, blistering/vesicants, and riot control chemicals.[13] Any suspicion of an attack using chemical weapons would mandate the use of personal protective equipment by all rescue and medical personnel. Some chemical weapons, such as neurotoxins, may not be easily detectable and may have a disastrous impact on facilities and response personnel who may inadvertently become secondarily contaminated before decontamination procedures. Similarly, biologic agents may also be difficult to detect, and an outbreak may be well underway before the presence of the agents is realized. Surveillance is critical to the identification of a biologic event. The Centers for Disease Control and Prevention, as well as state and local public health officials and emergency departments, continually monitor police, fire, and hospital admissions for occult biologic environmental spread, looking for spikes in illness or symptom presentation consistent with a biologic attack. These would include school absenteeism, an increase in hospital admissions for fevers of unknown origin, and increased sales of over-the-counter pharmaceutical agents. The Centers for Disease Control and Prevention categories of biologic threats are based on such factors as ease of dissemination, potential for high mortality, and impact on the public. Category A threats include pathogens believed to have the highest potential for use as weapons, category B are only moderately easy to disseminate, and category C threats are those that require bioengineering techniques to develop or may also include emerging viruses (such as H1N1 influenza).[14]

Nuclear agents and radiation exposure pose unique threats to the civilian population, whether caused by nuclear detonation, industrial facility intentional or accidental destruction, dispersal as a "dirty bomb," or dispersal without a bomb component. Victims are not radioactive unless they have a contaminating film or dust on their skin or clothing. Clothing can be removed, and radioactive dust can usually be washed off with soap and lukewarm water. Medical and surgical care need not necessarily be delayed. Ionizing radiation exposure and lethality is determined by the source type (for example, x-ray versus gamma rays versus α particles), the distance from the source, and the amount of shielding available as protection. The absorbed dose can be calculated; when taken in context with radiation type, it will determine the amount of biologic damage. These calculations made by a radiation physicist can aid in the treatment and the prognosis of the exposed patient. A rough estimate of radiation exposure is made by assessing time to emesis. Emesis within 1 hour carries a grave prognosis. The prodromal symptoms of significant radiation exposure include nausea, vomiting, diarrhea, central nervous system signs, and skin tingling. Time to symptom onset is the most important factor in determining whether the amount of radiation exposure has been serious. If there are no symptoms within 24 hours and the patient's blood count remains stable, exposure can be considered minimal and probably not life threatening. In the face of significant exposure, required emergency surgery should be performed in the first 48 hours before the onset of marrow suppression.[15]

Current Barriers to a Coordinated Orthopaedic Response for Mass Casualties

Based on the response to the January 2010 earthquake in Haiti, it appears that a two-pronged approach should be considered for an orthopaedic response to mass casualty situations. The first would be an acute phase response in which orthopaedic trauma surgeons would become initially involved. Following this would be the sustaining or recovery phase response that would more likely be populated by a broader group of orthopaedic surgical volunteers. This phase would include those with restorative, reconstructive, and rehabilitation experience. The acute phase response group would most likely be drawn from members of the Orthopaedic Trauma Association (OTA), whereas the recovery phase responders could be drawn more broadly from the general membership of the American Academy of Orthopaedic Surgeons (AAOS), perhaps being organized by individual specialty societies. These considerations are currently under review by the AAOS Haiti Disaster Project Team; recommendations would be applicable to both US and offshore disaster responses.

Key areas for consideration include the concept of credentialing and tracking of individual surgeons who either by training or experience may be in a position to become a responder. The difficulty lies in creating a system for overseeing the credentialing process and establishing a database that is continually updated. By necessity, this database would include personal information, licensing and board certification information, national practitioner database information, educational benchmarks in disaster management, areas of expertise, and health status (including updated immunization status). Liability issues also need to be considered, including personal liability, such as health, life, disability, and professional malpractice insurance status. There are also liabilities that might be applicable to individual societies, such as the AAOS or the OTA, which may assume the position as a clearinghouse for coordinating surgeon responders. Many physicians may not know if their health, life, disability, and malpractice insurance policies are in full force for providing this type of service. Ideally, a cadre of legitimate and credentialed responders would best be organized under some type of federal umbrella, whereby if a physician is "activated," he or she would become a federal employee or contractor and be covered under a federal umbrella. Also, memorandums of understanding should be developed prospectively with the Department of Defense, whereby the Department of Defense would be able to tap into subspecialty organizations such as the OTA and the AAOS to assist with any military-based component of a disaster response.

The potential for such cooperation between the Department of Defense and civilian volunteers was embodied with the deployment of the USNS *Comfort* for the Haiti disaster. The *Comfort* provided the most sophisticated medical facility available in Haiti, with sterile operating rooms, advanced imaging capabilities, and intensive care units. The active duty Navy medical staff, like all other facilities on the island, was overwhelmed by the number of complex musculoskeletal injuries that resulted from the earthquake. The OTA offered its membership to assist in the care of the injured. An arrangement was worked out in only 3 weeks to allow civilians to work alongside their military colleagues at this navy facility in providing the most sophisticated level of care to the severely injured. For future disasters, the delays in making these cooperative arrangements can be eliminated by working out a memorandum of understanding in advance. It also would be helpful to have a civilian liaison office within the Department of Defense to assist with managing the multitude of questions that arise in the time of crisis when the military is trying to coordinate activity with civilian organizations.

Summary

The ability to respond to large-scale disasters, such as the terrorist attacks of September 11, 2001, Hurricane Katrina in 2005, the 2004 tsunami in Indonesia, and the 2010 earthquake in Haiti have underscored the need for physicians and surgeons to have the requisite knowledge, education, preparation, affiliations, and credentialing for disaster response. To improve the coordination of disaster incident response between all levels of government, NIMS under the NRF provides the standard for emergency management under a unified command structure (the ICS). Most disasters have predictable, common elements whether natural, man-made, intentional or unintentional. Planning can be performed with an all-hazards approach, a single overall response structure, and one plan that is modular, flexible, and scalable. Risks can be identified using a HVA before disaster plans are developed. Response to a disaster starts with chaos and moves through phases in which command and control are established. The integration of emergency management, public health, and medical care is requisite. After the safety of victims and rescuers is secured, casualties are triaged to collection sites, sent to hospitals, or evacuated. Communication is essential, but it is also the most common pitfall in disaster response. Hospital response requires an emergency operations plan and a deployable hospital incident command system framework. Disaster response must include some level of education on the pathophysiology of weaponry. Knowledge of blast physics and the pattern of injury from explosives allows for diagnostic and treatment strategies, as does a basic understanding of chemical, ordnance, biologic, and radiologic weaponry along with clinical symptoms and recommended treatment strategies. Credentialing and affiliation with designated specialty organizations under a coordinated federal umbrella can provide orthopaedic surgeons with access to disaster response systems or response planning.

Acknowledgment

The authors thank Joann J. Mead, MA, for her assistance in preparing this manuscript.

References

1. FEMA: Department of Homeland Security: National Response Framework Document. National Response Framework (NRF) Resource Center. January 2008. http://www.fema.gov/pdf/emergency/nrf/nrf-core.pdf. Accessed March 5, 2010.
2. FEMA: Department of Homeland Security: Emergency Support Function Annexes. National Response Framework (NRF) Resource Center. January 2008. http://www.fema.gov/emergency/nrf/. Accessed March 5, 2010.
3. U.S. Geological Survey: Magnitude 7.0—Haiti Region: 2010 January 12 21:53:10 UTC. http://earthquake.usgs.gov/earthquakes/recenteqsww/Quakes/us2010rja6.php. Accessed March 5, 2010.
4. Halpern P, Tsai MC, Arnold JL, Stok E, Ersoy G: Mass-casualty, terrorist bombings: Implications for emergency department and hospital emergency response (Part II). *Prehosp Disaster Med* 2003;18(3):235-241.
5. Auf der Heide E: *Disaster Response: Principles of Preparation and Coordination*. St. Louis, MO, CV Mosby, 1989.
6. OSHA: Best Practices for Hospital-Based First Receivers: Appendix F. Example 1: Kaiser Permanente Hazard Vulnerability Analysis. http://www.osha.gov/dts/osta/bestpractices/html/docs/appf_example1.pdf. Accessed March 5, 2010.
7. Edsall L, Keyes D: Personal protection and decontamination for radiation emergencies, in Keyes D, Burstein J, Schwartz R, Swienton R, eds: *Medical Response to Terrorism: Preparedness and Clinical Practice*. Philadelphia, PA, Lippincott Williams & Wilkins, 2005.
8. Mohammed AB, Mann HA, Nawabi DH, Goodier DW, Ang SC: Impact of London's terrorist attacks on a major trauma center in London. *Prehosp Disaster Med* 2006;21(5):340-344.
9. Reshaur LM, Luongo RP: Lessons learned in business continuity planning: One hospital's response to disaster. *Disaster Recovery J* 2000:12-13.
10. Born CT, Briggs SM, Ciraulo DL, et al: Disasters and mass casualties: I. General principles of response and management. *J Am Acad Orthop Surg* 2007;15(7):388-396.
11. Hull JB: Blast: Injury patterns and their recording. *J Audiov Media Med* 1992;15(3):121-127.
12. Born CT, Briggs SM, Ciraulo DL, et al: Disasters and mass casualties: II. Explosive, biologic, chemical, and nuclear agents. *J Am Acad Orthop Surg* 2007;15(8):461-473.
13. Centers for Disease Control and Prevention (CDC): Chemical Categories. http://www.bt.cdc.gov/chemical/. Accessed March 30, 2010.
14. Centers for Disease Control and Prevention (CDC): Bioterrorism Agents/Diseases. http://www.bt.cdc.gov/agent/agentlist-category.asp. Accessed February 17, 2010.
15. Centers for Disease Control and Prevention (CDC): Radiation Emergencies. www.bt.cdc.gov/radiation. Accessed March 5, 2010.

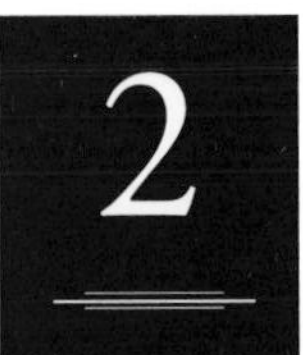

Soft-Tissue Management After Trauma: Initial Management and Wound Coverage

Nirmal C. Tejwani, MD
Lawrence X. Webb, MD
Edward J. Harvey, MD, FRCSC
Philip R. Wolinsky, MD, FACS

Abstract

Before proceeding with treatment, it is necessary to recognize that bony injuries are always associated with soft-tissue disruption and damage. A good soft-tissue envelope is essential to fracture healing and overall extremity function. Injury management begins by recognizing and classifying the injury. Wound débridement with irrigation fluid at low pressure and the administration of antibiotics are essential aspects of treatment. Wound treatment starts with applying dressing material using negative suction and can be guided by the tenets of an algorithm modeled on the reconstructive ladder.

Instr Course Lect 2011;60:15-25.

It is important to recognize that bony injuries are always associated with soft-tissue disruption and damage.[1-3] A good soft-tissue envelope is essential to fracture healing and overall extremity function. An unrecognized soft-tissue injury can result in the development of compartment syndrome with lifetime morbidity. The outcome of any attempt at managing bony injuries or limb salvage is often determined by the amount of soft-tissue loss.[4,5] Understanding and appreciating the complexity of soft-tissue injuries is crucial to determining the appropriate approach in managing a traumatized limb.

At the initial patient presentation, soft-tissue injury may be obvious in the form of an open fracture with an exposed soft-tissue disruption. In closed injuries, external manifestations in the form of skin abrasions, road rash, ecchymosis, and palpable hematomas may be present. In a patient with a severe soft-tissue traumatic injury to an extremity, the goal of treatment is to restore near-normal function in a reasonable period of time while limiting morbidity.

Classification Schemes

Many classification schemes have been proposed to describe soft-tissue injury patterns after bony injury and increase interobserver and intraobserver reliability. Gustilo and Anderson[6] classified open fractures in an attempt to guide treatment protocols and combat the high rates of infection seen with these injuries. A type I fracture is described as an open fracture with a wound smaller than 1 cm, and a type

Dr. Tejwani or an immediate family member serves as a board member, owner, officer, or committee member of the American Academy of Orthopaedic Surgeons; has received royalties from Biomet; is a member of a speakers' bureau or has made paid presentations on behalf of Zimmer and Stryker; and serves as a paid consultant to or is an employee of Zimmer and Stryker. Dr. Webb or an immediate family member serves as a board member, owner, officer, or committee member of the Orthopaedic Trauma Association and the Southeastern Fracture Consortium; is a member of a speakers' bureau or has made paid presentations on behalf of the Musculoskeletal Transplant Foundation; serves as a paid consultant to or is an employee of Zimmer; and has received nonincome support (such as equipment or services), commercially derived honoraria, or other non–research-related funding (such as paid travel) from Synthes, Smith & Nephew, Stryker, and Kinetic Concepts. Dr. Harvey or an immediate family member serves as a board member, owner, officer, or committee member of the American Academy of Orthopaedic Surgeons, the Orthopaedic Trauma Association, the Canadian Orthopaedic Association, and the Orthopaedic Research Society; has received research or institutional support from Synthes; and owns stock or stock options in Pfizer. Dr. Wolinsky or an immediate family member is a member of a speakers' bureau or has made paid presentations on behalf of Zimmer; serves as a paid consultant to or is an employee of Biomet; and has received research or institutional support from Zimmer, AO, and Biomet.

Table 1
Orthopaedic Trauma Association Proposed Classification of Open Fractures

Category for Assessing Fracture Severity	Factors
Skin	1. Can be approximated 2. Cannot be approximated 3. Extensive degloving
Muscle	1. No muscle in area, no appreciable muscle necrosis, some muscle injury with intact muscle function 2. Loss of muscle, but the muscle remains functional; some localized necrosis in the zone of injury that requires excision; intact muscle-tendon unit 3. Dead muscle, loss of muscle function, partial or complete compartment excision, complete disruption of the muscle-tendon unit, muscle defect does not approximate
Arterial	1. No injury 2. Artery injury without ischemia 3. Artery injury with distal ischemia
Contamination	1. None or minimal contamination 2. Surface contamination (easily removed, not embedded in bone or deep soft tissues 3. a. Embedded in bone or deep soft tissues b. High-risk environmental conditions (barnyard, fecal, dirty water, etc.)
Bone Loss	1. None 2. Bone missing or devascularized but still some contact between proximal and distal fragments 3. Segmental bone loss

Reproduced with permission from Orthopaedic Trauma Association: Open Fracture Study Group: A new classification scheme for open fractures. *J Orthop Trauma* 2010;24(8):457-464.

II fracture is an open fracture with a wound size greater than 1 cm without extensive soft-tissue damage. Type III fractures are divided into three subtypes. A type IIIA fracture is an open fracture with a wound more than 10 cm long resulting from a high-energy injury. A type IIIB fracture is an open, high-energy fracture necessitating the use of a soft-tissue flap for coverage. A type IIIC fracture is an open fracture with vascular injury requiring repair.[7]

In the late 1980s, Tscherne and Oestern[8] proposed a classification system for closed fractures. Grade 0 are closed fractures with no apparent soft-tissue injury. Grade I fractures are characterized by indirect injury and a superficial laceration. Grade II fractures result from direct injury and are characterized by significant blistering, edema, and impending compartment syndrome. Grade III fractures have extensive crushing, muscle damage, compartment syndrome, or vascular injury.

Based on the AO/ASIF classification system, the components of the soft tissue are divided into three groups—the integument, the muscles and tendons, and the neurovascular bundles. These groups are further subdivided into five grades depending on injury severity.

The Orthopaedic Trauma Association has recently proposed a new classification system for open fractures that focuses on the injury characteristics defined by the pathoanatomy of the open fracture[9] (**Table 1**).

Initial Management

The Advanced Trauma Life Support (ATLS) protocol must be initiated in all patients with high-energy traumatic injuries. After life-threatening injuries have been addressed and the cervical spine stabilized, trauma to the extremities is evaluated. The initial evaluation of the extremities consists of a vascular examination, including assessment of the pulse, color, and capillary refill. Assessment of the ankle-brachial index is needed for vascular evaluation when the pulse is not well felt or for fracture patterns that have a high association with vascular injuries, such as medial tibial plateau fractures. The patient's history and the mechanism of injury are determined. The fracture pattern; the extent of skin shear or damage; and the presence of periosteal stripping, muscle crushing, contamination, and compartment syndrome also are assessed. The urge to initially classify open injuries should be resisted because surgical débridement is needed to delineate the complete extent of the soft-tissue injury and determine future treatment plans.

Open Fractures

When a patient with an open fracture presents in the emergency department, the presence of life-threatening bleeding is evaluated first. In cases of life-threatening bleeding, which are often seen in pelvic or femoral fractures, urgent management in the operating room includes exploration and vascular repair or angiography with embolization. For vascular injury at or below the knee, emergent application of a tourniquet is useful in temporarily managing bleeding until the patient is stabilized for exploration and repair of the vascular injury.

If no life-threatening bleeding is present, all loose gross contamination is removed with gentle irrigation. The wound is then covered with a sterile dressing. The extremity is stabilized with a splint. Tetanus toxoid and intravenous antibiotics and fluids are administered as needed. If the patient's general condition permits, formal surgical débridement and stabilization of the bony injury is performed emergently in the operating room.

Principles of Tissue Management

Débridement

The basic surgical principle used in the management of traumatic wounds is débridement—the surgical removal of all dead tissues and contaminants from the wound. A lack of complete débridement leads to a feedback loop that is detrimental to tissue healing (**Figure 1**). The initial débridement allows an accurate assessment of the extent of the soft-tissue injury and the patient's reconstructive needs. The size and location of the defect, the type of tissue that is exposed, the condition of the local tissues, and patient comorbidities should be considered.[10,11]

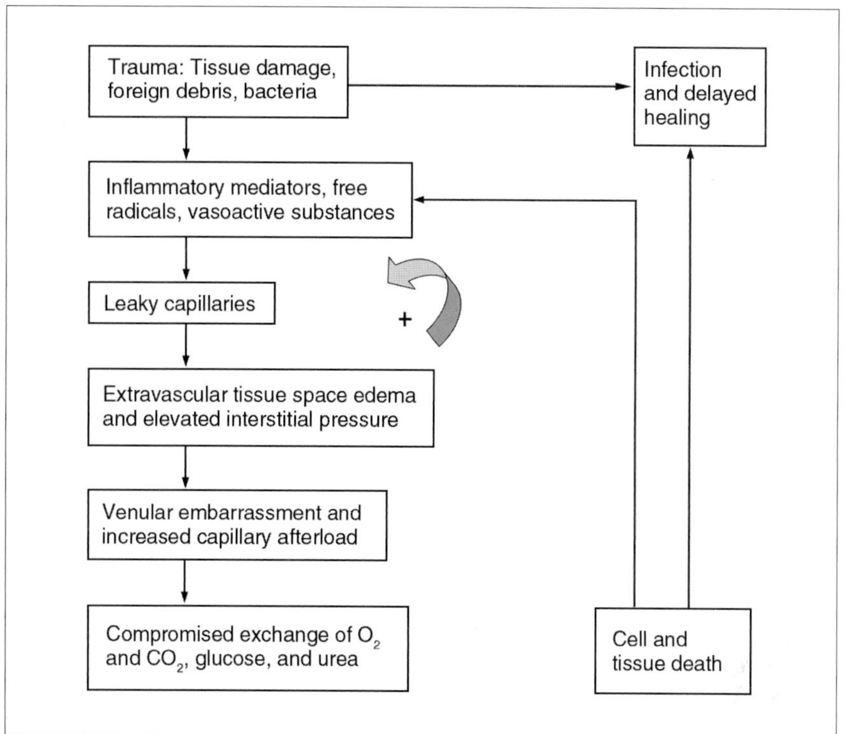

Figure 1 This algorithm shows how the persistence of necrotic tissues and foreign debris can lead to cell death and potential infection with delayed healing.

Ideally, débridement should be done in the sterile environment of the operating room. All viable tissue in the injured area must be preserved, while an aggressive excision of nonviable tissue is performed. The wound should be extended to gain maximum access to the injury. The surgical extensions are usually done along tissue planes and are traditionally closed at the conclusion of the procedure. The surgical extensions allow the surgeon to determine if any dead tissue remains in the wound that warrants excision. An open wound may be extended with incisions made at less than a 45° angle, with full-thickness flaps raised to avoid tissue necrosis.

Starting with the skin and proceeding deeper, all tissue that lacks a blood supply is excised, including bony fragments. Articular pieces, if large enough to be necessary for joint stability, are usually retained and may be cleaned using copious amounts of irrigating fluid. Skin that is likely to demarcate the area between living and dead tissue may be useful in covering desiccation-prone tissue if it is used early as a split-thickness skin graft after it is defatted and pie crusted. Pie crusting is a technique of making multiple skin incisions, usually measuring 1 cm or less, covering the flap. These incisions extend from the skin to and including the fascia and are spaced 1 to 2 cm apart. The advantage of this technique is that it allows the skin to stretch, allows retained fluid and hematoma to escape, and requires no wound coverage with either a skin graft or flap because the incisions will heal by secondary intention. When a wound is associated with a high-energy mechanism of injury and/or a high level of contamination, a second look at the wound in the operating room setting at 24 to 96 hours after injury can be helpful in some situations.

Irrigation

After viable, normal tissue is visualized, copious amounts of irrigation will help decrease the infection rate. Topical antibiotics in the irrigation fluid are toxic to local tissues, and no significant benefit is achieved by using such antibiotics in the irrigation.[12,13] Recent information has called into question the use of high-pressure pulsatile lavage because of the possibilities of causing additional soft-tissue trauma and driving the contaminants deeper into the wound (hence the need for a thorough débridement before lavage), the potential for damage to superficial neurovascular structures, and the effect on bone healing. For these reasons, many surgeons prefer low-pressure pulsatile lavage or irrigation with a bulb syringe.[12-15] The effectiveness of the irrigation fluid in removing contaminants is contingent on the nature of the solute and solvent. In most

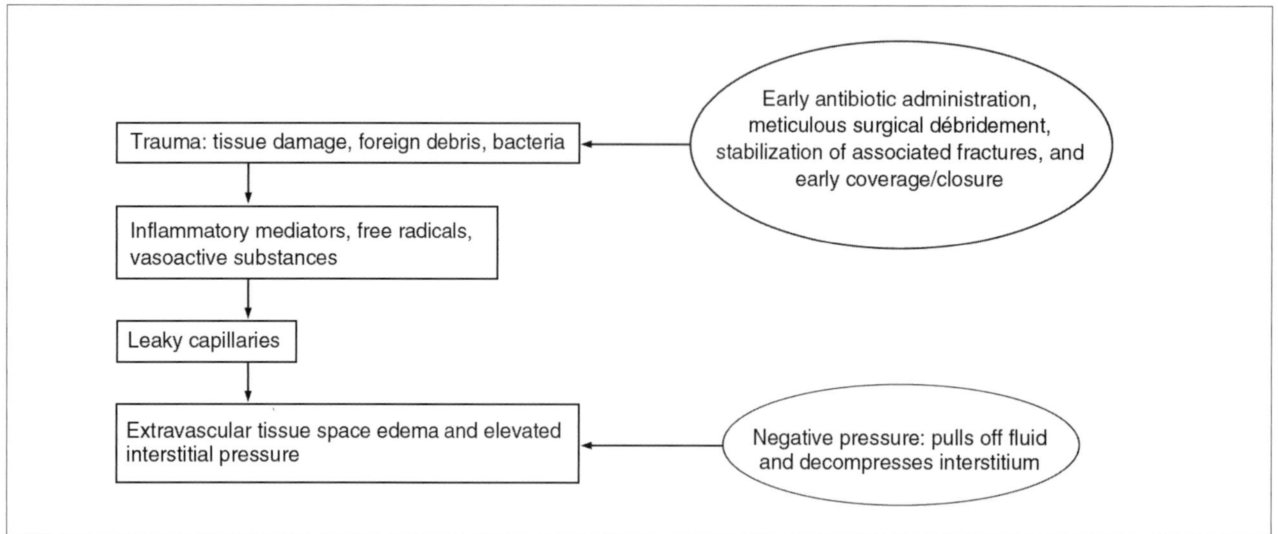

Figure 2 This algorithm gives the keys to management and assurance of rapid healing. It shows the relationship between the use of antibiotics, débridement, fracture stabilization and decreased tissue death, which is also potentiated by decreased edema as achieved with a negative pressure dressing.

settings, normal saline is used, but additives such as antibiotics and nontoxic levels of antiseptic, as well as soaps and detergents, have been advocated.[16-24] This chapter's authors recommend using saline alone or saline with soap at low pressure.

Antibiotics

The use, type, and duration of antibiotic administration remain a subject of debate. Prophylactic antibiotics have been shown to reduce the risk of infection in open fractures.[25] Administering a cephalosporin to a patient with an open fracture upon arrival in the emergency department is recommended. Gram-negative coverage in the form of aminoglycosides may be used in type IIIB open fractures and those with severe contamination. Penicillin coverage is recommended for farm injuries (**Figure 2**). This chapter's authors recommend administering one antibiotic (usually cephalosporin) for 48 hours for type I and II open fractures, and administering two antibiotics (usually aminoglycoside with a single daily dose) for type III open fractures.

Timing of Wound Closure

Current opinion is that primary wound closure is the better option for most wounds.[3,26,27] Primary closure of wounds can avoid the need for a second visit to the operating room. Primary coverage or closure may also minimize the desiccation of exposed tendon or bone, which may become necrotic and foster bacterial growth and the release of vasoactive substances and propagate the cycle. Early closure is usually possible in type I up to type IIIA injuries, with minimal to no contamination and limited soft-tissue devitalization. At the New York University Hospital for Joint Diseases, the use of free tissue and flap transfer has been decreased by appropriately using the simplest procedures first. The treatment algorithm used is modeled on the original thinking of the reconstructive ladder[28,29] (**Figure 3**).

The disadvantages of early wound closure are the retention of nonviable tissue, the potential for infection, and the risk of too tight a closure leading to flap necrosis. If the surgeon is unsure of the status of the wound with respect to potentially retained contaminants or tissue necrosis, open wound management is recommended. Early consultation with a plastic surgeon is recommended for patients with extensive, contaminated wounds with loss of skin and deeper tissue. The treatment goal should be early soft-tissue coverage, which should be done as soon as feasible, preferably within 7 to 10 days.[30]

Wound dressings should be capable of absorbing exudates, provide an effective barrier against bacterial contamination, and have no deleterious effect on wound healing. Currently, negative pressure wound systems are gaining popularity as a dressing and for promoting granulation tissue. The contaminants, bacteria, and traumatized tissue trigger the release of vasoactive substances that cause capillary leakage and result in an outpouring of fluid from the vascular space to the interstitium. This causes tissue swelling and, in extreme circumstances, elevates the interstitial compartment pressure and thereby elevates capillary afterload. When the afterload approximates the pressure on the venular side of a capillary, capillary flow is arrested; the exchange of oxygen, carbon dioxide, glucose, and urea ceases; and "watershed" tissues die. These effects may be one of the causes of the secondary necrosis seen in high-energy traumatic wounds. The use of a negative pressure dressing in this setting is based on the idea of inducing an interstitial fluid flow gradient and decompressing the otherwise embarrassed interstitium by actively pulling the excess interstitial fluid from the tissue space.

Vacuum-assisted negative suction devices help with wound management; however, there are no data to suggest that this may allow delayed soft-tissue coverage. The advantage of having a sealed dressing to prevent hospital-acquired infection should be considered in using this type of device, but no literature is available to support this hypothesis.

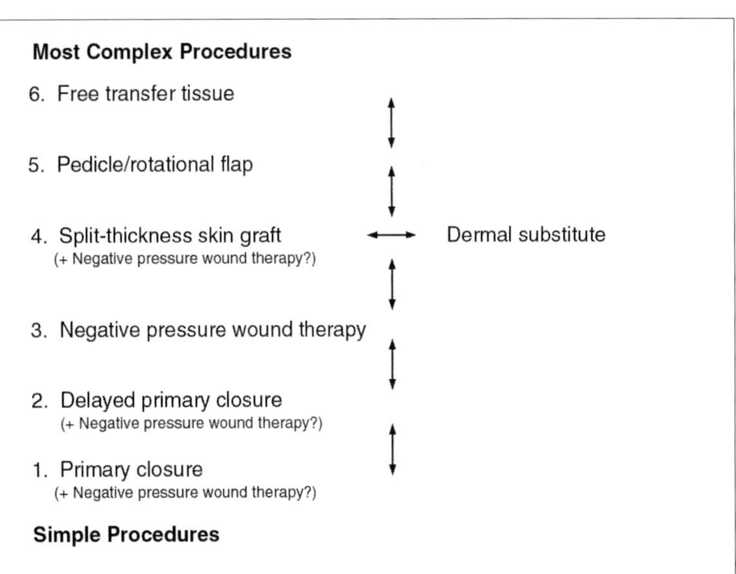

Figure 3 Algorithm based on the new reconstructive ladder for treating soft-tissue injuries caused by high-energy trauma.

Bony Stabilization

High-energy injuries leading to open fractures are usually associated with unstable fracture patterns. Once viable tissues have been reached and a thorough débridement performed, the bony injury is stabilized by using one of the many available fixation devices. Any injury caused by a high-velocity mechanism or with a fracture pattern compatible with high-energy injury is best treated in a staged procedure. Stabilization of associated fractures should maximally preserve the viability of tissue, particularly in the zone of injury. The benefit of a reduced and stable fracture is that, theoretically, the surrounding tissues and their capillary beds are neither unduly tensioned nor compressed, as would be the case with an unstable fracture.

Applying an external fixator allows the fracture to be spanned while the soft tissues are treated; it then may be continued as definitive treatment or converted to internal fixation. In tibial or femoral fractures, intramedullary nailing is a safe option. Studies have shown that type IIIA open fractures can be safely treated with a reamed nail.[31]

If the leg is too swollen to support even limited internal fixation, the procedure should not be attempted. A possible exception is a situation in which a portion of the fracture is tenting the skin and will result in necrosis of the tissue envelope. Pressure can be alleviated with a smaller incision and near-anatomic placement of the fracture piece if the soft tissue is too swollen to support a larger incision for open reduction and internal fixation. All future incisions should be drawn on the patient to allow planning for all eventualities. If the incision used for limited fixation at the time of surgery hinders these plans or endangers the limb in the future, then limited fixation should not be performed. If the surgeon does not have the ability to obtain an anatomic result after limited fixation, then it should not be attempted. The use of small or mini-fragment plates to aid in reduction along with external fixators may help in holding the fragments together. These plates can be removed, if necessary, at the time of definitive fixation. Such plates should be used with caution because exposed and colonized hardware can result in infection.

Free Flaps

In some instances, only free tissue transfer provides appropriate treatment. The advantages of free flaps include the abundant donor tissue available that supplies composite tissues to treat bone defects. The major disadvantage of free flaps is the need for microsurgical techniques requiring longer and more complicated surgery. Muscle and fasciocutaneous free flaps are now commonly used for covering orthopaedic injuries. Although fasciocutaneous free flaps, such as the anterolateral thigh flap,[32] are gaining in popularity, the muscle flap remains the gold standard.[11,33] Muscle probably provides increased vascularity resulting in better oxygen, neutrophil, and antibiotic delivery and is better at contouring and filling dead space. Once it has been decided that a free flap is necessary, combined internal fixation with application of the flap is recommended.

This will prevent colonization of the hardware if used with an open wound prior to definitive coverage.

Avoiding Free Tissue Transfer

The primary goal in wound closure is to avoid more complex procedures (such as free tissue transfer) if possible. The simplest technique for wound closure is shortening the underlying skeleton. Bony shortening for wound closure can be used in some circumstances when using an external fixator for definitive treatment. Shortening of 2 to 3 cm may allow wound closure in some wounds without the use of a free flap but will then require gradual lengthening of the bone using a multiplane external fixator. In patients with complex wounds, early involvement of a microsurgery specialist is important to facilitate the design of a coordinated management plan. Levin and Condit[10] popularized the "orthoplastic approach" between the microsurgeon and trauma surgeon. This approach is intimately connected to the reconstructive ladder.[29] This algorithm is constantly changing, but the basic tenet remains—start simple and proceed to more complex reconstruction only if the simple procedure is insufficient. This approach may facilitate early wound coverage, shorten the overall reconstructive time, and minimize mistakes that can jeopardize limb salvage.[34-37]

Negative Pressure Wound Therapy and Dermal Substitutes

New developments such as negative pressure wound therapy and the use of dermal substitutes have added more rungs to the reconstructive ladder. Negative pressure wound therapy uses subatmospheric pressure applied to a wound to increase the proliferation of granulation tissue and wound healing.[38]

Dermal substitutes used with or without vacuum-assisted wound closure can permit the coverage of large wounds. These substitutes are typically composed of collagen and other extracellular matrix proteins that provide a scaffold for tissue ingrowth.[39,40] Dermal substitutes provide a layer of tissue that adds bulk underneath split-thickness skin grafts and minimizes adhesions between the skin graft and underlying tendon or neurovascular structures. The bulk provided by this tissue also results in improved appearance of the graft as well as a decrease in wound contractures. Dermal substitutes have been particularly useful across joints or in full-thickness burns with tissue loss. The use of dermal substitutes as a strategy for coverage in concert with topical negative pressure is a relatively new concept. Further clinical experience will determine whether the strategy is valid.

The Integra Dermal Regeneration Template (Integra Life Sciences, Plainsboro, NJ) has two layers, a silicone layer and a layer consisting of type I cross-linked bovine collagen and glycosaminoglycan. The bilayer is fenestrated by the technique of pie crusting on its silicone side. It is cut to conform to the surface area of the wound and applied over the appropriately prepared (clean with living vascularized tissue) wound bed. The template is then anchored to the wound edges with sutures or staples, and topical negative pressure is applied with a vacuum-assisted closure system set at a continuous –50 mm Hg and left in place for 5 to 7 days. At that point, the "take" is assessed by removing the topical negative pressure sponge and gently lifting the silicone layer off the now-host cell-laden collagen/glycosaminoglycan layer, which should be adherent to the tissue bed. A thin (dermatome setting at 0.012) skin graft harvest (meshed 3 to 1) is applied to replace the silicone, anchored to the periphery of the wound with sutures, and dynamically bolstered at a continuous pressure of –50 mm Hg for another 5 to 7 days. At that point, the grafted area is inspected. If small areas of exposed tissue remain, these may be successfully managed with moist saline dressing changes.

Dermal substitutes are useful for open wounds with uncovered bone (with an intact periosteum and for areas with minimal muscle coverage, such as the foot). Silicone bilayer dressing allows a base for skin grafting and is durable to shear forces.

Local Flaps

In some patients with lower extremity traumatic injuries, pedicle flaps are a suitable treatment option rather than free tissue transfer. The use of fasciocutaneous principles of dissecting a flap off tendons or deep muscle while preserving the skin and underlying fascia allows closure of even complex wounds.[41] The rule of thirds—which recommends gastrocnemius flaps for defects involving the proximal third of the tibia, soleus flaps for the middle third, and free flaps for the distal third—holds true for most injuries. Gastrocnemius and soleal flaps are advantageous because they are familiar to many orthopaedic surgeons and do not require microsurgical techniques. Orthopaedic surgeons also use other types of pedicle flaps, including classic simple flaps that are extended to increase their reach. Innovative flaps and new uses for commonly used pedicle flaps also have been described.[10,37] The reverse sural artery flap, posterior tibial artery perforator flap, dorsalis pedis flap, and others are now used to cover the distal third of the tibia, an area where only free flaps were traditionally used. Local flaps are bulky, sometimes located in the zone of injury, and limited by the size of the area that needs to be covered. Complications such as flap necrosis and venous congestion are possible. Care must be taken in using local flaps, but they can be useful in averting

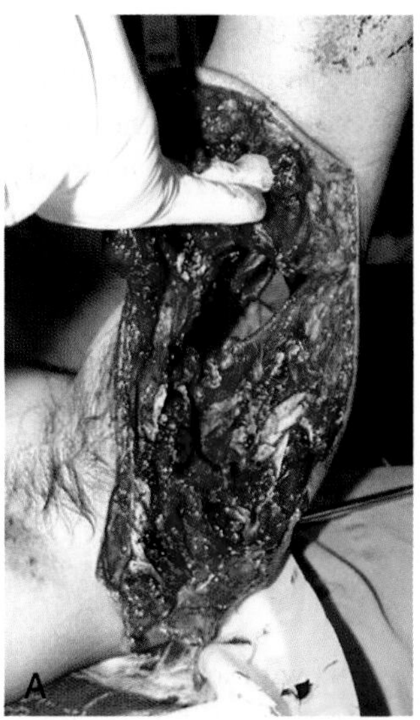

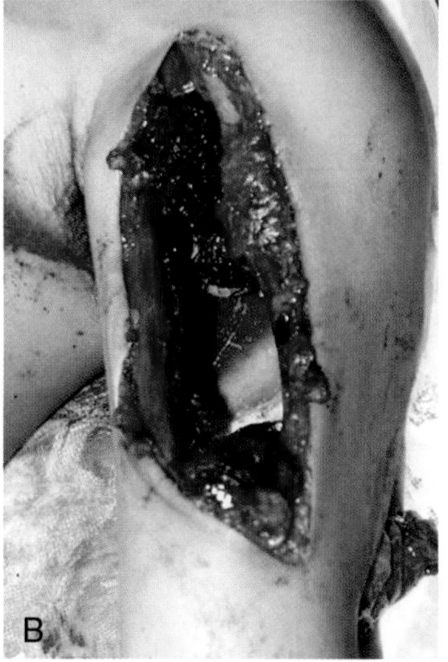

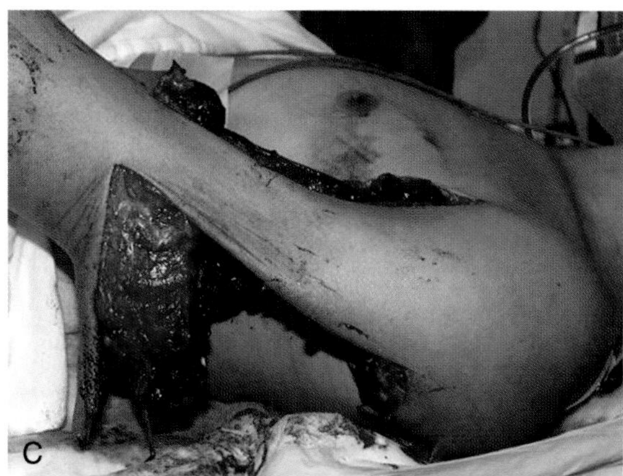

Figure 4 Clinical photographs of the proximal left arm of a 24-year-old man who was injured by a self-inflicted high-energy rifle wound. Posterior (**A**), anterior (**B**), and lateral (**C**) views of the open wound.

morbidity and amputation in some lower extremity wounds and do not have the same donor site morbidity as free tissue transfer. New techniques (modern flaps) and technologies (grafting options) have allowed successful limb salvage with less complex and invasive techniques.

Closed Fractures

Closed, high-energy injuries can be as devastating as open fractures. Segmental fractures, fracture comminution, and potential compartment syndrome are markers of high-energy injury mechanisms. Closed fractures with significant soft-tissue trauma (such as high-energy injuries, especially around the knee or ankle) should be treated in a staged fashion. Early application of a spanning external fixator will allow bony alignment to be regained while managing soft-tissue injuries such as compartment syndrome. When the soft tissues allow (no blisters, wrinkled skin, resolved blisters), definitive fixation of the fracture can proceed.

Morel-Lavallee Lesions

Morel-Lavallee lesions are serious injuries and represent an internal degloving of the affected region. These lesions are commonly associated with fractures of the acetabulum and pelvis. Clinically, a boggy, fluid-filled, ballotable swelling is palpable over the affected buttock and proximal thigh and can also be visualized on CT or MRI scans. If necessary, these lesions can be débrided with open or percutaneous methods.

Blister Management

The treatment of blisters has been dictated by only two published articles, one of which involved cadaver limbs.[42,43] The condition of the underlying skin determines the timing of surgery. If the skin is wrinkled, an extensile incision can usually be performed. If there is a blister in the area, it may be avoided if choosing a different location for the incision will not endanger the vascularity of the soft-tissue envelope or make fracture fixation unduly difficult. However, if the incision must be made through an area of blister, it may not be problematic. Whether the blister is blood filled has little bearing on the safety of the incision. If the underlying skin is wrinkled, an incision can be made that goes straight down to bone and keeps the underlying dermofascial planes intact. Larger blisters (> 1 cm) are more difficult to treat. If large blisters are placed under a dressing they will break, creating an area for potential bacterial colonization and superinfection. If a 10- to 14-day surgical delay is expected to allow soft-tissue stabilization, blisters can be initially decompressed, allowing reepithelialization to occur.

Case Example

A case example of soft-tissue management of a high-energy injury with bony and soft-tissue defects illustrates some of the treatment principles discussed in this chapter. A 24-year-old man was injured by a self-inflicted high-energy rifle wound through the proximal left arm. He presented to the hospital in shock from significant blood loss. The wound is shown in **Figure 4**, and a radiographic view is shown in **Figure 5**. With blood and fluid replacement underway, the patient was taken to the operating room for meticulous wound débridement. Except for the radial nerve, the other major nerves and the brachial artery were anatomically intact. Skeletal stabilization was provided by placing a

Steinmann pin to align the major proximal and distal humeral fragments (**Figure 6**) as well as a transfixing olecranon pin to permit skeletal traction (**Figure 7**). A topical negative pressure dressing was applied with sponges placed anteriorly and posteriorly. The sponges were contiguous at the depth of the wound, enabling the negative pressure sponge to be in contact with the entire wound surface. The negative pressure was set at a continuous −50 mm Hg. Following two subsequent return trips to the operating room for dressing changes, the posterior portion of the wound was amenable to closure with suture (**Figure 8**), leaving just the anterior portion open; the tissue remained clean and viable. This facilitated subsequent negative pressure dressing changes, which occurred at bedside. The skeletal defect was treated by the placement of an allograft stabilized with a blade plate (**Figure 9**). Negative pressure dressing changes every 48 to 72 hours were used with good resolution of local swelling. Stable wound coverage was achieved with a combination of closure and skin grafting. Views of the healed anterior wound and posterior wound are shown in **Figure 10, A** and **B**, respectively. The patient was fitted with a wrist splint with dynamic outriggers because of a radial nerve deficit (**Figure 10, C**).

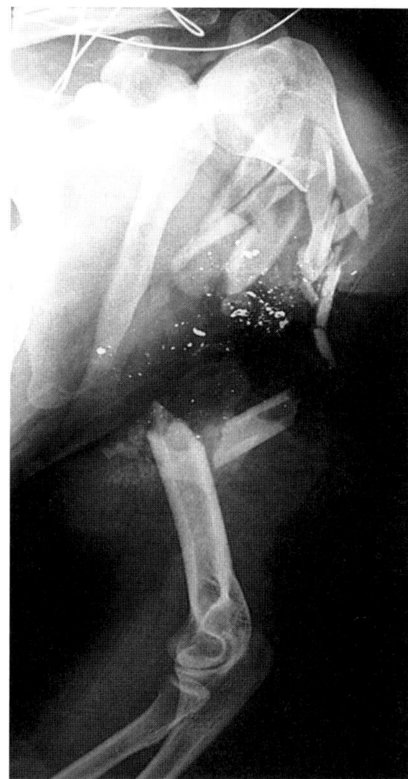

Figure 5 Radiograph of the injured left arm of the patient in Figure 4.

Summary

The successful management of soft-tissue loss is critical in the treatment of high-energy extremity traumatic injuries. The damaged tissue should be treated in the same manner as a locally aggressive tumor, sparing the neurovascular and cartilage elements while resecting all other involved tissue. Bony stabilization is integral to soft-tissue management and should be performed using tissue-friendly techniques. The reconstructive ladder is a good guide for the orthopaedic surgeon. When possible, it is advisable to use the least invasive technique that can provide an acceptable outcome. Dermal substitutes are helpful along with negative pressure dressings to aid in soft-tissue coverage. When the simpler techniques fail, or if the size or location of the defect necessitates it, more complex procedures are warranted, with free tissue transfer as the ultimate solution.

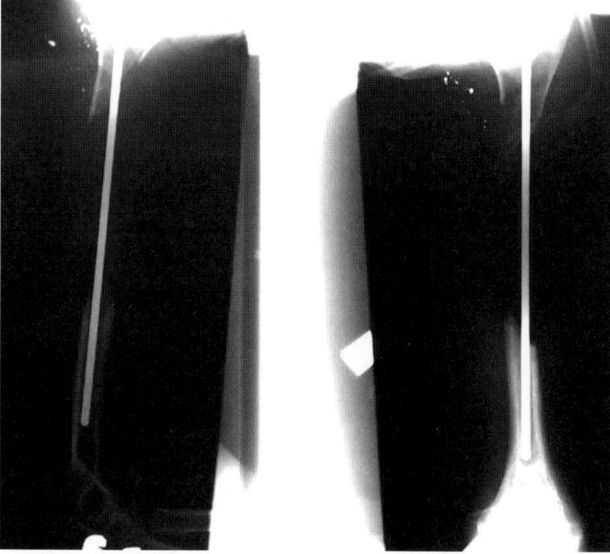

Figure 6 Radiograph of the injured left arm after surgical débridement and provisional fracture stabilization.

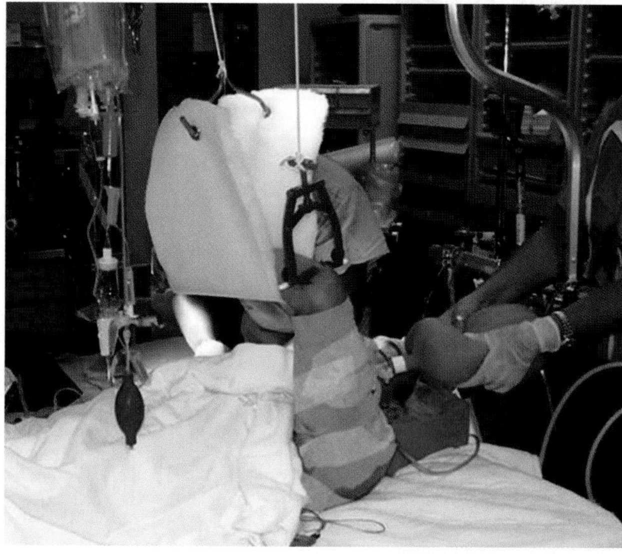

Figure 7 Clinical photograph of the left arm in traction via the transolecranon pin.

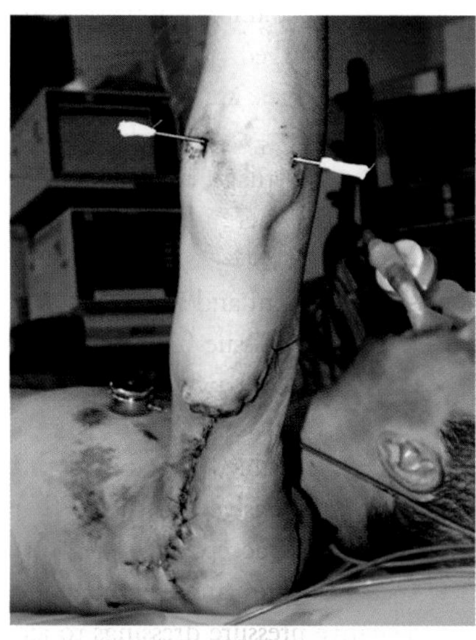

Figure 8 Clinical photograph of the arm after closure of the posterior portion of the wound.

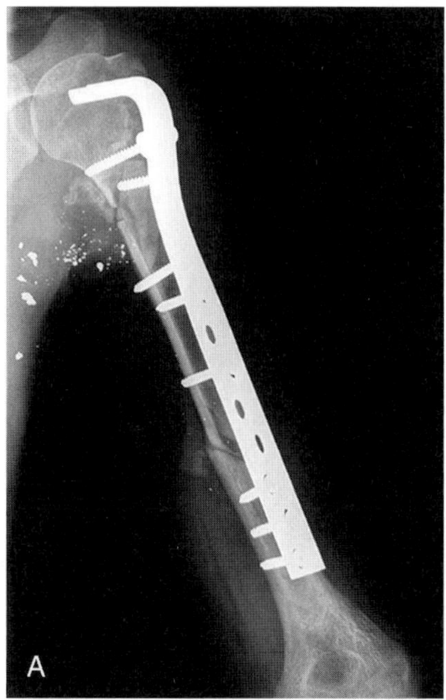

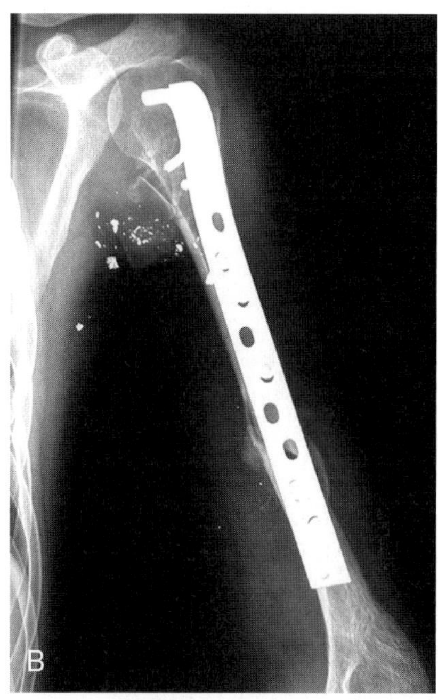

Figure 9 AP (**A**) and lateral (**B**) radiographs of the humerus following placement of an allograft in the void and stabilization with a blade plate.

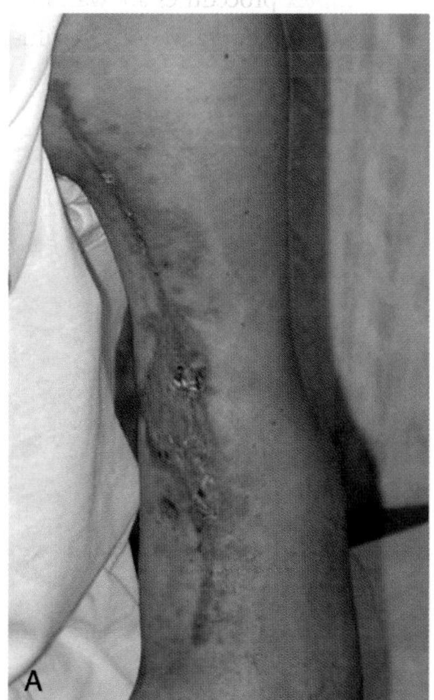

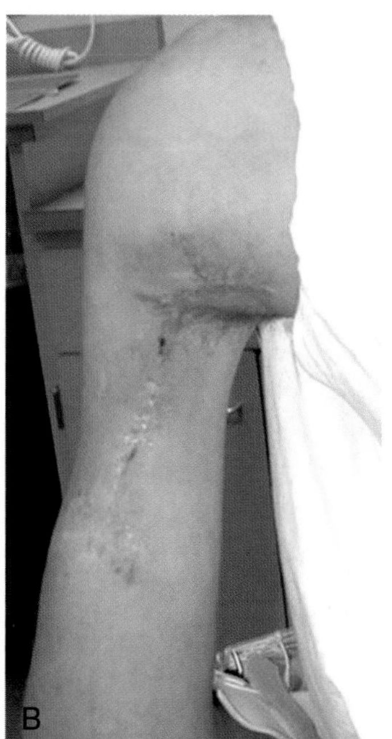

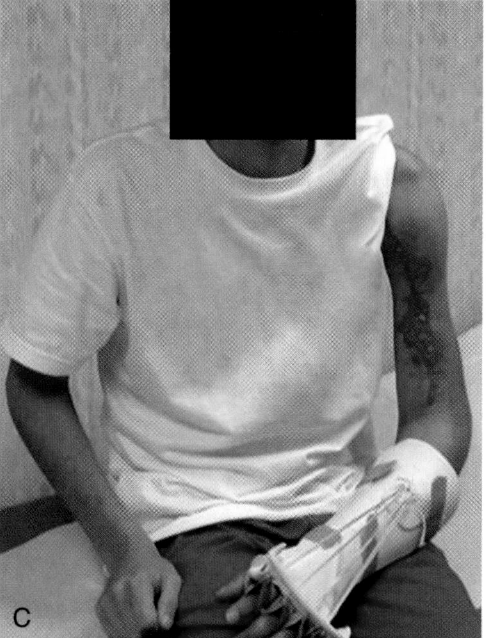

Figure 10 Anterior (**A**) and posterior (**B**) clinical photographs of the arm following the epithelialization of the wound, which was hastened by a split thickness skin graft and a negative pressure dressing. **C,** The patient wore a splint with outriggers for finger extension because of a radial nerve injury.

References

1. Cierny G III, Byrd HS, Jones RE: Primary versus delayed soft tissue coverage for severe open tibial fractures: A comparison of results. *Clin Orthop Relat Res* 1983;178: 54-63.
2. DeLong WG Jr, Born CT, Wei SY, Petrik ME, Ponzio R, Schwab CW: Aggressive treatment of 119 open fracture wounds. *J Trauma* 1999;46(6):1049-1054.
3. Hohmann E, Tetsworth K, Radziejowski MJ, Wiesniewski TF: Comparison of delayed and primary wound closure in the treatment of open tibial fractures. *Arch Orthop Trauma Surg* 2007; 127(2):131-136.
4. Sanders R, Swiontkowski M, Nunley J, Spiegel P: The management of fractures with soft-tissue disruptions. *J Bone Joint Surg Am* 1993;75(5):778-789.
5. Olson S: Open fractures of the tibial shaft: Current treatment. *J Bone Joint Surg Am* 1996;78: 1428-1437.
6. Gustilo RB, Anderson JT: Prevention of infection in the treatment of one thousand and twenty-five open fractures of long bones: Retrospective and prospective analyses. *J Bone Joint Surg Am* 1976; 58(4):453-458.
7. Gustilo RB, Mendoza RM, Williams DN: Problems in the management of type III (severe) open fractures: A new classification of type III open fractures. *J Trauma* 1984;24(8):742-746.
8. Tscherne H, Oestern HJ: [A new classification of soft-tissue damage in open and closed fractures (author's transl)]. *Unfallheilkunde* 1982;85(3):111-115.
9. Orthopaedic Trauma Association: Open Fracture Study Group: A new classification scheme for open fractures. *J Orthop Trauma* 2010; 24(8):457-464.
10. Levin LS, Condit DP: Combined injuries: Soft tissue management. *Clin Orthop Relat Res* 1996;327: 172-181.
11. Hampton OP Jr: Management of open fractures and open wounds of joints: 1968. *Clin Orthop Relat Res* 1997;345:4-7.
12. Keblish DJ, DeMaio M: Early pulsatile lavage for the decontamination of combat wounds: Historical review and point proposal. *Mil Med* 1998;163(12):844-846.
13. Lee EW, Dirschl DR, Duff G, Dahners LE, Miclau T: High-pressure pulsatile lavage irrigation of fresh intraarticular fractures: Effectiveness at removing particulate matter from bone. *J Orthop Trauma* 2002;16(3):162-165.
14. Polzin B, Ellis T, Dirschl DR: Effects of varying pulsatile lavage pressure on cancellous bone structure and fracture healing. *J Orthop Trauma* 2006;20(4):261-266.
15. Dirschl DR, Duff GP, Dahners LE, Edin M, Rahn BA, Miclau T: High pressure pulsatile lavage irrigation of intraarticular fractures: Effects on fracture healing. *J Orthop Trauma* 1998;12(7): 460-463.
16. Adili A, Bhandari M, Schemitsch EH: The biomechanical effect of high-pressure irrigation on diaphyseal fracture healing in vivo. *J Orthop Trauma* 2002; 16(6):413-417.
17. Anglen JO: Wound irrigation in musculoskeletal injury. *J Am Acad Orthop Surg* 2001;9(4):219-226.
18. Conroy BP, Anglen JO, Simpson WA, et al: Comparison of castile soap, benzalkonium chloride, and bacitracin as irrigation solutions for complex contaminated orthopaedic wounds. *J Orthop Trauma* 1999;13(5):332-337.
19. Gainor BJ, Hockman DE, Anglen JO, Christensen G, Simpson WA: Benzalkonium chloride: A potential disinfecting irrigation solution. *J Orthop Trauma* 1997; 11(2):121-125.
20. Moussa FW, Gainor BJ, Anglen JO, Christensen G, Simpson WA: Disinfecting agents for removing adherent bacteria from orthopaedic hardware. *Clin Orthop Relat Res* 1996;329:255-262.
21. Tarbox BB, Conroy BP, Malicky ES, et al: Benzalkonium chloride: A potential disinfecting irrigation solution for orthopaedic wounds. *Clin Orthop Relat Res* 1998;346:255-261.
22. Bhandari M, Adili A, Schemitsch EH: The efficacy of low-pressure lavage with different irrigating solutions to remove adherent bacteria from bone. *J Bone Joint Surg Am* 2001;83-A(3):412-419.
23. Anglen J, Apostoles PS, Christensen G, Gainor B, Lane J: Removal of surface bacteria by irrigation. *J Orthop Res* 1996;14(2): 251-254.
24. Marberry KM, Kazmier P, Simpson WA, et al: Surfactant wound irrigation for the treatment of staphylococcal clinical isolates. *Clin Orthop Relat Res* 2002;403: 73-79.
25. Patzakis MJ, Harvey JP Jr, Ivler D: The role of antibiotics in the management of open fractures. *J Bone Joint Surg Am* 1974; 56(3):532-541.
26. Russell GG, Henderson R, Arnett G: Primary or delayed closure for open tibial fractures. *J Bone Joint Surg Br* 1990;72(1):125-128.
27. Weitz-Marshall AD, Bosse MJ: Timing of closure of open fractures. *J Am Acad Orthop Surg* 2002;10(6):379-384.
28. Levin LS: The reconstructive ladder: An orthoplastic approach. *Orthop Clin North Am* 1993; 24(3):393-409.
29. Mathes SJ, Alpert BS: Advances in muscle and musculocutaneous flaps. *Clin Plast Surg* 1980;7(1): 15-26.

30. Fischer MD, Gustilo RB, Varecka TF: The timing of flap coverage, bone-grafting, and intramedullary nailing in patients who have a fracture of the tibial shaft with extensive soft-tissue injury. *J Bone Joint Surg Am* 1991; 73(9):1316-1322.

31. Finkemeier CG, Schmidt AH, Kyle RF, Templeman DC, Varecka TF: A prospective, randomized study of intramedullary nails inserted with and without reaming for the treatment of open and closed fractures of the tibial shaft. *J Orthop Trauma* 2000;14(3): 187-193.

32. Wang HT, Erdmann D, Fletcher JW, Levin LS: Anterolateral thigh flap technique in hand and upper extremity reconstruction. *Tech Hand Up Extrem Surg* 2004;8(4):257-261.

33. Gopal S, Majumder S, Batchelor AG, Knight SL, De Boer P, Smith RM: Fix and flap: The radical orthopaedic and plastic treatment of severe open fractures of the tibia. *J Bone Joint Surg Br* 2000;82(7):959-966.

34. Byrd HS, Cierny G III, Tebbetts JB: The management of open tibial fractures with associated soft-tissue loss: External pin fixation with early flap coverage. *Plast Reconstr Surg* 1981;68(1): 73-82.

35. Ostermann PA, Henry SL, Seligson D: Timing of wound closure in severe compound fractures. *Orthopedics* 1994;17(5):397-399.

36. Hertel R, Lambert SM, Müller S, Ballmer FT, Ganz R: On the timing of soft-tissue reconstruction for open fractures of the lower leg. *Arch Orthop Trauma Surg* 1999; 119(1-2):7-12.

37. Heller L, Levin LS: Lower extremity microsurgical reconstruction. *Plast Reconstr Surg* 2001;108(4): 1029-1042.

38. Webb LX: New techniques in wound management: Vacuum-assisted wound closure. *J Am Acad Orthop Surg* 2002;10(5):303-311.

39. Chu CS, McManus AT, Matylevich NP, Goodwin CW, Pruitt BA Jr: Integra as a dermal replacement in a meshed composite skin graft in a rat model: A one-step operative procedure. *J Trauma* 2002;52(1):122-129.

40. De Vries HJ, Mekkes JR, Middelkoop E, Hinrichs WL, Wildevuur CR, Westerhof W: Dermal substitutes for full-thickness wounds in a one-stage grafting model. *Wound Repair Regen* 1993; 1(4):244-252.

41. Cole JD, Ansel LJ, Schwartzberg R: A sequential protocol for management of severe open tibial fractures. *Clin Orthop Relat Res* 1995;315:84-103.

42. Strauss EJ, Petrucelli G, Bong M, Koval KJ, Egol KA: Blisters associated with lower-extremity fracture: Results of a prospective treatment protocol. *J Orthop Trauma* 2006;20(9):618-622.

43. Giordano CP, Koval KJ: Treatment of fracture blisters: A prospective study of 53 cases. *J Orthop Trauma* 1995;9(2):171-176.

The Mangled Limb: Salvage Versus Amputation

Philip R. Wolinsky, MD, FACS
Lawrence X. Webb, MD
Edward J. Harvey, MD, FRCSC
Nirmal C. Tejwani, MD

Abstract

A mangled extremity is defined as a limb with injury to three of four systems in the extremity. The decision to salvage or amputate the injured limb has generated much controversy in the literature, with studies to support advantages of each approach. Various scoring systems have proved unreliable in predicting the need for amputation or salvage; however, a recurring theme in the literature is that the key to limb viability seems to be the severity of the soft-tissue injury. Factors such as associated injuries, patient age, and comorbidities (such as diabetes) also should be considered. Attempted limb salvage should be considered only if a patient is hemodynamically stable enough to tolerate the necessary surgical procedures and blood loss associated with limb salvage. For persistently hemodynamically unstable patients and those in extremis, life comes before limb.

Recently, the Lower Extremity Assessment Project study attempted to answer the question of whether amputation or limb salvage achieves a better outcome. The study also evaluated other factors, including return-to-work status, impact of the level of and bilaterality of the amputation, and economic cost. There appears to be no significant difference in return to work, functional outcomes, or the cost of treatment (including the prosthesis) between the two groups. A team approach with different specialties, including orthopaedics, plastic surgery, vascular surgery and trauma general surgery, is recommended for treating patients with a mangled extremity.

Instr Course Lect 2011;60:27-34.

This chapter will discuss the absolute and relative indications for limb salvage versus amputation, as well as review expected postoperative rehabilitation and outcomes after limb salvage or amputation for the treatment of a mangled extremity.

A mangled extremity is defined as a limb with an injury to three of four systems. The systems of the lower extremity are the soft tissues, the nerves, the blood supply, and the bone.[1] These are the most severe types of injuries, with extensive involvement of structures, and are more severe than a simple open fracture. Attempted limb salvage should be considered only if a patient is hemodynamically stable enough to tolerate the surgical procedures and blood loss. For persistently hemodynamically unstable patients and those in extremis, the preservation of life supersedes the preservation of limb.

Dr. Wolinsky or an immediate family member is a member of a speakers' bureau or has made paid presentations on behalf of Zimmer; serves as a paid consultant to or is an employee of Biomet; and has received research or institutional support from Zimmer, AO, and Biomet. Dr. Webb or an immediate family member serves as a board member, owner, officer, or committee member of the Orthopaedic Trauma Association and the Southeastern Fracture Consortium; is a member of a speakers' bureau or has made paid presentations on behalf of the Musculoskeletal Transplant Foundation; serves as a paid consultant to or is an employee of Zimmer; and has received nonincome support (such as equipment or services), commercially derived honoraria, or other non–research-related funding (such as paid travel) from Synthes, Smith & Nephew, Stryker, and Kinetic Concepts. Dr. Harvey or an immediate family member serves as a board member, owner, officer, or committee member of the American Academy of Orthopaedic Surgeons, the Orthopaedic Trauma Association, the Canadian Orthopaedic Association, and the Orthopaedic Research Society; has received research or institutional support from Synthes; and owns stock or stock options in Pfizer. Dr. Tejwani or an immediate family member serves as a board member, owner, officer, or committee member of the American Academy of Orthopaedic Surgeons; has received royalties from Biomet; is a member of a speakers' bureau or has made paid presentations on behalf of Zimmer and Stryker; and serves as a paid consultant to or is an employee of Zimmer and Stryker.

It has been questioned why an attempt is not made to salvage every mangled limb, with a revision to amputation if the salvage is problematic. One potential issue with this approach is that patients often become emotionally attached to their injured limb and will not consider a delayed amputation. The patient may rationalize that if the injury were severe enough to require an amputation, the limb would have been amputated at the time of the first surgery. However, failed limb salvage has potentially severe consequences: "Two to three years of hospitalizations, surgeries, complications from infections, nonunions, and inevitable amputations ..." Patients lose their jobs, families, savings, self-image, and respect; although their limbs were saved, their lives were ruined.[2]

Indications for Amputation

Unfortunately, there are few useful clinical indications for amputation detailed in the literature. Some helpful indications for amputation include total or near-total amputation of the limb at the time of the initial injury, a complete anatomic sciatic or tibial nerve transection (rather than simply a lack of sensation), and/or loss of plantar skin and soft tissues. Some less helpful indications include an "extremely mangled" limb (with no clear definition of what constitutes extremely mangled versus not so extremely mangled), massive amounts of nonviable soft tissue (with "massive" not clearly defined), and unreconstructible bone or vascular injuries (involving a fairly subjective decision regarding what is and is not reconstructible).

In a classic 1989 article, Lange[3] described the decision-making processs for limb salvage versus amputation for a severely injured limb. He emphasized the need to evaluate the entire patient, including variables such as occupation, age, underlying disease processes (such as diabetes), and the needs of the patient and family. Associated variables, including other injuries and the severity and duration of shock (if present) should then be considered. The physician should evaluate the extremity, including the fracture pattern, the level of the vascular injury, the warm ischemia time, the anatomic status of nerves that are not clinically functioning, and the status of the ipsilateral foot. Lange's absolute indications for amputation included anatomic nerve disruption, warm ischemia time of more than 6 hours, hemodynamic instability, and/or a smashed ipsilateral foot. He emphasized that most patients will not have an absolute indication for an amputation but will be classified into an indeterminate gray zone.[3]

Importance of the Magnitude of the Soft-Tissue Injury

A recurring theme in the orthopaedic literature is that the key to limb viability (determining if a limb is salvageable) seems to be the severity of the soft-tissue injury. Lange[3] reported that the magnitude of the soft-tissue injury was the most important factor in determining limb viability.[3] McNamara et al,[4] in a study using the Mangled Extremity Severity Score, found that a soft-tissue injury combined with a skeletal injury was the only significant predictor of amputation (P = 0.011). Hafez et al[5] performed a multivariate analysis of risk factors for amputation after the repair of arterial injuries and found that graft occlusion was predictive of failure (odds ratio, 16.7) and that failed revascularization most often occurred because of either a technical error or a severe muscle injury with microcirculatory damage leading to limited outflow and proximal thrombosis.

Patient Outcomes

A patient with a mangled extremity wants to know if limb salvage or amputation will result in a better outcome. The answer is difficult because of the conflicting results in the literature. Studies can be found that support limb salvage as the better option, whereas other studies support amputation as the superior choice.

Limb Salvage as the Better Option

A study of patients after limb salvage or amputation to treat grade IIIB and IIIC open tibial fractures reported that there was no difference between the two groups in terms of the length of hospital stay (25 days after successful limb salvage, 28 days after a primary amputation, and 33 days after a secondary amputation).[6] Successful limb salvage surgery required an average of 5.39 procedures (SD, 2.22), and unsuccessful salvage procedures required an average of 7.6 procedures (SD, 1.52). Ninety-two percent of the patients with successful limb salvage preferred their salvaged leg to an amputation. The salvage group had higher scores than the amputation group on the physical function portion of the Medical Outcomes Study 36-Item Short Form (38 versus 28, respectively), and there were no significant difference in mental health outcome scores (52 versus 47). All the patients considered themselves more disabled than patients affected by heart attacks, chronic obstructive pulmonary disease, diabetes, cancer, angina, or back pain. The same percentage of patients in each group returned to work (in those patients working before the injury); however, there was a difference in the length of absence from work. Patients with successful limb salvage took 17.6 months to return to work, whereas patients in the primary and secondary amputation groups took 9 months to return to work. The authors of the study concluded that limb salvage was a better treatment option, but patients have a longer recovery than those treated with amputation. All of the patients had significant physical disabilities.

In a Swiss study by Hertel et al[7] of patients with type IIIB and IIIC open tibial fractures, patients treated with early amputation needed fewer surgical procedures than those treated with limb salvage (3.5 versus 8, respectively), as well as less rehabilitation time (12 months versus 30 months, respectively). However, more amputees changed jobs, and all amputees had to change to a less physically demanding job, whereas 10 of 21 limb-salvage patients were able to adapt their prior jobs. More amputees received a disability pension than those treated with limb salvage (54% versus 16%, respectively), and there was a greater lifestyle change for amputees. Phantom limb pain occurred in 50% of amputees, with a median visual analog pain score of 3.4 of 10. Pain occurred in 19% of the limb-salvage patients with prolonged standing, with a median visual analog pain score of 0.9 of 10. Amputees walked less (average distance per day, 5.25 km) than salvage patients (average distance per day, 12 km), wore their prosthesis for an average of 13 hours per day, and 50% had chronic ulcers. The authors concluded that limb-salvage patients had better functional outcomes than amputees; however, when compared with amputation, limb salvage requires a longer recovery period and more surgeries.[7]

Amputation as the Better Option

In a study by Georgiadis et al[8] comparing patients with type IIIB and IIIC tibial fractures, 20 patients (2 with type IIIC injuries) were treated with limb salvage with free flaps and 18 patients (15 with type IIIC injuries) were treated with amputation. Patients were excluded from the study if they had major foot or ankle injuries, did not have an intact heel pad or intact plantar sensation, had vascular injuries without a soft-tissue injury, or had wounds that were treated with a local flap. The limb salvage group had 70 complications (89%) with an average of 3 complications per patient, whereas the amputation group had 17 complications. Osteomyelitis developed in 56% of the limb salvage patients; these patients required more surgical procedures and had longer hospital stays than the amputation group.

Time to full weight bearing was 13 months in the limb salvage group compared with 6 months in the amputation group. Fewer patients in this group were working (3 of 16 working, with 1 more willing to work) than in the amputation group (9 of 18 working, with 5 more willing to work). Twelve of 16 patients in the limb-salvage group considered themselves disabled, whereas only 4 of 18 amputees considered themselves disabled. Using Quality of Life scoring, the amputees did better than the salvage group, although neither group had scores close to the healthy reference population.[8]

All Amputees Do Well: Truth or Perception?

There is a perception among some orthopaedic surgeons that all amputees have favorable outcomes. It is important to examine if this is just a perception because of the lack of long-term follow-up or has a basis in truth. One study followed 42 patients treated with traumatic amputations for a mean of 2 years. Two to three procedures were required to close the stump in most patients, stump complications occurred in 40% of the patients, and 50% returned to work (only two patients who performed manual labor were able to return to work). Twelve patients (48%) with a below-knee amputation were able to return to work, whereas none of the patients with above-knee amputations were able to return to work.[9]

Dillingham et al[10] reported on 78 traumatic amputees followed for 10 years. Eighty-seven percent of the patients were male, and 66% were young (ages 21 to 39 years). In the 95% of amputees with prostheses, it took an average of 6 months from the time of injury to the time they received their first prosthesis, and a new prosthesis was needed at a mean of every 2 years. The prosthesis was used for an average of 80 hours per week; 43% were satisfied with the comfort of the prosthesis. Thirteen percent of the amputees used crutches all or most of the time, and 12% used a wheelchair all or most of the time. Fifty-eight percent were satisfied with the appearance of the amputation, 24% had skin irritation, 24% had some type of wound on the affected extremity, and 25% had phantom limb pain. Each patient visited a prosthetist an average of four times a year. Factors associated with prosthetic use and satisfaction were being male and having a lower Injury Severity Score.[10]

The longest follow-up period of traumatic amputations in the literature found by this chapter's authors was a 28-year follow-up of unilateral below-knee amputees from the Vietnam War. These patients required an average of 1.94 surgeries, the average time to permanent prosthesis fitting was 6.57 months, the average prosthesis wear was 15.9 hours per day, and the average number of prostheses needed was 8.31, or one every 3 years. Patients with isolated injuries had no difference in Medical Outcomes Study 36-Item Short Form scores compared with a

Table 1
Patients in the LEAP Study Compared With the General Population

Factor	LEAP Study Patients	General Population
Education	70% high school graduates nationally	86% high school graduates nationally
Economic status	25% below the federal poverty line	20% below the federal poverty line
Health insurance status	38% have no health insurance	20% have no health insurance
Heavy alcohol drinker	27%	11%
Smoker	37%	29%
Personality traits	More neurotic and extroverted Less open to new experiences	Less neurotic and extroverted More open to new experiences

LEAP = Lower Extremity Assessment Project.

control group at 28 years from injury. This finding suggests that young patients with isolated below-knee amputations have a chance to lead normal productive lives with regard to work and families.[11]

Costs Associated With Amputation

Because limb salvage requires more surgeries and more time in the hospital than an amputation, it would be logical to believe that limb salvage costs more than amputation, and patients with limited resources may fare better financially if treated with amputation rather than limb salvage. However, this logic does not account for the long-term costs of prosthetic devices. One estimation of the long-term costs of amputation was calculated based on the amputee requiring two prostheses for the first 2 years after amputation, and one new prosthesis every 5 years thereafter, which is probably an underestimation.[12] The costs for a below-knee amputation were $4,218 for 1 year and $42,180 over a 30-year period. The costs for an above-knee amputation were $5,695 for 1 year and $56,850 over a 30-year period.

Lower Extremity Assessment Project

The National Institutes of Health funded a multicenter study of mangled limbs called the Lower Extremity Assessment Project (LEAP). The LEAP study enrolled patients treated at eight level I trauma centers. This prospective, observational study was designed to follow outcomes after either amputation or limb-salvage treatment for a severely injured lower extremity. The remainder of this chapter describes the results of various studies based on LEAP data.

LEAP Study Questions

The LEAP study tried to answer several questions. Who gets severe lower extremity injuries? What are the characteristics of patients enrolled in the study? What are the characteristics of patients treated with lower limb salvage compared with those treated with leg amputation? Seventy-seven percent of the patients were male, 71% were young (age 20 to 45 years), 77% were white, and 77% were working at the time of injury. Of those working, 75% had jobs that involved moderate to heavy physical demands. Differences between these patients and the general population are shown in **Table 1**.

There were no differences between study patients treated with amputation or limb salvage. The clinical relevance of these findings is that the LEAP study patients in general had fewer resources, which could potentially limit their access to rehabilitation services and/or prosthetics; had poorer health habits than the general population; had physically demanding jobs; and had personality traits that could predispose them to a more difficult recovery.[13]

Determinants of Disability

The LEAP study tried to determine which factors influence the progression from physical impairment to patient-perceived disability. Impairment was defined as abnormalities of body structure and/or appearance, whereas disability was defined as the consequence(s) of impairment that lead to difficulty performing everyday activities. Physical impairment was assessed by measuring range of motion, strength, pain (assessed using a visual analog pain score) and by using the American Medical Association guides for evaluating permanent impairment. Disability was assessed using the Sickness Impact Profile (SIP) at admission and at 12-month follow-up. After a multivariate analysis, the nine factors listed in **Table 2** correlated with the 12-month SIP score; however, these factors accounted for only 52% of the variance.[14]

Functional Outcomes After 2 Years

Bosse et al[15] analyzed patient outcomes after salvage or amputation to determine if the functional results of limb salvage and amputation for a severely injured limb were different. The working hypothesis was that amputees would do better than limb salvage patients. The authors found that the injuries in the two groups differed in that patients treated with amputation had more severe injuries with a greater frequency of bone loss, had more soft-tissue damage, and were more likely to have an initial pulse deficit and/or lack of plantar sensation than those in the limb salvage group. At 2-year follow-up, the SIP scores were the same in the two groups: 12.6 versus 11.8 ($P = 0.53$). These scores reflect high levels of disability (norm, 2 to 3). More than 40% of the patients in both groups had scores greater than 10, which indicated a severe disability. Similar proportions of amputees and limb salvage patients were able to return to work by 2 years (53% versus 49.4%, respectively). The predictors of a poor SIP score included rehospitalization for a complication, less than a high school education, nonwhite race, income below the federal poverty line, no insurance or Medicaid, smoking, a poor social support network, low self-efficacy, and involvement with the legal system regarding injury compensation.

The authors commented that major outcome improvements may require nonclinical interventions, such as psychosocial specialists or vocational specialists. The authors also recommended that "patients with limbs at high risk for amputation can be advised that reconstruction typically results in two-year outcomes equivalent to those of amputation."[15] Reconstruction, however, was associated with a higher risk of complications, additional surgeries, rehospitalizations, and psychological issues.

Table 2

Factors That Correlated With the LEAP Participants' SIP Scores Indicating Disability at 12-Month Follow-up

Impairment score (range of motion, strength) and visual analog pain score
Age: Patients younger than 25 years did better than older study participants.
Poverty status strongly correlated with a worse SIP score.
Score on the baseline SIP (at the time of hospital admission): A worse score on the baseline SIP was predictive of a worse outcome. The worse baseline SIP score was not likely caused by chronic medical problems because most of the patients were young (mean age, 34 years; range, 18 to 63 years) but was more likely the result of psychosocial and emotional disorders.
Educational status: Not having a high school degree was predictive of a lower SIP score.
Type of health insurance: Private insurance was predictive of the best outcome; having no insurance was predictive of an intermediate outcome; having Medicaid was predictive of the worst outcome.
Level of social support: Lack of social support was predictive of a worse outcome.
Legal representation: Representation by an attorney was predictive of a worse outcome.
Workers' compensation status: Being a recipient of workers' compensation was predictive of a worse outcome.

LEAP = Lower Extremity Assessment Project, SIP = sickness impact profile.

Psychological Distress

A study by McCarthy et al[16] determined the incidence of psychological distress in the LEAP study patients by administering the Brief System Inventory at 3, 6, 12, and 24 months after injury. A likely psychological disorder was found in 48% of the patients at 2-month follow-up and in 42% at 2-year follow-up. Relatively few patients had any mental health services (12% at 3 months and 22% at 4 months). The predictors of psychological distress included poorer physical function, younger age, nonwhite race, poverty, alcohol abuse, neuroticism, a poor sense of self-efficacy, and limited social support. Most of these risk factors are beyond the control of the treating surgeon.

Complications at 2-Year Follow-up

In an analysis of the LEAP study patients by Harris et al,[17] the type and incidence of complications at 2 years after injury were examined. This study evaluated 149 patients treated with amputation, with 5% of them requiring a revision. Most complications occurred at 3 months after injury, and the most frequent complication was a wound infection (34% of the patients). In 371 patients treated with limb salvage, 4% required a late amputation. Most complications in this group occurred at 6 months after injury, and the most frequent complication was a wound infection (23% of the patients). Osteomyelitis developed in 9% of the patients and nonunions in 31%. One third of all the patients had to be rehospitalized; patients treated with limb salvage were more likely to require hospitalization for complications.[17]

Outcomes at 7-Year Follow-up

A study by MacKenzie el al[18] analyzed the long-term effects of disability. The authors hypothesized that outcomes may improve between 2 and 7 years because nonunions may have resolved in the limb salvage group, and those with amputations may have gained increased comfort and confidence with their prosthesis. However, at an average 7-year follow-up, there was a long-term persistence of disability, and the

SIP subscores were worse at 84 months than at 24 months ($P < 0.05$). This worsening of disability was consistent across all treatment groups. Thirty-four percent of patients had a normal physical SIP subscore (≤ 5), 49% had a score consistent with a severe disability, and 26% had a score consistent with a very severe disability. There were two significant differences between the treatment groups. Patients with a severe soft-tissue injury were 3.1 times more likely to have a SIP subscore of 5 or greater, and patients with a through-knee amputation were 11.5 times more likely to have a low SIP subscore. Predictors of a better outcome included male sex, younger age at the time of injury, having a higher socioeconomic status, being a nonsmoker at the time of injury, and having better self-efficacy (confidence to perform certain tasks). In addition, 39% of limb salvage patients and 33% of amputees required rehospitalization between 2 and 7 years.[18]

Surgical Decision Making

A bivariate study by MacKenzie et al[19] showed that all limb injury characteristics (bony, soft-tissue, neurologic, and vascular) were significantly associated ($P < 0.01$) with decision making regarding amputation or reconstruction after a severe traumatic lower extremity injury, but the Injury Severity Score was not a predictor of the treatment choice. Higher-energy injuries, such as motor vehicle crashes or gunshot wounds, had a greater likelihood of amputation ($P < 0.01$), as did a patient presenting in shock ($P < 0.05$). There were no statistical differences between different institutions; however, all the surgeons in this study worked at level I trauma centers.

The multivariate analysis showed a hierarchy of importance of the injuries to the limb in the following order: soft tissue, nerve, bone, and artery. One reason why most limb injury scoring systems are not useful is because similar weighting systems are not used.[19]

Importance of Intact Plantar Sensation

A study by Bosse et al[20] emphasized the importance of using the anatomic status of the tibial nerve, not just the clinical examination finding when making a decision regarding limb salvage or amputation in a severely injured limb. Outcomes at 2 years did not differ between the insensate salvage group, the sensate salvage group, or the insensate amputation group. An equal number of patients who had presented with or without plantar sensation in the limb salvage group had normal plantar sensation (55%) at 2-year follow-up. Only one patient in the insensate salvage group had absent plantar sensation at 2 years. The authors stated that "the findings ... do not support the belief that the initial plantar sensory status... is correlated with poor late outcome ...," and "tibial nerve dysfunction on clinical examination cannot be assumed to be equivalent to nerve disruption." The authors also reported that in patients with absent plantar sensation at the initial examination, substantial impairment was present at 12- and 24-month follow-up. The impairment did not appear to be related to the choice of treatment with amputation or limb salvage.

The Effect of the Amputation Level on Patient Satisfaction

In a study examining and comparing the functional outcomes of below-knee amputations, through-knee amputations, and above-knee amputations at 2-year follow-up, the working hypothesis was that patients with above-knee amputations would have worse outcomes than patients with through-knee or below-knee amputations.[21] Using SIP scores, the authors found no differences between below-knee and above-knee amputations. Speed of walking was better for patients with below-knee amputations than for those with above-knee amputations, but SIP scores indicated that the patients believed there was no difference. Walking speed of both above-knee and below-knee amputees was faster than in those with a through-knee amputation. A regression-adjusted analysis of the SIP scores showed that through-knee amputees had the worst scores (37% higher SIP scores; $P = 0.05$). The authors stressed that the reason for the poor results of the through-knee amputees may have resulted from the fact that most through-knee amputations were performed through the level of the soft-tissue injury in an effort to save limb length. Overall, the SIP scores were higher (worse) than norms, and the functional outcomes were poor at 2-year follow-up, with no differences between below-knee and above-knee amputations.

For all amputation levels, the initial length of hospital stay averaged 17.7 days, it took 100 days until the first permanent prosthesis was fitted, 30% of patients were rehospitalized for a complication, 15% needed a stump revision during the first 2 years, patients required an average of 2.3 surgical procedures during the first 2 years, 6.5% had soft-tissue wounds that had not healed, 4.8% still needed additional surgery, and 54% returned to work. Other predictors of a poorer SIP score included preexisting medical conditions, smoking, an ipsilateral limb injury, having less than a college education, having low self-efficacy, and nonwhite race. Again, orthopaedic surgeons have no control over these variables.

Cost Considerations for Limb Salvage and Amputation

A 2007 study looked at 2-year health costs and projected lifetime costs of amputation and limb salvage.[22] Costs included the initial hospitalization, all rehospitalizations, inpatient rehabilitation, outpatient physician visits, outpatient physical and occupational therapy, and prosthetics. At 2 years, if only the costs of hospitalizations and post-acute care are included, the costs of limb salvage and amputation are equal. If the costs of the prostheses are included, an amputation costs $91,106, and limb salvage costs $81,316. Using an assumption of needing a new prosthesis every 2.3 years, the projected lifetime cost of an amputation was $509,275, and the projected lifetime cost of limb salvage was $163,282. However, limb salvage patients may incur additional costs if future surgeries or orthotics are needed.

The length of hospital stay of the initial care and number of surgical procedures were the same for both groups, but 61% of limb salvage patients and 35% of amputees required rehospitalization. Eighteen percent of amputees and 10% of limb salvage patients required admission to an inpatient rehabilitation facility.

Scoring Systems for Predicting Outcomes After Limb Salvage

Although scoring systems are not good predictors of which patients should be treated with salvage versus amputation, a study by Ly et al[23] evaluated the ability to predict functional outcomes after limb salvage. Using five limb salvage scores, 407 patients were analyzed at 6 months and 24 months. No score was found to be predictive of the SIP score at 6 or 24 months, and scores were nonpredictive of any improvement between 6 and 24 months.

Bilateral Severe Lower Extremity Injuries

A study by Smith et al[24] analyzed 32 patients with severe bilateral lower extremity injuries to see if different decision-making factors should be applied to patients with bilateral limb-threatening injuries. Patients were followed for 2 years. All possible treatment combinations resulted in severe disability at 2 years. Patients treated with bilateral limb salvage were most improved from their baseline condition at the time of hospital discharge over the 2 years, and those with bilateral amputations had the worst outcomes at 2 years. Better outcomes occurred in the following rank order: bilateral salvages, unilateral salvage, bilateral amputations. Salvage procedures were associated with a higher rehospitalization rate for complications than the amputations. The return-to-work rate at 2 years was 67% in the unilateral salvage and unilateral amputation groups, 21% in the bilateral salvage group, and 16% in the bilateral amputation group. The authors concluded that severe disability results from bilateral injuries, but not more severe than from unilateral injuries; SIP scores improve over time; and treatment decisions should be made based on the larger unilateral limb data.

Summary

There are few absolute indications for lower extremity limb amputations after traumatic injuries. The decision-making process for choosing limb salvage or amputation requires global limb assessment, with the extent of the soft-tissue damage taking precedence. The patient is best treated with a team approach, which includes plastic, vascular, trauma, and orthopaedic surgeons. Orthopaedic surgeons should take the lead in decision making because they will administer long-term care to the patient.

References

1. Gregory RT, Gould RJ, Peclet M, et al: The mangled extremity syndrome (M.E.S.): A severity grading system for multisystem injury of the extremity. *J Trauma* 1985; 25(12):1147-1150.
2. Hansen ST Jr: Overview of the severely traumatized lower limb: Reconstruction versus amputation. *Clin Orthop Relat Res* 1989; 243:17-19.
3. Lange RH: Limb reconstruction versus amputation decision making in massive lower extremity trauma. *Clin Orthop Relat Res* 1989;243:92-99.
4. McNamara MG, Heckman JD, Corley FG: Severe open fractures of the lower extremity: A retrospective evaluation of the Mangled Extremity Severity Score (MESS). *J Orthop Trauma* 1994; 8(2):81-87.
5. Hafez HM, Woolgar J, Robbs JV: Lower extremity arterial injury: Results of 550 cases and review of risk factors associated with limb loss. *J Vasc Surg* 2001;33(6):1212-1219.
6. Dagum AB, Best AK, Schemitsch EH, Mahoney JL, Mahomed MN, Blight KR: Salvage after severe lower-extremity trauma: Are the outcomes worth the means? *Plast Reconstr Surg* 1999; 103(4):1212-1220.
7. Hertel R, Strebel N, Ganz R: Amputation versus reconstruction in traumatic defects of the leg: Outcome and costs. *J Orthop Trauma* 1996;10(4):223-229.
8. Georgiadis GM, Behrens FF, Joyce MJ, Earle AS, Simmons AL: Open tibial fractures with severe soft-tissue loss: Limb salvage compared with below-the-knee amputation. *J Bone Joint Surg Am* 1993; 75(10):1431-1441.
9. Livingston DH, Keenan D, Kim D, Elcavage J, Malangoni MA: Extent of disability following traumatic extremity amputation. *J Trauma* 1994;37(3): 495-499.
10. Dillingham TR, Pezzin LE, MacKenzie EJ, Burgess AR: Use

and satisfaction with prosthetic devices among persons with trauma-related amputations: A long-term outcome study. *Am J Phys Med Rehabil* 2001;80(8): 563-571.

11. Dougherty PJ: Transtibial amputees from the Vietnam War: Twenty-eight-year follow-up. *J Bone Joint Surg Am* 2001; 83-A(3):383-389.
12. Dirschl DR, Dahners LE: The mangled extremity: When should it be amputated? *J Am Acad Orthop Surg* 1996;4(4):182-190.
13. MacKenzie EJ, Bosse MJ, Kellam JF, et al: Characterization of patients with high-energy lower extremity trauma. *J Orthop Trauma* 2000;14(7):455-466.
14. Mock C, MacKenzie E, Jurkovich G, et al: Determinants of disability after lower extremity fracture. *J Trauma* 2000;49(6): 1002-1011.
15. Bosse MJ, MacKenzie EJ, Kellam JF, et al: An analysis of outcomes of reconstruction or amputation after leg-threatening injuries. *N Engl J Med* 2002; 347(24):1924-1931.
16. McCarthy ML, MacKenzie EJ, Edwin D, Bosse MJ, Castillo RC, Starr A; LEAP study group: Psychological distress associated with severe lower-limb injury. *J Bone Joint Surg Am* 2003;85-A(9): 1689-1697.
17. Harris AM, Althausen PL, Kellam J, Bosse MJ, Castillo R; Lower Extremity Assessment Project (LEAP) Study Group: Complications following limb-threatening lower extremity trauma. *J Orthop Trauma* 2009; 23(1):1-6.
18. MacKenzie EJ, Bosse MJ, Pollak AN, et al: Long-term persistence of disability following severe lower-limb trauma: Results of a seven-year follow-up. *J Bone Joint Surg Am* 2005;87(8):1801-1809.
19. MacKenzie EJ, Bosse MJ, Kellam JF, et al; LEAP Study Group: Factors influencing the decision to amputate or reconstruct after high-energy lower extremity trauma. *J Trauma* 2002;52(4): 641-649.
20. Bosse MJ, McCarthy ML, Jones AL, et al; Lower Extremity Assessment Project (LEAP) Study Group: The insensate foot following severe lower extremity trauma: An indication for amputation? *J Bone Joint Surg Am* 2005; 87(12):2601-2608.
21. MacKenzie EJ, Bosse MJ, Castillo RC, et al: Functional outcomes following trauma-related lower-extremity amputation. *J Bone Joint Surg Am* 2004;86-A(8):1636-1645.
22. MacKenzie EJ, Jones AS, Bosse MJ, et al: Health-care costs associated with amputation or reconstruction of a limb-threatening injury. *J Bone Joint Surg Am* 2007;89(8):1685-1692.
23. Ly TV, Travison TG, Castillo RC, Bosse MJ, MacKenzie EJ; LEAP Study Group: Ability of lower-extremity injury severity scores to predict functional outcome after limb salvage. *J Bone Joint Surg Am* 2008;90(8):1738-1743.
24. Smith JJ, Agel J, Swiontkowski MF, Castillo R, Mackenzie E, Kellam JF; LEAP Study Group: Functional outcome of bilateral limb threatening: Lower extremity injuries at two years postinjury. *J Orthop Trauma* 2005;19(4): 249-253.

Review of Treatment and Diagnosis of Acute Compartment Syndrome of the Calf: Current Evidence and Best Practices

John T. Gorczyca, MD
Craig S. Roberts, MD, MBA
Kevin J. Pugh, MD
David Ring, MD, PhD

Abstract

Compartment syndrome of the calf has received a great deal of attention in the literature. A MEDLINE search was conducted to identify English-language publications pertaining to compartment syndrome of the leg and calf so that principles, recent evidence, and best practices for the diagnosis and treatment of this syndrome could be reviewed. Clinical series that reported outcomes and diagnostic criteria were reviewed and summarized. The currently available evidence is limited to level IV and V studies.

Early diagnosis and treatment of compartment syndromes is associated with better results; however, many patients have chronic symptoms after treatment, even when the diagnosis is made promptly and fasciotomy is performed early. Although compartment syndrome of the leg and calf often has been described in the literature, prospective clinical series are lacking, and meaningful outcomes data are scarce. There is a need for further study on functional outcomes of acute compartment syndrome of the calf, with particular attention to diagnosis and treatment.

Instr Course Lect 2011;60:35-42.

Dr. Gorczyca or an immediate family member serves as a paid consultant to or is an employee of Zimmer. Dr. Roberts or an immediate family member serves as a board member, owner, officer, or committee member of the RRC, Orthopaedic Trauma Association, Mid-America Orthopaedic Association, Kentucky Orthopaedic Association, and Orthopaedic Incubator; has received research or institutional support from Stryker and Synthes; and has received nonincome support (such as equipment or services), commercially derived honoraria, or other non–research-related funding (such as paid travel) from Saunders/Mosby-Elseiver. Dr. Pugh or an immediate family member is a member of a speakers' bureau or has made paid presentations on behalf of Medtronic and Smith & Nephew and serves as a paid consultant to or is an employee of Medtronic and Smith & Nephew. Dr. Ring or an immediate family member has received royalties from DePuy and Wright Medical Technology; is a member of a speakers' bureau or has made paid presentations on behalf of Acumed and Wright Medical Technology; serves as a paid consultant to or is an employee of Acumed and Wright Medical Technology; has received research or institutional support from Acumed, Biomet, Stryker, Tornier, and Joint Active Systems; and owns stock or stock options in Mimedex and Illuminoss.

Although compartment syndrome of the leg and calf has been frequently described in the literature, prospective clinical series are lacking, and meaningful outcomes data are scarce. The currently available evidence is limited to level IV and V studies. Of the various compartment syndromes of the upper and lower extremities, compartment syndrome of the calf has historically received the most attention in the medical literature. This chapter will present a review of the principles, current evidence, and best practices in the diagnosis and treatment of compartment syndrome of the calf.

Early diagnosis and treatment of compartment syndromes is associated with better results; however, even when the diagnosis is made promptly and fasciotomy is performed early, many patients have chronic symptoms after treatment. This supports the need for further study on the functional outcomes of calf compartment syndrome, with particular reference to diagnosis and treatment.

The challenge in treating compartment syndrome of the calf is obtaining

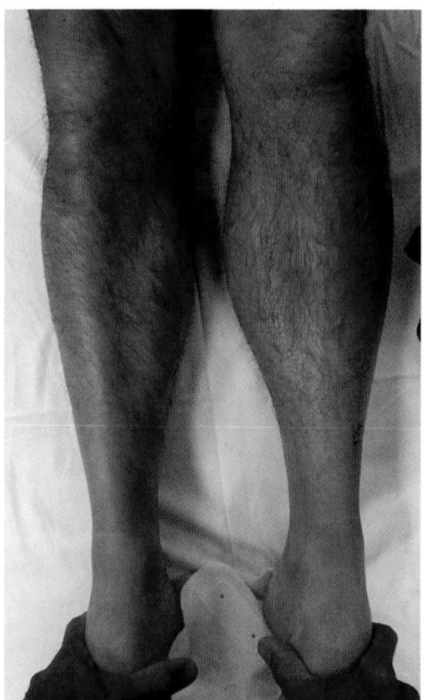

Figure 1 Photograph showing compartment syndrome in the left leg of a patient after a relatively minor injury. The patient was receiving anticoagulation therapy. The left leg has significant swelling, and the compartments are firm.

an early diagnosis that allows timely fasciotomy to prevent tissue necrosis and functional loss.[1] Most compartment syndromes are caused by trauma. McQueen et al[2] reported that 69% of the patients in their study had sustained a fracture, with a tibial fracture occurring in 36%. The corresponding traumatic injury made it difficult to distinguish the symptoms of compartment syndrome from symptoms related to the fracture. The authors also reported that 10% of the patients had coagulopathy; the prevalence this condition appears to be increasing as more elderly trauma patients are treated with anticoagulants for medical disorders. The patient receiving anticoagulation therapy is at a higher risk for compartment syndrome caused by bleeding within the compartments (**Figure 1**).

Clinical Findings

The most common symptom in a patient with compartment syndrome in the calf is pain. In an alert patient, the diagnosis is clinical. As the compartment syndrome progresses, the pain becomes more difficult to treat with analgesics and is out of proportion compared with the severity of the injury.

On physical examination, the compartment feels swollen and is often tense. Pressure applied to the compartment causes pain. Passive stretching of the muscles will also produce pain in the area of the compartment syndrome. Paralysis occurs late in the course of compartment syndrome and will manifest as an inability to use or contract muscles in the compartment.

Sensory nerves that pass through the compartment may have paresthesias caused by ischemia of the nerve or sensory loss, although this condition may not occur and can be misleading if absent. The patient may have palpable pulses and good capillary refill distal to a compartment syndrome.

Patients may be unable to comply with a physical examination because of sedation or head, spinal, or peripheral nerve injuries. If the patient has a swollen, firm extremity, it will be difficult for the examining physician to rule out compartment syndrome without measuring compartment pressures. Similarly, patients with significant trauma to the leg may have unbearable pain, paresis, and pain with passive stretching caused by the traumatic injury itself. In the presence of complicating factors, establishing a diagnosis of compartment syndrome that requires emergent fasciotomy is best done by measuring compartment pressure.

In patients in a cast who have symptoms that are suggestive of compartment syndrome, the cast should be bivalved, the cast padding split, and the extremity placed in a neutral ankle position or slight plantar flexion at heart level for 10 to 15 minutes. Often, the symptoms will significantly subside as tissue perfusion improves with release of the confining structure. If there is no clinical change, pressure measurement or fasciotomy is indicated. Compartment syndrome may also be caused by soft dressings on the leg that are too tight. The dressing should be loosened, with the patient evaluated for improvement before further intervention.

When traction is applied to a fractured leg, compartment pressures will rise.[3,4] Thus, prolonged and excessive traction of a leg with a tibial fracture should be avoided, especially in an anesthetized or neurologically impaired patient who is unable to provide feedback. Ankle dorsiflexion is associated with higher posterior compartment pressure. A neutral position or slightly plantar-flexed position of the ankle is more desirable.[5] The well leg holder and the lithotomy position have been associated with compartment syndrome, most likely resulting from external pressure on compartments, positioning of the hip and knee that impairs arterial perfusion, and sedation or anesthesia that interferes with patient feedback.[6]

Schatzer type VI plateau fractures and medial tibial plateau fracture-dislocations have a higher incidence of compartment syndrome[7] as do tibia fracture-dislocations and tibial shaft fractures in adolescent soccer players. External fixators are useful in providing provisional stabilization of these high-energy fractures and fracture-dislocations but have been shown to be associated with transient elevations in compartment pressure.[8] Because this effect is likely the result of soft-tissue tension, which effectively decreases the volume of the compartments,[9] care should be taken to avoid overdistraction in fractures or fracture-dislocations. Placing external fixators will improve patient comfort and facilitate ongoing evaluation of the extremity for compartment syndrome and neurovascular complications.

There is a paucity of published data from which to determine the predictive value of clinical findings in diagnosing compartment syndrome. In a review of the literature by Ulmer et al,[10] only four studies were found that correlated clinical findings with compartment syndrome. The sensitivity of clinical findings for diagnosing compartment syndrome was low, ranging from 13% to 19%. The authors concluded that the absence of clinical findings was more useful in excluding the diagnosis of compartment syndrome than was the presence of clinical findings in confirming the diagnosis. Although this conclusion may be correct and supports cautious evaluation of symptomatic patients, it should be noted that the diagnosis of compartment syndrome in the investigation was not strict, and very few patients actually had compartment syndrome; therefore, the authors' conclusion may be misleading.[11-14]

Compartment Pressure Measurements

In most patients, the diagnosis of compartment syndrome is either confirmed or ruled out based on the physical examination alone. When the diagnosis is unclear, compartment pressures should be measured to clarify the issue.[1,15] Common indications include obtunded, anesthetized, or sedated patients; those with a nerve injury; unclear clinical examination findings; and patients with prolonged hypotension and extremity injury. In patients who have progressive exacerbation of symptoms but in whom pressure measurements do not indicate compartment syndrome, an indwelling catheter may be placed for ongoing monitoring of compartment pressures.

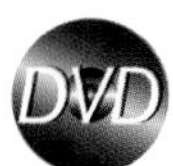

Video 4.1: Compartment Syndrome of the Leg: Compartment Pressure Measurements. Carol Copeland, MD; Alan Jones, MD (3 min)

The perfusion of tissue within a compartment is related to both the arterial pressure and compartment pressure. Therefore, the diagnosis of compartment syndrome should incorporate both pressures. Most surgeons believe that when the difference between the patient's diastolic pressure and the compartment pressure (delta P) is less than 30 mm Hg, tissue perfusion is inadequate, so emergent fasciotomy should be performed.[12] Studies have shown that muscle in nontraumatized canine legs will tolerate a delta P as low as 20 mm Hg.[16] However, after ischemia, a delta P of 40 mm Hg may be insufficient to maintain perfusion.[17] Therefore, using delta P less than 30 mm Hg as an indication for fasciotomy appears to be a safe threshold in the traumatized leg and has solid clinical support in patients with compartment syndrome of the leg.[2]

Recently, it has become clear that during surgery patients often have transient diastolic hypotension while under anesthesia.[18] Therefore, patients with normal or high-normal compartment pressures with diastolic hypotension may have delta P less than 30 mm Hg. In most instances, the diastolic hypotension will be corrected when the effects of anesthesia subside; therefore, fasciotomy should not be performed unless justified by the clinical examination. The patient's preoperative diastolic pressure is a good predictor of the diastolic pressure obtained in the recovery room.

Because compartment pressure syndrome may occur in any or all of the compartments in the leg, measurements should be taken in all four compartments. It is recommended that compartment pressure measurements be made within 5 cm of a fracture (if present), as the pressure will be closer to normal at longer distances from the fracture site.[15] Only a small amount of fluid (enough to clear the catheter of tissue) should be injected through the catheter into the compartment, and the monitor should be allowed to completely equilibrate before determining the pressure.

Treatment

Once the diagnosis of compartment syndrome of the calf is made, surgery should proceed emergently. In general, all four compartments should be released.[1] These releases are most easily performed through two skin incisions: a longitudinal medial incision 1 cm posterior to the medial tibia through which the superficial posterior and the deep posterior compartments are released, and a longitudinal anterolateral incision approximately 2 cm anterior to the fibula through which the anterior and lateral compartments are released (**Figure 2**). Alternatively, all four compartments may be released through a single lateral incision that leaves the fibula intact, but this is a more technically demanding approach.[19]

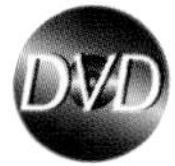

Video 4.2: Compartment Syndrome of the Leg: Anatomic Landmarks. Carol Copeland, MD; Alan Jones, MD (2 min)

If compartment syndrome of the calf is associated with a tibial fracture, the fracture should be stabilized to facilitate soft-tissue monitoring and management. Depending on the fracture type and the character of the soft tissues, bony stabilization can be

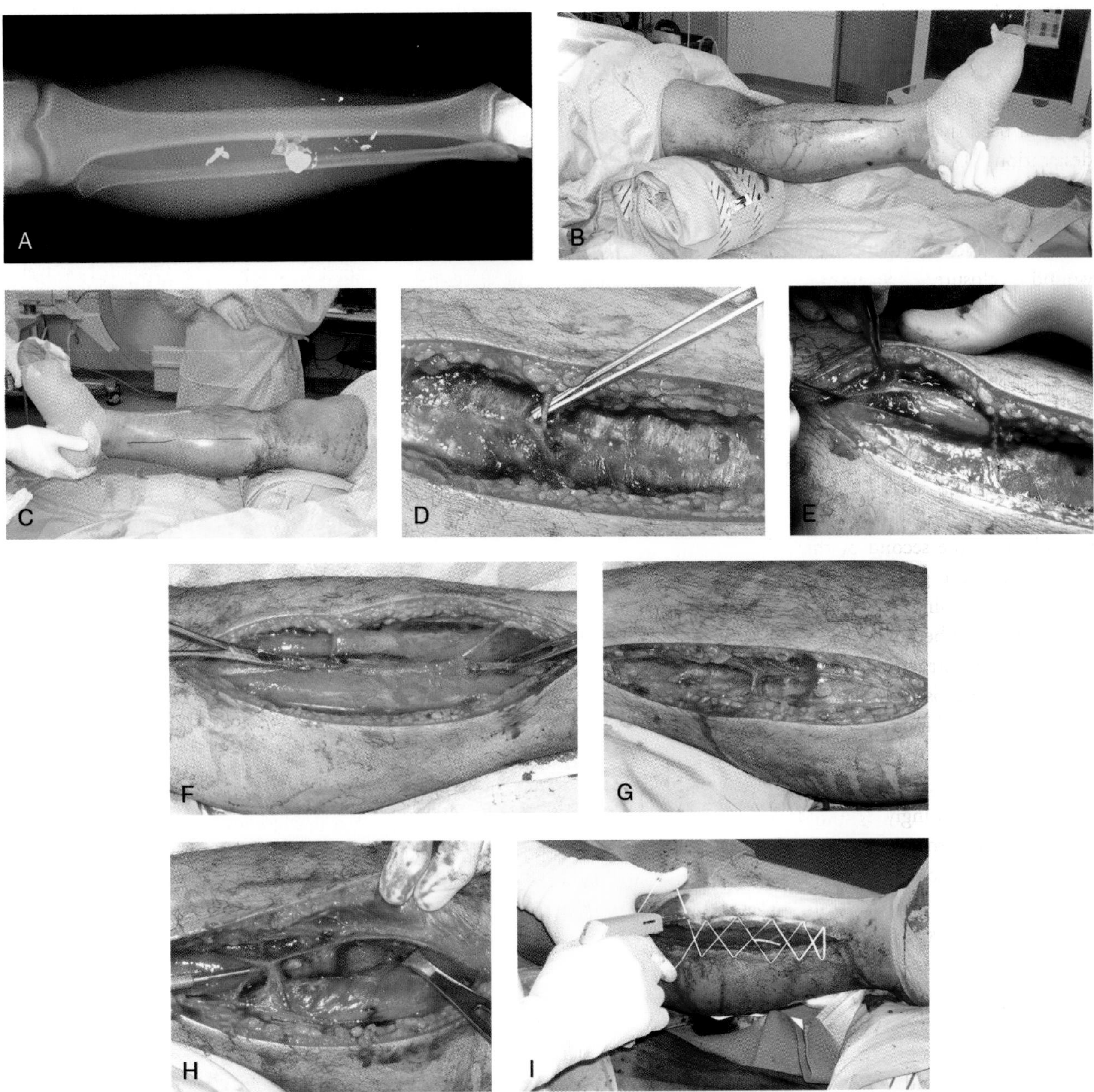

Figure 2 Compartment syndrome was diagnosed in all four compartments of the right leg of a 19-year-old man after a gunshot wound. **A,** AP radiograph shows bullet fragments in the leg but no obvious fracture. Intraoperative lateral (**B**) and medial (**C**) photographic views show the markings for the dual-incision fasciotomy technique. **D,** A close-up view of the lateral incision shows bulging in the anterior and lateral compartments and perforating vessels at the fascial interval. **E,** After partial release of the anterior compartment, the muscle appears discolored and swollen but viable. **F,** After completion of the anterior and lateral compartment fasciotomies, the anterior compartment musculature appears healthy and well perfused. The fascia between the anterior and lateral compartments is held by clamps; the perforating vessels to the superficial tissues have been preserved. **G,** The superficial medial incision shows the swollen posterior compartments. **H,** After release of the superficial posterior compartment fascia, the deep posterior compartment fascia is easily identified distally (left) and is shown partially incised. **I,** After evacuating any hematoma and irrigating the tissue, gentle tension is placed on the skin using vessel loops, which are stapled to the skin in a crisscross fashion.

achieved by intramedullary nailing, open reduction and internal fixation, or external fixation.

The tissues should be covered with moist or occlusive dressings to prevent desiccation. Using crisscross elastic bands or vessel loops to gently pull the skin edges together will prevent skin retraction and facilitate secondary wound closure. Vacuum-assisted wound closure can be used to reduce postoperative edema, which may improve wound closure with or without negative pressure therapy. The patient should be returned to the operating room in 2 to 3 days for irrigation, débridement, and a "second look" at the calf musculature. If skin closure is not possible after the second or third débridement, skin grafting should be considered. Closing the medial side first is preferred because the bone and neurovascular structures are more likely to be exposed in this incision than in the lateral incision.

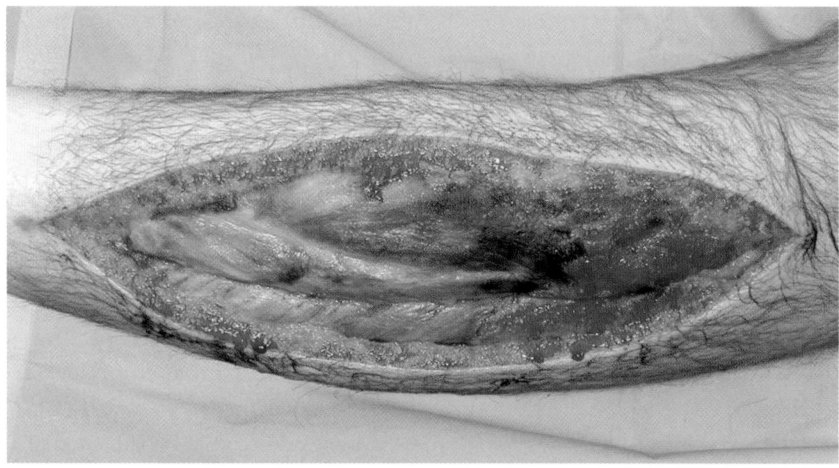

Figure 3 Intraoperative photograph showing a lateral fasciotomy incision 2 days after delayed fasciotomies for compartment syndrome. The muscle is discolored, avascular, and noncontractile.

Outcomes

There are surprisingly few data on functional outcomes of compartment syndrome of the calf, with no level I, II, or III studies published to date. Sheridan and Matsen[20] reported on 44 patients with 66 acute compartment syndromes. A review of the outcomes of patients treated with fasciotomy within 12 hours of symptom onset showed that 68% had normal function and 4.5% had complications. In patients treated with fasciotomy more than 12 hours after symptom onset, only 8% had normal function and 54% had complications, including infection, amputation, renal failure, and death. This level IV study showed a clear relationship between delayed fasciotomy and poorer functional results (**Figure 3**).

Fitzgerald et al[21] evaluated 60 patients with compartment syndrome over an 8-year period and reported that most had long-term sequelae, including altered sensation (77%), dry scaly skin (40%), pruritus (33%), swollen limbs (15%), wound pain (10%), and recurrent ulceration (8%).

Frink et al[22] reported on results over a 5-year period in 55 patients with multiple trauma and compartment syndrome. The patients in this study had a reduction in strength and range of motion and an increase in pain; however, there was no association between multiple injuries and poor results.

Giannoudis et al[23] evaluated 39 patients with compartment syndrome at 12 months using the EuroQol self-reported health-related quality of life instrument. The results were worse in patients with skin grafts than in those without skin grafts and worse in patients with delayed closure/coverage of fasciotomy wounds than in patients with earlier wound closure. Patients who reported problems with the appearance of the wound also had a reduced quality of life.

Heemskerk and Kitslaar[24] reported the outcomes of 40 patients with compartment syndrome of the lower leg treated with a fasciotomy. The authors did not analyze the timing of surgery. The rates for mortality, amputation, and nerve injury were 15%, 25%, and 15%, respectively. Only 45% of patients had a good functional result. A multivariate analysis showed that patients younger than 50 years had better outcomes.

Finkelstein et al[25] reported on five patients treated with fasciotomy more than 35 hours after the onset of compartment syndrome. One patient died from multisystem failure, and the remaining four patients had amputation, three of which were performed for infection. This level IV study concluded that the benefits of fasciotomy should be reconsidered if there is considerable delay in performing the procedure.

Tremblay et al[26] described secondary extremity compartment syndrome, which is a rare occurrence (10 of 11,996 trauma patients [0.1%] in 6 years). The unique feature of this syndrome is that it occurred in nontraumatized extremities of hemodynamically unstable patients with systemic inflammatory response syndrome. Each patient had an average of 3.1 extremities involved, and the mortality rate was 70%. The authors recommended checking compartment pressures in patients with severe diffuse edema after resuscitation for injury.

In a review article, Olson and Glasgow[1] concluded that if compartment syndrome was present for more than 8 hours in a patient with intact cognitive and neurologic function, and the patient was unable to contract muscles within the compartment, irreversible necrosis had already occurred, so it was too late to perform a fasciotomy.

Thus, there are limited data on functional outcomes of compartment syndromes. Level IV evidence shows complications involving muscle strength, functional loss, and skin symptoms. These complications are more common in older patients and may occur even when fasciotomy is performed early. There is weak (level IV and V) evidence showing high morbidity and mortality rates with late fasciotomy.

Discussion and Best Practices

This chapter focuses on the principles, evidence, and best practices used in diagnosing and treating compartment syndrome of the calf. Best practices have been defined as "a technique (or method, process, activity, etc) that is more effective at delivery of a particular outcome than any other techniques (or method, process, activity, etc)" or the "most efficient (least effort) and most effective (best results) method of accomplishing a task."[27] The definition of best practices is changing to mean "rules," a change that has been termed "linguistic drift."[27]

The standard treatment of compartment syndrome of the calf remains surgical fasciotomy of all four compartments. The role of selective compartment releases (release of some but not all osteofascial compartments) for compartment syndrome of the calf is still experimental. There has been a resurgence of interest in this topic particularly with regard to compartment syndrome of the calf. A recent study reported an algorithm for selective anterior and lateral compartment fasciotomies, followed by intraoperative measurement of superficial and deep posterior compartment pressures before performing fasciotomies of these compartments.[28] In some patients, posterior compartment pressures were normal after release of the anterior and lateral compartments, so a fasciotomy of the posterior compartments was not performed. However, some patients had to be returned to the operating room a second time for posterior compartment syndrome that occurred in the postoperative period.

The Current Procedural Terminology (CPT) codes set by the American Medical Association for procedural reimbursement include three different options for various combinations of releases of the calf compartments, which suggest that selective releases are an acceptable practice. CPT 27600 includes anterior and/or lateral fasciotomy, CPT code 27601 includes posterior fasciotomy only, and CPT code 27602 includes four-compartment fasciotomy. Isolated anterior or lateral compartment syndrome is uncommon, especially when significant trauma to the extremity has occurred. If release of just the anterior and/or lateral compartments is performed, close intraoperative and postoperative evaluation of the other compartments is essential, and the surgeon must remain on high alert to return the patient to the operating room on short notice for fasciotomy of the posterior compartments. In this regard, the leg contrasts with the forearm in which the three compartments (volar, dorsal, and mobile wad) lack firm fascial divisions; therefore, release of the volar compartment only is more likely to decompress the entire forearm.[29]

Fasciotomy, even if performed correctly and early, does not ensure an excellent outcome or completely mitigate the possibility of morbidity and disability caused by compartment syndrome. Outcomes appear to be linked to many factors, including self-reported quality of life scores and the cosmesis of the fasciotomy site.[23] Advances in new technology, such as ultrafiltration[30] and a better understanding of genetic polymorphisms, may lead to treatment breakthroughs and better outcomes for patients with compartment syndrome of the calf.

Summary

The linchpin for successful outcomes in patients with compartment syndrome of the calf is timely diagnosis. Clinical evaluation for compartment syndrome is sufficient for most awake and alert patients. Measuring compartment pressures has value in the obtunded patient. Because currently available evidence on functional outcomes after compartment syndrome of the calf is limited, there is a tremendous need for prospective, multicenter studies to increase understanding and scientific knowledge concerning the best treatment for this condition.

References

1. Olson SA, Glasgow RR: Acute compartment syndrome in lower extremity musculoskeletal trauma. *J Am Acad Orthop Surg* 2005; 13(7):436-444.
2. McQueen MM, Gaston P, Court-Brown CM: Acute compartment syndrome. Who is at risk? *J Bone Joint Surg Br* 2000;82(2): 200-203.
3. Tornetta P III, French BG: Compartment pressures during nonreamed tibial nailing without traction. *J Orthop Trauma* 1997; 11(1):24-27.

4. Shakespeare DT, Henderson NJ: Compartmental pressure changes during calcaneal traction in tibial fractures. *J Bone Joint Surg Br* 1982;64(4):498-499.
5. Weiner G, Styf J, Nakhostine M, Gershuni DH: Effect of ankle position and a plaster cast on intramuscular pressure in the human leg. *J Bone Joint Surg Am* 1994;76(10):1476-1481.
6. Slater RR Jr, Weiner TM, Koruda MJ: Bilateral leg compartment syndrome complicating prolonged lithotomy position. *Orthopedics* 1994;17(10):954-959.
7. Stark E, Stucken C, Trainer G, Tornetta P III: Compartment syndrome in Schatzker type VI plateau fractures and medial condylar fracture-dislocations treated with temporary external fixation. *J Orthop Trauma* 2009;23(7): 502-506.
8. Egol KA, Bazzi J, McLaurin TM, Tejwani NC: The effect of knee-spanning external fixation on compartment pressures in the leg. *J Orthop Trauma* 2008;22(10): 680-685.
9. Kenny C: Compartment pressures, limb length changes and the ideal spherical shape: A case report and in vitro study. *J Trauma* 2006;61(4):909-912.
10. Ulmer WH, Silvestri L, Pearson SE, Beach WR: Two- to 6-year results of Fulkerson osteotomy: Retrospective evaluation. *75th Annual Meeting Proceedings*. Rosemont, IL, American Academy of Orthopaedic Surgeons, 2008, p 482.
11. Triffitt PD, König D, Harper WM, Barnes MR, Allen MJ, Gregg PJ: Compartment pressures after closed tibial shaft fracture. Their relation to functional outcome. *J Bone Joint Surg Br* 1992;74(2):195-198.
12. McQueen MM, Court-Brown CM: Compartment monitoring in tibial fractures. The pressure threshold for decompression. *J Bone Joint Surg Br* 1996;78(1): 99-104.
13. Gibson MJ, Barnes MR, Allen MJ, Chan RN: Weakness of foot dorsiflexion and changes in compartment pressures after tibial osteotomy. *J Bone Joint Surg Br* 1986;68(3):471-475.
14. Allen MJ, Stirling AJ, Crawshaw CV, Barnes MR: Intracompartmental pressure monitoring of leg injuries. An aid to management. *J Bone Joint Surg Br* 1985; 67(1):53-57.
15. Heckman MM, Whitesides TE Jr, Grewe SR, Rooks MD: Compartment pressure in association with closed tibial fractures. The relationship between tissue pressure, compartment, and the distance from the site of the fracture. *J Bone Joint Surg Am* 1994;76(9): 1285-1292.
16. Matava MJ, Whitesides TE Jr, Seiler JG III, Hewan-Lowe K, Hutton WC: Determination of the compartment pressure threshold of muscle ischemia in a canine model. *J Trauma* 1994;37(1): 50-58.
17. Bernot M, Gupta R, Dobrasz J, Chance B, Heppenstall RB, Sapega A: The effect of antecedent ischemia on the tolerance of skeletal muscle to increased interstitial pressure. *J Orthop Trauma* 1996; 10(8):555-559.
18. Kakar S, Firoozabadi R, McKean J, Tornetta P III: Diastolic blood pressure in patients with tibia fractures under anaesthesia: Implications for the diagnosis of compartment syndrome. *J Orthop Trauma* 2007;21(2):99-103.
19. Maheshwari R, Taitsman LA, Barei DP: Single-incision fasciotomy for compartmental syndrome of the leg in patients with diaphyseal tibial fractures. *J Orthop Trauma* 2008;22(10):723-730.
20. Sheridan GW, Matsen FA III: Fasciotomy in the treatment of the acute compartment syndrome. *J Bone Joint Surg Am* 1976;58(1): 112-115.
21. Fitzgerald AM, Gaston P, Wilson Y, Quaba A, McQueen MM: Long-term sequelae of fasciotomy wounds. *Br J Plast Surg* 2000; 53(8):690-693.
22. Frink M, Klaus AK, Kuther G, et al: Long term results of compartment syndrome of the lower limb in polytraumatised patients. *Injury* 2007;38(5):607-613.
23. Giannoudis PV, Nicolopoulos C, Dinopoulos H, Ng A, Adedapo S, Kind P: The impact of lower leg compartment syndrome on health related quality of life. *Injury* 2002; 33(2):117-121.
24. Heemskerk J, Kitslaar P: Acute compartment syndrome of the lower leg: Retrospective study on prevalence, technique, and outcome of fasciotomies. *World J Surg* 2003;27(6):744-747.
25. Finkelstein JA, Hunter GA, Hu RW: Lower limb compartment syndrome: course after delayed fasciotomy. *J Trauma* 1996; 40(3):342-344.
26. Tremblay LN, Feliciano DV, Rozycki GS: Secondary extremity compartment syndrome. *J Trauma* 2002;53(5):833-837.
27. Best practice, Wikipedia Website, 2009. http://en.wikipedia.org/wiki/Best_practices. Accessed June 16, 2010.
28. Tornetta P III, Puskas B, Wang K: Compartment syndrome of the leg associated with fracture: An algorithm to avoid releasing the posterior compartment. *Orthopaedic Trauma Association 24th Annual Meeting*, Rosemont, IL, Orthopaedic Trauma Association, 2008, pp 147-148.
29. Gelberman RH, Garfin SR, Hergenroeder PT, Mubarak SJ, Menon J: Compartment syndromes of the forearm: Diagnosis

and treatment. *Clin Orthop Relat Res* 1981;161:252-261.

30. Odland R, Schmidt AH, Hunter B, et al: Use of tissue ultrafiltration for treatment of compartment syndrome: A pilot study using porcine hindlimbs. *J Orthop Trauma* 2005;19(4): 267-275.

Video References

4.1 and 4.2: Copeland C, Jones A: Video. Excerpt. *Compartment Syndrome of the Leg: Diagnosis and Fasciotomy*. Aurora, CO, Touch of Life Technologies, 2008.

Diagnosis and Treatment of Less Common Compartment Syndromes of the Upper and Lower Extremities: Current Evidence and Best Practices

Craig S. Roberts, MD, MBA
John T. Gorczyca, MD
David Ring, MD, PhD
Kevin J. Pugh, MD

Abstract

Compartment syndromes of the forearm, gluteal region, thigh, and foot have not been extensively studied. To provide best-practice recommendations, the available evidence from four systematic reviews of English-language reports with two or more patients with compartment syndromes of the forearm, gluteal region, thigh, and foot were reviewed and compared. For each case of compartment syndrome, the cause, method of diagnosis, treatment options, and outcomes were determined. Most compartment syndromes were caused by trauma, with the exception of gluteal compartment syndrome, which usually resulted from prolonged immobilization and postarthroplasty analgesia. The diagnosis was often based on clinical findings, with compartment pressure measurements performed in approximately 50% of the patients. Compartment pressure measurements of the foot were more commonly obtained (in 64% of the patients). Compartment syndrome of the forearm and thigh were treated surgically in 73% and 100% of patients, respectively. Complications occurred with all four compartment syndromes, with nerve deficits and stiffness being the most common problems. Reports on functional outcomes lacked uniformity and did not allow for meaningful comparisons.

Management principles for the less common compartment syndromes are the same as those used in treating compartment syndrome of the calf. Gluteal compartment syndrome usually has a nontraumatic etiology and is less likely to be surgically treated, probably because of major systemic complications and late presentation. Complications are common after these four types of compartment syndrome, but outcomes data are lacking.

Instr Course Lect 2011;60:43-50.

Compartment syndromes of the forearm, the gluteal region, the thigh, and the foot have not been studied as extensively as compartment syndrome of the calf despite the fact that they are equally significant. This chapter presents a review of the causes, diagnoses, treatment methods, complications, and functional outcomes of compartment syndromes of the forearm, gluteal region, thigh, and foot and compares these five parameters among the four compartments to provide best-practice recommendations based on the available evidence.

Compartment Syndrome of the Forearm

A systematic literature review was performed using an Ovid MEDLINE (Wolters Kluwer Health–Ovid, New York, NY) database search of the available evidence on compartment syndrome of the forearm. Twelve articles met the search criteria of a study in the English-language literature, with a minimum of two patients with the condition. The 86 patients in the studies ranged in age from birth to 67 years.[1-12]

Causes

The most common causes of compartment syndrome of the forearm were fractures (31%), narcotic overdoses (9.5%), intravenous infiltrations (8%), neonatal origins (8%), snake bites (6%), crush injuries (5%), and penetrating trauma (gunshot and stab wounds; 15.4%).[1-12] Injuries at specific risk for compartment syndrome of the forearm were high-energy distal radius fractures, gunshot fractures of the proximal third of the forearm, crush injuries, pressure injuries from prolonged lying on an upper extremity in comatose patients, burn injuries with circumferential eschar, high-pressure injection injuries, floating elbow in children, and any dual-level injury (such as wrist and forearm or wrist and elbow injuries) in adults.[4,13-15]

Diagnosis

The diagnosis of compartment syndrome of the forearm in the 12 reviewed studies was based on clinical findings alone in 40 of 84 extremities (48%) and on both clinical findings and compartment pressure measurements in 44 of 84 extremities (52%).[1-12] Compartment pressure measurements were obtained using either a wick catheter, the Whiteside technique, or a slit catheter. In awake, alert patients without peripheral nerve injuries, the hallmark of the compartment syndrome diagnosis was disproportionate pain, particularly severe forearm pain with passive motion of the digits. In the arm and forearm, decreased threshold sensibility (light touch measured with monofilaments using the Semmes-Weinstein technique) was followed by decreased discriminate sensibility (measured as two-point discrimination) in the digits and later by weakness of the intrinsic hand musculature.[4,16]

In awake and alert patients, the diagnosis of compartment syndrome of the forearm can be established with clinical findings alone; patients who are comatose, intoxicated, intubated, or cognitively impaired or who have central nervous system or peripheral nerve injuries may be better evaluated with measurements of intracompartmental pressures.[4,16] As at other sites, the need for compartment release is indicated by elevated or rising pressures.[4,6,16,17] The pressure at which fasciotomy is indicated has been debated, but pressures higher than 30 mm Hg are a cause for concern.[4,17] At pressures higher than 45 mm Hg, forearm fascial release should be strongly considered.[13] A difference between the diastolic blood pressure and the compartment pressure of less than 30 mm Hg may be the best criterion but that has not yet been definitely established.[13,16,17]

Treatment

In the reviewed studies, 63 patients (73%) were treated surgically. Fifty-one of these patients (81%) were treated with a fasciotomy of the volar compartment alone, whereas 11 patients (17%) required fasciotomies of the volar and dorsal compartments. Thirty-four patients (54%) also had a carpal tunnel release at the time of the forearm fasciotomy. Eaton and Green[2] reported excellent results in 75% of cases, fair results in 6.2%, and poor results in 18.8%.

In the setting of a forearm fracture, the incisions used to repair radius and/or ulna fractures may be extended so that a complete forearm fascial release can be accomplished. The standard Henry exposure is extensile and may be used.[18] Textbooks often show a curvilinear incision that is intended to provide access to the mobile wad, but such an incision can compromise venous and lymphatic drainage and places more cutaneous nerves at risk. When there is no fracture (for example, in burns, vascular injuries, and crush injuries), an ulnar McConnell exposure may be useful.[18,19]

Eight reports (37 patients) documented details of wound management. In 17 patients (46%), the fasciotomy wounds were treated with delayed primary closure; 20 patients (54%) required skin grafting.

Complications

Complications occurred in 18 of 64 patients (28%). The most common reported complication was a neurologic deficit that occurred in nine patients (14%), followed by contracture in four patients (6%). Other complications included crush syndrome in two patients, gangrene in one, Volkmann ischemic contracture in one, and Sudeck algodystrophy in one. Unsightly scars were common. Irreversible ischemic nerve injury, myoglobinuria, and acute renal injury may also occur.[6]

Outcomes

Limited outcome information was reported for 39 patients. Decreased wrist flexibility occurred in 10 patients

Dr. Roberts or an immediate family member serves as a board member, owner, officer, or committee member of the RRC, Orthopaedic Trauma Association, Mid-America Orthopaedic Association, Kentucky Orthopaedic Association, and Orthopaedic Incubator; has received research or institutional support from Stryker and Synthes; and has received nonincome support (such as equipment or services), commercially derived honoraria, or other non–research-related funding (such as paid travel) from Saunders/Mosby-Elsevier. Dr. Gorczyca or an immediate family member serves as a paid consultant to or is an employee of Zimmer. Dr. Ring or an immediate family member has received royalties from DePuy and Wright Medical Technology; is a member of a speakers' bureau or has made paid presentations on behalf of Acumed and Wright Medical Technology; serves as a paid consultant to or is an employee of Acumed and Wright Medical Technology; has received research or institutional support from Acumed, Biomet, Stryker, Tornier, and Joint Active Systems; and owns stock or stock options in Mimedex and Illuminoss. Dr. Pugh or an immediate family member is a member of a speakers' bureau or has made paid presentations on behalf of Medtronic and Smith & Nephew and serves as a paid consultant to or is an employee of Medtronic and Smith & Nephew.

(26%), and sensory loss was reported in 8 patients (21%).

Gelberman et al[4] reported on 31 patients with suspected compartment syndrome of the forearm, which was diagnosed in 12 patients on the basis of compartment pressures greater than 30 mm Hg. The loss of two-point discrimination was the most useful clinical factor in distinguishing patients with true compartment syndrome. The time from injury to fasciotomy averaged 21 hours (range, 6 to 48 hours). All but two patients had residual wrist and digital stiffness and weakness. Poor outcomes were associated with crush injuries, but the study did not show an association between results and the interval from injury to decompression.

Compartment syndromes of the forearm associated with fractures of the distal radius may have a delayed onset; many do not become evident for 12 to 48 hours after injury.[9,11,20] It is possible for patients to regain full nerve function, but wrist and digital stiffness, probably resulting in part from the fracture and in part from its treatment, are common.

Compartment Syndrome of the Gluteal Region

The gluteal region is compartmentalized and therefore is susceptible to the effects of increased pressure within an enclosed anatomic space. A systematic review of the available evidence on compartment syndrome of the gluteal region was done by one of this chapter's authors (CSR).[21] PubMed and Ovid databases were searched for published evidence on the causes, diagnosis, treatments, and functional outcomes of this syndrome. Selected studies were original articles in the English language that contained two or more cases. Seven studies with 28 patients were reviewed.[22-28] Compartment syndrome of the gluteal region mainly affects middle-age men; 82% of the patients were male, and the average age was 45 years (range, 25 to 72 years).

Causes

The most common cause of compartment syndrome of the gluteal region was prolonged immobilization, with pressure from the patient's body weight implicated in 14 of 28 patients (50%). Trauma was reported as a cause in six patients (21%), with postoperative epidural analgesia after arthroplasty with immobility in six patients (21%). Infection was reported in two patients (7.1%), which occurred as a result of necrotizing fasciitis.

Diagnosis

The review reported that 46% of cases were diagnosed by compartment pressure measurements. The remaining cases (54%) were diagnosed by clinical signs and symptoms.

Treatment

Surgical decompression was used to treat 20 patients (71.4%). Three compartments have been described in the gluteal region: the maximus, the minimus, and the tensor compartments.[23,24] There was a lack of consistency in the decompression procedures reported in the studies; however, the surgical skin incision was similar to the incision for a posterior approach to the hip, with the incision on the anterior edge of the gluteus maximus running distally to the greater trochanter. Decompression of the gluteus medius and gluteus minimus compartments has been noted to be the decisive factor in the adequacy of the decompression because of the location in the osteofibrous sheath.[22] In four patients with a mean follow-up of 29 months, all of the patients showed decreased gluteal muscle force on ergometric tests, and three showed decreased muscle volume. Some authors[25] recommend multiple epimysiotomies within the gluteus maximus. If there are sciatic nerve symptoms, the tensor fascia compartment should be separately decompressed.[22] A posterior approach with multiple epimysiotomies has been described.[25] Nonsurgical treatment, which was often the result of late diagnosis, was reported in eight patients (28.6%).

Functional Outcomes

Seven studies[22-28] in this review reported on the functional outcomes of 28 patients with compartment syndrome of the gluteal region; however, there was a lack of uniformity in the method of assessing outcomes. One study[25] reported on three patients; one had a mild abductor limp and two fully recovered. Lachiewicz and Latimer[24] reported that four of six patients fully recovered, whereas two had paresthesias along the dorsum of the foot with normal muscle strength. Yoshioka[28] reported that three of four patients fully recovered, whereas one patient had a normal gait but mild weakness of the hip external rotators with foot numbness. Bosch and Tscherne[22] used more rigorous assessment methods and noted that three patients reported a reduced state of health. Three patients had some form of dysesthesia, and two patients had decreased ankle flexion or extension strength. Schmalzried et al[27] reported that all three of the patients in their review had decreased function. Pacheco et al[26] reported that one of two patients reported gluteal discomfort; the other patient was not evaluated. Kumar et al[23] reported that three of four patients made a complete recovery, whereas one patient had weak abductors and a Trendelenburg gait. Prompt decompression when the clinical presentation is consistent with compartment syndrome and knowledge of the anatomy of the compartments appear to be associated with better outcomes for patients.

Compartment Syndrome of the Thigh

The osteofascial compartment of the thigh is vulnerable to the deleterious effects of elevated compartment pressures. Ojike et al[29] performed a systematic review in which PubMed and Ovid databases in the English language were searched for case series involving two or more patients. Nine articles met the search criteria.[30-38] The authors reported that 76 of 89 patients (85%) were male and 13 (15%) were female, and that the average age was 38 years (range, 12 to 81 years).

Causes

The reported causes of compartment syndrome of the thigh were femoral fractures in 49% of cases, motor vehicle crashes in 36%, motorcycle crashes in 9%, train derailment injuries in 2%, and external compression in 4%.

Surgical Treatment

A single skin incision was used for the fasciotomy in 31 of 36 patients (86%), and two-incision fasciotomies were used in 5 patients (14%). Thirty-one of 53 patients (59%) had delayed primary wound closure. Fourteen patients (26%) were treated with a split-thickness skin graft. Early primary closure was performed in eight patients (15%).

Complications

The most common complication was neurologic deficit (16%), followed by infection (14%), renal failure (11%), heterotopic ossification (10%), limp (9%), and pain (7%). Less common complications were deep venous thrombosis and muscle necrosis, both of which occurred in 1% of patients.

Outcomes

Outcomes were measured in 38 patients from six studies by assessing muscle strength and/or knee range of motion.[31,32,34,35,37,38] Poor outcomes were defined as a 10% reduction in quadriceps strength, permanent muscle weakness, persistent sensory deficits, the presence of a limp, and knee range of motion less than 110°. Good functional outcomes were reported in 25 patients (66%). The authors of one study reported that full thigh muscle strength was not recovered in 8 of 18 patients (44%), and 57% had long-term functional deficits.[33]

Compartment Syndrome of the Foot

Before the 1980s, compartment syndrome of the foot was largely unrecognized.[39] This fact is compelling because some authors report that 4.7% to 17% of patients with calcaneus fractures have compartment syndrome of the foot.[40,41] The available published evidence in the English-language literature on compartment syndrome of the foot was recently compiled by Ojike et al[42] who performed PubMed and Ovid database searches. Original articles discussing compartment syndrome of the foot caused by trauma were included. Four articles[40,43-45] describing 35 patients with 39 cases of compartment syndrome of the foot met the search criteria. There were 27 males and 8 females in the studies. Of the 30 patients whose age was specified, the average age was 32 years (range, 10 to 58 years). The average clinical follow-up was 21 months (range, 3 to 60 months).

Causes

The most common causes of compartment syndrome of the foot were crush injuries (28%), falls from a height (26%), motor vehicle crashes (26%), and motorcycle crashes (7.5%).[40,43-45] The various bony injuries causing compartment syndrome were calcaneal fractures (23%), Lisfranc fracture-dislocations (21%), metatarsophalangeal fractures (18%), and lower leg and upper leg fractures without foot fractures (18%).

Diagnosis

The diagnosis of compartment syndrome of the foot was made by tissue compartment pressure measurements in 64% of the cases, clinical findings and compartment syndrome measurements in 31%, and clinical findings alone in 5%.[40,43-45] Clinical examination alone appeared to be less sensitive and less specific than compartment pressure measurements.

Surgical Treatment

Controversy exists about whether decompression is always necessary for compartment syndrome of the foot. Arguments against surgery include the fact that systemic complications of compartment syndrome of the foot are rare, the local morbidity of claw toes is well tolerated and potentially correctable at a later date, and the morbidity of the surgical procedure of decompression of compartment syndrome of the foot is significant and potentially worse than the natural history of the untreated condition.

In the studies reviewed, one skin incision was needed for the fasciotomies in 33% of patients, two incisions in 39%, three incisions in 23%, and four incisions in 5%.[40,43-45] The question of how many incisions are necessary for fasciotomies of the foot is complicated by the debate about how many anatomic compartments actually exist. Whereas older studies describe only four compartments of the foot, more contemporary studies describe as many as nine. Because of the ability to access multiple compartments through a single incision and the fact that foot compartment syndromes often do not involve all of the compartments, there are a variety of acceptable options for surgical incisions to perform decompression.

The techniques of wound closure were recorded in 31 cases. Of these, delayed primary closure was used in 11 cases (35%) and split-thickness skin grafting in 20 (65%). All of the cases requiring skin grafting had been treated with fracture fixation. The data in the studies regarding which incisions were the most likely to require skin grafting were incomplete. However, in the experience of this chapter's authors, medial incisions are more likely to require skin grafting than dorsal incisions.

Complications

Complications were reported in 17 of 39 cases (44%), and most of the complications (52%) were neurologic. Clawfoot was reported in 2 of 39 cases (5%), representing 12% of the complications (2 of 17); muscle necrosis occurred in 1 of 39 cases (3%), representing 6% of the complications (1 of 17); amputation occurred in 2 of 39 cases (5%), representing 12% of the complications; marked scarring in 2 of 39 cases (5%), representing 12% of the complications; and varus-valgus deformity in 1 of 39 cases (3%), representing 6% of the complications.[40,43-45] The data on infection rates were limited and did not allow for a meaningful comparison.

Functional Outcomes

Outcomes were reported based on the ability of the patient to walk or wear shoes, the need for arthrodesis, the patient's ability to return to work, or the presence of symptoms and limitations. Four of 35 patients (11%) were able to return to work. Only five patients (14%) were able to walk and wear shoes without symptoms, whereas 15 (43%) were able to walk or wear shoes with mild symptoms.

Cross-Comparison of the Four Compartment Syndromes

The cross-comparison of the data from the reviewed studies on the four types of compartment syndromes is shown in **Table 1**. There was nearly an equal number of reported cases of forearm compartment syndrome (84) as thigh compartment syndrome (89). A smaller number of cases for compartment syndrome of the foot (39) and the gluteal region (28) was reported.

The causes of these four compartment syndromes varied. There were many causes of compartment syndrome of the forearm, with fractures accounting for 31%. In contrast, femoral fractures caused 49% of the compartment syndromes of the thigh.

Compartment pressure measurements in conjunction with the patient's clinical evaluation results were used to diagnose approximately 50% of the cases of forearm, gluteal, and thigh compartment syndromes. Pressure measurements appeared to be more important in diagnosing compartment syndrome of the foot; those measurements were used in 95% of cases.

The reported treatment of acute compartment syndromes is largely surgical. Interestingly, the number of incisions through which the fasciotomy was performed varied according to the anatomic region. Most forearm, gluteal, and thigh fasciotomies were performed through a single incision. Foot fasciotomies were performed through multiple incisions in 67% of cases.

The complication rate was significant in all four compartment syndromes. Nerve deficits appeared to be the most frequently occurring complication in compartment syndromes of the forearm, the thigh, and the foot. Conclusions could not be obtained regarding complications in patients with compartment syndrome of the gluteal region. The reports on functional outcomes lacked uniformity and did not allow for meaningful comparisons.

Discussion and Best Practices

The available evidence regarding forearm, gluteal, thigh, and foot compartment syndromes was reviewed to provide guidance on choosing the optimal clinical applications to daily orthopaedic practice (best practices) for treating patients with these syndromes. Best practices have been defined as "a technique (or method, process, activity, etc) that is more effective at the delivery of a particular outcome than any other techniques (or method, process, activity, etc)."[46] Best practices have also been defined as "the most efficient (least effort) and most effective (best results) method of accomplishing a task."[46] A new term, used by the Accreditation Council for Graduate Medical Education[47] is notable practices, which has been defined as "a unique approach or practical tool."

The linchpin of treating compartment syndromes is a timely diagnosis. Compartment syndrome of the forearm can usually be diagnosed based on the clinical findings in an awake and alert patient. In contrast, the diagnosis of compartment syndromes of the gluteal region, thigh, and foot is best made in conjunction with measurements of compartment pressure. These measurements, however, are imperfect and should be interpreted in the context of the limitations of the technique and clinical findings. Because most data regarding compartment pressure measurements are from literature regarding compartment syndrome of the calf, the applicability and translation of these data to the other compartment syndromes is not fully defined. Determining the absolute measurements that constitute a compartment syndrome is

Table 1

Cross-Comparison of Systematic Review Data for Compartment Syndromes of the Forearm, Gluteal Region, Thigh, and Foot

	Published Reports	Causes	Method of Diagnosis	Treatment	Complications	Outcomes
Forearm	12 papers 84 cases	31% fractures (high-energy distal radius) 15.4% penetrating trauma 9.5% drug overdose 8% intravenous infiltration 8% neonatal origins 6% snake bites 5% crush injuries	48% clinical 52% clinical + pressure measurements	73% surgery 17% had two incisions	28% overall 14% nerve deficit 6% contracture	26% decreased wrist motion 21% sensory loss
Gluteal Region	7 papers 28 cases	50% prolonged immobilization 21% trauma 21% epidural analgesia after arthroplasty with immobility 7.1% infection	54% clinical 46% pressure measurements	71.4% surgery (all single incision)	No good data available	Reports too variable to allow accurate summary
Thigh	9 papers 89 cases	49% with femoral fracture (22% open femoral fracture) 36% motor vehicle crashes 9% motorcycle crashes 4% external compression 2% train derailments	26% clinical 52% clinical + pressure measurements 22% pressure measurements alone	86% one-incision fasciotomy 14% two-incision fasciotomy	16% nerve deficit 14% infection 11% renal failure 10% heterotopic ossification	66% good results
Foot	4 papers 39 cases	28% crush injuries 26% falls from a height 26% motor vehicle crashes 7.5% motorcycle crashes	5% clinical 31% clinical + pressure measurements 64% pressure measurements alone	33% one-incision fasciotomy 39% two-incision fasciotomy 23% three-incision fasciotomy 5% four-incision fasciotomy	44% overall 52% neurologic 12% clawfoot 12% amputation 12% marked scarring 6% muscle necrosis 6% varus-valgus deformity	No good data available

not as important as the delta P measurement (the difference between the diastolic pressure and the compartment pressure). A delta P measurement of less than 30 mm Hg in a traumatized calf, 20 mm Hg in a nontraumatized calf, or 40 mm Hg in a postischemic limb[48] are believed to indicate compartment syndrome. More information on calf compartment syndrome can be found in chapter 4.

The principles of treatment are the same for compartment syndromes of the forearm, gluteal region, thigh, and foot. Open fasciotomy to restore tissue perfusion is the most common treatment. Concerns remain regarding the morbidity of foot compartment releases, but surgical treatment is recommended in nearly all patients with acute compartment syndrome of this region. For compartment syndrome of the forearm, in the absence of a fracture, fasciotomy through an ulnar-sided McConnell exposure should be strongly considered to decrease morbidity and improve outcomes. The initial enthusiasm for this approach emphasized access to the deep volar compartment and the entire median and ulnar nerves in the forearm; however, neurolysis and epimysiotomy are not believed to be necessary. The carpal tunnel should be released when treating compartment syndrome of the forearm, either by extending the ulnar-sided McConnell incision or with a second incision.

Selective compartment releases (for example, releasing some but not all osteofascial compartments) have a role in compartment syndrome of the forearm. The role of selective releases in compartment syndromes of the gluteal region, thigh, and foot has not yet been determined. Fasciotomy wound closure is usually successfully treated with delayed primary wound closure or skin grafting. Even if fasciotomies are performed well and early, excellent outcomes are not assured, and the morbidity and disability from compartment syndrome may not be completely mitigated.

Advances in new technology, such as ultrafiltration[49] or understanding genetic polymorphisms, should lead to treatment breakthroughs in the future.

In the less common compartment syndromes of the lower extremity (gluteal region, thigh, and foot), diagnosis is often difficult to make on clinical grounds alone, and compartment pressure measurements are often required.

Summary

Compartment syndromes of the forearm, gluteal region, thigh, and foot have not been studied extensively. The available evidence on these four compartment syndromes was reviewed and cross-compared to provide best-practice recommendations. There is a tremendous need for prospective, multicenter studies to increase understanding of these less common compartment syndromes and improve the science of treatment.

References

1. Caouette-Laberge L, Bortoluzzi P, Egerszegi EP, Marton D: Neonatal Volkmann's ischemic contracture of the forearm: A report of five cases. *Plast Reconstr Surg* 1992;90(4):621-628.
2. Eaton RG, Green WT: Volkmann's ischemia: A volar compartment syndrome of the forearm. *Clin Orthop Relat Res* 1975;113: 58-64.
3. Geary N: Late surgical decompression for compartment syndrome of the forearm. *J Bone Joint Surg Br* 1984;66(5):745-748.
4. Gelberman RH, Garfin SR, Hergenroeder PT, Mubarak SJ, Menon J: Compartment syndromes of the forearm: Diagnosis and treatment. *Clin Orthop Relat Res* 1981;161:252-261.
5. Kline SC, Moore JR: Neonatal compartment syndrome. *J Hand Surg Am* 1992;17(2):256-259.
6. Mubarak SJ, Owen CA, Hargens AR, Garetto LP, Akeson WH: Acute compartment syndromes: Diagnosis and treatment with the aid of the wick catheter. *J Bone Joint Surg Am* 1978;60(8): 1091-1095.
7. Peters CL, Scott SM: Compartment syndrome in the forearm following fractures of the radial head or neck in children. *J Bone Joint Surg Am* 1995;77(7):1070-1074.
8. Seiler JG III, Valadie AL III, Drvaric DM, Frederick RW, Whitesides TE Jr: Perioperative compartment syndrome: A report of four cases. *J Bone Joint Surg Am* 1996;78(4):600-602.
9. Simpson NS, Jupiter JB: Delayed onset of forearm compartment syndrome: A complication of distal radius fracture in young adults. *J Orthop Trauma* 1995;9(5): 411-418.
10. Sneyd JR, Lau W, McLaren ID: Forearm compartment syndrome following intravenous infusion with a manual "bulb" pump. *Anesth Analg* 1993;76(5): 1160-1161.
11. Stockley I, Harvey IA, Getty CJ: Acute volar compartment syndrome of the forearm secondary to fractures of the distal radius. *Injury* 1988;19(2):101-104.
12. Morin RJ, Swan KG, Tan V: Acute forearm compartment syndrome secondary to local arterial injury after penetrating trauma. *J Trauma* 2009;66(4):989-993.
13. Moed BR, Fakhouri AJ: Compartment syndrome after low-velocity gunshot wounds to the forearm. *J Orthop Trauma* 1991;5(2): 134-137.
14. Ring D, Waters PM, Hotchkiss RN, Kasser JR: Pediatric floating elbow. *J Pediatr Orthop* 2001;21(4):456-459.
15. Hwang RW, de Witte PB, Ring D: Compartment syndrome associated with distal radial fracture and ipsilateral elbow injury. *J Bone Joint Surg Am* 2009;91(3): 642-645.
16. Whitesides TE, Haney TC, Morimoto K, Harada H: Tissue pressure measurements as a determinant for the need of fasciotomy. *Clin Orthop Relat Res* 1975;113: 43-51.
17. McQueen MM, Court-Brown CM: Compartment monitoring in tibial fractures: The pressure threshold for decompression. *J Bone Joint Surg Br* 1996;78 (1):99-104.
18. Henry AK: *Extensile Exposure*, ed 2. Edinburgh, United Kingdom, Churchill Livingstone, 1973.
19. McConnell A: Approach to the median nerve in the forearm. *Dublin J Med Science* 1920;149: 90-92.
20. Shall J, Cohn BT, Froimson AI: Acute compartment syndrome of the forearm in association with fracture of the distal end of the radius: Report of two cases. *J Bone Joint Surg Am* 1986;68(9):1451-1454.
21. Henson JT, Roberts CS, Giannoudis PV: Gluteal compartment syndrome. *Acta Orthop Belg* 2009; 75(2):147-152.
22. Bosch U, Tscherne H: The pelvic compartment syndrome. *Arch Orthop Trauma Surg* 1992;111 (6):314-317.
23. Kumar V, Saeed K, Panagopoulos A, Parker PJ: Gluteal compartment syndrome following joint arthroplasty under epidural anaesthesia: A report of 4 cases. *J Orthop Surg (Hong Kong)* 2007;15 (1):113-117.
24. Lachiewicz PF, Latimer HA: Rhabdomyolysis following total hip arthroplasty. *J Bone Joint Surg Br* 1991;73(4):576-579.
25. Owen CA, Woody PR, Mubarak SJ, Hargens AR: Gluteal compartment syndromes: A report of three cases and management utilizing the Wick catheter. *Clin Orthop Relat Res* 1978;132:57-60.

26. Pacheco RJ, Buckley S, Oxborrow NJ, Weeber AC, Allerton K: Gluteal compartment syndrome after total knee arthroplasty with epidural postoperative analgesia. *J Bone Joint Surg Br* 2001; 83(5):739-740.
27. Schmalzried TP, Neal WC, Eckardt JJ: Gluteal compartment and crush syndromes: Report of three cases and review of the literature. *Clin Orthop Relat Res* 1992;277: 161-165.
28. Yoshioka H: Gluteal compartment syndrome: A report of 4 cases. *Acta Orthop Scand* 1992;63(3): 347-349.
29. Ojike NI, Roberts CS, Giannoudis PV: Compartment syndrome of the thigh: A systematic review. *Injury* 2010;41(2): 133-136.
30. Hsieh M, Ko J, Liu H: Acute thigh compartment syndrome following thigh trauma: A report of three cases. *Formos J Surg* 2003; 36:82-87.
31. Klasson SC, Vander Schilden JL: Acute anterior thigh compartment syndrome complicating quadriceps hematoma: Two case reports and review of the literature. *Orthop Rev* 1990;19(5):421-427.
32. Mithöfer K, Lhowe DW, Vrahas MS, Altman DT, Altman GT: Clinical spectrum of acute compartment syndrome of the thigh and its relation to associated injuries. *Clin Orthop Relat Res* 2004; 425:223-229.
33. Mithoefer K, Lhowe DW, Vrahas MS, Altman DT, Erens V, Altman GT: Functional outcome after acute compartment syndrome of the thigh. *J Bone Joint Surg Am* 2006;88(4):729-737.
34. Rööser B, Bengtson S, Hägglund G: Acute compartment syndrome from anterior thigh muscle contusion: A report of eight cases. *J Orthop Trauma* 1991;5(1):57-59.
35. Schwartz JT Jr, Brumback RJ, Lakatos R, Poka A, Bathon GH, Burgess AR: Acute compartment syndrome of the thigh: A spectrum of injury. *J Bone Joint Surg Am* 1989;71(3):392-400.
36. Suzuki T, Moirmura N, Kawai K, Sugiyama M: Arterial injury associated with acute compartment syndrome of the thigh following blunt trauma. *Injury* 2005;36(1): 151-159.
37. Tarlow SD, Achterman CA, Hayhurst J, Ovadia DN: Acute compartment syndrome in the thigh complicating fracture of the femur: A report of three cases. *J Bone Joint Surg Am* 1986; 68(9):1439-1443.
38. Winternitz WA Jr, Metheny JA, Wear LC: Acute compartment syndrome of the thigh in sports-related injuries not associated with femoral fractures. *Am J Sports Med* 1992;20(4):476-477.
39. Fulkerson E, Razi A, Tejwani N: Review: Acute compartment syndrome of the foot. *Foot Ankle Int* 2003;24(2):180-187.
40. Myerson MS: Management of compartment syndromes of the foot. *Clin Orthop Relat Res* 1991; 271:239-248.
41. Myerson M, Manoli A: Compartment syndromes of the foot after calcaneal fractures. *Clin Orthop Relat Res* 1993;290:142-150.
42. Ojike NI, Roberts CS, Giannoudis PV: Foot compartment syndrome: A systematic review of the literature. *Acta Orthop Belg* 2009;75(5):573-580.
43. Fakhouri AJ, Manoli A II: Acute foot compartment syndromes. *J Orthop Trauma* 1992;6(2):223-228.
44. Manoli A II, Fakhouri AJ, Weber TG: Concurrent compartment syndromes of the foot and leg. *Foot Ankle* 1993;14(6):339.
45. Ziv I, Mosheiff R, Zeligowski A, Liebergal M, Lowe J, Segal D: Crush injuries of the foot with compartment syndrome: Immediate one-stage management. *Foot Ankle* 1989;9(4):185-189.
46. Best practice, Wikipedia. http://en.wikipedia.org/wiki/Best_practices. Accessed June 21, 2010.
47. Accreditation Council for Graduate Medical Education. Glossary of Terms 2009. http://www.acgme.org/acWebsite/about/ab_ACGMEglossary.pdf. Accessed June 21, 2010.
48. McQueen MM, Gaston P, Court-Brown CM: Acute compartment syndrome: Who is at risk? *J Bone Joint Surg Br* 2000;82(2): 200-203.
49. Odland R, Schmidt AH, Hunter B, et al: Use of tissue ultrafiltration for treatment of compartment syndrome: A pilot study using porcine hindlimbs. *J Orthop Trauma* 2005;19(4):267-275.

Clavicle and Scapula Fracture Problems: Functional Assessment and Current Treatment Strategies

Kyle J. Jeray, MD
Peter A. Cole, MD

Abstract

Historically, nonsurgical treatment was recommended for both clavicle and scapula fractures. Good functional outcomes were reported with nonsurgical treatment, whereas surgical treatment had a high complication rate. Recent studies have shown that the functional outcomes of nonsurgically treated fractures may not be as acceptable as had been previously believed. These studies also support the surgical treatment of clavicle and scapula fractures in certain circumstances. Relative indications for surgical treatment of clavicle fractures include skin compromise, neurologic or vascular injury, open fractures, high-energy closed fractures with greater than 15 to 20 mm of shortening, fractures with 100% displacement, and fractures with comminution. Relative indications for the surgical treatment of scapula fractures include displaced acromion or coracoid process fractures (> 10 mm), displaced intra-articular glenoid fractures (> 5 mm), and those associated with humeral subluxation.

Instr Course Lect 2011;60:51-71.

Traditional beliefs supported the nonsurgical treatment of both clavicle and scapula fractures. Nonsurgical treatment of these injuries was believed to achieve good functional outcomes, whereas surgical treatment resulted in high complication rates. However, recent studies have shown that the functional outcomes of nonsurgical treatment of these fractures may not be as acceptable as had been previously believed.[1-5] These studies also support the surgical treatment of clavicle and scapula fractures in certain circumstances.

Clavicle Fractures

In approximately AD 400, Hippocrates first described the treatment of midshaft clavicle fractures using "benign neglect."[6] This treatment approach remained the mainstay for many years. Two large studies in the 1960s supported the use of nonsurgical treatment.[7,8] Data from these studies showed that nonunions were rare and suggested that even displaced fractures healed without complications. More recently, however, these findings have been questioned. Retrospective, prospective cohort studies and randomized controlled trials have reported that fracture comminution, fracture displacement (usually > 15 to 20 mm of distraction or shortening or complete loss of apposition), advancing age, and female sex are associated with poorer outcomes and a notably increased risk of nonunion and malunion after nonsurgical treatment.[1-5] Therefore, midshaft clavicle fractures should be considered a spectrum of injuries with varying outcomes that require careful assessment and individualized treatments.[9]

Epidemiology

The clavicle is one of the most commonly fractured bones and represents 2.6% to 5% of all fractures.[10,11] The incidence of clavicle fractures in adults

Dr. Jeray or an immediate family member serves as a board member, owner, officer, or committee member of the American Academy of Orthopaedic Surgeons, the Orthopaedic Trauma Association, the South Carolina Orthopaedic Association, the American Orthopaedic Association, and the Southeastern Fracture Consortium; is a member of a speakers' bureau or has made paid presentations on behalf of AONA; serves as a paid consultant to or is an employee of Zimmer; and has received research or institutional support from Synthes and Zimmer. Dr. Cole or an immediate family member serves as a paid consultant to or is an employee of Synthes and has received research or institutional support from Zimmer, Synthes, DePuy, and Acumed.

has been estimated to be 71/100,000 in men and 30/100,000 in women. Midshaft clavicle fractures have a bimodal age distribution, with peaks occurring in those younger than 40 years and older than 70 years. Midshaft fractures account for approximately 69% to 82% of all clavicle fractures.[7,10-13] Midshaft fractures are more common in children and young adults and typically represent higher-energy fractures with comminution, displacement, and shortening.[11] In patients older than 70 years, these fractures tend to result from lower-energy injuries or can be insufficiency fractures caused by a simple fall.[7,12] Patients with midshaft clavicle fractures often present with a bruise or abrasion over the point or midline of the shoulder, depending on the mechanism of injury. The shoulder generally droops and appears shortened compared with the contralateral side, with the scapula appearing slightly internally rotated (**Figure 1**).

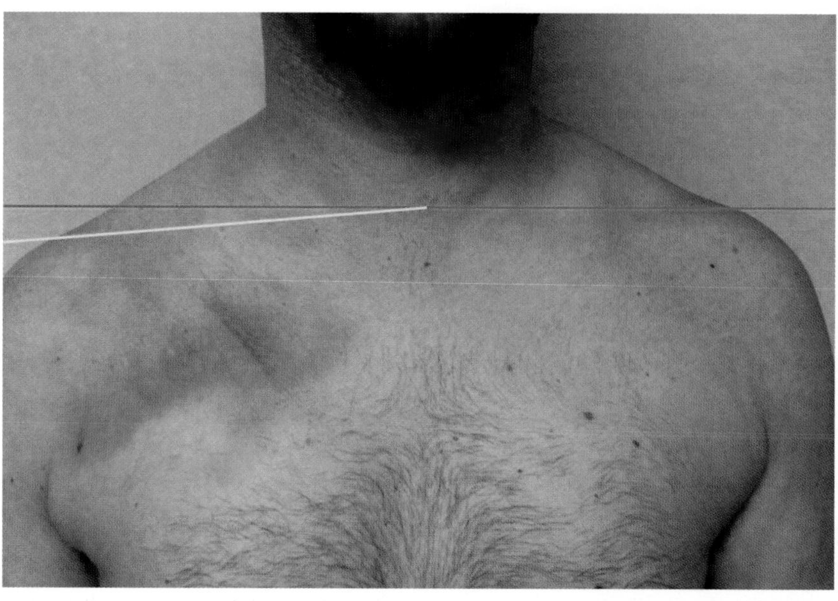

Figure 1 Clinical photograph of a patient with an acute right displaced clavicle shaft fracture with a drooped shoulder and bruising.

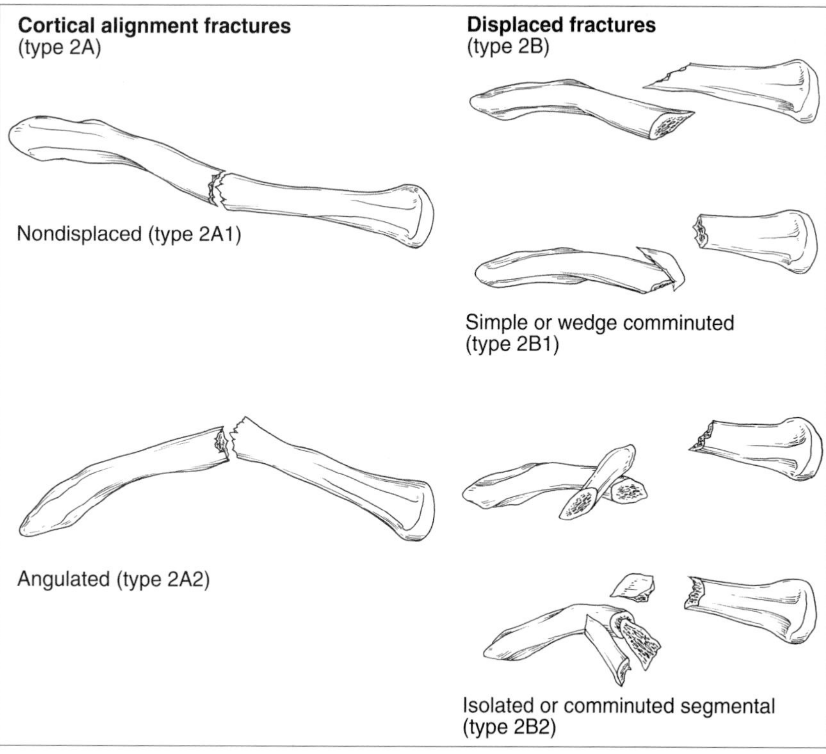

Figure 2 The Robinson classification system for midshaft clavicular fractures. (Reproduced with permission from Robinson CM: Fractures of the clavicle in the adult: Epidemiology and classification. *J Bone Joint Surg Br* 1998; 80:576-484.)

Classification

Allman[14] used location to classify clavicle fractures into three anatomic regions, with group I representing middle-third fractures, group II representing lateral-third fractures, and group III representing medial-third fractures. Other systems include the Orthopaedic Trauma Association classification system, which assigns clavicle fractures to anatomic regions: medial end (15-A), diaphysis (15-B), and lateral end (15-C).[15] Diaphyseal clavicle fractures are then further divided into simple (15-B1), wedge (15-B2), and complex (15-B3) fractures. These types are then further divided into three subtypes. In an effort to produce a system that demonstrates satisfactory levels of interobserver and intraobserver reliability and reproducibility and is useful in directing treatment and prognosis, Robinson[12] proposed another classification system (**Figure 2**). This system divides midshaft clavicle fractures into type 2A (cortical alignment fractures) and type 2B (displaced fractures). These types are then divided into subgroups: type 2A1 (nondisplaced), type 2A2 (angulated), type 2B1 (simple or wedge comminuted), and type 2B2 (isolated or comminuted segmental). Robinson's system has shown satisfactory levels of intraobserver and interobserver reliability, making it at least equal to other systems; however, it has not yet proved to be reliable in guiding treatment or predicting functional outcomes.

Nonsurgical Indications and Treatment

The primary goal in treating clavicle fractures is to restore shoulder function to the preinjury level. The objective is to allow the clavicle to heal with minimal deformity, thus minimizing loss of motion and pain while maximizing muscle strength and endurance. There is general agreement that indications for nonsurgical treatment include nondisplaced or minimally displaced (< 15 mm) fractures. Many nonsurgical treatment methods have been described,[16] but the two most frequently used techniques involve immobilization with a sling or figure-of-8 bandage. In two prospective, randomized or quasi-randomized controlled studies, the patients treated with a sling reported less discomfort compared with those treated with a figure-of-8 bandage; however, there was no difference in overall healing and fracture alignment.[17-19] Neither method helped to obtain or maintain reduction.[17] With either device, the shoulder is typically immobilized for 2 to 6 weeks based on the patient's comfort level. Return to light work with restricted overhead activity can begin when allowed by the patient's comfort level, usually at 2 to 4 weeks. Overhead activities, including athletics and heavy labor, are started only after clinical and radiographic union has occurred.

Lubbert et al[20] evaluated the effect of low-intensity pulsed ultrasound on fracture healing in 101 patients with nonsurgically treated clavicle shaft fractures. Fifty-two patients were treated with ultrasound stimulation, and 49 received a placebo transducer. The authors reported no outcome differences between the groups and concluded that low-intensity pulsed ultrasound does not accelerate fracture healing in nonsurgically treated clavicle shaft fractures.

Surgical Indications and Treatment

Historically, indications for the surgical fixation of clavicle fractures included those with skin compromise, neurologic or vascular injury, and open fractures. Relative indications for the surgical treatment of acute fractures have included "floating shoulder" fractures or those occurring in patients with multiple injuries. Surgery also has been indicated for symptomatic malunions or nonunions. More recently, relative indications for surgical treatment have been expanded to include high-energy closed fractures with greater than 15 to 20 mm of shortening, fractures with 100% displacement, and comminuted fractures.[2,21-23]

In a large epidemiologic study, Robinson[12] reported that the risk of nonunion for midshaft clavicle fractures is significantly increased in older patients, female patients, fractures with increasing displacement, and fractures with comminution. In 2007, a prospective randomized multicenter study of displaced midshaft clavicle fractures in 132 patients reported superior Disabilities of the Arm, Shoulder and Hand (DASH) scores and Constant shoulder scores in surgically treated patients compared with nonsurgically treated patients.[5] There were also significantly fewer nonunions and malunions in the surgically treated group. Additionally, increased fracture displacement was directly correlated with worse DASH scores. More recently, Davies et al[24] retrospectively reviewed 56 patients managed with closed treatment of clavicle fractures at 1- to 2-year follow-ups, specifically evaluating the ability of patients to perform activities of daily living. Most patients perceived a cosmetic deformity, and 22 of 56 patients had impaired function, suggesting that surgery may help to avoid these poorer outcomes. Nowak et al[23] evaluated 208 patients with clavicle fractures at 9- to 10-year follow-ups. Results showed a 15% nonunion rate with 100% displacement; 46% of patients had continued symptoms. The authors recommended that surgical treatment should be considered for patients with displaced clavicle fractures. In an attempt to summarize the data on surgical versus nonsurgical treatment of displaced clavicle fractures, a meta-analysis of studies from 1975 to 2005 was performed. The meta-analysis reviewed 2,144 clavicle fractures.[4] The authors reported that the nonunion rate for the closed treatment of displaced clavicle fractures was 15.1% compared to 2.2% and 2.0% for surgical treatment with compression plating and intramedullary (IM) pinning, respectively. Based on the reviewed studies in the meta-analysis, surgical fixation of displaced clavicle fractures is supported. These data should be interpreted with caution, however, because most of the reviewed data were taken from level III through V studies.

Patient-based outcome measures have shown deficits in shoulder strength and endurance after closed treatment of displaced clavicle fractures.[25] Lenza et al[26] also attempted to summarize the data on surgical versus nonsurgical outcomes in treating clavicle fractures. The authors suggested that additional level I data are needed before surgical treatment can definitively be recommended.

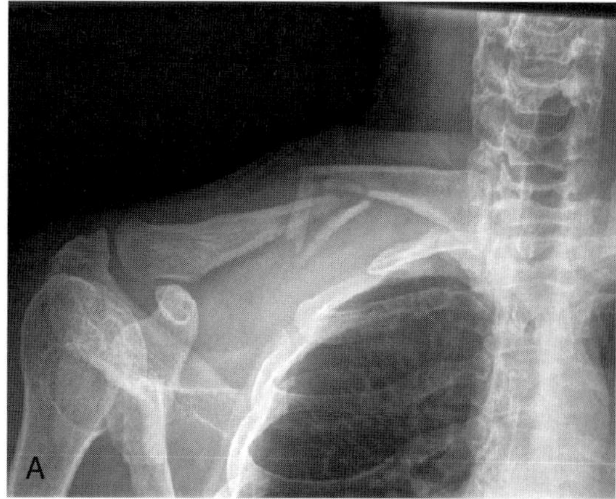

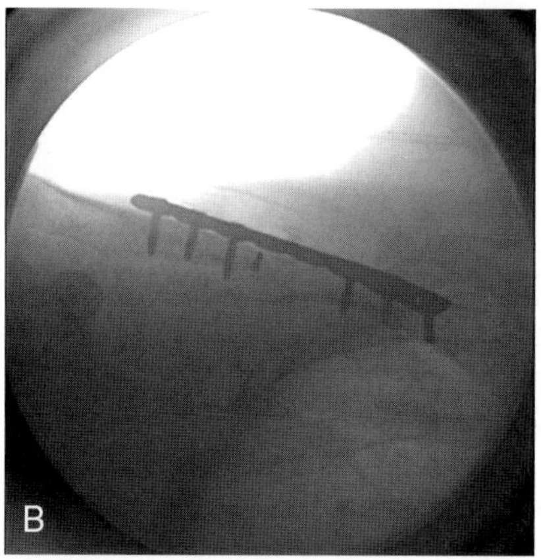

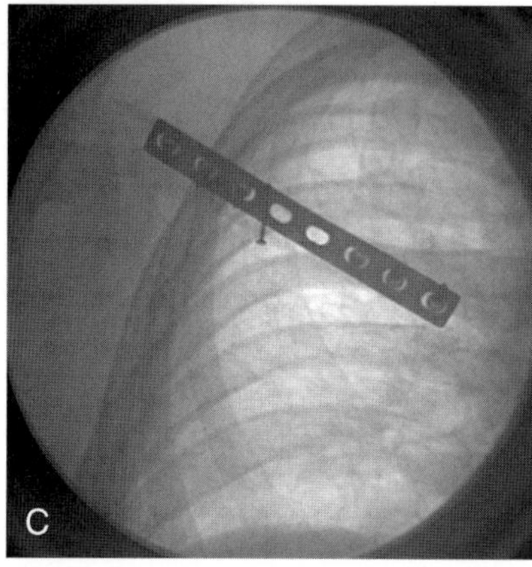

Figure 3 Radiographs of the patient shown in Figure 1. **A,** AP radiograph showing a displaced midshaft clavicle fracture. AP (**B**) and 45° oblique (**C**) views of the superior placement of a 3.5-mm dynamic compression plate.

Surgical Fixation Techniques

Open reduction and internal fixation using plates and screws or IM pinning can be done with the patient supine or in the beach chair position, with the head and neck tilted away from the operative site. A bump placed behind the scapula is sometimes used to aid in the reduction or allow access to the posterolateral shoulder for some pinning techniques. The arm can be prepped into the field to allow traction or manipulation to assist in the reduction, but this is often unnecessary. A skin incision is made following the lines of Langer over the clavicle as the skin permits. The incision also can be made inferior to the clavicle in an effort to minimize scar irritation and for easier exposure if anteroinferior plating will be used.[27] Identifying and preserving the supraclavicular nerves with the initial dissection may help avoid neuroma formation; however, the nerves can be sacrificed if necessary.

Plate Fixation

Placing the plate in the anterosuperior position (on the tension side of the bone) provides greater biomechanical stability[28] (**Figure 3**). Clinically successful treatment with anteroinferior plate placement has also been described.[29,30] The advantages of anteroinferior placement include drilling away from the lung and subclavian vessels (**Figure 4**). Theoretically, this placement may be less likely to cause hardware irritation, therefore decreasing the need for hardware removal. However, anteroinferior placement demands additional soft-tissue stripping and makes it more difficult to contour the plate, although precontoured plates are now readily available for all plate positions. Ideally, a 3.5-mm dynamic compression plate or a plate of similar strength should be used with at least six cortices on each side. Semitubular plates or similarly thin plates are not as rigid and should not be used.[31] Reconstruction plates are more easily contoured and have been used with success; however, several failures have been reported.[31] Locked plates are not typically needed for acute plating because they have no significant advantage over conventional plating and are more expensive. However, a prospective study of 64 patients older than 60 years showed a 17% complication rate with nonlocked plating compared with a 3.4% rate for locked plating.[32] Four patients treated with nonlocked plating had plate loosening that required additional surgery. The nonunion rate of 3.4% was the same in both groups. Patients with osteoporotic bone may benefit from locked plating.

With a sufficiently stable construct, unrestricted motion is allowed, with the exception of overhead lifting for 4 to 6 weeks until radiographic union is achieved. Because pain relief associated with stabilizing the fracture is often dramatic (even at 5 to 7 days), the patient should be cautioned to limit activities. Pain relief is cited as a potential benefit for surgical treatment along with earlier return to work; however, neither benefit has been validated with level I or II evidence.

Intramedullary Fixation

An alternative to plating is IM fixation. Many variations of IM implants have been described over the past 40 years, including Hagie pins, modified Hagie pins, Knowles pins, Her-

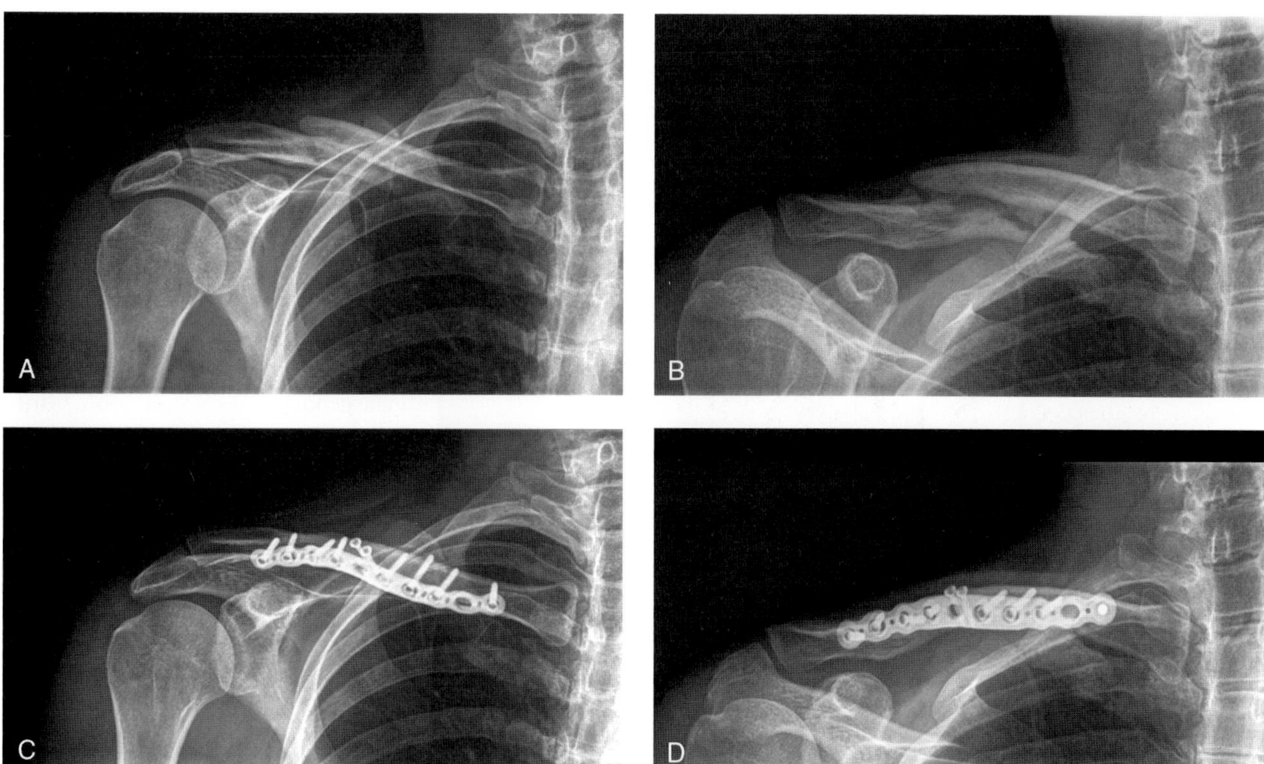

Figure 4 Radiographs of a clavicular fracture malunion/nonunion. AP view (**A**) and 30° cephalic tilt view (**B**) of malunion/nonunion at 12 months after injury. Note the significant shortening of the clavicle and the lack of callus formation. AP view (**C**) and 30° cephalic tilt view (**D**) of the anteroinferior placement of a precontoured plate for fixation of the malunion/nonunion. Note that the clavicle length is restored with fixation.

bert screws, Steinmann pins, elastic nails, cancellous screws, and Kirschner wires.[33-39] Modifications in the techniques and devices have led to a resurgence of interest in IM fixation of clavicle fractures. The potential benefits of IM fixation compared with plate fixation include less soft-tissue stripping at the fracture site, better cosmesis with a smaller skin incision, easier hardware removal, and less bone weakness after hardware removal. Biomechanically, plates provide a stronger construct because IM devices have less ability to resist torsional forces.[40] Historically, because of the risk of medial pin migration, IM fixation lost favor; however, newer designs and techniques, such as lateral-end locking nuts, avoid medial fragment cortex penetration and prevent medial migration of the devices.[41]

Patient positioning for IM fixation is similar to that for plate fixation, either supine or in the beach chair position. The techniques vary based on the type of IM device used, so techniques will not be discussed in detail. It is worth mentioning that IM fixation requires a much smaller incision over the fracture site to expose the fracture ends if any incision is needed. **Figure 5** shows fixation with a clavicle pin. Alternatively, the use of elastic titanium nails from the anteromedial aspect of the clavicle passed across the fracture in a closed manner also has been described.[37,42]

Postoperatively, shoulder motion is allowed, but forward elevation is usually restricted to 90° and abduction to 90° for the first 4 weeks if rotational stability is a concern. It is recommended that some IM devices be removed at 8 to 14 weeks. Other IM devices do not require removal unless hardware irritation is a problem. As with plating, a major theoretic benefit of IM fixation is earlier return to activities compared with nonsurgical treatment.

Malunions

The sequela of malunions and nonunions include shoulder girdle weakness; loss of endurance; ptosis and/or scapular winging; thoracic outlet syndrome; and neurologic changes, which are often related to brachial plexopathy. However, the two most common symptoms that motivate surgery are pain and cosmetic deformity.[3,43-47]

Malunion is not clearly defined in the literature. The deformity is a three-dimensional complication with the most consistent characteristics of

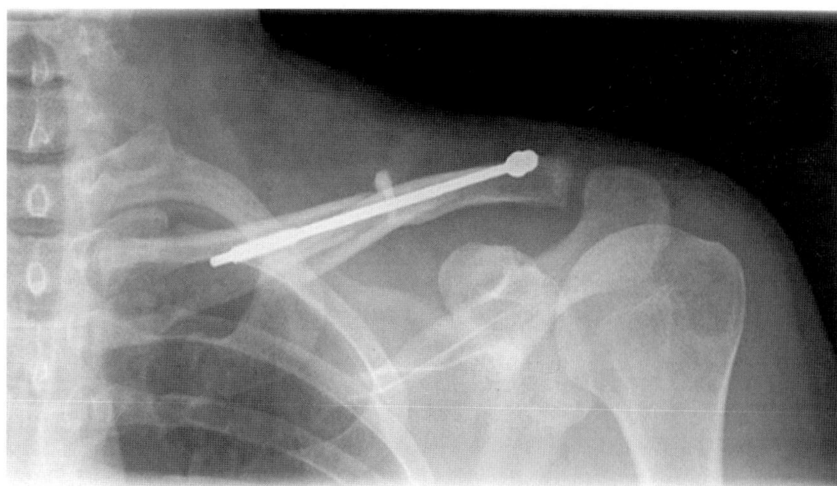

Figure 5 Radiograph of fracture fixation using a clavicle pin.

shortening, with inferior displacement of the lateral fragment; superior and posterior displacement of the medial fragment; and internal rotation of the shoulder. The incidence of symptomatic malunion is also unclear, with the most recent studies suggesting rates of 18% to 35% in nonsurgically treated patients.[5,46,48] Many studies have indicated that shortening of as little as 12 mm to 20 mm leads to poor patient satisfaction and unsatisfactory outcomes, including pain and cosmetic deformity.[2,21,46,49]

Ledger et al[50] found that more than 15 mm of shortening of the sternoclavicular joint on the injured side compared with the uninjured side resulted in a significant increase in upward angulation (mean, 10.7°), and the muscle torque of the injured arm was significantly weaker than the uninjured arm in extension, adduction, and internal rotation.[50]

Functional outcomes based on DASH and Constant scores were notably inferior in patients with clavicle malunions compared with the general population.[3,25] The authors concluded that fractures with greater than 2 cm of shortening tended to be associated with decreased abduction strength and greater patient dissatisfaction. Further investigation is needed to clearly define the type of fracture deformities that are likely to result in symptomatic clavicular malunion so that acute surgical treatment can be offered to patients who are at the greatest risk for this complication.

The treatment of a symptomatic malunion consists of surgical correction to restore length, angular deformity, and rotation of the clavicle. The approach is similar to that used to fix an acute clavicle fracture. Both IM devices and plates have been used successfully to treat malunions.[44,45,51] In simple fractures, it is often possible to identify the proximal and distal fragments after removing the callus of the malunion to anatomically reconstruct the clavicle.[44,45,51] If it is anticipated that it will be difficult to determine the proper length of the fractured clavicle, a preoperative radiographic image of both clavicles is recommended. Preoperative planning also includes a discussion with the patient about the potential need for a bone graft if it is suspected that is will be difficult to restore clavicular length. A tricortical wedge of bone often is used to restore clavicular length. Restoration of the deformity (especially length) with a corrective osteotomy will improve patient satisfaction, outcome scores, and cosmesis and will lessen pain.[3,43,44]

Nonunions

Although the time frame for defining a clavicular nonunion is not clearly specified in the literature, most authors consider a clavicular nonunion as the absence of healing at 16 weeks.[45,51,53] Risk factors for nonunion include fracture fragment displacement, female gender, and comminution. Other risk factors identified in clavicular nonunions are advancing age, lack of cortical apposition, more severe initial trauma, a greater extent of fracture fragment displacement, and soft-tissue interposition.[1,2,4,52,53] Early mobilization has not been associated with nonunion in surgically or nonsurgically treated patients. The traditional belief that surgical treatment was the major cause of nonunion has been proved false.[4] Most of the prior discussion in this chapter on malunions also applies to nonunions because malpositioning is often involved. The exception is a postoperative surgical nonunion in which there is no deformity, but hardware failure and/or pain may be present.

The surgical treatment of clavicle nonunions has a high success rate. Techniques are the same as those described for malunions, including plating with bone graft, IM pin fixation with bone graft, and external fixation. Union rates with each method have been reported to be higher than 92%, with some studies reporting a 100% rate of union.[53-55] As with malunions, preoperative planning is key to ensuring restoration of clavicular length, rotation, and displacement matching the contralateral side. In atrophic nonunions, autologous bone grafting helps to achieve union. If there is bone loss, a tricortical graft may be indicated to restore length. Few data exist regarding the use of bone morphogenetic proteins and other bone graft substitutes in patients with clavicular nonunion. In terms of treatment choice, plate fixation has the most support in the literature and, in the experience of this chapter's authors, is the most predictable option for treating symptomatic clavicular nonunion. Other techniques, including IM pinning, have been successful when used by experienced surgeons.

Scapula Fractures

The scapula provides distinctive and complex linkage for the entire forequarter, transitioning the musculoskeletal anatomy from the axial to the appendicular skeleton between the clavicle and humerus and over the thoracic cage. In the opinion of this chapter's authors, it would not be surprising if increasing levels of malalignment of the glenoid joint in scapular fractures was associated with increasing levels of dysfunction or symptoms based on its intrinsic linkage. The present challenge is to understand how the type and level of displacement associated with specific scapular fracture patterns affects function. Because most available studies on scapula fractures are retrospective studies without comparative cohorts, there are still many unanswered questions regarding the diagnosis and treatment of these fractures.

Epidemiology and Associated Injuries

Scapula neck and body fractures, as well as fractures of the glenoid fossa, are associated with high-energy trauma and occur most commonly in the third and fourth decades of life.[56,57] Because of the high-energy mechanisms associated with these fractures, approximately 90% of the fractures are associated with injuries to other organ systems, including the cervicocranium in approximately 33% of patients and the ipsilateral extremity in approximately 50% of patients.[58-61] A lower mortality rate has been reported in polytrauma patients with scapula fractures compared with those without scapula fractures. Vital organs may be protected from injury because of the energy absorbed by the clavicle and ribs.[59,60] The clinician should be alert for limb- and life-threatening conditions in patients with these complex shoulder injuries.

Diagnosis and Classification

Although the AO/Orthopaedic Trauma Association classification of scapular fractures has recently been modified,[15] there are few published studies on treatment outcomes based on this classification system. Comparing outcomes is difficult because clinicians do not have validated methods to measure and interpret scapular displacement; there is also no established agreement on what constitutes the scapular neck. The Ideberg classification and its modifications[62,63] are helpful in diagnosing intra-articular fractures because they are based on clinical findings; this is also true of the more comprehensive classification system by Ada and Miller.[64]

A recent study with 90 patients described scapula fracture patterns of highly displaced scapula fractures detected with three-dimensional CT scans.[65] The authors found highly reproducible patterns for extra-articular fractures and highly variable fracture patterns when the glenoid fossa was involved. In almost 70% of patients, the fracture coursed from the lateral border just below the glenoid process and exited the vertebral border just caudal to the spine of the scapula. Approximately 20% of the fractures involved the spinoglenoid notch, and 20% involved the articular surface.[65] This mapping of scapula fracture patterns may potentially aid surgeons in choosing the best approach for treating the most common patterns of injury.

Three standard radiographic views (AP, scapula Y, and axillary) are warranted if a shoulder injury is suspected; however, imaging of these fractures is challenging, and radiographs are often difficult to interpret, especially when the scapula is fractured and displaced, rendering the scapula body and/or glenohumeral joint out of plane with the x-ray beam. The role of two-dimensional CT does not add diagnostic value when imaging extra-articular fractures;[66] however, this modality should be used for interpreting intra-articular fractures. The role of three-dimensional CT reconstructions was elucidated in a study by Tadros et al.[67] The authors reported that standard radiographs of the shoulder were adequate for assessing scapula body and acromion fractures but were not suitable for evaluating glenoid, coracoid, or scapula neck fractures. Three-dimensional CT detected all fractures in the study group, thus demonstrating a high sensitivity.

There is still a knowledge deficit regarding terms and definitions of scapular displacement and angular deformity, specifically because angulation is generally not ascribed to a particular plane and displacement is not ascribed to a particular direction. This controversy is highlighted by the disagreement in the meaning of "medialization" in scapula fractures.

Outcomes

All studies to date on scapula fractures have been retrospective and noncomparative. One systematic review analyzed 22 studies that included 520 surgically and nonsurgically treated patients.[56] The authors reported that 80% of isolated glenoid fractures were surgically treated, with 82% good to excellent results according to varying

Table 1
Published Scapula Fracture Studies: Combined Patient Cohorts (Intra-articular and Extra-articular Fractures)

Authors (Year)	Total Number of Patients	Treatment: Surgical (S), Nonsurgical (N)	Intra-articular	Extra-articular
Wilber and Evans[69] (1977)	30	N		X
	10	S	X	
Hardegger et al[70] (1984)	37	S	X	X
McGinnis and Denton[71] (1989)	39	N	X	X
Ada and Miller[64] (1991)[a]	113	N	X	X
	8	S		X
Bauer et al[72] (1995)	25	S	X	X
Zhou et al[73] (2006)	21	S	X	X
Schofer et al[68] (2009)	137	N	X	X

[a]Of these authors, only Ada and Miller included surgical indications of medial displacement > 1 cm and angular deformity > 40°.

(often soft) outcome criteria. It is noteworthy that although 99% of scapula body fractures were treated conservatively, 14% of patients with these fractures had fair to poor outcomes. Eighty-three percent of scapula neck fractures were treated nonsurgically; more than 20% of these patients had fair to poor outcomes.[56]

The second systematic review included 17 studies with 243 patients with surgically treated scapula fractures.[57] Most fractures were treated with a posterior approach; 22% of the patients also had clavicle fractures. Good to excellent results were reported in 83.4% of patients; complication rates were exceptionally low. Infection, nonunion, and wound problems are rarely reported in surgical procedures involving the scapula, probably because of the robust musculature and a rich blood supply around the scapula. The few documented poor outcomes seemed to be associated with brachial plexus or peripheral nerve pathology.[57]

Table 1 summarizes the results of reported studies of scapula fracture outcomes with mixed patient cohorts, including surgical and nonsurgical treatment of intra-articular and/or extra-articular fractures.[64,68-73] **Table 2** summarizes results from studies of only intra-articular scapula fractures.[63,74-77] **Table 3** presents the results of studies of extra-articular fractures, with and without ipsilateral clavicle fractures.[78-97] Maquieira et al[98] reported on a retrospective review

Table 1 (cont)
Published Scapula Fracture Studies: Combined Patient Cohorts (Intra-articular and Extra-articular Fractures)

Mean Follow-up (Range) Follow-up/Total Patients (%) Union Rate	Functional Outcomes	Complications
F/U: 6-12 mo Patients: 30/30 Union: 100%	Nonsurgical patients did well	None reported
F/U: 12-144 mo Patients: 6/10 (60%) Union: 100%	Good: 1, fair: 3, poor: 2	
F/U: 6.5 yr (1.5-15 yr) Patients: 33/37 (89%) Union: 100%	No pain: 25; minimal pain: 3; moderate pain: 4; severe pain: 1 Glenohumeral osteoarthritis leading to arthrodesis: 1 Brachial plexus: 1	2 superficial infections, both healed after being drained 2 hematomas, which required evacuation 1 reoperation for instability, which healed uneventfully 8 shoulder manipulations under anesthesia; no second procedures needed
F/U: 15.8 mo (2-48 mo) Patients: 26/ 39 (67%) Union: 100%	Excellent: 16; good: 3; fair: 2; poor: 3 Brachial plexus: 1 Unable to grade (comatose): 1	1 readmission for acromioclavicular joint fixation 1 readmission for missed pneumothorax
F/U: Not stated Patients: 24/113 (21%) Union: 112/113 (99%)	Displaced neck fractures: 20% decreased range of motion 50% residual pain 40% pain and weakness Intra-articular fractures: 100% decreased range of motion 100% residual pain 66% pain and weakness	1 nonunion 2 malunions
F/U: ≥ 15 mo Patients: 8/8 (100%) Union: 100%	All patients achieved > 85° glenohumeral abduction No night pain or pain at rest	None reported
F/U: 6.1 yr Patients: 20/25 (80%) Union: 100%	13 patients obtained very good outcomes	None reported
F/U: 21 mo (6-48 mo) Patients: 18/21 (86%) Union: 100%	Rowe score: Excellent: 12; good: 3; fair: 2; poor: 1	None reported
F/U: 65 mo (13-120 mo) Patients: 50/137 (37%) Union: 100%	Constant and Murley score: 78.8 ± 4.45 Very good: 23%; good: 51%; satisfactory: 20%; poor: 6%	None reported

F/U = follow-up

of conservatively treated low-energy shoulder dislocations associated with a glenoid rim (Ideberg type 1 fracture) in 14 patients (mean age, 53 years). Thirteen of the 14 shoulders had a centered glenohumeral joint at final follow-up, and 1 shoulder was anteriorly subluxated. All patients had excellent functional outcomes at a mean of 5.6 years after injury, although three patients had radiographic signs of osteoarthritis. Eight patients were excluded, some because of the loss of glenohumeral joint concentricity on postreduction radiographs, which underscores the question of whether surgical treatment is appropriate for an isolated, partial articular glenoid injury. The authors concluded that shoulder immobilization for 6 weeks to maintain reduction during early healing is warranted for patients (especially elderly patients) who meet these injury parameters.[98] Arthroscopic methods for treating bony Bankart lesions should be considered in younger populations; various techniques have been described.[74,99-102]

Schandelmaier et al[75] reported on long-term functional outcomes in higher-energy surgically treated glenoid fractures (Ideberg types II through V) in 22 consecutive patients. At a mean 10-year follow-up, the median Constant and Murley score was 94%, and the mean Constant and Murley score was 79%. Four patients had a Constant and Murley score lower than 50%, including two with

Table 2
Published Scapula Fracture Studies: Intra-articular Patient Cohorts

Authors (Year)	Total Number of Patients	Treatment: Surgical (S), Nonsurgical (N)	Surgical Indications (Displacement)	Mean Follow-up (Range) Follow-up/Total Patients (%) Union Rate
Kavanagh et al[76] (1993)	10	S	> 2 mm	F/U: 4 yr (2-10 yr) Patients: 9/10 (90%) Union: 100%
Leung et al[77] (1993)	14	S	Displaced (amount not specified)	F/U: 30.5 mo (18-68 mo) Patients: 14/14 (100%) Union: 100%
Mayo et al[63] (1998)	31	S	> 5 mm	F/U: 43 mo (25-75 mo) Patients: 27/31 (87%) Union: 100%
Adam[74] (2002)	10	S	Displaced (amount not specified)	F/U: 18-84 mo Patients: 10/10 (100%) Union: 100%
Schandelmaier et al[75] (2002)	22	S	Displaced (amount not specified)	F/U: 10 yrs (5-23 yrs) Patients: 22/22 (100%) Union: 100%

F/U = follow-up

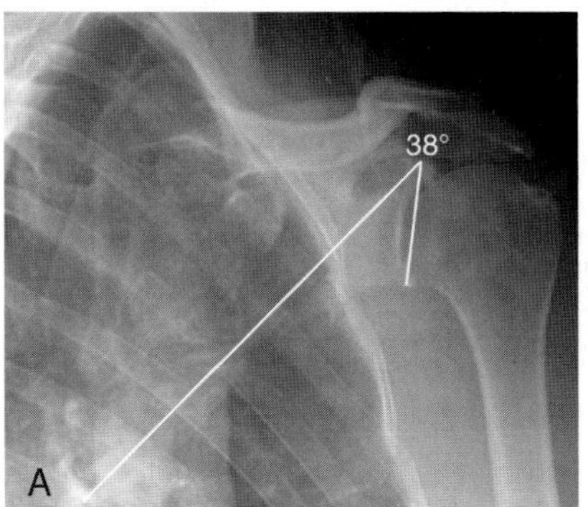

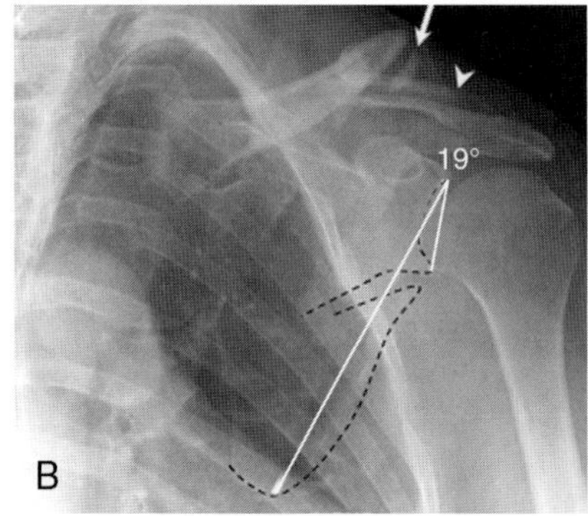

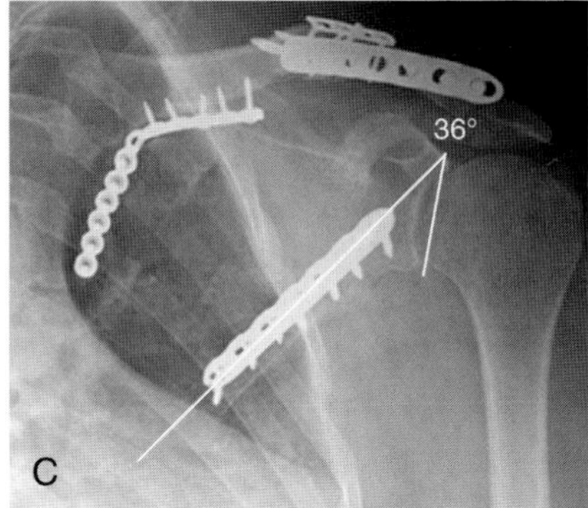

Figure 6 Radiographs of a patient with a scapula fracture malunion. **A,** AP radiograph of the uninjured shoulder with a glenopolar angle of 38°. The image is inverted to facilitate comparison with the injured shoulder. **B,** Radiograph of the malunited scapular fracture 9 months after the initial injury. The patient presented with chronic pain and decreased range of motion and strength. The proximal and distal fragments are outlined (dashed lines) to show the severity of the mediolateral displacement of the lateral border and the glenopolar angle of 19°. A segmental clavicle fracture nonunion is also present (arrow). The arrowhead points to the distal clavicle fracture that was better appreciated on a two-dimensional CT scan. **C,** AP radiograph of the shoulder 18 months after surgery. Note the significant improvement in the lateral border offset and the reconstructed glenopolar angle of 36°.

deep infections. An additional two patients had an associated complete palsy of the brachial plexus not attributed to surgical treatment.[75] Other smaller studies of intra-articular fractures with shorter-term follow-up have described generally good to excellent outcomes.

In a study of 18 nonsurgically treated patients with scapula neck fractures, a statistically significant positive correlation was reported between the Constant and Murley scores and the glenopolar angles[78,103] (**Figure 6**). In a similar study, the authors showed a positive correlation in the Constant and Murley scores and glenopolar angles in 16 patients at a mean follow-up

Table 2 (cont)
Published Scapula Fracture Studies: Intra-articular Patient Cohorts

Functional Outcomes	Complications
No patients reported pain	1 heterotopic bone; no reoperation needed
Rowe score: excellent: 9; good: 5 Pain: none: 7; slight pain during activity: 7 Function: normal: 2; minimal limitation: 12	None reported
Excellent: 6; good: 16; fair: 3; poor: 2	1 wound dehiscence; healed uneventfully 2 marked infraspinatus weakness; positive electromyogram for suprascapular nerve lesion 3 hardware removal
Excellent: 5; good: 3; fair: 1; poor: 1	1 superficial infection, resolved 1 hematoma requiring evacuation 1 implant failure; deep infection resulting in glenohumeral arthritis
Constant and Murley score (injured reported as a % of uninjured): Mean = 79% (range, 17%-100%)	1 superficial infection resolved 1 hardware failure with delayed healing and infection 1 deep infection 1 manipulation under anesthesia for stiffness 1 impingement treated with subacromial decompression 1 hardware failure

F/U = follow-up

of 32 months.[79] A significant difference ($P < 0.05$) in outcomes also was found among patients with glenopolar angles of more than 30° compared with those with glenopolar angles of less than 30°.

In a study of 50 patients treated nonsurgically for scapula fractures, forward flexion, abduction, and external rotation was found to be significantly compromised at a mean follow-up of 65 months.[68] It is interesting to note that these findings of restricted motion did not necessarily correlate with lower functional outcomes, even though there was a positive relationship between decreased range of motion and decreased strength. In contrast, a study by Pace et al[80] reported poor outcomes in nine patients with glenoid neck fractures who were treated conservatively with immobilization and early active motion. All patients had pain associated with scapula malunion; five patients reported pain when at rest. Chadwick et al[104] performed a biomechanical analysis on the effects of scapular malunion and described the reasons for increased muscle effort needed to execute glenohumeral constraint. Patients with severe deformity reported a slumped or drooped shoulder appearance (**Figure** 7); however, this complication has not been generally acknowledged in the literature.

Often, there is a delay in treating scapula fractures because other injuries are being managed and the need to refer these patients to specialists for fracture treatment. Herrera et al[81] evaluated 22 patients with highly displaced fractures of the scapula neck (11 with concomitant glenoid involvement) treated between 21 to 90 days after injury. The patients had good functional outcomes approaching normative values based on DASH scores and the Medical Outcomes Study 36-Item Short Form survey. Eleven of 16 patients who were available for follow-up at a mean of 27 months had returned to their original occupations (2 patients did not return to their original occupations because of associated injuries rather than as a result of the scapula neck fracture).[81]

Surgical Indications

The surgical treatment of certain patients with scapula fractures is supported by evidence showing poor outcomes in some nonsurgically treated patients. Because no level I or II studies are available to support surgical treatment for specific indications, recommendations for surgical management vary and are likely based on the treating surgeon's individual experience, training, and practice setting.

Among those surgeons who favor surgical treatment of scapula fractures, it is generally agreed that an acromion or coracoid process fracture displaced 1 cm or more has a high risk for symptomatic nonunion or malunion and should be considered for surgical fixation. Displaced intra-articular glenoid fractures (> 5 mm), as well as those associated with humeral subluxation, also should be considered for surgical treatment (**Figure 8**). The more

Table 3
Published Scapula Fracture Series: Extra-articular Patient Cohorts

Authors (Year)	Total Number of Patients	Treatment: Surgical (S), Nonsurgical (N)	Concomitant Double Superior Shoulder Suspensory Complex (SSSC)	Surgical Indications[a]
Herscovici[83] (1992)	2	N	Double SSSC	N/A
	7	S	Double SSSC	C
Nordqvist and Petersson[84] (1992)	129	N	N/A	N/A
Leung and Lam[85] (1993)	15	S	Double SSSC	A
Rikli et al[86] (1995)	12	S	Double SSSC	A
Ramos et al[87] (1997)	16	N	Double SSSC	N/A
Edwards et al[88] (2000)	36	N	Double SSSC	N/A
Low and Lam[89] (2000)	4	S	Double SSSC	A
Egol et al[90] (2001)	12	N	Double SSSC	A
	7	S	Double SSSC	A
Romero et al[91] (2001)	16	N	N/A	N/A
	3	S	Double SSSC	A

[a]Surgical indications: A = unstable shoulder girdle or displaced double lesion, B = medial displacement, angular deformity or articular step-off, C = no surgical indications reported in this studyt

F/U = follow-up; N/A = not available; DASH = Disabilities of the Arm, Shoulder and Hand; ASES = American Shoulder and Elbow Surgeons; UCLA = University of California at Los Angeles; ADL = activities of daily living, ROM = range of motion; ORIF = open reduction and internal fixation

Table 3 (cont)
Published Scapula Fracture Series: Extra-articular Patient Cohorts

Mean Follow-up (Range) Follow-up/Total Patients (%) Union Rate	Functional Outcomes	Complications
F/U: 48.5 mo (2-132 mos) Patients: 9/9 (100%) Union: 100%	Good:1; poor: 1	None reported
	No pain: 5; pain only with exertion: 2 Function, excellent: 7	
F/U: (10-20 yr) Patients: 84/129 (65%) Union: 100%	Returned to original job: 68 Retired because of age or disease unrelated to shoulder: 12 Persistent shoulder impairment and unable to return to work: 4 Clinical evaluation of 68 patients: good: 51; fair: 15; poor: 2	None reported
F/U: 25 mo (14-47 mo) Patients: 15/15 (100%) Union: 100%	Rowe score: mean = 84 excellent: 8; good: 6; fair: 1 Pain: no pain: 9; slight: 5; moderate: 1	1 hardware removal
F/U: 6 yr (0.5-10 yr) Patients: 12/12 (100%) Union: 100%	Constant and Murley score: mean = 96% (range, 69%-113%) Pain: no pain: 9; cold sensitivity: 2; pain with mobilization: 1 Function: normal ADL: 5; sleeplessness when lying on injured side: 4; increased fatigability with overhead work: 2; apprehension in using arm: 1	1 wound infection leading to frozen shoulder requiring manipulation under anesthesia
F/U: 7.5 yr (2-18 yr) Patients: 13/16 (81%) Union: 100%	Excellent: 11; good: 1; fair: 1 Pain: no pain: 11; pain with severe stress: 1; pain with normal activity: 1 Function: returned to previous activity: 11; required lifestyle change: 2	None reported
F/U: 28 mo (9-79 mo) Patients: 20/36 (56%) Union: 19/20 (95%)	Herscovici score: excellent 17; good: 3 Rowe score: mean = 95 excellent: 18; good: 1; fair: 1 Constant and Murley score: mean = 96	1 clavicular nonunion
F/U: 3.3 yr (2-4 yr) Patients: 4/4 (100%) Union: 100%	Rowe score: excellent: 3; good: 1	None reported
F/U: 53 mo (12-81 mo) Patients: 19/19 (100%) Union: 11/12 (92%)	DASH score: mean = 52.7 ASES: mean = 80.2	1 clavicular nonunion
F/U: 36 mo (12-78 mo) Patients: 19/19 (100%) Union: 7/7 (100%)	DASH score: mean = 46.1 ASES score: mean = 88.7	2 persistent infraclavicular nerve palsies 1 iatrogenic brachial plexus injury, resolved
F/U: 6 yr (2-23 yr) Patients: 19/19 Union: 100%	Pain: moderate-severe: 7; mild-none: 12 Impairment: moderate-severe: 5; mild-none: 14	None reported

Table 3 (cont)
Published Scapula Fracture Series: Extra-articular Patient Cohorts

Authors (Year)	Total Number of Patients	Treatment: Surgical (S), Nonsurgical (N)	Concomitant Double Superior Shoulder Suspensory Complex (SSSC)	Surgical Indications[a]
van Noort et al[92] (2001)	31	N	Double SSSC	N/A
	4	S	Double SSSC	A
Oh et al[93] (2002)	10	N	N/A	N/A
	3	S	Double SSSC	A
Hashiguchi and Ito[94] (2003)	5	S	Double SSSC	A
Labler et al[95] (2004)	8	N	Double SSSC	N/A
	9	S	Double SSSC	C
Bozkurt et al[78] (2005)	18	N	N/A	N/A
Pace et al[80] (2005)	11	N	N/A	N/A
	1	S	Double SSSC	C
van Noort and van Kampen[96] (2005)	23	N	N/A	N/A
	1	S	N/A	C
Khallaf et al[97] (2006)	14	S	N/A	B
Kim et al[79] (2008)	7	N	Double SSSC	N/A
	9	S	Double SSSC	C
Herrera et al[81] (2009)	22	S	N/A	B
Jones et al[82] (2009)	37	S	N/A	B

[a]Surgical indications: A = unstable shoulder girdle or displaced double lesion, B = medial displacement, angular deformity or articular step-off, C = no surgical indications reported in this studyt

F/U = follow-up; N/A = not available; DASH = Disabilities of the Arm, Shoulder and Hand; ASES = American Shoulder and Elbow Surgeons; UCLA = University of California at Los Angeles; ADL = activities of daily living, ROM = range of motion; ORIF = open reduction and internal fixation

Table 3 (cont)
Published Scapula Fracture Series: Extra-articular Patient Cohorts

Mean Follow-up (Range) Follow-up/Total Patients (%) Union Rate	Functional Outcomes	Complications
F/U: 35 mo (8-80 mo) Patients: 35/46 (76%) Union: 29/31 (94%)	Constant and Murley score: mean = 76 (range, 30-10) Pain: at rest: 3; during ADL: 13	1 clavicle nonunion; 3 secondary ORIF (1 clavicle nonunion and 2 malunion corrections); 1 posttraumatic dystrophy caused by brachial plexus lesion
F/U: 35 mo (8-80 mo) Patients: 35/46 (76%) Union: 4/4 (100%)	Constant and Murley score: mean = 71 (range, 43-100) Pain: at rest: 3; during ADL: 4	1 posttraumatic dystrophy caused by a brachial plexus lesion
F/U: 20 mo (12-40 mo) Patients: 13/13 (100%) Union: 100%	Rowe score: mean = 85.7 excellent: 7, good: 5, fair: 1	2 implant failures requiring reoperation
F/U: 57.4 mo (21-79 mo) Patients: 5/5 (100%) Union: 100%	UCLA score: mean = 34.2 (range, 33-35) Satisfactory outcomes for all patients	None reported
F/U: (30-118 mo) Patients: 17/17 (100%) Union: 100%	Constant and Murley score: excellent: 5; fair: 3	None reported
F/U: (9-117 mo) Patients: 17/17 (100%) Union: 100%	Constant and Murley score: excellent: 5; fair to bad: 4	None reported
F/U: 25 mo Patients: 18/18 (100%) Union: 100%	Constant and Murley score: mean = 78.8 (range, 68-94)	None reported
F/U: > 1 yr Patients: 9/12 (75%) Union: 100%	Pain: no patients completely free of pain Function: reported disability in normal ADL caused by pain: 6; significant disability: 1	None reported
F/U: 5.5 yr (1.6-12 yr) Patients: 13/24 (54%) Union: 100%	Constant and Murley score: mean = 90 (range, 64 - 100) Good to excellent: 11 Function: returned to original employment: 8; did not return to original employment because of shoulder problem: 1; retired or not working at time of injury: 4	None reported
F/U: 1.5 yr (0.5-2.5 yr) Patients: 14/14 (100%) Union: 100%	UCLA score: excellent: 12; good: 2 No patients reported pain during ADL	1 heterotopic bone formation
F/U: 32 mo (13-84 mo) Patients: 16/20 (80%) Union: 100%	Constant and Murley score: mean = 64.7	None reported
	Constant and Murley score: mean = 73.6	
F/U: 26.4 mo (12-72 mo) Patients: 16/22 (73%) Union: 100%	DASH score: mean = 14 (range, 0-41) Pain: none: 12; mild: 1; moderate with prolonged activity: 1 Function: returned to former employment: 11; did not return to preinjury ADL because of associated injuries: 2	1 required manipulation under anesthesia
F/U: ≥ 1 yr Patients: 37/37 (100%) Union: 100%	ROM in forward flexion: mean = 158° (range 90°-180°)	3 patients (4 scapula fractures) required manipulation under anesthesia

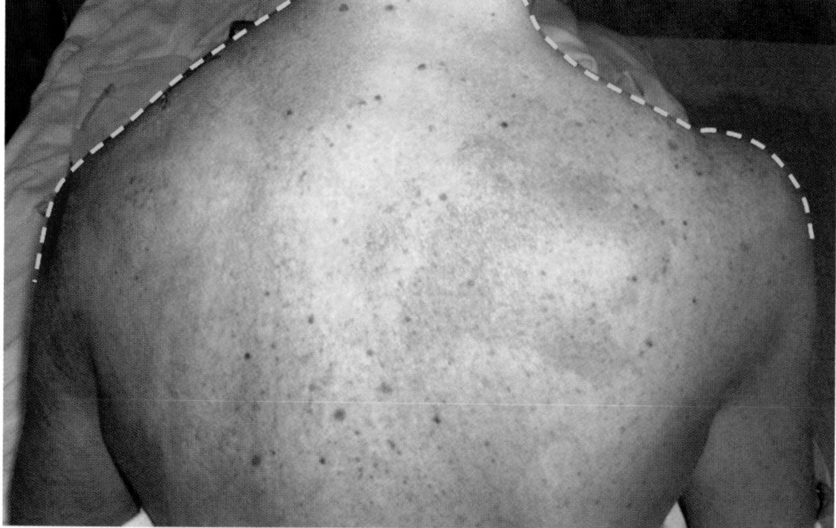

Figure 7 Clinical photograph of a patient with left-sided ipsilateral scapula and clavicle fractures. The normal contour (dashed line) of the right shoulder is significantly altered on the injured left side (dashed line). Extensive skin abrasions on the left shoulder were allowed to heal before open reduction and internal fixation of the fractures.

controversial scapula neck or body fractures in which the fracture is located medial to the coracoid should be considered for surgery if there is 2 cm of lateral border offset (medialization), 40° of angular deformity on a scapular Y radiograph, or a glenopolar angle of less than 20°. The threshold for considering surgery should be even lower if the scapula neck fracture enters the spinoglenoid notch or in patients with an ipsilateral displaced clavicle fracture or acromioclavicular dislocation because of the possibility of an unstable floating shoulder.

Surgical Approach

Lambotte[105] was the first to describe internal fixation of a scapula fracture in 1910,[106] and Judet described an

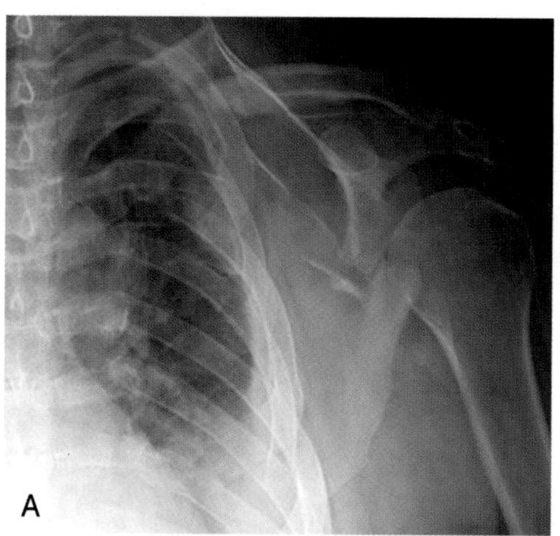

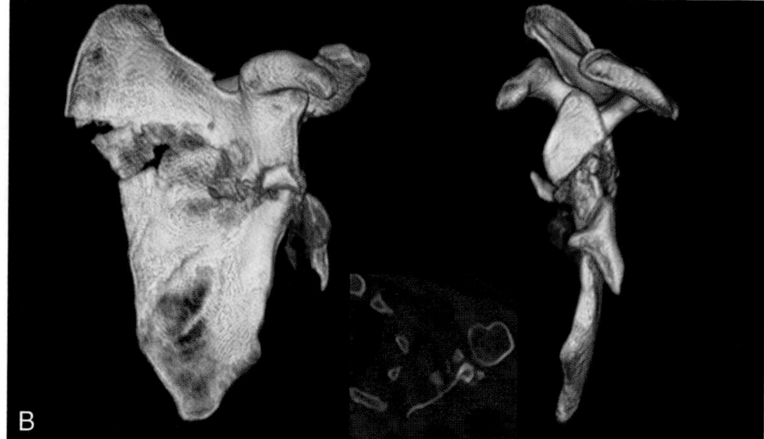

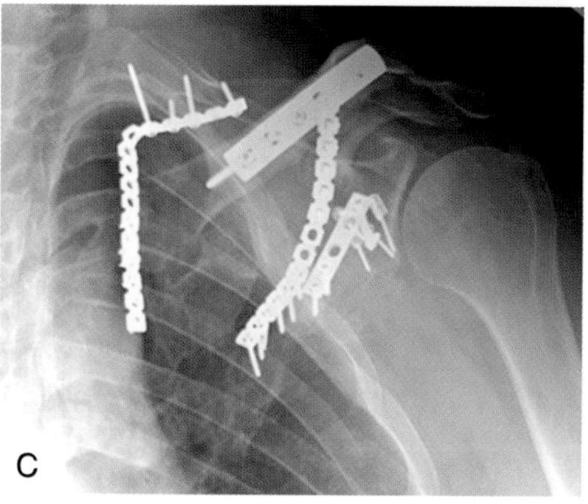

Figure 8 Intra-articular glenoid fracture with extension into the scapula body. **A,** The initial AP radiograph of the shoulder shows a highly displaced clavicle fracture, multiple rib fractures, and an intra-articular glenoid fracture. **B,** Three-dimensional CT reconstructions aid in classifying and measuring the fracture and determining the surgical approach. The inset shows an axial two-dimension CT image of the glenoid fracture. **C,** AP radiograph of the shoulder after open reduction and internal fixation of the scapula and clavicle fractures.

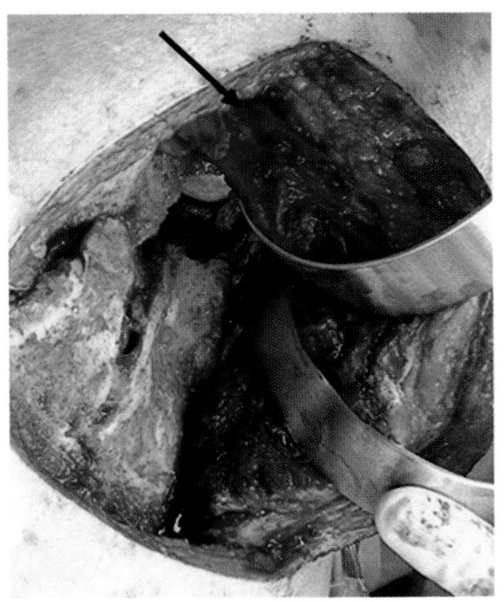

Figure 9 Intraoperative photograph showing the surgical exposure through a posterior approach. The scapula neck and body are fractured. Access to the entire posterior scapula is obtained using the Judet approach. This approach is most often used for complex or late presenting fractures. Note that the rotator cuff is elevated on the neurovascular pedicle of the suprascapular artery and the nerve emanating from the base of the acromion (arrow).

extensile posterior approach in 1964[106,107] (**Figure 9**). Recently, iterations of the posterior approach have been described by other authors.Obremskey and Lyman[108] reported a modification of the Judet approach using intermuscular windows to access the scapula borders. Nork et al[109] emphasized mobilization of the infraspinatus fascia with the deltoid during its detachment from the spine of the scapula after making a Judet incision. Wirbel et al[110] and van Noort et al[111] advocated sparing the deltoid completely when treating intra-articular fractures by using an abducted arm position, thus allowing retraction of the deltoid and access to the rotator cuff interval. Jones et al[82] reported on 37 scapula fractures treated through a modified Judet approach and detailed the use of 2.7- and 2-mm implants for fixation. No complications were related to the surgical approach. Although prolonged shoulder stiffness was reported in four patients, the stiffness resolved in all patients after manipulation under anesthesia. Wijdicks et al[112] highlighted the critical structures and landmarks used in posterior approaches, illustrating the relationship of the suprascapular nerve in the spinoglenoid notch and defining the anterior circumflex artery off the lateral border.

Summary

Patients presenting for treatment with scapula and clavicle fractures are becoming increasingly more common, especially in trauma centers that treat a large number of patients with high-energy injuries. Because of the universal motion of the glenohumeral joint and the compensatory motion of the sternoclavicular, acromioclavicular, and scapulothoracic joints, scapula and clavicle deformity is usually well tolerated; however, there is increasing awareness of the risk of dysfunction in patients with severe malunions or nonunions. The need to better define deformity and displacement has been aided by the availability and use of three-dimensional CT, which is useful in measuring fracture angulation and displacement in an attempt to establish criteria for the surgical treatment of these injuries.

Acknowledgments

The authors would like to acknowledge Stephanie L. Tanner, MS; Lisa K. Schroder, BS, MBA; and Erich M. Gauger, MD, for their assistance in preparing this manuscript.

References

1. Robinson CM, Court-Brown CM, McQueen MM, Wakefield AE: Estimating the risk of nonunion following nonoperative treatment of a clavicular fracture. *J Bone Joint Surg Am* 2004; 86-A(7):1359-1365.
2. Hill JM, McGuire MH, Crosby LA: Closed treatment of displaced middle-third fractures of the clavicle gives poor results. *J Bone Joint Surg Br* 1997;79(4): 537-539.
3. McKee MD, Wild LM, Schemitsch EH: Midshaft malunions of the clavicle. *J Bone Joint Surg Am* 2003;85-A(5): 790-797.
4. Zlowodzki M, Zelle BA, Cole PA, Jeray K, McKee MD; Evidence-Based Orthopaedic Trauma Working Group: Treatment of acute midshaft clavicle fractures: Systematic review of 2144 fractures. *J Orthop Trauma* 2005; 19(7):504-507.
5. Canadian Orthopaedic Trauma Society: Nonoperative treatment compared with plate fixation of displaced midshaft clavicular fractures: A multicenter, randomized clinical trial. *J Bone Joint Surg Am* 2007;89(1):1-10.
6. Adams F: *The Genuine Works of Hippocrates*. New York, NY, William Wood, 1886.
7. Rowe CR: An atlas of anatomy and treatment of midclavicular fractures. *Clin Orthop Relat Res* 1968;58:29-42.
8. Neer CS II: Nonunion of the clavicle. *J Am Med Assoc* 1960; 172:1006-1011.
9. Khan LA, Bradnock TJ, Scott C, Robinson CM: Fractures of the clavicle. *J Bone Joint Surg Am* 2009;91(2):447-460.
10. Postacchini F, Gumina S, De Santis P, Albo F: Epidemiology of clavicle fractures. *J Shoulder Elbow Surg* 2002;11(5):452-456.
11. Nordqvist A, Petersson C: The incidence of fractures of the clavicle. *Clin Orthop Relat Res* 1994; 300:127-132.
12. Robinson CM: Fractures of the clavicle in the adult: Epidemiol-

ogy and classification. *J Bone Joint Surg Br* 1998;80(3):476-484.

13. Nowak J, Mallmin H, Larsson S: The aetiology and epidemiology of clavicular fractures: A prospective study during a two-year period in Uppsala, Sweden. *Injury* 2000;31(5):353-358.
14. Allman FL Jr: Fractures and ligamentous injuries of the clavicle and its articulation. *J Bone Joint Surg Am* 1967;49(4):774-784.
15. Marsh JL, Slongo TF, Agel J, et al: Fracture and dislocation classification compendium 2007: Orthopaedic Trauma Association classification, database and outcomes committee. *J Orthop Trauma* 2007;21(10, Suppl): S1-S133.
16. Lester CW: The treatment of fractures of the clavicle. *Ann Surg* 1929;89(4):600-606.
17. Andersen K, Jensen PO, Lauritzen J: Treatment of clavicular fractures: Figure-of-eight bandage versus a simple sling. *Acta Orthop Scand* 1987;58(1):71-74.
18. Hoofwijk AG, van der Werken C: Conservative treatment of clavicular fractures. *Z Unfallchir Versicherungsmed Berufskr* 1988; 81(3):151-156.
19. Cheung A, Van Rensburg L, Tytherleigh-Strong GM: Surgical versus conservative interventions for treating fractures of the middle third of the clavicle. *Cochrane Database Syst Rev* 2008;3: CD007314.
20. Lubbert PH, van der Rijt RH, Hoorntje LE, van der Werken C: Low-intensity pulsed ultrasound (LIPUS) in fresh clavicle fractures: A multi-centre double blind randomised controlled trial. *Injury* 2008;39(12):1444-1452.
21. Wick M, Müller EJ, Kollig E, Muhr G: Midshaft fractures of the clavicle with a shortening of more than 2 cm predispose to nonunion. *Arch Orthop Trauma Surg* 2001;121(4):207-211.
22. Oroko PK, Buchan M, Winkler A, Kelly IG: Does shortening matter after clavicular fractures? *Bull Hosp Jt Dis* 1999;58(1):6-8.
23. Nowak J, Holgersson M, Larsson S: Can we predict long-term sequelae after fractures of the clavicle based on initial findings? A prospective study with nine to ten years of follow-up. *J Shoulder Elbow Surg* 2004;13(5):479-486.
24. Davies D, Longworth A, Amirfeyz R, Fox R, Bannister G: The functional outcome of the fractured clavicle. *Arch Orthop Trauma Surg* 2009;129(11): 1557-1564.
25. McKee MD, Pedersen EM, Jones C, et al: Deficits following nonoperative treatment of displaced midshaft clavicular fractures. *J Bone Joint Surg Am* 2006; 88(1):35-40.
26. Lenza M, Belloti JC, Gomes Dos Santos JB, Matsumoto MH, Faloppa F: Surgical interventions for treating acute fractures or nonunion of the middle third of the clavicle. *Cochrane Database Syst Rev* 2009;4:CD007428.
27. Coupe BD, Wimhurst JA, Indar R, Calder DA, Patel AD: A new approach for plate fixation of midshaft clavicular fractures. *Injury* 2005;36(10):1166-1171.
28. Iannotti MR, Crosby LA, Stafford P, Grayson G, Goulet R: Effects of plate location and selection on the stability of midshaft clavicle osteotomies: A biomechanical study. *J Shoulder Elbow Surg* 2002;11(5):457-462.
29. Collinge C, Devinney S, Herscovici D, DiPasquale T, Sanders R: Anterior-inferior plate fixation of middle-third fractures and nonunions of the clavicle. *J Orthop Trauma* 2006;20(10): 680-686.
30. Kloen P, Sorkin AT, Rubel IF, Helfet DL: Anteroinferior plating of midshaft clavicular nonunions. *J Orthop Trauma* 2002;16(6): 425-430.
31. Böstman O, Manninen M, Pihlajamäki H: Complications of plate fixation in fresh displaced midclavicular fractures. *J Trauma* 1997;43(5):778-783.
32. Pai HT, Lee YS, Cheng CY: Surgical treatment of midclavicular fractures in the elderly: A comparison of locking and nonlocking plates. *Orthopedics* 2009;32(4):ii.
33. Neer CS: Fractures of the clavicle, in Rockwood CA, Green DP, eds: *Fractures in Adults,* ed 2. Philadelphia, PA, JB Lippincott Company, 1981, pp 707-713.
34. Ngarmukos C, Parkpian V, Patradul A: Fixation of fractures of the midshaft of the clavicle with Kirschner wires: Results in 108 patients. *J Bone Joint Surg Br* 1998;80(1):106-108.
35. Poigenfürst J, Rappold G, Fischer W: Plating of fresh clavicular fractures: Results of 122 operations. *Injury* 1992;23(4):237-241.
36. Grassi FA, Tajana MS, D'Angelo F: Management of midclavicular fractures: Comparison between nonoperative treatment and open intramedullary fixation in 80 patients. *J Trauma* 2001;50(6): 1096-1100.
37. Jubel A, Andemahr J, Bergmann H, Prokop A, Rehm KE: Elastic stable intramedullary nailing of midclavicular fractures in athletes. *Br J Sports Med* 2003; 37(6):480-484.
38. Basamania CJ: Claviculoplasty. *J Shoulder Elbow Surg* 1999; 8(5):540.
39. Strauss EJ, Egol KA, France MA, Koval KJ, Zuckerman JD: Complications of intramedullary Hagie pin fixation for acute midshaft clavicle fractures. *J Shoulder Elbow Surg* 2007;16(3):280-284.
40. Golish SR, Oliviero JA, Francke EI, Miller MD: A biomechanical study of plate versus intramedullary devices for midshaft clavicle fixation. *J Orthop Surg Res* 2008;3:28.

41. Leppilahti J, Jalovaara P: Migration of Kirschner wires following fixation of the clavicle: A report of 2 cases. *Acta Orthop Scand* 1999; 70(5):517-519.

42. Frigg A, Rillmann P, Perren T, Gerber M, Ryf C: Intramedullary nailing of clavicular midshaft fractures with the titanium elastic nail: Problems and complications. *Am J Sports Med* 2009;37(2): 352-359.

43. Bosch U, Skutek M, Peters G, Tscherne H: Extension osteotomy in malunited clavicular fractures. *J Shoulder Elbow Surg* 1998;7(4): 402-405.

44. Chan KY, Jupiter JB, Leffert RD, Marti R: Clavicle malunion. *J Shoulder Elbow Surg* 1999;8(4): 287-290.

45. Kuhne JE: Symptomatic malunions of the middle clavicle. *J Shoulder Elbow Surg* 1999; 8(5):539.

46. Lazarides S, Zafiropoulos G: Conservative treatment of fractures at the middle third of the clavicle: The relevance of shortening and clinical outcome. *J Shoulder Elbow Surg* 2006;15(2):191-194.

47. Craig EV: Fractures of the shoulder: Part II. Fractures of the clavicle, in Rockwood CA, Green DP, Bucholz RW, eds: *Rockwood and Green's Fractures in Adults*, ed 3. Philadelphia, PA, JB Lippincott Company, 1991, pp 928-990.

48. Nowak J, Holgersson M, Larsson S: Sequelae from clavicular fractures are common: A prospective study of 222 patients. *Acta Orthop* 2005;76(4):496-502.

49. Eskola A, Vainionpää S, Myllynen P, Pätiälä H, Rokkanen P: Outcome of clavicular fracture in 89 patients. *Arch Orthop Trauma Surg* 1986;105(6):337-338.

50. Ledger M, Leeks N, Ackland T, Wang A: Short malunions of the clavicle: An anatomic and functional study. *J Shoulder Elbow Surg* 2005;14(4):349-354.

51. Simpson NS, Jupiter JB: Clavicular nonunion and malunion: Evaluation and surgical management. *J Am Acad Orthop Surg* 1996; 4(1):1-8.

52. Brinker MR, Edwards TB, O'Connor DP: Estimating the risk of nonunion following nonoperative treatment of a clavicular fracture. *J Bone Joint Surg Am* 2005;87(3):676-677.

53. Manske DJ, Szabo RM: The operative treatment of mid-shaft clavicular non-unions. *J Bone Joint Surg Am* 1985;67(9):1367-1371.

54. Wu CC, Shih CH, Chen WJ, Tai CL: Treatment of clavicular aseptic nonunion: Comparison of plating and intramedullary nailing techniques. *J Trauma* 1998;45(3): 512-516.

55. Boehme D, Curtis RJ Jr, DeHaan JT, Kay SP, Young DC, Rockwood CA Jr: Non-union of fractures of the mid-shaft of the clavicle: Treatment with a modified Hagie intramedullary pin and autogenous bone-grafting. *J Bone Joint Surg Am* 1991;73(8): 1219-1226.

56. Zlowodzki M, Bhandari M, Zelle BA, Kregor PJ, Cole PA: Treatment of scapula fractures: Systematic review of 520 fractures in 22 case series. *J Orthop Trauma* 2006;20(3):230-233.

57. Lantry JM, Roberts CS, Giannoudis PV: Operative treatment of scapular fractures: A systematic review. *Injury* 2008;39(3): 271-283.

58. Baldwin KD, Ohman-Strickland P, Mehta S, Hume E: Scapula fractures: A marker for concomitant injury? A retrospective review of data in the National Trauma Database. *J Trauma* 2008;65(2):430-435.

59. Weening B, Walton C, Cole PA, Alanezi K, Hanson BP, Bhandari M: Lower mortality in patients with scapular fractures. *J Trauma* 2005;59(6):1477-1481.

60. Veysi VT, Mittal R, Agarwal S, Dosani A, Giannoudis PV: Multiple trauma and scapula fractures: So what? *J Trauma* 2003;55(6): 1145-1147.

61. Tadros AM, Lunsjo K, Czechowski J, Abu-Zidan FM: Multiple-region scapular fractures had more severe chest injury than single-region fractures: A prospective study of 107 blunt trauma patients. *J Trauma* 2007;63(4): 889-893.

62. Ideberg R, Grevsten S, Larsson S: Epidemiology of scapular fractures: Incidence and classification of 338 fractures. *Acta Orthop Scand* 1995;66(5):395-397.

63. Mayo KA, Benirschke SK, Mast JW: Displaced fractures of the glenoid fossa: Results of open reduction and internal fixation. *Clin Orthop Relat Res* 1998;347: 122-130.

64. Ada JR, Miller ME: Scapular fractures: Analysis of 113 cases. *Clin Orthop Relat Res* 1991;269: 174-180.

65. Armitage BM, Wijdicks CA, Tarkin IS, et al: Mapping of scapular fractures with three-dimensional computed tomography. *J Bone Joint Surg Am* 2009;91(9):2222-2228.

66. McAdams TR, Blevins FT, Martin TP, DeCoster TA: The role of plain films and computed tomography in the evaluation of scapular neck fractures. *J Orthop Trauma* 2002;16(1):7-11.

67. Tadros AM, Lunsjo K, Czechowski J, Corr P, Abu-Zidan FM: Usefulness of different imaging modalities in the assessment of scapular fractures caused by blunt trauma. *Acta Radiol* 2007;48(1): 71-75.

68. Schofer MD, Sehrt AC, Timmesfeld N, Störmer S, Kortmann HR: Fractures of the scapula: Long-term results after conservative treatment. *Arch Orthop Trauma Surg* 2009;129(11):1511-1519.

69. Wilber MC, Evans EB: Fractures of the scapula: An analysis of forty cases and a review of the literature. *J Bone Joint Surg Am* 1977; 59(3):358-362.
70. Hardegger FH, Simpson LA, Weber BG: The operative treatment of scapular fractures. *J Bone Joint Surg Br* 1984;66(5):725-731.
71. McGinnis M, Denton JR: Fractures of the scapula: A retrospective study of 40 fractured scapulae. *J Trauma* 1989;29(11):1488-1493.
72. Bauer G, Fleischmann W, Dussler E: Displaced scapular fractures: Indication and long-term results of open reduction and internal fixation. *Arch Orthop Trauma Surg* 1995;114(4):215-219.
73. Zhou DS, Li LX, Wang LB, Wang BM, Xu SH, Mu WD: Operative treatment of the scapular fractures through modified Judet approach. *Zhonghua Wai Ke Za Zhi* 2006;44(24):1686-1688.
74. Adam FF: Surgical treatment of displaced fractures of the glenoid cavity. *Int Orthop* 2002;26(3): 150-153.
75. Schandelmaier P, Blauth M, Schneider C, Krettek C: Fractures of the glenoid treated by operation: A 5- to 23-year follow-up of 22 cases. *J Bone Joint Surg Br* 2002;84(2):173-177.
76. Kavanagh BF, Bradway JK, Cofield RH: Open reduction and internal fixation of displaced intra-articular fractures of the glenoid fossa. *J Bone Joint Surg Am* 1993;75(4):479-484.
77. Leung KS, Lam TP, Poon KM: Operative treatment of displaced intra-articular glenoid fractures. *Injury* 1993;24(5):324-328.
78. Bozkurt M, Can F, Kirdemir V, Erden Z, Demirkale I, Başbozkurt M: Conservative treatment of scapular neck fracture: The effect of stability and glenopolar angle on clinical outcome. *Injury* 2005; 36(10):1176-1181.
79. Kim KC, Rhee KJ, Shin HD, Yang JY: Can the glenopolar angle be used to predict outcome and treatment of the floating shoulder? *J Trauma* 2008;64(1):174-178.
80. Pace AM, Stuart R, Brownlow H: Outcome of glenoid neck fractures. *J Shoulder Elbow Surg* 2005; 14(6):585-590.
81. Herrera DA, Anavian J, Tarkin IS, Armitage BA, Schroder LK, Cole PA: Delayed operative management of fractures of the scapula. *J Bone Joint Surg Br* 2009; 91(5):619-626.
82. Jones CB, Cornelius JP, Sietsema DL, Ringler JR, Endres TJ: Modified Judet approach and minifragment fixation of scapular body and glenoid neck fractures. *J Orthop Trauma* 2009;23(8): 558-564.
83. Herscovici D Jr: Open reduction and internal fixation of ipsilateral fractures of the scapular neck and clavicle. *J Bone Joint Surg Am* 1994;76(7):1112-1113.
84. Nordqvist A, Petersson C: Fracture of the body, neck, or spine of the scapula: A long-term follow-up study. *Clin Orthop Relat Res* 1992;283:139-144.
85. Leung KS, Lam TP: Open reduction and internal fixation of ipsilateral fractures of the scapular neck and clavicle. *J Bone Joint Surg Am* 1993;75(7):1015-1018.
86. Rikli D, Regazzoni P, Renner N: The unstable shoulder girdle: Early functional treatment utilizing open reduction and internal fixation. *J Orthop Trauma* 1995; 9(2):93-97.
87. Ramos L, Mencía R, Alonso A, Ferrández L: Conservative treatment of ipsilateral fractures of the scapula and clavicle. *J Trauma* 1997;42(2):239-242.
88. Edwards SG, Whittle AP, Wood GW II : Nonoperative treatment of ipsilateral fractures of the scapula and clavicle. *J Bone Joint Surg Am* 2000;82(6): 774-780.
89. Low CK, Lam AW: Results of fixation of clavicle alone in managing floating shoulder. *Singapore Med J* 2000;41(9):452-453.
90. Egol KA, Connor PM, Karunakar MA, Sims SH, Bosse MJ, Kellam JF: The floating shoulder: Clinical and functional results. *J Bone Joint Surg Am* 2001; 83-A(8):1188-1194.
91. Romero J, Schai P, Imhoff AB: Scapular neck fracture: The influence of permanent malalignment of the glenoid neck on clinical outcome. *Arch Orthop Trauma Surg* 2001;121(6):313-316.
92. van Noort A, te Slaa RL, Marti RK, van der Werken C: The floating shoulder: A multicentre study. *J Bone Joint Surg Br* 2001;83(6):795-798.
93. Oh W, Jeon IH, Kyung S, Park C, Kim T, Ihn C: The treatment of double disruption of the superior shoulder suspensory complex. *Int Orthop* 2002;26(3):145-149.
94. Hashiguchi H, Ito H: Clinical outcome of the treatment of floating shoulder by osteosynthesis for clavicular fracture alone. *J Shoulder Elbow Surg* 2003;12(6): 589-591.
95. Labler L, Platz A, Weishaupt D, Trentz O: Clinical and functional results after floating shoulder injuries. *J Trauma* 2004;57(3): 95-602.
96. van Noort A, van Kampen A: Fractures of the scapula surgical neck: Outcome after conservative treatment in 13 cases. *Arch Orthop Trauma Surg* 2005;125(10): 696-700.
97. Khallaf F, Mikami A, Al-Akkad M: The use of surgery in displaced scapular neck fractures. *Med Princ Pract* 2006;15(6): 443-448.
98. Maquieira GJ, Espinosa N, Gerber C, Eid K: Non-operative treatment of large anterior glenoid rim

fractures after traumatic anterior dislocation of the shoulder. *J Bone Joint Surg Br* 2007;89(10):1347-1351.

99. Bauer T, Abadie O, Hardy P: Arthroscopic treatment of glenoid fractures. *Arthroscopy* 2006;22(5): 569e1-569e6.

100. Millett PJ, Braun S: The "bony Bankart bridge" procedure: A new arthroscopic technique for reduction and internal fixation of a bony Bankart lesion. *Arthroscopy* 2009;25(1):102-105.

101. Tauber M, Moursy M, Eppel M, Koller H, Resch H: Arthroscopic screw fixation of large anterior glenoid fractures. *Knee Surg Sports Traumatol Arthrosc* 2008;16(3): 326-332.

102. Sugaya H, Kon Y, Tsuchiya A: Arthroscopic repair of glenoid fractures using suture anchors. *Arthroscopy* 2005;21(5):635.

103. Bestard E, Schvene H, Bestard E: Glenoplasty in the management of recurrent shoulder dislocation. *Contemp Orthop* 1986;12:47-55.

104. Chadwick EK, van Noort A, van der Helm FC: Biomechanical analysis of scapular neck malunion: A simulation study. *Clin Biomech (Bristol, Avon)* 2004; 19(9):906-912.

105. Lambotte A: *Chirurgie Opératoire des Fractures*. Paris, France, Masson, 1913.

106. Bartoníček J, Cronier P: History of the treatment of scapula fractures. *Arch Orthop Trauma Surg* 2009.

107. Judet R: Surgical treatment of scapular fractures. *Acta Orthop Belg* 1964;30:673-678.

108. Obremskey WT, Lyman JR: A modified judet approach to the scapula. *J Orthop Trauma* 2004; 18(10):696-699.

109. Nork SE, Barei DP, Gardner MJ, Schildhauer TA, Mayo KA, Benirschke SK: Surgical exposure and fixation of displaced type IV, V, and VI glenoid fractures. *J Orthop Trauma* 2008;22(7): 487-493.

110. Wirbel R, Pohlemann T, Braun C: A modified judet approach to the scapula. *J Orthop Trauma* 2005;19(5):365.

111. van Noort A, van Loon CJ, Rijnberg WJ: Limited posterior approach for internal fixation of a glenoid fracture. *Arch Orthop Trauma Surg* 2004;124(2): 140-144.

112. Wijdicks CA, Armitage BM, Anavian J, Schroder LK, Cole PA: Vulnerable neurovasculature with a posterior approach to the scapula. *Clin Orthop Relat Res* 2009; 467(8):2011-2017.

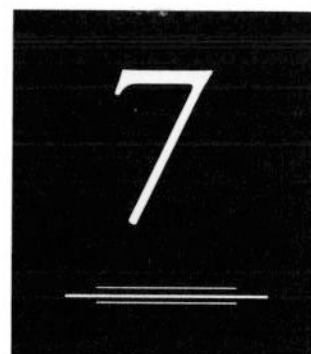

The "Not So Simple" Ankle Fracture: Avoiding Problems and Pitfalls to Improve Patient Outcomes

David J. Hak, MD, MBA
Kenneth A. Egol, MD
Michael J. Gardner, MD
Andrew Haskell, MD

Abstract

Ankle fractures are among the most common injuries managed by orthopaedic surgeons. Many ankle fractures are simple, with straightforward management leading to successful outcomes. Some fractures, however, are challenging, and debate arises regarding the best treatment to achieve an optimal outcome. Some patients have medical comorbidities that increase the risk for complications or may require modifications to standard surgical techniques and fixation methods.

Several recent investigations have highlighted the pitfalls in accurately reducing syndesmotic injuries. Controversy remains regarding the number and diameter of screws, the duration of weight-bearing limitations, and the need or timing of screw removal. Open reduction may allow more accurate reduction than standard closed methods. Direct fixation of associated posterior malleolus fractures may provide improved syndesmotic stability. Posterior malleolus fractures vary in size and can be classified based on the orientation of the fracture line. As the size of the posterior malleolus fracture fragment increases, the load pattern in the ankle is altered. Direct or indirect reduction and surgical fixation may be required to prevent posterior talar subluxation and restore articular congruency.

The supination-adduction fracture pattern is also important to recognize. Articular depression of the medial tibial plafond may require reduction and bone grafting. Optimal fixation requires directing screws parallel to the ankle joint or using a buttress plate.

Identifying ankle fractures that may present additional treatment challenges is essential to achieving a successful outcome. A careful review of radiographs and CT scans, a thorough patient assessment, and detailed preoperative planning are needed to improve patient outcomes.

Instr Course Lect 2011;60:73-88.

Although the nonsurgical or surgical treatment of many ankle fractures is considered to be simple and straightforward, certain ankle fracture patterns and fractures in patients with specific comorbidities can add significant challenges to achieving successful outcomes. It is important to understand potential problems to avoid complications and technical difficulties that may result in a poor outcome.

Ankle Fractures in Diabetic Patients

The public health burden of caring for diabetic patients with ankle fractures is substantial and increasing.[1-3] Diabetic patients are more prone to complications and poor outcomes and have higher rates of in-hospital mortality and longer hospital stays compared with nondiabetic patients.[4,5] Recognizing the higher risk involved, appropriately screening patients, collaborating on care, and tailoring management strategies will achieve the best possible outcomes in this challenging patient population.

Dr. Hak or an immediate family member is a member of a speakers' bureau or has made paid presentations on behalf of Medtronic; serves as a paid consultant to or is an employee of Medtronic; and has received research or institutional support from Synthes and Stryker. Dr. Egol or an immediate family member serves as a board member, owner, officer, or committee member of the Orthopaedic Trauma Association; serves as an unpaid consultant to Exactech; has received research or institutional support from Biomet, Smith & Nephew, Stryker, and Synthes; owns stock or stock options in Johnson & Johnson; and has received nonincome support (such as equipment or services), commercially derived honoraria, or other non–research-related funding (such as paid travel) from Surgix. Dr. Gardner or an immediate family member serves as a paid consultant to or is an employee of Synthes, DGIMed, and Expanding Orthopedics and has received research or institutional support from Axial Biotech, Biomet, Breg, Cerapedics, K2M, Medtronic, Midwest Stone Institute, Smith & Nephew, Stryker, Synthes Spine, Wright Medical Technology, and Wyeth. Dr. Haskell or an immediate family member is a member of a speakers' bureau or has made paid presentations on behalf of Tornier and Smith & Nephew.

The chronic hyperglycemia of diabetes causes disruptions in cellular functions and alters extracellular tissue properties. Diabetes causes poor oxygen delivery to tissues, poor wound healing, susceptibility to infection, and delayed fracture healing.[6,7] It can also lead to peripheral neuropathy and neuropathic arthropathy, a destructive, noninfectious, periarticular process that often has devastating consequences.[8]

Risk Stratification

Risk stratification helps predict the chances of developing complications, guides preoperative risk reduction strategies, and may help focus the decision for surgery. Glycemic control should be addressed because reducing glycated hemoglobin levels by just 1% can reduce complications by 25% to 30%.[9,10] Patients with diabetic comorbidities, such as retinopathy, nephropathy, and neuropathy, have a higher risk of surgical complications.[11,12] In one study, the rate of complications in diabetic patients without comorbidities was identical to that of nondiabetic patients matched by age, sex, fracture type, and treatment.[12] In contrast, the rate of complications in diabetic patients with comorbidities was significantly increased compared with matched nondiabetic patients (47% versus 14%, respectively; $P = 0.034$). The lack of distal pulses, ankle-brachial indices less than 0.9, and transcutaneous oxygen pressure less than 30 mm Hg suggest the need for further vascular studies and possible revascularization before ankle surgery; however, ankle-brachial indices are often spuriously elevated in patients with diabetes. The risk of neuropathic arthropathy is associated with the loss of protective sensation, poor glucose control, the duration of diabetes, and a prior history of neuropathic arthropathy.[11-13] Screening for neuropathy can include testing with a 5.07 (10 g) Semmes-Weinstein monofilament, testing for vibration sensation, or performing nerve conduction velocity studies. Other risk factors include the duration of diabetes, insulin use, smoking, hypertension, dyslipidemia, older age, delayed treatment, and an increased body mass index.

Patient Evaluation

The initial management of an ankle fracture begins with a thorough patient history, with particular attention to medical comorbidities such as peripheral neuropathy, neuropathic arthropathy, nephropathy, retinopathy, and the duration of diabetes. Appropriate consultation for managing comorbidities can help avoid complications.[14] The physical examination should evaluate the skin, the vascular status, and the peripheral neurologic systems and inspect the midfoot or the contralateral foot for signs of neuroarthropathic changes.

Treatment and Outcomes

Fractures and dislocations should be reduced and splinted; joint-spanning external fixation can be applied if soft tissues will not tolerate splinting.

Stable ankle fractures can be treated with casting and a strict non–weight-bearing protocol. These fractures include isolated distal fibular fractures or nondisplaced medial malleolus fractures with no talar displacement or syndesmosis widening. The patient does not bear weight for 6 to 12 weeks, after which protected weight bearing is instituted for 4 to 8 weeks. Healing may take two to three times longer than expected in these patients.[11] Follow-up radiographs should be obtained, with intervention in cases of fracture displacement. In a study by Schon and Marks,[15] 15 nondisplaced ankle fractures in patients with diabetes and neuropathy healed with non–weight-bearing casting for 3 to 9 months.

Unstable ankle fractures in patients without diabetes-associated comorbidities can be treated in the same manner as ankle fractures in nondiabetic patients.[12] When comorbidities are present, open reduction and internal fixation is indicated for unstable fractures if vascular status and soft tissues allow and there is no ongoing neuroarthropathic joint destruction. Unstable fractures include displaced medial malleolus fractures, fibula fractures with talar displacement, bimalleolar or trimalleolar fractures, posterior malleolus fractures, and fractures with syndesmosis widening. Surgery may be delayed for 1 to 3 weeks to optimize the patient's medical management and allow soft-tissue swelling to subside, fracture blisters to resolve, and wrinkles to return to the skin.

The principles of reduction and fixation of ankle fractures in diabetic patients follow those used in nondiabetic patients; however, more rigid fixation should be used. A variety of techniques, including locked plating, fibula into tibia (syndesmosis) screws, supplementary intramedullary Kirschner wires, and posterolateral antiglide fibula plating allow more rigid fixation.[15-19] Extraperiosteal contoured medial, lateral, and posterior plates help limit iatrogenic soft-tissue injury.[20] Internal fixation can be augmented or replaced by joint-spanning external fixation if the condition of the soft tissues will not allow open surgery (**Figure 1**). Even a simple transcalcaneal pin can provide stability.[21] Postoperative care should include longer immobilization and prolonged weight-bearing restrictions. A good rule in treating diabetic patients is to increase the degree of immobilization (cast rather than removable boot), increase the degree of protected weight bearing (not bearing weight rather than par-

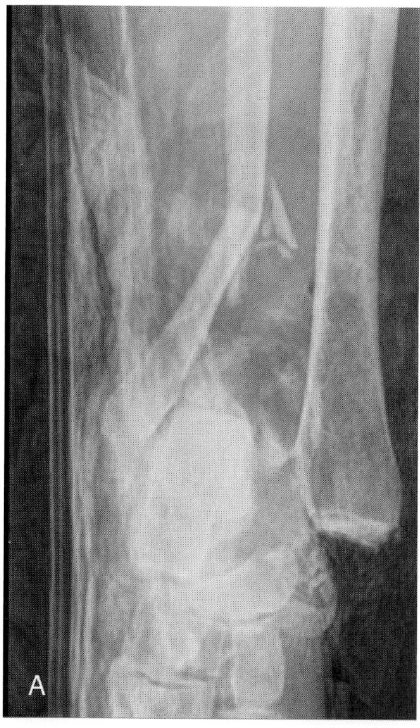

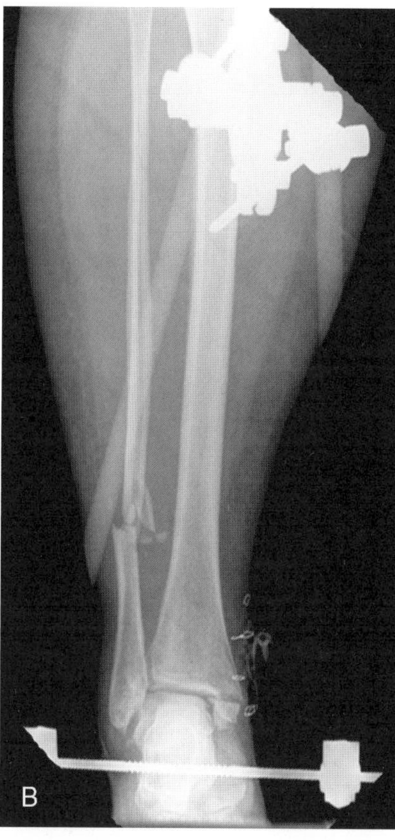

Figure 1 **A,** AP radiograph of an open ankle fracture in a diabetic patient. The condition of the soft tissue would not safely allow open reduction and internal fixation. **B,** AP radiograph after débridement, fracture reduction, and stabilization with joint-spanning external fixation, which was used for definitive treatment along with a posterior splint.

tially or fully bearing weight), and at least double the duration of the limited weight-bearing period. Long-term bracing can be considered, especially when a fibrous union develops. Adjuvant treatments, including ultrasound, platelet-rich plasma, and internal electrical stimulation may speed bone healing.[22-24]

Unfortunately, there are no prospective or randomized trials to guide surgical decision making for unstable ankle fractures in diabetic patients. The surgical treatment of unstable ankle fractures in diabetic patients with comorbidities has a high complication rate, but closed treatment also results in frequent complications. In one small case series of neuropathic patients with unstable ankle fractures treated with casting, neuroarthropathy developed in 40% of the patients, and nonunion or malunion was reported in 100% of the patients.[8,15] Closed treatment may avoid some complications of surgical treatment, including wound complications, infection, and amputation.[25]

The results of surgical fixation of unstable ankle fractures in diabetic patients are limited to case series and case-controlled studies of patients with diabetes of varying severities and mixed fracture types. Overall complication rates in diabetic patients ranged from 14% to 44%.[15,26] Complications include poor wound healing, infection, malunion, loss of reduction, delayed union or nonunion, neuropathic arthropathy, noncompliance-related problems, and the need for further surgery or amputation (**Figure 2**). Risk factors for infection include peripheral vascular disease, neuropathy, and poor glucose control. In a study by Flynn et al,[27] infections in patients with surgically treated ankle fractures were reported in 4 of 19 diabetic patients (21%) compared with 6 of 68 nondiabetic patients (9%). Open ankle fractures in diabetic patients are particularly devastating, with infection in 67% of patients, wound complications in 64%, and below-knee amputation in 36% reported in a 2003 study.[28]

If neuroarthropathic changes are present, internal fixation may not be beneficial, and salvage procedures may be required. Conservative care begins with serial total contact casts. This care is followed by long-term bracing for a well-aligned ankle and foot or fusion for an unbraceable deformity. Amputation is a reasonable treatment option for patients with nonreconstructible deformities, failed reconstructions, or deep infection.

Revision surgery should be considered for delayed fixation failure, syndesmosis widening, and instability or when additional fractures are discovered early and are not associated with neuroarthropathic joint destruction (**Figure 3**).

Understanding the additional risks of caring for diabetic patients with ankle fractures will reinforce the need for stratifying risks, treating medical comorbidities, and appropriately selecting patients for surgical treatment. Careful technique and a more conservative postoperative course will help to maximize the probability for a successful outcome.

Ankle Fractures in Elderly Patients With Severe Osteoporosis

The demographic predictors of ankle fractures in elderly patients include fe-

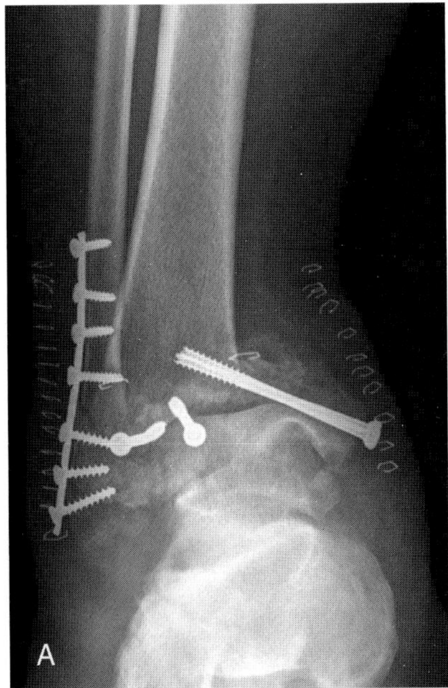

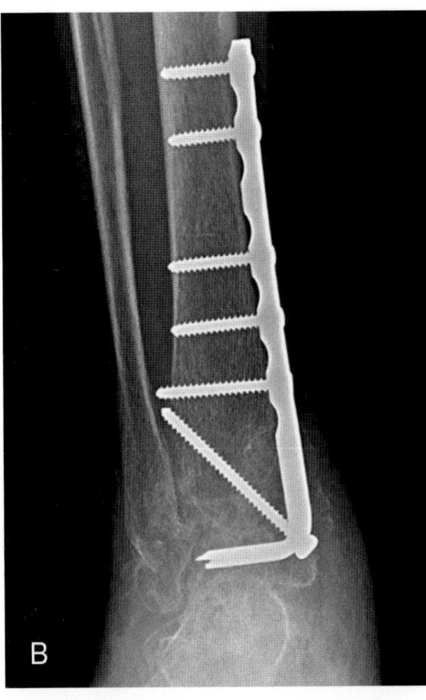

Figure 2 **A,** AP radiograph of the ankle of a diabetic patient treated with open reduction and internal fixation. Neuropathic arthropathy subsequently developed. **B,** AP radiograph after ankle fusion with a medial blade plate.

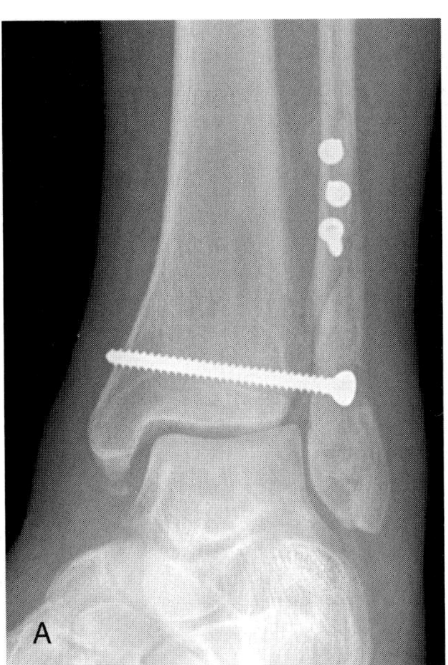

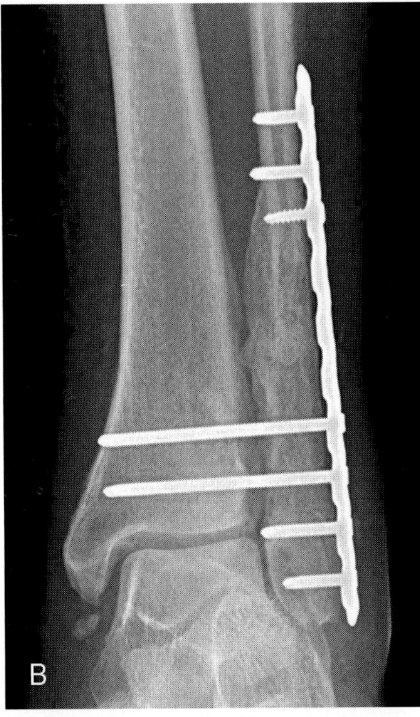

Figure 3 **A,** AP radiograph showing interfragmentary fibular fixation with early syndesmosis screw failure in a patient with diabetic neuropathy. **B,** AP radiograph after revision surgery with locked fibular plating and fibula into tibia screws to stabilize the syndesmosis and augment fibular fixation. Satisfactory healing occurred.

male sex, obesity, and diabetes.[29,30] The frequency of fractures observed in postmenopausal women has led several investigators to classify ankle fractures as osteoporotic fragility fractures.[30,31] However, clinical studies suggest that the incidence of ankle fractures increases until age 65 years and then the occurrence either plateaus or declines; this finding contradicts the association between fracture risk and bone strength.[32-36]

In a study comparing 103 women (age 50 to 80 years) with ankle fractures with 375 women of a similar age without ankle fractures, Greenfield and Eastell[30] used dual-energy x-ray absorptiometry scanning and quantitative ultrasound to evaluate the presence of osteoporosis and its relationship to ankle fracture risk. The authors reported no significant difference in bone mineral density in the patient cohorts, except in the trochanteric region where the patients with ankle fractures had a higher bone density than the population-based group. Based on these findings, the authors concluded that an ankle fracture is not a typical osteoporotic fracture, and patients with an ankle fracture are not at an increased risk for fragility fractures. Because the patients with ankle fractures were significantly heavier with a higher body mass index than the population-based cohort, the authors believe that increased body weight increases the forces applied to the ankle during a fall and therefore contributes to the development of ankle fractures.

Treatment Options and Techniques

The goal of managing ankle fractures in elderly patients centers on providing a functionally stable ankle joint, which will allow patients to return to their preinjury functional levels. Currently, there is a lack of consensus within the orthopaedic community regarding the appropriate surgical indications for this patient population. Treatment goals have been reevaluated because of the growing number of older adults who are more physically active and have greater expectations for functional recovery.

In recent clinical investigations to evaluate the efficacy of surgical versus nonsurgical treatment of ankle fractures in elderly patients, results have varied. In general, the clinical results of the surgical treatment of ankle fractures in elderly patients have been favorable, with higher American Orthopaedic Foot and Ankle Society scores. The major problem with surgical treatment has been the need for reoperation. The results of nonsurgical treatment have been less favorable, with higher rates of nonunion.[37,38] Davidovitch et al[39] reported a steady improvement in functional recovery during the first postoperative year in elderly patients surgically treated for an ankle fracture; however, the rate of improvement was slower than that seen in a younger patient cohort. Based on these findings, the authors concluded that surgical fixation of unstable ankle fractures in elderly patients provides a reasonable postoperative functional result.

Because it can be challenging to surgically manage ankle fractures in osteoporotic bone, modifications of the standard surgical treatments have been advocated.[40] Koval et al[18] reported on the surgical treatment of 20 patients older than 50 years with comminuted or osteopenic ankle fractures. Two intramedullary Kirschner wires were used to augment fracture fixation with a contoured lateral plate (**Figure 4**). All the fractures healed without loss of reduction, with approximately 90% of the patients reporting either no pain or mild pain. Biomechanical evaluation of Kirschner wire augmented fibular fixation showed 81% greater resistance to bending and twice the resistance to torsional loading compared with lateral fibular plate fixation alone.

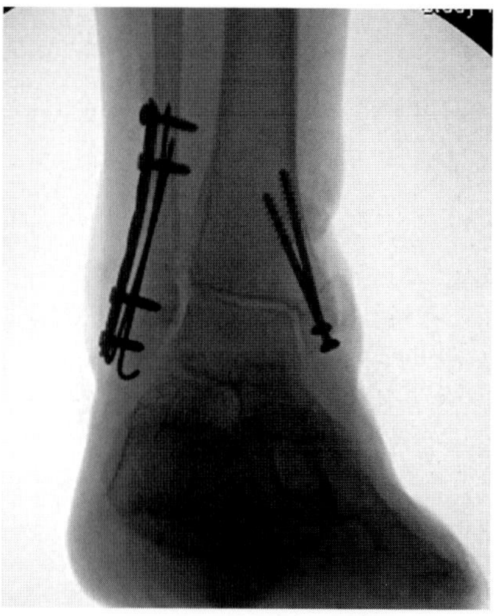

Figure 4 Lateral radiograph showing adjunctive intramedullary Kirschner wires placed anterior and posterior to the fibular plate screws to improve fixation stability in a severely osteoporotic patient with an ankle fracture. Kirschner wires also have been used for the tension band fixation of the medial malleolus. Heavy radiolucent suture has been used instead of cerclage wire.

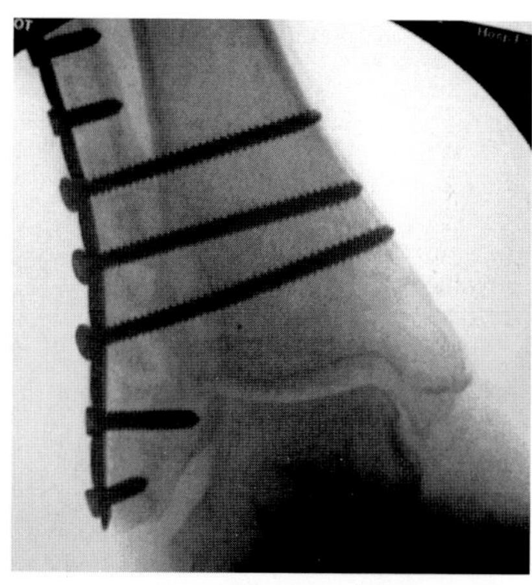

Figure 5 Lateral radiograph showing quadricortical screw fixation into the tibia. Improved fixation can be achieved with tricortical or quadricortical screw fixation into the tibia, even in the absence of syndesmotic injury.

Intramedullary fibular fracture stabilization can be accomplished through a small incision without a significant amount of soft-tissue stripping. In a review of 11 Weber type B ankle fractures in elderly osteoporotic patients treated with fibular nailing, Ramasamy and Sherry[41] reported no wound complications and good to excellent results in 88% of patients.

Modifications of traditional plate and screw constructs have been advocated for these fractures as a method of addressing fixation concerns in osteoporotic bone. Using multiple syndesmosis screws or tricortical and quadricortical fixation of fibula fractures have been described to improve fixation in osteoporotic ankle fractures (**Figure 5**). Using multiple plates on the fibula is another strategy that may allow capture of multifragmented fracture patterns. Locked plating systems improve fixation in osteoporotic bone and can be useful in treating elderly patients with ankle fractures. The advantages of locked plates include better resistance to bending and torsional forces associated with the toggling and pullout of conventional screws and the preservation of the periosteal blood supply because the plate is not firmly compressed against the cortex.[42]

Screw purchase in osteoporotic bone may be improved with cement augmentation. Calcium phosphate cement augmentation has been used successfully in the management of hip and calcaneus fractures in patients with poor bone quality. Recent animal studies have shown that calcium phosphate cement augmentation of orthopaedic hardware significantly increases the screw pullout strength and the load required for failure.[43,44] By improving fixation strength and stability, the addition of cement augmentation may allow a more rapid return to weight bearing and improve the overall outcome after surgical repair.

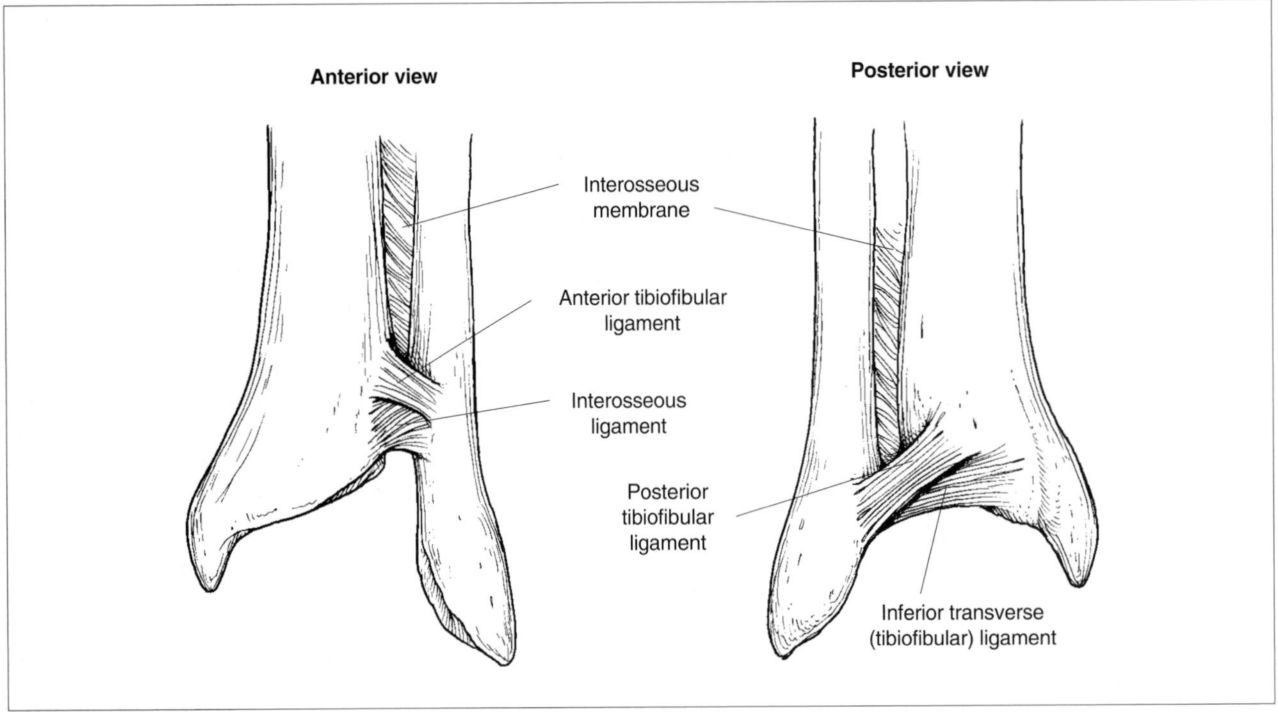

Figure 6 Illustrations showing the ligaments of the distal syndesmosis. (Adapted from Wuest TK: Injuries to the distal lower extremity syndesmosis. *J Am Acad Orthop Surg* 1997;5:172-181.)

When formal open surgery is precluded (such as in patients with severe soft-tissue compromise, poor vascularity, or brittle diabetes), external fixation, with or without limited internal fixation, is an option for maintaining reduction in an unstable ankle mortise. The frame will hold the joint reduced until internal fixation is possible; in certain patients, the frame may be used definitively until healing is complete, with or without the addition of percutaneously placed screws.

Complications

Complications following the surgical treatment of ankle fractures in elderly patients can be devastating and significantly impact treatment outcomes. Common complications include painful prominent hardware, wound healing problems, infection, and malunion. Diabetes mellitus, discussed previously, is one of the most common comorbidities in elderly patients. Medical comorbidities play an important role in both the incidence and type of postoperative complications in elderly patients with ankle fractures.

Ankle Syndesmosis

Anatomy

The ankle syndesmosis is the ligamentous complex that stabilizes the distal articulation between the fibula and tibia. The medial aspect of the distal fibula normally resides within the concave posteromedial fibular notch of the distal tibia (incisura fibularis tibiae). Because of the minimal bony stability inherent in the tibial incisura, ligamentous integrity is necessary for syndesmotic stability. The four main ligaments that contribute to the syndesmotic complex are the anterior inferior tibiofibular ligament, the posterior inferior tibiofibular ligament, the transverse ligament, and the interosseous ligament (**Figure 6**). The anterior inferior tibiofibular ligament is situated obliquely between the anterolateral tibial (Chaput) tubercle and the anteromedial distal fibula. The posterior inferior tibiofibular ligament joins the posterolateral tibial (Volkmann) tubercle and the posteromedial distal fibula. The transverse ligament represents a deep, thickened zone of the most distal portion of the posterior inferior tibiofibular ligament and functions like a labrum, deepening and stabilizing the tibiotalar joint. The posterior inferior tibiofibular ligament and associated transverse ligament provide nearly 50% of the overall syndesmotic strength.[45] The interosseous ligament is the distal aspect of the tibiofibular interosseous membrane and joins the tibia to the fibula several centimeters above the articular surface. The syndesmosis is normally a mobile articulation, allowing slight motion in the coronal, sagittal, and rotational axes.[46] Injury to the syndesmosis alters the normal relationship and motion between the fibula and the tibia and between the tibia and the talus.

Avoiding Pitfalls

Diagnosis

Ankle fractures are frequently accompanied by injury to one or more of the syndesmotic ligaments. The severity of syndesmotic injury can result in varying degrees of instability. The ultimate goal of ankle injury treatment is to maintain the normal relationships between the ankle mortise and the syndesmosis until healing. This requires accurate diagnosis of syndesmotic injuries and appropriate treatment.

The main potential pitfall in treating syndesmotic injuries involves the diagnosis. The Lauge-Hansen classification system was devised to provide mechanistic insight of ligamentous injuries based on the fracture patterns; however, this classification does not accurately correlate the mechanism of injury with the soft-tissue injury pattern.[47,48] In 1989, Boden et al[49] recommended that syndesmotic fixation was required only when rigid medial fixation was not possible and the fibular fracture was greater than 3 to 4.5 mm proximal to its tip. Since that report, it has become clear that rigid medial and lateral malleoli fixation is not sufficient to stabilize the syndesmosis in an unstable injury. The first flawed assumption is that rigid medial malleolar fixation obviates medial instability. In fact, up to 25% of medial malleolus fractures, particularly of the anterior colliculus, may have a concomitant deep deltoid injury.[50] MRI data have demonstrated that the level of the fibular fracture is not an accurate indicator of the level of the syndesmotic injury.[51] Clinical evidence has corroborated the high incidence of syndesmotic injuries in Weber type B injuries, which would not be predicted by the Boden criteria or the Lauge-Hansen or Weber fracture classification systems.[52]

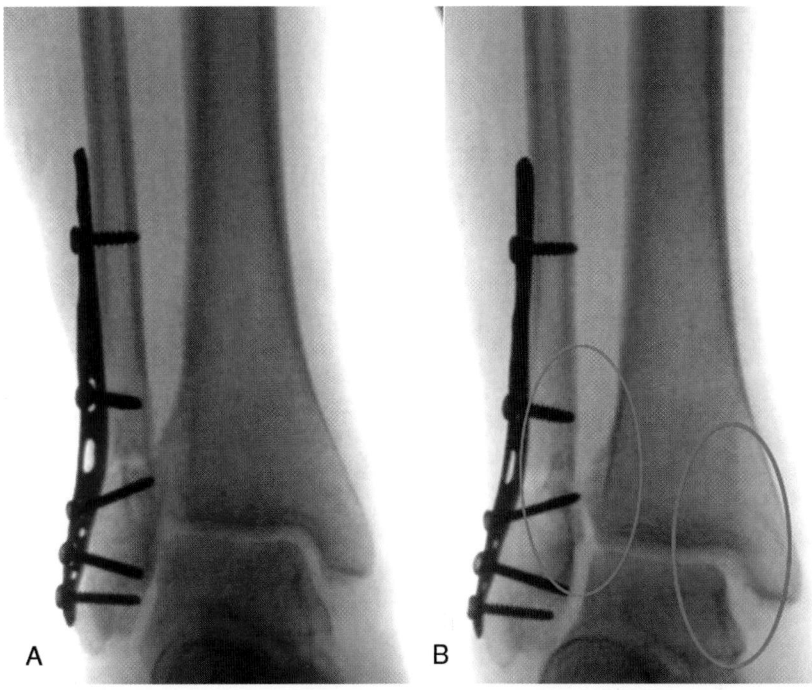

Figure 7 **A,** Radiograph showing fixation of a Weber type B lateral malleolus fracture. **B,** Gentle external rotation stress led to widening of the syndesmotic space, with loss of radiographic tibiofibular overlap and medial clear-space widening (area in red ovals).

Traditional radiographic measurement criteria for syndesmotic injuries include the tibiofibular clear space and tibiofibular overlap, with specific thresholds for both the AP and mortise views. Unfortunately, these static radiographic measurements have a poor correlation with syndesmotic injury.[53] Dynamic stress testing is necessary for the diagnosis of a syndesmotic injury; however, because the syndesmosis cannot be adequately stressed until the fibula is stabilized, dynamic stress testing cannot be performed preoperatively. Given the high incidence of ankle fractures with concomitant syndesmotic injuries and the difficulty in making a preoperative diagnosis, every surgically treated ankle fracture should undergo intraoperative dynamic stress testing after malleolar fixation. This testing can be done with the Cotton test (lateral fibular translation), the external rotation stress test, and the sagittal plane stress test or by placing a Hohmann retractor directly in the syndesmotic space (**Figure** 7).

Malreduction

Once the appropriate diagnosis has been made, it is necessary to avoid syndesmotic malreduction. Based on CT data, the rate of malreduction with the use of standard techniques is higher than previously recognized.[54] Achieving anatomic syndesmotic reduction is critical for optimizing a patient's outcome. Syndesmotic malreduction is a significant predictor of a poor functional outcome.[55] Many factors can lead to syndesmotic malreduction. Fibular malreduction may be the main source of malreduction. Substantial anatomic variability of the tibial incisura predisposes some patients to malreduction, particularly those with flatter articulations compared with those with more concave articulations (**Fig-**

ure 8). In these patients, the vector of the clamp or other reduction instrument is critical for appropriately positioning the fibula within the incisura. The posterolateral Volkmann tibial tubercle, which is involved in fractures of the posterior malleolus, is critical for incisura competence. A large or displaced posterior malleolar fragment that remains malreduced may also lead to syndesmotic malreduction. Because the posterior inferior tibiofibular ligament is universally intact when the posterior malleolus is avulsed, anatomic reduction and stable fixation of the posterior malleolus may achieve reduction and stabilization of the syndesmosis[56] (**Figure 9**).

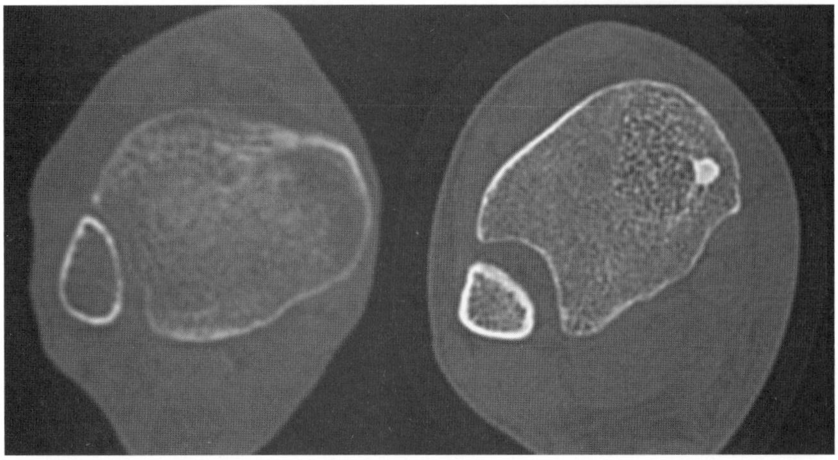

Following reduction, it is critical to use a reliable method to assess the accuracy of the reduction. Assessing reduction on a mortise fluoroscopic view is necessary, but it is insufficient when used alone. A true talar dome lateral view is vital to assess the sagittal position of the fibula; however, because of the high regional anatomic variability, comparison with the contralateral limb is necessary. Open reduction with direct anterior visualization of the syndesmotic articulation may also have a role in assessing reduction, but whether this is necessary when using a true lateral fluoroscopic view and contralateral comparison remains controversial.

Figure 8 Axial CT scans. Patients with flatter incisura anatomy (left) are more prone to syndesmotic malreduction compared with those with more concave incisurae (right).

Fixation

Several implants and configurations are available for syndesmotic fixation. Larger screw diameters (4.5 mm) do not appear to provide a clinically significant mechanical advantage over

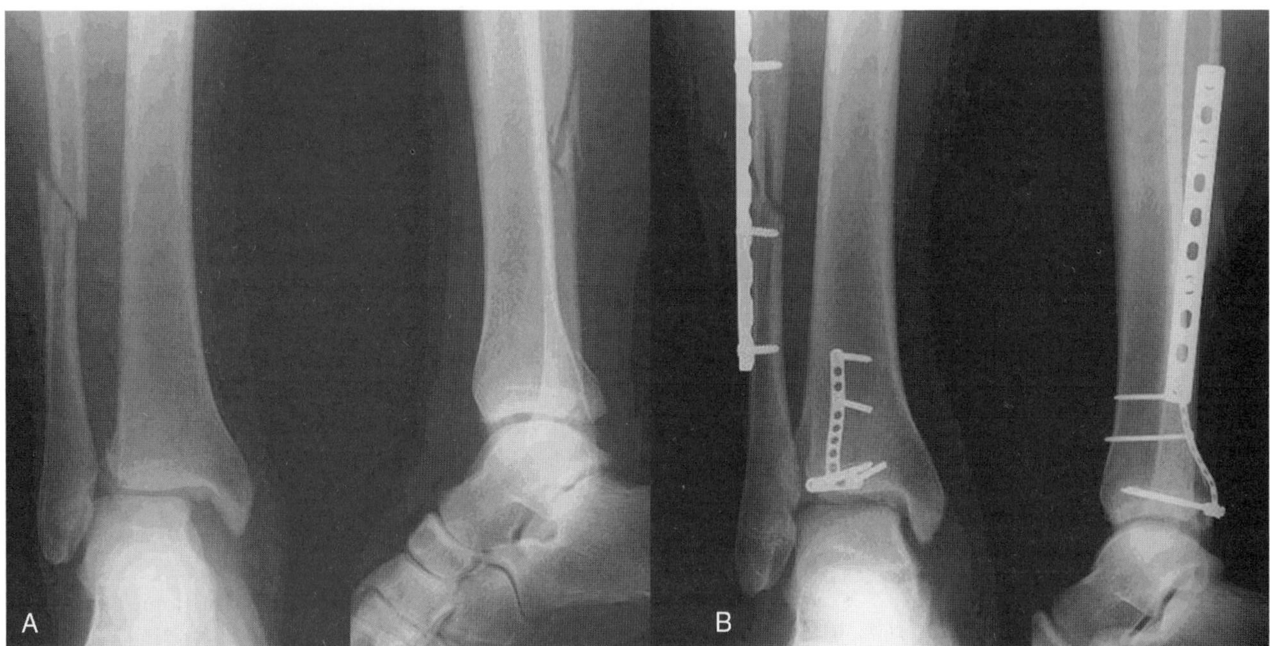

Figure 9 **A,** Preoperative AP (left) and lateral (right) radiographs of a patient with a Weber type C fibula fracture and clear syndesmotic injury. **B,** AP (left) and lateral (right) radiographs after reduction and fixation of the posterior malleolus fracture led to anatomic reduction of the syndesmosis and provided adequate syndesmotic stability so that independent syndesmotic fixation was not required.

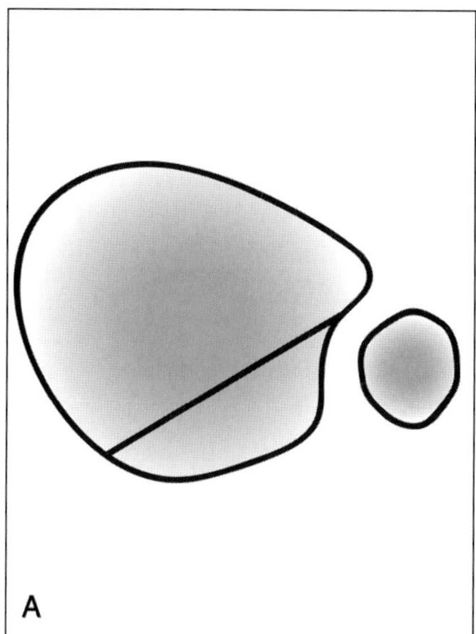

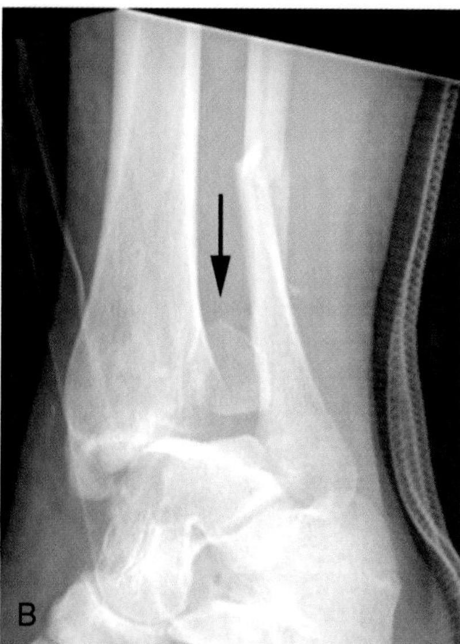

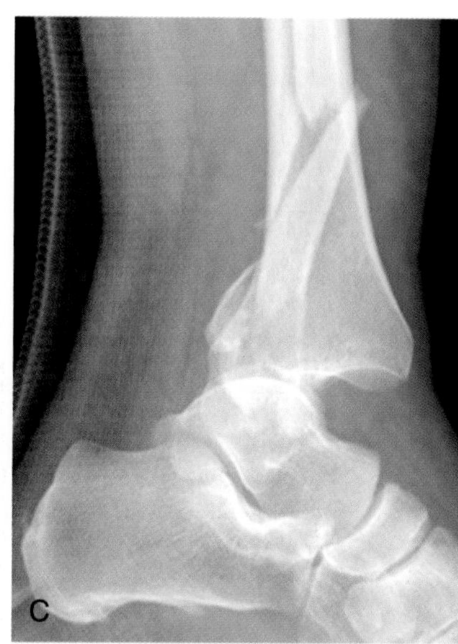

Figure 10 **A,** Cross-sectional diagram of the distal tibia and fibula showing a posterior malleolus fracture with a typical posterolateral fracture pattern. AP (**B**) and lateral (**C**) radiographs of a trimalleolar ankle fracture with a posterolateral fracture pattern. The AP view shows the posterior fragment (arrow), which travels with the fibula by its attachment to the posterior inferior tibiofibular ligament.

small fragment screws, and their heads are often prominent.[57] A prospective, randomized study reported no difference in functional outcomes at 1 year when comparing tricortical with quadricortical fixation.[58] This finding was confirmed by a subsequent randomized study.[59] Early clinical data on suture fixation of syndesmotic injuries are promising, although biomechanical data have implied poor fixation strength compared with screws.[60,61]

Postoperative management of syndesmotic injuries also remains controversial, specifically regarding the time to weight bearing and screw removal. Moore et al[59] reported the outcomes of 120 syndesmotic injuries in which weight bearing was initiated between 6 and 10 weeks and screw removal was not routinely performed. Although screw breakage was common, very few patients were symptomatic. The authors recommended against routine screw removal. A study by Hamid et al[62] analyzed 1 year outcomes of patients with syndesmotic injuries and found no benefit to screw removal.

Posterior Malleolus Fractures

Incidence

Posterior malleolus fractures have been reported in 14% to 44% of all ankle fractures.[63,64] These fractures are differentiated from tibial plafond fractures by their recognizable fracture patterns and sparing of the anterior distal tibial articular surface. Most are associated with other fractures or ligament injuries around the ankle, with less than 1% of posterior malleolar fractures occurring as isolated injuries.[65]

Classification

Posterior malleolus fractures can be classified into three patterns.[66] The most common pattern involves an oblique fracture of the posterolateral corner of the distal tibia[66] (**Figure 10**). The fracture is an avulsion of the tibial insertion of the posterior inferior tibiofibular ligament and typically occurs with a rotational injury. An external rotation lateral radiograph will show the true fracture size and may aid in assessing fracture reduction[67,68] (**Figure 11**). The second common fracture pattern is a large transverse fracture of the posterior distal tibia, often with a separate posteromedial fragment or impaction injury to the articular surface[66,69] (**Figure 12**). This pattern occurs with rotation, an axial load with posterior shear, or hyperplantar flexion. Standard radiographs show the large posterior fragment and often the presence of a double contour or flake fragment above the medial malleolus. Posterior lip fractures are the least common type, appearing as one or multiple shell-like avulsion fragments of the far posterior distal tibial surface.[66] A CT scan may better define the size and orientation of the fracture fragments.

Treatment

Surgical indications for open reduction and internal fixation remain controversial. Criteria based on the fracture characteristics include fragments greater than 25% to 33% of the joint surface area or with greater than 2 mm articular incongruity. Cadaver studies

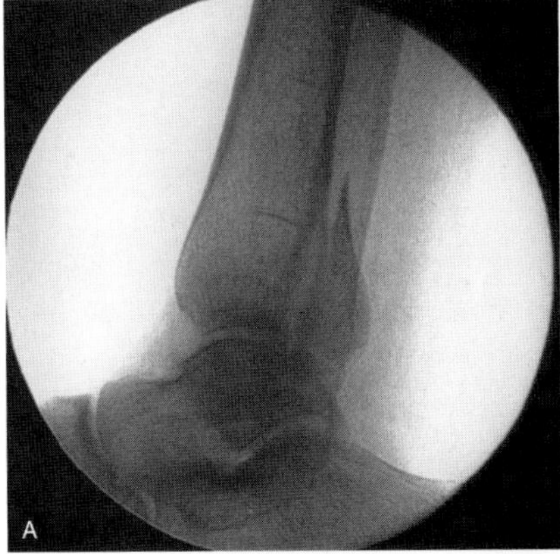

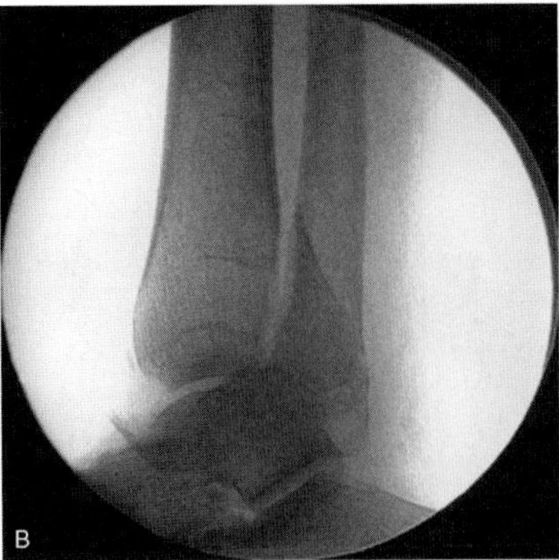

Figure 11 Lateral (**A**) and external rotation lateral (**B**) radiographs of a posterolateral posterior malleolus fracture. The external rotation lateral view shows the true size and position of the posterior malleolar fracture fragment.

have shown increasing alterations in the joint-loading pattern with an increase in the fragment size and degree of articular step-off.[70,71] Clinical studies have reported mixed recommendations regarding the fragment size that requires fixation.[63,72] These studies do not address the fracture pattern or the adequacy of syndesmosis fixation. Fibular or syndesmosis reduction and fixation often reduces and stabilizes the posterior malleolus in posterolateral oblique fractures but not transverse fractures.[73] Conversely, reduction and fixation of a posterolateral fracture restores syndesmosis stability more rigidly than does syndesmosis fixation.[56,74] Residual posterior subluxation of the talus after reduction of the medial and lateral malleoli is an absolute indication for posterior malleolus fixation.[74] A displaced posterior malleolus with posterior talar subluxation should be repaired with corrective osteotomy even after fracture healing.[75]

A variety of surgical approaches, reduction techniques, and fixation methods are available for treating the posterior malleolus. The lateral approach between the fibula and peroneal tendons allows access to the posterolateral fracture fragment but is limiting for larger transverse fractures or when posterior plating is planned. Attention must be given to the superficial peroneal nerve if this approach is extended proximally. A posterolateral approach between the peroneal and Achilles tendons allows better access to the medial aspect of the posterior malleolus and allows more direct access for plating. The sural nerve is at risk with this approach. A medial approach may be made between the posterior tibial and flexor digitorum longus tendons. This approach is well suited for posteromedial fractures or split posterolateral and posteromedial fragments that are not easily accessed with the lateral approaches or when there is posteromedial marginal impaction.[69,76] Experience with medial ankle approaches is helpful because the posterior tibial neurovascular bundle is adjacent to the incision.

Posterior malleolar fragment reduction may be evaluated with palpation, direct visualization, fluoroscopy, or arthroscopy.[77] A periosteal elevator assists with elevating the flexor hallucis longus muscle off the posterior tibia and can help disimpact a fragment that is reluctant to move. A large tenaculum clamp helps reduce and hold the fragment (**Figure 13**). The choice of fixation depends on the size of the fragments, the comminution present, and the stability required. Anterior to posterior or posterior to anterior interfragmentary screw fixation is useful for noncomminuted fragments. Posterior plating may provide additional stability for comminuted or transverse-type fractures. The addition of syndesmosis fixation can help augment stability in posterolateral fractures.

Postoperative Care and Outcomes

Postoperative care depends on fixation stability. Early motion is acceptable for sensate patients with rigid fixation. Although avoiding weight bearing for 4 to 6 weeks is the prudent approach, no loss of reduction was reported in 15 patients with fixation of small posterior malleolus fractures who were allowed to bear weight in a cast within 7 days of surgery.[78]

Reported clinical results of posterior malleolar fractures are limited to case-controlled and case studies; outcomes have been mixed. Large posterior malleolar fractures did better with internal fixation but still had worse 5-year outcomes in a study of 62 fractures matched to similar fractures without posterior malleolar involvement.[63] Large posterior malleolar fractures or those with talar subluxation had fair to poor outcomes in a series of 51 trimalleolar ankle fractures followed for 42 months; however, 44 of the fractures were not internally fixed.[72] In a series of 612 fractures with 1-year follow-up, posterior malleolar fractures of more than one third of the cross-sectional area had worse outcomes than those with small unfixed fragments.[79] In a series of 57 trimalleolar fractures with more than a 4-year follow-up, posterior malleolus fractures with joint incongruity of more than 10% had worse outcomes.[80] Failure to reduce posterior fragments smaller than 25% of the cross-sectional area did not affect results.[72] Other large studies have failed to find a

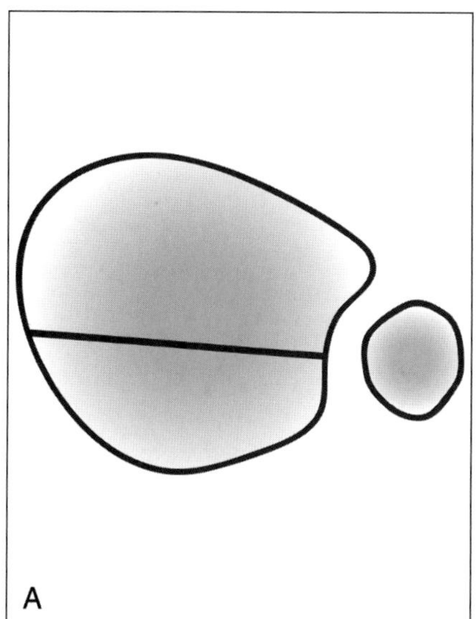

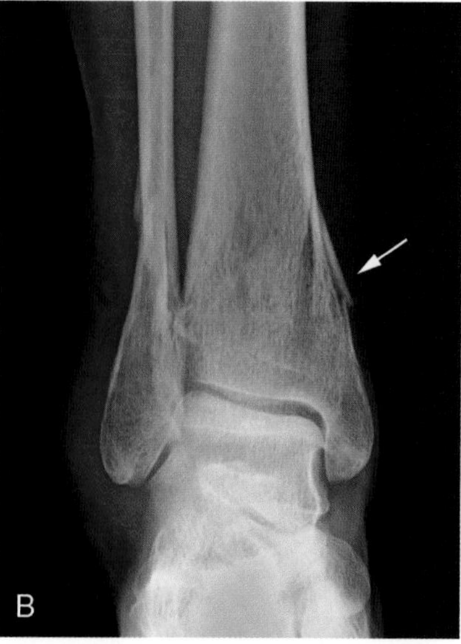

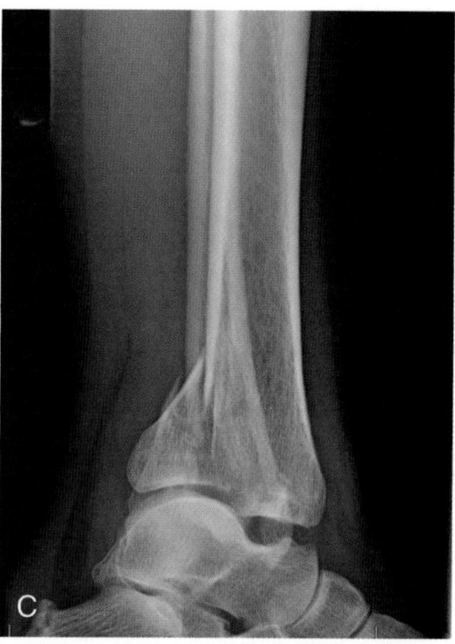

Figure 12 **A,** Cross-sectional diagram of the distal tibia and fibula showing a posterior malleolus fracture with a typical transverse fracture pattern. AP (**B**) and lateral (**C**) radiographs of a trimalleolar ankle fracture with a transverse fracture pattern. Note the medial flake fragment (arrow) on the AP view.

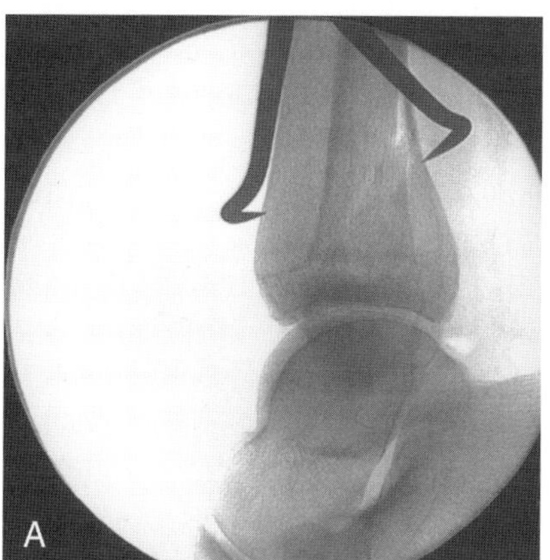

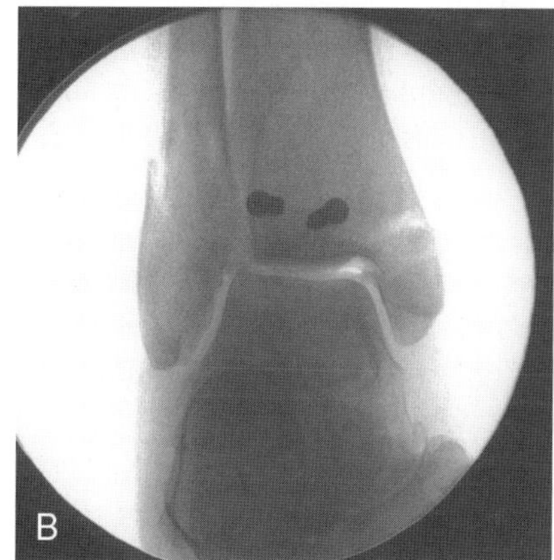

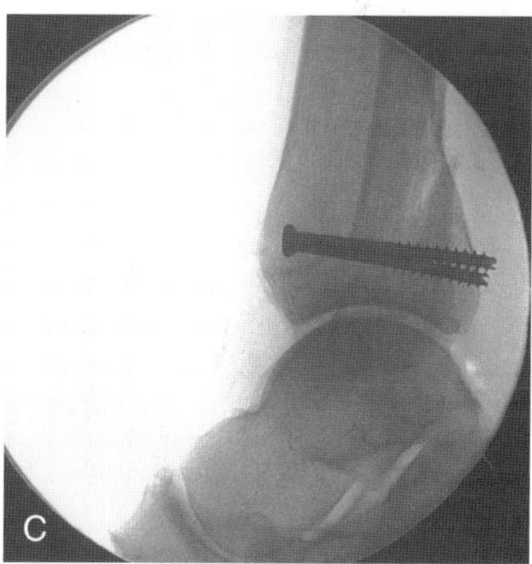

Figure 13 **A,** Intraoperative lateral fluoroscopic image showing reduction of a posterior malleolus fracture with a large tenaculum clamp. Intraoperative AP (**B**) and lateral (**C**) fluoroscopic images showing fixation of a posterior malleolus fracture with two partially threaded cannulated screws placed from anterior to posterior.

relationship between fragment size or fixation of posterior malleolar fractures and outcomes.[81,82]

Posterior malleolus fractures should be treated as part of the overall ankle fracture management to ensure optimal outcomes. Small posterolateral fractures typically reduce and are stable after fibular reduction and fixation. Larger posterolateral fragments, transverse-type fractures, or fragments that do not reduce with fibular reduction should be reduced and fixed. Fixation of the syndesmosis may provide indirect stability to the posterolateral fragment; however, anatomic reduction and internal fixation of the fragment itself is more stable and will typically aid in syndesmosis reduction and stability.

The Supination-Adduction Fracture Pattern

The supination-adduction fracture pattern occurs in 5% to 20% of ankle fractures.[83,84] This type of fracture occurs when a foot in supination undergoes a forceful adduction moment without a rotational component. The first structure injured is either the lateral collateral ligament or the fibula. A fibular fracture created by this mechanism appears on radiographs or intraoperatively as a low transverse fracture line at a level below the syndesmosis. As the severity of the adduction moment increases, the talus displaces toward the medial malleolus, and a vertical fracture line is created extending

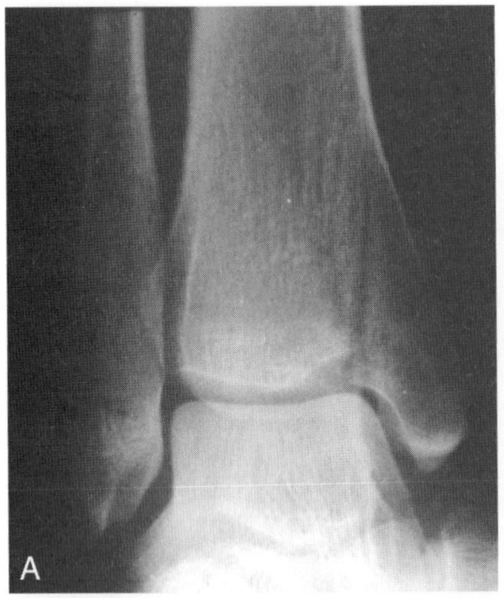

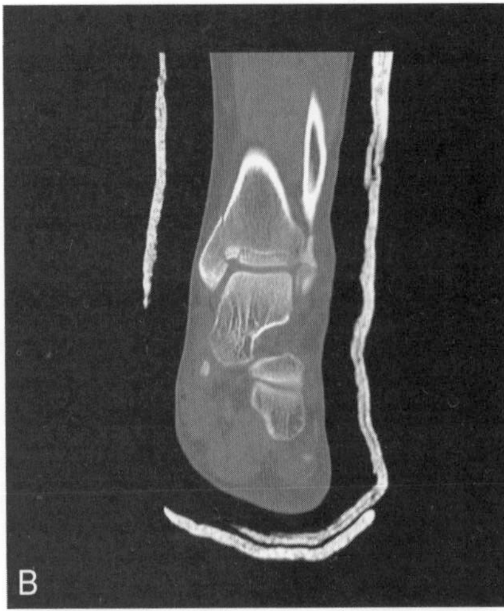

Figure 14 **A,** AP radiographic view of a supination-adduction fracture pattern. Note the vertical fracture line of the medial malleolus and the articular impaction of the tibial surface at the border of the malleolus fracture line. **B,** CT coronal reconstruction scan allows optimal visualization of the degree of articular impaction.

from the medial axilla of the joint and proximally into the metaphyseal cortex of the tibia (**Figure 14**). This fracture mechanism tends to result in a large vertical shear fragment and is rarely associated with comminution at the medial malleolus. Usually the medial tibial plafond will sustain an impaction injury, which is not always easily recognized on plain radiographs, although a CT scan will clearly show this injury (**Figure 14, B**).

It is important to note that the presence of a vertical shear fracture pattern of the medial malleolus is the essential component of this injury pattern and may be the only osseous injury, with the lateral-sided injury being purely ligamentous. It is important for the treating surgeon to have a high index of suspicion for this injury when assessing this fracture pattern. A failure to adequately assess articular impaction will lead to inadequate reduction of the articular surface and may potentially lead to poor results.

Most of these injuries require surgical fixation. The procedure usually begins on the medial side of the ankle. Following exposure, the medial malleolus should be "booked open" to allow visualization of the medial aspect of the talar dome and tibial plafond. Copious irrigation is used to remove fracture hematoma and any loose fragments of bone and cartilage. The periosteum is elevated 1 to 2 mm from the fracture edges to aid in anatomic reduction. The area of articular impaction is disimpacted and may be provisionally stabilized with Kirschner wires placed in an anterior to posterior direction. The void left following disimpaction may require grafting with some type of osteoconductive material. The malleolar fragment is then anatomically reduced. Vertically oriented fractures of the medial malleolus benefit from the use of either a buttress plate or screws inserted parallel to the ankle joint (perpendicular to the fracture line).

The transverse fracture pattern of the fibula is amenable to intramedullary fixation, which can be achieved with several different implants. The benefit of this technique is the relative sparing of the soft-tissue envelope associated with percutaneous placement. Under fluoroscopic control, the tip of the lateral malleolus is identified on the AP and lateral views. This chapter's authors prefer using an intramedullary screw. A small incision is made, and either a guidewire or drill bit is used to enter the distal fibular metaphysis. Once entry is confirmed, the wire is either advanced up the canal across the fracture site, or a partially threaded screw of appropriate length is inserted retrograde to gain purchase on the proximal intramedullary cortex. Formal open reduction with plate and screw fixation is an alternative method (**Figure 15**).

Complications specifically related to this fracture pattern include pain from the hardware and the development of posttraumatic arthrosis. Prominent hardware is common around the medial ankle. When hardware is removed for pain relief about the ankle, the results are somewhat better than for hardware removal at other locations in the body. Jacobsen et al[85] reported on 66 patients who had hardware removal as part of their standard treatment protocol following a malleolar fracture. The authors reported improvement in pain symptoms following hardware removal.

Summary

An increasing percentage of patients presenting with ankle fractures have significant comorbidities that increase the risk of complications and provide technical challenges in achieving stable fixation. Diabetic patients, with the associated comorbidities of retinopathy, nephropathy, and neuropathy, are at especially high risk for complications. The duration of weight-bearing limitations and immobilization should be increased in patients with diabetes, but care must be exercised to monitor insensate patients for potential skin breakdown. If surgical treatment is re-

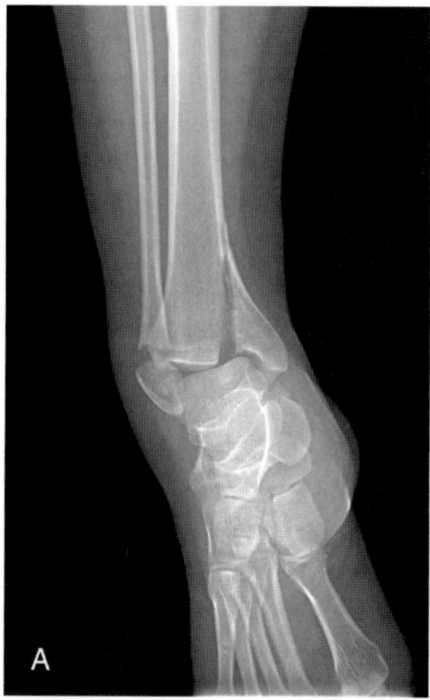

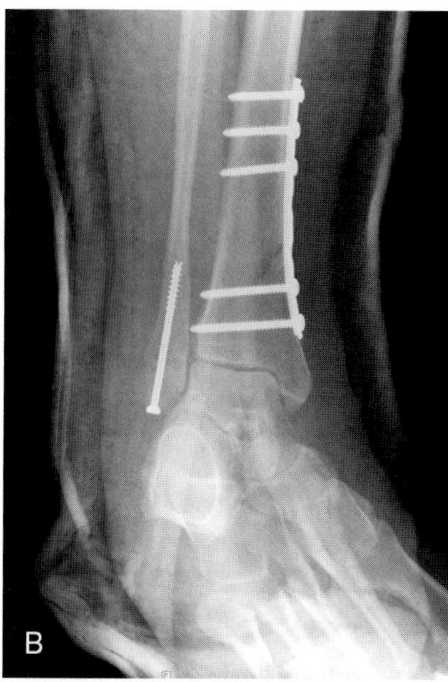

Figure 15 **A,** AP radiograph of a supination-adduction fracture pattern. **B,** Fixation of the vertical shear medial malleolus has been achieved with a one third tubular plate placed as a buttress. Intramedullary screw fixation has been used for the fibula.

quired, more fixation should be used than in nondiabetic patients. Elderly patients with severe osteoporosis also present challenges in achieving stable fixation. Bone clamps should be used judiciously and with caution. Locked plate fixation offers a mechanical advantage in osteoporotic bone. Other techniques include the use of transtibial tricortical or quadricortical screw fixation (even in the absence of syndesmotic injury) and supplementary Kirschner wire fixation.

There are numerous pitfalls in accurately reducing and fixing syndesmotic injuries, especially in patients with a shallow incisura. Direct fixation of an associated posterior malleolus fracture may provide improved syndesmotic stability because the posterior inferior tibiofibular ligament is very strong and usually intact. Open reduction of the syndesmosis may allow more accurate reduction than standard closed methods. Careful intraoperative radiographic assessment is required but still may not identify subtle malreduction, which can be best assessed with CT.

Posterior malleolus fractures vary in size and fracture orientation. Oblique radiographs can be used to estimate the fragment size, but a CT scan can more accurately evaluate the fragment size. Fixation is recommended when the fragment involves more than 25% to 33% of the joint surface and when there is any posterior subluxation of the talus. Although the supination-adduction injury pattern occurs in a minority of ankle fractures, it is important to recognize because of the associated medial tibial articular impaction and the need to alter the standard orientation of the medial malleolar screws.

Identifying ankle fractures that may present additional treatment challenges is essential for achieving a successful outcome. A careful review of radiographs, the addition of CT, a thorough patient assessment, and detailed preoperative planning are needed to improve patient outcomes.

References

1. Kannus P, Palvanen M, Niemi S, Parkkari J, Järvinen M: Increasing number and incidence of low-trauma ankle fractures in elderly people: Finnish statistics during 1970-2000 and projections for the future. *Bone* 2002;31(3): 430-433.
2. Mokdad AH, Ford ES, Bowman BA, et al: Prevalence of obesity, diabetes, and obesity-related health risk factors, 2001. *JAMA* 2003;289(1):76-79.
3. Prisk VR, Wukich DK: Ankle fractures in diabetics. *Foot Ankle Clin* 2006;11(4):849-863.
4. Egol KA, Tejwani NC, Walsh MG, Capla EL, Koval KJ: Predictors of short-term functional outcome following ankle fracture surgery. *J Bone Joint Surg Am* 2006;88(5):974-979.
5. Ganesh SP, Pietrobon R, Cecílio WA, Pan D, Lightdale N, Nunley JA: The impact of diabetes on patient outcomes after ankle fracture. *J Bone Joint Surg Am* 2005;87(8):1712-1718.
6. Loder RT: The influence of diabetes mellitus on the healing of closed fractures. *Clin Orthop Relat Res* 1988;232:210-216.
7. Macey LR, Kana SM, Jingushi S, Terek RM, Borretos J, Bolander ME: Defects of early fracture-healing in experimental diabetes. *J Bone Joint Surg Am* 1989;71(5): 722-733.
8. Connolly JF, Csencsitz TA: Limb threatening neuropathic complications from ankle fractures in patients with diabetes. *Clin Orthop Relat Res* 1998;348:212-219.
9. Goodson WH III, Hung TK: Studies of wound healing in experimental diabetes mellitus. *J Surg Res* 1977;22(3):221-227.
10. Hoogwerf BJ, Sferra J, Donley BG: Diabetes mellitus: Overview. *Foot Ankle Clin* 2006;11(4): 703-715.

11. Bibbo C, Lin SS, Beam HA, Behrens FF: Complications of ankle fractures in diabetic patients. *Orthop Clin North Am* 2001;32(1): 113-133.

12. Jones KB, Maiers-Yelden KA, Marsh JL, Zimmerman MB, Estin M, Saltzman CL: Ankle fractures in patients with diabetes mellitus. *J Bone Joint Surg Br* 2005;87(4):489-495.

13. Olmos PR, Cataland S, O'Dorisio TM, Casey CA, Smead WL, Simon SR: The Semmes-Weinstein monofilament as a potential predictor of foot ulceration in patients with noninsulin-dependent diabetes. *Am J Med Sci* 1995;309(2):76-82.

14. The Diabetes Control and Complications Trial Research Group: The effect of intensive treatment of diabetes on the development and progression of long-term complications in insulin-dependent diabetes mellitus. *N Engl J Med* 1993;329(14): 977-986.

15. Schon LC, Marks RM: The management of neuroarthropathic fracture-dislocations in the diabetic patient. *Orthop Clin North Am* 1995;26(2):375-392.

16. Dunn WR, Easley ME, Parks BG, Trnka HJ, Schon LC: An augmented fixation method for distal fibular fractures in elderly patients: A biomechanical evaluation. *Foot Ankle Int* 2004;25(3): 128-131.

17. Kim T, Ayturk UM, Haskell A, Miclau T, Puttlitz CM: Fixation of osteoporotic distal fibula fractures: A biomechanical comparison of locking versus conventional plates. *J Foot Ankle Surg* 2007; 46(1):2-6.

18. Koval KJ, Petraco DM, Kummer FJ, Bharam S: A new technique for complex fibula fracture fixation in the elderly: A clinical and biomechanical evaluation. *J Orthop Trauma* 1997;11(1): 28-33.

19. Minihane KP, Lee C, Ahn C, Zhang LQ, Merk BR: Comparison of lateral locking plate and antiglide plate for fixation of distal fibular fractures in osteoporotic bone: A biomechanical study. *J Orthop Trauma* 2006;20(8): 562-566.

20. Siegel J, Tornetta P III: Extraperiosteal plating of pronation-abduction ankle fractures. *J Bone Joint Surg Am* 2007;89(2): 276-281.

21. Jani MM, Ricci WM, Borrelli J Jr, Barrett SE, Johnson JE: A protocol for treatment of unstable ankle fractures using transarticular fixation in patients with diabetes mellitus and loss of protective sensibility. *Foot Ankle Int* 2003;24(11): 838-844.

22. Gandhi A, Doumas C, O'Connor JP, Parsons JR, Lin SS: The effects of local platelet rich plasma delivery on diabetic fracture healing. *Bone* 2006;38(4):540-546.

23. Gebauer GP, Lin SS, Beam HA, Vieira P, Parsons JR: Low-intensity pulsed ultrasound increases the fracture callus strength in diabetic BB Wistar rats but does not affect cellular proliferation. *J Orthop Res* 2002;20(3): 587-592.

24. Hockenbury RT, Gruttadauria M, McKinney I: Use of implantable bone growth stimulation in Charcot ankle arthrodesis. *Foot Ankle Int* 2007;28(9):971-976.

25. McCormack RG, Leith JM: Ankle fractures in diabetics: Complications of surgical management. *J Bone Joint Surg Br* 1998;80(4): 689-692.

26. Costigan W, Thordarson DB, Debnath UK: Operative management of ankle fractures in patients with diabetes mellitus. *Foot Ankle Int* 2007;28(1):32-37.

27. Flynn JM, Rodriguez-del Rio F, Pizá PA: Closed ankle fractures in the diabetic patient. *Foot Ankle Int* 2000;21(4):311-319.

28. White CB, Turner NS, Lee GC, Haidukewych GJ: Open ankle fractures in patients with diabetes mellitus. *Clin Orthop Relat Res* 2003;414:37-44.

29. Daly PJ, Fitzgerald RH Jr, Melton LJ, Ilstrup DM: Epidemiology of ankle fractures in Rochester, Minnesota. *Acta Orthop Scand* 1987;58(5):539-544.

30. Greenfield DM, Eastell R: Risk factors for ankle fracture. *Osteoporos Int* 2001;12(2):97-103.

31. Kröger H, Huopio J, Honkanen R, et al: Prediction of fracture risk using axial bone mineral density in a perimenopausal population: A prospective study. *J Bone Miner Res* 1995;10(2):302-306.

32. Baron JA, Barrett J, Malenka D, et al: Racial differences in fracture risk. *Epidemiology* 1994;5(1): 42-47.

33. Bengnér U, Johnell O, Redlund-Johnell I: Epidemiology of ankle fracture 1950 and 1980: Increasing incidence in elderly women. *Acta Orthop Scand* 1986;57(1): 35-37.

34. Nilsson BE: Age and sex incidence of ankle fractures. *Acta Orthop Scand* 1969;40(1):122-129.

35. Riggs BL, Melton LJ III: Clinical review 8: Clinical heterogeneity of involutional osteoporosis: Implications for preventive therapy. *J Clin Endocrinol Metab* 1990; 70(5):1229-1232.

36. Seeley DG, Kelsey J, Jergas M, Nevitt MC; The Study of Osteoporotic Fractures Research Group: Predictors of ankle and foot fractures in older women. *J Bone Miner Res* 1996;11(9):1347-1355.

37. Salai M, Dudkiewicz I, Novikov I, Amit Y, Chechick A: The epidemic of ankle fractures in the elderly: Is surgical treatment warranted? *Arch Orthop Trauma Surg* 2000;120(9):511-513.

38. Ali MS, McLaren CA, Rouholamin E, O'Connor BT: Ankle fractures in the elderly: Nonopera-

tive or operative treatment. *J Orthop Trauma* 1987;1(4):275-280.

39. Davidovitch RI, Walsh M, Spitzer A, Egol KA: Functional outcome after operatively treated ankle fractures in the elderly. *Foot Ankle Int* 2009;30(8):728-733.
40. Cole PA, Craft JA: Treatment of osteoporotic ankle fractures in the elderly: Surgical strategies. *Orthopedics* 2002;25(4):427-430.
41. Ramasamy PR, Sherry P: The role of a fibular nail in the management of Weber type B ankle fractures in elderly patients with osteoporotic bone: A preliminary report. *Injury* 2001;32(6): 477-485.
42. Wagner M: General principles for the clinical use of the LCP. *Injury* 2003;34(Suppl 2):B31-B42.
43. Hutchinson GS, Griffon DJ, Siegel AM, et al: Evaluation of an osteoconductive resorbable calcium phosphate cement and polymethylmethacrylate for augmentation of orthopedic screws in the pelvis of canine cadavers. *Am J Vet Res* 2005;66(11):1954-1960.
44. Leung KS, Siu WS, Li SF, et al: An in vitro optimized injectable calcium phosphate cement for augmenting screw fixation in osteopenic goats. *J Biomed Mater Res B Appl Biomater* 2006;78(1): 153-160.
45. Ogilvie-Harris DJ, Reed SC, Hedman TP: Disruption of the ankle syndesmosis: Biomechanical study of the ligamentous restraints. *Arthroscopy* 1994;10(5):558-560.
46. McCullough CJ, Burge PD: Rotatory stability of the load-bearing ankle: An experimental study. *J Bone Joint Surg Br* 1980; 62-B(4):460-464.
47. Haraguchi N, Armiger RS: A new interpretation of the mechanism of ankle fracture. *J Bone Joint Surg Am* 2009;91(4):821-829.
48. Gardner MJ, Demetrakopoulos D, Briggs SM, Helfet DL, Lorich DG: The ability of the Lauge-Hansen classification to predict ligament injury and mechanism in ankle fractures: An MRI study. *J Orthop Trauma* 2006; 20(4):267-272.
49. Boden SD, Labropoulos PA, McCowin P, Lestini WF, Hurwitz SR: Mechanical considerations for the syndesmosis screw: A cadaver study. *J Bone Joint Surg Am* 1989;71(10):1548-1555.
50. Tornetta P III: Competence of the deltoid ligament in bimalleolar ankle fractures after medial malleolar fixation. *J Bone Joint Surg Am* 2000;82(6):843-848.
51. Nielson JH, Sallis JG, Potter HG, Helfet DL, Lorich DG: Correlation of interosseous membrane tears to the level of the fibular fracture. *J Orthop Trauma* 2004; 18(2):68-74.
52. Stark E, Tornetta P III, Creevy WR: Syndesmotic instability in Weber B ankle fractures: A clinical evaluation. *J Orthop Trauma* 2007;21(9):643-646.
53. Nielson JH, Gardner MJ, Peterson MG, et al: Radiographic measurements do not predict syndesmotic injury in ankle fractures: An MRI study. *Clin Orthop Relat Res* 2005;436:216-221.
54. Gardner MJ, Demetrakopoulos D, Briggs SM, Helfet DL, Lorich DG: Malreduction of the tibiofibular syndesmosis in ankle fractures. *Foot Ankle Int* 2006; 27(10):788-792.
55. Weening B, Bhandari M: Predictors of functional outcome following transsyndesmotic screw fixation of ankle fractures. *J Orthop Trauma* 2005;19(2):102-108.
56. Gardner MJ, Brodsky A, Briggs SM, Nielson JH, Lorich DG: Fixation of posterior malleolar fractures provides greater syndesmotic stability. *Clin Orthop Relat Res* 2006;447:165-171.
57. Thompson MC, Gesink DS: Biomechanical comparison of syndesmosis fixation with 3.5- and 4.5-millimeter stainless steel screws. *Foot Ankle Int* 2000;21(9):736-741.
58. Høiness P, Strømsøe K: Tricortical versus quadricortical syndesmosis fixation in ankle fractures: A prospective, randomized study comparing two methods of syndesmosis fixation. *J Orthop Trauma* 2004;18(6):331-337.
59. Moore JA Jr, Shank JR, Morgan SJ, Smith WR: Syndesmosis fixation: A comparison of three and four cortices of screw fixation without hardware removal. *Foot Ankle Int* 2006;27(8):567-572.
60. Cottom JM, Hyer CF, Philbin TM, Berlet GC: Treatment of syndesmotic disruptions with the Arthrex Tightrope: A report of 25 cases. *Foot Ankle Int* 2008;29(8):773-780.
61. Forsythe K, Freedman KB, Stover MD, Patwardhan AG: Comparison of a novel FiberWire-button construct versus metallic screw fixation in a syndesmotic injury model. *Foot Ankle Int* 2008;29(1):49-54.
62. Hamid N, Loeffler BJ, Braddy W, Kellam JF, Cohen BE, Bosse MJ: Outcome after fixation of ankle fractures with an injury to the syndesmosis: The effect of the syndesmosis screw. *J Bone Joint Surg Br* 2009;91(8):1069-1073.
63. Jaskulka RA, Ittner G, Schedl R: Fractures of the posterior tibial margin: Their role in the prognosis of malleolar fractures. *J Trauma* 1989;29(11):1565-1570.
64. Koval KJ, Lurie J, Zhou W, et al: Ankle fractures in the elderly: What you get depends on where you live and who you see. *J Orthop Trauma* 2005;19(9): 635-639.
65. Nugent JF, Gale BD: Isolated posterior malleolar ankle fractures. *J Foot Surg* 1990;29(1):80-83.

66. Haraguchi N, Haruyama H, Toga H, Kato F: Pathoanatomy of posterior malleolar fractures of the ankle. *J Bone Joint Surg Am* 2006; 88(5):1085-1092.

67. Ebraheim NA, Mekhail AO, Haman SP: External rotation-lateral view of the ankle in the assessment of the posterior malleolus. *Foot Ankle Int* 1999;20(6): 379-383.

68. Ferries JS, DeCoster TA, Firoozbakhsh KK, Garcia JF, Miller RA: Plain radiographic interpretation in trimalleolar ankle fractures poorly assesses posterior fragment size. *J Orthop Trauma* 1994;8(4): 328-331.

69. Bois AJ, Dust W: Posterior fracture dislocation of the ankle: Technique and clinical experience using a posteromedial surgical approach. *J Orthop Trauma* 2008; 22(9):629-636.

70. Fitzpatrick DC, Otto JK, McKinley TO, Marsh JL, Brown TD: Kinematic and contact stress analysis of posterior malleolus fractures of the ankle. *J Orthop Trauma* 2004;18(5):271-278.

71. Macko VW, Matthews LS, Zwirkoski P, Goldstein SA: The joint-contact area of the ankle: The contribution of the posterior malleolus. *J Bone Joint Surg Am* 1991;73(3):347-351.

72. McDaniel WJ, Wilson FC: Trimalleolar fractures of the ankle: An end result study. *Clin Orthop Relat Res* 1977;122:37-45.

73. Raasch WG, Larkin JJ, Draganich LF: Assessment of the posterior malleolus as a restraint to posterior subluxation of the ankle. *J Bone Joint Surg Am* 1992;74(8): 1201-1206.

74. Miller AN, Carroll EA, Parker RJ, Helfet DL, Lorich DG: Posterior malleolar stabilization of syndesmotic injuries is equivalent to screw fixation. *Clin Orthop Relat Res* 2010;468(4):1129-1135.

75. Weber M, Ganz R: Malunion following trimalleolar fracture with posterolateral subluxation of the talus: Reconstruction including the posterior malleolus. *Foot Ankle Int* 2003;24(4):338-344.

76. Weber M: Trimalleolar fractures with impaction of the posteromedial tibial plafond: Implications for talar stability. *Foot Ankle Int* 2004;25(10):716-727.

77. Holt ES: Arthroscopic visualization of the tibial plafond during posterior malleolar fracture fixation. *Foot Ankle Int* 1994;15(4): 206-208.

78. Papachristou G, Efstathopoulos N, Levidiotis C, Chronopoulos E: Early weight bearing after posterior malleolar fractures: An experimental and prospective clinical study. *J Foot Ankle Surg* 2003; 42(2):99-104.

79. Broos PL, Bisschop AP: Operative treatment of ankle fractures in adults: Correlation between types of fracture and final results. *Injury* 1991;22(5):403-406.

80. Langenhuijsen JF, Heetveld MJ, Ultee JM, Steller EP, Butzelaar RM: Results of ankle fractures with involvement of the posterior tibial margin. *J Trauma* 2002; 53(1):55-60.

81. De Vries JS, Wijgman AJ, Sierevelt IN, Schaap GR: Long-term results of ankle fractures with a posterior malleolar fragment. *J Foot Ankle Surg* 2005;44(3): 211-217.

82. Harper MC, Hardin G: Posterior malleolar fractures of the ankle associated with external rotation-abduction injuries: Results with and without internal fixation. *J Bone Joint Surg Am* 1988;70(9): 1348-1356.

83. McConnell T, Tornetta P III: Marginal plafond impaction in association with supination-adduction ankle fractures: A report of eight cases. *J Orthop Trauma* 2001;15(6):447-449.

84. Hamilton W: *Traumatic Disorders of the Ankle*. New York, NY, Springer-Verlag, 1984.

85. Jacobsen S, Honnens de Lichtenberg M, Jensen CM, Tørholm C: Removal of internal fixation: The effect on patients' complaints. A study of 66 cases of removal of internal fixation after malleolar fractures. *Foot Ankle Int* 1994; 15(4):170-171.

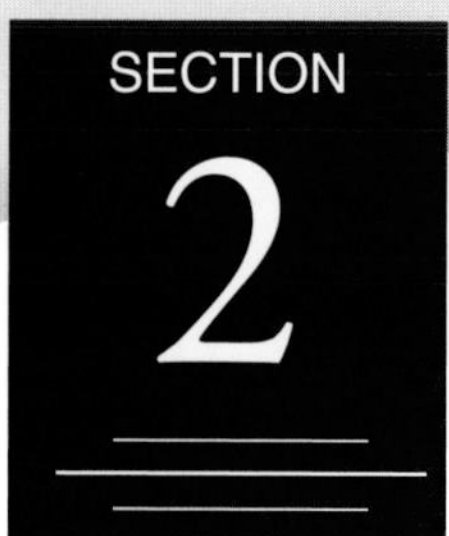

SECTION 2

Shoulder

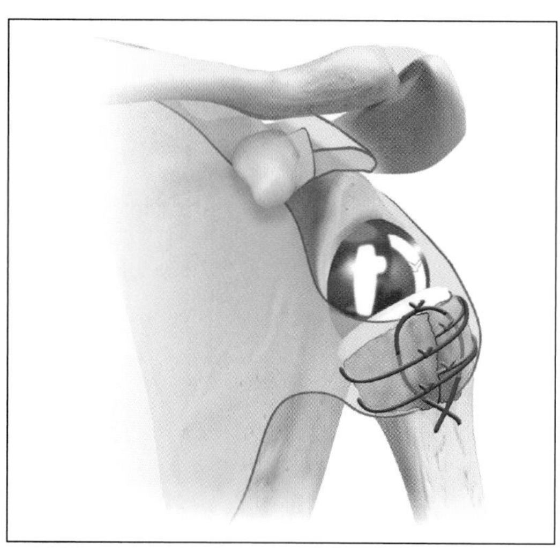

Surgical Approach and Techniques for Total Shoulder Arthroplasty: Tips and Tricks

Justin W. Chandler, MD
Gerald R. Williams Jr, MD

Abstract

In patients treated with total shoulder arthroplasty, it is beneficial to be aware of several tips and tricks to optimize patient outcomes. Prior to surgery, appropriate preoperative planning is essential to ensure a smooth procedure with no unexpected intraoperative findings. The procedure begins with appropriate patient positioning to allow for safety and ease of shoulder manipulation. The approach using the deltopectoral interval is described, with emphasis on the proper use of retractors and adequate soft-tissue releases. Appropriate handling of the subscapularis and lesser tuberosity during both exposure and closure is imperative for a good surgical outcome. Other portions of the procedure also can be less problematic if the surgeon is familiar with certain techniques.

Instr Course Lect 2011;60:91-97.

Certain tips and tricks can help optimize the outcomes of patients treated with total shoulder arthroplasty. Understanding proper preoperative planning, patient positioning, and intraoperative techniques are useful in preventing complications and improving outcomes.

Preoperative Planning

Prior to surgery, appropriate preoperative planning is essential to ensure a smooth procedure without unexpected intraoperative findings. Recommended preoperative radiographs include AP views in internal and external rotation as well as axillary views. These images will allow preoperative templating, which can be helpful in determining needed modifications to the standard surgical technique. Radiographic findings may show significant varus or valgus neck-shaft angles as well as variation in the humeral head and canal size. These factors may alter the surgeon's selection of an implant or the level and angle of the head cut made during surgery.

Depending on the shoulder pathology, more advanced imaging methods may be useful. Glenoid deformity may be visible on routine radiographs but may be more accurately characterized on two- or three-dimensional CT scans. The glenoid classification system described by Walch et al[1] is useful in surgical planning in patients with a posterior glenoid deformity (**Table 1**). Although rotator cuff tears are not common in patients with osteoarthritis, MRI can be used if a tear is clinically suspected or in patients with rheumatoid arthritis in whom erosive loss of cuff integrity is more common.[2-4]

Anesthesia and Patient Positioning

Many patients elect regional anesthesia with an interscalene block combined with general anesthesia. This method provides excellent pain relief and can make early postoperative motion easier for the patient.[5,6] It is important to have an experienced team of anesthesiologists because interscalene blocks can increase the risk of neurologic, pulmonary, and vascular complications.[7-9]

Dr. Williams or an immediate family member serves as a board member, owner, officer, or committee member of the American Shoulder and Elbow Surgeons, Pennsylvania Orthopaedic Society, American Academy of Orthopaedic Surgeons, The Rothman Institute, and Philadelphia Human Performance Laboratory; has received royalties from DePuy; is a member of a speakers bureau or has made paid presentations on behalf of DePuy and Mitek; serves as a paid consultant to or is an employee of DePuy; and has stock or stock options held in Invivo Therapeutics. Neither Dr. Chandler nor an immediate family member has received anything of value from or owns stock in a commercial company or institution related directly or indirectly to the subject of this chapter.

Table 1
Glenoid Classification System as Described by Walch et al

Type	Description
A1	Humeral head is well centered in glenoid with minor erosion.
A2	Humeral head is well centered in glenoid with major central erosion.
B1	Humeral head is subluxated posteriorly with narrowing of the posterior joint space.
B2	Humeral head is subluxated posteriorly with a biconcave glenoid.
C	Glenoid retroversion > 25°, regardless of erosion.

The interscalene block is administered in the preoperative holding area, and the patient is then brought to the operating room where general anesthesia is induced. The patient is placed in the beach chair position with the back elevated 30° to 45° from the floor. There are several systems to ensure that the head and body are well stabilized; it is essential to ensure that all pressure points and potential sites of nerve compression are well padded. The operative arm must be completely unsupported by the table and should hang off the edge so that complete extension, adduction, and external rotation are permitted to allow delivery of the humeral head. After the patient is properly positioned and before the patient is prepped and draped, an examination of preoperative range of motion should be completed, with special attention to external rotation. This chapter's authors prefer using a mechanical arm-holding device to assist in positioning the arm during surgery; however, an assistant or padded Mayo stand can be used to position the arm.

Surgical Approach

The deltopectoral approach is most commonly used in shoulder arthroplasty. Superficially, the cephalic vein is identified and taken either medially or laterally depending on the surgeon's preference. This chapter's authors prefer to routinely take the vein laterally because of the larger tributaries from the deltoid muscle. The interval is opened from the clavicle to the insertion of the deltoid. A Cobb elevator is a useful instrument for developing the plane between the surgical neck of the humerus and the overlying deltoid muscle. Care must be taken to keep the instruments and electrocautery close to bone to avoid injury to the axillary nerve on the undersurface of the deltoid. The coracoid tip is used as a landmark to identify the conjoined tendon. If necessary, the upper 1 cm of the insertion of the pectoralis major can be incised to improve exposure. A Kolbel self-retaining retractor can be used with one limb under the deltoid laterally and one limb medially under the pectoralis major to allow deep exposure.

After the lateral edge of the conjoined tendon is identified, the clavipectoral fascia is incised along the lateral edge proximally to the anterior border of the coracoacromial ligament and distally to the most inferior extent of the subscapularis. Although incision or excision of the coracoacromial ligament can improve visualization of the superior glenoid, it should be preserved whenever possible to minimize the risk of anterosuperior subluxation.[10,11] Rotator cuff tears in patients with osteoarthritis are uncommon[2,3] but can develop after shoulder arthroplasty; exposure is almost always adequate without dividing the coracoacromial ligament.

The location of the axillary and musculocutaneous nerves should be identified by palpation and noted when possible to minimize the risk of injury from dissection or retraction. The musculocutaneous nerve usually penetrates the conjoined tendon distal to the surgical field; however, in some instances, it can insert closer to the coracoid and should be recognized to avoid injury with retractors beneath the conjoined tendon.[12] The anterior circumflex vessels are ligated or coagulated. The long head of the biceps tendon is then exposed in the bicipital groove. This chapter's authors routinely suture the biceps tendon to the upper border of the pectoralis major using two nonabsorbable sutures. The tendon proximal to the site of tenodesis is then transected and excised at the supraglenoid tubercle.

Subscapularis Reflection

The subscapularis tendon is reflected to expose the glenohumeral joint. Although no data are available from randomized controlled trials, recent literature suggests that better postoperative subscapularis function is achieved with a lesser tuberosity osteotomy than with soft-tissue reflection and repair.[13,14] A recent study by Caplan et al[15] reported good subscapularis function with tenotomy and direct tendon-to-tendon repair.

This chapter's authors prefer a lesser tuberosity osteotomy with anatomic repair in all primary shoulder arthroplasties with the exception of shoulders with rheumatoid arthritis and significant bony erosions, those treated with a prior procedure that shortened the subscapularis (for example, a Putti-Platt or Magnuson-Stack procedure), or in shoulders with severe internal rotation contracture (passive external rotation < –40°). In these cases, the subscapularis is taken off the lesser tuberosity and then repaired medially to the cut surface of the humeral osteotomy. Although rarely needed, a coronal Z-lengthening of the subscapularis can be performed in shoulders with severe internal rotation contracture. The need for subscapularis advancement or lengthening may occur much less frequently than traditionally believed if the capsular contracture is adequately treated and the subscapularis is adequately released.

This chapter's authors perform the lesser tuberosity osteotomy using a 2-inch curved osteotome in a manner similar to that described by Gerber et al[16] (**Figure 1**). The lesser tuberosity fragment reflected with the subscapularis will ideally be a solid noncomminuted piece that is 0.5 to 1.0 cm thick. The osteotomy is done by first clearing the bicipital groove of soft tissue to expose the lateral edge of the lesser tuberosity. The osteotome is then placed in the base of the bicipital groove and directed medially. The surgeon can direct the osteotome with one hand and palpate the anterior tuberosity with the other hand to gauge the depth of the osteotomy while an assistant strikes the osteotome. A straight osteotome and a Cobb elevator can then be used to further elevate the fragment and separate it from the underlying soft-tissue attachments. Once the fragment is sufficiently freed and mobile, three 1-mm nonabsorbable sutures are passed through the bone-tendon junction at the superior, central, and inferior aspect of the tuberosity fragment. These sutures will be used for traction and then for reattachment of the fragment at the conclusion of the procedure. The inferior muscle belly of the subscapularis is then incised longitudinally in line with its fibers approximately 1 cm superior to the inferior edge of the muscular attachment. The subscapularis is then further elevated off the underlying capsule using a blunt elevator and a scalpel, while the lesser tuberosity is retracted anteriorly. A blunt Hohmann retractor can then be placed between the capsule and remaining inferior border of the subscapularis to protect the axillary nerve.

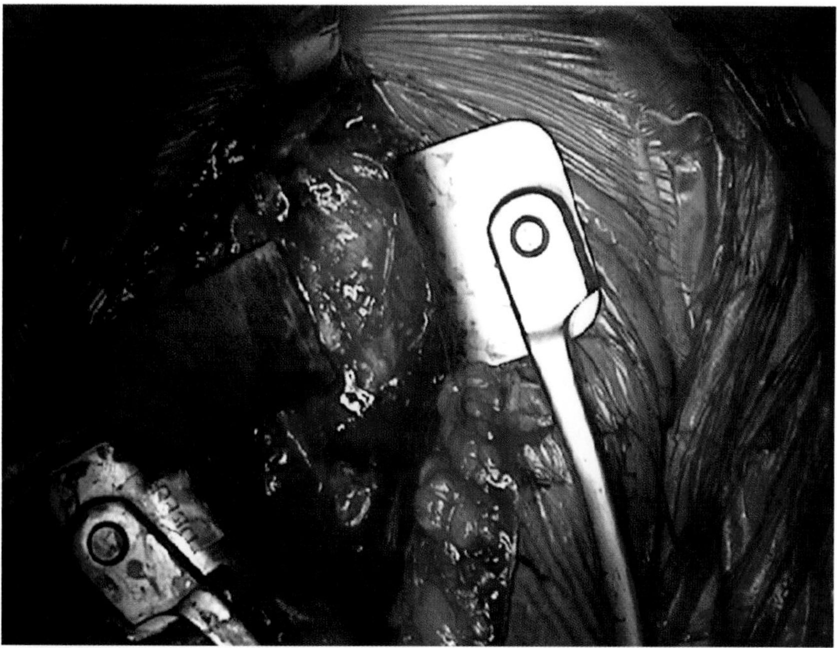

Figure 1 Intraoperative photograph of a lesser tuberosity osteotomy using a 2-inch curved osteotome starting at the floor of the bicipital groove.

When the subscapularis attachment is of poor quality (such as in patients with rheumatoid arthritis), or the subscapularis has been shortened from prior surgery (such as a Putti-Platt procedure), or the internal contracture is severe (external rotation of < –40°), the subscapularis tendon is released from the lesser tuberosity as far laterally as possible and is reflected with the capsule in a single layer.

Capsular Release

The anterior capsule is released from the anatomic neck of the humerus while gently externally rotating and flexing the adducted humerus. The release progresses superiorly to inferiorly and extends well past the 6 o'clock position. When Z-lengthening is planned, which is rare (if external rotation is less than –60°), the capsule is released from the glenoid and incised laterally to medially, starting at the inferior portion of the humerus. The capsule inferior to this lateral to medial incision is then released from the humerus. This technique produces a laterally based capsular flap on the humerus that can be used in the deep layer of the Z-lengthening. As stated, this lengthening is rarely required.

After appropriate release, the humeral head can be delivered into the wound with external rotation, adduction, and extension. All osteophytes are then removed circumferentially from the humeral head with rongeurs and osteotomes. This step is important for anatomic component placement and also decreases the anteroposterior dimensions of the humeral head, making glenoid exposure easier.

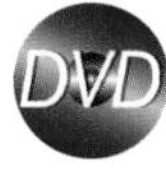

Video 8.1: Deltopectoral Exposure and Glenoid Preparation for Total Shoulder Replacement. Christian Gerber, MD (14 min)

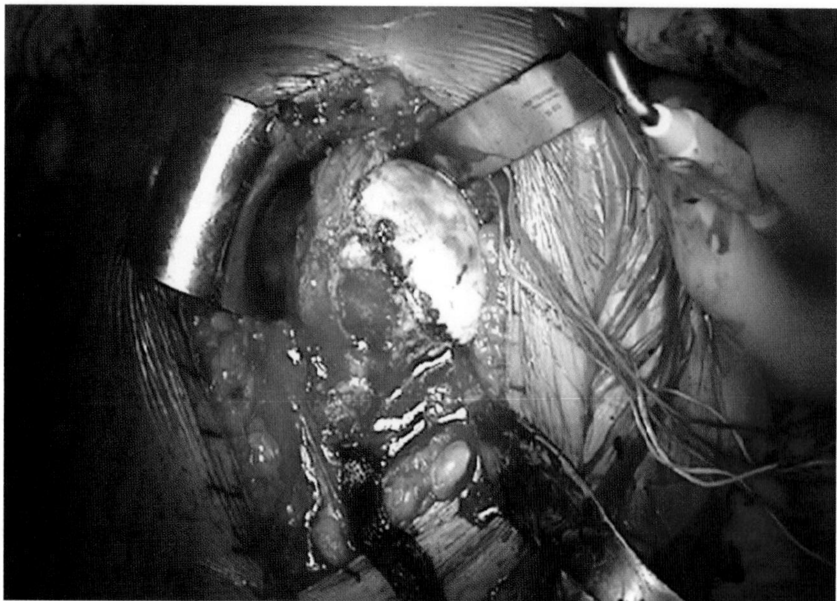

Figure 2 Retractors used during humeral head resection include a large Darrach retractor in the glenohumeral joint, a Browne deltoid retractor under the deltoid, and a blunt Hohmann retractor at the inferior humeral neck.

Humeral Head Resection

Retractors used during humeral head resection include a large Darrach retractor in the glenohumeral joint; a modified Taylor, blunt Hohmann, or Browne deltoid retractor (Innomed, Savannah, GA) in the subacromial space; and a blunt Hohmann retractor at the inferior humeral neck, taking care to note the location of the axillary nerve and keeping the retractor directly on bone (**Figure 2**). The humeral head is then resected using a saw. The method of humeral head resection is based on whether the implant used has a fixed or a variable neck-shaft angle. If using a fixed neck-shaft angle implant, an intramedullary or extramedullary cutting guide typically will be used to ensure that the cut matches the angle of the implant. If an implant with a variable neck-shaft angle is used, a freehand resection of the humeral head can be performed using the anatomic neck or articular margin as a guide. This technique allows the surgeon to match the native neck-shaft angle, which is variable in normal humeri.[17,18] It should be noted that using the flexibility of a variable neck-shaft angle implant to conform to a nonanatomic freehand cut is possible but should be avoided.

The humeral cut can be made to match native retroversion by cutting in the plane of the periphery of the native articular cartilage after the removal of osteophytes. As previously mentioned, preoperative templating can be helpful in detecting humeri with excessive varus or valgus neck-shaft angles. This is important in planning the humeral cut when using a fixed-angle cementless stem because a more varus or valgus cut will be needed, and the native anatomy cannot be relied on to determine the proper osteotomy angle. This is not as important in variable-angle devices, which can match the native neck-shaft angle. Great care should be taken to preserve the rotator cuff reflection during humeral head resection. After humeral head size is estimated by placing trial implants over the cut surface of the osteotomy, attention is turned to the glenoid.

Glenoid Exposure and Preparation

Exposing the glenoid is often the most challenging part of the procedure. Soft-tissue releases are not only necessary for adequate exposure for glenoid resurfacing but are also important in obtaining maximal postoperative range of motion. Proper arm positioning and retractor placement are essential to allow maximal posterior humeral displacement. With the arm in abduction, external rotation, and extension, the posterior and superior capsule are relaxed and allow more posterior displacement. However, the ideal position for glenoid exposure varies among patients. Humeral positioning should be tested and optimized in each patient. Placing the arm so that the osteotomy surface is nearly parallel to the glenoid surface is often a good place to begin; the arm position is then adjusted until exposure is maximized.

The humerus is retracted posteriorly with a Fukuda ring retractor cupping the posterior glenoid rim. Anteriorly, a reverse double-pronged Bankart retractor is used between the anterior capsule and subscapularis on the scapular neck. A blunt Hohmann retractor is used anteroinferiorly on the scapular neck to protect the axillary nerve. A moist, folded sponge can be placed beneath the Fukuda retractor to protect the cephalic vein and the deltoid muscle. These three retractors are usually sufficient to provide excellent glenoid exposure (**Figure 3**); however, it is helpful to have more than one type of glenoid retractor available in instances when the Fukuda retractor is not ideal.

When the subscapularis is in good condition and Z-lengthening is not anticipated, the anterior and inferior capsule is excised at this point. In instances of poor or questionable subscapularis quality (such as in patients with rheumatoid arthritis), the capsule is released from the glenoid anteriorly and inferiorly past the 6 o'clock position and is left attached to the subscapularis laterally for tendon reinforcement.

If significant posterior subluxation (> 25%) was not noted preoperatively, the posterior capsule is released. If preoperative posterior subluxation was noted, the posterior capsule is preserved to prevent posterior instability. The labrum is then circumferentially excised, exposing the periphery of the glenoid, which is then sized with a sizing disk. The center of the glenoid is marked, and a centering hole is drilled. The central hole must be perpendicular to the planned glenoid surface. Preoperative imaging is helpful in guiding this angle based on the amount of posterior glenoid bone loss. If there is significant posterior glenoid wear, it can be helpful to use a reamer without a tip to preferentially ream anteriorly to correct version before placing a central drill hole. The glenoid is then reamed using the central hole until a concentric surface is obtained. This is often one of the most difficult steps in glenoid preparation because the presence of the retractors can make it difficult to position the reamer straight so that it is flush with the surface of the glenoid. In such instances, the Fukuda ring retractor can be removed, and the shaft of the reamer can be used to retract the humeral head posteriorly during reaming.

After concentric reaming, anchoring holes for either a keeled or a pegged glenoid component are created. If peripheral peg holes are used, they should be probed after drilling to evaluate cortical penetration. If penetration occurs, bone plugs from the humeral head can be used to prevent cement extravasation. Even if bone plugs are used in a hole with cortical penetration, cement pressurization should be avoided. A trial glenoid is placed, which ensures adequate seating and also provides a "rehearsal" for the final implant to ensure that the exposure is adequate for glenoid placement. The holes are then irrigated and dried, and cement is placed in the peripheral holes using a syringe for pressurization. The glenoid component is then impacted in place. The same process is used for a keeled component.

Research into the development of an uncemented glenoid continues; however, few long-term follow-up data are available. The few available studies have reported unfavorable outcomes.[19,20]

Humeral Component Placement

Attention is then turned back to the humerus, which is again delivered into the wound. Sequentially larger intramedullary reamers are then used by hand until appropriate cortical contact is appreciated. The box osteotome corresponding to the last size reamer selected is then used to open the proximal humerus to accept the implant. An appropriately sized broach is then placed in the canal. If a fixed-angle device is being used, a calcar planar can be used at this point to plane the surface to the correct neck-shaft angle, assuming that this is permissible based on the rotator cuff attachment. A trial humeral head is then placed. An eccentric offset head is used that is rotated to provide the most complete coverage of the humeral metaphysis and then locked to the broach in the appropriate position. At this point, any remaining humeral osteophytes can be removed around the periphery of the implant.

The humerus is then reduced and assessed for adequate soft-tissue tension and stability. If the trial is acceptable, it is removed and the final implant is assembled. Prior to impacting the implant into the humerus, a nonabsorbable suture, which will be used in repairing the lesser tuberosity osteotomy, is placed around the neck of the prosthesis. The implant is then impacted flush with the humeral cut. If bone is of poor quality or the proximal humeral anatomy prevents proper implant positioning, cement may be needed.

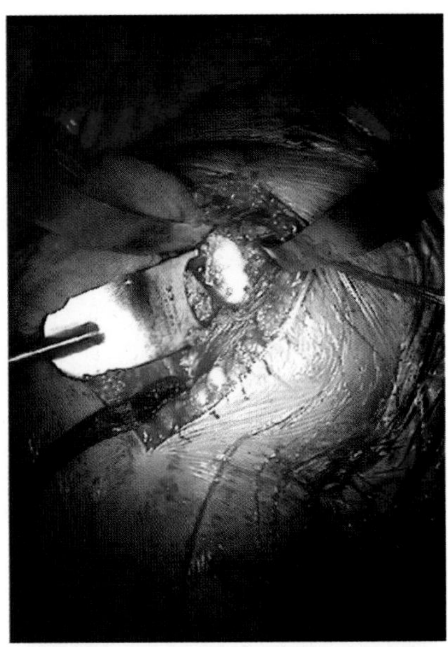

Figure 3 Intraoperative photograph showing excellent glenoid exposure using a Fukuda ring retractor between the glenoid and the humerus, a single pronged Bankart retractor posterosuperiorly, and a large Darrach retractor anteriorly.

Lesser Tuberosity and Subscapularis Repair and Closure

After copious irrigation of the joint, the lesser tuberosity osteotomy or subscapularis is repaired. For repair of the lesser tuberosity osteotomy, the nonabsorbable suture that was placed around the neck of the implant is passed in a mattress configuration at the bone-tendon junction through the subscapularis from deep to superficial. These sutures are clamped. With the arm in neutral position, the deep limb of the three sutures that were initially passed around the fragment are passed

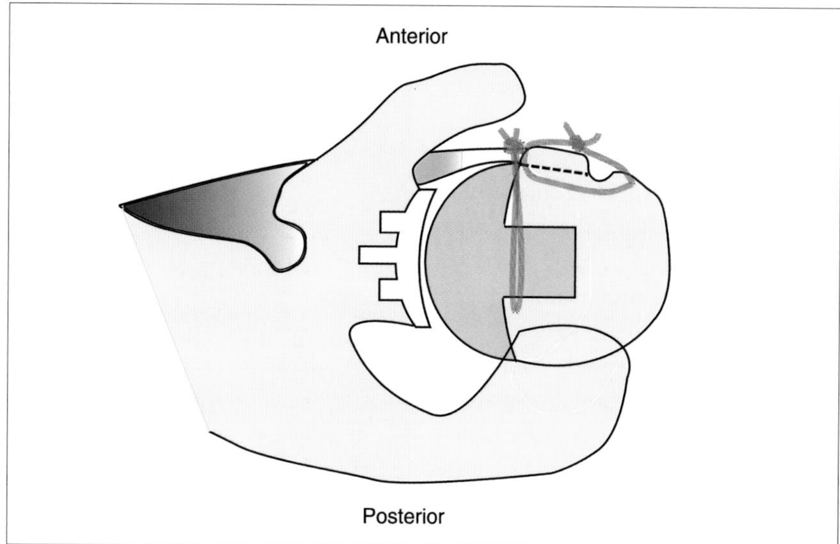

Figure 4 Illustration showing the suture configuration for repair of the lesser tuberosity osteotomy.

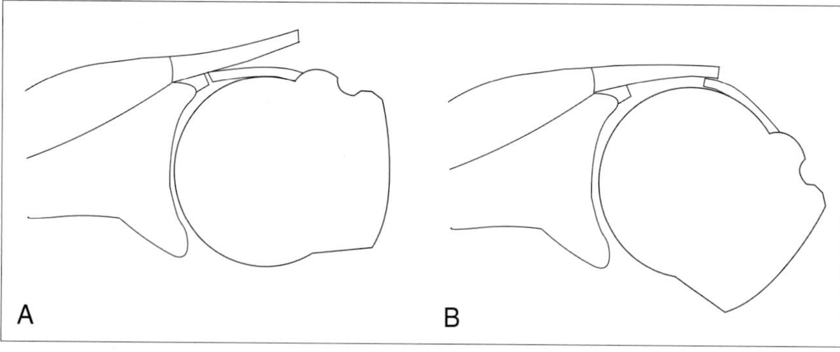

Figure 5 **A,** Illustration showing a subscapularis tenotomy with laterally based capsular flap. **B,** The tendon is sutured to the flap at a point that allows 35° to 40° of external rotation.

through the lateral aspect of the osteotomy site, under the bicipital groove, and out the lateral cortex of the humerus. This chapter's authors use a large cutting free needle to pass the sutures; a new needle is used for each pass. Each suture is clamped to its corresponding superficial limb and then pulled laterally to reduce the lesser tuberosity anatomically. One nonabsorbable 1-mm suture is then placed in the most lateral aspect of the rotator interval and tied to set the position of the tuberosity. The three sutures around the tuberosity are then tied, followed by the mattress suture at the bone-tendon junction around the implant (**Figure 4**). Passive external rotation is then tested within the limits of undue tension on the repair to provide a guide for postoperative rehabilitation early motion parameters.

In rare instances, the subscapularis is released from the lesser tuberosity and needs to be reattached to the bone of the anterior humeral metaphysis. If there is poor tendon quality, the repair will include the tendon and the attached anterior capsule. Using a grasping configuration (such as a Mason-Allen stitch), 1-mm tapes are passed through the tendon. The ends are then passed through bone and tied over the lateral cortex.

In the rare instances when Z-lengthening of the subscapularis is needed, the laterally based capsular flap that was created during the exposure is used as the deep limb of the repair. The tendon is sutured to this flap at a point that allows 35° to 40° of external rotation (**Figure 5**). After copious irrigation, a drain is placed beneath the deltoid and exiting distal to the axillary nerve, and the wound is closed in layers.

Postoperative Rehabilitation

The postoperative rehabilitation protocol is divided into three stages: early rehabilitation, midterm rehabilitation, and late rehabilitation. In the early rehabilitation period (the first 6 weeks after surgery), the goals are to maximize passive range of motion within parameters set intraoperatively based on subscapularis tension, and allow healing of the lesser tuberosity osteotomy or the subscapularis tendon. Generally, with a good subscapularis or lesser tuberosity repair, passive elevation and external rotation are allowed to 140° and 40°, respectively. These parameters are modified appropriately if tissue quality is poor or if there is concern about the subscapularis repair. Seven to 10 days postoperatively, the patient discontinues use of a sling when at home; the arm may be used at waist level for light activities.

From 7 to 12 weeks after surgery, after the subscapularis has healed, rehabilitation focuses on more active range of motion as well as passive stretching exercises. Strengthening exercises for the deltoid, the rotator cuff, and the scapular stabilizers also are performed during this period. Active range of motion is initially assisted with a pulley and a stick, with progression to full active motion as tolerated.

Late rehabilitation (from 13 to 24 weeks after surgery) involves continued strengthening and a gradual return to activities as strength and range of motion allow. Strength and motion will continue to improve up to 1 year postoperatively, but generally the benefits of formal rehabilitation will be realized in the first 6 months.

Summary

Anatomic implant placement is critical, but total shoulder arthroplasty is also largely a soft-tissue surgery. When careful attention is paid to proper preoperative planning, patient positioning, appropriate retractor placement, and adequate soft-tissue release, the most difficult aspects of shoulder replacement surgery can be made significantly less problematic.

References

1. Walch G, Badet R, Boulahia A, Khoury A: Morphologic study of the glenoid in primary glenohumeral osteoarthritis. *J Arthroplasty* 1999;14(6):756-760.
2. Edwards TB, Boulahia A, Kempf JF, Boileau P, Nemoz C, Walch G: The influence of rotator cuff disease on the results of shoulder arthroplasty for primary osteoarthritis: Results of a multicenter study. *J Bone Joint Surg Am* 2002;84-A(12):2240-2248.
3. Neer CS II: Replacement arthroplasty for glenohumeral osteoarthritis. *J Bone Joint Surg Am* 1974; 56(1):1-13.
4. Hawkins RJ, Bell RH, Jallay B: Total shoulder arthroplasty. *Clin Orthop Relat Res* 1989;242(242): 188-194.
5. Brown AR, Weiss R, Greenberg C, Flatow EL, Bigliani LU: Interscalene block for shoulder arthroscopy: Comparison with general anesthesia. *Arthroscopy* 1993;9(3):295-300.
6. Tetzlaff JE, Yoon HJ, Brems J: Interscalene brachial plexus block for shoulder surgery. *Reg Anesth* 1994;19(5):339-343.
7. Plit ML, Chhajed PN, Macdonald P, Cole IE, Harrison GA: Bilateral vocal cord palsy following interscalene brachial plexus nerve block. *Anaesth Intensive Care* 2002;30(4):499-501.
8. Walton JS, Folk JW, Friedman RJ, Dorman BH: Complete brachial plexus palsy after total shoulder arthroplasty done with interscalene block anesthesia. *Reg Anesth Pain Med* 2000;25(3): 318-321.
9. Weber SC, Jain R: Scalene regional anesthesia for shoulder surgery in a community setting: An assessment of risk. *J Bone Joint Surg Am* 2002;84-A(5):775-779.
10. Flatow EL, Wang VM, Kelkar R, et al: The coracoacromial ligament restrains anterosuperior humeral subluxation in the rotator cuff deficient shoulder. *Trans Orthop Res Soc* 1996;21:229.
11. Wiley AM: Superior humeral dislocation: A complication following decompression and debridement for rotator cuff tears. *Clin Orthop Relat Res* 1991;263: 135-141.
12. Flatow EL, Bigliani LU, April EW: An anatomic study of the musculocutaneous nerve and its relationship to the coracoid process. *Clin Orthop Relat Res* 1989;244:166-171.
13. Gerber C, Yian EH, Pfirrmann CA, Zumstein MA, Werner CM: Subscapularis muscle function and structure after total shoulder replacement with lesser tuberosity osteotomy and repair. *J Bone Joint Surg Am* 2005;87(8): 1739-1745.
14. Qureshi S, Hsiao A, Klug RA, Lee E, Braman J, Flatow EL: Subscapularis function after total shoulder replacement: Results with lesser tuberosity osteotomy. *J Shoulder Elbow Surg* 2008;17(1): 68-72.
15. Caplan JL, Whitfield B, Neviaser RJ: Subscapularis function after primary tendon to tendon repair in patients after replacement arthroplasty of the shoulder. *J Shoulder Elbow Surg* 2009;18(2): 193-196, discussion 197-198.
16. Gerber C, Pennington SD, Yian EH, Pfirrmann CA, Werner CM, Zumstein MA: Lesser tuberosity osteotomy for total shoulder arthroplasty: Surgical technique. *J Bone Joint Surg Am* 2006;88(Suppl 1 Pt 2): 170-177.
17. Boileau P, Walch G: The three-dimensional geometry of the proximal humerus: Implications for surgical technique and prosthetic design. *J Bone Joint Surg Br* 1997;79(5):857-865.
18. Iannotti JP, Gabriel JP, Schneck SL, Evans BG, Misra S: The normal glenohumeral relationships: An anatomical study of one hundred and forty shoulders. *J Bone Joint Surg Am* 1992;74(4): 491-500.
19. Boileau P, Avidor C, Krishnan SG, Walch G, Kempf JF, Molé D: Cemented polyethylene versus uncemented metal-backed glenoid components in total shoulder arthroplasty: A prospective, double-blind, randomized study. *J Shoulder Elbow Surg* 2002;11(4):351-359.
20. Martin SD, Zurakowski D, Thornhill TS: Uncemented glenoid component in total shoulder arthroplasty: Survivorship and outcomes. *J Bone Joint Surg Am* 2005;87(6):1284-1292.

Video Reference

8.1: Gerber C: Video. *Deltopectoral Exposure and Glenoid Preparation for Total Shoulder Replacement.* Zurich, Switzerland, 2005.

Shoulder Arthroplasty for the Young, Active Patient

Ryan M. Tibbetts, MD
Michael A. Wirth, MD

Abstract

Patients younger than 55 years with degenerative conditions of the glenohumeral joint represent a unique population that can be treated with shoulder arthroplasty. Certain challenges related to this cohort may include greater patient expectations, higher functional demands, soft-tissue contracture from previous surgery, and glenoid bone loss. Surgical treatment options include unconstrained total shoulder arthroplasty; hemiarthroplasty; humeral head resurfacing alone; hemiarthroplasty with concentric reaming of the glenoid; and hemiarthroplasty with adjunctive biologic glenoid resurfacing with autogenous fascia lata, Achilles tendon allograft, or meniscal allograft.

Instr Course Lect 2011;60:99-104.

Shoulder arthroplasty in young (age 55 years or younger), active patients is challenging because of higher patient expectations and functional demands, soft-tissue contracture from previous surgery, and glenoid bone loss. Surgical treatment options include hemiarthroplasty; unconstrained total shoulder arthroplasty (TSA); humeral head resurfacing alone; hemiarthroplasty with concentric reaming of the glenoid; and hemiarthroplasty with adjunctive biologic glenoid resurfacing with autogenous fascia lata, Achilles tendon allograft, or meniscal allograft.[1-4]

Humeral hemiarthroplasty in young patients has historically been favored over TSA for the management of specific shoulder conditions, such as humeral head osteonecrosis with an intact glenoid cartilaginous surface, posttraumatic sequelae, capsulorrhaphy arthropathy, glenohumeral arthritis secondary to recurrent instability, and primary glenohumeral arthrosis.[3,5-9] Despite good early and midterm results with humeral hemiarthroplasty, progressive glenoid erosion and painful glenoid arthrosis are the most common reasons for implant failure and revision surgery.[10-12] In a recent review of 33 studies (2,540 shoulders) pertaining to unconstrained TSA with a mean follow-up of 5 years, glenoid component loosening was the leading cause of complications (39%).[13] Persistent concerns regarding the long-term durability of glenoid prostheses in terms of wear and loosening have prompted some surgeons to favor hemiarthroplasty in young patients with glenohumeral arthrosis. However, clinical outcome studies and meta-analyses have indicated that, overall, TSA provides better results than hemiarthroplasty alone with regard to pain relief, motion, and level of activity.[10,14-16]

When conservative treatment fails, proponents of shoulder arthroplasty in younger patients have advocated TSA or humeral head resurfacing alone, hemiarthroplasty with concentric reaming of the glenoid, and adjunctive biologic glenoid resurfacing with autogenous fascia lata, Achilles tendon allograft, or meniscal allograft.[1-4]

Surgical Options and Results

Unconstrained TSA and Hemiarthroplasty

In 2004, Sperling et al[17] described the results of hemiarthroplasty and TSA in patients 50 years or younger with a mean follow-up of 17 years. Diagnoses

Neither Dr. Tibbetts nor an immediate family member has received anything of value from or owns stock in a commercial company or institution related directly or indirectly to the subject of this chapter. Dr. Wirth or an immediate family member has received royalties from DePuy; is a member of a speakers bureau or has made paid presentations on behalf of DePuy; has received research or institutional support from DePuy; and has stock or stock options held in Tornier.

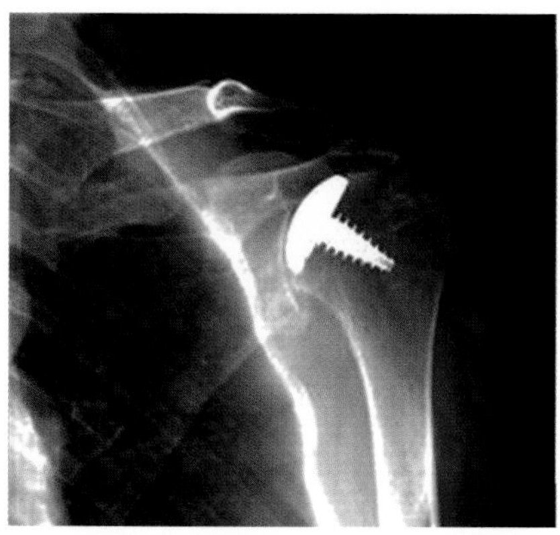

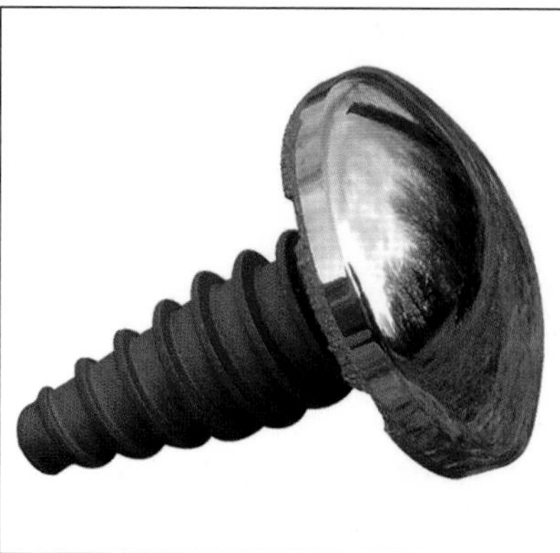

Figure 1 Postoperative radiograph (*left*) and photograph (*right*) of a partial resurfacing prosthesis consisting of a tapered post and a cobalt-chromium surface component. (Reproduced with permission from Burgess DL, McGrath MS, Bonutti PM, Marker DR, Delanois RE, Mont MA: Shoulder resurfacing. *J Bone Joint Surg Am* 2009;91(5):1228-1238.)

included posttraumatic sequelae, inflammatory arthritis, osteonecrosis, osteoarthritis, and previous septic arthritis. Patients in both the hemiarthroplasty and TSA groups showed significant improvement in long-term pain relief and active motion; however, unsatisfactory results were reported in 37 patients treated with hemiarthroplasty (60%) and 14 patients with TSA (48%). Seventeen patients treated with hemiarthroplasty (22%) and 5 patients with TSA (14%) had a revision procedure. Twelve of the 17 patients in the hemiarthroplasty group were treated with revision secondary to painful glenoid arthrosis. In comparison with midterm results in this same cohort of patients, the percentage of unsatisfactory results among those treated with hemiarthroplasty increased from 47% to 60%, whereas the rate of unsatisfactory results among TSA patients remained unchanged.[11] Using a Kaplan-Meier survival analysis with revision as the end point, the estimated 20-year implant survival rate was 74% for hemiarthroplasty and 84% percent for TSA, with no significant difference reported between the two groups.[17]

In a midterm follow-up (mean, 5.6 years) of 22 shoulders in 19 patients with a mean age of 39 years treated with shoulder arthroplasty, Burroughs et al[18] reported unsatisfactory results in 3 patients (14%) treated with hemiarthroplasty. These results were associated with persistent pain and limited function. Two patients (9%) required revision surgery secondary to painful glenoid erosion and humeral head "overstuffing." Patient diagnoses included rheumatoid arthritis, osteonecrosis, trauma, and hemophilic-related shoulder arthropathy.

In 2002, Parsons et al[19] evaluated outcomes with TSA in a series of 24 young patients (mean age, 50 years) treated for capsulorrhaphy arthropathy. A significant reduction in functional deficits was reported at a mean follow-up of 5 years; however, these results showed less improvement than previous reports of functional outcomes with TSA for primary glenohumeral arthritis.

Sperling et al[5] reported the results of TSA and hemiarthroplasty for arthritis after instability surgery in young patients. There was a significant improvement in pain relief and range of motion at 7-year follow-up; however, unsatisfactory results were reported in 17 patients (55%), and 11 shoulders (35%) required revision surgery. Eight of the revisions were in the TSA group, with most performed for component failure and instability. The estimated Kaplan-Meier implant survivorship, with revision as the end point, was 61% at 10 years.

In contrast to most studies pertaining to TSA in young patients, Raiss et al[20] reported more predictable outcomes with TSA when the diagnosis was limited to primary glenohumeral arthritis. Significant improvements were reported in pain relief, power, activity, and range of motion. Twenty patients (95%) were satisfied with their outcomes at a mean follow-up of 7 years, with no patients requiring revision surgery.

Humeral Head Resurfacing

Humeral head resurfacing was initially proposed as a treatment for glenohumeral arthritis in an attempt to preserve the original anatomy and proximal humeral bone stock.[21] This procedure provides a theoretic benefit for the younger patient who may require revision to a TSA with a stemmed prosthesis later in life (**Figure 1**). Resurfacing also has the potential advantage of decreasing the risk of periprosthetic fracture that occurs with a stemmed prosthesis secondary to reaming or broaching of the proximal humerus.[22] Indications for resurfacing include pain and decreased function related to osteoarthritis, rheumatoid arthritis, osteonecrosis, posttraumatic arthritis, and chronic instability of the joint.[22] In a recent prospective study of cementless humeral resurfacing arthroplasty in patients younger than 55 years, significant improvement was reported in pain relief and functional outcomes at short-term follow-up (mean, 38 months).[21] Thirty-five of 36 patients reported satisfactory outcomes and had returned to their desired level of activity. Longer follow-up is needed to determine the durability and implant survivorship in a young patient population with high functional demands.[21]

Hemiarthroplasty With Nonprosthetic Glenoid Arthroplasty

In 2004, Weldon et al[23] first described nonprosthetic glenoid arthroplasty coupled with humeral hemiarthroplasty, also known as the "ream and run" procedure. The procedure involves humeral hemiarthroplasty performed in conjunction with concentric, spherical reaming of the glenoid subchondral bone.[24,25] The premise for this procedure was based on a canine study that was performed to characterize the healing response of the glenoid after spherical reaming and prosthetic humeral head replacement. Histologic results showed a consistent, contoured, fibrocartilaginous interface articulating with the humeral prosthesis.[26] A recent cadaver study confirmed that spherical, concentric reaming of the glenoid could restore shoulder stability to a level equivalent to that of glenoid resurfacing with a polyethylene component.[23]

In a recent case-matched control study of 35 patients, Clinton et al[24] compared the functional outcomes of hemiarthroplasty with nonprosthetic glenoid arthroplasty and conventional TSA in patients with a mean age of 56 years. Those treated with TSA showed significantly better improvement at 12 months postoperatively; however, no significant difference was reported between the two groups at 2-year follow-up. The authors attributed the delay in functional recovery to the time required for healing and remodeling of the reamed glenoid bone.

At short-term follow-up (mean, 3 years), 32 shoulders (91%) showed significant improvement in shoulder comfort and function after hemiarthroplasty with concentric glenoid reaming.[25] Twenty-two shoulders (63%) showed regenerated joint space as seen by radiographic lucency between the humeral prosthesis and the reamed glenoid bone at final follow-up. Functional outcome was significantly greater for patients with regenerated joint space ($P < 0.017$). Although early results are promising for hemiarthroplasty with concentric glenoid reaming, long-term studies are needed to evaluate the efficacy and durability of this procedure.

Hemiarthroplasty With Biologic Resurfacing of the Glenoid

Biologic glenoid resurfacing in conjunction with prosthetic humeral head replacement has been described using anterior glenohumeral capsule, autogenous fascia lata, Achilles tendon allograft, and meniscal allograft.[1-4,27] Krishnan et al[4] analyzed the results of 2- to 15-year outcomes of humeral hemiarthroplasty with biologic resurfacing in patients with a mean age of 51 years (range, 30 to 75 years). Anterior capsule, autogenous fascia lata, and Achilles tendon allograft were used as resurfacing substrate. Significant improvement was reported in function and relief of pain, with 29 patients (85%) returning to their premorbid level of activity. The authors concluded that autogenous tissue was not the optimal resurfacing tissue because of unsatisfactory results in 5 of 18 shoulders (28%). Of concern, radiographs indicated that overall glenoid erosion averaged 7.2 mm (range, 3 to 9 mm); however, this erosion appeared to stabilize at 5 years in patients with longer radiographic follow-up. In contrast to this study, Elhassan et al[28] evaluated the results of soft-tissue interposition arthroplasty in active patients with a mean age of 34 years. The results were uniformly poor, with an overall failure rate of 92% (12 of 13 patients) at 48-month follow-up. Complete loss of joint space was reported in 11 patients (85%), with 10 of these patients requiring revision TSA (77% revision rate).

In a recent study, Nicholson et al[27] reported favorable preliminary results (mean follow-up of 18 months) of lateral meniscal allograft resurfacing of the glenoid with hemiarthroplasty in young patients with a mean age of 42 years. Radiographic analysis at 1 year showed no significant decrease in the glenohumeral joint space and no erosion of the glenoid.

With longer follow-up (2 to 5 years) in a similar cohort of patients with a mean age of 43 years, Wirth[3] reported comparable results with significant pain relief, improved function, glenohumeral stability, and absence of glenoid erosion (**Figures 2** and **3**). These findings were particularly significant because a large multicenter clinical trial showed that humeral head subluxation and glenoid erosion had an adverse effect on the outcome of TSA[29] (**Figure 4**). In contrast to the study by Nicholson et al,[27] a progressive decrease in glenohumeral joint space was reported radiographically, ranging from a mean of 3.5 mm postoperatively to a mean of 1.7 mm at most recent follow-up (51% decrease). Some of the cited potential benefits of meniscal allograft compared to other means of glenoid resurfacing include the compliance of the lateral meniscus and the concavity of the superior surface, which complements the convex surface of the prosthetic humeral head; the short-term results of meniscal allograft transplantation in the knee, which indicate a reduction in pain and increased function, even in patients with pain and swelling caused by early arthritis; and the load-bearing function of the lateral meniscus, which has been studied extensively in the knee and more recently in the shoulder. The effect of a lateral meniscal allograft on

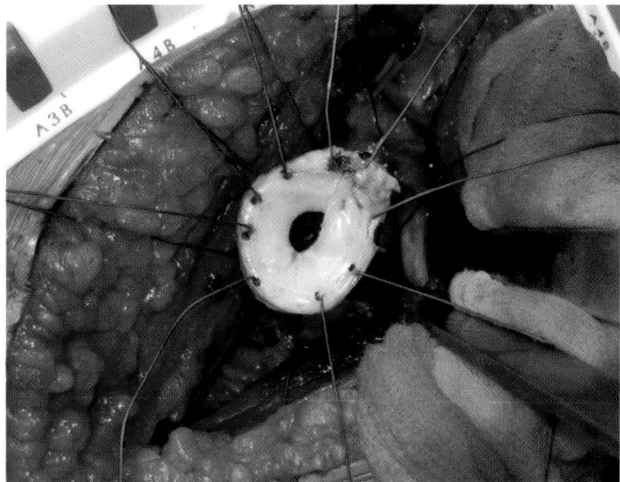

Figure 2 The lateral meniscus is suspended anterior to the glenohumeral joint before sliding the allograft to the glenoid articular surface. (Reproduced with permission from Wirth MA: Humeral head arthroplasty and meniscal allograft resurfacing of the glenoid. *J Bone Joint Surg Am* 2009;91(5):1109-1119.)

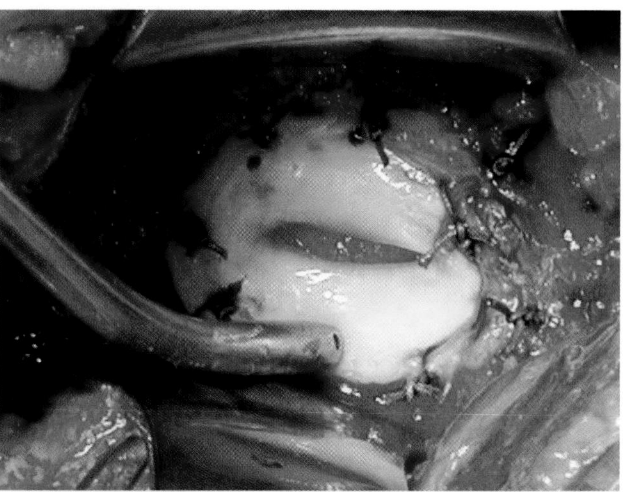

Figure 3 Intraoperative photograph showing a fixated meniscal allograft. (Reproduced with permission from Wirth MA: Humeral head arthroplasty and meniscal allograft resurfacing of the glenoid. *J Bone Joint Surg Am* 2009;91(5):1109-1119.)

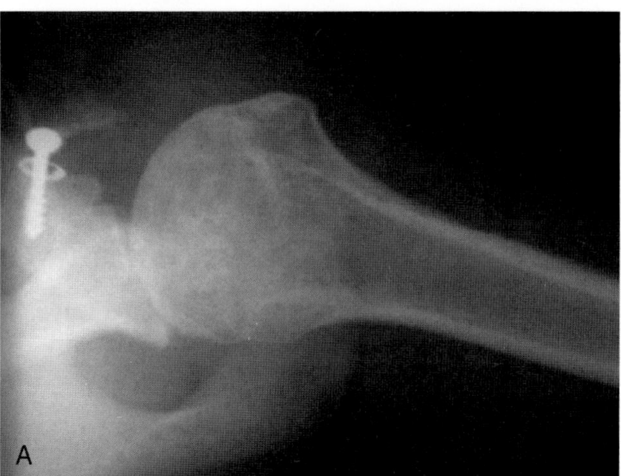

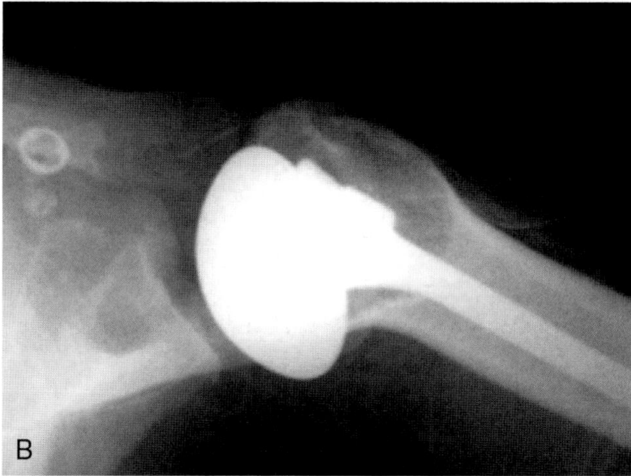

Figure 4 Comparison of preoperative (**A**) and postoperative (**B**) axillary radiographs of the shoulder of a patient with glenohumeral arthropathy shows the postoperative gain in glenohumeral joint space and glenohumeral registry after hemiarthroplasty and meniscal allograft resurfacing. (Reproduced with permission from Wirth MA: Humeral head arthroplasty and meniscal allograft resurfacing of the glenoid. *J Bone Joint Surg Am* 2009;91(5):1109-1119.)

the shoulder articular contact area and pressures was evaluated by Creighton et al[30] in a fresh-frozen cadaver model. The specimens that had a lateral meniscal allograft showed a substantial decrease in total force and glenoid contact area, which suggests that a meniscal allograft may decrease both pain and progression of glenoid arthritis.

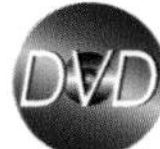

Video 9.1: Humeral Head Replacement Arthroplasty and Meniscal Allograft Resurfacing of the Glenoid in Young Patients. Michael A. Wirth, MD (13 min)

Summary

Patients younger than 55 years with degenerative conditions of the glenohumeral joint represent a unique population of individuals being treated with shoulder arthroplasty. Higher levels of activity and an increased life expectancy put these patients at increased risks for midterm and long-term complications. At the present time, the literature shows inferior functional results with TSA and hemiarthroplasty in these patients; however, more promising results have been reported at midterm follow-up with TSA when the diagnosis was limited to primary glenohumeral arthritis. Also, glenoid component loosening and polyethylene wear remain a long-term concern. Alternative treatment methods to TSA, including humeral head resurfacing, hemiarthroplasty with nonprosthetic glenoid arthroplasty, and hemiarthroplasty with biologic resurfacing, have shown favorable results in most studies. Nonetheless, longitudinal follow-up and randomized, prospective controlled studies are needed to determine the durability and effectiveness of these procedures.

References

1. Burkhead WZ Jr, Hutton KS: Biologic resurfacing of the glenoid with hemiarthroplasty of the shoulder. *J Shoulder Elbow Surg* 1995;4(4):263-270.
2. Ball C, Galatz L, Yamaguchi K: Meniscal allograft interposition arthroplasty for the arthritic shoulder: Description of a new technique. *Tech Shoulder Elbow Surg* 2001;2:247-254.
3. Wirth MA: Humeral head arthroplasty and meniscal allograft resurfacing of the glenoid. *J Bone Joint Surg Am* 2009;91(5):1109-1119.
4. Krishnan SG, Nowinski RJ, Harrison D, Burkhead WZ Jr: Humeral hemiarthroplasty with biologic resurfacing of the glenoid for glenohumeral arthritis: Two to fifteen-year outcomes. *J Bone Joint Surg Am* 2007;89(4):727-734.
5. Sperling JW, Antuna SA, Sanchez-Sotelo J, Schleck C, Cofield RH: Shoulder arthroplasty for arthritis after instability surgery. *J Bone Joint Surg Am* 2002; 84-A(10):1775-1781.
6. Matsen FA III, Rockwood CA Jr, Wirth MA, Lippitt SB, Parsons IM: Glenohumeral arthritis and its management, in Rockwood CA Jr, Matsen FA III, Wirth MA, Lippitt SB, eds: *The Shoulder*, ed 3. Philadelphia, PA, WB Saunders, 2004, pp 879-1008.
7. Visotsky JL, Basamania C, Seebauer L, Rockwood CA Jr, Jensen KL: Cuff tear arthropathy: Pathogenesis, classification, and algorithm for treatment. *J Bone Joint Surg Am* 2004;86-A(Suppl 2):35-40.
8. Pearl ML, Romeo AA, Wirth MA, Yamaguchi K, Nicholson GP, Creighton RA: Decision making in contemporary shoulder arthroplasty. *Instr Course Lect* 2005;54: 69-85.
9. Klimkiewicz JJ, Iannotti JP, Rubash HE, Shanbhag AS: Aseptic loosening of the humeral component in total shoulder arthroplasty. *J Shoulder Elbow Surg* 1998;7(4):422-426.
10. Gartsman GM, Roddey TS, Hammerman SM: Shoulder arthroplasty with or without resurfacing of the glenoid in patients who have osteoarthritis. *J Bone Joint Surg Am* 2000;82(1):26-34.
11. Sperling JW, Cofield RH, Rowland CM: Neer hemiarthroplasty and Neer total shoulder arthroplasty in patients fifty years old or less: Long-term results. *J Bone Joint Surg Am* 1998;80(4): 464-473.
12. Levine WN, Djurasovic M, Glasson JM, Pollock RG, Flatow EL, Bigliani LU: Hemiarthroplasty for glenohumeral osteoarthritis: Results correlated to degree of glenoid wear. *J Shoulder Elbow Surg* 1997;6(5):449-454.
13. Bohsali KI, Wirth MA, Rockwood CA Jr: Complications of total shoulder arthroplasty. *J Bone Joint Surg Am* 2006;88(10):2279-2292.
14. Edwards TB, Kadakia NR, Boulahia A, et al: A comparison of hemiarthroplasty and total shoulder arthroplasty in the treatment of primary glenohumeral osteoarthritis: Results of a multicenter study. *J Shoulder Elbow Surg* 2003;12(3):207-213.
15. Bishop JY, Flatow EL: Humeral head replacement versus total shoulder arthroplasty: Clinical outcomes. A review. *J Shoulder Elbow Surg* 2005;14(1, Suppl S): 141S-146S.
16. Bryant D, Litchfield R, Sandow M, Gartsman GM, Guyatt G, Kirkley A: A comparison of pain, strength, range of motion, and functional outcomes after hemiarthroplasty and total shoulder arthroplasty in patients with osteoarthritis of the shoulder: A systematic review and meta-analysis. *J Bone Joint Surg Am* 2005;87(9):1947-1956.
17. Sperling JW, Cofield RH, Rowland CM: Minimum fifteen-year follow-up of Neer hemiarthroplasty and total shoulder arthroplasty in patients aged fifty years or younger. *J Shoulder Elbow Surg* 2004;13(6):604-613.
18. Burroughs PL, Gearen PF, Petty WR, Wright TW: Shoulder arthroplasty in the young patient. *J Arthroplasty* 2003;18(6): 792-798.
19. Parsons IM IV, Buoncristiani AM, Donion S, Campbell B, Smith KL, Matsen FA III: The effect of total shoulder arthroplasty on self-assessed deficits in shoulder function in patients with capsulorrhaphy arthropathy. *J Shoulder Elbow Surg* 2007;16(3, Suppl):S19-S26.
20. Raiss P, Aldinger PR, Kasten P, Rickert M, Loew M: Total shoulder replacement in young and middle-aged patients with glenohumeral osteoarthritis. *J Bone Joint Surg Br* 2008;90(6): 764-769.

21. Bailie DS, Llinas PJ, Ellenbecker TS: Cementless humeral resurfacing arthroplasty in active patients less than fifty-five years of age. *J Bone Joint Surg Am* 2008; 90(1):110-117.

22. Burgess DL, McGrath MS, Bonutti PM, Marker DR, Delanois RE, Mont MA: Shoulder resurfacing. *J Bone Joint Surg Am* 2009;91(5):1228-1238.

23. Weldon EJ III, Boorman RS, Smith KL, Matsen FA III: Optimizing the glenoid contribution to the stability of a humeral hemiarthroplasty without a prosthetic glenoid. *J Bone Joint Surg Am* 2004;86-A(9):2022-2029.

24. Clinton J, Franta AK, Lenters TR, Mounce D, Matsen FA III: Nonprosthetic glenoid arthroplasty with humeral hemiarthroplasty and total shoulder arthroplasty yield similar self-assessed outcomes in the management of comparable patients with glenohumeral arthritis. *J Shoulder Elbow Surg* 2007;16(5):534-538.

25. Lynch JR, Franta AK, Montgomery WH Jr, Lenters TR, Mounce D, Matsen FA III: Self-assessed outcome at two to four years after shoulder hemiarthroplasty with concentric glenoid reaming. *J Bone Joint Surg Am* 2007;89(6):1284-1292.

26. Matsen FA III, Clark JM, Titelman RM, et al: Healing of reamed glenoid bone articulating with a metal humeral hemiarthroplasty: A canine model. *J Orthop Res* 2005;23(1):18-26.

27. Nicholson GP, Goldstein JL, Romeo AA, et al: Lateral meniscus allograft biologic glenoid arthroplasty in total shoulder arthroplasty for young shoulders with degenerative joint disease. *J Shoulder Elbow Surg* 2007;16:S261-S266.

28. Elhassan B, Ozbaydar M, Diller D, Higgins LD, Warner JJ: Soft-tissue resurfacing of the glenoid in the treatment of glenohumeral arthritis in active patients less than fifty years old. *J Bone Joint Surg Am* 2009;91(2):419-424.

29. Iannotti JP, Norris TR: Influence of preoperative factors on outcome of shoulder arthroplasty for glenohumeral osteoarthritis. *J Bone Joint Surg Am* 2003; 85-A(2):251-258.

30. Creighton RA, Cole BJ, Nicholson GP, Romeo AA, Lorenz EP: Effect of lateral meniscus allograft on shoulder articular contact areas and pressures. *J Shoulder Elbow Surg* 2007;16(3):367-372.

Video Reference

9.1: Wirth MA: Video. Humeral head replacement arthroplasty and meniscal allograft resurfacing of the glenoid in young patients, in Green A, Blaine TA, eds: *Surgical Techniques in Orthopaedics: Total Shoulder Arthroplasty,* ed 2. DVD. Rosemont, IL, American Academy of Orthopaedic Surgeons, 2009.

Arthroplasty for Fractures of the Proximal Part of the Humerus

James E. Voos, MD
Joshua S. Dines, MD
David M. Dines, MD

Abstract

Proximal humeral fractures account for 4% to 5% of all fractures. Most of these fractures are nondisplaced or minimally displaced and amenable to nonsurgical treatment or open reduction and internal fixation. Complex proximal humeral fractures with displaced three- and four-part fragments, fracture-dislocations, and humeral head splits are more difficult to treat. In older patients, hemiarthroplasty or reverse shoulder arthroplasty is often the indicated treatment. Arthroplasty in this patient cohort is very technique-dependent and relies on preserving deltoid function, proper component placement and fixation, and tuberosity healing. Complications include tuberosity nonunion, instability, heterotopic ossification, and infection. Although pain relief is predictable, it is often difficult to achieve functional improvement. Results depend on the patient's age, timing of the surgery, tuberosity healing, and adequate rehabilitation. Recently, successful outcomes for reverse total shoulder arthroplasty have been reported in older, low-demand patients with cuff deficiency, deficient bone in the tuberosity, or compromised healing of the tuberosity.

Instr Course Lect 2011;60:105-112.

Proximal humeral fractures represent nearly 50% of all shoulder girdle injuries, and the incidence has been increasing in the elderly population in recent decades.[1-4] Overall, proximal humeral fractures account for 4% to 5% of all fractures.[5] Most of these fractures occur in women as the result of a low-impact fall, although high-velocity trauma is often involved in younger patients.[1,6] Most proximal humeral fractures are either nondisplaced or minimally displaced and do not require surgical treatment.[7,8] The treatment of displaced fractures presents a more difficult challenge. Complex displaced three- and four-part fractures, fracture-dislocations, and fractures with a humeral head split are at risk for the development of malunion and osteonecrosis, especially after internal fixation.[9-12] Shoulder hemiarthroplasty or, recently, reverse total shoulder arthroplasty is indicated for the treatment of some of these complex fractures. Strict attention to preoperative planning and surgical technique are paramount for a successful outcome and to avoid complications.

Patient Assessment

History and Physical Examination

It is important to obtain a thorough history to determine the mechanism of injury and any concomitant injuries that may have occurred during the trauma. Head injuries are common in elderly patients after a fall. An

Dr. J.S. Dines or an immediate family member has received royalties from Biomet; is a member of a speakers' bureau or has made paid presentations on behalf of Arthrex; and serves as a paid consultant to or is an employee of Biomimetic and Tornier. Dr. D.M. Dines or an immediate family member serves as a board member, owner, officer, or committee member of the American Shoulder and Elbow Surgeons; has received royalties from Biomet and Biomimetic; serves as a paid consultant to or is an employee of Biomet, Biomimetic, and Tornier; has received research or institutional support from Biomet and Biomimetic; owns stock or stock options in Biomimetic; and has received nonincome support (such as equipment or services), commercially derived honoraria, or other non–research-related funding (such as paid travel) from Biomet. Neither Dr. Voos nor any immediate family member has received anything of value from or owns stock in a commercial company or institution related directly or indirectly to the subject of this chapter.

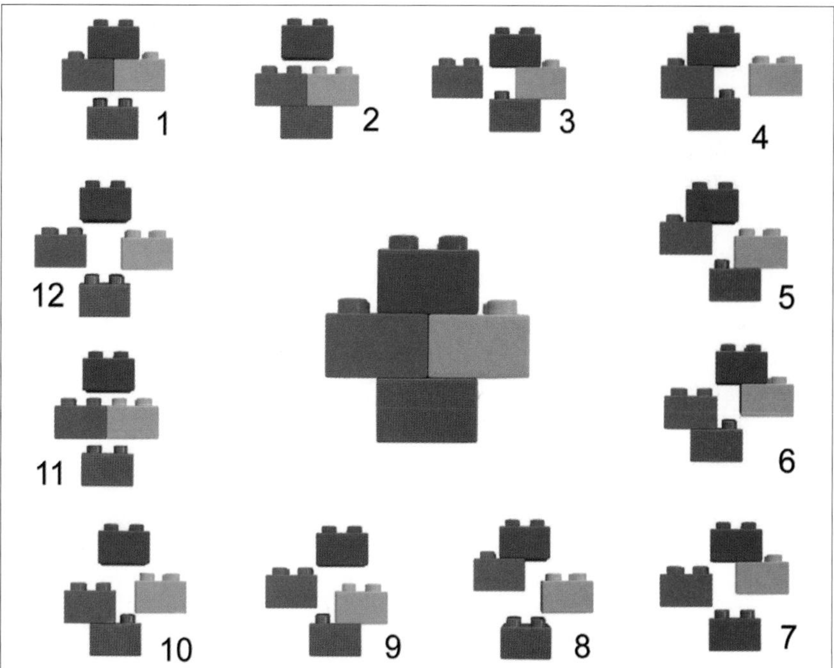

Figure 1 Binary (LEGO) description system for proximal humeral fractures as developed by Hertel et al.[14] Each LEGO segment represents the humeral head (red), the humeral shaft (green), the lesser tuberosity (yellow), or the greater tuberosity (blue). Five basic fracture planes are possible, which result in 12 basic fracture patterns as shown here. (Reprinted with permission from Elsevier from Hertel R, Hempfing A, Stiehler M, Leunig M: Predictors of humeral head ischemia after intracapsular fracture of the proximal humerus. *J Shoulder Elbow Surg* 2004;13:427-433.)

assessment to determine if there are cardiac or neurologic reasons for the fall and to detect any additional fractures can be performed at the initial evaluation. Inquiry about the patient's preinjury shoulder function and comorbidities provides valuable information that may impact the surgical procedure or postoperative rehabilitation. Important additional information includes any history of a fracture, rotator cuff deficiency, limited walking ability, and the presence of osteoporosis.

The physical examination often reveals a swollen shoulder, which may have extensive ecchymosis extending to the elbow. Shoulder motion is painful, and crepitus from the fracture fragments may be noted on gentle manipulation of the shoulder. Documentation of neurovascular status is important, as axillary nerve injuries are common.

Radiographic Assessment

Standard radiographs include an AP view of the shoulder, a transscapular Y view, and an axillary view. AP and lateral views of the entire humerus and elbow may provide additional information about the full extent of the injury if a more extensive injury is clinically suspected. In most instances, these plain radiographs are sufficient to classify the fracture pattern. When there is uncertainty about whether the fracture is displaced, bone quality is poor, or there is extensive comminution, CT with three-dimensional reconstructions can help to further define the fracture configuration. A head-splitting or articular component can also be detected with CT. A full-length view of the contralateral humerus is used to template the proper height and length of the implants when arthroplasty options are considered. In some instances of severe proximal comminution, scanograms facilitate surgical planning and the determination of proper humeral length.

Fracture Classification

The fracture pattern and its relationship to the humeral head blood supply are important for determining treatment and predicting the risk of osteonecrosis.[13-15] The Neer[7] and AO/ASIF[16] classifications are the systems most commonly used for the radiographic evaluation of proximal humeral fractures. The Neer classification is based on the number of fracture parts (with displacement of > 1 cm or angulation of > 45°), the direction of dislocation, and the involvement of the articular surface.[7,8] The AO/ASIF classification system for proximal humeral fractures broadly groups fractures on the basis of the degree of articular involvement and the potential for humeral head ischemia.[16] Recently, Hertel et al[14] developed a binary description system (LEGO; LEGO Systems, Enfield, CT) as shown in **Figure 1**. In this system, the most relevant predictors of ischemia were the length of the dorsomedial metaphyseal extension, the integrity of the medial hinge, and the basic fracture type as determined with the binary description system. Although this system provides guidance for precise fracture description, the Neer classification is still used because of its widespread use throughout the literature and its simplicity.

Indications for Arthroplasty

Hemiarthroplasty and reverse total shoulder arthroplasty are indicated in patients who are medically stable, can

Table 1
Indications for Hemiarthroplasty and Reverse Total Shoulder Arthroplasty for Proximal Humeral Fractures

Hemiarthroplasty	Reverse Total Shoulder Arthroplasty
Displaced three- and four-part fractures	Age > 70 years
Age > 70 years	Low functional demands
Severe osteoporosis	Cuff tear arthropathy/massive rotator cuff tear with fatty atrophy
Humeral head osteonecrosis	Severe osteoporosis
Motivated patient	Irreparable tuberosity fractures
Failure to maintain open reduction and internal fixation/malunion	Failed hemiarthroplasty
Head-splitting fracture	Comorbidities that prohibit tuberosity healing
Fracture-dislocation	Chronic fracture

tolerate extensive surgery, and are able to participate in a postoperative rehabilitation program. In young patients with a displaced proximal humeral fracture and some patients with an impacted four-part valgus fracture, an attempt at open reduction and internal fixation is indicated to try to avoid prosthetic replacement and its potential complications.[8,17-21] Even if osteonecrosis or nonunion does occur in these fractures, the tuberosities may be better positioned for conversion to a prosthesis.[22]

Indications for hemiarthroplasty include displaced three- and four-part fractures (according to the Neer classification) not amenable to open reduction and internal fixation, fracture-dislocations, and head-splitting fracture patterns[7,12,17,18,22-25] (**Figure 2**). Severely osteoporotic bone, a failure to maintain open reduction and internal fixation, and osteonecrosis are also indications (**Table 1**). Krishnan et al[2] outlined four factors guiding the choice of treatment: age, bone quality, fracture pattern, and timing of the surgery. Patients older than 70 years are candidates for arthroplasty,[2,12,22] but it is important to note that chronologic age is not an indication in itself. Patient activity level, the presence of osteoporosis, and the fracture pattern are of greater importance.

Although hemiarthroplasty is the procedure of choice in most patients, indications for reverse total shoulder arthroplasty include age older than 70 years combined with low demands, a fracture with severe tuberosity and metaphyseal comminution, severe osteoporosis, cuff tear arthropathy or fatty infiltration of a massive rotator cuff tear, a failed hemiarthroplasty, and comorbidities that would affect tuberosity healing[22,26,27] (**Table 1**). Arthroplasty is contraindicated for patients who cannot undergo surgery because they are medically unstable, are young and active, or have infection or axillary nerve palsy.

Surgical Technique

After proper induction of anesthesia, the patient is placed in the beach chair position with the head of the bed elevated approximately 40° to 45°. The patient is shifted to the side of the table so that the freely draped arm that is to be operated on can be extended while it is at the patient's side. An extended deltopectoral exposure is used, and the subdeltoid space is exposed.

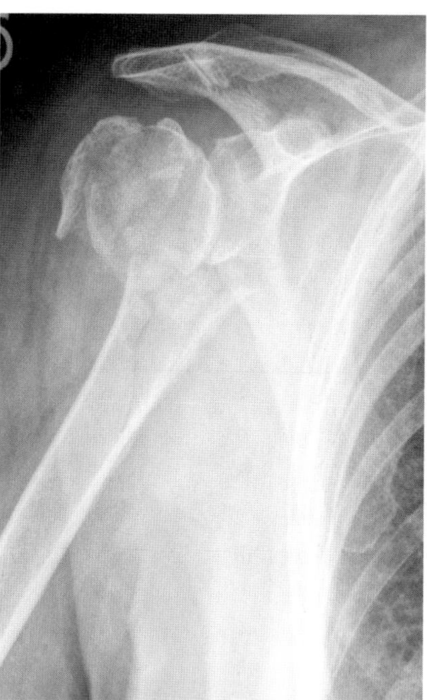

Figure 2 AP radiograph showing a four-part proximal humeral fracture. There are displacements of the greater tuberosity, the lesser tuberosity, the humeral shaft, and the humeral head exceeding 1 cm.

The distal portion of the bicipital groove is a critical landmark to identify. From there, assessment of the fracture pattern can begin; it often occurs less than 1 cm posterior to the groove. An osteotome or a periosteal elevator is used to separate the tuberosities and the humeral head, which is then excised. The greater and lesser tuberosities are tagged with heavy sutures at the bone-tendon interface. Three or four sutures are placed in the greater tuberosity to be used later for the reconstruction.

Next, the humeral canal is exposed and prepared with sequential reaming. Then either an intramedullary or an extramedullary positioning device is placed. This chapter's authors often use an intramedullary device at this point to ensure that the component is at the proper height.[28] The correct height can also be determined by using preoperative radiographs, and the

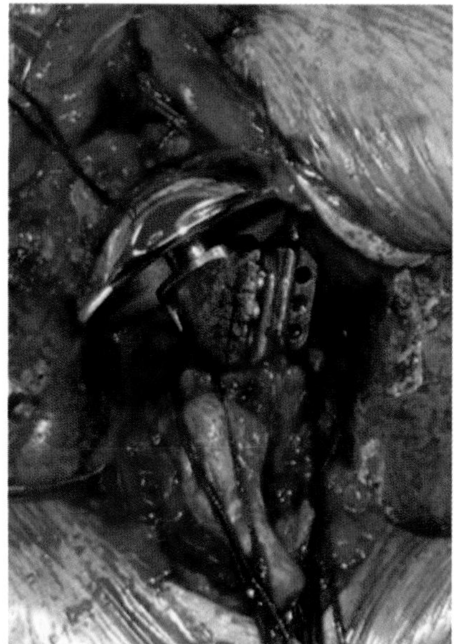

Figure 3 Intraoperative photograph of a left shoulder with the humeral stem in place. The calibrated measurement lines on the implant have been used to achieve the proper height.

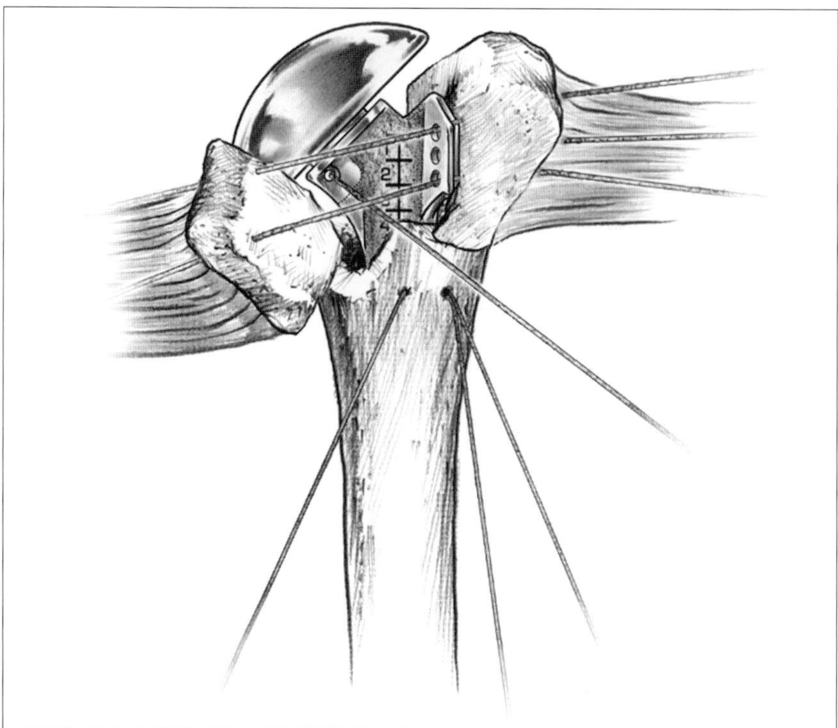

Figure 4 A diagram of the left shoulder depicting the proper suture configuration for tuberosity reconstruction to the humeral shaft and implant. The sutures are placed through the greater tuberosity and the fin of the implant. The sutures are then passed through the lesser tuberosity, and both tuberosities are reduced to the implant and the humeral shaft. The sutures that have been placed through drill holes in the humeral shaft are then tied over the top in a figure-of-8 fashion. (Reprinted with permission from Abrutyn DA, Dines DM: Secure tuberosity fixation in shoulder arthroplasty for fractures. *Tech Shoulder Elbow Surg* 2004;5:177-183.)

measurements on the implant are used for proper placement of the component (**Figure 3**). Another described internal landmark is the distance between the top of the pectoralis major tendon and the top of the humeral head, which is 5.6 cm on average.[29]

Before the fracture-specific humeral component is cemented, anterolateral and posterolateral drill holes are created 1 to 1.5 cm distal to the fracture site in the humeral shaft. Sutures are placed through these holes before cementing, to be used later in the tuberosity reconstruction. At this point, a fracture-specific humeral component of proper size is cemented in place at the predetermined height. The humeral head should be in 20° to 30° of retroversion in most cases. Boileau et al[30] showed that more than 40° of retroversion compromises tuberosity healing. After the humeral component is cemented in position, a closed reduction with the selected trial humeral head is performed. The head should translate 50% anteriorly, posteriorly, and inferiorly on the glenoid surface. There should be 160° of forward elevation and stable internal and external rotation of the arm.

The most critical portion of the procedure is tuberosity reconstruction.[31] The success of the surgery depends on the ability of the tuberosities to heal to themselves and to the humeral shaft in anatomic positions surrounding the implant. This involves both longitudinal and transverse fixation with use of the sutures that were previously placed through the tuberosities and the shaft (**Figure 4**). The greater tuberosity is secured to the shaft and the implant first, and this is followed by fixation of the lesser tuberosity.

The sutures through the greater tuberosity are brought around the proximal portion of the implant and through the slots in the implant fins. The middle sutures are then used for fixation of the greater tuberosity, while the top and bottom sutures are brought inside-out through the lesser tuberosity for later repair. The final humeral head component is placed after these sutures have been passed, and the tuberosity reconstruction commences.

The greater tuberosity is then placed against the anterior fin of the

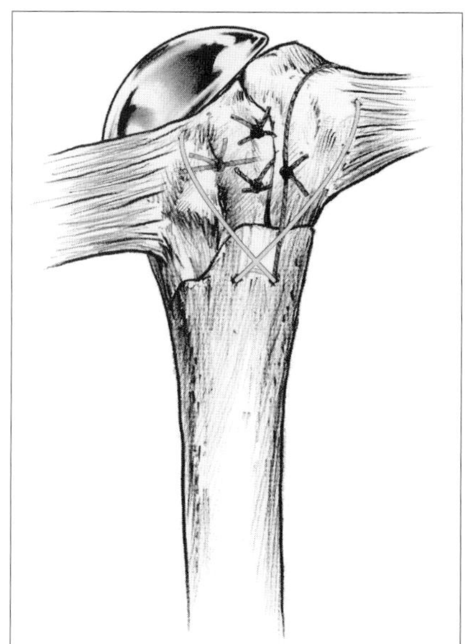

Figure 5 Diagram of the left shoulder depicting a completed tuberosity reconstruction. (Reprinted with permission from Abrutyn DA, Dines DM: Secure tuberosity fixation in shoulder arthroplasty for fractures. *Tech Shoulder Elbow Surg* 2004;5:177-183.)

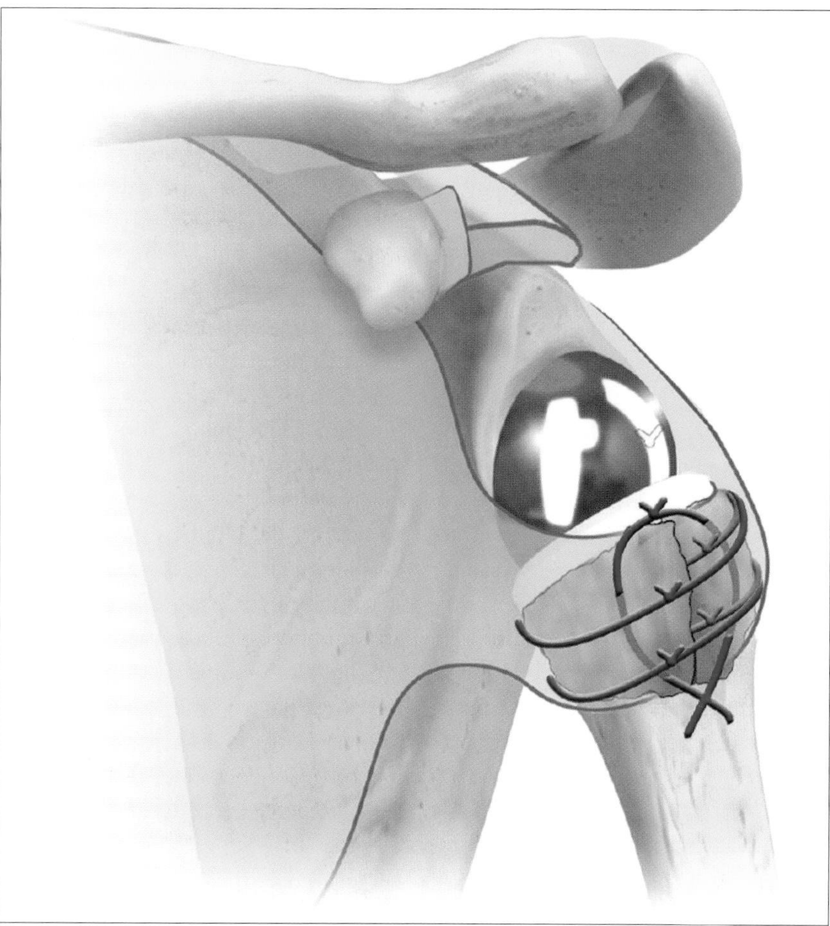

Figure 6 A diagram depicting tuberosity reconstruction around a reverse total shoulder prosthesis. In this figure, the supraspinatus is deficient. The subscapularis, connected to the lesser tuberosity, and the infraspinatus and teres minor, connected to the posterior portion of the greater tuberosity, have been repaired to the shaft. (Reprinted with permission from Sirveaux F, Navez G, Roche O, Molé D, Williams MD: Reverse prosthesis for proximal humerus fracture, technique and results. *Tech Shoulder Elbow Surg* 2008;9:15-22.)

implant, shingled over the humeral shaft, and fixed 0.5 cm distal to the top of the humeral head. The one or two middle sutures that had been previously placed transversely and the posterolateral shaft suture are securely tied in place. The lesser tuberosity is approximated to the greater tuberosity and fixed with the previously placed transverse sutures. Finally, the suture that was placed through the humeral shaft from front to back is now used as a figure-of-8 suture over the top of the tuberosities to secure the reconstruction (**Figure 5**).

The security of the repair is assessed with closed reduction and a range-of-motion trial. At this point, postoperative rehabilitation can be planned on the basis of the security of the reconstruction. A portable radiograph is obtained immediately postoperatively to confirm the implant and tuberosity positions.

The surgical technique for fracture treatment with a reverse total shoulder arthroplasty follows principles similar to those for a hemiarthroplasty regarding proper implant height and tuberosity fixation when possible[27] (**Figure 6**).

Postoperative Rehabilitation

The success of a hemiarthroplasty for fracture treatment depends on a proper rehabilitation program.[22,24] A sling is used for the first 4 to 6 weeks. A physician-directed program is begun immediately after surgery. Shoulder shrugs and elbow, wrist, and hand motion are begun in the hospital. Early pendulum exercises are performed with the shoulder in the sling. For the first 6 weeks, only passive range-of-motion exercises are performed with the aid of a therapist, and are defined by the parameters of stable external rotation and forward flexion achieved in the operating room. The goal during this period is to achieve 140° of elevation in the scapular plane and 30° of external rotation.[22] In patients with severe osteoporosis or tenuous tuberosity fixation, immobilization may be continued, and the regimen may be limited to passive range-of-motion exercises for a longer period. Active-assisted range-of-motion exercises are begun at 6 weeks if tuberosity healing is evident radiographically. Strengthening is begun at 8 to 12 weeks. The exercises should be continued for up to 1 year as improvement in function can be expected during that time.

After reverse total shoulder arthroplasty, the sling is worn for at least 6 weeks. Active rotation is avoided for the first 6 weeks to provide an environment conducive to tuberosity healing if a tuberosity repair has been performed. Passive motion, consisting of pendulum exercises only, is performed during this time period, and strengthening is delayed until 12 weeks postoperatively.[26,27]

Complications

Complications, including tuberosity nonunion, component malposition, instability, heterotopic ossification, rotator cuff failure, periprosthetic fracture, glenoid erosion, infection, and nerve injury, are common after hemiarthroplasties for fractures, and overall complication rates as high as 35% have been reported.[2,17,20,22,23,25,32,33] Although neurovascular complications have been reported, complications related to surgical technique are the most common causes of a poor result.

Kontakis et al[25] recently reviewed the results of 810 hemiarthroplasties performed primarily for acute four-part fractures. Complications associated with tuberosity healing were observed in 11% of the patients. The rate of heterotopic ossification was 9%, and the rate of proximal migration of the humeral head was 7%. The rates of superficial and deep infection were less than 2% and less than 1%, respectively.

Instability may result if the humeral component is placed too high or too low, resulting in secondary impingement or poor soft-tissue tension, respectively. Improper placement of the component in excessive anteversion or retroversion may lead to dislocation and tuberosity failure.[2,22,34]

Healing of the tuberosity to the humeral shaft as well as healing of the tuberosities to each other and to the prosthesis is critical for regaining rotator cuff function. The tuberosities must be placed below the top of the humeral head prosthesis to create a normal offset and restore deltoid tension.[22] Tuberosity placement above the head can result in impingement on the acromion.

Complication rates after reverse total shoulder arthroplasty for fracture treatment have been higher than those after reverse total shoulder arthroplasty for the treatment of cuff tear arthropathy.[27] Reported complications include dislocation, tuberosity nonunion, nerve injury, infection, reflex sympathetic dystrophy, scapular notching, proximal bone resorption, and glenoid loosening.[26,27,35]

Bufquin et al[35] reported an overall complication rate of 28% in a series of 43 patients treated with reverse total shoulder arthroplasty. Based on the knowledge of this chapter's authors, all studies thus far have included only short-term follow-up. These studies indicate that tuberosity reconstruction is critical for function after either type of arthroplasty for fracture treatment.

Results

The results of hemiarthroplasty for the treatment of complex proximal humeral fractures include good pain relief but varying outcomes with regard to function, motion, and strength.[2,17,22-25,33]

Bastian and Hertel[23] reported on 100 proximal humeral fractures treated with either open reduction and internal fixation (51 fractures; average patient age, 54 years) or hemiarthroplasty (49 fractures; average patient age, 66 years). They concluded that open reduction and internal fixation and hemiarthroplasty yield similar functional results and comparable patient satisfaction. Open reduction and internal fixation with preservation of the humeral head should be considered when an adequate reduction and stable conditions for revascularization can be obtained. Hemiarthroplasty is a viable alternative for patients with osteopenic bone and/or a comminuted fracture.

Kontakis et al[25] reported an average duration of follow-up of 3.7 years in their review of 16 studies with a total of 810 hemiarthroplasties for acute proximal humeral fractures in patients with an average age of 67.7 years. The mean active anterior elevation was 105.7°, the mean abduction was 92.4°, and the mean Constant score was 56 points. Most patients experienced no pain or only mild pain at the time of final follow-up, but marked limitations of function often persisted.

Krishnan et al[2] reported an average of 2 years of follow-up of 130 hemiarthroplasties for fractures reconstructed with the Gothic arch technique; 88% of the tuberosities healed anatomically. The mean active anterior elevation was 129°, and pain scores averaged 1.2 points on a 10-point scale.

Boileau et al[30] described the "unhappy triad," in which a prosthesis has excessive height and retroversion and the greater tuberosity is positioned too low. This combination of factors was frequently associated with poor functional results and persistent pain and stiffness.[30]

Studies have also shown that acute reconstruction (less than 4 weeks after the injury) results in better functional outcomes because of the ease of tuberosity reconstruction.[2,24,25]

Bufquin et al[35] reported the short-term follow-up results (at a mean of

22 months) of 43 reverse total shoulder arthroplasties performed for acute three- and four-part fractures. The average patient age was 78 years. At the time of the most recent follow-up, active anterior elevation averaged 97° and external rotation in abduction averaged 30°. The mean Constant and modified Constant scores were 44 points and 66%, respectively. The authors concluded that satisfactory mobility was obtained despite frequent migration of the tuberosities, and they cautioned that an assessment of long-term results is required before reverse shoulder arthroplasty can be recommended as a routine procedure for complex fractures of the proximal part of the humerus in elderly patients.

In a study of 45 patients treated with the Grammont reverse prosthesis, Boileau et al[36] reported that five of the patients were treated with arthroplasty because of fracture sequelae. Three patients reported that they were satisfied, and two stated that they were no better or worse. The authors concluded that, although the Grammont prosthesis offers a solution for severe fracture sequelae, the revision rates are higher than those in patients treated for cuff tear arthropathy.

On the basis of the current literature, arthroplasties for the treatment of complex proximal humeral fractures can be listed in descending order with regard to their clinical success as follows: (1) hemiarthroplasty in a patient with reconstructible tuberosities, (2) reverse total shoulder arthroplasty in a patient with reconstructible tuberosities, (3) reverse total shoulder arthroplasty in a patient without reconstructible tuberosities, and (4) hemiarthroplasty in a patient without reconstructible tuberosities.[27]

References

1. Court-Brown CM, Garg A, McQueen MM: The epidemiology of proximal humeral fractures. *Acta Orthop Scand* 2001;72(4): 365-371.
2. Krishnan SG, Bennion PW, Reineck JR, Burkhead WZ: Hemiarthroplasty for proximal humeral fracture: Restoration of the Gothic arch. *Orthop Clin North Am* 2008;39(4):441-450, vi.
3. Nordqvist A, Petersson CJ: Incidence and causes of shoulder girdle injuries in an urban population. *J Shoulder Elbow Surg* 1995; 4(2):107-112.
4. Palvanen M, Kannus P, Niemi S, Parkkari J: Update in the epidemiology of proximal humeral fractures. *Clin Orthop Relat Res* 2006; 442:87-92.
5. Green A, Norris T: Proximal humerus fractures and fracture dislocations, in Browner B, Jupiter J, Levine A, Trafton P, eds: *Skeletal Trauma: Basic Science, Management and Reconstruction*, ed 3. Philadelphia, PA, Saunders, 2003, pp 1532-1624.
6. Kannus P, Palvanen M, Niemi S, Sievänen H, Parkkari J: Rate of proximal humeral fractures in older Finnish women between 1970 and 2007. *Bone* 2009;44(4): 656-659.
7. Neer CS II: Displaced proximal humeral fractures: I. Classification and evaluation. *J Bone Joint Surg Am* 1970;52(6):1077-1089.
8. Nho SJ, Brophy RH, Barker JU, Cornell CN, MacGillivray JD: Innovations in the management of displaced proximal humerus fractures. *J Am Acad Orthop Surg* 2007;15(1):12-26.
9. Connor PM, Flatow EL: Complications of internal fixation of proximal humeral fractures. *Instr Course Lect* 1997;46:25-37.
10. Edelson G, Safuri H, Salami J, Vigder F, Militianu D: Natural history of complex fractures of the proximal humerus using a three-dimensional classification system. *J Shoulder Elbow Surg* 2008;17(3): 399-409.
11. Gerber C, Werner CM, Vienne P: Internal fixation of complex fractures of the proximal humerus. *J Bone Joint Surg Br* 2004;86(6): 848-855.
12. Hertel R: Fractures of the proximal humerus in osteoporotic bone. *Osteoporos Int* 2005; 16(Suppl 2):S65-S72.
13. Gerber C, Schneeberger AG, Vinh TS: The arterial vascularization of the humeral head: An anatomical study. *J Bone Joint Surg Am* 1990;72(10):1486-1494.
14. Hertel R, Hempfing A, Stiehler M, Leunig M: Predictors of humeral head ischemia after intracapsular fracture of the proximal humerus. *J Shoulder Elbow Surg* 2004;13(4):427-433.
15. Laing PG: The arterial supply of the adult humerus. *J Bone Joint Surg Am* 1956;38-A(5):1105-1116.
16. Müller ME: Appendix A: The comprehensive classification of fractures of long bones, in Müller ME, Allgöwer M, Schneider R, Willenegger H, eds: *Manual of Internal Fixation: Techniques Recommended by the AO-ASIF Group*, ed 3. Berlin, Germany, Springer, 1991, pp 118-125.
17. DeFranco MJ, Brems JJ, Williams GR Jr, Iannotti JP: Evaluation and management of valgus impacted four-part proximal humerus fractures. *Clin Orthop Relat Res* 2006;442:109-114.
18. Moeckel BH, Dines DM, Warren RF, Altchek DW: Modular hemiarthroplasty for fractures of the proximal part of the humerus. *J Bone Joint Surg Am* 1992;74(6): 884-889.
19. Ricchetti ET, DeMola PM, Roman D, Abboud JA: The use of precontoured humeral locking plates in the management of dis-

placed proximal humerus fracture. *J Am Acad Orthop Surg* 2009; 17(9): 582-590.

20. Sperling JW, Cuomo F, Hill JD, Hertel R, Chuinard C, Boileau P: The difficult proximal humerus fracture: Tips and techniques to avoid complications and improve results. *Instr Course Lect* 2007;56: 45-57.
21. Thanasas C, Kontakis G, Angoules A, Limb D, Giannoudis P: Treatment of proximal humerus fractures with locking plates: A systematic review. *J Shoulder Elbow Surg* 2009;18(6):837-844.
22. Dines DM, Warren RF: Arthroplasty for proximal humerus fractures, in Dines DM, Lorich DG, Helfet DL, eds: *Solutions for Complex Upper Extremity Trauma.* New York, NY, Thieme, 2008, pp 79-87.
23. Bastian JD, Hertel R: Osteosynthesis and hemiarthroplasty of fractures of the proximal humerus: Outcomes in a consecutive case series. *J Shoulder Elbow Surg* 2009;18(2):216-219.
24. Dines DM, Warren RF: Modular shoulder hemiarthroplasty for acute fractures: Surgical considerations. *Clin Orthop Relat Res* 1994;307(307):18-26.
25. Kontakis G, Koutras C, Tosounidis T, Giannoudis P: Early management of proximal humeral fractures with hemiarthroplasty: A systematic review. *J Bone Joint Surg Br* 2008;90(11): 1407-1413.
26. Frankle MA, Chacon-Balados A, Cuff D: Reverse shoulder prosthesis for acute and chronic fractures, in Dines DM, Laurencin CT, Williams GR, eds: *Arthritis and Arthroplasty: The Shoulder.* Philadelphia, PA, Saunders, 2009, pp 218-231.
27. Sirveaux F, Navez G, Roche O, Molé D, Williams MD: Reverse prosthesis for proximal humerus fracture, technique and results. *Tech Shoulder Elbow Surg* 2008;9: 15-22.
28. Dines DM, Warren RF, Craig EV, Lee D, Dines JS: Intramedullary fracture positioning sleeve for proper placement of hemiarthroplasty in fractures of the proximal humerus. *Tech Shoulder Elbow Surg* 2007;8:69-74.
29. Murachovsky J, Ikemoto RY, Nascimento LG, Fujiki EN, Milani C, Warner JJ: Pectoralis major tendon reference (PMT): A new method for accurate restoration of humeral length with hemiarthroplasty for fracture. *J Shoulder Elbow Surg* 2006;15(6): 675-678.
30. Boileau P, Walch G, Krishnan SG: Tuberosity osteosynthesis and hemiarthroplasty for four-part fractures of the proximal humerus. *Tech Shoulder Elbow Surg* 2000;1:96-109.
31. Abrutyn DA, Dines DM: Secure tuberosity fixation in shoulder arthroplasty for fractures. *Tech Shoulder Elbow Surg* 2004;5: 177-183.
32. Zuckerman JD, Cuomo F, Koval KJ: Proximal humeral replacement for complex fractures: Indications and surgical technique. *Instr Course Lect* 1997;46: 7-14.
33. Tanner MW, Cofield RH: Prosthetic arthroplasty for fractures and fracture-dislocations of the proximal humerus. *Clin Orthop Relat Res* 1983;179(179):116-128.
34. Hempfing A, Leunig M, Ballmer FT, Hertel R: Surgical landmarks to determine humeral head retrotorsion for hemiarthroplasty in fractures. *J Shoulder Elbow Surg* 2001;10(5):460-463.
35. Bufquin T, Hersan A, Hubert L, Massin P: Reverse shoulder arthroplasty for the treatment of three- and four-part fractures of the proximal humerus in the elderly: A prospective review of 43 cases with a short-term follow-up. *J Bone Joint Surg Br* 2007; 89(4): 516-520.
36. Boileau P, Watkinson D, Hatzidakis AM, Hovorka I: The Grammont reverse shoulder prosthesis: Results in cuff tear arthritis, fracture sequelae, and revision arthroplasty. *J Shoulder Elbow Surg* 2006;15(5):527-540.

Shoulder Arthroplasty for the Treatment of Rotator Cuff Insufficiency

Jon J.P. Warner, MD
Anup Shah, MD

Abstract

Irreparable rotator cuff tendon tears result from chronic tears, failed cuff repairs, and fracture sequelae and occur in patients with rheumatoid arthritis. The management of patients with cuff tear arthropathy can be challenging. When pain is severe and function is poor, surgical options include hemiarthroplasty, bipolar arthroplasty, extended head arthroplasty, arthroplasty with tendon transfer, reverse shoulder arthroplasty, and fusion. A review of the literature shows good pain relief with hemiarthroplasty in carefully selected patients; however, the reverse prosthesis has been found to better restore motion in patients with pseudoparalysis, failed fracture treatment, or a failed prosthesis.

Instr Course Lect 2011;60:113-121.

Irreparable rotator cuff tendon tears may occur in the setting of chronic tears with or without prior surgery, fracture sequelae, and in patients with rheumatoid arthritis. When chronic irreparable rotator cuff tears are associated with progressive glenohumeral joint deterioration, characteristic changes include static superior displacement of the humeral head combined with superior glenoid erosion. These changes have been termed rotator cuff tear arthropathy. Pain typically results, along with superior humeral head migration and deltoid retraction. These scenarios usually do not respond to conservative treatment with physical therapy and anti-inflammatory medications. When poor function and severe pain are chronic and refractory, various surgical options are available, including hemiarthroplasty, bipolar arthroplasty, extended head arthroplasty (or cuff tear arthropathy head), arthroplasty with tendon transfer, reverse shoulder arthroplasty, or fusion.

Pathophysiology of Cuff Tear Arthropathy

The rotator cuff muscles provide dynamic stabilization of the glenohumeral joint through a mechanism called concavity compression, which is the result of a force couple balance between the anterior and posterior rotator cuff muscles and the superior rotator cuff and deltoid.[1-3] The role of the biceps as a joint stabilizer is still controversial. In most of these patients, a torn biceps tendon is part of the pathology; however, at the current time, the preponderance of evidence favors the conclusion that the long head of the biceps tendon plays no role in stabilizing the humeral head in the glenoid in patients with massive rotator cuff tears.[4] Most surgeons believe that if the long head of the biceps is present, it acts as a source of pain that can be relieved through either tenotomy or tenodesis.[5,6]

Loss of humeral head containment and superior migration occurs when the anteroposterior force couple of the infraspinatus and subscapularis tendons is disrupted (**Figure 1**). When these cuff muscles are involved, the proximal pull of the deltoid is unopposed, resulting in eventual progressive superior displacement of the humeral head. Superior glenoid erosion and possibly acromial erosion may eventually develop. The acromioclavicular

Dr. Warner or an immediate family member has received royalties from Zimmer; and has received research or institutional support from Aircast (DJ), Arthrex, Mitek, Smith & Nephew, and Arthrocare. Neither Dr. Shah nor any immediate family member has received anything of value from or owns stock in a commercial company or institution related directly or indirectly to the subject of this chapter.

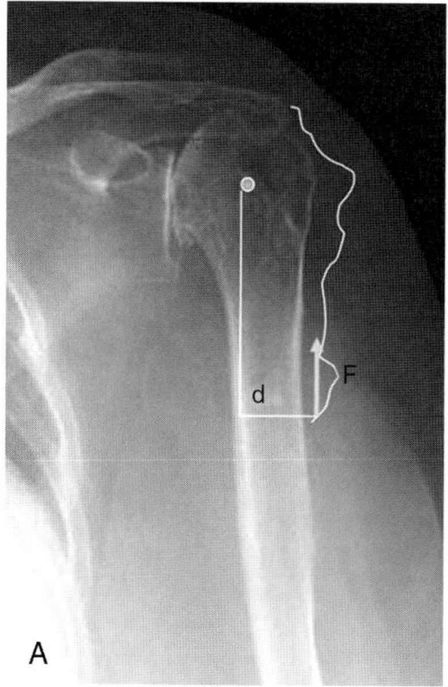

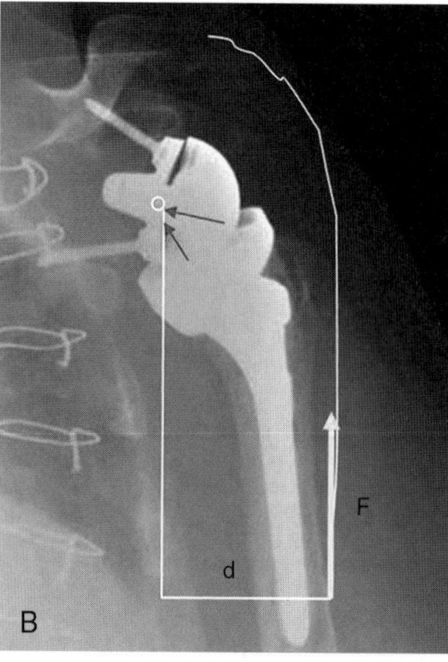

Figure 1 **A,** Radiograph showing rotator cuff tear arthropathy. When the humeral head moves superiorly in association with superior glenoid erosion, the lever arm of the deltoid (d) and the deltoid force (F) is reduced. **B,** When an Inverse Prosthesis (Zimmer, Warsaw, IN) is placed, the center of rotation is moved downward and medially so that the lever arm of the deltoid (d) and the force of the deltoid (F) are increased.

joint can become involved as well. When the humeral head moves superiorly, the deltoid loses its mechanical advantage, and the patient has pain and is unable to elevate his or her arm. Seebauer[7] classified rotator cuff-deficient arthritis based on the position and stability of the humeral head (**Table 1**).

History and Physical Examination

Patients with rotator cuff tear arthropathy are primarily elderly and female. Patients mainly report pain, night pain, limited motion, and occasional swelling. On examination, some degree of atrophy of the supraspinatus and infraspinatus is often evident. Patients usually have decreased passive and active range of motion as well as pseudoparalysis, a term that describes the inability to lift the arm despite a functioning deltoid muscle. Other sit-

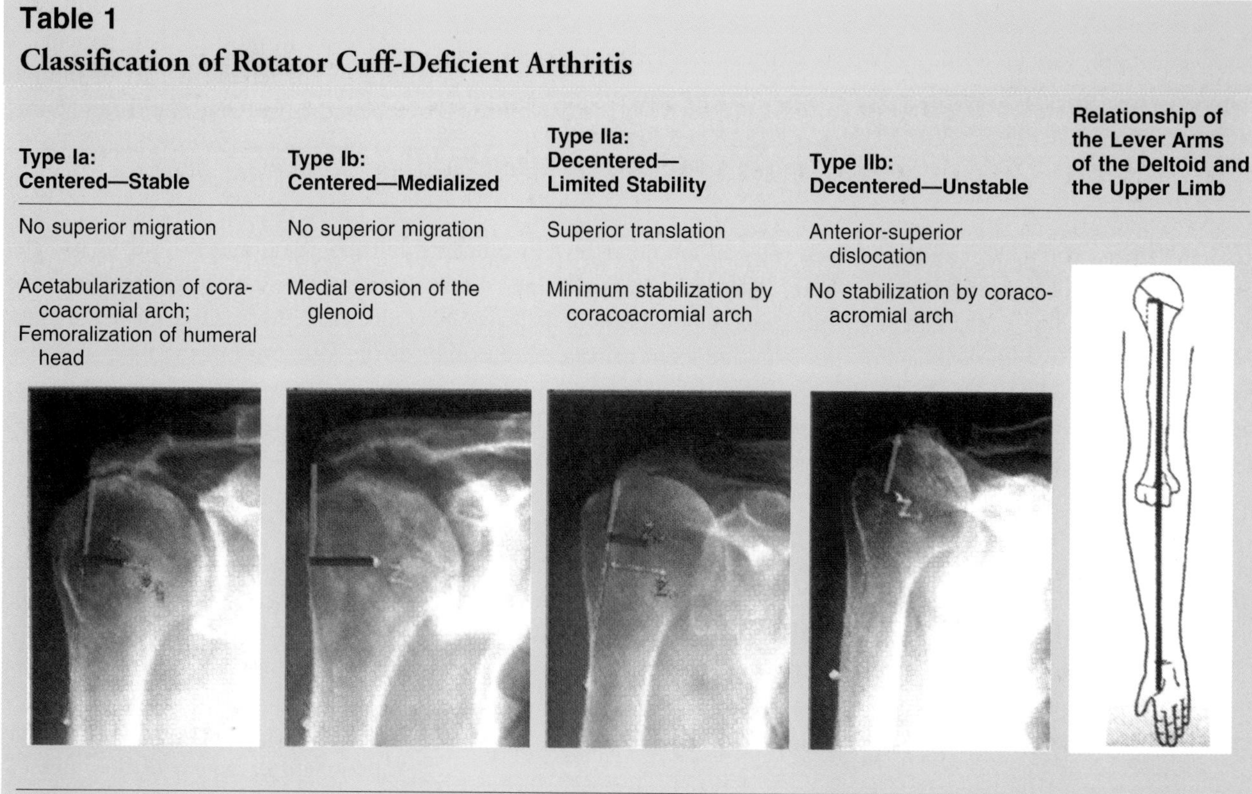

Table 1
Classification of Rotator Cuff-Deficient Arthritis

Type Ia: Centered—Stable	Type Ib: Centered—Medialized	Type IIa: Decentered—Limited Stability	Type IIb: Decentered—Unstable	Relationship of the Lever Arms of the Deltoid and the Upper Limb
No superior migration	No superior migration	Superior translation	Anterior-superior dislocation	
Acetabularization of coracoacromial arch; Femoralization of humeral head	Medial erosion of the glenoid	Minimum stabilization by coracoacromial arch	No stabilization by coracoacromial arch	

(Reproduced with permission from Safran O, Iannotti JP: Rotator cuff arthroplasty: The unconstrained arthroplasty, in Warner JJP, Iannotti JP, Flatow EL, eds: *Complex and Revision Problems in Shoulder Surgery*, ed 2. Philadelphia, PA, Lippincott Williams and Wilkins, 2005, p 490.)

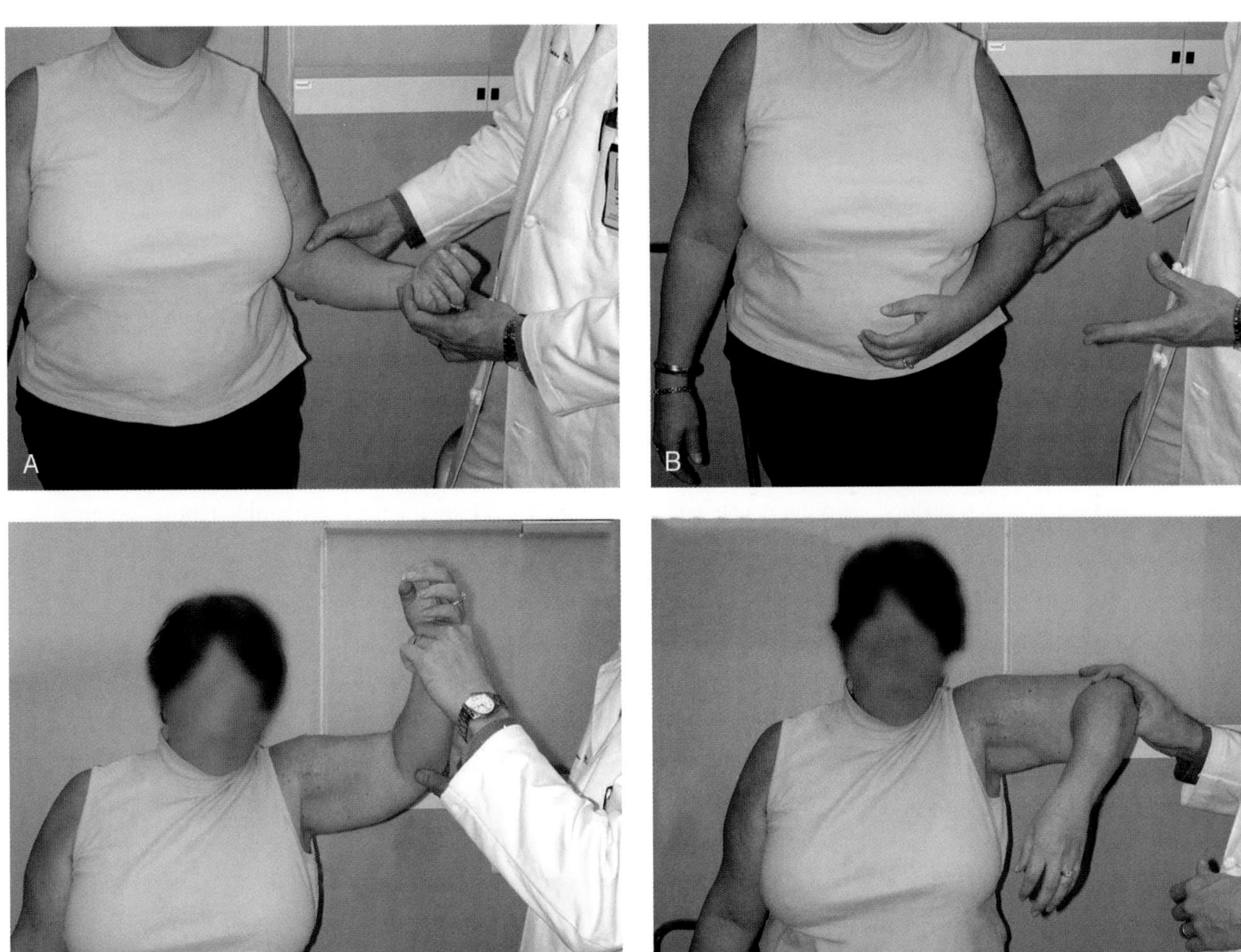

Figure 2 The external rotation lag signs demonstrate profound loss of the teres minor in a patient with severe rotator cuff tear arthropathy. **A,** Passive external rotation with the arm at the side. **B,** When the patient is asked to maintain this external rotation, the arm falls back toward the midline. The difference between the passive external rotation and the position the patient is able to maintain is the magnitude of the external rotation lag. **C,** When the arm is abducted and the elbow is supported by the examiner, the shoulder is externally rotated passively. **D,** The magnitude of the external rotation lag in this position is evident as the shoulder falls into internal rotation with the absence of both infraspinatus and teres minor function.

uations in which chronic loss of rotator cuff function may occur include failed prior surgery, hemiarthroplasty for fracture with loss of tuberosity position, and failed prior arthroplasty with subscapularis insufficiency with or without insufficiency of the superior rotator cuff.

In patients with profound rotator cuff deficiency, the function of the teres minor is important to observe. The specific finding of an external rotation lag sign is pathognomonic for teres minor insufficiency and demonstrates a profound inability to externally rotate the arm into a position required for daily functions (such as hair grooming)[8] (**Figure 2**).

Imaging

Plain radiography, CT, and other imaging modalities are recommended for evaluating patients with arthritis and rotator cuff deficiency. Biplanar radiographs will show decentering of the humeral head not only in the superior direction but also anteriorly or posteriorly depending on the extent of the rotator cuff insufficiency and the glenoid erosion. Arthritic changes, such as subchondral cysts, sclerosis, joint irregularity, and osteophytes, will also be seen. With advanced disease, progressive bone loss may result in protrusion of the femoral head into the glenoid and severe loss of humeral head contour. Glenoid erosion with cuff tear arthropathy or a failed prior arthroplasty may be problematic when reconstruc-

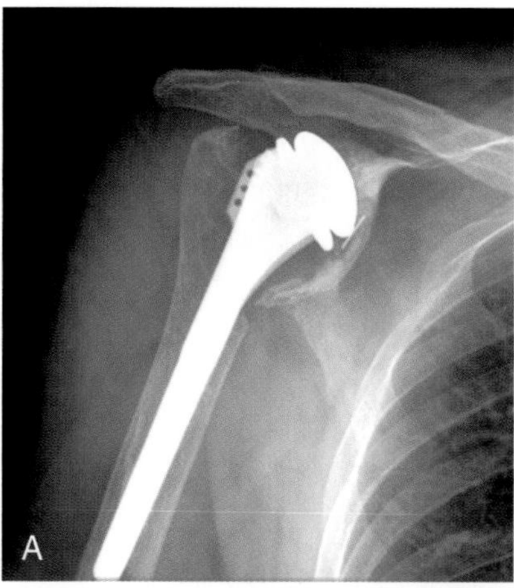

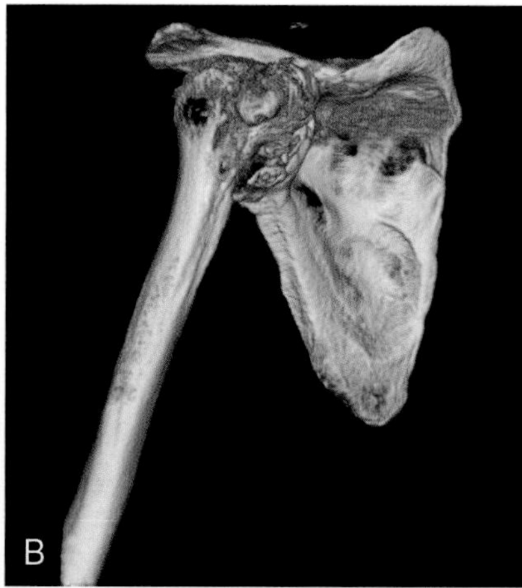

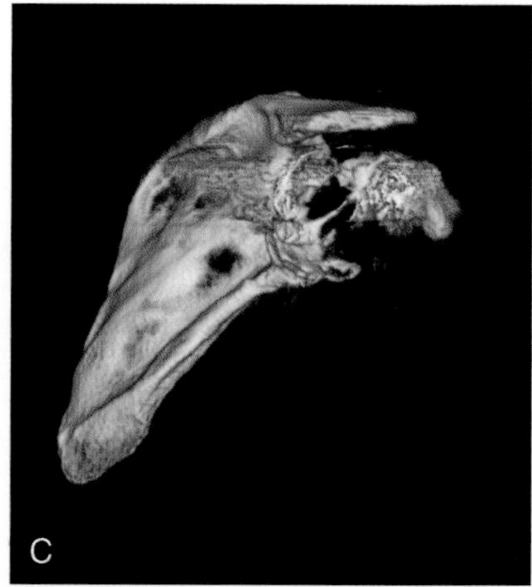

Figure 3 **A,** Radiograph showing hemiarthroplasty with rotator cuff insufficiency, which has resulted in severe superior and central glenoid erosion. **B,** Three-dimensional CT scan shows the extent of the glenoid bone loss. **C,** Three-dimensional CT scan with subtraction of the humeral head further illustrates the extent of the glenoid bone loss.

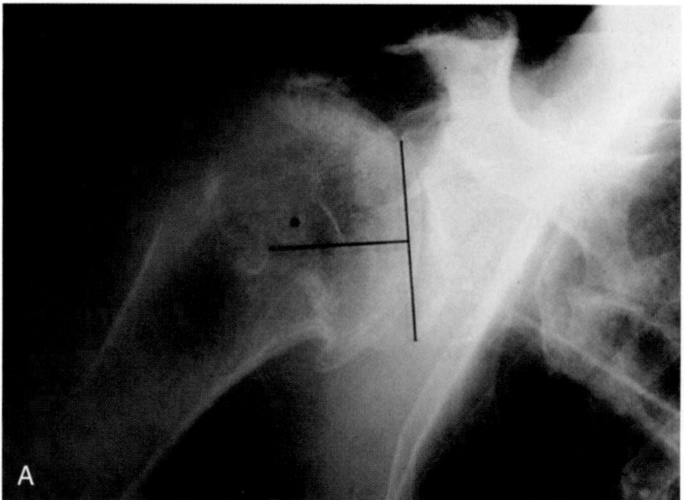

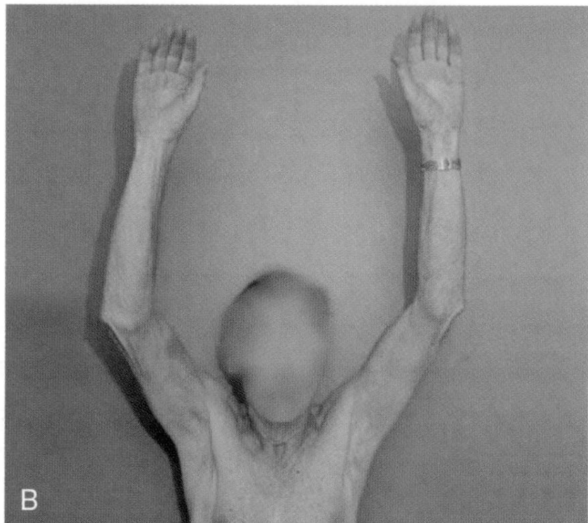

Figure 4 **A,** True AP radiograph shows superior displacement of the humeral head with arthritis typically seen with rotator cuff tear arthropathy. **B,** The patient has well-maintained motion and mild pain.

tion is being considered (**Figure 3**). Determining the magnitude of the decentered humeral head and the extent of bony erosion is critical for selecting the correct surgical option for each patient.

CT allows for the assessment of glenoid bone stock, glenoid version, humeral head position (static versus dynamic subluxation), and the degree of fatty infiltration (assessment of the teres minor). MRI may also be helpful in some patients when the status of rotator cuff muscle atrophy and fatty degeneration is unclear.[9,10]

Nonsurgical Treatment

A nonsurgical approach is recommended if the patient has mild pain and some functional limitation (**Figure 4**). If the patient is able to maintain strength of the deltoid muscle and glenohumeral joint motion (prevents capsular contracture that often accompanies the disease process), a conservative approach is also favored. If a patient is unable to tolerate surgery because of associated health comorbidities, nonsurgical treatment is also used. Anti-inflammatory medications, analgesics, and the judicious use of steroid injections can be beneficial.

Shoulder Arthroplasty for Rotator Cuff Deficiency

Unconstrained Total Shoulder Arthroplasty

Unconstrained total shoulder arthroplasty is not currently favored for cuff tear arthropathy because of the high rate of early glenoid component loosening. Conventional total shoulder arthroplasty failed in the past because of eccentric forces from the subluxated humeral head onto the superior glenoid component, resulting in the "rocking horse" phenomenon.[9-11]

Shoulder Hemiarthroplasty

Shoulder hemiarthroplasty was popularized because of early glenoid loosening with conventional total shoulder arthroplasty. Neer et al[12,13] originally called this "limited goals surgery" because he believed the functional outcome was limited, although pain relief was realistic for such patients. Although using a large humeral head in hemiarthroplasty was traditionally believed to be a good solution, this approach places the subscapularis at risk for rupture caused by overstuffing the joint (**Figure 5**). If hemiarthroplasty is the selected treatment, it is important not to oversize the humeral head.

Indications for hemiarthroplasty include a competent coracoacromial arch (superior containment) and an intact subscapularis tendon. Patients meeting these criteria usually do not have severe joint distortion and are able to elevate the arm to at least the shoulder level. Hemiarthroplasty is contraindicated in patients with profound external rotation weakness and pseudoparalysis because functional recovery and pain relief is unlikely. In rare cases, tendon transfers may also be performed at the time of hemiarthroplasty if limited external rotation is a functional factor.

Improvement in pain and elevation have been reported with conventional hemiarthroplasty.[14-18] According to Neer's limited goals criteria, Field et al[14] reported successful outcomes in 10 of 12 patients, with good deltoid function and an intact coracoacromial arch. Williams and Rockwood[16] observed an improvement in forward flexion and external rotation by 50° and 19°, respectively. Goldberg et al[17] reported that patients with more than 90° of forward flexion preoperatively did better at 43 months after surgery. Zuckerman et al[18] also reported an increase in forward flexion and external rotation, commenting that patients in the study showed an increase in their ability to perform activities of daily living at 28 months.

Although studies have reported positive results, a larger humeral head component can result in overstuffing the joint, which is believed to cause increased glenoid and acromial erosion and place the subscapularis at risk for failure. The most common complication of hemiarthroplasty in this population is superior instability with loss of contact with the coracoacromial arch. This can be seen in patients treated with prior acromioplasty. Therefore, Williams and Rockwood[16] recommend hemiarthroplasty only if there is a balanced anteroposterior cuff, fixed-fulcrum kinematics, an intact deltoid, and an intact coracoacromial arch.

Extended head hemiarthroplasty extends the superior arc of the humeral head posteriorly so that it theoretically improves contact of the humeral head against the acromion. This is accomplished without increasing the size of the humeral head. Proponents of extended head hemiarthroplasty believe there is an improvement in kinematics with a pain-free fulcrum provided by the extended humeral head surface; however, no clinical or biomechanical data show any advantage of the extended head hemiarthroplasty prosthesis over conventional hemiarthroplasty. Visotsky et al[19] reported improved pain relief, a 60° increase in forward flexion, and decreased greater tuberosity impingement in 60 patients at an average follow-up of 32 months.

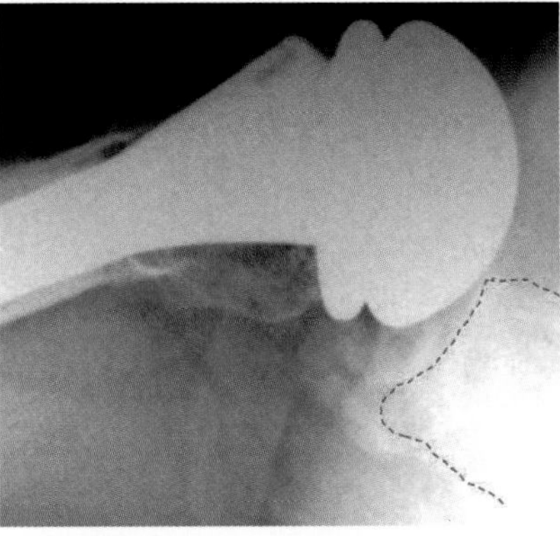

Figure 5 Radiograph of hemiarthroplasty with a large humeral head that resulted in failure of the subscapularis tendon and anterior subluxation. The dashed line represents the glenoid.

The bipolar humeral prosthesis also has been advocated as a potential option in the treatment of patients with deficient rotator cuffs and arthritis. Swanson et al[20] reported good to excellent pain relief in 31 of 35 patients at 60-month follow-up. Worland et al[21] also reported good pain relief with an increase in forward flexion and external rotation by 29° and 39°, respectively, at 24- to 48-month follow-up. At 27-month follow-up, Sarris et al[22] reported increased forward flexion and external rotation by 53° and 27°, respectively. Contrary to the results reported in these studies, Vrettos et al[23] reported poor pain relief and no identifiable glenohumeral or intrinsic bipolar motion. Although initial reports showed results similar to hemiarthroplasty, complications associated with the bipolar prosthesis include joint overstuffing, causing progressive glenoid bone erosion and subscapularis rupture. With excessive bone removal and soft-tissue loss (especially in revision cases), treatment with a bipolar prosthesis has largely been abandoned because of the associated complications and the advent of the reverse prosthesis. In summary, the problems associated with the bipolar humeral

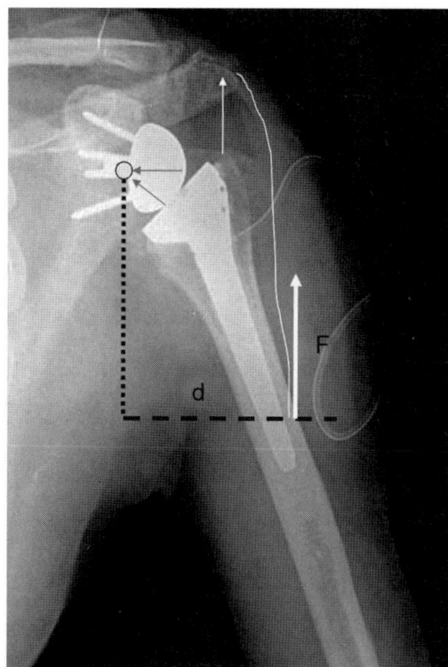

Figure 6 Radiograph showing a Delta Reverse Shoulder Prosthesis. The center of rotation is medialized (d), allowing for improved deltoid lever arm force (F). Arrows point to the circle representing the medialized center of rotation.

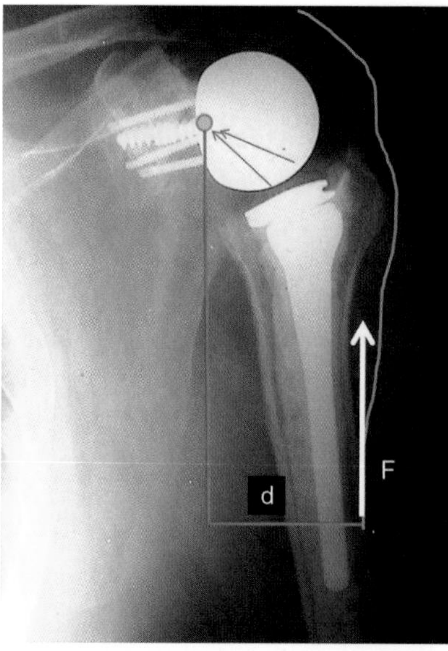

Figure 7 The RSP device lateralizes the center of rotation (d), allowing for improved deltoid lever arm force (F). The yellow dot with red arrows pointing to it represents the lateralized center of rotation.

prosthesis and advancements of the reverse prosthesis have prevented the bipolar prosthesis from gaining more recognition.

Constrained Shoulder Arthroplasty

The reverse shoulder prosthesis, originally proposed by Grammont et al,[24] resulted in a high failure rate because of design issues. The final version of the Delta Reverse Shoulder Prosthesis (DePuy, Warsaw, IN) was used effectively by many European Surgeons.[25-27] The reverse prosthesis creates a fixed fulcrum without a functioning rotator cuff. This enables the deltoid muscle to become the primary elevator of the arm. Depending on the type of reverse prosthesis, the center of rotation can vary. For example, with the Delta prosthesis, the center of rotation is medialized while lengthening the deltoid lever arm (**Figure 6**). The Encore Reverse Shoulder Prosthesis (RSP; DJO Surgical, Austin, TX) lateralizes the point of rotation (**Figure 7**), whereas the Inverse Prosthesis moves the center of rotation inferiorly and medially. Distal displacement of the center of rotation of the joint increases the lever arm and force of the deltoid muscle, resulting in compression of the humeral cup during elevation. These fixed-fulcrum devices are most commonly used in patients with cuff tear arthropathy, pseudoparalysis, failed fracture management, and those needing revision arthroplasty. Contraindications to this procedure include active or latent infection, deltoid dysfunction, significant bone loss, younger patients with heavy physical demands, and patients who are unable to tolerate surgery or comply with postoperative restrictions. Infection is particularly important to rule out in revision cases; this can often be done with joint aspiration and the evaluation of inflammatory markers, such as C-reactive protein and the erythrocyte sedimentation rate. If an infection is present, a two-stage approach is recommended. This approach consists of the initial removal of the infected prosthesis, extensive irrigation, placement of an antibiotic cement spacer device (prosthesis with antibiotic-loaded acrylic cement [PROSTALAC]), and subsequent second-stage revision to a reverse prosthesis when the infection is resolved.

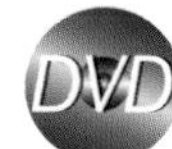

Video 11.1: Infected Total Shoulder Arthroplasty: A Novel Method for PROSTALAC Construction. Laurence D. Higgins, MD; Monica L. Morman, MD; Benjamin A. Sanofsky, BA; et al (9 min)

Deltoid function can be difficult to evaluate secondary to pain; however, it must be evaluated in patients treated with revision surgery. Axillary nerve function can be assessed with preoperative electrodiagnostic studies. The glenoid bone stock must also be evaluated with CT during preoperative planning to determine if there is sufficient bone for fixation of the glenosphere or if bony augmentation is required (**Figure 3**).

Although the reverse prosthesis has been used extensively in Europe over the past two decades, its use in the United States began in 2004 after approval by the Food and Drug Administration. Outcomes in patients treated with the reverse prosthesis for rotator cuff arthropathy, pseudoparesis, revision arthroplasty, and fractures have shown promising results; however, complications are more frequent compared with conventional unconstrained shoulder replacement.

Most studies report an improvement in various outcome scoring measures as well as increased motion. Boileau et al[28] reported improved

Constant scores, an increase in forward flexion by 66°, and a 76% overall satisfaction rate in 45 patients treated with a reverse prosthesis for cuff tear arthropathy, fracture, and failed arthroplasty. Boileau et al[29] also published results specific to patients with failed rotator cuff surgery and found a greater increase in forward flexion in pseudoparalytic shoulders when compared with painful shoulders. It was concluded that the results were not as good as those achieved in primary reverse total shoulder arthroplasty. Werner et al[30] and Frankle et al[31] also reported results in patients with painful pseudoparesis and found improvements in Constant and American Shoulder and Elbow Surgeon scores, subjective shoulder values, and forward flexion.

The degree of involvement of the teres minor has also been shown to affect outcomes in patients with cuff tear arthropathy. Simovitch et al[32] and Boileau et al[33] reported worse outcomes when the fatty infiltration of the teres minor was grade III or IV. Based on these studies, some investigators have proposed teres major tendon transfer at the time of the reverse prosthesis to help restore external rotation and improve outcomes in these patients[33,34] (**Figure 8**).

In studies of the reverse prosthesis in fracture management, Bufquin et al[35] and Wall et al[27] reported improved Constant scores and improved motion. Results, however, were not as good as those achieved in patients treated for rotator cuff-deficient shoulders. In the setting of revision arthroplasty, improved scores and motion were also seen but not to the extent seen in primary reverse arthroplasty for patients with a rotator cuff deficieny.[36,37]

Despite favorable results with the reverse prosthesis, the procedure is associated with a higher complication rate when compared to other forms of shoulder arthroplasty. The literature reports complication rates ranging from 9% to 50% (**Table 2**). Complications include infection, dislocation, loosening, hematoma, acromion or glenoid fracture, axillary nerve palsy, and scapular notching. Scapular notching in patients treated with the reverse prosthesis has been associated with poorer outcomes when compared with patients without radiographic evidence of notching.[38] Simovitch et al[38] found notching with the Delta III design occurs within the first 14 months after surgery and determined that superior placement and less inferior tilt of the glenosphere were predictors of notching. Other investigators have observed inferior scapular notching to be

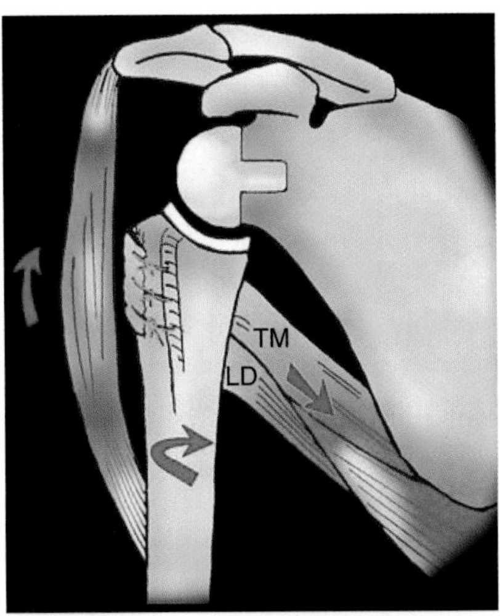

Figure 8 Illustration showing the technique of latissimus dorsi (LD) and teres major (TM) transfer for profound external rotation weakness according to the method of Boileau et al.[33] In this technique, the pectoralis major is tenotomized, and the latissimus dorsi and teres major tendons are sharply dissected off the humerus. The latissimus dorsi is first visualized, and the teres major is identified with its short tendon length and large muscle belly. The muscle-tendon units are mobilized with great care to prevent injury to the radial nerve. The tendons are transferred posteriorly around the humerus and attached to the humerus just lateral to the biceps groove with a transosseous technique. The arrows represent the line of pull of each muscle.

Table 2
Outcomes With the Reverse Prosthesis

Authors	No. of Patients	Forward Flexion Gain (degrees)	External Rotation Gain (degrees)	Constant Score	Subjective Shoulder Values	Complication Rate
Werner et al[30]	58	58	NR	64	56	50%
Frankle et al[31]	60	50	NR	NR	NR	17%
Boileau et al[28]	45	66	0	41	NR	31%
Wall et al[27]	240	NR	NR	60	NR	12%
Harvard Reverse[a]	81	40	10	NR	70	17%
Harvard Inverse[a]	75	45	10	NR	75	9%

[a] Results from an unpublished study by Jon J.P. Warner, MD, Boston, MA.
NR = not reported

less common with the RSP and the Inverse designs;[31] however, there is no evidence that notching affects the ultimate outcome of the procedure and the durability of the prosthesis.

Overall, the complication rate of a reverse prosthesis using any one of the available designs is at least three times that of unconstrained conventional arthroplasty.

Summary

A careful physical examination and radiographic imaging are required to determine the most effective treatment of rotator cuff insufficiency in each patient who presents with a painful and weak shoulder. Although hemiarthroplasty may offer good pain relief, the evidence supports the observation that treatment with a reverse shoulder prosthesis restores better motion in patients who present with profound weakness (pseudoparalysis) in the setting of rotator cuff tear arthropathy, failed fracture treatment, or a failed prosthesis. Reverse shoulder prosthetic designs create a fixed fulcrum; this allows the deltoid to function and elevate the arm in the absence of a rotator cuff. A small percentage of patients may also require tendon transfers to restore severe external rotation deficits. The reverse shoulder prosthesis, however, has a higher complication rate than conventional unconstrained shoulder arthroplasty.

References

1. Hsu HC, Boardman ND III, Luo ZP, An KN: Tendon-defect and muscle-unloaded models for relating a rotator cuff tear to glenohumeral stability. *J Orthop Res* 2000;18(6):952-958.
2. Lee SB, Kim KJ, O'Driscoll SW, Morrey BF, An KN: Dynamic glenohumeral stability provided by the rotator cuff muscles in the mid-range and end-range of motion: A study in cadavera. *J Bone Joint Surg Am* 2000;82(6): 849-857.
3. Karduna AR, Williams GR, Williams JL, Iannotti JP: Kinematics of the glenohumeral joint: Influences of muscle forces, ligamentous constraints, and articular geometry. *J Orthop Res* 1996; 14(6):986-993.
4. Sethi N, Wright R, Yamaguchi K: Disorders of the long head of the biceps tendon. *J Shoulder Elbow Surg* 1999;8(6):644-654.
5. Walch G, Edwards TB, Boulahia A, Nové-Josserand L, Neyton L, Szabo I: Arthroscopic tenotomy of the long head of the biceps in the treatment of rotator cuff tears: Clinical and radiographic results of 307 cases. *J Shoulder Elbow Surg* 2005;14(3): 238-246.
6. Lam F, Mok D: Treatment of the painful biceps tendon: Tenotomy or tenodesis? *Curr Orthop* 2006; 20(5):370-375.
7. Seebauer L: Optimierung der endoprothetischen versorgung der omarthritis und defektarhropathie-konventionelle, bipolare oder inverse prothese. *Z Orthop Ihre Grenzgeb* 2002; 140S:121.
8. Hertel R, Ballmer FT, Lombert SM, Gerber CH: Lag signs in the diagnosis of rotator cuff rupture. *J Shoulder Elbow Surg* 1996; 5(4):307-313.
9. Franklin JL, Barrett WP, Jackins SE, Matsen FA III: Glenoid loosening in total shoulder arthroplasty: Association with rotator cuff deficiency. *J Arthroplasty* 1988;3(1):39-46.
10. Barrett WP, Franklin JL, Jackins SE, Wyss CR, Matsen FA III: Total shoulder arthroplasty. *J Bone Joint Surg Am* 1987;69(6): 865-872.
11. Lohr JF, Cofield RH, Uhthoff HK: Glenoid component loosening in cuff tear arthropathy. *J Bone Joint Surg Br* 1991; 73(suppl 2):106.
12. Neer CS II, Craig EV, Fukuda H: Cuff-tear arthropathy. *J Bone Joint Surg Am* 1983;65(9):1232-1244.
13. Neer CS II, Watson KC, Stanton FJ: Recent experience in total shoulder replacement. *J Bone Joint Surg Am* 1982;64(3):319-337.
14. Field LD, Dines DM, Zabinski SJ, Warren RF: Hemiarthroplasty of the shoulder for rotator cuff arthropathy. *J Shoulder Elbow Surg* 1997;6(1):18-23.
15. Sanchez-Sotelo J, Cofield RH, Rowland CM: Shoulder hemiarthroplasty for glenohumeral arthritis associated with severe rotator cuff deficiency. *J Bone Joint Surg Am* 2001;83-A(12):1814-1822.
16. Williams GR Jr, Rockwood CA Jr: Hemiarthroplasty in rotator cuff-deficient shoulders. *J Shoulder Elbow Surg* 1996;5(5): 362-367.
17. Goldberg SS, Bell JE, Kim HJ, Bak SF, Levine WN, Bigliani LU: Hemiarthroplasty for the rotator cuff-deficient shoulder. *J Bone Joint Surg Am* 2008;90(3): 554-559.
18. Zuckerman JD, Scott AJ, Gallagher MA: Hemiarthroplasty for cuff tear arthropathy. *J Shoulder Elbow Surg* 2000;9(3):169-172.
19. Visotsky JL, Basamania C, Seebauer L, Rockwood CA, Jensen KL: Cuff tear arthropathy: Pathogenesis, classification, and algorithm for treatment. *J Bone Joint Surg Am* 2004;86-A (Suppl 2):35-40.
20. Swanson AB, de Groot Swanson G, Sattel AB, Cendo RD, Hynes D, Jar-Ning W: Bipolar implant shoulder arthroplasty: Long-term results. *Clin Orthop Relat Res* 1989;249(249):227-247.
21. Worland RL, Jessup DE, Arredondo J, Warburton KJ: Bipolar shoulder arthroplasty for rotator cuff arthropathy. *J Shoulder Elbow Surg* 1997;6(6):512-515.

22. Sarris IK, Papadimitriou NG, Sotereanos DG: Bipolar hemiarthroplasty for chronic rotator cuff tear arthropathy. *J Arthroplasty* 2003;18(2):169-173.

23. Vrettos BC, Wallace WA, Neumann L: Bipolar hemiarthroplasty of the shoulder for the elderly patient with rotator cuff arthropathy (abstract): In proceedings of the British Elbow and Shoulder Society. *J Bone Joint Surg* 1998; 80(Suppl I):106.

24. Grammont P, Trouilloud P, Laffay J, Deries X: Etude et realization d'une nouvelle prothese d'epaule. *Rhumatologie* 1987;39: 407-418.

25. Nyffeler RW, Werner CM, Simmen BR, Gerber C: Analysis of a retrieved delta III total shoulder prosthesis. *J Bone Joint Surg Br* 2004;86(8):1187-1191.

26. Grassi FA, Murena L, Valli F, Alberio R: Six year experience with the Delta III reverse shoulder prosthesis. *J Orthop Surg (Hong Kong)* 2009;17(2):151-156.

27. Wall B, Nové-Josserand L, O'Connor DP, Edwards TB, Walch G: Reverse total shoulder arthroplasty: A review of results according to etiology. *J Bone Joint Surg Am* 2007;89(7):1476-1485.

28. Boileau P, Watkinson D, Hatzidakis AM, Hovorka I: Neer Award 2005: The Grammont reverse shoulder prosthesis. Results in cuff tear arthritis, fracture sequelae, and revision arthroplasty. *J Shoulder Elbow Surg* 2006;15(5): 527-540.

29. Boileau P, Gonzalez JF, Chuinard C, Bicknell R, Walch G: Reverse total shoulder arthroplasty after failed rotator cuff surgery. *J Shoulder Elbow Surg* 2009;18(4): 600-606.

30. Werner CM, Steinmann PA, Gilbart M, Gerber C: Treatment of painful pseudoparesis due to irreparable rotator cuff dysfunction with the Delta III reverse-ball-and-socket total shoulder prosthesis. *J Bone Joint Surg Am* 2005; 87(7):1476-1486.

31. Frankle M, Siegal S, Pupello D, Saleem A, Mighell M, Vasey M: The Reverse Shoulder Prosthesis for glenohumeral arthritis associated with severe rotator cuff deficiency: A minimum two-year follow-up study of sixty patients. *J Bone Joint Surg Am* 2005;87(8): 1697-1705.

32. Simovitch RW, Helmy N, Zumstein MA, Gerber C: Impact of fatty infiltration of the teres minor muscle on the outcome of reverse total shoulder arthroplasty. *J Bone Joint Surg Am* 2007;89(5): 934-939.

33. Boileau P, Chuinard C, Roussanne Y, Bicknell RT, Rochet N, Trojani C: Reverse shoulder arthroplasty combined with a modified latissimus dorsi and teres major tendon transfer for shoulder pseudoparalysis associated with dropping arm. *Clin Orthop Relat Res* 2008;466(3):584-593.

34. Gerber C, Pennington SD, Lingenfelter EJ, Sukthankar A: Reverse Delta-III total shoulder replacement combined with latissimus dorsi transfer: A preliminary report. *J Bone Joint Surg Am* 2007;89(5):940-947.

35. Bufquin T, Hersan A, Hubert L, Massin P: Reverse shoulder arthroplasty for the treatment of three- and four-part fractures of the proximal humerus in the elderly: A prospective review of 43 cases with a short-term follow-up. *J Bone Joint Surg Br* 2007;89(4):516-520.

36. Levy JC, Virani N, Pupello D, Frankle M: Use of the reverse shoulder prosthesis for the treatment of failed hemiarthroplasty in patients with glenohumeral arthritis and rotator cuff deficiency. *J Bone Joint Surg Br* 2007;89(2): 189-195.

37. Levy J, Frankle M, Mighell M, Pupello D: The use of the reverse shoulder prosthesis for the treatment of failed hemiarthroplasty for proximal humeral fracture. *J Bone Joint Surg Am* 2007;89(2): 292-300.

38. Simovitch RW, Zumstein MA, Lohri E, Helmy N, Gerber C: Predictors of scapular notching in patients managed with the Delta III reverse total shoulder replacement. *J Bone Joint Surg Am* 2007; 89(3):588-600.

Video Reference

11.1: Higgins LD, Morman ML, Sanofsky BA, et al: Video. *Infected Total Shoulder Arthroplasty: A Novel Method for PROSTALAC Construction.* Boston, MA, 2009.

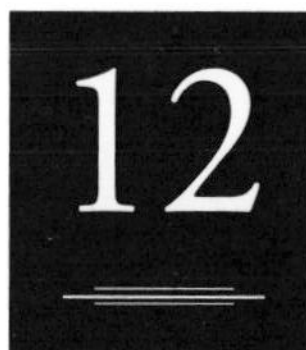

Evolution of Rotator Cuff Repair Techniques: Are Our Patients Really Benefiting?

CDR Matthew T. Provencher, MD, MC, USN
James S. Kercher, MD
Leesa M. Galatz, MD
Neal S. ElAttrache, MD
Rachel M. Frank, BS
Brian J. Cole, MD, MBA

Abstract

The repair integrity of rotator cuff tears, which are a common disorder, is influenced by many biologic, environmental, and surgical factors. Surgery for rotator cuff repairs has evolved significantly over the past decade. The technical goals of rotator cuff repair include achieving high initial fixation strength, minimizing gap formation, and maintaining mechanical stability until biologic healing occurs. A variety of surgical techniques have been established to capitalize on certain aspects of these tenets and have been shown to provide biomechanical and biologic benefits; however, overall clinical outcomes may be dependent on certain tear characteristics. It is important for orthopaedic surgeons to be familiar with the natural history of rotator cuff disease to understand the various repair strategies and techniques and the outcomes associated with these procedures.

Instr Course Lect 2011;60:123-136.

Rotator cuff repair is one of the most common orthopaedic shoulder procedures. The primary goal of rotator cuff repair is to successfully reconstitute glenohumeral joint function by restoring normal rotator cuff kinematics. It is well known that rotator cuff repairs are at risk for failure, with 20% to 40% of primary repairs resulting in failure. Even higher rates of failure have been reported in revision cases.[1-6] Outcome studies following rotator cuff repair have shown that patients report high satisfaction ratings,[5,7,8] often despite the failure of complete anatomic healing. Recent data have shown that healing and the anatomic integrity of the rotator cuff repair site correlates with improved outcomes, particularly with regard to strength and functional recovery.[1-4,8,9] Repair methods have significantly evolved over the past decade to allow improvement in

Dr. Provencher or an immediate family member serves as a board member, owner, officer, or committee member of the American Academy of Orthopaedic Surgeons, the American Orthopaedic Society for Sports Medicine, the Arthroscopy Association of North America, and the Society of Military Orthopaedic Surgeons. Dr. Galatz or an immediate family member serves as a board member, owner, officer, or committee member of the American Shoulder and Elbow Surgeons. Dr. ElAttrache or an immediate family member serves as a board member, owner, officer, or committee member of the American Orthopaedic Society for Sports Medicine; has received royalties from Arthrex; is a member of a speakers' bureau or has made paid presentations on behalf of Arthrex; serves as a paid consultant to or is an employee of Arthrex; has received research or institutional support from Arthrex; owns stock or stock options in Arthrex; and has received nonincome support (such as equipment or services), commercially derived honoraria, or other non–research-related funding (such as paid travel) from Arthrex. Dr. Cole or an immediate family member has received royalties from Arthrex, DJ Orthopaedics, Lippincott, and Elsevier; is a member of a speakers' bureau or has made paid presentations on behalf of Genzyme; serves as a paid consultant to or is an employee of Zimmer, Arthrex, Carticept, Biomimmetic, and Allosource; and has received research or institutional support from Regentis, Arthrex, Smith & Nephew, and DJ Orthopaedics. Neither of the following authors nor any immediate family member has received anything of value from or owns stock in a commercial company or institution related directly or indirectly to the subject of this chapter: Dr. Kercher and Dr. Frank.

The views expressed in this article are those of the authors and do not reflect the official policy or position of the Department of the Navy, the Department of Defense, or the US Government.

postoperative cuff integrity, strength, and overall outcomes.

Recent biomechanical and clinical research has focused on the numerous variables that are known to influence repair integrity and clinical outcomes. The natural history of rotator cuff disease, with a focus on the important examination and presentation findings that have a known association with repair success, are discussed in this chapter. Various rotator cuff repair strategies are also reviewed, including the evolving repair constructs, guidelines for using repair techniques, and an overview of the outcomes associated with the evolving repair techniques.

Tendon Healing and the Natural History of the Disease

The incidence of rotator cuff disease increases naturally with age.[10] Yamaguchi et al[10] examined bilateral shoulders using ultrasound in a large group of patients with unilateral shoulder pain. Contralateral asymptomatic tears were present in a large percentage of patients and occurred in an age-dependent fashion. The mean age of the patients with no tear on the contralateral side was 49 years, with unilateral tears, 59 years, and with bilateral tears, 68 years. These results strongly suggest that rotator cuff disease is a progressive, age-related, degenerative process.

Full-thickness tears of the rotator cuff initiate a cascade of alterations that compromise the muscle-tendon unit. These include atrophy, degeneration, retraction, fibrosis, and decreased collagen expression,[11-14] which play significant roles in the success of repairs. Outcomes following rotator cuff repair are primarily dependent on factors such as patient age, tear size, muscle atrophy, fatty change, and chronicity.[1,2,4,7,8,11,12,15] In one of the first studies to identify age as a significant factor affecting healing, Boileau et al[1] evaluated cuff integrity after arthroscopic repair of the supraspinatus tendon. The authors reported a 70% healing rate, although healing occurred in only 45% of patients older than 65 years. Similar results were reported by Lichtenberg et al[16] in a study of 53 patients in whom the overall healing rate was 75%. The average age of the patients with healed repairs was 59 years compared with an average age of 65 years for patients in whom healing did not occur. Age as an independent variable related to retearing following rotator cuff repair has recently been challenged by Oh et al.[17] Based on a multivariate analysis, the authors determined that advanced age did not act independently of tendon retraction and the degree of fatty degeneration as a factor in retearing after repair.

The classification system defining fatty degeneration of the rotator cuff was first described by Goutallier et al;[18] it was subsequently determined that degenerative changes are indicative of the size and chronicity of the tear.[19-22] The amount of fatty degeneration is an important factor relating to outcomes after repair.[23-25] Using MRI to correlate muscle atrophy and fatty degeneration to patient outcomes, Gladstone et al[26] evaluated 38 patients 1 year after rotator cuff repair. It was found that muscle atrophy and fatty degeneration of the rotator cuff were independent predictors of American Shoulder and Elbow Surgeons and Constant scores.[26]

In addition to biologic factors, environmental factors such as smoking or other chemical exposure may have significant affects on healing. In an evaluation of a population of patients with shoulder pain, a highly statistically significant association, which demonstrated a time- and dose-dependent response, was reported between smoking and the presence of a rotator cuff tear.[27] More recent smoking and heavier smoking were also associated with the presence of a tear.[27] Smoking also has been shown to be detrimental to rotator cuff healing.[10] In an animal model, the administration of nicotine resulted in decreased cell proliferation and extracellular matrix production in the healing tendon.[28] Biomechanical testing showed inferior material properties of the repair tissue exposed to nicotine when compared with a control group.[10]

Basic science research on tendon biology and healing has proliferated in the past several years. In general, a tendon heals by scar formation rather than by tendon regeneration. The healing process is largely (but not independently) modulated by transforming growth factor beta-1 rather than by transforming growth factor beta-3, which leads to scar-free healing in skin and tendon in fetal models of soft-tissue injury. In animal models of rotator cuff healing, most repairs attain only 50% of the structural properties and 10% of the material properties compared with normal tendon.[29,30] The challenge going forward is to integrate the use of growth factor and tissue engineering strategies to enhance healing in a cost-effective and reliable manner.

Biomechanical Rationale

The technical goals of rotator cuff repair include achieving high initial fixation strength, minimizing gap formation, and maintaining mechanical stability until biologic healing. The important characteristics of rotator cuff repair at time zero are shown in **Table 1**. It is well documented that healing of the rotator cuff repair site correlates with superior outcomes, particularly regarding the recovery of function and strength.[1-4,8,9]

Bone-to-tendon healing begins with the formation of a fibrovascular tissue interface between the tendon and bone.[29,30] Early on, bone will grow into the interface tissue,[31] which is followed by a gradual increase in collagen fiber continuity created between the tendon and bone.[29] The fibrovascular tissue interface is an important consideration regarding the improved surface area for healing afforded by restoration of the anatomic footprint.[32-34] Traditional single-row repairs result in persistent tear rates ranging from 29% to 90%.[1,7,8,35] These tears may be caused in part by the prolonged and complex biologic process of rotator cuff tendon healing, the lack of footprint restoration, and biomechanical considerations. Typically, after a rotator cuff tear, the tissue is relatively avascular for several months. To incite a vascular response, biologic factors necessary for healing must originate from bone; however, these factors are impeded by the synovial environment because the synovial fluid and other factors are believed to be an impediment to healing at the tendon-bone interface. The repaired tendon must remain relatively still for long periods of time over as large an area of the healing zone as possible to maintain the healing response; this is difficult to achieve because of tendon-bone interface motion and is the reason why increasing tissue compression on bone potentially enhances the healing process.[36] An ideal rotator cuff repair should be strong and gap-resistant with compression forces that protect the endosteal healing factors. In an attempt to address these considerations, rotator cuff repair configurations have evolved considerably over the past decade.

Technical failures related to technique, implants, and suture selection are becoming less commonplace because of recent technologic advancements in implant materials. More concerning is the concept of anatomic failure, which takes into consideration the rotator cuff tendon footprint, biomechanics, and resting tension on the repair. The footprint of the supraspinatus rotator cuff tendon is two-dimensional and measures approximately 12 to 14 mm medial to lateral and 25 mm anterior to posterior.[37,38] Pressure on the rotator cuff tendon should be considered as a third dimension, taking into account compression on the tendon and contact area. Many biomechanical studies have established that double-row configurations significantly increase the amount of native footprint covered with the repaired tendon.[33,39,40] In a cadaver study, Meier and Meier[34] reported that a double-row repair restores the supraspinatus tendon footprint more closely than a single-row technique. Brady et al[33] reported on a clinical intraoperative study of patients treated with repair of full-thickness rotator cuff tears using double-row fixation. The authors compared the footprint coverage of repairs after an initial lateral-row repair and after the double-row repair and determined that single-row repairs left an average of 52.7% of the rotator cuff footprint uncovered. After a double-row repair in which the medial-row sutures were secured, there was complete (100%) footprint coverage in all patients, representing a mean increase in footprint coverage of 119%.

Table 1
Ideal Rotator Cuff Repair Construct Characteristics at Time Zero

Restoration of anatomic footprint
Resistance to gap formation
Ultimate tensile strength
Resistance to cyclic elongation
Number of cycles to failure

Double-row repairs also have shown improved strength, less gap formation, and significantly increased resistance to cyclic displacement.[41-46] A meta-analysis[47] compared the biomechanical properties of single-row and double-row constructs in 15 studies using animal and human models. Nine studies demonstrated a statistically significant advantage to a double-row repair with regard to biomechanical strength, repair failure, and gap formation. Additionally, five of the studies demonstrated the double-row repair was superior to single-row repairs with respect to anatomic restoration.[47]

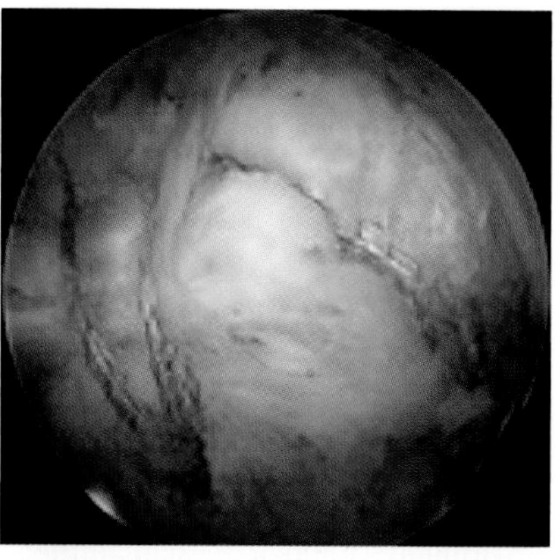

Figure 1 Arthroscopic image of a transosseous equivalent (TOE) rotator cuff repair.

Transosseous Equivalent Repairs

When discussing double-row rotator cuff repairs, a differentiation must be made between first-generation constructs and newer constructs containing bridging sutures between the medial and lateral rows, known as the modified double-row or transosseous equivalent (TOE) repair[48-50] (**Figure 1**). First-generation, double-row repair constructs consist of a medial row of mattress-type sutures with simple sutures placed at the lateral edge of the cuff without linkage between the two rows.[51] This configuration has been shown to mechanically outperform single-row suture anchor techniques in the laboratory in terms of footprint restoration and construct strength.[34,44] However, anchor crowding can occur on the tuberosity, and biomechanical testing also has shown that first-generation, double-row configurations fail to prevent repair site gapping during humeral rotation, especially at the anterior anchor point.[41] TOE repairs perform better than single-row repairs under cyclic loading and ultimate failure testing while providing biologic containment and tissue-to-bone compression.[33,34,44,49,50,52] Anatomic anchor crowding is diminished because the lateral fixation is placed more distally on the lateral wall of the greater tuberosity rather than proximally on the lateral crest of the tuberosity. Biomechanical testing that emphasized internal and external rotation during high loading conditions showed the TOE construct was superior because of self-reinforcing properties, allowing for solid tendon fixation during rotational testing.[53]

Bisson and Manohar[54] compared open transosseous repair (considered the gold standard) with the bridging TOE construct for supraspinatus tears in paired cadaver shoulders. The authors reported no significant difference between the two techniques with respect to elongation, load to failure, or stiffness. In addition, these repair methods demonstrated failure loads of approximately 400 to 450 N, which is approximately 50% of the strength of an intact supraspinatus tendon.[55] However, failure loads were higher than those previously reported for earlier-generation techniques.[39,44,45,56-58] Gerber et al[57] reported that the single-row configuration produces an ultimate tensile strength of 208 N, which is barely sufficient to resist the physiologic rotator cuff load of the supraspinatus. The repair strength at time zero was reported to be 336 N for double-row[59] and 443 N for TOE repairs.[50]

Mini-Open and Arthroscopic Repairs: Making the Transition

Advancements in arthroscopy have dramatically changed rotator cuff surgery and have facilitated the evolution from open to mini-open to complete arthroscopic repairs. Arthroscopically assisted rotator cuff repair is a hybrid technique, which combines the benefits of mini-open and arthroscopic techniques and is useful for certain repairs and by surgeons transitioning to complete arthroscopic procedures. The mini-open technique, first described by Levy et al[60] in 1990, uses arthroscopy to treat intra-articular pathology and subacromial decompression and is followed by rotator cuff repair through a limited deltoid-splitting approach. The approach, which is an extension of the anterior portal, allows the deltoid fibers to be split in line for access to the repair and avoids deltoid takedown from its origin. The addition of arthroscopic inspection permits a detailed examination of the glenohumeral joint for possible concomitant disorders such as degenerative biceps lesions, labral pathology, cartilage defects, and glenohumeral arthritis. Several studies have documented the high incidence of intra-articular pathology found during arthroscopy; knowledge of this pathology provides important prognostic details.[61-64]

The main advantages of the arthroscopically assisted mini-open technique over traditional open surgery are lower perioperative morbidity, improved cosmesis, accelerated rehabilitation, improved identification of intra-articular pathology, and preservation of the deltoid. The open repair allows the use of transosseous repair sutures, which are considered the gold standard;[8] however, the results of this technique have not been fully elucidated. A disadvantage of the mini-open technique is increased subdeltoid scarring, which leads to higher rates of stiffness. There are also a variety of tears that are difficult to treat using this technique, including massive tears with a posterior-to-anterior and U-shape orientation, as well as retracted tears.

The indications for mini-open and arthroscopic rotator cuff repairs are the same as those for open repairs and include persistent pain or weakness and a documented tear of the rotator cuff. Specific indications for the mini-open repair include tears with minimal retraction and those that are primarily limited to the supraspinatus tendon. Relative contraindications to arthroscopic repair include active or recent infection, medical comorbidities making anesthesia unsafe, massive tears with fixed tendon retraction, and those with superior escape.

Arthroscopic Rotator Cuff Repair

Arthroscopic rotator cuff repair represents a notable improvement with regard to morbidity associated with deltoid takedown and postoperative rehabilitation. In comparison to the open or mini-open methods, the complete arthroscopic procedure is more technically demanding and requires a steep learning curve before it can be done proficiently. The arthroscopic rotator cuff repair technique has unique complications, including fluid extravasation, device failure, thermal injury, longer surgical times, and concerns about higher cost.[65] The advantages of the arthroscopic technique include a marked improvement in cuff tear visualization, an expedited postoperative phase, the ability to identify and treat all concomitant pathologies, and the ability to repair the rotator cuff with minimal surgical insult to the deltoid. Most notably, the arthroscopic technique offers greater versatility in recognizing and anatomically reducing a va-

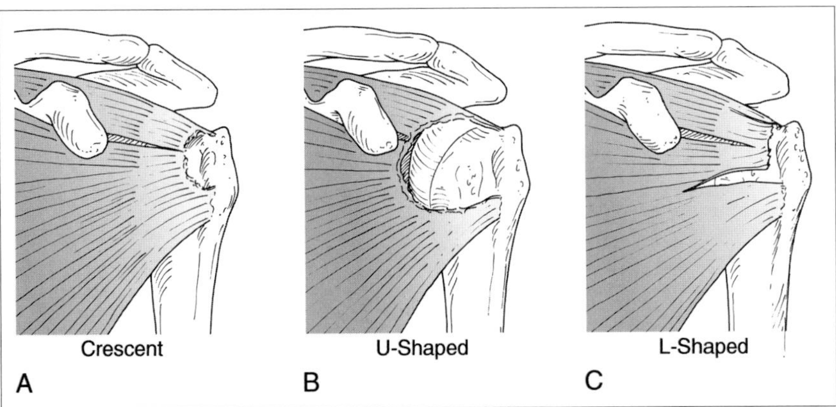

Figure 2 Illustration of the basic rotator cuff tear patterns. **A,** The crescent tear is the most basic pattern and may be approached with a variety of techniques. **B,** The U-shaped tear is usually more chronic and degenerative in nature and can require margin before footprint. **C,** The L-shaped tear consists of an anterior-to-posterior component at the footprint in conjunction with a medial-to-lateral component, which can be either anterior or posterior at the supraspinatus-infraspinatus junction.

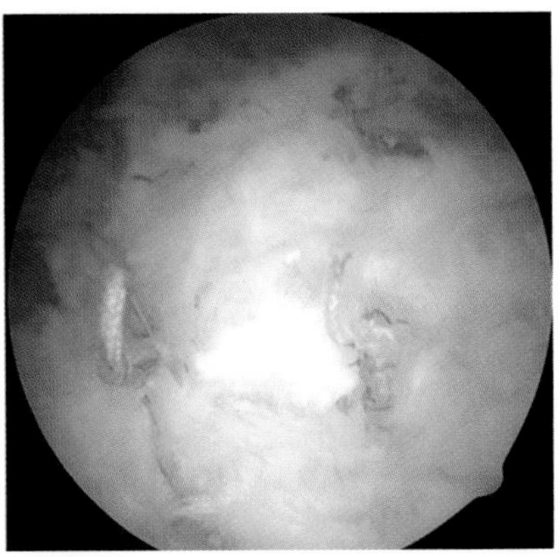

Figure 3 Arthroscopic image showing an intact single-row rotator cuff repair.

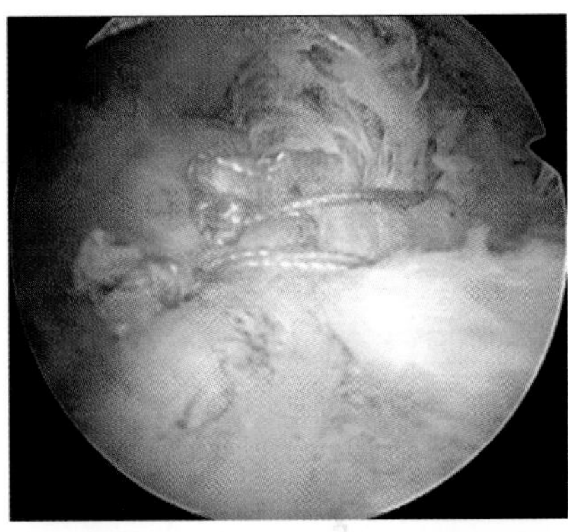

Figure 4 Arthroscopic image showing margin convergence of a large U-shaped rotator cuff tear before footprint repair. These tears are typically chronic and/or degenerative in nature.

riety of partial- and full-thickness tear patterns. Patients should be advised that a more minimally invasive approach to repair does not equate with improved tendon healing and faster recovery from a functional standpoint, and differences at 1 year postoperatively, except the incision size, are indistinguishable.

Arthroscopic Strategy

Successful arthroscopic rotator cuff repair begins by determining the tear pattern. Although several classification systems exist, the most valuable is a straightforward description of the tear pattern as crescent, U-shaped, or L-shaped (**Figure 2**).[66,67] The crescent tear is typically an avulsion injury and is the most basic pattern. The crescent tear is unique because it is typically acute and has excellent biologic healing potential. This pattern may be treated with a variety of techniques; however, an acceptable result may be achieved using a single-row configuration with multiple anchors as needed[67] (**Figure 3**). To assist with reducing the tear, it may be helpful to repair the posterior margin first, followed by the anterior portion and then the central portion of the tear. The U-shaped tear is usually more chronic and degenerative in nature. In general, this type of repair may require margin convergence or side-to-side repair (**Figure 4**) before the footprint repair and begins at the apex of the tear progressing medially to laterally. Using this technique will help reduce tension and repair length at the repair site. The repair is completed using a single- or double-row technique, depending on the surgeon's preference.

One of the most common configurations is the L-shaped tear, which consists of an anterior-to-posterior component at the footprint in conjunction with a medial-to-lateral component. The medial-to-lateral component is almost always one of the limbs of the L and extends upward into the weaker tissue of the rotator interval; however, the L (or reverse L) may extend into the junction between the supraspinatus and infraspinatus. The lateral limb of the L-shaped tear is usually located along the rotator cuff cable or where the infraspinatus comes around laterally to envelop the supraspinatus (**Figure 5**). The apex of the L-shaped tear should be anatomically reduced to the exact area in which it was torn to reduce the risk of postoperative failure (**Figure 5, C**). Arthroscopic visualization of these tear patterns greatly facilitates anatomic reduction and a tension-minimized repair construct.

Surgical Technique: Critical Steps

Complete arthroscopic repair begins in the same manner as that previously de-

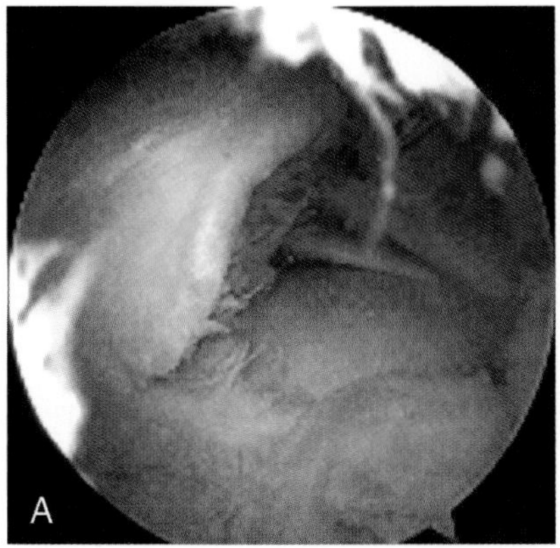

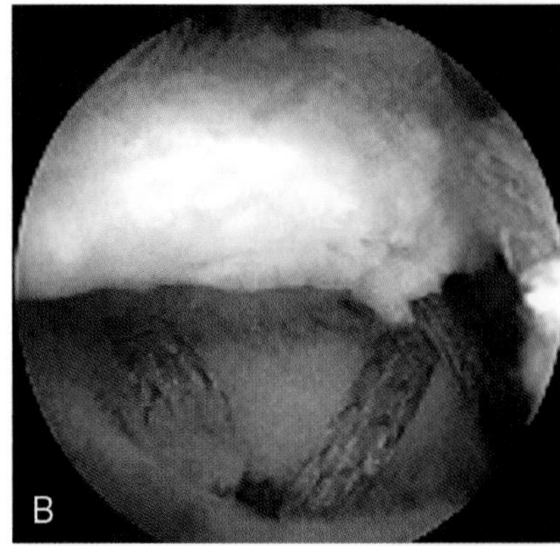

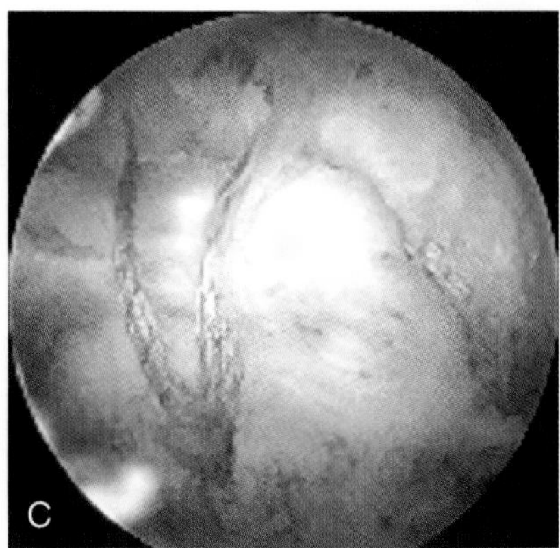

Figure 5 Arthroscopic images showing the pathology and repair of an L-shaped tear consisting of an anterior-to-posterior component at the footprint in conjunction with a medial-to-lateral component. **A,** L-shaped tear. **B,** Anatomic reduction of the tear. **C,** Final intact repair.

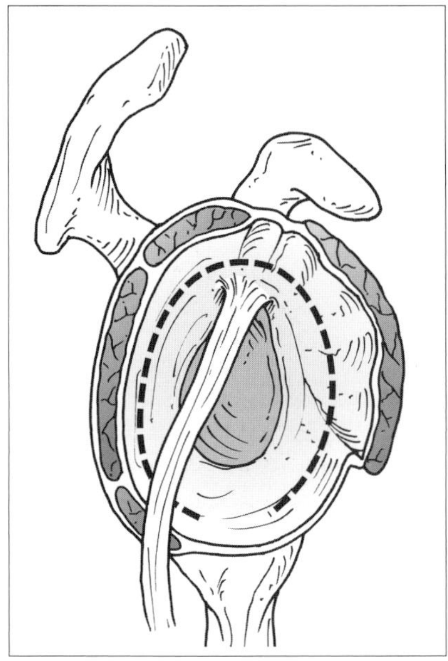

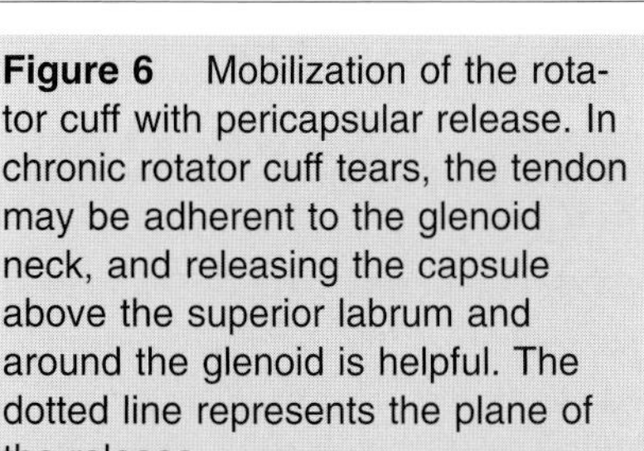
Figure 6 Mobilization of the rotator cuff with pericapsular release. In chronic rotator cuff tears, the tendon may be adherent to the glenoid neck, and releasing the capsule above the superior labrum and around the glenoid is helpful. The dotted line represents the plane of the release.

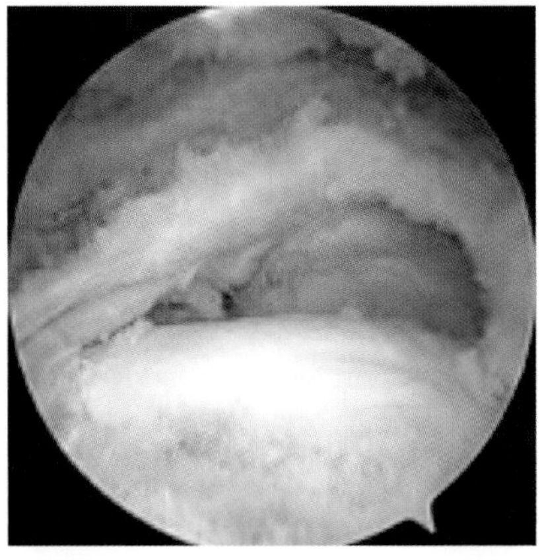

Figure 7 Arthroscopic image showing visualization of rotator cuff pathology through the lateral portal.

scribed for mini-open repairs; however, there are a few key steps that are critical to success. Tendon releases are crucial and can be performed with arthroscopic hand instruments, an electrothermal device, or an arthroscopic elevator to obtain mobilization of the rotator cuff tissue and prevent undue tension on the repair. Initially, releases should be performed between the rotator cuff tendon and the undersurface of the acromion. Anteriorly, releases are performed to separate adhesions in the rotator interval (interval slide) region between the supraspinatus and subscapularis, with releases performed to the base of the coracoid. A posterior release or slide will separate the supraspinatus and the infraspinatus, although this is rarely required. In chronic rotator cuff tears, the tendon may adhere to the glenoid neck; releasing the capsule above the superior labrum and around the glenoid is helpful (**Figure 6**).

Tendon footprint reconstruction can be performed using a variety of configurations; however, the surgeon must be aware of appropriate portals and the benefits of each in facilitating suture passing. Although viewing from the posterior portal and working through the lateral portal is possible, viewing through the lateral portal and working through the posterior, anterior, and accessory anterolateral portals improves suture passing capabilities and direct visualization (**Figure 7**). To establish the accessory anterolateral portal, an 18-gauge spinal needle is used to determine the proper trajectory for anchor placement and suture passing (**Figure 8**). Footprint preparation also is performed through this portal. When preparing the footprint, it is important to create a bleeding surface by removing only minimal cortical bone to improve suture anchor pull-out strength. However, with TOE fixation constructs, more cortical bone may be removed with the burr during preparation to obtain a viable bleeding bony surface of the greater tuberosity.

The anchor position is dependent on the suture repair configuration. When performing a single-row repair,

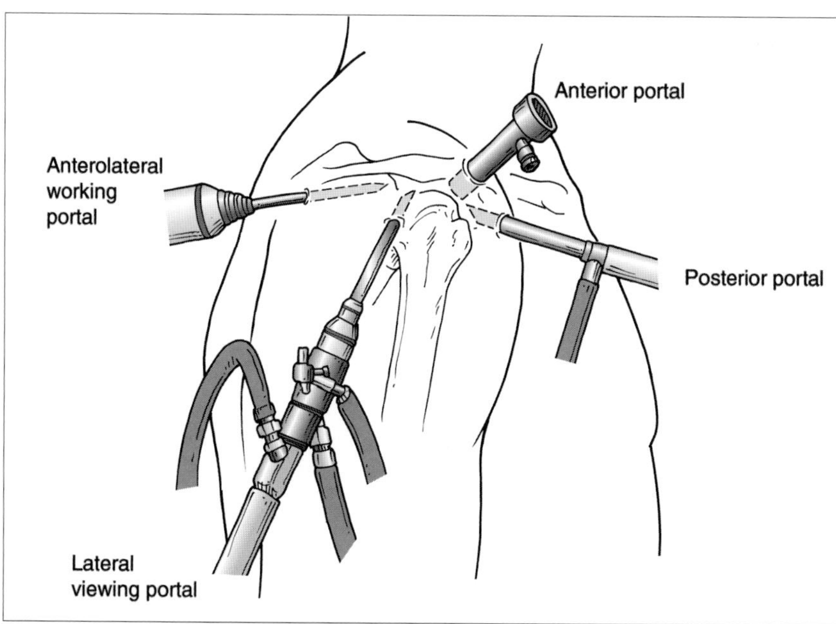

Figure 8 Illustration showing standard portal placement for an arthroscopic rotator cuff repair.

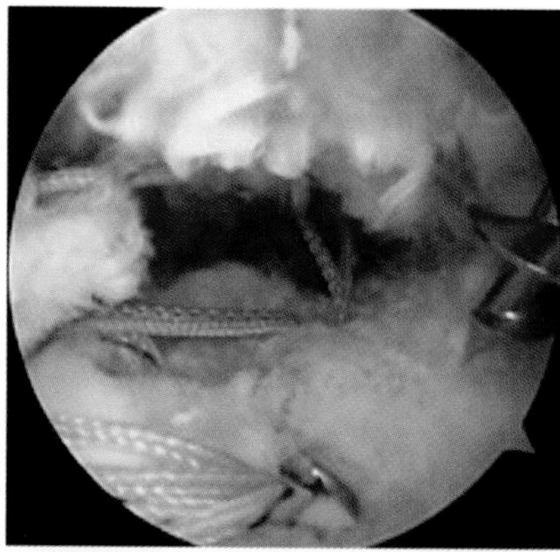

Figure 9 Arthroscopic image showing the placement of medial row anchors just off the articular margin of the footprint in a double-row rotator cuff repair.

the anchor is placed at or near the lateral edge of the greater tuberosity. In a double-row repair, the medial row of anchors (**Figure 9**) is placed just off the articular margin of the footprint. Lateral row anchors are placed after medial knots are tied and are positioned lateral to the footprint just off the greater tuberosity. Following anchor placement, sutures are passed through the rotator cuff tendon using a variety of suture passing devices, tissue penetrators, or suture shuttle devices. Arthroscopic knot tying is crucial to a successful repair. Although many sliding and nonsliding knots have been described (including the Roeder, the midshipman, the Revo, and the western), using simple half-hitch knots passed on alternating posts tied from posterior to anterior is a reliable and simple technique. There are now numerous devices, anchors, and suture configurations to replicate the TOE, both with and without knots.

Several authors have reported the clinical outcomes of complete arthroscopic repairs that are comparable to the results achieved with open and arthroscopically assisted techniques.[68-75] A brief summary of the results comparing mini-open to all-arthroscopic rotator cuff repairs is found in **Table 2**.

Evolution of Techniques: Clinical Outcomes

The clinical outcomes of the newer suture repair constructs have yet to be fully defined. It is important to note that not all of the reported data can be generalized to a particular repair construct. When evaluating the literature on repair techniques and outcomes, there are numerous contributing factors to consider, such as the number of anchors used, the chronicity of the tear, and patient age. Although reports will typically describe the basic repair configuration (single-row, double-row, or TOE), it is important to note the total number of anchors involved in the repair, the number of anchors that are used for the medial and lateral rows in double-row repairs, and the configuration of the sutures as they bridge the tissue from medial to lateral (such as straight medial to lateral, sutures crossed over one another to create interconnectivity, or knotless or knotted medial row). The number of anchors represents the number of fixation points; therefore, it may be possible that, regardless of how the repair is configured, more fixation points may ultimately result in a stronger repair.[44] This may also be true in studies involving larger rotator cuff repairs because more anchors are used in large repairs, and outcomes may be dependent on this factor. Chronicity and the number of tendons involved should also be considered. In certain situations, chronic tears can be less amenable to double-row constructs because the tissue may not allow full reapproximation to re-create the anatomic footprint. Patient age should be noted because younger patients may place higher loads on the repair site despite the fact that their tissue quality is often superior.

Currently, prospective results have suggested that rotator cuff repair tendon healing occurs more frequently in patients treated with double-row repairs compared with single-row repairs.[6,76-78] Sugaya et al[79] compared

Table 2
Summary of Results Comparing All-Arthroscopic to Mini-Open Rotator Cuff Repairs

Authors (Year)	Number of Patients	Mean Follow-up	Reported Outcomes
Kose et al[68] (2008)	25 all-arthroscopic, 25 mini-open	26 months	Preoperative and postoperative Constant-Murley and University of California at Los Angeles scores and satisfaction not significantly different between groups
Pearsall et al[69] (2007)	27 all-arthroscopic, 25 mini-open	50.6 months	No statistical difference in outcome between the two groups
Verma et al[70] (2006)	38 all-arthroscopic, 33 mini-open	minimum 2 years	No difference in clinical outcomes between the two techniques
Sauerbrey et al[71] (2005)	28 all-arthroscopic, 26 mini-open	33 months	All improved; the difference in scores between the two techniques not statistically significant
Warner et al[72] (2005)	9 all-arthroscopic, 12 mini-open	minimum 27 months	No differences in outcomes
Youm et al[73] (2005)	42 all-arthroscopic, 42 mini-open	minimum 2 years	Arthroscopic and mini-open rotator cuff repairs produced similar results for small, medium, and large rotator cuff tears with equivalent patient satisfaction rates
Severud et al[74] (2003)	35 all-arthroscopic, 29 mini-open	44.6 months	Shoulders in the all-arthroscopic group showed better motion at 6 and 12 weeks
Kim et al[75] (2003)	42 all-arthroscopic, 34 mini-open	39 months	No difference in shoulder scores, pain, and return to activity between the groups

39 patients treated with a single-row repair to 41 patients treated with standard double-row suture anchor repair at an average follow-up of 35 months. Using MRI, the authors found a 25.6% retear rate in the single-row constructs compared with a 9.8% retear rate in the double-row repairs. Similarly, Charousset et al[76] used CT to assess healing at 6 months in both single- and standard double-row repairs. Double-row fixation resulted in a significantly greater healing rate (19 of 31 repairs; 61%) compared with single-row fixation (14 of 35 repairs; 40%). Duquin et al[77] performed a systematic review of more than 1,100 rotator cuff repairs described in studies that compared single-row to double-row constructs. A statistically significant decrease in anatomic retear rates was found for true double-row repairs when compared with single-row repairs for all tears larger than 1 cm.

Although double-row repairs appear to be superior in the laboratory and on imaging exhibit improved healing rates over single-row repairs, similar clinical outcomes between the two techniques have been reported in most studies. Franceschi et al[80] performed a randomized controlled trial comparing 30 patients with single-row repairs and 30 patients with standard double-row fixation. Although the authors believed that the double-row technique produced a mechanically superior construct as evidenced by better cuff integrity on postoperative MRI, they found no significant difference in postoperative clinical scores or range of motion between the two groups at 2-year follow-up.[80] Similarly, in a randomized clinical trial comparing 40 patients (20 single-row and 20 double-row constructs), Burks et al[81] reported no significant differences in clinical outcomes or physical examination results. There were no significant differences in MRI measurements of footprint coverage, tendon thickness, and tendon signal between the groups.[81] Many of these studies may be underpowered, which presents a significant challenge in interpreting the data and applying the information clinically. Researchers at Rush University in Chicago recently determined that to detect a 10% difference in healing rates based on an estimated 30% failure rate for single-row repairs and a 20% failure rate for double-row repairs, 219 patients in each group would be needed for the study to be considered appropriately powered. A summary of the studies comparing single- to double-row repairs and the results of double-row outcome studies are found in **Tables 3** and **4**, respectively.[6,76,79-86]

The TOE bridging construct was developed to provide increased contact and compression on the footprint to enhance healing potential. The medial row of anchors theoretically may provide a barrier between the synovial environment and the healing zone to contain healing factors. Although there are limited clinical data on TOE constructs, early results have been promising. To evaluate the healing rate of TOE repairs, Frank et al[78] examined a cohort of 25 patients with a minimum 1-year follow-up. Postoperative

Table 3
Summary of Results Comparing Single-Row to Double-Row Rotator Cuff Repairs

Authors (Year)	Number of Patients	Mean Age (years)	Mean Anchors	Reported Outcomes
Burks et al[81] (2009)	20 SR, 20 DR	56.5	SR: 2.2 DR: 3.2	No clinical or MRI differences between SR or DR repairs
Park et al[84] (2008)	40 SR, 38 DR	56	Not given	No difference between SR and DR for all, but DR had better outcome scores and Shoulder Strength Index for tears > 3 cm
Franceschi et al[80] (2007)	30 SR, 30 DR	61	SR: 1.9 DR: 2.3	Both had comparable clinical outcome at 2 years; DR repairs produced mechanically superior construct compared with SR repairs
Charousset et al[76] (2007)	35 SR, 31 DR	59	Not given	No significant difference in clinical results, but tendon healing rates were better with DR repairs
Sugaya et al[79] (2005)	39 SR, 41 DR	57.9	SR: 2.4 DR: 3.2	No statistical difference between the groups in the postoperative scores; DR repairs had improved structural outcomes

SR = single row, DR = double row

Table 4
Summary of Results Following Arthroscopic Double-Row Rotator Cuff Repairs

Authors (Year)	Number of Patients	Mean Follow-up	Reported Outcomes
Vaishnav and Millet[85] (2010)	17 with knotless self-reinforcing DR system	1.5 years	Average pain scores decreased; average SANE scores increased; satisfaction 9.8 of 10
Lafosse et al[83] (2008)	105 with DR of SS or SS + IS	Prospective (minimum 2 years)	12 failed repairs (11%); intact RCR associated with significantly increased strength and ROM; postoperative Constant score 80.1 ± 11.1
Sugaya et al[6] (2007)	86 with full-thickness RCT using suture anchors	Prospective, average 31 months (14 months for MRI)	All clinical outcomes scores significantly improved ($P < 0.05$); retear rate higher for larger/massive tears
Huijsmans et al[82] (2007)	242 with DR suture anchor technique	22 months (minimum 12 months)	VAS improved from 7.4 to 0.7; good to excellent outcome in 220 (91%); intact RCR in 174 (83%) via US; improved strength and ROM in intact repairs
Anderson et al[86] (2006)	52 with DR suture anchor technique	30 months (minimum 24 months)	L'Insalata shoulder ratings improved from 42 to 93 ($P < 0.001$); active ROM improved in all planes ($P < 0.001$); strength increased in ER and FE ($P < 0.001$) and IR ($P = 0.033$); failure rate of 17%

DR = double row, SANE = single assessment numeric evaluation, SS = supraspinatus, IS = infraspinatus, RCR = rotator cuff repair, ROM = range of motion, US = ultrasound, ER = external rotation, FE = forward elevation, IR = internal rotation, VAS = visual analog scale

MRIs showed intact rotator cuff repairs in 22 of 25 patients (88%). In tears that were limited to the supraspinatus tendon, 16 of 18 patients (89%) had intact repairs. Healing was noted in three tears that were considered massive.[78]

With the development of these second-generation double-row repair constructs, a new failure mode has been reported. Historically, recognized failure modes for arthroscopic rotator cuff repairs included failure at the bone-anchor interface, the anchor-suture interface, and the suture-tendon interface.[87-89] However, repair failure at the musculotendinous junction following double-row and TOE repairs are now being reported. Trantalis et al[90] identified a subset of five patients who showed an atypical mechanism of tendon failure after a double-row repair. The tendon footprint appeared well fixed in these patients; however, medial to the intact footprint, the tendon was torn through the rotator cuff. Other investigators have reported similar failure modes.[91,92] Cho et al[91] reported on 46 retears following either single-row or TOE repairs. Most of the TOE repairs (74.1%) had a retear pattern that had remnant cuff tissue at the rotator cuff footprint, with the tear occurring more medially. The authors concluded that the TOE technique tended to better preserve the footprint, but retear occurred mainly in the musculotendinous junction. This information may have significant implications in revision surgery following failed bridging repairs. There are several considerations related to this failure mode. If healing rates are superior in double-row or TOE repairs, advocating the implementation of these techniques should be weighed against the potential mechanism of failure. This finding has not been appreciated by most studies that used MRI or ultrasound to evaluate retear rates following double-row or TOE repairs.[1,6,78,80-83] Certainly, there are technical precautions that will minimize this failure mode, and it should be assumed that this failure mode could occur with either standard double-row or TOE repairs. Preventive measures, such as avoiding overtensioning of the medial row by performing an anatomic cuff tear reduction, will reduce stress at the musculotendinous junction. Placing the medial suture lateral to the musculotendinous junction and closer to the rotator cuff cable entirely within the tendon may also minimize this type of failure.

Clinical Decision Making: Single-Row Versus Double-Row Techniques

With such a large amount of data available in the literature and the similarities of the various results, it is prudent to consider patients individually before generalizing the use of a certain construct to all patients. Factors such as patient characteristics, length of the procedure, surgical cost, and technical demands are important when weighing the benefits of the different techniques. Churchill and Ghorai[65] examined the total cost and operating room time of mini-open compared with all-arthroscopic rotator cuff repair techniques at low-, intermediate-, and high-volume centers using the 2006 New York State Ambulatory Surgery Database. The authors reported that the surgical time was significantly shorter in the mini-open group (103 minutes) compared with the all-arthroscopic group (113 minutes). Surgical costs were also significantly less in the mini-open group ($7,841) compared with the all-arthroscopic group ($8,985), resulting in an additional cost of $1,144 more per patient when an arthroscopic repair was performed.[65] Although a breakdown in cost was not reported between the different arthroscopic techniques, it can be assumed that the cost would be higher when a double-row construct is used rather than a single-row repair. Similar surgical time differences were found by Franceschi et al[80] in a study comparing single-row to double-row outcomes. It was reported that the average surgical time for single-row procedures was 42 ± 18.9 minutes and that double-row repair averaged 65 ± 23.4 minutes. These studies did not consider the financial burden associated with anatomic failure following rotator cuff repair (such as time off work or the cost of revision surgery).

Decision making must also take into account certain clinical factors. Probably the most important of these is the size of the rotator cuff tear. Most studies to date examining outcomes from single- and double-row repairs typically have enrolled most patients with tears that are less than 3 cm.[6,41,76,81,93] Park et al[84] compared 40 patients with single-row fixation to 38 patients treated with double-row fixation. The mean age of the patients was 56 years, and outcomes were measured at 2 years postoperatively using the American Shoulder and Elbow Surgeons and Constant scoring systems and the Shoulder Strength Index. The authors reported improvement in functional outcome in both groups, but there was no significant difference between the groups. When patient results were stratified by tear size, no difference was found between the repair techniques in patients with small to medium (< 3 cm) tears; however, in patients with large to massive tears (> 3 cm), all outcome measures were significantly improved in the group that had been treated with a double-row repair.[84] This may be evidence to support the use of single-row fixation in small to medium rotator cuff tears while reserving double-row techniques for large and massive tears.

Summary

Many factors play a vital role in obtaining a successful result after a rotator cuff repair. Patient factors such as age, biology, and environmental influences are beyond the control of the treating surgeon; however, the surgeon does influence the technique of cuff reduction and the repair construct. Recently, many advances have been made in rotator cuff repair. Despite these improvements, it is important to keep in mind the basic tenets of achieving a strong repair, including minimizing motion, achieving an anatomic repair, and preventing gaps. Although second-generation techniques appear to be biomechanically superior to single-row repairs, additional research is needed to define the patient characteristics and type of rotator cuff tear that would benefit from a double-row or TOE repair construct.

References

1. Boileau P, Brassart N, Watkinson DJ, Carles M, Hatzidakis AM, Krishnan SG: Arthroscopic repair of full-thickness tears of the supraspinatus: Does the tendon really heal? *J Bone Joint Surg Am* 2005;87(6):1229-1240.
2. Cole BJ, McCarty LP III, Kang RW, Alford W, Lewis PB, Hayden JK: Arthroscopic rotator cuff repair: Prospective functional outcome and repair integrity at minimum 2-year follow-up. *J Shoulder Elbow Surg* 2007;16(5):579-585.
3. DeFranco MJ, Bershadsky B, Ciccone J, Yum JK, Iannotti JP: Functional outcome of arthroscopic rotator cuff repairs: A correlation of anatomic and clinical results. *J Shoulder Elbow Surg* 2007;16(6):759-765.
4. Flurin PH, Landreau P, Gregory T, et al: Arthroscopic repair of full-thickness cuff tears: A multicentric retrospective study of 576 cases with anatomical assessment. *Rev Chir Orthop Reparatrice Appar Mot* 2005;91(S8):31-42.
5. Klepps S, Bishop J, Lin J, et al: Prospective evaluation of the effect of rotator cuff integrity on the outcome of open rotator cuff repairs. *Am J Sports Med* 2004;32(7):1716-1722.
6. Sugaya H, Maeda K, Matsuki K, Moriishi J: Repair integrity and functional outcome after arthroscopic double-row rotator cuff repair: A prospective outcome study. *J Bone Joint Surg Am* 2007;89(5):953-960.
7. Galatz LM, Ball CM, Teefey SA, Middleton WD, Yamaguchi K: The outcome and repair integrity of completely arthroscopically repaired large and massive rotator cuff tears. *J Bone Joint Surg Am* 2004;86-A(2):219-224.
8. Harryman DT II, Mack LA, Wang KY, Jackins SE, Richardson ML, Matsen FA III: Repairs of the rotator cuff: Correlation of functional results with integrity of the cuff. *J Bone Joint Surg Am* 1991;73(7):982-989.
9. Wilson F, Hinov V, Adams G: Arthroscopic repair of full-thickness tears of the rotator cuff: 2- to 14-year follow-up. *Arthroscopy* 2002;18(2):136-144.
10. Yamaguchi K, Ditsios K, Middleton WD, Hildebolt CF, Galatz LM, Teefey SA: The demographic and morphological features of rotator cuff disease: A comparison of asymptomatic and symptomatic shoulders. *J Bone Joint Surg Am* 2006;88(8):1699-1704.
11. Coleman SH, Fealy S, Ehteshami JR, et al: Chronic rotator cuff injury and repair model in sheep. *J Bone Joint Surg Am* 2003;85-A(12):2391-2402.
12. Gerber C, Meyer DC, Frey E, et al: Neer Award 2007: Reversion of structural muscle changes caused by chronic rotator cuff tears using continuous musculotendinous traction: An experimental study in sheep. *J Shoulder Elbow Surg* 2009;18(2):163-171.
13. Kannus P, Józsa L: Histopathological changes preceding spontaneous rupture of a tendon: A controlled study of 891 patients. *J Bone Joint Surg Am* 1991;73(10):1507-1525.
14. Thomopoulos S, Hattersley G, Rosen V, et al: The localized expression of extracellular matrix components in healing tendon insertion sites: An in situ hybridization study. *J Orthop Res* 2002;20(3):454-463.
15. Liu SH, Baker CL: Arthroscopically assisted rotator cuff repair: Correlation of functional results with integrity of the cuff. *Arthroscopy* 1994;10(1):54-60.
16. Lichtenberg S, Liem D, Magosch P, Habermeyer P: Influence of tendon healing after arthroscopic rotator cuff repair on clinical outcome using single-row Mason-Allen suture technique: A prospective, MRI controlled study. *Knee Surg Sports Traumatol Arthrosc* 2006;14(11):1200-1206.
17. Oh JH, Kim SH, Kang JY, Oh CH, Gong HS: Effect of age on functional and structural outcome after rotator cuff repair. *Am J Sports Med* 2010;38(4):672-678.
18. Goutallier D, Bernageau J, Patte D: L'évaluation par le scanner de la trophicité des muscles de la coiffe ayant une rupture tendineuse. *Rev Chir Orthop Repar Appar Mot* 1989;75:126-127.
19. Melis B, DeFranco MJ, Chuinard C, Walch G: Natural history of fatty infiltration and atrophy of the supraspinatus muscle in rotator cuff tears. *Clin Orthop Relat Res* 2010;468(6):1498-1505.
20. Melis B, Nemoz C, Walch G: Muscle fatty infiltration in rotator cuff tears: Descriptive analysis of 1688 cases. *Orthop Traumatol Surg Res* 2009;95(5):319-324.
21. Melis B, Wall B, Walch G: Natural history of infraspinatus fatty infiltration in rotator cuff tears. *J Shoulder Elbow Surg* 2010;19(5):757-763.
22. Rubino LJ, Stills HF Jr, Sprott DC, Crosby LA: Fatty infiltration of the torn rotator cuff worsens over time in a rabbit model. *Arthroscopy* 2007;23(7):717-722.
23. Goutallier D, Postel JM, Bernageau J, Lavau L, Voisin MC: Fatty infiltration of disrupted rotator cuff muscles. *Rev Rhum Engl Ed* 1995;62(6):415-422.
24. Goutallier D, Postel JM, Bernageau J, Lavau L, Voisin MC: Fatty muscle degeneration in cuff ruptures: Pre- and postoperative evaluation by CT scan. *Clin Orthop Relat Res* 1994;304:78-83.
25. Jost B, Zumstein M, Pfirrmann CW, Gerber C: Long-term outcome after structural failure of

rotator cuff repairs. *J Bone Joint Surg Am* 2006;88(3):472-479.

26. Gladstone JN, Bishop JY, Lo IK, Flatow EL: Fatty infiltration and atrophy of the rotator cuff do not improve after rotator cuff repair and correlate with poor functional outcome. *Am J Sports Med* 2007; 35(5):719-728.
27. Baumgarten KM, Gerlach D, Galatz LM, et al: Cigarette smoking increases the risk for rotator cuff tears. *Clin Orthop Relat Res* 2010;468(6):1534-1541.
28. Galatz LM, Silva MJ, Rothermich SY, Zaegel MA, Havlioglu N, Thomopoulos S: Nicotine delays tendon-to-bone healing in a rat shoulder model. *J Bone Joint Surg Am* 2006;88(9):2027-2034.
29. Rodeo SA, Arnoczky SP, Torzilli PA, Hidaka C, Warren RF: Tendon-healing in a bone tunnel: A biomechanical and histological study in the dog. *J Bone Joint Surg Am* 1993;75(12):1795-1803.
30. St Pierre P, Olson EJ, Elliott JJ, O'Hair KC, McKinney LA, Ryan J: Tendon-healing to cortical bone compared with healing to a cancellous trough: A biomechanical and histological evaluation in goats. *J Bone Joint Surg Am* 1995; 77(12):1858-1866.
31. Aoki M, Oguma H, Fukushima S, Ishii S, Ohtani S, Murakami G: Fibrous connection to bone after immediate repair of the canine infraspinatus: The most effective bony surface for tendon attachment. *J Shoulder Elbow Surg* 2001;10(2):123-128.
32. Apreleva M, Ozbaydar M, Fitzgibbons PG, Warner JJ: Rotator cuff tears: The effect of the reconstruction method on three-dimensional repair site area. *Arthroscopy* 2002; 18(5):519-526.
33. Brady PC, Arrigoni P, Burkhart SS: Evaluation of residual rotator cuff defects after in vivo single- versus double-row rotator cuff repairs. *Arthroscopy* 2006;22(10): 1070-1075.
34. Meier SW, Meier JD: Rotator cuff repair: The effect of double-row fixation on three-dimensional repair site. *J Shoulder Elbow Surg* 2006;15(6):691-696.
35. Gazielly DF, Gleyze P, Montagnon C: Functional and anatomical results after rotator cuff repair. *Clin Orthop Relat Res* 1994;304: 43-53.
36. Weiler A, Peine R, Pashmineh-Azar A, Abel C, Südkamp NP, Hoffmann RF: Tendon healing in a bone tunnel: Part I. Biomechanical results after biodegradable interference fit fixation in a model of anterior cruciate ligament reconstruction in sheep. *Arthroscopy* 2002;18(2):113-123.
37. Dugas JR, Campbell DA, Warren RF, Robie BH, Millett PJ: Anatomy and dimensions of rotator cuff insertions. *J Shoulder Elbow Surg* 2002;11(5):498-503.
38. Ruotolo C, Fow JE, Nottage WM: The supraspinatus footprint: An anatomic study of the supraspinatus insertion. *Arthroscopy* 2004;20(3):246-249.
39. Mazzocca AD, Millett PJ, Guanche CA, Santangelo SA, Arciero RA: Arthroscopic single-row versus double-row suture anchor rotator cuff repair. *Am J Sports Med* 2005;33(12):1861-1868.
40. Nelson CO, Sileo MJ, Grossman MG, Serra-Hsu F: Single-row modified mason-allen versus double-row arthroscopic rotator cuff repair: A biomechanical and surface area comparison. *Arthroscopy* 2008;24(8):941-948.
41. Ahmad CS, Kleweno C, Jacir AM, et al: Biomechanical performance of rotator cuff repairs with humeral rotation: A new rotator cuff repair failure model. *Am J Sports Med* 2008;36(5):888-892.
42. Baums MH, Buchhorn GH, Spahn G, Poppendieck B, Schultz W, Klinger HM: Biomechanical characteristics of single-row repair in comparison to double-row repair with consideration of the suture configuration and suture material. *Knee Surg Sports Traumatol Arthrosc* 2008; 16(11):1052-1060.
43. Domb BG, Glousman RE, Brooks A, Hansen M, Lee TQ, ElAttrache NS: High-tension double-row footprint repair compared with reduced-tension single-row repair for massive rotator cuff tears. *J Bone Joint Surg Am* 2008; 90(Suppl 4):35-39.
44. Kim DH, Elattrache NS, Tibone JE, et al: Biomechanical comparison of a single-row versus double-row suture anchor technique for rotator cuff repair. *Am J Sports Med* 2006;34(3):407-414.
45. Ma CB, Comerford L, Wilson J, Puttlitz CM: Biomechanical evaluation of arthroscopic rotator cuff repairs: Double-row compared with single-row fixation. *J Bone Joint Surg Am* 2006;88(2): 403-410.
46. Milano G, Grasso A, Zarelli D, Deriu L, Cillo M, Fabbriciani C: Comparison between single-row and double-row rotator cuff repair: A biomechanical study. *Knee Surg Sports Traumatol Arthrosc* 2008;16(1):75-80.
47. Wall LB, Keener JD, Brophy RH: Double-row vs single-row rotator cuff repair: A review of the biomechanical evidence. *J Shoulder Elbow Surg* 2009;18(6):933-941.
48. Adams JE, Zobitz ME, Reach JS Jr, An KN, Steinmann SP: Rotator cuff repair using an acellular dermal matrix graft: An in vivo study in a canine model. *Arthroscopy* 2006;22(7):700-709.
49. Park MC, ElAttrache NS, Tibone JE, Ahmad CS, Jun BJ, Lee TQ: Part I: Footprint contact characteristics for a transosseous-equivalent rotator cuff repair technique compared with a double-row repair technique. *J Shoulder Elbow Surg* 2007;16(4):461-468.

50. Park MC, Tibone JE, El-Attrache NS, Ahmad CS, Jun BJ, Lee TQ: Part II: Biomechanical assessment for a footprint-restoring transosseous-equivalent rotator cuff repair technique compared with a double-row repair technique. *J Shoulder Elbow Surg* 2007;16(4):469-476.
51. Lo IK, Burkhart SS: Double-row arthroscopic rotator cuff repair: Re-establishing the footprint of the rotator cuff. *Arthroscopy* 2003; 19(9):1035-1042.
52. Park MC, Pirolo JM, Park CJ, Tibone JE, McGarry MH, Lee TQ: The effect of abduction and rotation on footprint contact for single-row, double-row, and modified double-row rotator cuff repair techniques. *Am J Sports Med* 2009;37(8):1599-1608.
53. Burkhart SS, Adams CR, Burkhart SS, Schoolfield JD: A biomechanical comparison of 2 techniques of footprint reconstruction for rotator cuff repair: The SwiveLock-FiberChain construct versus standard double-row repair. *Arthroscopy* 2009;25(3):274-281.
54. Bisson LJ, Manohar LM: A biomechanical comparison of transosseous-suture anchor and suture bridge rotator cuff repairs in cadavers. *Am J Sports Med* 2009;37(10):1991-1995.
55. Itoi E, Berglund LJ, Grabowski JJ, et al: Tensile properties of the supraspinatus tendon. *J Orthop Res* 1995;13(4):578-584.
56. Busfield BT, Glousman RE, McGarry MH, Tibone JE, Lee TQ: A biomechanical comparison of 2 technical variations of double-row rotator cuff fixation: The importance of medial row knots. *Am J Sports Med* 2008;36(5):901-906.
57. Gerber C, Schneeberger AG, Beck M, Schlegel U: Mechanical strength of repairs of the rotator cuff. *J Bone Joint Surg Br* 1994; 76(3):371-380.
58. Lorbach O, Bachelier F, Vees J, Kohn D, Pape D: Cyclic loading of rotator cuff reconstructions: Single-row repair with modified suture configurations versus double-row repair. *Am J Sports Med* 2008;36(8):1504-1510.
59. Cummins CA, Appleyard RC, Strickland S, Haen PS, Chen S, Murrell GA: Rotator cuff repair: An ex vivo analysis of suture anchor repair techniques on initial load to failure. *Arthroscopy* 2005; 21(10):1236-1241.
60. Levy HJ, Uribe JW, Delaney LG: Arthroscopic assisted rotator cuff repair: Preliminary results. *Arthroscopy* 1990;6(1):55-60.
61. Altchek DW, Warren RF, Wickiewicz TL, Skyhar MJ, Ortiz G, Schwartz E: Arthroscopic acromioplasty: Technique and results. *J Bone Joint Surg Am* 1990;72(8): 1198-1207.
62. Gartsman GM: Arthroscopic acromioplasty for lesions of the rotator cuff. *J Bone Joint Surg Am* 1990;72(2):169-180.
63. Kim TK, Rauh PB, McFarland EG: Partial tears of the subscapularis tendon found during arthroscopic procedures on the shoulder: A statistical analysis of sixty cases. *Am J Sports Med* 2003; 31(5):744-750.
64. Paulos LE, Franklin JL: Arthroscopic shoulder decompression development and application: A five year experience. *Am J Sports Med* 1990;18(3):235-244.
65. Churchill RS, Ghorai JK: Total cost and operating room time comparison of rotator cuff repair techniques at low, intermediate, and high volume centers: Mini-open versus all-arthroscopic. *J Shoulder Elbow Surg* 2010;19(5): 716-721.
66. Burkhart SS, Athanasiou KA, Wirth MA: Margin convergence: A method of reducing strain in massive rotator cuff tears. *Arthroscopy* 1996;12(3):335-338.
67. Burkhart SS, Lo IK: Arthroscopic rotator cuff repair. *J Am Acad Orthop Surg* 2006;14(6):333-346.
68. Kose KC, Tezen E, Cebesoy O, et al: Mini-open versus all-arthroscopic rotator cuff repair: Comparison of the operative costs and the clinical outcomes. *Adv Ther* 2008;25(3):249-259.
69. Pearsall AW, Ibrahim KA, Madanagopal SG: Abstract: The results of arthroscopic versus mini-open repair for rotator cuff tears at mid-term follow-up. *J Orthop Surg Res* 2007;2:24.
70. Verma NN, Dunn W, Adler RS, et al: All-arthroscopic versus mini-open rotator cuff repair: A retrospective review with minimum 2-year follow-up. *Arthroscopy* 2006;22(6):587-594.
71. Sauerbrey AM, Getz CL, Piancastelli M, Iannotti JP, Ramsey ML, Williams GR Jr: Arthroscopic versus mini-open rotator cuff repair: A comparison of clinical outcome. *Arthroscopy* 2005;21: 1415-1420.
72. Warner JJ, Tetreault P, Lehtinen J, Zurakowski D: Arthroscopic versus mini-open rotator cuff repair: A cohort comparison study. *Arthroscopy* 2005;21:328-332.
73. Youm T, Murray DH, Kubiak EN, Rokito AS, Zuckerman JD: Arthroscopic versus mini-open rotator cuff repair: A comparison of clinical outcomes and patient satisfaction. *J Shoulder Elbow Surg* 2005;14:455-459.
74. Severud EL, Ruotolo C, Abbott DD, Nottage WM: All-arthroscopic versus mini-open rotator cuff repair: A long-term retrospective outcome comparison. *Arthroscopy* 2003;19:234-238.
75. Kim SH, Ha KI, Park JH, Kang JS, Oh SK, Oh I: Arthroscopic versus mini-open salvage repair of the rotator cuff tear: Outcome analysis at 2 to 6years' follow-up. *Arthroscopy* 2003;19: 746-754.

76. Charousset C, Grimberg J, Duranthon LD, Bellaiche L, Petrover D: Can a double-row anchorage technique improve tendon healing in arthroscopic rotator cuff repair? A prospective, nonrandomized, comparative study of double-row and single-row anchorage techniques with computed tomographic arthrography tendon healing assessment. *Am J Sports Med* 2007;35(8):1247-1253.

77. Duquin TR, Buyea C, Bisson LJ: Which method of rotator cuff repair leads to the highest rate of structural healing? A systematic review. *Am J Sports Med* 2010; 38(4):835-841.

78. Frank JB, ElAttrache NS, Dines JS, Blackburn A, Crues J, Tibone JE: Repair site integrity after arthroscopic transosseous-equivalent suture-bridge rotator cuff repair. *Am J Sports Med* 2008; 36(8):1496-1503.

79. Sugaya H, Maeda K, Matsuki K, Moriishi J: Functional and structural outcome after arthroscopic full-thickness rotator cuff repair: Single-row versus dual-row fixation. *Arthroscopy* 2005;21(11): 1307-1316.

80. Franceschi F, Ruzzini L, Longo UG, et al: Equivalent clinical results of arthroscopic single-row and double-row suture anchor repair for rotator cuff tears: A randomized controlled trial. *Am J Sports Med* 2007;35(8):1254-1260.

81. Burks RT, Crim J, Brown N, Fink B, Greis PE: A prospective randomized clinical trial comparing arthroscopic single- and double-row rotator cuff repair: Magnetic resonance imaging and early clinical evaluation. *Am J Sports Med* 2009;37(4):674-682.

82. Huijsmans PE, Pritchard MP, Berghs BM, van Rooyen KS, Wallace AL, de Beer JF: Arthroscopic rotator cuff repair with double-row fixation. *J Bone Joint Surg Am* 2007;89(6):1248-1257.

83. Lafosse L, Brzoska R, Toussaint B, Gobezie R: The outcome and structural integrity of arthroscopic rotator cuff repair with use of the double-row suture anchor technique: Surgical technique. *J Bone Joint Surg Am* 2008;90(Suppl 2, Pt 2):275-286.

84. Park JY, Lhee SH, Choi JH, Park HK, Yu JW, Seo JB: Comparison of the clinical outcomes of single- and double-row repairs in rotator cuff tears. *Am J Sports Med* 2008;36(7):1310-1316.

85. Vaishnav S, Millett PJ: Arthroscopic rotator cuff repair: Scientific rationale, surgical technique, and early clinical and functional results of a knotless self-reinforcing double-row rotator cuff repair system. *J Shoulder Elbow Surg* 2010;19(2, Suppl): 83-90.

86. Anderson K, Boothby M, Aschenbrener D, van Holsbeeck M II: Outcome and structural integrity after arthroscopic rotator cuff repair using 2 rows of fixation: Minimum 2-Year follow-up. *Am J Sport Med* 2006;34(12):1899-1905.

87. Mahar A, Allred DW, Wedemeyer M, Abbi G, Pedowitz R: A biomechanical and radiographic analysis of standard and intracortical suture anchors for arthroscopic rotator cuff repair. *Arthroscopy* 2006;22(2):130-135.

88. Bardana DD, Burks RT, West JR, Greis PE: The effect of suture anchor design and orientation on suture abrasion: An in vitro study. *Arthroscopy* 2003;19(3):274-281.

89. Burkhart SS, Diaz Pagàn JL, Wirth MA, Athanasiou KA: Cyclic loading of anchor-based rotator cuff repairs: Confirmation of the tension overload phenomenon and comparison of suture anchor fixation with transosseous fixation. *Arthroscopy* 1997;13(6): 720-724.

90. Trantalis JN, Boorman RS, Pletsch K, Lo IK: Medial rotator cuff failure after arthroscopic double-row rotator cuff repair. *Arthroscopy* 2008;24(6):727-731.

91. Cho NS, Yi JW, Lee BG, Rhee YG: Retear patterns after arthroscopic rotator cuff repair: Single-row versus suture bridge technique. *Am J Sports Med* 2010; 38(4):664-671.

92. Yamakado K, Katsuo S, Mizuno K, Arakawa H, Hayashi S: Medial-row failure after arthroscopic double-row rotator cuff repair. *Arthroscopy* 2010;26(3): 430-435.

93. Grasso A, Milano G, Salvatore M, Falcone G, Deriu L, Fabbriciani C: Single-row versus double-row arthroscopic rotator cuff repair: A prospective randomized clinical study. *Arthroscopy* 2009;25(1): 4-12.

13

Glenohumeral Arthritis in the Young Adult

CDR Matthew T. Provencher, MD, MC, USN
Joseph U. Barker, MD
Eric J. Strauss, MD
Rachel M. Frank, BS
Anthony A. Romeo, MD
Frederick A. Matsen III, MD
Brian J. Cole, MD, MBA

Abstract

Treating glenohumeral arthritis in the young adult remains a significant challenge. There are a variety of etiologies that can lead to this condition, and the diagnosis is often not straightforward. With advances in both surgical techniques and biologic options, the treatment algorithm for patients with glenohumeral arthritis is constantly evolving. When nonsurgical treatment fails, there are a variety of possible surgical options, each with potential benefits. It is helpful to review the diagnostic challenges presented by these patients and understand the palliative, reparative, restorative, and reconstructive surgical options and their associated clinical outcomes, which provide a framework for clinical and surgical decision making.

Instr Course Lect 2011;60:137-153.

Dr. Provencher or an immediate family member serves as a board member, owner, officer, or committee member of the American Academy of Orthopaedic Surgeons, the American Orthopaedic Society for Sports Medicine, the Arthroscopy Association of North America, and the Society of Military Orthopaedic Surgeons. Dr. Romeo or an immediate family member serves as a board member, owner, officer, or committee member of the American Orthopaedic Society for Sports Medicine, the American Shoulder and Elbow Surgeons, and the Arthroscopy Association of North America; has received royalties from Arthrex and Saunders/Mosby-Elsevier; is a member of a speakers' bureau or has made paid presentations on behalf of Arthrex and DJ Orthopaedics; serves as a paid consultant to or is an employee of Arthrex; has received research or institutional support from Arthrex, Ossur, and Smith & Nephew; and has received nonincome support (such as equipment or services), commercially derived honoraria, or other non–research-related funding (such as paid travel) from Arthrex and DJ Orthopaedics. Dr. Matsen or an immediate family member has received royalties from Kinamed. Dr. Cole or an immediate family member has received royalties from Arthrex, DJ Orthopaedics, Lippincott, and Elsevier; is a member of a speakers' bureau or has made paid presentations on behalf of Genzyme; serves as a paid consultant to or is an employee of Zimmer, Arthrex, Carticept, Biomimetic, and Allosource; and has received research or institutional support from Regentis, Arthrex, Smith & Nephew, and DJ Orthopaedics. None of the following authors or any immediate family member has received anything of value from or owns stock in a commercial company or institution related directly or indirectly to the subject of this chapter: Dr. Barker, Dr. Strauss, and Ms. Frank.

The views expressed in this chapter are those of the authors and do not reflect the official policy or position of the Department of the Navy, the Department of Defense, or the US government.

Glenohumeral arthritis in young, active patients presents a growing challenge for the orthopaedic surgeon. Diagnosing symptomatic cartilage lesions can be difficult, and a thorough understanding of shoulder anatomy as well as the available surgical techniques is critical for effective treatment. Localized articular cartilage lesions of the glenohumeral joint are rare; however, such lesions can become painful and may limit shoulder function when symptomatic. Often, the diagnosis is initially unclear, and patients continue to present with substantial pain despite previous surgical or nonsurgical treatments. Young adult patients may also present with more global glenohumeral degenerative changes because of a variety of etiologic factors.[1-3] Although total joint arthroplasty offers a definitive solution for resolving symptoms, this remains a less than ideal option in the young, high-demand patient population. Other cartilage treatment options range from palliative arthroscopy to reparative, restorative, and reconstructive surgical techniques. Currently, there are limited

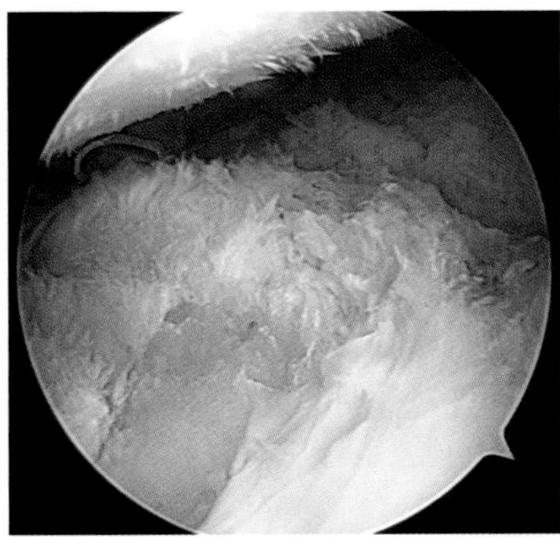

Figure 1 Arthroscopic view of a grade IV lesion of the glenoid in the dominant shoulder in a 27-year-old man.

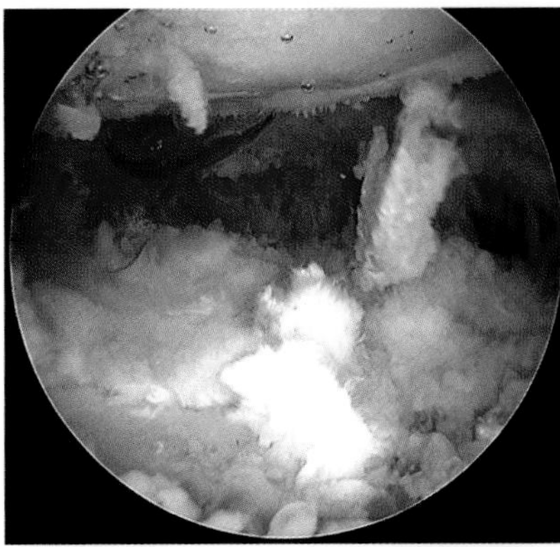

Figure 2 Arthroscopic view of diffuse degenerative disease in the shoulder of a 23-year-old man following the placement of an intra-articular pain pump after labral repair.

data and recommendations to guide treatment decisions for patients with symptomatic chondral lesions of the shoulder. However, with the increasing prevalence of young patients with symptomatic shoulder arthritis, joint-preserving treatments will continue to evolve. This chapter provides an overview of glenohumeral cartilage pathology, discusses patient evaluation and appropriate clinical decision making, and describes the various surgical treatment options for these challenging clinical situations.

Anatomic Considerations

The unique anatomic features of the glenohumeral joint make it challenging to evaluate and treat chondral lesions within this area. There are significant differences in the thickness of the glenohumeral articular cartilage compared with other joints, such as the knee or ankle. Specifically, the mean articular depth of the humerus is 1.24 mm, whereas the mean depth of the glenoid fossa is 1.88 mm.[4] The humeral head cartilage is thickest in the center (1.2 to 1.3 mm thick) but thins to less than 1 mm along the periphery.[5] In the glenoid, the articular cartilage is thickest along the periphery but tapers toward the center with an area that is completely devoid of cartilage (known as the bare area). From a biologic standpoint, the layout of the articular cartilage along both the glenoid surface and the humeral head may make it difficult to diagnose and treat symptomatic chondral lesions. It is important, for example, to avoid inadvertently attributing the bare areas on the glenoid or the humerus to pathologic chondral defects because this may lead to inappropriate treatment recommendations.

The geometry of the glenohumeral joint is also important when considering symptomatic cartilage defects. Specifically, the glenoid radius of curvature is within 2 to 3 mm of the humeral head and is relatively congruent with the humeral head when soft tissues, including the cartilage and labrum, are included.[6] Glenoid version typically varies, with an average of 1.5° of retroversion; notably, retroversion is considerably increased (approximately 11°) with advanced cartilage damage (such as the damage resulting from glenohumeral osteoarthritis). Glenoid inclination also varies, with an average of 4.2° in the superior direction.[6]

Classification of Glenohumeral Chondral Defects

Currently, there is no specific classification scheme for articular cartilage defects of the glenohumeral joint. The Outerbridge classification system,[7] which is commonly used for chondral defects in the knee, can be applied to similar defects in the shoulder. In this system, grade 0 refers to normal articular cartilage, grade I to cartilage softening, grade II to fibrillation involving half the depth of the cartilage, grade III to fissuring involving more than half the depth of the cartilage, and grade IV to full-thickness loss reaching to or through the subchondral bone (**Figure 1**). It is equally important to document the location of the defect, the depth of bony involvement, and the size of the defect relative to the entire dimension of the articular surface. If there are bipolar defects, it should be determined if these defects articulate with one another when bipolar disease exists.

Incidence and Etiology of Glenohumeral Chondral Defects

Injury to the glenohumeral articular cartilage can occur through a variety of mechanisms. Because cartilage lesions are often incidental findings, more common shoulder pathologic entities must be considered and evaluated. Overall, the diagnosis of a symptomatic chondral injury is one of exclusion.[1] Potential etiologies of chondral defects in the shoulder are varied and include genetic and/or degenerative changes to the joint, posttraumatic lesions, postoperative changes, osteonecrosis (commonly from corticosteroid use, alcohol use, or iatrogenic), and defects caused by intra-articular pain pump placement, radiofrequency therapy, and infection[2,3,8-10] (**Figure 2**). Because the etiology of the articular disease can affect disease progression, it is crucial for the clinician to obtain as much information as possible concerning the patient's symptoms. Specifically, the clinician should note previous surgeries, the nature and onset of symptoms, and the rate of symptom progression. The qualitative nature of symptoms (such as pain and mechanical and neurologic symptoms) should be assessed to help the clinician weigh options relative to the magnitude of the patient's clinical disorders and treatment expectations.

The overall incidence and natural history of glenohumeral chondral defects is unknown. As diagnostic modalities for symptomatic cartilage lesions continue to advance, an improved understanding of glenohumeral articular cartilage pathology can be expected. As previously mentioned, lesions are often found incidentally during imaging and/or the treatment of other shoulder pathologies. In a study of magnetic resonance arthrography (MRA), glenohumeral chondral lesions were found in up to one third of all patients.[11] In a cadaver study analyzing rotator cuff tears, an increase in chondral injury was seen in shoulders with cuff tears compared with those without rotator cuff pathology. Specifically, in shoulders with rotator cuff tears, defects in the glenoid were found in 32% of specimens, and defects in the humeral head were found in 36% compared with 6% and 7%, respectively, in shoulders without cuff tears.[12] Another study found a 4.5% incidence of significant cartilage lesions (Outerbridge type grade IV) in shoulders with rotator cuff tears.[13]

Chondral injuries also have been associated with shoulder instability. In a clinical study of patients with first-time traumatic dislocations, Taylor et al[14] reported that 57 of 63 patients (90%) had Hill-Sachs lesions, with 40% classified as chondral lesions and 60% classified as osteochondral lesions. Hintermann and Gächter[15] prospectively studied the arthroscopic findings of 212 patients with unstable shoulders and reported an increased incidence of chondral damage in patients with multiple dislocation events. Specifically, the authors found a 23% incidence of glenoid defects and an 8% incidence of humeral head degenerative arthritis in patients who sustained only one dislocation, and a 27% incidence of glenoid degenerative arthritis and a 36% incidence of humeral head arthritis in patients who sustained two or more dislocations.[15] Importantly, information related to the prevalence of symptoms associated with these traumatic chondral injuries is largely lacking.

Although focal chondral defects, whether found as primary lesions or as incidental findings, are challenging to treat, it is perhaps even more difficult to treat patients with progressive and/or diffuse disease. These patients present with varying etiologies, including rheumatoid arthritis, traumatic arthrosis, and osteoarthritis. Patients can also present after one or more failed treatment attempts, especially in the case of postoperative glenohumeral chondrolysis.[2,3,8-10,16] In 1998, Sperling et al[17] described long-term survivorship of total shoulder arthroplasty or hemiarthroplasty in 114 shoulders in patients younger than 50 years with painful glenohumeral arthritis or arthrosis. The authors described long-term improvement in motion as well as substantial pain relief but noted that approximately 50% of the patients were dissatisfied with their treatment, indicating the significant challenge in managing this disease. Although advances in the diagnosis and treatment of isolated chondral defects are certainly areas of focus, increased consideration of more diffuse glenohumeral chondral pathology is also warranted.

Patient Evaluation

Because articular cartilage defects are often incidental findings, it can be difficult to determine which chondral defects are truly symptomatic and which are simply incidental. Especially in patients with multiple shoulder pathologies who had several prior surgical treatments, it is often impossible to ascertain if the articular defects were responsible for their preoperative symptoms. To avoid treating asymptomatic injuries and ignoring truly symptomatic lesions, it is crucial for the surgeon to obtain as much information as possible from the patient during the initial history and physical examination. During the initial clinical visit, the patient should be asked about the original mechanism of injury as well as previous nonsurgical and surgical treatment of the shoulder, including the response to therapy. Specific questions about the activity level of the patient and his or her postoperative treatment goals are important initial considerations to address any potential unrealistic expectations of the patient before discussing potential treatment strategies.

Physical Examination

In addition to a thorough history, a complete physical examination of both shoulders is important for evaluating symptomatic chondral defects and any coexisting pathology, including rotator cuff tears and/or instability. The structure, function, neurologic status, and strength of the injured shoulder should be compared with that of the contralateral shoulder.[16] Loss of motion and stiffness must be noted at the preoperative examination to allow the patient time to restore any deficit before surgically treating the chondral defect. Stability, scapulothoracic dyskinesis, and manual muscle testing should be assessed. If necessary, special shoulder tests should be performed to evaluate any potential comorbidity or primary etiology for the patient's symptoms. Of note, in patients who have previously been treated with open shoulder surgery, subscapularis dysfunction may be present and should be documented and addressed before any surgical treatment.

Imaging Studies

Imaging studies are a routine component in the evaluation of symptomatic chondral lesions and are especially helpful in analyzing bone loss. Standard views should include AP, scapular-Y, and axillary views; the addition of a Stryker notch view is helpful for evaluating Hill-Sachs lesions, whereas the West Point view is useful in determining glenoid bone loss.[16] CT studies, especially those conducted using three-dimensional reconstruction software, are especially helpful for evaluating glenohumeral joint alignment, glenoid version, and glenoid bone loss. This can be helpful in patients who require more invasive osteochondral reconstruction for full-thickness cartilage defects that include subchondral bone. CT arthrography is quite helpful in evaluating joints and soft tissues without MRI artifact in the setting of prior hardware placement, such as metal glenoid or humeral head anchors.

MRI and MRA are the imaging modalities of choice for evaluating the glenoid and humeral head articular surfaces and are especially helpful in evaluating changes in subchondral bone and associated soft-tissue comorbidities,[18,19] including ligamentous, labrum, and rotator cuff pathologies. Typically, the T2-weighted image, with and without fat suppression, and the T1-weighted fat-suppressed three-dimensional spoiled gradient-echo technique are used. However, the sensitivity and specificity of MRI in evaluating glenohumeral chondral lesions is relatively poor,[11] and up to 45% of grade IV chondral lesions can be missed.[20] Glenohumeral arthroscopy, although clearly more invasive than MRI and MRA, remains the gold standard for diagnosing glenohumeral chondral defects.

Summary of Patient Evaluation

A global evaluation of the patient with symptomatic glenohumeral chondral lesions involves the patient presentation, physical examination, and imaging studies. After considering all the information from the initial patient evaluation, the surgeon must consider several important factors before deciding on an appropriate treatment plan. The patient's age and desired activity level are both crucial factors in the decision process. In addition, the global location of the defect (glenoid surface, humeral head, or bipolar "kissing" lesions); local location of the defect (central, periphery); size, depth, and containment of the defect; and any coexisting shoulder pathologies must be considered in the evaluation of a patient with glenohumeral arthritis. Special attention must be given to any patient presenting with more global or progressive chondral disease because the clinical decision-making process is not as clear in this patient population.

Nonsurgical Treatment

In most patients with symptomatic glenohumeral articular cartilage lesions, nonsurgical treatment should be initially attempted to relieve symptoms. The nonsurgical treatment options for shoulder cartilage defects are similar to those for other joints. A course of oral nonsteroidal anti-inflammatory drugs is often helpful in patients who are able to tolerate the medication and are compliant with the dosing regimen.[21] Physical therapy, with a focus on scapulothoracic and glenohumeral strengthening, is an excellent option for most patients. Stretching the joint and improving range of motion are two important aspects of physical therapy because there is usually some restriction in motion in patients with glenohumeral cartilage damage. Patients usually have relief of symptoms after a course of physical therapy. In instances when future surgery is indicated, preoperative strengthening of the shoulder joint will help to improve postoperative outcomes.

Injecting the glenohumeral joint with corticosteroids or a lidocaine pain challenge may be helpful in some patients; however, this treatment is usually not effective in high-demand, athletic patients because symptoms often return after the patient returns to the sports activity.[22] Often, steroid injections (the efficacy is still unknown) can be more useful as a diagnostic modality rather than as a treatment that provides significant long-term relief of symptoms.[23] Recently, off-label viscosupplementation via hyaluronic acid injections, which has been approved for use in the knee, has been shown to be potentially beneficial in patients with symptomatic glenohumeral arthritis.[24] This type of injection needs further investigation before specific recommendations can be made regarding its efficacy. Explicit informed consent is needed for any patient receiving this type of injection because it is not currently approved by the Food and Drug Administration for use in the shoulder.

Surgical Treatment

Palliative Arthroscopic Débridement

After conservative treatment modalities have been exhausted without success in the active patient with glenohumeral arthritis, arthroscopic débridement is generally considered as the next treatment choice. Arthroscopic débridement is considered a palliative treatment and aims to reduce pain and potentially increase functional range of motion. An arthroscopic débridement may postpone the need for a total joint arthroplasty, which has been shown to have higher incidences of component failure and worse outcomes scores in younger patients.[25,26] Shoulder arthroscopy also can be used as a diagnostic tool to address other pathologies that may coexist with glenohumeral arthritis.

Arthroscopic débridement is generally considered a first-line surgical option in the patient with glenohumeral arthritis if treatment with conservative modalities has failed. In patients older than 65 years or in patients with lower physical demands, an arthroscopic débridement is often used in an attempt to avoid more invasive options. Arthroscopic débridement is especially indicated for patients with significant comorbidities who may not tolerate total shoulder arthroplasty. Younger patients with advanced or diffuse chondral disease are not ideal candidates for arthroplasty because of issues related to glenoid component wear; therefore, débridement may be warranted in an attempt to delay arthroplasty. Patients who have significantly decreased range of motion can potentially benefit from a capsular release to decrease the capsular contracture often associated with glenohumeral arthritis.

Palliative treatment attempts to ameliorate symptoms by decreasing the intra-articular mechanical and biologic milieu.[27] There are a variety of standard techniques used in arthroscopic débridement, including complete synovectomy, the removal of loose bodies, and defect management (**Figure 3**). For cartilage injury, the removal of chondral flaps can be performed with a combination of motorized shavers and arthroscopic curets. In grade IV lesions, a stable, vertical transition zone should be created between the defect and the surrounding cartilage. This was shown to be beneficial in a canine model in which converting cartilage edges with gradual zones to vertical margins led to slower disease progression.[28] With arthroscopic débridement, capsular contractures can be managed with either targeted capsular releases or a complete 360° release. Two studies have reported that complete capsular release is effective for pain relief and patient satisfaction.[29,30] In addition to treating cartilage lesions and capsular contractures, other potential procedures that can be performed based on symptomatic pathology include subacromial decompression, distal clavicle excision, and biceps tenotomy or tenodesis.

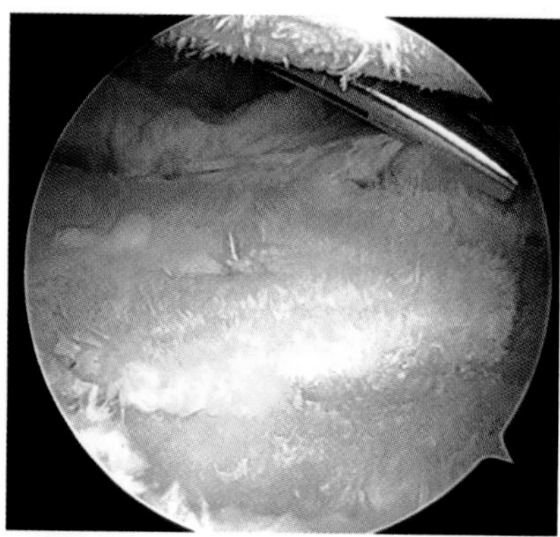

Figure 3 Arthroscopic view of palliative treatment of a grade IV chondral lesion of the glenoid. The motorized shaver is used to create a stable, vertical, transition zone between the defect and the surrounding cartilage.

Limited data in the literature are available on the outcomes of arthroscopic débridement for glenohumeral arthritis. The few available studies show that symptomatic relief can often be achieved but is usually incomplete and of short duration.[31,32] In general, 80% good or excellent results can be achieved at short-term follow-up.[20,32] In 2002, Cameron et al[20] reported on 61 patients with grade IV osteochondral lesions treated with arthroscopic débridement. Thirty-six percent of these patients were treated with capsular release, and 48% were treated with concomitant arthroscopic procedures other than capsular release. At an average follow-up of 28 months, 88% reported significant pain relief (average time to maximal pain relief, 11 weeks), and 87% were satisfied with the procedure. The authors reported worse outcomes with cartilage degeneration greater than 2 × 2 cm^2. Weinstein et al[32] reported on 25 patients, with an average age of 46 years and an average follow-up of 34 months, treated with arthroscopic débridement for early glenohumeral arthritis. In this group, all patients were treated with chondral débridement, synovectomy, and loose body removal as needed. Twenty-three of 25 patients were treated with subacromial bursectomy, and 12 of 25 had capsular release for preoperative stiffness. All the patients had good or excellent results, with 10 of 12 reporting improvement in range of motion after capsular release. In a study of patients treated with arthroscopic débridement, 16 of 71 patients (23%) required arthroplasty at an average of 10.1 months, with 55 of 71 patients (77%) showing significant improvement in American Shoulder and Elbow Surgeons (ASES) scores, simple shoulder test (SST) scores, the visual analog scale (VAS), and range of motion at an average follow-up of 27 months (A Romeo et al, Chicago IL, unpublished data).

Reparative: Microfracture

Even in patients with comorbidities, reparative options are used to treat superficial defects believed to be associated with symptoms. The goal of reparative strategies is to resurface a defect with fibrocartilage using a marrow stimulation technique. Steadman et al[33] initially described the technique

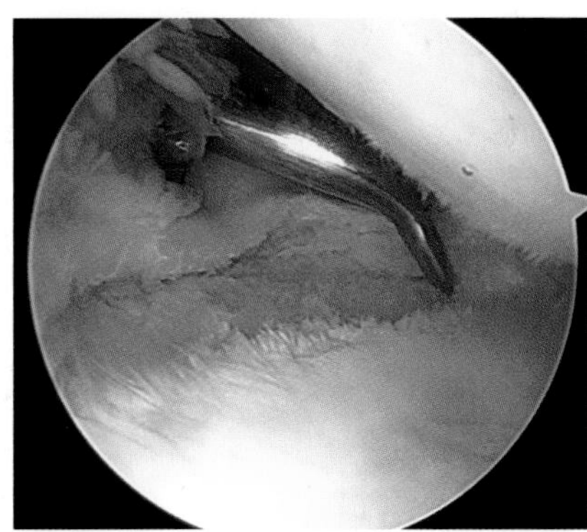

Figure 4 Arthroscopic view of microfracture of a grade IV glenoid lesion using specifically designed awls to penetrate the subchondral bone plate every 2 to 3 mm.

of microfracture to treat cartilage lesions in the knee; this technique has remained the preferred marrow stimulation procedure of this chapter's authors. Other potential reparative strategies include abrasion chondroplasty and drilling. Microfracture has a theoretic advantage over drilling because of the decreased risk of thermal damage to bone and cartilage.[33,34] Reparative techniques do not compromise a surgeon's ability to perform future restorative surgeries and can be performed entirely arthroscopically with little associated morbidity. Rudd et al[28] reported that smaller, well-shouldered lesions should perform better clinically than larger unshouldered lesions with gradual transition zones. Reparative treatment is contraindicated in any osteochondral defects in which the subchondral plate has been violated and in any patient with bone and cartilage loss.[34-36]

The surgical technique for microfracture of glenohumeral cartilage lesions stems from the technique described in the knee.[33,36] The initial step is to débride the lesion to the level of calcified cartilage. This portion of the procedure can be done with a combination of motorized shavers and arthroscopic curets. Next, it is critical to establish vertical walls so that the lesion is contained with normal or near-normal cartilage. Specifically designed awls are then used to penetrate the subchondral plate every 2 to 3 mm (**Figure 4**). This penetration allows mesenchymal marrow elements to form a fibrin scaffold that is gradually replaced by fibrocartilage.

Currently, there are only a limited number of published studies of patients treated with microfracture for glenohumeral cartilage defects. In a recent study by Frank et al,[37] 16 patients (17 shoulders) treated with arthroscopic microfracture of the humeral head and/or glenoid surface were retrospectively reviewed and examined by an independent, blinded examiner. All patients with concomitant labral or rotator cuff repairs were excluded. The mean age of patients was 37 years, and the average follow-up was 27.8 months (minimum follow-up, 12 months). Two shoulders were lost to follow-up, leaving 14 patients (15 shoulders). The average size of humeral and glenoid defects was 5.07 cm^2 and 1.66 cm^2, respectively. Twelve of 14 patients (86%) stated they would have the procedure again, and there was a significant improvement in VAS, ASES, and SST outcomes scores. Based on this small series, the authors concluded that microfracture can provide significant improvement in pain relief and shoulder function in patients with isolated chondral lesions. Yen et al[38] performed a similar study of 31 shoulders in 30 patients treated with microfracture of the glenohumeral joint. Shoulders with rotator cuff tears and patients older than 60 years were excluded. The mean patient age was 43 years, and the average follow-up was 47 months (minimum follow-up, 25 months). In the 6 of 31 shoulders requiring additional surgery, microfracture was considered a failed procedure. Mean ASES scores showed significant postoperative improvement ($P < 0.05$) in ability to work, perform the activities of daily living, and participate in sports activities. The authors concluded that microfracture can be a successful procedure in the glenohumeral joint, with the greatest success achieved in patients with isolated, small, humeral lesions.

Cartilage Restorative Options

Restorative treatment options for glenohumeral defects include osteochondral autografts, osteochondral allografts, and autologous chondrocyte implantation (an off-label indication). These techniques can be used as the primary procedure to treat patients with chondral pathology or as a secondary procedure after failed reparative treatment. These procedures involve significantly greater surgical morbidity than reparative techniques, and all are typically performed through a shoulder arthrotomy. Proper patient selection is critical for success. The ideal candidate is a young, active individual with an isolated focal cartilage defect of the humerus or glenoid in whom nonsurgical treatment options have been exhausted. Although autologous chondrocyte implantation can be used only with isolated cartilage defects, osteochondral autografts and allografts can be used to treat lesions with combined cartilage and bone loss.

Osteochondral Autograft Transfer

Osteochondral autograft transfer traditionally has been used to treat knee and talar lesions with successful results.[39,40] This technique is generally reserved for smaller humeral lesions (1 to 1.5 cm^2) in which first-line treatment has failed. The advantages of this procedure are the ability to restore the glenohumeral architecture with a viable "organ" of bone and cartilage with a single-stage procedure and the ability to achieve osseous integration and preserve the articular tidemark. A unique disadvantage of this procedure is donor-site morbidity, with the autograft usually harvested from the lateral trochlea of the knee. An arthroscopic procedure is technically challenging, and the current standard procedure is an arthrotomy. The literature has only limited reports of osteochondral autograft transfer to the shoulder. Scheibel et al[41] reported on eight traumatic grade IV chondral lesions of the humeral head treated with osteochondral autograft transfer and followed for a mean of 32.6 months. At this short-term follow-up, six patients were pain free, and two had a reduction in pain compared with the preoperative level. Postoperative MRI showed graft incorporation and congruent articular surfaces in seven of eight patients. One patient required two additional procedures at the donor knee for recurrent effusions. Connor et al[42] described a case report of a patient with bilateral posterior fracture-dislocations of the glenohumeral joint in which one side was treated with hemiarthroplasty and the other side with local autograft taken from the shoulder treated with arthroplasty. This same procedure was used by Ivkovic et al[43] to treat a patient with bilateral locked posterior dislocations, with excellent clinical and radiographic results at 3-year follow-up.

Osteochondral Allograft

The goal of osteochondral allograft implantation is to restore the congruency of an articular surface with an intact osteochondral segment. With increasing availability, improved donor screening and procurement protocols, and rapidly evolving surgical techniques, the use of these grafts in the shoulder is increasing.[44] Fresh osteochondral allografts are composite tissues with viable cartilage layers attached to nonviable subchondral bone.[45] Recent studies have shown that the success of fresh osteochondral allograft implants depends on the number of viable chondrocytes that remain after implantation.[46-48] Currently, osteochondral allografts are being used to treat both humeral and glenoid defects, most commonly associated with postdislocation combined bone and cartilage pathology; however, lesser tuberosity transfer is an available option for reverse Hill-Sachs defects. Fresh osteochondral allografts are the current standard of care because these grafts have higher chondrocyte viability, improved maintenance of the cartilage matrix, and better long-term results compared with cryopreserved grafts.[47,48] Although disease transmission remains a concern, since screening standards were introduced in 1985, there have been no reported cases of human immunodeficiency virus transmission from an allogeneic graft.[49,50]

The surgical technique for osteochondral allograft placement is adapted from clinical experiences with knee procedures. The surgeon's preferred standard exposure method is used to visualize the lesion. For the humerus, commercial allograft transplantation systems are available. The usual goal is to create a socket with a healthy bed of subchondral bone that is typically 7 to 8 mm deep. This can be accomplished using either the dowel technique to create a circular socket, or a wedge-shaped defect can be created in a freehand manner. The graft is usually placed with either a press-fit technique or press-fit with screw fixation for augmentation (**Figure 5**). For the glenoid, a fresh distal tibial osteochondral allograft can be used for glenoid deficiency, and is most commonly indicated for patients with significant bony Bankart lesions after recurrent dislocations. Typically, the graft is fashioned to re-create the normal contour and shape of the glenoid and is fixed with two 3.5-mm fully treated cortical screws in a lag fashion.[51] This technique can be used as a substitute for Latarjet and Bristow procedures and is advantageous because it creates a viable cartilage surface on the glenoid.

The published data on treating glenohumeral defects with osteochondral allografts are limited to case reports and a single case series. Yagishita and Thomas[52] recently described a patient with a chronic anterior shoulder dislocation secondary to a large Hill-Sachs lesion that was treated with a femoral head allograft. At 2-year follow-up, the patient was symptom free with no episodes of recurrent instability. Chapovsky and Kelly[18] used three osteochondral allograft plugs placed arthroscopically to treat a 16-year-old boy with recurrent instability secondary to an engaging Hill-Sachs lesion. One year after surgery, the patient had returned to athletic activity and was symptom free. Gerber and Lambert[53] treated four patients with chronic, locked posterior shoulder dislocations using osteochondral allografts to fill the reverse Hill-Sachs lesion. In all four patients the humeral head defect was at least 40% of the articular surface. At a mean follow-up of 68 months, good to excellent results were reported in three patients; osteonecrosis in the remainder of the humeral head developed postoperatively in the fourth patient. Osteochondral allograft humeral head resurfacing in combination with a lateral meniscal allograft glenoid resurfacing was described by McCarty and Cole[54] in a case report involving a 16-year-old girl with symptomatic bipolar glenohumeral chondrolysis subsequent to arthroscopic thermal capsulorrhaphy. At 2-year follow-up, the patient reported complete resolution of her shoulder pain, and radiographs showed maintenance of the glenohumeral joint space

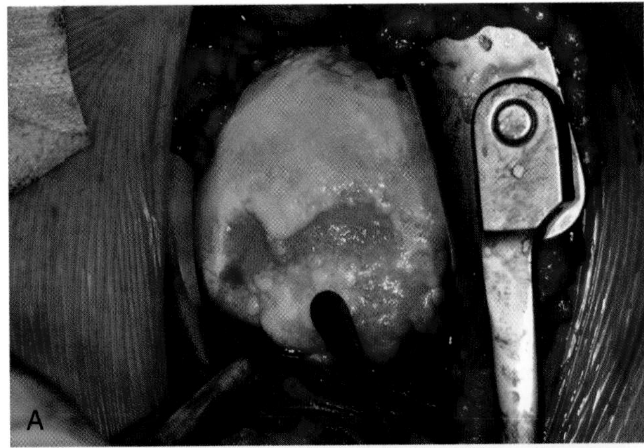
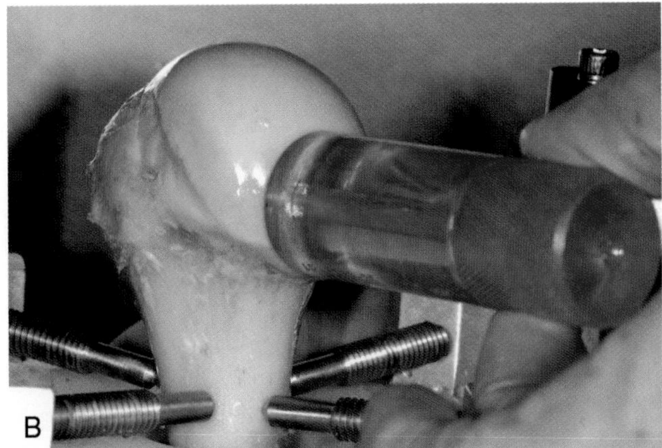
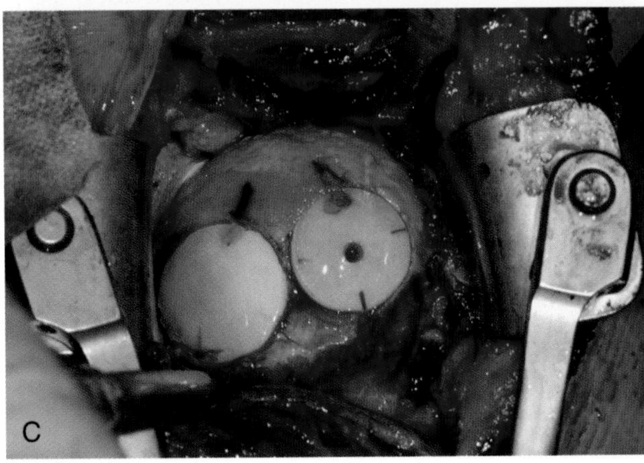

Figure 5 Reconstruction of the articular surface in a 25-year-old man with 9 months of activity-limiting shoulder pain. **A,** Photograph of grade IV changes (approximately 25 × 20 mm) in the anteroinferior area of the humeral head. **B,** Fresh humeral head allograft is sized in a site-matched donor area. **C,** Two fresh humeral head allograft plugs (20 mm and 18 mm) are used to reconstruct the defect.

with no evidence of allograft collapse or hardware migration. The patient's postoperative ASES score was 83 (preoperative = 50), and her SST score was 8 (preoperative = 1). Glenohumeral forward flexion and external rotation improved from 90° and 40° to 160° and 50°, respectively. Kropf and Sekiya[55] used arthroscopic management of the anterior capsulolabral pathology combined with a limited, open, posterior approach to place an osteochondral allograft to fill a large Hill-Sachs lesion. At 1-year follow-up, the patient was on active military duty without restrictions. In a study of 20 young patients (mean age, 19.7 years) with extensive postoperative surgical glenohumeral arthritis, McNickle et al[2] described the use of biologic resurfacing with osteochondral allografts for the humeral head and lateral meniscal allografts for the glenoid in seven patients; one patient was treated with osteochondral allograft resurfacing of the humeral head alone. At a mean follow-up of 3.1 years (range, 1.9 to 6.5 years), improvements were reported with respect to SST, ASES and VAS scores.

Three case series report on the treatment of anterior glenoid defects with osteochondral allografts. Weng et al[56] describes a study of nine consecutive patients with anterior instability associated with glenoid bone loss. Patients were treated with an anteroinferior capsular shift combined with a bone buttress femoral head osteochondral allograft. One patient had a repeat dislocation, and one had subluxation (both events occurred following a seizure). At mean follow-up of 4.5 years, all grafts had radiographic evidence of bony union with the native glenoid. Hutchinson et al[57] performed a similar procedure with a femoral head osteochondral allograft bone buttress to treat nine epileptic patients with recurrent instability. In this study, there were no recurrences. Provencher et al[51] reported using a distal tibial allograft for anterior glenoid reconstruction with a mean glenoid bone loss of 30%. The advantages of this graft include a viable cartilage surface, a dense weight-bearing corticocancellous bone, a radius of curvature that nearly matches the normal glenoid contour, and increased availability compared with glenoid allografts (**Figure 6**). Further research, including clinical studies, of this promising treatment option for anterior glenoid bone loss is currently being performed.

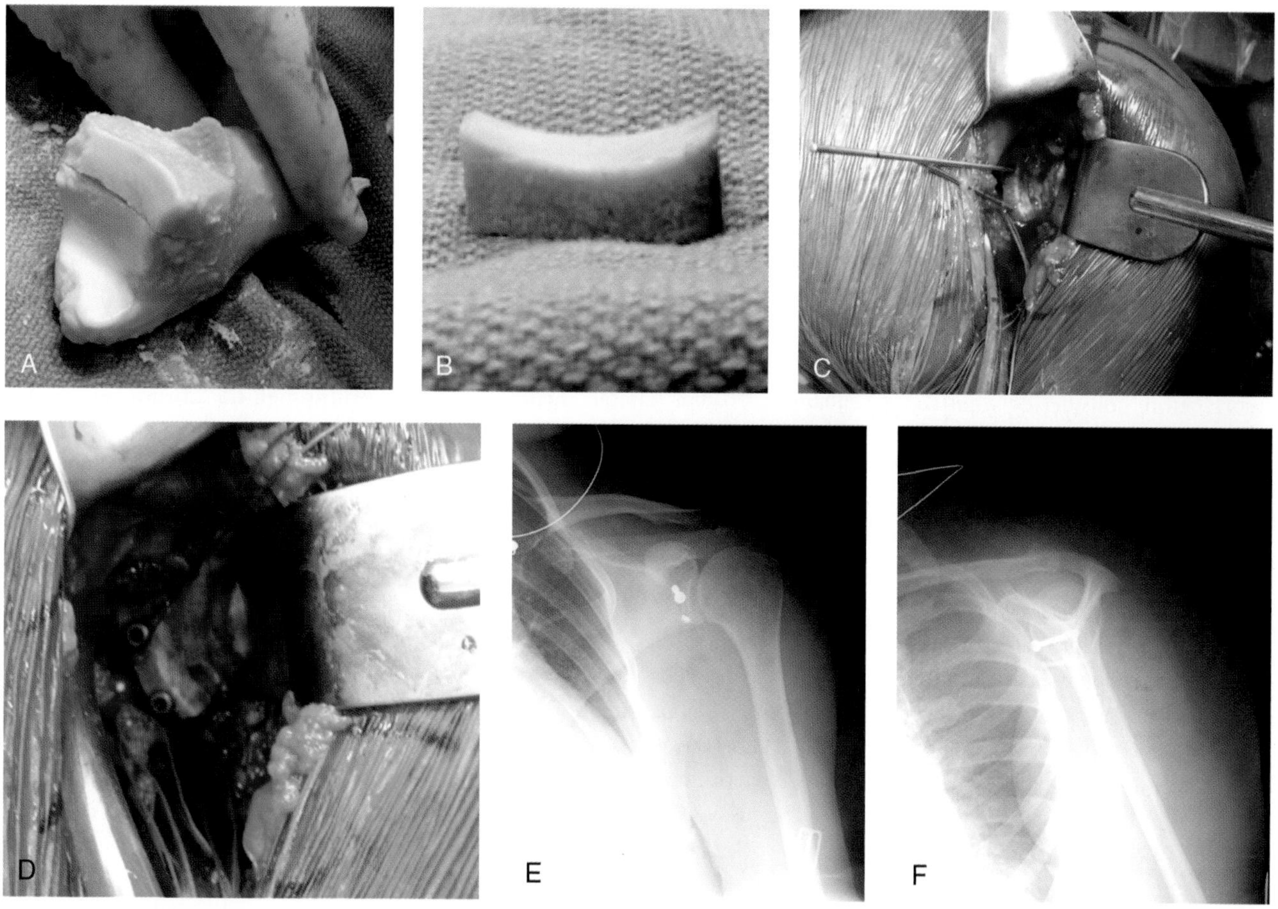

Figure 6 A distal tibial allograft is used to reconstruct the anterior glenoid with significant bone loss. **A,** The lateral aspect of the distal tibia provides a good fitting allograft for the anterior or posterior glenoid. **B,** The donor fresh distal tibial graft is harvested. It is approximately 30 mm superior to inferior, 10 mm anterior to posterior, and 10 mm deep. **C,** Intraoperative photograph of the fresh distal tibial graft in place and temporarily fixed with Kirschner wires. The native anterior glenoid was prepared with a high-speed burr to remove the defect (8 mm anterior to posterior). **D,** The fresh distal tibial allograft is affixed with two 3.5-mm cortical screws and small washers. **E,** AP radiograph shows the allograft in place. **F,** Postoperative supraspinatus outlet radiographic view of the allograft in place.

Autologous Chondrocyte Implantation

Autologous chondrocyte implantation remains investigational and is an off-label use of this technique in the glenohumeral joint. The basic principle of autologous chondrocyte implantation stems from its use in the knee and includes harvesting of healthy articular cartilage, subsequent culturing and expansion of cells over a 3- to 4-week period, and implantation. This technique may have potential use in a contained unipolar superficial defect greater than 2 cm^2 of the humerus in a young patient in whom first-line treatment has failed (**Figure** 7). The current literature is limited to a case report of a 16-year-old baseball player with a focal defect of the humeral head, which developed following arthroscopic capsulorrhaphy using a radiofrequency device.[58] The standard autologous chondrocyte implantation technique was performed, including harvesting cartilage from the intercondylar notch, growing the cells for 1 month, and using a periosteal graft from the proximal tibia. At 1-year follow-up, the patient had full range of painless motion.

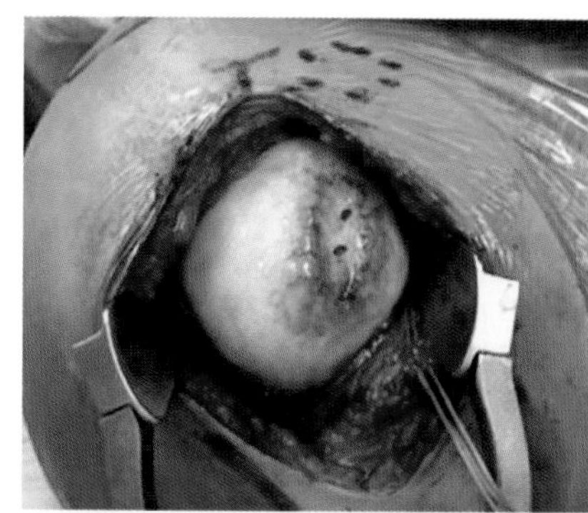

Figure 7 Intraoperative view of a focal humeral head chondral defect treated with autologous chondrocyte implantation.

Glenohumeral Reconstructive Options

In an effort to decrease pain and restore long-lasting shoulder function, biologic reconstructive techniques have been developed for young patients with glenohumeral degenerative arthritis. These techniques are indicated for patients with advanced unipolar or bipolar disease because biologic reconstructive surgery is a last resort before considering total shoulder arthroplasty. Reconstructive surgical options typically include biologic resurfacing of the glenoid coupled with either biologic or nonbiologic resurfacing of the humeral head.

Biologic resurfacing of the humeral head may be performed using an osteochondral allograft or autologous chondrocyte implantation.[1] As stated previously, at the present time, these treatment options remain investigational with limited clinical evidence available in the orthopaedic literature. More commonly, humeral head implant resurfacing or hemiarthroplasty is used in combination with biologic resurfacing of the glenoid. First proposed by Burkhead and Hutton[59] in 1988, biologic resurfacing of the glenoid combined with hemiarthroplasty has been used with variable results in treating young patients with glenohumeral arthritis. In their initial clinical series, interposition of soft tissue (local articular capsule or autogenous fascia lata) between the humeral head implant and the native glenoid provided consistent pain relief and improvement in shoulder range of motion at 2-year follow-up. As experience with biologic glenoid resurfacing has increased, other interposition options have been used, including Achilles tendon allografts; lateral meniscal allografts; and processed tissue grafts; such as the dermal patch regenerative tissue matrix (dermis) and porcine small intestine submucosa.[59-66]

The use of lateral meniscal allografts for soft-tissue glenoid resurfacing has been described using both open and arthroscopic techniques.[60,67] As an interposition material, the lateral meniscus has been shown to provide more complete coverage of the glenoid compared with the medial meniscus; this coverage significantly reduces the peak force and contact area across the glenohumeral joint during physiologic loading.[1,68] For lateral meniscal allograft resurfacing, the allograft tissue should be requested from a male donor younger than 30 years to maximize the size and quality of the material for glenoid coverage. Dermal patch regenerative tissue matrix resurfacing of the glenoid has similarly been described using both open and arthroscopic methods.[69] This processed human skin retains the native collagen structure, bioactive components, and vascular channels of the dermis, providing a framework to support cellular repopulation and vascularization after implantation.[1] Available in 4 × 4 cm^2 sheets, 1 to 2 mm thick, the dermal patch matrix can be fashioned to the size and shape of each patient's glenoid.

Open Lateral Meniscal Allograft or Dermal Patch Resurfacing

With the patient in the beach chair position under a combination of regional interscalene anesthesia and general anesthesia, a deltopectoral surgical approach is used. Preparation of the humeral head along with the necessary soft-tissue and/or capsular releases is routinely first performed to provide adequate access to the glenoid. The glenoid labrum is left in situ to serve as an anchor for fixation of either the interposition lateral meniscal allograft or the dermal patch matrix. Any remaining articular cartilage on the glenoid surface is removed with a curet, and concentric reaming is performed starting with a small reamer to avoid damage to the native labral tissue. Reaming creates a concentric surface with punctate bleeding to allow adhesion and healing of the interposed lateral meniscal allograft or the dermal patch matrix and provides the opportunity to correct glenoid version if any orientation abnormalities have developed during the disease course. When reaming is completed, nonabsorbable sutures are placed through the labrum, allowing 6 to 8 points of circumferential fixation to the glenoid (**Figure 8**). When necessary for supplemental graft fixation, suture anchors are inserted into the glenoid rim, and/or transosseous sutures are placed.

In patients treated with lateral meniscal allograft resurfacing, sutures from the labrum are passed through the lateral meniscal allograft, orienting the graft so that the anterior and posterior horns face anteriorly and the thickest portion of the graft covers the posterior portion of the glenoid. The horns are sutured together to provide stability during peripheral fixation. Each circumferential suture is then tied, leaving the fixation of the horns to the anterior aspect of the glenoid as the last step. Final suturing of the two horns of the meniscal allograft is then performed allowing for adjustment (as needed) for stability and sizing. Once the lateral meniscal allograft is placed, the humerus is carefully dislocated forward, which allows the hemiarthroplasty prosthesis to be implanted. The shoulder is then reduced to allow assessment of the conformity of the humeral head component, the implanted lateral meniscal allograft, and glenohumeral range of motion and stability. The subscapularis is then anatomically repaired, and the surgical incision is closed in layers.

In contrast to the lateral meniscal allograft resurfacing procedure, in dermal patch resurfacing, preparation and implantation of the humeral head hemiarthroplasty is completed before approaching the glenoid. After the hemiarthroplasty is implanted, the shoulder is reduced, and the conformity of the implant with the patient's native articular surface is evaluated. Retractors are then inserted, which allows the humeral head implant to be displaced posteriorly, providing a straight-on approach to the glenoid. After the glenoid is prepared, its size and shape are noted; this allows the thawed, hydrated, dermal patch matrix to be fashioned accordingly. After cutting to the proper size and shape, the thickest available dermal patch matrix (2 mm in thickness) is secured to the glenoid by individually passing the sutures from the labrum through the edges of the material. This sequential suture passage and tying allows the dermal patch to be tensioned over the glenoid surface. The shoulder is then reduced, allowing glenohumeral range of motion and stability to be assessed. The subscapularis is then anatomically repaired, and the surgical incision is closed in layers.

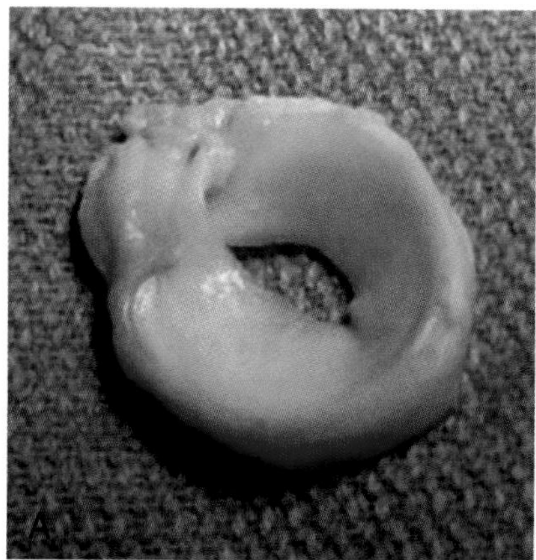

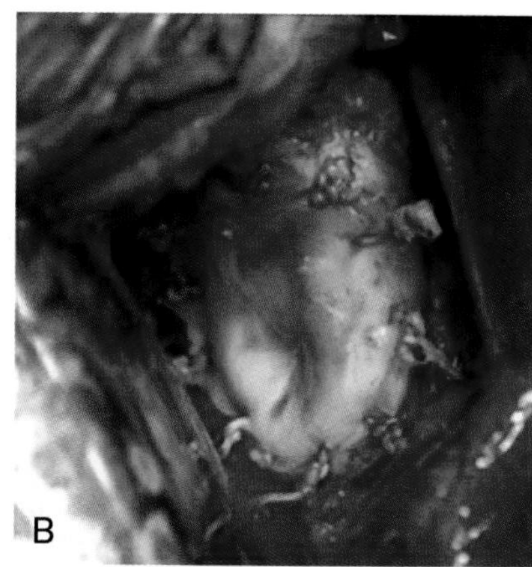

Figure 8 Biologic resurfacing of the glenoid using a lateral meniscal allograft (**A**) in combination with hemiarthroplasty in a 44-year-old patient with symptomatic glenohumeral arthrosis. **B,** View of the lateral meniscal allograft in place. It is affixed with suture to the remaining glenoid labral rim.

Outcomes

In the initial clinical series of Burkhead and Hutton,[59] 14 patients were treated with humeral head hemiarthroplasty and biologic resurfacing of the glenoid using either autogenous fascia lata or anterior shoulder capsule. Six patients with a mean age of 48 years (range, 33 to 54 years) were available for evaluation at a minimum 2-year follow-up. At a mean of 28 months postoperatively, the authors reported a reduction in pain in all patients and improvements in glenohumeral forward elevation, external rotation, and internal rotation of 57°, 45°, and six spinal segments, respectively. According to Neer's criteria, five of the six patients had excellent outcomes, with the remaining results classified as satisfactory. Lee et al[70] retrospectively evaluated 18 shoulders (mean patient age, 54.8 years) treated with soft-tissue resurfacing of the glenoid (anterior capsule) coupled with humeral head surface replacement. At a mean follow-up of 4.8 years, the authors reported a mean ASES score of 74.4; a mean Constant score of 71.4; and glenohumeral forward flexion, abduction, and external rotation of 130°, 122°, and 39°, respectively. Although 83% of the patients were satisfied with their postoperative clinical outcome, radiographic analysis showed moderate to severe glenoid erosion in 56% of the shoulders.

Long-term follow-up was reported by Krishnan et al[71] in their retrospective evaluation of 36 shoulders in 34 patients treated over a 15-year period. Biologic glenoid resurfacing was performed using autologous fascia lata (11 shoulders), anterior articular capsule (7 shoulders), and Achilles tendon allograft (18 shoulders). At a mean follow-up of 7 years, the authors reported an improvement in ASES scores from 39 preoperatively to 91 at the most recent evaluations. According to Neer's criteria, good to excellent results were seen in 86% of the shoulders. Radiographic evaluation of this cohort showed a mean 7.2 mm of glenoid erosion over the observation period, which appeared to stabilize at 5 years postoperatively.

Significantly worse outcomes following biologic resurfacing were reported by Elhassan et al[63] in a retrospective review of 13 patients younger than 50 years treated with hemiarthroplasty combined with soft-tissue interposition (Achilles tendon allograft, autogenous fascia lata, or anterior shoulder capsule). Ten of the 13 patients required conversion to total shoulder arthroplasty at a mean of 14 months postoperatively (range, 6 to 34 months). Combined with postoperative infection that developed in two patients, the authors found a 92.3% failure rate. Based on their findings, the authors concluded that soft-tissue resurfacing of the glenoid combined with humeral head arthroplasty is unreliable as a treatment in young, active patients with glenohumeral arthritis.

Lateral meniscal allograft interposition performed in conjunction with humeral head implant resurfacing was reviewed by Nicholson et al[64] in a study of 30 patients with a mean age of 42 years (range, 18 to 52 years). At a mean follow-up of 18 months, the authors reported significant improvements in ASES scores (38 preoperatively to 69 postoperatively), SST scores (3.3 to 7.8), VAS pain scores (6.4 to 2.3), and shoulder range-of-motion parameters (forward elevation, 96° to 139°; external rotation, 26° to 53°). Complications requiring revision surgery occurred in five patients (17%) within the first postoperative year; however, despite this incidence, 94% of study patients reported satisfaction with their clinical outcome and would have the procedure again if needed.

Wirth[72] recently reported the outcomes for 30 patients treated with humeral head arthroplasty and lateral meniscus allograft interposition of the glenoid. Ninety percent of the patients were available for follow-up at a mean of 35 months. Overall, there was a 16% reoperation rate, with 50% of those procedures performed secondary to failure of the meniscal portion of the construct. The author did not report significant improvement in ASES, SST, and VAS scores for the patients in the study.

The use of dermal patch regenerative matrix in interposition resurfacing of the glenoid was reported by Huijsmans et al[73] in a clinical study of six patients with a mean age of 47 years. At 6-month follow-up, the authors reported preliminary improvement with overall good results. Savoie et al[74] recently reported outcomes following arthroscopic glenoid resurfacing using a biologic patch (Restore; DePuy Orthopaedics, Warsaw, IN) in 23 consecutive patients with a mean age of 32 years (range, 15 to 58 years) treated for severe glenohumeral arthritis. At 3- to 6-year follow-ups, 75% of patients in the cohort remained satisfied with their surgical results. Significant improvements were reported with respect to ASES scores (22 preoperatively to 78 postoperatively), University of California at Los Angeles scores (15 to 29), Rowe scores (55 to 81), and Constant-Murley scores (26 to 79). Five patients required conversion to arthroplasty during the follow-up period; however, four of the five reported that they would undergo the arthroscopic resurfacing again if necessary.

Glenoid Ream and Run Procedure

The ream and run procedure involves humeral head implant resurfacing coupled with concentric reaming of the glenoid to a radius of curvature 1 to 2 mm greater than that of the humeral head prosthesis.[75] The ream and run procedure attempts to achieve glenohumeral stability by spherical reaming about the centerline of the glenoid to correct eccentric wear and minimize the potential progressive erosion and instability that has been reported with humeral hemiarthroplasty alone.[76]

In a cadaver model, Weldon et al[77] showed that denuding the glenoid of its cartilaginous surface reduced its contribution to glenohumeral stability, and spherical reaming restored stability to values seen in both the native glenoid and those reconstructed with a polyethylene implant. The potential for a healing response or remodeling at the reamed glenoid surface was reported by Matsen et al[78] in a canine model using the ream and run technique. The authors reported that at 24 weeks following the procedure, a thick, firmly attached fibrocartilaginous tissue layer completely covered the glenoid surface and articulated with the prosthetic humeral head.

In a recent case-controlled study comparing the ream and run procedure with standard total shoulder arthroplasty, Clinton et al[75] reported significant and comparable functional improvement in both patient groups. At 12-month follow-up, patients in the total shoulder arthroplasty cohort had significantly higher SST scores; however, at both 2 and 3 years after surgery, the SST scores were similar between the two treatment groups. Based on these results, the authors concluded that although a longer recovery time was required, the ream and run procedure provided the opportunity for a comparable functional outcome without the potential risk of glenoid component failure.

Arthroplasty in the Young, Active Patient

For appropriately selected patients, total shoulder arthroplasty has been shown to reliably decrease pain and improve shoulder function.[79,80] Other options include osteotomies of the glenoid, humerus, or both; a double osteotomy of the neck of the glenoid and humerus (without displacement has been described in 13 patients with good results at approximately 3 years after surgery.[81]

In a recent meta-analysis of 23 clinical studies comparing total shoulder arthroplasty with humeral head replacement for the treatment of primary glenohumeral osteoarthritis, Radnay et al[82] reported that total shoulder arthroplasty resulted in significantly better pain relief, postoperative range of motion, and patient satisfaction, along with a lower revision rate. However, in younger active patients, the longevity of a total shoulder arthroplasty has been questioned, secondary to increased rates of glenoid component failure reported in several clinical studies.[83-85] In the younger patient population, the results of total shoulder arthroplasty have been shown to be variable, with recent studies reporting outcomes inferior to those seen in the typical patient older than 60 years.[17,86-88]

Humeral head hemiarthroplasty alone has been reported to provide pain relief and improved short-term function, but studies with longer follow-up have shown progressive joint-space narrowing, glenoid erosion, and diminishing outcomes.[89-92] In a retrospective review of 78 hemiarthroplasties performed in patients younger than 50 years, Sperling et al[17] reported that at 15-year follow-up, the procedure had unsatisfactory results in 45% of their patients. Radiographic analysis demonstrated significant glenoid erosions in 68% of hemiarthroplasties. Radiolucent lines around the humeral component were reported in 24% of patients, perhaps indicating some degree of loosening. Survival estimates performed on data from this cohort found that 92% of the hemiarthroplasties survived to 5 years, 83% to 10 years, and 73% to 15 years. Based on their findings, the authors concluded that care should be exercised when hemiarthroplasty is offered to patients who are 50 years or younger. The outcomes after the conversion of a hemiarthroplasty to a total shoulder replacement with a polyethylene resurfaced glenoid are much less predictable than outcomes after a primary total shoulder arthroplasty. Patients treated in this fashion have increased residual pain, a higher risk for subsequent surgeries, and less predictable postoperative range of motion.[93,94]

Saltzman et al[86] recently evaluated 1,045 consecutive total shoulder arthroplasties and compared the surgical diagnoses between patients younger than 50 years and those older than 50 years. The authors found that the younger patients in their study had more complex pathologic conditions leading to shoulder arthroplasty compared with the older patients, adding a level of difficulty to the surgical procedure and potentially contributing to the poorer outcomes seen in the younger patient population. In a 1998 study, Sperling et al[17] reviewed the long-term results of Neer hemiarthroplasty (78 cases) and Neer total shoulder replacement (36 cases) performed in patients 50 years or younger who were followed for a mean of 12.3 years. Both total shoulder replacement and hemiarthroplasty in this series resulted in significant long-term pain relief and active shoulder abduction and external rotation. Based on their data, estimated implant survivorship for total shoulder replacement in this patient population was 97% at 10 years and 84% at 15 years. However, despite the high percentage of implant survivorship, unsatisfactory outcomes were reported in 17 of the total shoulder patients (47.2%). In a 2002 study by Sperling et al,[87] the authors retrospectively reviewed 33 patients with a mean age of 46 years managed with shoulder arthroplasty (10 hemiarthroplasties and 21 total shoulder replacements) for symptomatic glenohumeral arthritis after instability surgery. They found that while the procedures were associated with significant pain relief and improvement in active range of motion, high rates of revision surgery and unsatisfactory results occurred. According to the Neer criteria, at a mean follow-up of 7 years, patients treated with total shoulder arthroplasty had 3 excellent, 5 satisfactory, and 13 unsatisfactory outcomes. Eight total shoulder arthroplasty patients (38%) required revision surgery secondary to component failure and instability during the follow-up period. Better outcomes were reported by Raiss et al[95] in their prospective study of 21 patients with a mean age of 55 years (range, 37 to 60 years) with glenohumeral arthritis treated with total shoulder arthroplasty. At a mean follow-up of 7 years, 20 patients (95%) were either very satisfied (18 patients) or satisfied (2 patients) with their postoperative results. Significant improvement in the Constant-Murley score was reported (24.1 to 64.5). No patients had clinical or radiographic evidence of implant loosening, and at most recent follow-up, no revision surgeries had been necessary.

An alternative to arthroplasty, the Arthrosurface HemiCap (Arthrosurface, Franklin, MA) can also be used as a treatment option for pain relief and restoration of function in the shoulder with both focal and diffuse chondral damage. Using the Arthrosurface HemiCap on the diseased humeral head is similar in theory to hemiarthroplasty; however, instead of an entire stem positioned into the humeral shaft, the cap is attached to the humeral head with a smaller, central post. Only a single case report describing the use of the Arthrosurface HemiCap on the humerus is available in the literature, which was performed in conjunction with a Latarjet coracoid transfer procedure with successful results in a patient with recurrent shoulder dislocation.[96]

Based on the available data in the orthopaedic surgery literature, hemiarthroplasty and total shoulder arthroplasty in young, active patients represent viable treatment options. However, the potential for variable postoperative outcomes and concerns for glenoid erosion with hemiarthroplasty as well as glenoid component loosening with total shoulder arthroplasty must be acknowledged. Although a few recent follow-up studies have legitimized some of these concerns, these potential postoperative complications seem to occur over the long term, providing the patient with years of symptom-free, improved function. With improved implant designs, more durable biomaterials, and innovations in surgical technique, shoulder arthroplasty may become the procedure of choice for the young, active patient with glenohumeral degenerative disease.

Summary

Young patients with symptomatic degenerative disease of the glenohumeral joint represent a challenge for the treating orthopaedic surgeon. Secondary to the variety of etiologies that can lead to glenohumeral arthritis in the young adult, a thorough understanding of the appropriate workup and initial management of the disease is vital. Palliative, reparative, restorative, and reconstructive surgical options are available, with variable indications and outcomes. The development of a workable treatment algorithm based on the individual patient's pathology and physical demands will help guide the surgeon in the decision-making process. Continued research with an emphasis on correlating new surgical techniques with clinical outcomes is ongoing in an effort to optimize the treatment of patients with symptomatic degenerative disease of the glenohumeral joint.

References

1. Cole BJ, Yanke A, Provencher MT: Nonarthroplasty alternatives for the treatment of glenohumeral arthritis. *J Shoulder Elbow Surg* 2007;16(5, Suppl): S231-S240.
2. McNickle AG, L'Heureux DR, Provencher MT, Romeo AA, Cole BJ: Postsurgical glenohumeral arthritis in young adults. *Am J Sports Med* 2009;37(9): 1784-1791.
3. Solomon DJ, Navaie M, Stedje-Larsen ET, Smith JC, Provencher MT: Glenohumeral chondrolysis after arthroscopy: A systematic review of potential contributors and causal pathways. *Arthroscopy* 2009;25(11):1329-1342.
4. Yeh LR, Kwak S, Kim YS, et al: Evaluation of articular cartilage thickness of the humeral head and the glenoid fossa by MR arthrography: Anatomic correlation in cadavers. *Skeletal Radiol* 1998; 27(9):500-504.
5. Fox JA, Cole BJ, Romeo AA, et al: Articular cartilage thickness of the humeral head: An anatomic study. *Orthopedics* 2008;31(3):216.
6. Bicos J, Mazzocca A, Romeo AA: The glenoid center line. *Orthopedics* 2005;28(6):581-585.
7. Outerbridge RE: The etiology of chondromalacia patellae. *J Bone Joint Surg Br* 1961;43-B:752-757.
8. Busfield BT, Romero DM: Pain pump use after shoulder arthroscopy as a cause of glenohumeral chondrolysis. *Arthroscopy* 2009; 25(6):647-652.
9. Saltzman M, Mercer D, Bertelsen A, Warme W, Matsen F: Postsurgical chondrolysis of the shoulder. *Orthopedics* 2009;32(3):215.
10. Bailie DS, Ellenbecker TS: Severe chondrolysis after shoulder arthroscopy: A case series. *J Shoulder Elbow Surg* 2009;18(5):742-747.
11. Guntern DV, Pfirrmann CW, Schmid MR, et al: Articular cartilage lesions of the glenohumeral joint: Diagnostic effectiveness of MR arthrography and prevalence in patients with subacromial impingement syndrome. *Radiology* 2003;226(1):165-170.
12. Hsu HC, Luo ZP, Stone JJ, Huang TH, An KN: Correlation between rotator cuff tear and glenohumeral degeneration. *Acta Orthop Scand* 2003;74(1):89-94.
13. Gartsman GM, Taverna E: The incidence of glenohumeral joint abnormalities associated with full-thickness, reparable rotator cuff tears. *Arthroscopy* 1997;13(4): 450-455.
14. Taylor DC, Arciero RA: Pathologic changes associated with shoulder dislocations. Arthroscopic and physical examination findings in first-time, traumatic anterior dislocations. *Am J Sports Med* 1997;25(3):306-311.
15. Hintermann B, Gächter A: Arthroscopic findings after shoulder dislocation. *Am J Sports Med* 1995;23(5):545-551.
16. Kang RW, Frank RM, Nho SJ, et al: Complications associated with anterior shoulder instability repair. *Arthroscopy* 2009;25(8): 909-920.
17. Sperling JW, Cofield RH, Rowland CM: Neer hemiarthroplasty and Neer total shoulder arthroplasty in patients fifty years old or less: Long-term results. *J Bone Joint Surg Am* 1998;80(4): 464-473.
18. Chapovsky F, Kelly JD IV: Osteochondral allograft transplantation for treatment of glenohumeral instability. *Arthroscopy* 2005; 21(8):1007.
19. Gold GE, Reeder SB, Beaulieu CF: Advanced MR imaging of the shoulder: Dedicated cartilage techniques. *Magn Reson Imaging Clin N Am* 2004;12(1):143-159, vii.
20. Cameron BD, Galatz LM, Ramsey ML, Williams GR, Iannotti JP: Non-prosthetic management of grade IV osteochondral lesions of the glenohumeral joint. *J Shoulder Elbow Surg* 2002;11(1): 25-32.
21. Millett PJ, Gobezie R, Boykin RE: Shoulder osteoarthritis: Diagnosis and management. *Am Fam Physician* 2008;78(5):605-611.
22. Buchbinder R, Green S, Youd JM: Corticosteroid injections for shoulder pain. *Cochrane Database Syst Rev* 2003;1:CD004016.
23. Bell AD, Conaway D: Corticosteroid injections for painful shoulders. *Int J Clin Pract* 2005; 59(10):1178-1186.
24. Silverstein E, Leger R, Shea KP: The use of intra-articular hylan G-F 20 in the treatment of symptomatic osteoarthritis of the shoulder: A preliminary study. *Am J Sports Med* 2007;35(6):979-985.

25. Green A, Norris TR: Shoulder arthroplasty for advanced glenohumeral arthritis after anterior instability repair. *J Shoulder Elbow Surg* 2001;10(6):539-545.

26. Matsoukis J, Tabib W, Guiffault P, et al: Shoulder arthroplasty in patients with a prior anterior shoulder dislocation: Results of a multicenter study. *J Bone Joint Surg Am* 2003;85-A(8):1417-1424.

27. Hsieh YS, Yang SF, Chu SC, et al: Expression changes of gelatinases in human osteoarthritic knees and arthroscopic debridement. *Arthroscopy* 2004;20(5):482-488.

28. Rudd RG, Visco DM, Kincaid SA, Cantwell HD: The effects of beveling the margins of articular cartilage defects in immature dogs. *Vet Surg* 1987;16(5): 378-383.

29. Nicholson GP: Arthroscopic capsular release for stiff shoulders: Effect of etiology on outcomes. *Arthroscopy* 2003;19(1):40-49.

30. Warner JJ, Allen A, Marks PH, Wong P: Arthroscopic release for chronic, refractory adhesive capsulitis of the shoulder. *J Bone Joint Surg Am* 1996;78(12):1808-1816.

31. Ellman H, Harris E, Kay SP: Early degenerative joint disease simulating impingement syndrome: Arthroscopic findings. *Arthroscopy* 1992;8(4):482-487.

32. Weinstein DM, Bucchieri JS, Pollock RG, Flatow EL, Bigliani LU: Arthroscopic debridement of the shoulder for osteoarthritis. *Arthroscopy* 2000;16(5):471-476.

33. Steadman JR, Rodkey WG, Rodrigo JJ: Microfracture: surgical technique and rehabilitation to treat chondral defects. *Clin Orthop Relat Res* 2001;(391, Suppl): S362-S369.

34. Salata MJ, Bajaj S, Verma NN, Cole BJ: Glenohumeral microfracture. *Cartilage* 2010;1(2): 121-126.

35. McCarty LP III, Cole BJ: Nonarthroplasty treatment of glenohumeral cartilage lesions. *Arthroscopy* 2005;21(9):1131-1142.

36. Frank RM, Romeo AA, Verma NN, Cole BJ: Resurfacing of isolated articular cartilage defects in the glenohumeral joint with microfracture: Surgical technique and case report. *Am J Orthop* 2010;39(7):326-332.

37. Frank RM, Van Thiel GS, Slabaugh MA, Romeo AA, Cole BJ, Verma NN: Clinical outcomes after microfracture of the glenohumeral joint. *Am J Sports Med* 2010;38(4):772-781.

38. Yen YM, Cascio B, O'Brien L, Stalzer S, Millett PJ, Steadman JR: Treatment of osteoarthritis of the knee with microfracture and rehabilitation. *Med Sci Sports Exerc* 2008;40(2):200-205.

39. Hangody L, Feczkó P, Bartha L, Bodó G, Kish G: Mosaicplasty for the treatment of articular defects of the knee and ankle. *Clin Orthop Relat Res* 2001;391(Suppl): S328-S336.

40. Hangody L, Kish G, Módis L, et al: Mosaicplasty for the treatment of osteochondritis dissecans of the talus: Two to seven year results in 36 patients. *Foot Ankle Int* 2001;22(7):552-558.

41. Scheibel M, Bartl C, Magosch P, Lichtenberg S, Habermeyer P: Osteochondral autologous transplantation for the treatment of full-thickness articular cartilage defects of the shoulder. *J Bone Joint Surg Br* 2004;86(7): 991-997.

42. Connor PM, Boatright JR, D'Alessandro DF: Posterior fracture-dislocation of the shoulder: Treatment with acute osteochondral grafting. *J Shoulder Elbow Surg* 1997;6(5):480-485.

43. Ivkovic A, Boric I, Cicak N: One-stage operation for locked bilateral posterior dislocation of the shoulder. *J Bone Joint Surg Br* 2007; 89(6):825-828.

44. Ho JY, Miller SL: Allografts in the treatment of athletic injuries of the shoulder. *Sports Med Arthrosc* 2007;15(3):149-157.

45. Görtz S, Bugbee WD: Fresh osteochondral allografts: Graft processing and clinical applications. *J Knee Surg* 2006;19(3):231-240.

46. Williams RJ III, Dreese JC, Chen CT: Chondrocyte survival and material properties of hypothermically stored cartilage: An evaluation of tissue used for osteochondral allograft transplantation. *Am J Sports Med* 2004;32(1):132-139.

47. Wingenfeld C, Egli RJ, Hempfing A, Ganz R, Leunig M: Cryopreservation of osteochondral allografts: Dimethyl sulfoxide promotes angiogenesis and immune tolerance in mice. *J Bone Joint Surg Am* 2002;84-A(8): 1420-1429.

48. Czitrom AA, Keating S, Gross AE: The viability of articular cartilage in fresh osteochondral allografts after clinical transplantation. *J Bone Joint Surg Am* 1990;72(4): 574-581.

49. Simonds RJ, Holmberg SD, Hurwitz RL, et al: Transmission of human immunodeficiency virus type 1 from a seronegative organ and tissue donor. *N Engl J Med* 1992;326(11):726-732.

50. Buck BE, Malinin TI, Brown MD: Bone transplantation and human immunodeficiency virus: An estimate of risk of acquired immunodeficiency syndrome (AIDS). *Clin Orthop Relat Res* 1989;240:129-136.

51. Provencher MT, Ghodadra N, LeClere L, Solomon DJ, Romeo AA: Anatomic osteochondral glenoid reconstruction for recurrent glenohumeral instability with glenoid deficiency using a distal tibia allograft. *Arthroscopy* 2009; 25(4):446-452.

52. Yagishita K, Thomas BJ: Use of allograft for large Hill-Sachs lesion

associated with anterior glenohumeral dislocation: A case report. *Injury* 2002;33(9):791-794.

53. Gerber C, Lambert SM: Allograft reconstruction of segmental defects of the humeral head for the treatment of chronic locked posterior dislocation of the shoulder. *J Bone Joint Surg Am* 1996; 78(3):376-382.
54. McCarty LP III, Cole BJ: Reconstruction of the glenohumeral joint using a lateral meniscal allograft to the glenoid and osteoarticular humeral head allograft after bipolar chondrolysis. *J Shoulder Elbow Surg* 2007;16(6): e20-e24.
55. Kropf EJ, Sekiya JK: Osteoarticular allograft transplantation for large humeral head defects in glenohumeral instability. *Arthroscopy* 2007;23(3):322, e1-e5.
56. Weng PW, Shen HC, Lee HH, Wu SS, Lee CH: Open reconstruction of large bony glenoid erosion with allogeneic bone graft for recurrent anterior shoulder dislocation. *Am J Sports Med* 2009;37(9):1792-1797.
57. Hutchinson JW, Neumann L, Wallace WA: Bone buttress operation for recurrent anterior shoulder dislocation in epilepsy. *J Bone Joint Surg Br* 1995;77(6): 928-932.
58. Romeo AA, Cole BJ, Mazzocca AD, Fox JA, Freeman KB, Joy E: Autologous chondrocyte repair of an articular defect in the humeral head. *Arthroscopy* 2002; 18(8):925-929.
59. Burkhead WZ Jr, Hutton KS: Biologic resurfacing of the glenoid with hemiarthroplasty of the shoulder. *J Shoulder Elbow Surg* 1995;4(4):263-270.
60. Ball CG, Yamaguchi K: Meniscal allograft interposition arthroplasty for the arthritic shoulder: Description of a new surgical technique. *Tech Shoulder Elbow Surg* 2001;2: 247-254.
61. Baumgarten KM, Lashgari CJ, Yamaguchi K: Glenoid resurfacing in shoulder arthroplasty: Indications and contraindications. *Instr Course Lect* 2004;53:3-11.
62. Burkhead WZ Jr, Krishnan SG, Lin KC: Biologic resurfacing of the arthritic glenohumeral joint: Historical review and current applications. *J Shoulder Elbow Surg* 2007;16(5, Suppl):S248-S253.
63. Elhassan B, Ozbaydar M, Diller D, Higgins LD, Warner JJ: Soft-tissue resurfacing of the glenoid in the treatment of glenohumeral arthritis in active patients less than fifty years old. *J Bone Joint Surg Am* 2009;91(2):419-424.
64. Nicholson GP, Goldstein JL, Romeo AA, et al: Lateral meniscus allograft biologic glenoid arthroplasty in total shoulder arthroplasty for young shoulders with degenerative joint disease. *J Shoulder Elbow Surg* 2007;16(5, Suppl): S261-S266.
65. Pearl ML, Romeo AA, Wirth MA, Yamaguchi K, Nicholson GP, Creighton RA: Decision making in contemporary shoulder arthroplasty. *Instr Course Lect* 2005;54: 69-85.
66. Brislin KJ, Field LD, Ramsey JR: Surgical treatment for glenohumeral arthritis in the young patient. *Tech Shoulder Elbow Surg* 2004;5:165-169.
67. Pennington WT, Bartz BA: Arthroscopic glenoid resurfacing with meniscal allograft: A minimally invasive alternative for treating glenohumeral arthritis. *Arthroscopy* 2005;21(12):1517-1520.
68. Creighton RA, Cole BJ, Nicholson GP, Romeo AA, Lorenz EP: Effect of lateral meniscus allograft on shoulder articular contact areas and pressures. *J Shoulder Elbow Surg* 2007;16(3):367-372.
69. Bhatia DN, van Rooyen KS, du Toit DF, de Beer JF: Arthroscopic technique of interposition arthroplasty of the glenohumeral joint. *Arthroscopy* 2006;22(5):570, e1-e5.
70. Lee KT, Bell S, Salmon J: Cementless surface replacement arthroplasty of the shoulder with biologic resurfacing of the glenoid. *J Shoulder Elbow Surg* 2009; 18(6):915-919.
71. Krishnan SG, Reineck JR, Nowinski RJ, Harrison D, Burkhead WZ: Humeral hemiarthroplasty with biologic resurfacing of the glenoid for glenohumeral arthritis: Surgical technique. *J Bone Joint Surg Am* 2008;90(Suppl 2, Pt 1):9-19.
72. Wirth MA: Humeral head arthroplasty and meniscal allograft resurfacing of the glenoid. *J Bone Joint Surg Am* 2009;91(5):1109-1119.
73. Huijsmans PR, van Rooyen K, du Toit DF, de Beer JF: The treatment of glenohumeral OA in the young and active patient with the graft jacket: Preliminary results. *J Bone Joint Surg Br* 2004; 87(suppl III):275.
74. Savoie FH III, Brislin KJ, Argo D: Arthroscopic glenoid resurfacing as a surgical treatment for glenohumeral arthritis in the young patient: Midterm results. *Arthroscopy* 2009;25(8):864-871.
75. Clinton J, Franta AK, Lenters TR, Mounce D, Matsen FA III: Nonprosthetic glenoid arthroplasty with humeral hemiarthroplasty and total shoulder arthroplasty yield similar self-assessed outcomes in the management of comparable patients with glenohumeral arthritis. *J Shoulder Elbow Surg* 2007;16(5):534-538.
76. Hasan SS, Leith JM, Campbell B, Kapil R, Smith KL, Matsen FA III: Characteristics of unsatisfactory shoulder arthroplasties. *J Shoulder Elbow Surg* 2002;11(5): 431-441.
77. Weldon EJ III, Boorman RS, Smith KL, Matsen FA III: Opti-

mizing the glenoid contribution to the stability of a humeral hemiarthroplasty without a prosthetic glenoid. *J Bone Joint Surg Am* 2004;86-A(9):2022-2029.

78. Matsen FA III, Clark JM, Titelman RM, et al: Healing of reamed glenoid bone articulating with a metal humeral hemiarthroplasty: A canine model. *J Orthop Res* 2005;23(1):18-26.

79. Iannotti JP, Norris TR: Influence of preoperative factors on outcome of shoulder arthroplasty for glenohumeral osteoarthritis. *J Bone Joint Surg Am* 2003; 85-A(2):251-258.

80. Norris TR, Iannotti JP: Functional outcome after shoulder arthroplasty for primary osteoarthritis: A multicenter study. *J Shoulder Elbow Surg* 2002;11(2): 130-135.

81. Benjamin A, Hirschowitz D, Arden GP: The treatment of arthritis of the shoulder joint by double osteotomy. *Int Orthop* 1979;3(3): 211-216.

82. Radnay CS, Setter KJ, Chambers L, Levine WN, Bigliani LU, Ahmad CS: Total shoulder replacement compared with humeral head replacement for the treatment of primary glenohumeral osteoarthritis: a systematic review. *J Shoulder Elbow Surg* 2007;16(4):396-402.

83. Torchia ME, Cofield RH, Settergren CR: Total shoulder arthroplasty with the Neer prosthesis: Long-term results. *J Shoulder Elbow Surg* 1997;6(6):495-505.

84. Wirth MA, Rockwood CA Jr: Complications of shoulder arthroplasty. *Clin Orthop Relat Res* 1994; 307:47-69.

85. Wirth MA, Rockwood CA Jr: Complications of total shoulder-replacement arthroplasty. *J Bone Joint Surg Am* 1996;78(4): 603-616.

86. Saltzman MD, Mercer DM, Warme WJ, Bertelsen AL, Matsen FA III: Comparison of patients undergoing primary shoulder arthroplasty before and after the age of fifty. *J Bone Joint Surg Am* 2010;92(1):42-47.

87. Sperling JW, Antuna SA, Sanchez-Sotelo J, Schleck C, Cofield RH: Shoulder arthroplasty for arthritis after instability surgery. *J Bone Joint Surg Am* 2002; 84-A(10):1775-1781.

88. Sperling JW, Cofield RH, Rowland CM: Minimum fifteen-year follow-up of Neer hemiarthroplasty and total shoulder arthroplasty in patients aged fifty years or younger. *J Shoulder Elbow Surg* 2004;13(6):604-613.

89. Levine WN, Djurasovic M, Glasson JM, Pollock RG, Flatow EL, Bigliani LU: Hemiarthroplasty for glenohumeral osteoarthritis: Results correlated to degree of glenoid wear. *J Shoulder Elbow Surg* 1997;6(5):449-454.

90. Parsons IM IV, Millett PJ, Warner JJ: Glenoid wear after shoulder hemiarthroplasty: Quantitative radiographic analysis. *Clin Orthop Relat Res* 2004;421:120-125.

91. Pfahler M, Jena F, Neyton L, Sirveaux F, Molé D: Hemiarthroplasty versus total shoulder prosthesis: Results of cemented glenoid components. *J Shoulder Elbow Surg* 2006;15(2):154-163.

92. Rispoli DM, Sperling JW, Athwal GS, Schleck CD, Cofield RH: Humeral head replacement for the treatment of osteoarthritis. *J Bone Joint Surg Am* 2006;88(12):2637-2644.

93. Sperling JW, Cofield RH: Revision total shoulder arthroplasty for the treatment of glenoid arthrosis. *J Bone Joint Surg Am* 1998;80(6):860-867.

94. Carroll RM, Izquierdo R, Vazquez M, Blaine TA, Levine WN, Bigliani LU: Conversion of painful hemiarthroplasty to total shoulder arthroplasty: Long-term results. *J Shoulder Elbow Surg* 2004;13(6):599-603.

95. Raiss P, Aldinger PR, Kasten P, Rickert M, Loew M: Total shoulder replacement in young and middle-aged patients with glenohumeral osteoarthritis. *J Bone Joint Surg Br* 2008;90(6): 764-769.

96. Moros C, Ahmad CS: Partial humeral head resurfacing and Latarjet coracoid transfer for treatment of recurrent anterior glenohumeral instability. *Orthopedics* 2009;32(8):602.

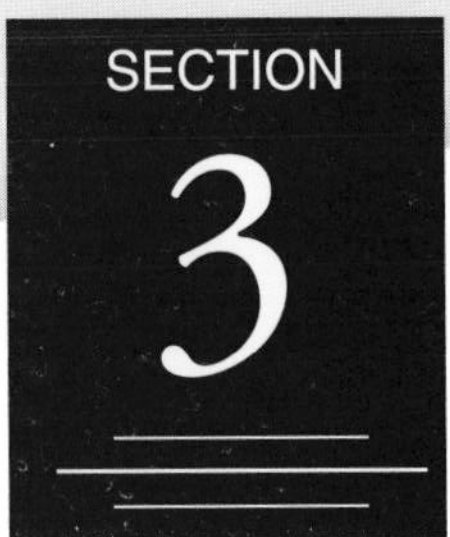

Elbow

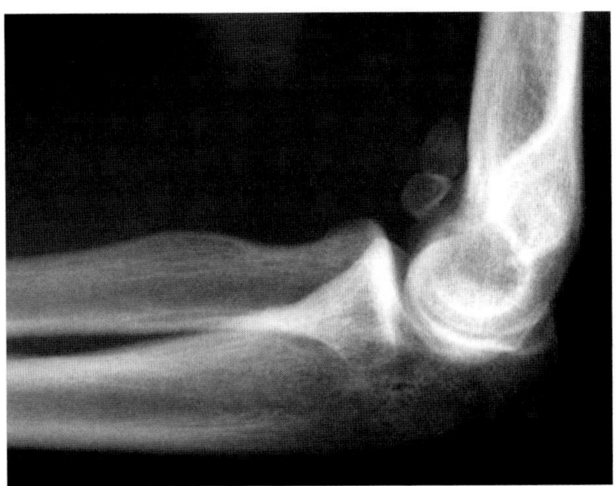

Elbow Arthroplasty: Lessons Learned From the Past and Directions for the Future

Joaquin Sanchez-Sotelo, MD, PhD
Matthew L. Ramsey, MD
Graham J.W. King, MD, FRCSC
Bernard F. Morrey, MD

Abstract

Joint arthroplasty in general has experienced tremendous advances over the past few decades. Numerous improvements in implant design, instrumentation, anesthesia, surgical techniques, intraoperative navigation, and materials have occurred in hip and knee arthroplasty. Although elbow arthroplasty also has seen continual improvements, much remains to be accomplished before elbow arthroplasty can be recommended to patients with the same level of confidence as hip or knee arthroplasty.

Instr Course Lect 2011;60:157-169.

Although the success rate of elbow arthroplasty is lower than that of hip and knee arthroplasty, decades of experience has provided insight into successful techniques and appropriate indications. Elbow arthroplasty can improve pain, motion, and function in most patients, but advances are still needed to resolve current deficiencies in the procedure.

Lessons Learned

Over the past two decades, several important lessons have been learned that have substantively improved the outcomes in prosthetic replacement of the elbow joint.[1] These lessons may be classified as those relating to fixation, instability, wear, and osteolysis, along with a recent focus on triceps function.

Lesson 1: Fixation

The failures that occurred in early elbow arthroplasties primarily resulted from implant loosening, with a failure rate of up to 25% at 5-year follow-up.[1] The addition of stems, anterior flanges, and loose-hinge articulations, along with fixation using bone cement, dramatically improved fixation reliability. The overall impact of these four improvements was an impressive increase in elbow implant survival rates for some prosthetic designs. The rate of loosening in one semiconstrained humeral component in rheumatoid patients was reported as less than 10%.[2]

Stems

Some early elbow replacement components attempted to replicate the natural anatomy and used the same concepts as other successful implants, such as the resurfacing-type designs that were so successful in knee arthroplas-

Dr. Sanchez-Sotelo or an immediate family member serves as a paid consultant to or is an employee of Stryker and has received research or institutional support from DePuy, Stryker, and Zimmer. Dr. Ramsey or an immediate family member serves as a board member, owner, officer, or committee member of the Philadelphia Orthopaedic Society; has received royalties from Zimmer and Ascension; is a member of a speakers' bureau or has made paid presentations on behalf of DePuy Mitek; serves as a paid consultant to or is an employee of Zimmer and Ascension; has received research or institutional support from Ortho-McNeil, Jansen Scientific Affairs, and Biomet; and owns stock or stock options in Johnson & Johnson, Norvartis, and Teva. Dr. King or an immediate family member has received royalties from Tornier, Wright Medical Technology, and Tenet Medical; serves as a paid consultant to or is an employee of Wright Medical Technology and Tornier; and has received research or institutional support from Wright Medical Technology. Neither Dr. Morrey nor any immediate family member has received anything of value from or owns stock in a commercial company or institution related directly or indirectly to the subject of this chapter.

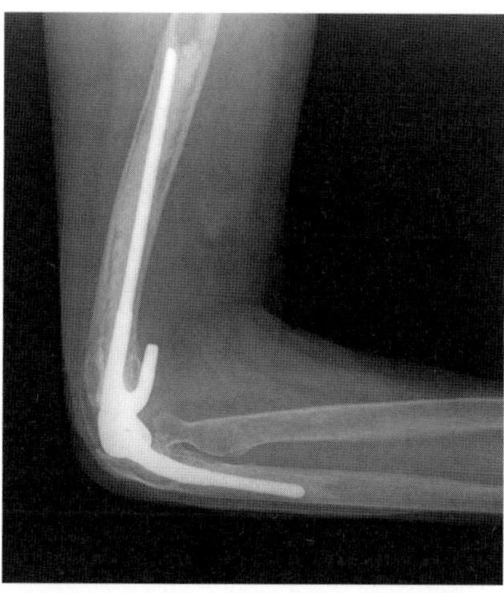

Figure 1 Lateral radiograph obtained 23 years after implantation of a semiconstrained total elbow arthroplasty shows a mature and fully incorporated bone graft behind the anterior humeral flange.

ties. In the elbow, however, unstemmed devices have high rates of loosening and fracture and provide unpredictable results. Since the late 1970s, most elbow joint arthroplasty systems have used some type of stemmed design.[1,3,4]

Anterior Flanges

Adjunct fixation was sought because of recognition of the significant forces transmitted across the elbow and the observation that some apparently well-fixed stemmed implants will ultimately loosen. Additional fixation is provided by an extracortical flange with a bone graft behind it. It has been shown that the graft matures and consolidates fixation of the implant in more than 90% of patients.[1] The anterior flange provides composite fixation of the humerus, with the cemented stem and osseous integration behind the flange providing extracortical fixation (**Figure 1**).

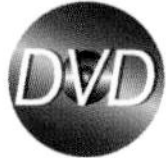

Video 14.1: Elbow Arthroplasty: Composite Fixation. Graham J.W. King, MD (1 min)

Loose-Hinge Articulation

The value of linked implants in eliminating instability and treating a broader range of pathology is well recognized. The linked articular mechanism allows approximately 7° of varus, valgus, and axial rotation, decreasing the stresses transferred to the bone-cement implant interfaces.

Cementation

The quality of bone cementation has been specifically studied and shown to be directly related to the decreased rate of stem loosening.[5] Specific nozzle and gun injection systems allow more uniform delivery of cement to further enhance fixation and lessen the likelihood of loosening.

Video 14.2: Elbow Arthroplasty: Cementation. Graham J.W. King, MD (5 min)

Lesson 2: Instability

Despite the theoretic attractiveness of anatomic implants, studies on various designs of unlinked devices reported instability rates averaging approximately 5%.[4,6,7] Unlinked elbow implant devices are not as reliable as linked implants in treating deformities or for revision procedures, and the anticipated lower revision rate with unlinked elbow implants has not been proven. A recent study reported that the failure rate of unlinked elbow implants because of instability or loosening was dramatically worse than the rate for linked implants.[7] Of additional significance is the fact that more than 90% of the unlinked devices were implanted in rheumatoid patients, and 50% of the linked implants were implanted in patients with posttraumatic arthritis. Currently available data indicate that linked devices provide more reliable long-term outcomes, even in patients with more severe elbow conditions such as a traumatic injury.[7]

Lesson 3: Wear

Problems with articular wear were not seen in early elbow arthroplasties because of early implant failures caused by stem loosening or dislocation. With improved stem fixation, implants survived longer, allowing time for deleterious wear of the articular surface. Lee et al[8] reviewed polyethylene wear in 919 semiconstrained linked elbow arthroplasties and reported 12 revisions (1.3%) caused by isolated articular bushing wear. An analysis showed that 9 of the 12 elbows had severe deformity at the time of revision and that an adequate soft-tissue release had not been performed. This study highlights the fact that linked devices also require soft-tissue balancing. Other studies on wear after elbow arthroplasty have prompted the introduction of new implant designs with more polyethylene at the articular surface to lessen the likelihood of failure caused by a worn articular bushing.[3] To date, there have been no reports of the long-term outcomes of these new devices.

Lesson 4: Osteolysis

The cause of osteolysis at the elbow after arthroplasty is debated. Although osteolysis has been implicated as secondary to polyethylene wear, a study by Goldberg et al[9] seems to indicate that the osteolysis at the elbow is much more likely caused by debris generated from a loose cemented implant. The abraded particles become embedded in the polyethylene bushing, further enhancing wear. However, osteolysis appears to be related more to wear caused by implant loosening than from polyethylene wear alone. This belief is supported by the experiences of one of this chapter's authors (JSS) and other surgeons at the Mayo Clinic with poly-

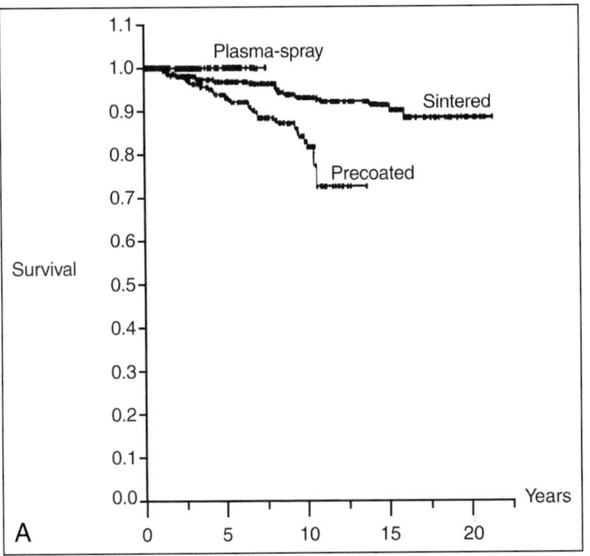

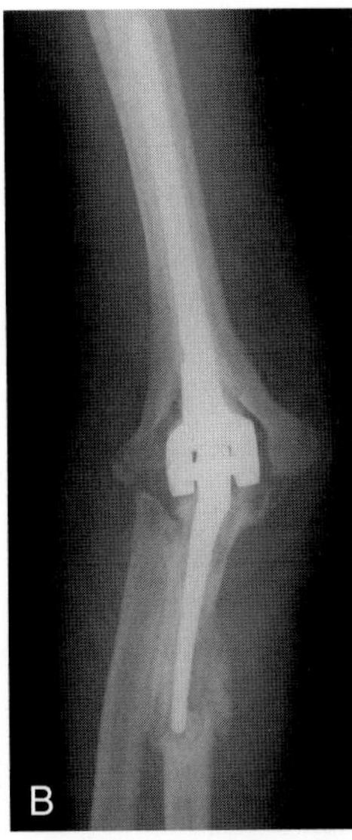

Figure 2 **A,** Graph showing comparative survivorships of semiconstrained total elbow arthroplasties with three different surface finishes on the ulnar component. **B,** The typical radiographic appearance of a failed, precoated, ulnar component shows loosening and severe osteolysis.

methylmethacrylate precoated ulnar component surfaces, which were known to cause osteolysis. A change was made to plasma-coated implants (**Figure 2**). Less debris resulted in a decrease in stem loosening, which decreased the likelihood of rapid third-body wear of the bushing.

Lesson 5: The Triceps

Triceps insufficiency has been a poorly documented complication of elbow replacement. Various methods of triceps management are being explored, including leaving the triceps attached to the ulna.[10,11] Because a detached triceps causes significant morbidity, great care is needed to securely repair the triceps.[12] Currently, the triceps-reflection, the triceps-splitting, and the triceps tongue are the most commonly used approaches. As the expectations of patients continue to increase, achieving a well-functioning triceps will be a paramount added benefit of elbow arthroplasty.

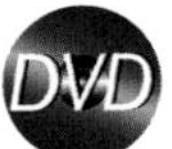

Video 14.3: Elbow Arthroplasty: Triceps Repair. Graham J.W. King, MD (4 min)

Outcomes

Total elbow arthroplasty is a relatively uncommon procedure compared to other joint arthroplasties. The literature supports the fact that appropriately selected patients have excellent functional outcomes and symptomatic relief with elbow arthroplasty.[1,2,13-17] In recent years, there has been a shift to using elbow arthroplasty to treat patients with traumatic conditions. Because of the pioneering work of several leaders in the field of orthopaedics, the pathology-specific results of elbow arthroplasty are well understood.

Rheumatoid Arthritis

Total elbow arthroplasty provides satisfactory pain relief and functional gains in patients with rheumatoid arthritis affecting the elbow.[2,13,18,19] In a 1998 study, Gill and Morrey[2] reported pain relief in more than 97% of the patients at 10- to 15-year follow-up, with functional range of motion and good objective and subjective results. The authors reported that 92.4% of implants survived and were free of revision at 10 to 12 years. However, the complication rate in total elbow arthroplasty for patients with rheumatoid arthritis is approximately 18%, with approximately 10% of patients requiring revision. Infection, mechanical failure, and triceps insufficiency are the most common causes of implant failure.[2]

Between 1982 and 2006, surgeons at the Mayo Clinic performed 461 consecutive total elbow arthroplasties on elbows with rheumatoid arthritis using semiconstrained total elbow prostheses (J Sanchez-Sotelo, MD, PhD, unpublished data presented at the American Academy of Orthopaedic Surgeons Annual Meeting, New Orleans, LA, 2010). At the most recent follow-up, 418 of the 461 implants (90.7%) had not been revised, 10 had been removed or revised for infection, 25 had been revised for component loosening (ulnar component, 21; humeral component, 3; and both components, 1), 8 had been revised for polyethylene wear; 3 elbows required internal fixation because of periprosthetic fractures. Seventeen additional elbows required débridement for deep infection (overall infection rate, 5.9%). In all but one of the eight elbows requiring revision for polyethylene wear, the revision was performed between 10 and 17 years after the initial total elbow arthroplasty. Twenty-year implant survivorship rates were as follows: 90% free of revision for loosening (95% confidence interval [CI]; range, 79% to 94%), 78% free of revision for mechanical failure (95% CI; range, 65% to 89%), and 72% free of revision for mechanical failure or deep

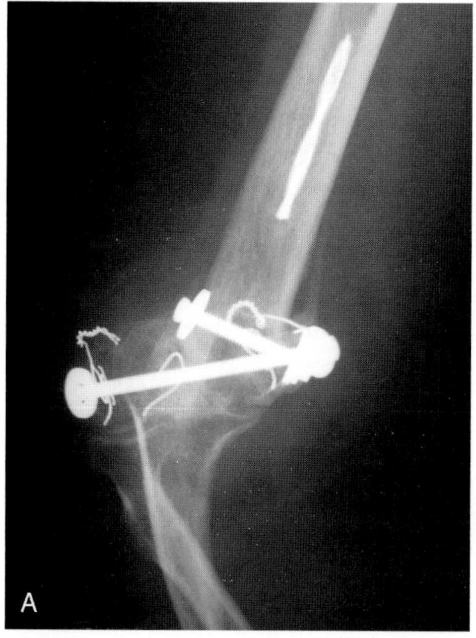

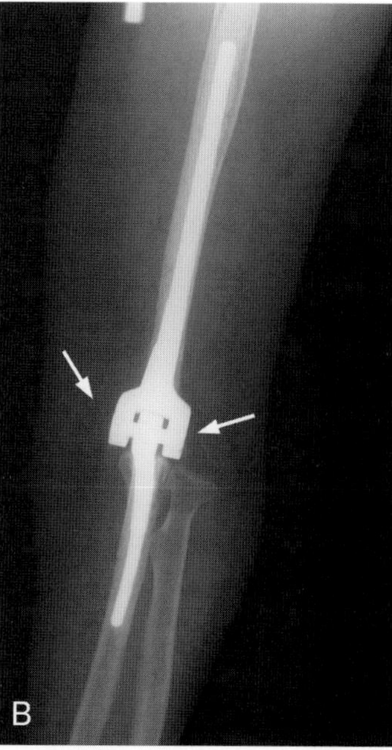

Figure 3 **A,** Preoperative radiograph of a distal humerus nonunion in an elderly patient. **B,** Elbow arthroplasty represents a predictable treatment option for patients with this condition; note the resected humeral condyles (arrows).

infection (95% CI; range, 58% to 85%).

Traumatic Conditions

The largest expansion in indications for elbow arthroplasty has occurred in posttraumatic and acute traumatic conditions of the elbow. The variability of the underlying pathologies makes it difficult to evaluate patients with posttraumatic conditions. Although the pathologic process can be isolated to the articular surface, some traumatic conditions, including acute fracture, humeral nonunions, and traumatic bone loss, involve the supracondylar region. In addition, chronic instability from dislocation or nonunion can result in significant disability. Although each of these pathologies presents unique challenges, total elbow arthroplasty is a commonly considered treatment option. A satisfactory medium-term outcome rate of approximately 90% has been reported in patients with posttraumatic elbow conditions.[14-17,20-24]

Posttraumatic Arthritis

Schneeberger et al[25] reported the results of total elbow arthroplasty in patients with posttraumatic arthritis. At a mean follow-up of approximately 6.5 years, postoperative range of motion was within the functional range, with good objective and subjective rates of patient satisfaction. However, the complication rate approached 31% in this group. Interestingly, complications were more mechanical in nature, including component fracture and bushing wear. Throckmorton et al[14] reported the results of total elbow arthroplasty for posttraumatic arthritis at one institution. Eighty-five consecutive arthroplasties were followed for a mean of 9 years or until failure. Sixteen primary arthroplasties (19%) failed, seven because of wear, four because of infection, three because of component fracture, and two because of loosening. Seven additional elbows had radiographic loosening or severe bone loss. Most failures occurred in patients younger than 60 years. The 15-year survivorship rates were as follows: 70% free of revision for any reason, 74% free of revision for mechanical failure, and 90% free of revision for aseptic loosening.

Distal Humerus Fractures

The successful use of total elbow arthroplasty for acute humeral fractures was first reported by Cobb and Morrey.[15] Several additional reports in the literature support the use of linked semiconstrained implants in distal humerus fractures, with excellent medium-term results.[20-23] Kamineni and Morrey[24] recently reported on 43 elbows followed for a mean of 7 years; the average Mayo Elbow Performance score was 93 points, and the average motion was 24° of extension and 132° of flexion; 5 elbows required revision surgery. A recent prospective randomized study comparing internal fixation versus arthroplasty (20 elbows in each group) reported decreased surgical time; better Mayo Elbow Performance scores; better early Disabilities of the Arm, Shoulder and Hand scores; better motion; and fewer reoperations with arthroplasty.[16]

Distal Humerus Nonunions

Total elbow arthroplasty is an attractive option for distal humerus nonunions because internal fixation can be challenging and unpredictable (**Figure 3**). As is the case with other traumatic indications, results are reasonable but the complication rate is high. Cil et al[17] reported on 92 elbows followed for a mean of 6.5 years. The Mayo Elbow Performance score was satisfactory in 78% of patients; however, the reoperation rate was 35%. Implant survivorship free of removal or revision for any reason was only 65%.

Special circumstances apply in elbows with distal humeral nonunions and traumatic bone loss in which dysfunctional instability results from the separation of the brachium from the forearm, such that no useful fulcrum can be established for elbow motion. A linked implant is used to reestablish the connection and align the extremity, which has substantial mechanical demands. Ramsey et al[26] reported on 19 arthroplasties for dysfunctional instability. Results were satisfactory in 16 elbows; complications included humeral loosening in 2 elbows and ulnar component fracture in 2 elbows.

Severe Stiffness or Ankylosis

Total elbow arthroplasty may also be a good option for selected patients with severe elbow stiffness, ankylosis, or fusion.[27,28] Range of motion generally increases, but a functional range is not always achieved, leading to unsatisfactory Mayo Elbow Performance scores secondary to persistent stiffness. In a study by Mansat and Morrey,[27] the average range of motion achieved was 67°; the main complications were infection (5 of 13 patients) and mechanical failure (2 of 13 patients).

Primary Osteoarthritis

Total elbow arthroplasty is rarely indicated for patients with primary elbow osteoarthritis. Symptoms in those patients are usually related to capsular fibrosis and osteophyte impingement and improve with arthroscopic or open débridement procedures. Two studies, with a total of 16 patients, reported overall satisfactory results.[29,30]

Complications and Revision Surgery

Many of the complications of total elbow arthroplasty can be successfully treated with revision surgery.

Infection

Infection after total elbow arthroplasty is a common cause of implant failure compared with other types of joint arthroplasties, with infection rates ranging from 2% to 10%.[31] Preventing infection involves not only soft-tissue management and perioperative antibiotic prophylaxis but also careful postoperative wound management. Most surgeons routinely use antibiotic-loaded cement in elbow arthroplasties.[1] Diagnosing infection after elbow arthroplasty requires a high clinical index of suspicion because the interpretation of laboratory findings remains unclear. Treatment considerations include timing of the infection, component fixation, and the type of infecting organism. Irrigation and débridement may be successful in selected patients, but certain glycocalyx-producing organisms are very difficult to eradicate despite aggressive measures to save the implant. In those circumstances, two-stage reimplantation or definitive resection is required.[31]

Aseptic Loosening and Osteolysis

As previously discussed, loosening was a common mode of failure with first-generation elbow implants. Loosening is now much less common in stemmed, cemented, semiconstrained implants. Improved cementing techniques, including low viscosity cement, appropriate canal preparation, and cement pressurization, have improved implant fixation. Ulnar components precoated with polymethylmethacrylate exhibit a much higher rate of mechanical failure, with loosening and osteolysis that is severe enough to cause periprosthetic fractures.

Instability

Instability following total elbow arthroplasty is predominantly a complication of unlinked and snap-fit articulations.[4] Instability is predominantly noted in extension but can occur throughout the range of motion. Component rotation can influence the development of instability and is difficult to correct without implant revision if component malrotation is identified.[6] Ligament reconstruction is seldom successful; most unstable unlinked implants require revision to a linked implant.

Wear

Polyethylene wear is an expected process in all joint arthroplasties. To date, there are no established minimum thickness standards for reducing contact stresses in polyethylene bearing surfaces. It should be noted that wear is not synonymous with osteolysis. Many implants that have been in place for decades have developed polyethylene wear with pristine bone cement and cement implant interfaces. Isolated polyethylene wear may be successfully treated with an exchange of the polyethylene bushings, provided the implants remain well fixed.[8]

Periprosthetic Fractures

The Mayo classification of periprosthetic elbow fractures considers fracture location, implant fixation, and bone loss.[32] Fractures of the condyles may be well tolerated, whereas olecranon fractures may require internal fixation. Most fractures around or beyond the stem are associated with loosening, often requiring both implant revision and fracture fixation.

Triceps Insufficiency

Triceps insufficiency is an underappreciated and underreported complication. Patients at risk for triceps insufficiency have compromised soft tissues, such as patients with rheumatoid arthritis or those who had multiple prior surgical procedures. Primary repair of a failed triceps may occasionally be successful, but other techniques such as anconeus rotationplasty or allograft reconstruction may be required.[33]

Revision Surgery

A failed elbow arthroplasty may occasionally be treated with relatively sim-

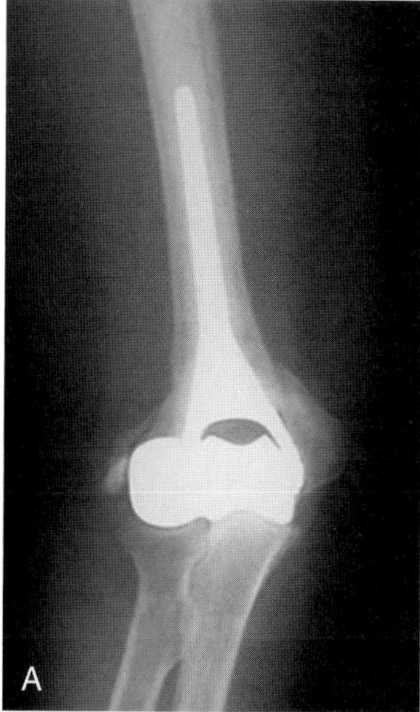

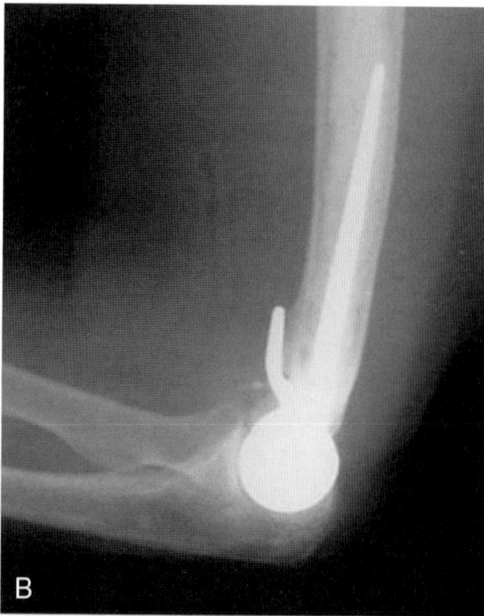

Figure 4 AP (**A**) and lateral (**B**) radiographs of an elbow treated with distal humerus hemiarthroplasty. This procedure may offer an attractive solution for selected patients with distal humerus fractures or nonunions, osteonecrosis, or posttraumatic osteoarthritis mostly affecting the distal humerus.

ple revision procedures, such as bushing exchange or cemented revision of the components.[34] However, the presence of bone loss often requires the use of more complex reconstructive techniques. Relatively good results have been reported with both impaction grafting and strut augmentation techniques.[32,35,36] In contrast, technique and results using allograft-prosthetic composites require improvements.[37]

The Future

Elbow arthroplasty has become an established treatment in managing low-demand patients with rheumatoid arthritis and some elderly patients with comminuted articular fractures of the distal humerus. However, the durability of implants and the occurrence of complications continue to be problematic, particularly in patients with greater physical demands. Future advances in elbow arthroplasty will likely include expanded implant options, more accurate positioning of the components, improved stability in unlinked implants, reduced bearing wear, better preservation of triceps strength, and a decrease in infections.

Expanded Implant Options

Implants designed for other joints now incorporate multiple options to replace separate joint compartments or different articulations on the same stems. Shoulder and elbow surgeons are familiar with such options for shoulder arthroplasty, which offers implant lines for resurfacing implants, anatomic implants, reverse implants, hemiarthroplasty, total shoulder arthroplasty, and dedicated fracture components. In the elbow, there is interest in the development and use of implants to separately replace the capitellum, the distal humerus, the proximal ulna, and the coronoid, as well as combining a capitellar implant with a radial head implant (unicompartmental radiocapitellar arthroplasty).

Distal Humerus Hemiarthroplasty

Isolated replacement of the distal humerus may offer an attractive solution for distal humerus fractures, nonunions, osteonecrosis, tumor resection, and posttraumatic osteoarthritis when the articular surfaces of the ulna and the radius are relatively well preserved (**Figure 4**). This type of implant would be ideal for younger patients to avoid ulnar violation or implantation of a polyethylene articulation.

Any distal humerus hemiarthroplasty design should be anatomic to articulate properly with the native radius and ulna. Ideally, it should be easily convertible to a total elbow arthroplasty if it becomes necessary because of progressive joint degeneration, instability, or other reasons.[3] The design should incorporate "fracture features" to facilitate healing of the columns in fractures or nonunions. It should also incorporate "ligament features" to facilitate stable reconstruction of the joint. Distal humerus hemiarthroplasty has been approved for use in multiple countries, but it is currently not approved for use in the United States.

Distal humerus hemiarthroplasty is not a new idea. Isolated case reports describe hemiarthroplasty using old designs. Shifrin and Johnson[38] reported on a single case of a custom-made, tumor-type implant that survived for 20 years. However, there is limited information about the outcome of distal humerus hemiarthroplasty in larger cohorts of patients. Swoboda and Scott[39] reported on seven rheumatoid patients who were treated with an isolated capitellocondylar humeral component implant. The patients ranged in age from 20 to 50 years. One implant was removed for infection; the six remaining elbows were followed for 2 to 9 years. At the most recent follow-up, four patients reported no pain and two reported mild pain; however, motion was poor with a mean flexion-extension arc of 53° to 136°.

Recent data seem to support the selective use of hemiarthroplasty for distal humerus fractures. Adolfsson and Hammer[40] reported good results in a study of four elderly women treated with a Kudo (Biomet, Warsaw, IN) distal humerus hemiarthroplasty for a distal humerus fracture. In a larger series using the Sorbie (Wright Medical, Arlington, TN) and the Latitude (Tornier, Edina, MN) distal humerus hemiarthroplasty implants, 29 elbows were followed for a minimum of 2 years.[41] Two elbows were revised to a linked total elbow arthroplasty; the overall instability rate was 12%. The mean American Shoulder and Elbow Surgeons and Mayo Elbow Performance scores were 84 and 77 points, respectively, with a mean range of motion of 22° to 129°. Better outcomes were reported in the acute setting and when the procedure was performed through an olecranon osteotomy.

Although it is a promising procedure and is already used by some surgeons, distal humerus hemiarthroplasty is not yet a well-established procedure. Limited range of motion remains a concern, and the optimal approach and the need for column or ligament reconstruction procedures are debated. Long-term outcomes are unknown.

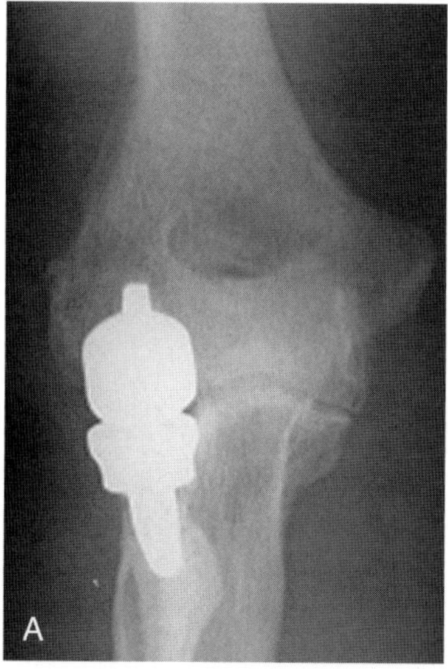

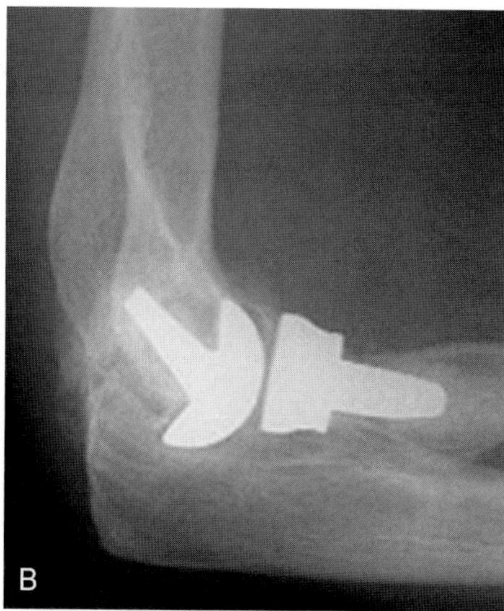

Figure 5 AP (**A**) and lateral (**B**) radiographic views of a radiocapitellar unicompartmental arthroplasty.

Capitellar Implants and Unicompartmental Radiocapitellar Arthroplasty

Isolated radial head replacement is a well-established procedure. Implants for replacing the capitellum may be attractive in patients with progressive cartilage degeneration of the radiohumeral compartment, capitellar shear fractures, focal cartilage defects secondary to osteochondritis dissecans, or osteonecrosis. The radiocapitellar compartment of the elbow lends itself to isolated replacement of either the radial head or capitellum or replacement of both[42] (**Figure 5**).

Capitellar and unicompartmental radiocapitellar implants are currently available. Capitellar implants are metallic and round and may have a stem for fixation. They may be combined with bipolar or monopolar radial head implants in which the head component is made completely of polyethylene or has a polyethylene articular surface. There is limited information concerning patient outcomes after this procedure. Heijink et al[42] reported on three patients treated with a unicompartmental radiocapitellar arthroplasty for longitudinal forearm dissociation associated with capitellar arthritis. Pain and function improved in all three patients although one radial head implant required revision because of loosening. Additional outcome studies are needed to better define the optimal design and role of these devices.

Implants for the Proximal Ulna

Isolated reconstruction of the proximal ulna may be required after traumatic injury or tumor resection. Posttraumatic coronoid deficiency is common in patients with persistent instability after trauma. Graft reconstruction of the coronoid in the chronic setting seems to be associated with a high failure rate.[43] A metal coronoid prosthesis with screw fixation and ingrowth properties would be an attractive solution. An anatomic replacement of the proximal third of the ulna has been used as a custom prosthesis in selected patients and would be attractive for patients with more extensive bone loss after high-energy fractures or tumor resection.

Convertible Implants, Cementless Fixation, and Revision Surgery

A total elbow arthroplasty system that can be converted from an unlinked to a linked arthroplasty is currently available for clinical use[3,44] (**Figure 6**). This system also can be used to convert a distal humerus hemiarthroplasty to a total elbow arthroplasty. This device simplifies the revision of an unstable unlinked arthroplasty to a linked arthroplasty, avoiding the need to remove the implant stems. Such a system may increase the use of unlinked arthroplasties and possibly improve the longevity of elbow arthroplasty relative to linked systems. Outcome studies are needed to test this hypothesis.

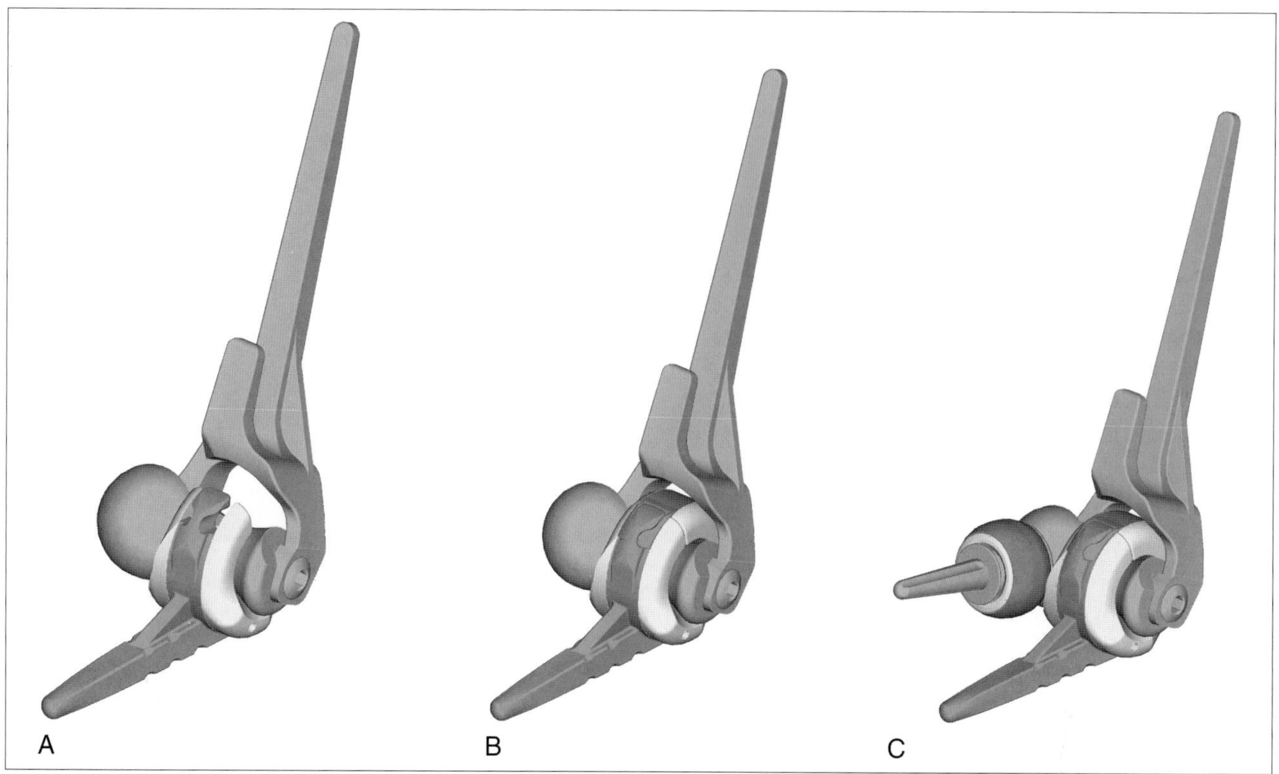

Figure 6 Modern convertible implants offer unlinked **(A)** and linked **(B)** options, as well as implants with radial head replacement **(C)**.

Cement fixation is used for most implanted elbow components. Cementless fixation remains very attractive in theory because it could facilitate revision surgery, especially in the setting of infection. Successful cementless fixation will depend on the development of more anatomic stems and the determination of the ideal surface finish and the extent of ingrowth required.

Revision arthroplasty systems for the elbow are in the very early stages of development. Many systems lack revision components or instrumentation. Although long-stem, cemented devices are commercially available, modular uncemented components are needed to permit easier revision surgery and improved outcomes, especially in patients with bone deficiency.

Precision Elbow Arthroplasty: Implant Design and Computer-Assisted Surgery

The inaccurate replication of the flexion axis of the elbow and malpositioning of the ulnar component may lead to premature wear and loosening in linked elbow arthroplasties, as well as instability in unlinked devices.[45] Humeral stem loading increases with malpositioning of a linked design; elbow maltracking and instability occurs when the elbow is unlinked.[46] In one study, surgeon error in estimating the flexion-extension axis of the elbow under optimal in vitro conditions was reported to be as high as 10°, thus making precise implant placement improbable with current in vivo techniques.[47] A cadaver study showed that stem collision within the medullary canal often precludes accurate placement, even in computer-assisted procedures.[48]

Future developments will include improved stem designs, which are more anatomic and will better fit the shape of the medullary canals.[48,49] Accurate reproduction of the normal kinematic axis of the elbow will be facilitated by modular, adjustable implants, similar to those commonly used in shoulder arthroplasty. Historically, most surgeons using total elbow arthroplasty systems have relied on visual cues to estimate component positioning and orientation. Considerable freehand bone work is typically used, which further compromises the accuracy and reproducibility of implant placement. Advances in implant instrumentation will make total elbow

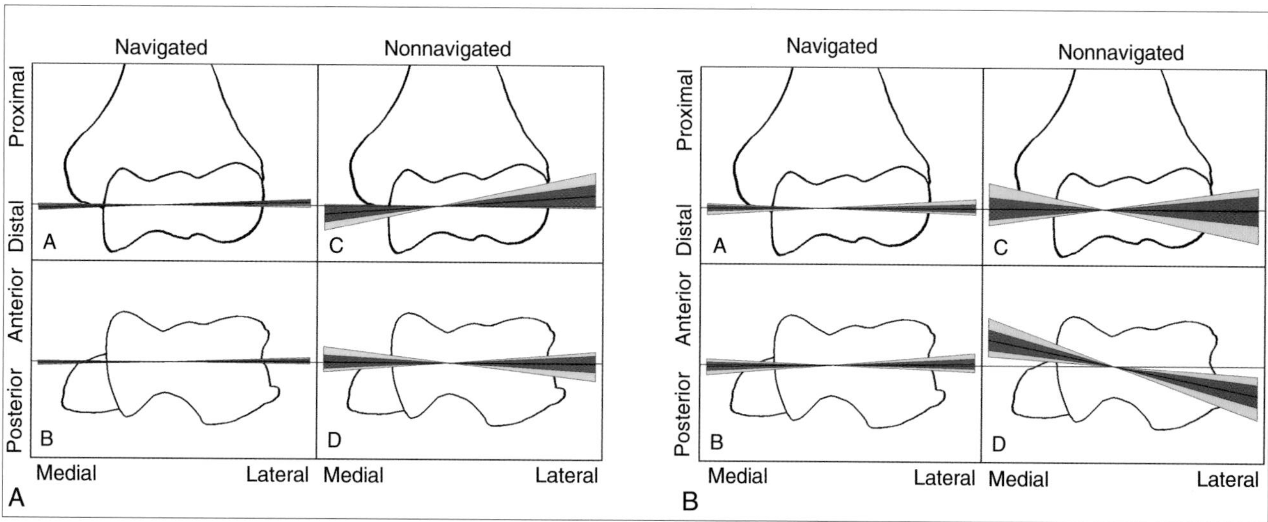

Figure 7 Diagrams comparing navigated and nonnavigated implant alignment. **A,** Implant alignment errors in intact bone structures. Navigation improves the accuracy of implant alignment compared with the nonnavigated traditional alignment methods. **B,** Implant alignment errors in the setting of humeral bone loss. High alignment accuracy is maintained with navigation. In nonnavigated alignment, a lack of anatomic landmarks results in a dramatic increase in alignment errors. (Reproduced with permission from McDonald CP, Johnson JA, Peters TM, King GJ: Image-based navigation improves the positioning of the humeral component in total elbow arthroplasty. *J Shoulder Elbow Surg* 2010; 19(4):533-543.)

arthroplasty a mechanized surgical procedure, similar to total knee arthroplasty. The relative infrequency of elbow arthroplasty limits surgeon experience, further emphasizing the need for well-designed instrument systems to make the procedure faster and more reproducible.

Future developments are likely to include the use of computer-assisted elbow arthroplasty systems, with or without image guidance.[50-52] Such systems will allow the accurate determination and replication of the flexion-extension axis of the elbow, using either preserved anatomic landmarks or via imaging of the contralateral normal elbow in patients with bone loss caused by trauma, tumors, or revision arthroplasty. These systems will not only allow for computer-guided bone resection but also computer-guided prosthesis insertion and positioning. Laboratory experience with prototype systems has shown markedly improved accuracy in implant positioning, even when the osseous structures are largely intact. Given that the morphology of the right and the left elbows are similar, image guidance using the contralateral normal elbow will likely become routine in patients with bone deficiency.[52] Only small amounts of remaining periarticular bone are needed to allow accurate CT registration of the elbow with bone deficiency to the contralateral elbow[51] (**Figure 7**).

Although computer-assisted systems have been shown to improve positioning accuracy and reduce outliers in hip and knee arthroplasty, these systems are not commonly used because computer-assisted surgery has not achieved superior clinical outcomes.[53] Because of the small number of elbow arthroplasties, the benefits of computer-assisted surgery will likely be greater than those reported for higher volume procedures, such as hip and knee arthroplasties. The advent of generic software and tracking platforms will make these systems cost-effective.

Improved Stability for Unlinked Elbow Arthroplasties

Because of the relatively high incidence of instability after unlinked elbow arthroplasty, many surgeons prefer linked designs.[4,7] Although linked elbow arthroplasties have been successful in low-demand patients with generalized rheumatoid arthritis, wear and mechanical failure have been problematic in higher-demand patients with pauciarticular disease and posttraumatic conditions.[14,17,24] Given the advent of improved disease-modifying antirheumatic drugs for inflammatory arthritis, most future elbow replacements will likely be performed for fractures and posttraumatic conditions. This trend to perform elbow arthroplasty in higher-demand patients with the need for greater implant loading has prompted a renewed interest in unlinked devices. Strategies to improve the reliability of unlinked devices will include new developments in implant design, a more secure initial ligament repair, the accurate replication of the flexion-extension axis, and, perhaps, ligament-preserving surgical approaches.

With respect to implant design, the development of an elbow arthroplasty system with optimal intrinsic constraint is needed.[54] Greater articular congruity results in higher loading of the bone-cement interface and increased aseptic loosening. A less conforming implant will result in a greater incidence of maltracking and instability. The optimal articular shape has not yet been determined but will require balancing the risk of instability, articular wear, and loosening. Future developments may also include the development of a more reliable radial head component to ensure better load balancing across the articulation.

More secure initial joint stability has been achieved in more recent designs by repairing the collateral ligaments directly to the implant rather than relying on drill holes through the epicondyles, which are prone to failure.[3,44] Future advances may include a resorbable linkage mechanism to allow reliable collateral ligament healing with early motion and a gradual transfer of the load away from the implant to the soft tissues as the linkage mechanism resorbs. More accurate replication of the flexion-extension axis using computer- and image-assisted approaches should allow better restoration of soft-tissue balance about the elbow and optimize muscle movement arms to improve stability and reduce implant wear. Alternative surgical approaches that retain one or both of the collateral ligaments may improve joint stability and the reliability of unlinked elbow arthroplasties.

Reduced Mechanical Failure

Wear, osteolysis, and aseptic loosening continue to be a common cause of failure of elbow arthroplasties in certain patient populations.[9,14] Wear of the coupling mechanism of linked total elbow implants generates particulate debris and is believed to be an important cause of aseptic loosening.[9] Reduced wear may be achieved by altering the design of the linkage mechanism, changing materials, and balancing forces across the elbow with the addition of a radial head implant.

With respect to linkage design, newer systems have focused on incorporating thicker polyethylene bearings and increasing the contact area; however, the effectiveness of these changes is not yet known.[3] The benefits of modified polyethylene implants, such as highly cross-linked polyethylene implants, have not been established in vitro or in vivo. Alternative bearing surfaces, such as ceramics, metal-on-metal, or those using other new polymers, may be used in future elbow arthroplasties. Radial head implants may reduce bearing wear of both linked and unlinked ulnohumeral arthroplasties by distributing some wear-producing loads to the radiocapitellar joint. Further laboratory and clinical studies are needed to confirm this hypothesis.

Advanced cement techniques have been shown to improve the initial fixation of elbow arthroplasty in vitro; the in vivo application of these techniques may increase implant longevity.[5] Improved cement restrictors and cement delivery and pressurization systems are needed for the elbow. Advances in stem design may also lower the rate of loosening. Cross-sectional shapes and surface treatments may influence the performance of cemented stems. Smooth, stemmed implants have fared poorly in the ulna, likely because of distraction forces that induce stem pullout.[55] Stress shielding of the surrounding bone and fatigue failure of the stems are also problematic, suggesting further efforts are needed to optimize stem design, perhaps using finite element studies and other in vitro testing approaches. Uncemented humeral stems were found to be highly successful in one implant system;[56] however, uncemented ulnar fixation has not been reliable. Further work is needed to improve uncemented stem designs, particularly for revision arthroplasty.

Preserving Triceps Strength

Alternative surgical approaches are needed to better maintain extension strength by respecting the integrity of the triceps mechanism. Leaving the triceps attached to the olecranon preserves extension strength but limits visualization, making the surgical procedure more difficult.[10,11] The development of improved instrumentation, the modification of implant designs, or the addition of computer assistance may allow more accurate component positioning, even with the triceps intact. If the triceps is detached, improved methods of repair to provide more secure fixation and more reliable healing are needed.

Lower Infection Rates

The incidence of infection in elbow arthroplasty continues to be high relative to other joint arthroplasties.[31] Although there are many factors contributing to this complication, future developments will likely include minimally invasive surgical approaches to reduce tissue trauma and allow for shorter surgical times. Alternative management of the ulnar nerve to avoid the need for transposition and user-friendly mechanistic instrumentation may further reduce the length of surgery and the incidence of infection. Sterile tourniquets may be helpful in avoiding contamination at the surgical site. Minimizing inflation times or completely avoiding the use of tourniquets could also prove beneficial.

Summary

Decades of experience with elbow arthroplasty have provided insight regarding the most effective techniques. Carefully documented outcomes show that elbow arthroplasty is successful in improving pain, motion, and function; however, implant durability varies depending on the underlying diagnosis and patient demands, and complications still occur. The knowledge and experience accumulated over the past few years has identified areas that require improvement.

Because elbow arthroplasty is less successful than other joint arthroplasties, future advances are needed to address the current deficiencies. An important limiting factor has been the relatively low volume of elbow arthroplasty procedures, resulting in little research support by peer-reviewed funding agencies and relatively modest investments by industry. Although it is important to remember that current elbow arthroplasties are highly effective in most patients, future developments should afford significant improvement in both short- and long-term patient outcomes. This should expand the indications for elbow arthroplasty to younger and more active patients.

References

1. Morrey BF: Linked elbow arthroplasty: Rationale, indications, and surgical technique, in Morrey BF, Sanchez-Sotelo J, eds: *The Elbow and Its Disorders*, ed 4. Philadelphia, PA, Saunders Elsevier, 2009, pp 765-781.
2. Gill DR, Morrey BF: The Coonrad-Morrey total elbow arthroplasty in patients who have rheumatoid arthritis: A ten to fifteen-year follow-up study. *J Bone Joint Surg Am* 1998;80(9): 1327-1335.
3. King GJ: Convertible total elbow arthroplasty, in Morrey BF, Sanchez-Sotelo J, eds: *The Elbow and Its Disorders*, ed 4. Philadelphia, PA, Saunders Elsevier, 2009, pp 754-764.
4. King GJ: Unlinked total elbow arthroplasty, in Morrey BF, Sanchez-Sotelo J, eds: *The Elbow and Its Disorders*, ed 4. Philadelphia, PA, Saunders Elsevier, 2009, pp 738-754.
5. Faber KJ, Cordy ME, Milne AD, Chess DG, King GJ, Johnson JA: Advanced cement technique improves fixation in elbow arthroplasty. *Clin Orthop Relat Res* 1997; 334:150-156.
6. Itoi E, King GJ, Neibur GL, Morrey BF, An KN: Malrotation of the humeral component of the capitellocondylar total elbow replacement is not the sole cause of dislocation. *J Orthop Res* 1994; 12(5):665-671.
7. Levy JC, Loeb M, Chuinard C, Adams RA, Morrey BF: Effectiveness of revision following linked versus unlinked total elbow arthroplasty. *J Shoulder Elbow Surg* 2009;18(3):457-462.
8. Lee BP, Adams RA, Morrey BF: Polyethylene wear after total elbow arthroplasty. *J Bone Joint Surg Am* 2005;87(5):1080-1087.
9. Goldberg SH, Urban RM, Jacobs JJ, King GJ, O'Driscoll SW, Cohen MS: Modes of wear after semiconstrained total elbow arthroplasty. *J Bone Joint Surg Am* 2008;90(3):609-619.
10. Pierce TD, Herndon JH: The triceps preserving approach to total elbow arthroplasty. *Clin Orthop Relat Res* 1998;354:144-152.
11. Prokopis PM, Weiland AJ: The triceps-preserving approach for semiconstrained total elbow arthroplasty. *J Shoulder Elbow Surg* 2008;17(3):454-458.
12. Bryan RS, Morrey BF: Extensive posterior exposure of the elbow: A triceps-sparing approach. *Clin Orthop Relat Res* 1982;166 :188-192.
13. Little CP, Graham AJ, Karatzas G, Woods DA, Carr AJ: Outcomes of total elbow arthroplasty for rheumatoid arthritis: Comparative study of three implants. *J Bone Joint Surg Am* 2005; 87(11):2439-2448.
14. Throckmorton T, Zarkadas P, Sanchez-Sotelo J, Morrey B: Failure patterns after linked semiconstrained total elbow arthroplasty for posttraumatic arthritis. *J Bone Joint Surg Am* 2010;92(6):1432-1441.
15. Cobb TK, Morrey BF: Total elbow arthroplasty as primary treatment for distal humeral fractures in elderly patients. *J Bone Joint Surg Am* 1997;79(6):826-832.
16. McKee MD, Veillette CJ, Hall JA, et al: A multicenter, prospective, randomized, controlled trial of open reduction-internal fixation versus total elbow arthroplasty for displaced intra-articular distal humeral fractures in elderly patients. *J Shoulder Elbow Surg* 2009;18(1):3-12.
17. Cil A, Veillette CJ, Sanchez-Sotelo J, Morrey BF: Linked elbow replacement: A salvage procedure for distal humeral nonunion. *J Bone Joint Surg Am* 2008;90(9): 1939-1950.
18. Landor I, Vavrik P, Jahoda D, Guttler K, Sosna A: Total elbow replacement with the Souter-Strathclyde prosthesis in rheumatoid arthritis: Long-term follow-up. *J Bone Joint Surg Br* 2006; 88(11):1460-1463.
19. Mori T, Kudo H, Iwano K, Juji T: Kudo type-5 total elbow arthroplasty in mutilating rheumatoid arthritis: A 5- to 11-year follow-up. *J Bone Joint Surg Br* 2006;88(7):920-924.
20. Frankle MA, Herscovici D Jr, DiPasquale TG, Vasey MB, Sanders RW: A comparison of open

reduction and internal fixation and primary total elbow arthroplasty in the treatment of intraarticular distal humerus fractures in women older than age 65. *J Orthop Trauma* 2003;17(7): 473-480.

21. Gambirasio R, Riand N, Stern R, Hoffmeyer P: Total elbow replacement for complex fractures of the distal humerus: An option for the elderly patient. *J Bone Joint Surg Br* 2001;83(7):974-978.
22. Garcia JA, Mykula R, Stanley D: Complex fractures of the distal humerus in the elderly: The role of total elbow replacement as primary treatment. *J Bone Joint Surg Br* 2002;84(6):812-816.
23. Ray PS, Kakarlapudi K, Rajsekhar C, Bhamra MS: Total elbow arthroplasty as primary treatment for distal humeral fractures in elderly patients. *Injury* 2000; 31(9):687-692.
24. Kamineni S, Morrey BF: Distal humeral fractures treated with noncustom total elbow replacement. *J Bone Joint Surg Am* 2004; 86-A(5):940-947.
25. Schneeberger AG, Adams R, Morrey BF: Semiconstrained total elbow replacement for the treatment of post-traumatic osteoarthrosis. *J Bone Joint Surg Am* 1997;79(8):1211-1222.
26. Ramsey ML, Adams RA, Morrey BF: Instability of the elbow treated with semiconstrained total elbow arthroplasty. *J Bone Joint Surg Am* 1999;81(1):38-47.
27. Mansat P, Morrey BF: Semiconstrained total elbow arthroplasty for ankylosed and stiff elbows. *J Bone Joint Surg Am* 2000;82(9): 1260-1268.
28. Peden JP, Morrey BF: Total elbow replacement for the management of the ankylosed or fused elbow. *J Bone Joint Surg Br* 2008;90(9): 1198-1204.
29. Kozak TK, Adams RA, Morrey BF: Total elbow arthroplasty in primary osteoarthritis of the elbow. *J Arthroplasty* 1998;13(7): 837-842.
30. Espag MP, Back DL, Clark DI, Lunn PG: Early results of the Souter-Strathclyde unlinked total elbow arthroplasty in patients with osteoarthritis. *J Bone Joint Surg Br* 2003;85(3):351-353.
31. Cheung EV, Adams RA, Morrey BF: Reimplantation of a total elbow prosthesis following resection arthroplasty for infection. *J Bone Joint Surg Am* 2008;90(3): 589-594.
32. Sanchez-Sotelo J, O'Driscoll S, Morrey BF: Periprosthetic humeral fractures after total elbow arthroplasty: Treatment with implant revision and strut allograft augmentation. *J Bone Joint Surg Am* 2002;84-A(9):1642-1650.
33. Sanchez-Sotelo J, Morrey BF: Surgical techniques for reconstruction of chronic insufficiency of the triceps: Rotation flap using anconeus and tendo Achillis allograft. *J Bone Joint Surg Br* 2002; 84(8):1116-1120.
34. King GJ, Adams RA, Morrey BF: Total elbow arthroplasty: Revision with use of a non-custom semiconstrained prosthesis. *J Bone Joint Surg Am* 1997;79(3): 394-400.
35. Kamineni S, Morrey BF: Proximal ulnar reconstruction with strut allograft in revision total elbow arthroplasty. *J Bone Joint Surg Am* 2004;86-A(6):1223-1229.
36. Loebenberg MI, Adams R, O'Driscoll SW, Morrey BF: Impaction grafting in revision total elbow arthroplasty. *J Bone Joint Surg Am* 2005;87(1):99-106.
37. Mansat P, Adams RA, Morrey BF: Allograft-prosthesis composite for revision of catastrophic failure of total elbow arthroplasty. *J Bone Joint Surg Am* 2004;86-A(4):724-735.
38. Shifrin PG, Johnson DP: Elbow hemiarthroplasty with 20-year follow-up study: A case report and literature review. *Clin Orthop Relat Res* 1990;254:128-133.
39. Swoboda B, Scott RD: Humeral hemiarthroplasty of the elbow joint in young patients with rheumatoid arthritis: A report on 7 arthroplasties. *J Arthroplasty* 1999; 14(5):553-559.
40. Adolfsson L, Hammer R: Elbow hemiarthroplasty for acute reconstruction of intraarticular distal humerus fractures: A preliminary report involving 4 patients. *Acta Orthop* 2006;77(5):785-787.
41. Hughes JF: Distal humeral hemiarthroplasty, in Morrey BF, Sanchez-Sotelo J, eds: *The Elbow and Its Disorders*, ed 4. Philadelphia, PA, Saunders Elsevier, 2009, pp 720-729.
42. Heijink A, Morrey BF, Cooney WP III: Radiocapitellar hemiarthroplasty for radiocapitellar arthritis: A report of three cases. *J Shoulder Elbow Surg* 2008; 17(2): e12-e15.
43. Papandrea RF, Morrey BF, O'Driscoll SW: Reconstruction for persistent instability of the elbow after coronoid fracture-dislocation. *J Shoulder Elbow Surg* 2007;16(1):68-77.
44. Gramstad GD, King GJ, O'Driscoll SW, Yamaguchi K: Elbow arthroplasty using a convertible implant. *Tech Hand Up Extrem Surg* 2005;9(3):153-163.
45. Brownhill JR, Ferreira LM, Pichora JE, Johnson JA, King GJ: Defining the flexion-extension axis of the ulna: Implications for intra-operative elbow alignment. *J Biomech Eng* 2009;131(2): 021005.
46. Brownhill JR, Pollock JW, Ferreira LM, Johnson JA, King GJ: The effect of humeral component malalignment on the loading of total elbow arthroplasty: An in-vitro study. *Trans ORS* 2008;33: 1561.

47. Brownhill JR, Furukawa K, Faber KJ, Johnson JA, King GJ: Surgeon accuracy in the selection of the flexion-extension axis of the elbow: An in vitro study. *J Shoulder Elbow Surg* 2006;15(4):451-456.

48. Brownhill JR, King GJ, Johnson JA: Morphologic analysis of the distal humerus with special interest in elbow implant sizing and alignment. *J Shoulder Elbow Surg* 2007;16(3, Suppl):S126-S132.

49. Brownhill JR, Mozzon JB, Ferreira LM, Johnson JA, King GJ: Morphologic analysis of the proximal ulna with special interest in elbow implant sizing and alignment. *J Shoulder Elbow Surg* 2009;18(1):27-32.

50. McDonald CP, Beaton BJ, King GJ, Peters TM, Johnson JA: The effect of anatomic landmark selection of the distal humerus on registration accuracy in computer-assisted elbow surgery. *J Shoulder Elbow Surg* 2008;17(5):833-843.

51. McDonald CP, Brownhill JR, King GJ, Johnson JA, Peters TM: A comparison of registration techniques for computer- and image-assisted elbow surgery. *Comput Aided Surg* 2007;12(4):208-214.

52. McDonald CP, Peters TM, King GJ, Johnson JA: Computer assisted surgery of the distal humerus can employ contralateral images for pre-operative planning, registration, and surgical intervention. *J Shoulder Elbow Surg* 2009;18(3):469-477.

53. Beringer DC, Patel JJ, Bozic KJ: An overview of economic issues in computer-assisted total joint arthroplasty. *Clin Orthop Relat Res* 2007;463:26-30.

54. Kamineni S, O'Driscoll SW, Urban M, et al: Intrinsic constraint of unlinked total elbow replacements: The ulnotrochlear joint. *J Bone Joint Surg Am* 2005;87(9):2019-2027.

55. Cheung EV, O'Driscoll SW: Total elbow prosthesis loosening caused by ulnar component pistoning. *J Bone Joint Surg Am* 2007;89(6):1269-1274.

56. Kudo H, Iwand K, Nishino J: Total elbow arthroplasty with use of a nonconstrained humeral component inserted without cement in patients who have rheumatoid arthritis. *J Bone Joint Surg Am* 1999;81(9):1268-1280.

Video Reference

14.1, 14.2, and 14,3: King GJW: Video. Excerpt. *Elbow Arthroplasty.* London, Ontario, Canada, 2008.

Elbow Arthroscopy: Setup, Portal Placement, and Simple Procedures

Christopher S. Ahmad, MD
Mark A. Vitale, MD, MPH

Abstract

Elbow arthroscopy has become an accepted treatment for numerous elbow conditions, including loose bodies, lateral epicondylitis, contractures, painful osteophytes, synovitis, osteochondritis dissecans, synovial plica, and osteoarthritis. It is absolutely necessary that the treating surgeon have complete knowledge of elbow anatomy. Three options exist for patient positioning: supine, prone, and lateral decubitus. Standard arthroscopic probes, grasping forceps, punches, and motorized shavers and burrs are used in the procedure. Retractors are essential for visualizing, exposing, and protecting nerves. Specially designed capsular biters can be used to develop a plane between the capsule and the surrounding soft tissues to facilitate capsulotomy and capsulectomy. Among elbow arthroscopists, the sequence of portal placement varies; however, there is little variation in the exact location of portal placement because of neurovascular constraints. Loose body removal and extensor carpi radialis brevis release for lateral epicondylitis are common procedures suitable for the beginning arthroscopist. For beginning and advanced procedures, the surgeon's skill and competence must be at a level consistent with the procedure to avoid complications.

Instr Course Lect 2011;60:171-180.

Elbow arthroscopy has significantly advanced because of an improved understanding of elbow anatomy, the development of enhanced equipment, and better surgeon education. These advancements in arthroscopy have led to safe and effective treatment of numerous elbow conditions with minimally invasive approaches, decreased morbidity, and accelerated recovery. Elbow arthroscopy began as a diagnostic tool for elbow disorders and experienced immediate success as a means for removing loose bodies.[1-4] Numerous disorders that previously required open approaches, including lateral epicondylitis, contractures, painful osteophytes, synovitis, osteochondritis dissecans, synovial plica, osteoarthritis, and some fractures, can now be treated safely and effectively with arthroscopy.[5-13] Despite rapid advancements in techniques and instrumentation, elbow arthroscopy remains a technically demanding procedure with the potential for serious complications. Special attention to proper elbow arthroscopic techniques is required to avoid complications and ensure predictable results. A complete knowledge of elbow anatomy is paramount, and the treating surgeon's skill and competence should be at a level consistent with the procedure. Safe and efficient elbow arthroscopy requires adequate training for the surgeon, selecting patients with the appropriate surgical indications, and proper execution of the desired procedure.

Anesthesia

General, regional, or a combination of both types of anesthesia may be used in elbow arthroscopy. General anesthesia has the advantages of complete muscle relaxation, patient comfort, and airway management, and allows for a postoperative neurologic examination. Regional blocks offer postoperative pain control but do not allow

Dr. Ahmad or an immediate family member has received research or institutional support from Acumed, Arthrex, and Zimmer. Neither Dr. Vitale nor any immediate family member has received anything of value from or owns stock in a commercial company or institution related directly or indirectly to the subject of this chapter.

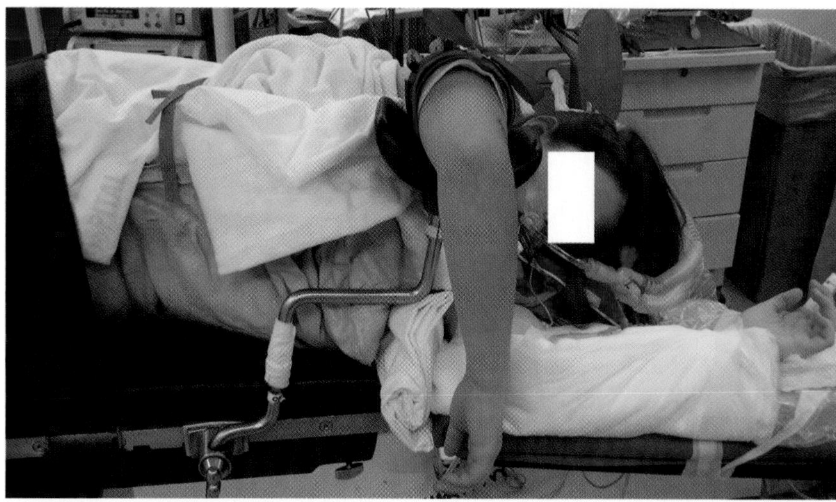

Figure 1 Photograph showing the lateral decubitus position. The shoulder is placed in 90° of flexion and maintained over a lateral arm support to allow ample room near the thorax for medial-sided work. The arm is free to allow flexion and extension.

an immediate postoperative nerve examination. A combined strategy is to use general anesthesia with a postoperative nerve examination followed by regional anesthesia for postoperative pain control. Patient and procedure requirements may dictate the type of anesthesia based on the risk of nerve injury and the need for postoperative pain control. For example, if a previous nerve injury or nerve transfer has occurred, general anesthesia in isolation is preferred.

Patient Positioning

Three options exist for patient positioning: supine, prone, and lateral decubitus.

Supine Positioning

In supine positioning, which was the first described method for elbow arthroscopy, the elbow is flexed to 90° and the arm is suspended with traction equipment.[1] The supine position offers several advantages. It provides easy access for airway management that facilitates the use of either regional or general anesthesia. The elbow anatomy is oriented in a manner familiar to the surgeon, with the anterior compartment facing upward and the posterior compartment facing downward. The supine position also permits easy conversion to an open procedure, such as medial collateral ligament reconstruction. Disadvantages include difficulty in accessing the posterior compartment and difficulty stabilizing the elbow while it is suspended in traction.

Prone Positioning

In the prone position, first described by Poehling et al,[4] the elbow is flexed to 90° in a stationary arm support, eliminating the need for a traction system. The advantages of the prone position include improved posterior compartment access and visualization and easy conversion to a posterior approach if necessary. The main disadvantages of the prone position are the relative difficulty in accessing the airway and the reversed orientation of elbow anatomy from the surgeon's perspective. General anesthesia is required for the patient.

Lateral Decubitus Positioning

This chapter's authors generally prefer the lateral decubitus position, a modification of the prone position, with the patient lying on the unaffected side with the affected elbow in an arm holder[4,14] (**Figure 1**). The arm is relatively stable, and traction is not needed. This position allows easy access to the posterior compartment, and a full range of elbow flexion-extension is easily achieved. Pulmonary function is less compromised in the lateral decubitus position than in the prone position. Regional or general anesthesia may be used. The operative shoulder is flexed forward to 90°, internally rotated 90°, and suspended over the arm holder with the forearm allowed to hang free. The shoulder must be forward flexed at least 90° and abducted slightly so that instrumentation does not interfere with the patient's chest. It is also important to minimize the bean bag and any other support structure for lateral positioning anterior to the patient to avoid obstructing the arthroscopic instrumentation to the elbow. Pressure or constriction of the antecubital fossa should be avoided because it will compress the neurovascular structures to the anterior capsule and can increase the risk of iatrogenic neurovascular injury. The shoulder and elbow of the contralateral arm should be flexed so they do not impede elbow flexion of the operative arm. After patient positioning is completed, the surgeon may simulate instruments entering the elbow from the various portals and at various elbow flexion angles to verify an optimal setup. The primary disadvantage of the lateral decubitus position is the need to reposition the patient if additional open procedures requiring supine positioning are necessary.

Instrumentation

A standard 4.0-mm, 30° arthroscope is used for most procedures, but a smaller 2.7-mm arthroscope may be necessary when working in the radiocapitellar joint or for young and/or small patients. Fluid management presents a challenge in elbow arthroscopy and can be improved with several methods. Side-vented inflow cannulas may cause fluid extravasation into the surrounding soft tissues if some vents remain superficial to the capsule; thus, side-vented inflow cannulas should be avoided. Outflow cannulas placed early in the procedure can help avoid excessive fluid extravasation into the soft tissues. Low pump pressures (30 mm Hg) can maintain distention of the joint and minimize fluid extravasation.

Standard arthroscopic probes, grasping forceps, punches, and motorized shavers and burrs are available. Specially designed capsular biters have been developed with an extended blunt tip that can develop a plane between the capsule and the surrounding soft tissues. Retractors are essential for visualizing, exposing, and protecting nerves.

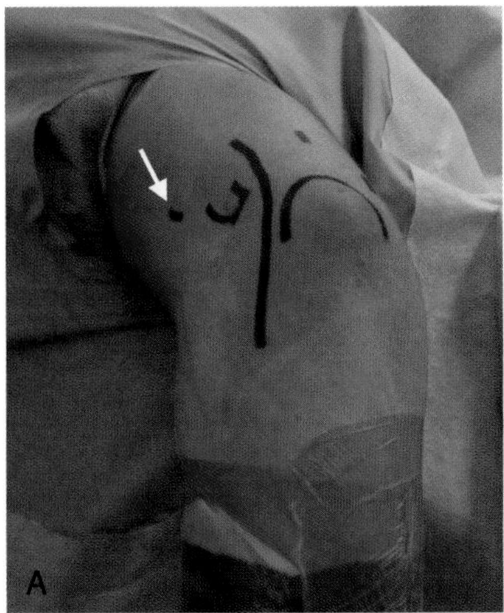

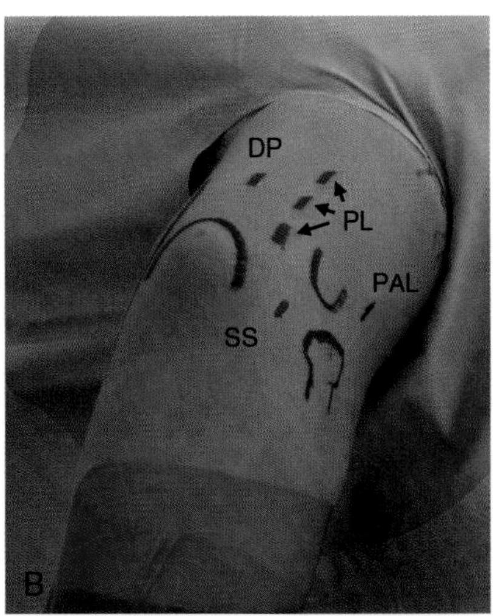

Figure 2 **A,** Photograph of the elbow with the medial elbow anatomy and portal placement markings. The ulnar nerve is outlined. The arrow points to the location for placing the proximal anteromedial portal. **B,** Portal placement markings on the lateral elbow. DP = direct posterior portal, PL = posterolateral portal, PAL = proximal anterolateral portal, SS = soft-spot portal.

Surgical Considerations

Anatomy

The bony anatomy of the elbow divides it into three arthroscopic compartments: anterior, posterior, and posterolateral. The anterior compartment is composed of the coronoid process, the anterior trochlea, the radial head, the capitellum, and the medial and lateral condyles. The posterior compartment contains the olecranon tip, the olecranon fossa, the posterior trochlea, and the medial and lateral gutters. The posterolateral compartment contains the radial head, the olecranon, the lateral gutter, and the capitellum.

The presence of a subluxating or previously transposed ulnar nerve must be identified. A transposed ulnar nerve requires a limited open medial exposure and protection during the creation of a medial portal, or alternatively, the medial portal can be avoided. A previous submuscular transposition is considered an absolute contraindication in using the medial portal for most procedures.

Portal Placement

Knowledge of elbow anatomy is essential to elbow arthroscopy to avoid nerve injury and properly execute the procedure. Among elbow arthroscopists, variations exist in the sequence of portal placement; however, fewer variations exist in establishing the exact locations of portal placement because of the need to respect the neurovascular anatomy. The proximal anteromedial portal is located 2 cm above the medial epicondyle and approximately 1 cm anterior to the intermuscular septum (**Figure 2, A**). Palpating the septum is usually possible and assists in accurately placing the portal. The medial antebrachial cutaneous nerve is at risk for injury and is located 2.3 mm (on average) from the portal. The ulnar nerve is located, on average, 12 to 23 mm from the portal. The proximal anteromedial portal is safer than a more distal anteromedial portal, in part because the arthroscope is directed distally and more parallel to the median nerve in the anteroposterior plane.[15] This portal facilitates systematic examination of the anterior compartment, including the capitellum, the radial head, and the anterior and lateral aspects of the capsule.

The proximal anterolateral portal is located 2 cm proximal to the lateral epicondyle and is placed directly on the anterior surface of the humerus[14,16] (**Figure 2, B**). The posterior antebrachial cutaneous nerve is, on average, 6.1 mm away but is in contact with the cannula 29% of the time.[14] The radial nerve lies 4.9 mm away in extension and 9.9 mm away in flexion. This portal allows visualization of the medial aspect of the anterior compartment, including the coronoid, the trochlea, and the anterior capsule. The risk of neurovascular injury decreases as the portal is moved more proximally.

It has been customary to locate the anterolateral portal 3 cm distal and 2 cm anterior to the lateral epicondyle;[1] however, this location poses significant risks of iatrogenic nerve injury.[17] The risk is decreased with more proximal positioning.

The posterolateral portal can be located anywhere from the tip of the olecranon to 3 cm proximal to it in the posterolateral gutter just lateral to the triceps tendon. The elbow is held in 30° of flexion to relax the triceps while establishing the portal. This portal poses little risk of nerve injury. It provides visualization of the entire posterior compartment and can be useful in débriding the olecranon fossa, the tip of the olecranon, and the lateral gutter when necessary.

The direct posterior portal splits the triceps in its midline 3 cm proximal to the olecranon tip (**Figure 2, B**). This portal allows visualization of the olecranon tip, olecranon fossa, and posterior trochlea. The medial and posterior antebrachial cutaneous nerves are at risk for injury and are located, on average, 25 mm from this portal.[17] The ulnar nerve is approximately 25 mm from this portal medially and is safe when instruments are placed lateral to the posterior midline.[2]

The posterolateral anatomy of the elbow allows portal placement anywhere from the proximal posterolateral portal to the lateral soft spot (**Figure 2, B**). A more distal position allows visualization of the posterior radiocapitellar joint.

The soft-spot portal is located in the center of the triangle formed by the lateral epicondyle, the tip of the olecranon, and the radial head. The closest neurovascular structure to the portal is the posterior antebrachial cutaneous nerve, which passes approximately 7 mm from the portal.[2] Because the soft-spot portal allows visualization of the inferior aspect of the capitellum and the inferior portion of the radioulnar articulation, it is useful in débriding posterolateral plica and osteochondritis dissecans lesions of the capitellum. Additional portals are made as necessary for retractor placement. See chapter 16 for more information on using arthroscopy for treating capitellar osteochondritis dissecans.)

Video 15.1: Elbow Arthroscopy: Portals. Champ L. Baker Jr, MD (11 min)

Technical Steps

After general or regional anesthesia is administered, the patient is positioned. In the lateral decubitus position, abuting the arthroscope and instruments against the patient and positioning devices should be avoided by placing the beanbag and supports away from the chest. The arm should be abducted 90° from the body, with the elbow positioned slightly higher than the shoulder. Once the patient is positioned, it is useful to simulate the instrumentation from the proximal medial and proximal anterolateral portals to ensure no abutment. A tourniquet is placed proximally on the arm with the pressure set at 250 mm Hg. The extremity is prepped and draped. The forearm is wrapped with an elastic bandage from the fingers to just below the elbow to reduce the effect of fluid extravasation into the forearm.

Surface landmarks are outlined, including the medial and lateral epicondyles, the radial head, and the olecranon. It is critically important to outline the ulnar nerve to preserve the mediolateral orientation and maintain constant awareness of the ulnar nerve to avoid injury. The initial portal for joint visualization is usually based on the surgeon's preference but may be chosen based on the type of procedure and the pathology. This chapter's authors prefer to visualize the anterior compartment of the elbow first, then the posterior compartment, and finally the posterolateral recess to complete the overall joint inspection. A medial portal is created first; the lateral portal is then established under direct visualization with the aid of a spinal needle.

An 18-gauge needle is inserted through the location of the lateral soft-spot portal. The elbow is then distended with 15 to 25 mL of sterile saline. Insufflation of fluid into the joint increases the distance between the neurovascular structures and the joint surfaces, helping to protect vessels and nerves from injury during joint entry. In a cadaver study with the elbow in 90° of flexion, Miller et al[18] showed that insufflation of 20 mL of saline increased the nerve-to-bone distance by a mean of 12 mm for the median nerve and by 6 mm for the radial nerve. Importantly, the capsule-to-nerve distance was minimally increased by insufflation and was as narrow as 6 mm in some specimens, highlighting the fact that insufflation of the joint does not protect the nerves from work performed against the joint capsule.

A superomedial portal is established first. A No. 11 blade is used to incise skin only, and a blunt clamp is used to spread the subcutaneous tissues to help avoid injury to the medial antebrachial cutaneous nerve. The blunt obturator and scope sheath is then placed on the anterior humerus anterior to the intermuscular septum. The sheath and obturator are then directed toward the radiocapitellar joint. A pump pressure of 30 mm Hg is used. Diagnostic arthroscopy proceeds with viewing the articular surface of the radial head and the superior and anterior portions of the capitellum (**Figure 3**). The elbow can be extended to better visualize the anterior capitellum. The radial fossa just superior to the capitellum is inspected for osteophytes. The arthroscope is withdrawn medially, and the anterior aspect of the proximal radioulnar articulation and the anterior ulnohumeral articulation are visualized.

The anterolateral portal is then created with an outside-in technique. A guidewire can assist in accurate placement (**Figure 4**). The joint is approached parallel to the capsule; often a blunt cannula will not easily penetrate the capsule. Working instruments are then introduced as necessary. The arthroscope is placed in this portal using switching sticks, and the coronoid process and its fossa are inspected for osteophytes and loose bodies (**Figure 5**). The trochlea then should be inspected using flexion and extension to assess its entire articular surface.

Creating space for visualization is a task unique to elbow arthroscopy. Synovectomy and the removal of fibrous adhesions must be done initially. Retractors to position the capsule anteriorly are held by an assistant through additional anteromedial and proximal anterolateral portals.

The posterior compartment is evaluated with a blunt trocar, which is introduced and aimed at the olecranon fossa through the posterolateral portal. Once the trocar is placed, bluntly elevating the posterior capsule off the distal humerus expands the joint space for better viewing. A cannula is then placed in the direct posterior portal. A shaver can be inserted into the posterolateral portal, and soft tissue can be safely débrided from the lateral olecranon fossa and lateral gutter. The posterior compartment should be thoroughly inspected because loose bodies will frequently migrate there. The posterior aspect of the trochlea, the olecranon fossa, and the tip of the olecranon can all be inspected from the posterolateral or posterocentral portal (**Figure 6**). By extending the arm, bony or soft-tissue impingement between the olecranon process and the olecranon fossa can be visualized. Advancement of the arthroscope into the lateral gutter allows further inspection of the capitellum by viewing its posterior surface.

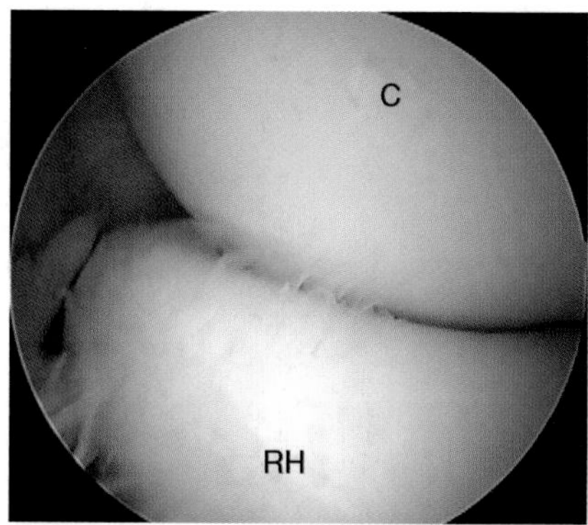

Figure 3 Arthroscopic view of the anterior compartment from the proximal anteromedial compartment, visualizing the radial head (RH) and the capitellum (C).

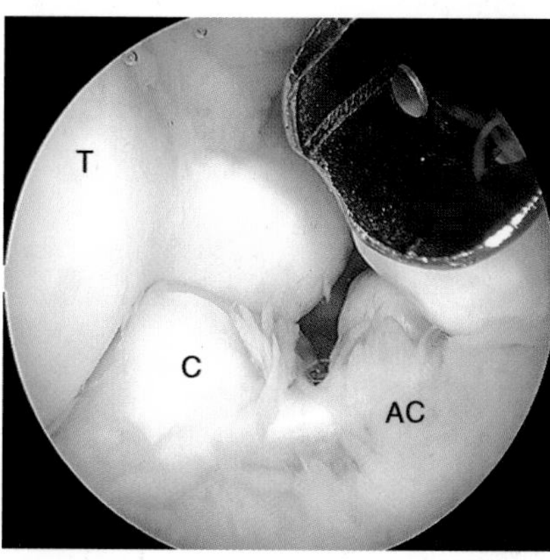

Figure 5 Arthroscopic view of the anterior compartment from the proximal anterolateral portal with the trochlea (T), coronoid (C), and anterior capsule (AC) visualized (note the arthroscope sheath from the proximal anteromedial portal).

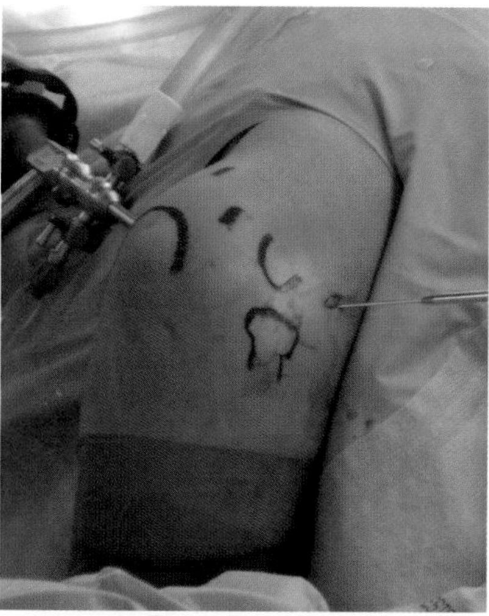

Figure 4 The proximal anterolateral portal is created using a cannulated dilator over a needle.

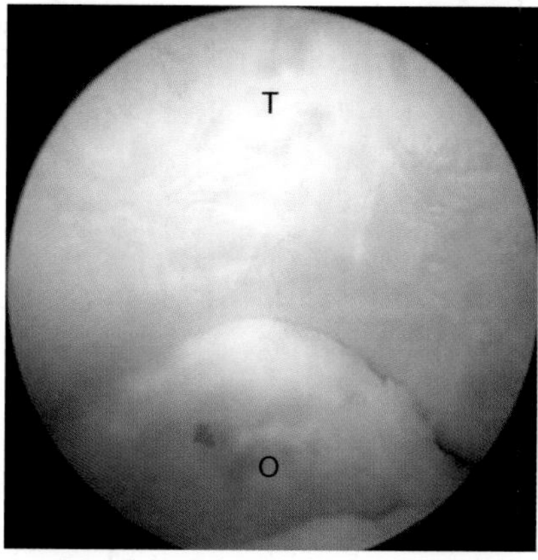

Figure 6 The posterior compartment with views of the trochlea (T) and the olecranon (O).

Diagnostic arthroscopy of the elbow is completed through the direct lateral portal. The capitellum, the semilunar fossa of the ulna, the trochlea, the undersurface of the radioulnar articulation, and the radial head articular margin are inspected through this portal.

Use of Retractors

Soft tissues in the elbow tend to obstruct visualization, particularly as tissues are taken down and fluid extravasation occurs as the procedure progresses. It is tempting to increase the pump pressure to distend soft tissues, but this will increase extravasations and should be avoided. Arthroscopic retractors provide visualization similar to retractors used in open surgery and have provided a tremendous technical advancement to elbow arthroscopic procedures. Arthroscopic retractors require accessory portals and an assistant to hold the retractor. Switching sticks, jokers, freers, and curved osteotomes may

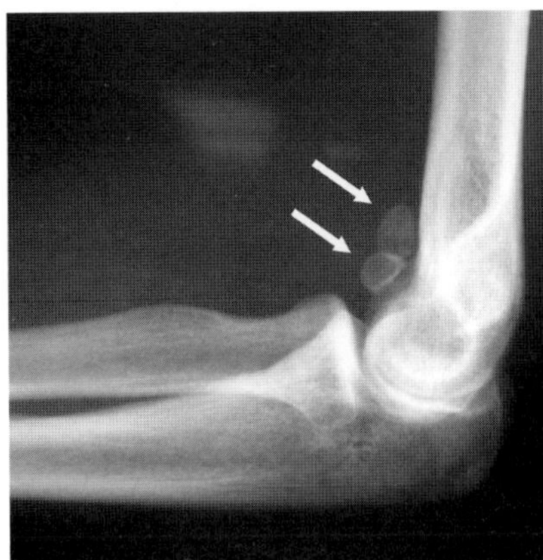

Figure 7 Lateral radiograph showing ossified loose bodies (arrows) in the anterior compartment.

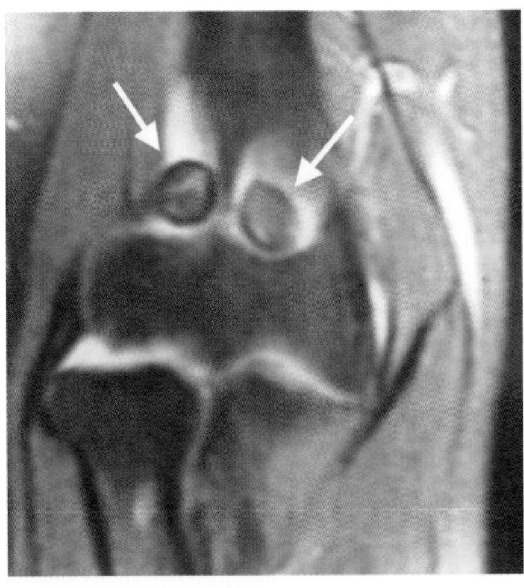

Figure 8 Coronal MRI scan showing loose bodies (arrows) in the anterior compartment.

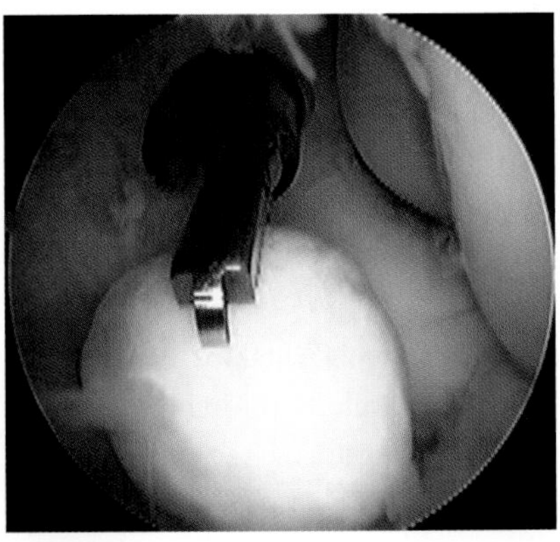

Figure 9 Arthroscopic view of the grasper from the lateral portal controlling a loose body for removal.

be used as retractors. A switching stick can be modified with a curve and used in the posterior compartment to protect the ulnar nerve (J Conway, MD, Las Vegas, NV, unpublished data presented at the American Academy of Orthopaedic Surgeons annual meeting, 2009).

The portal most typically used for retraction is the proximal anterolateral portal. This facilitates using the arthroscope through the proximal anteromedial portal and a working instrument through the anterolateral portal. In this position, the retractor can be used to lift away the capsule and the soft tissue, improving visualization and moving the radial nerve away from the bone.

Posteriorly, the retractor can be inserted through the proximal posterior or the proximal posterolateral portal and directed posteromedially to lift the ulnar nerve away from the bone.

Loose Bodies

Beginner elbow arthroscopists should start with simple procedures with limited technical challenges. Removal of loose bodies and extensor carpi radialis brevis (ECRB) release for lateral epicondylitis are two common procedures that are well suited for gaining experience and proficiency. The need to remove loose bodies is a common indication for elbow arthroscopy and can be associated with a variety of conditions, including osteochondritis dissecans, valgus extension overload, trauma, osteoarthritis, and synovial chondromatosis. It is important to determine the etiology of the loose body to ensure both adequate treatment of the loose body itself as well as the underlying condition.

Most patients with symptoms of loose bodies in the elbow are involved in activities such as throwing, gymnastics, or manual labor that require repetitive elbow motions. Symptoms include loss of motion and pain localized to the area of cartilage injury or osteophyte impingement. Locking or catching may result from intra-articular loose bodies. The arc of motion should be carefully assessed on examination.

Diagnosis

Loose bodies often can be identified with radiography (**Figure 7**). They are most commonly located anteriorly in the coronoid fossa or posteriorly in the olecranon fossa. Magnetic resonance or CT arthrography can identify cartilaginous and fibrous loose bodies not seen on plain radiographs and also allow loose-body donor site evaluation (**Figure 8**). After diagnosis, loose bodies should be removed to prevent chondral injury and relieve mechanical symptoms.

Complete diagnostic arthroscopy must be performed systematically to identify a loose body. Visualization of the medial and lateral recess must be obtained. Placing the arthroscope in both the anteromedial and anterolateral portals allows complete visualization of the anterior compartment. From the anterolateral portal, the medial capsule, the anterior portion of the medial collateral ligament, the coronoid process, the trochlea, and the medial aspect of the radiocapitellar joint can be viewed. Visualization from the anteromedial portal allows evaluation of the anterior radiocapitellar joint and the lateral capsule. During systematic diagnostic arthroscopy, loose bodies are sought, identified, and removed with grasping instruments (**Figure 9**). Once a loose body is localized, managing cannula inflow and outflow is helpful in directing the loose body. Outflow though the cannula will draw the loose body in that direction. Flow can be turned off to prevent turbulence. A needle can be used to control the loose body to help with grasping.

Removal

Removing large loose bodies may require enlarging the portal and removing the cannula. All compartments must be examined for loose bodies, including the medial and lateral gutters. The integrity of all articular surfaces should be carefully inspected for possible lesions. A direct soft-spot portal allows visualization of the posterior radiocapitellar joint. An accessory midlateral portal may be created 1 cm distal for removing loose bodies from the lateral compartment. The exact portal position can be established with spinal needle localization. The posterolateral gutter is a common location of loose bodies and is often difficult to visualize. Arthroscopic excision of hypertrophic synovium may be necessary for complete visualization.

Posterior loose bodies can be removed through the direct posterior portal but are often more easily removed through the posterolateral portal because the thick triceps are avoided. Soft tissue under the triceps should be débrided to improve visualization. The posterior compartment, including the posteromedial and posterolateral gutter, should be examined. The olecranon fossa is probed for loose fragments and examined for osteophytes as a source of loose bodies. The olecranon fossa is the most common location for loose bodies, which are often encased in soft tissue. A shaver can be used to débride hypertrophic synovium, allowing all potential sites of loose body entrapment to be explored. Because loose bodies migrate among the anterior, lateral, and posterior compartments, all compartments must be thoroughly examined in a systematic fashion.

Removing large loose bodies may require enlarging the portal. In general, removing large loose bodies in the anterior compartment through the anterolateral portal is preferred because of the thinner soft-tissue envelope in that area. Another useful technique is removing the cannula and the loose body simultaneously. Occasionally, the loose body must be cut and removed in a piecemeal fashion.

Loose bodies, which are often hidden in the coronoid and radial head fossae, are removed when encountered. A spinal needle is helpful for stabilizing a loose body when discovered. A larger-toothed grasper allows the loose body to be securely gripped to avoid incomplete removal or incarceration into the soft tissues. Larger loose bodies are broken into smaller pieces (with duckbill forceps or osteotomes) and removed with the shaver or the grasper. Unstable osteophytes are excised using a combination of small, curved osteotomes and a pituitary rongeur. Lowering the pump pressure; applying suction to a cannula, which is directed toward the loose body; enlarging the skin incision, and pushing the loose body and following it with the arthroscope out the portal are helpful techniques for successful and complete loose body removal. Loose bodies can usually be seen once the posterior fat pad, synovium, and fibrous adhesions are resected from the olecranon fossa.

Rehabilitation

Soft dressings are applied, and sutures are removed in 7 to 10 days. Strengthening and range-of-motion exercises are initiated as the incisions are healing. Postoperative management following isolated simple removal of loose bodies can be aggressive to return range of motion and strength with minimal restrictions. Arthroscopic removal of loose bodies has been reported to be the most successful of all the elbow arthroscopic procedures. Return to sports activities is expected when full range of motion and strength are achieved. Participation in a progressive throwing program is recommended for throwing athletes.

Results

Most studies report significant alleviation of pain, locking, and swelling, with good to excellent results in 75% to 97% of elbows after loose body removal. Andrews and Carson[1] reported that removing isolated loose bodies in the elbow is the most successful arthroscopic elbow procedure. Ogilvie-Harris and Schemitsch[3] reported on 34 patients with one or more loose bodies in the elbow with symptomatic locking and pain. Thirty-three of 34 loose bodies were removed arthroscopically; a small arthrotomy was needed to remove 1 large loose body. At an average follow-up of 2.7 years, pain improved in 85% of patients, locking symptoms improved in 92%, and swelling improved in 71%. Although the number of flexion contractures was reduced from 14 to 5, crepitus was improved in only 47% of patients. Overall, 89% of patients reported subjective improvement with arthroscopic treatment. Two patients had transient forearm numbness, but no lasting complications were observed.

Lateral Epicondylitis

Lateral epicondylitis is the most common elbow disorder in patients seeking medical treatment, affecting 50% of all recreational tennis players. It often occurs in the fourth decade of life. Risk factors for tennis players include heavy racquets, inappropriate grip size, high string tension, and poor swinging technique. The ECRB is most commonly involved, but the extensor digitorum communis, extensor radialis longus, and extensor carpi ulnaris may also be involved. Microtrauma from the repetitive activity results in histopathologic angiofibroblastic hyperplasia.[19,20]

Diagnosis

Affected patients are typically involved in a repetitive activity that requires

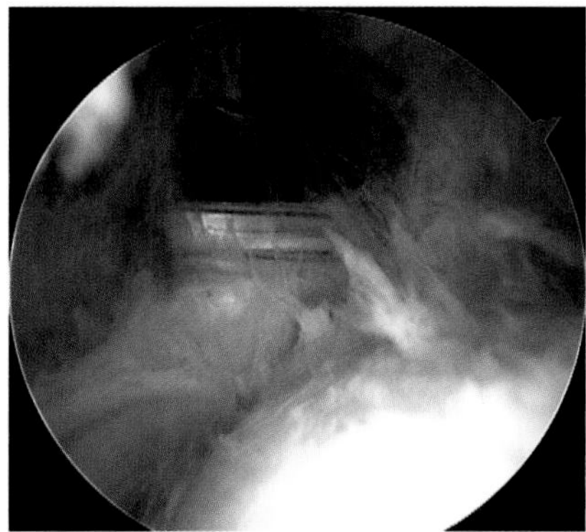

Figure 10 Arthroscopic view of the ECRB localized after capsular release.

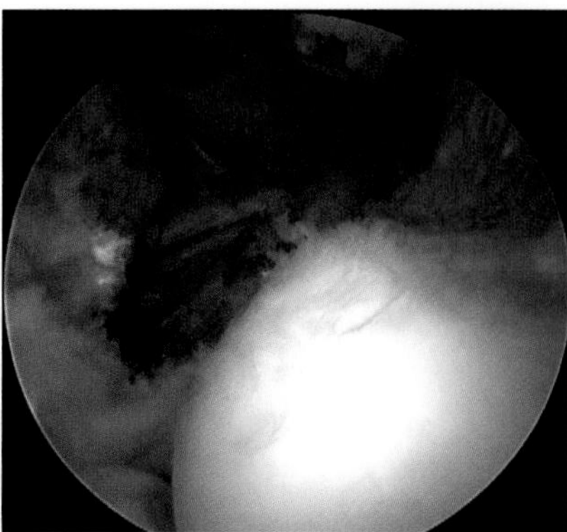

Figure 11 Arthroscopic view of the ECRB after release and débridement.

gripping (such as tennis). Pain is localized to just below the lateral epicondyle. Patients have tenderness over the ECRB insertion, and pain is reproduced with maximum passive wrist flexion, gripping, and resisted long-finger and wrist extension with the elbow fully extended. Grip strength is often decreased compared with the unaffected side. Radiographs are normal but occasionally show calcium deposits in the tendon, especially if prior treatment included cortisone injections. MRI may show increased signal and degeneration at the tendon origin but is not necessary for the diagnosis.

Nonsurgical Treatment

Nonsurgical treatment includes rest, nonsteroidal anti-inflammatory drugs, counterforce bracing, physical therapy, swinging technique or activity modifications, and cortisone injections. Physical therapy is directed at extensor stretching and strengthening. Counterforce bracing is believed to limit muscle fatigue and redistribute force into the muscle belly rather than the tendon origin.

Surgical Treatment

Indications for surgery include pain that interferes with daily activities and work, and failure of legitimate nonsurgical treatment of up to 6 months. There are a few contraindications to surgical intervention, including active infection or severe ankylosis of the elbow. Several surgical procedures have been described, including open ECRB release and removal of the degenerated portion of the tendon, with repair of the remainder of the tendon; and, more recently, arthroscopic release of the ECRB.

When using the arthroscopic method, the proximal medial portal is established first, and the radiocapitellar articulation and adjacent joint capsule are then examined. Pronation and supination of the forearm are performed to fully examine the radial head. The capsule is inspected for abnormalities. The condition of the capsule is classified as type 1 (intact capsule with fraying of the undersurface of the ECRB tendon), type 2 (linear capsular tears), or type 3 (complete capsular rupture).[6] The radiocapitellar joint should be examined for evidence of chondromalacia. Using an outside-in technique, the proximal anterolateral portal is established. A small motorized shaver is introduced into this portal, and the capsule is gently débrided and removed adjacent to the capitellum. The diseased ECRB tendon lies between the capsule and the overlying extensor digitorum communis (**Figure 10**). A radiofrequency probe also can be used to remove the capsule for exposure and release the ECRB from the lateral epicondyle. The release begins proximally and is carried distally. Care is taken to remain above the equator of the radial head anteriorly to prevent iatrogenic injury to the lateral ulnar collateral ligament and potential posterolateral rotatory instability of the elbow. Débridement of the ECRB is complete when all visible pathologic tissue has been removed and healthy overlying extensor digitorum communis and extensor radialis longus musculature can be seen (**Figure 11**).

Iatrogenic lateral ulnar collateral ligament injury results in pain and posterolateral rotatory instability. Other complications include missed concomitant radial nerve entrapment, which may occur in 5% of patients with lateral epicondylitis.[21]

Rehabilitation

Soft dressings are applied in the typical fashion. Sling immobilization is used for several days for comfort, and elbow motion exercises are then started. Wrist extension and flexion with the elbow in extension is avoided until the soft-tissue inflammation has subsided. Gentle stretching and strengthening is then initiated. Return-to-work status in these patients ranges from 1 day to a few months.

Results

Success rates as high as 93% to 100% have been reported for the arthroscopic treatment of lateral epicondylitis.[6,8,11] The average time to return to work was in as few as 11 days in some reports.[6,8,11] In a nonrandomized retrospective study, Szabo[22] reported no differences in arthroscopic (n = 41), open (n = 38), or percutaneous (n = 23) lateral epicondyle releases. Peart et al[12] reported nearly identical results for open versus arthroscopic treatment in a retrospective, comparative study.

Patients returned to work earlier following arthroscopic treatment. Baker and Baker[5] reported on 42 elbows (130-month follow-up) treated arthroscopically. The mean pain score at rest was 0, 1.0 with activities of daily living, and 1.9 with work or sports activities. The mean functional score was 11.7 of a possible 12 points, with 87% of patients reporting satisfaction with the procedure and 93% stating that they would have the surgery again if needed. The authors concluded that arthroscopic removal of pathologic tendinosis tissue is a reliable treatment of recalcitrant lateral epicondylitis.

Complications in Elbow Arthroscopy

Nerve injury is the most concerning complication of elbow arthroscopy and can be caused by direct laceration from the portal incisions, trauma from the cannula trocar, injury during débridement with a shaver, cutting with a basket instrument, or by the nerve becoming wrapped in a burring instrument.[1,10,21,23-27] Most nerve injuries are transient and are related to swelling, compression from retractors, or stretching injuries from increased postoperative motion.[1,17,28] As previously discussed, some portals described in the literature place the neurovascular structures at a higher relative risk for injury than other portals and should be avoided. Other risks include infection, articular cartilage injury, synovial fistula formation, instrument breakage, fluid extravasation, and tourniquet-related complications.

The largest study to date examining complications associated with elbow arthroscopy was a retrospective review of 473 consecutive elbow arthroscopies performed in 449 patients over an 18-year period by Kelly et al.[29] Major complications (joint infection) occurred in 4 of 473 elbows (0.8%); no permanent neurovascular injuries, hematomas, or compartment syndromes were documented. Minor complications occurred in 11% of the arthroscopic procedures. These included prolonged drainage or superficial infection at a portal site, persistent minor contractures of 20° or less, and transient nerve palsies (five ulnar nerve palsies, one posterior interosseous palsy, one medial antebrachial cutaneous palsy, and one anterior interosseous palsy). The authors identified risk factors for the development of transient nerve palsies, which included a diagnosis of rheumatoid arthritis and a flexion contracture of the elbow.

Summary

Elbow arthroscopy has become an accepted treatment option for numerous elbow conditions. Attention to patient positioning, proper instrumentation, and the use of retractors has helped expand the use of arthroscopic treatment. Proper indications and surgical planning remain critical. The surgeon's experience, skill level, and knowledge of local elbow anatomy should determine the complexity of attempted arthroscopic elbow procedures.

References

1. Andrews JR, Carson WG: Arthroscopy of the elbow. *Arthroscopy* 1985;1(2):97-107.
2. Baker CL, Brooks AA: Arthroscopy of the elbow. *Clin Sports Med* 1996;15(2):261-281.
3. Ogilvie-Harris DJ, Schemitsch E: Arthroscopy of the elbow for removal of loose bodies. *Arthroscopy* 1993;9(1):5-8.
4. Poehling GG, Whipple TL, Sisco L, Goldman B: Elbow arthroscopy: A new technique. *Arthroscopy* 1989;5(3):222-224.
5. Baker CL Jr, Baker CL III: Long-term follow-up of arthroscopic treatment of lateral epicondylitis. *Am J Sports Med* 2008;36(2):254-260.
6. Baker CL Jr, Murphy KP, Gottlob CA, Curd DT: Arthroscopic classification and treatment of lateral epicondylitis: Two-year clinical results. *J Shoulder Elbow Surg* 2000;9(6):475-482.
7. Morrey BF: Arthroscopy of the elbow. *Instr Course Lect* 1986;35:102-107.
8. Mullett H, Sprague M, Brown G, Hausman M: Arthroscopic treatment of lateral epicondylitis: Clinical and cadaveric studies. *Clin Orthop Relat Res* 2005;439:123-128.
9. O'Driscoll SW: Elbow arthroscopy for loose bodies. *Orthopedics* 1992;15(7):855-859.
10. O'Driscoll SW, Morrey BF: Arthroscopy of the elbow: Diagnostic and therapeutic benefits and hazards. *J Bone Joint Surg Am* 1992;74(1):84-94.
11. Owens BD, Murphy KP, Kuklo TR: Arthroscopic release for lateral epicondylitis. *Arthroscopy* 2001;17(6):582-587.
12. Peart RE, Strickler SS, Schweitzer KM Jr: Lateral epicondylitis: A comparative study of open and arthroscopic lateral release. *Am J Orthop (Belle Mead NJ)* 2004;33(11):565-567.
13. Savoie FH III, Nunley PD, Field LD: Arthroscopic management of the arthritic elbow: Indications, technique, and results. *J Shoulder Elbow Surg* 1999;8(3):214-219.
14. Stothers K, Day B, Regan WR: Arthroscopy of the elbow: Anatomy, portal sites, and a description of the proximal lateral portal. *Arthroscopy* 1995;11(4):449-457.
15. Lindenfeld TN: Medial approach in elbow arthroscopy. *Am J Sports Med* 1990;18(4):413-417.
16. Field LD, Altchek DW, Warren RF, O'Brien SJ, Skyhar MJ, Wickiewicz TL: Arthroscopic anatomy of the lateral elbow: A comparison of three portals. *Arthroscopy* 1994;10(6):602-607.

17. Lynch GJ, Meyers JF, Whipple TL, Caspari RB: Neurovascular anatomy and elbow arthroscopy: Inherent risks. *Arthroscopy* 1986; 2(3):190-197.

18. Miller CD, Jobe CM, Wright MH: Neuroanatomy in elbow arthroscopy. *J Shoulder Elbow Surg* 1995;4(3):168-174.

19. Kraushaar BS, Nirschl RP: Tendinosis of the elbow (tennis elbow): Clinical features and findings of histological, immunohistochemical, and electron microscopy studies. *J Bone Joint Surg Am* 1999; 81(2):259-278.

20. Nirschl RP, Pettrone FA: Tennis elbow: The surgical treatment of lateral epicondylitis. *J Bone Joint Surg Am* 1979;61(6A):832-839.

21. Thomas MA, Fast A, Shapiro D: Radial nerve damage as a complication of elbow arthroscopy. *Clin Orthop Relat Res* 1987;215: 130-131.

22. Szabo RM: Steroid injection for lateral epicondylitis. *J Hand Surg Am* 2009;34(2):326-330.

23. Dumonski ML, Arciero RA, Mazzocca AD: Ulnar nerve palsy after elbow arthroscopy. *Arthroscopy* 2006;22(5):577.e1-577.e3.

24. Gupta A, Sunil TM: Complete division of the posterior interosseous nerve after elbow arthroscopy: A case report. *J Shoulder Elbow Surg* 2004;13(5):566-567.

25. Haapaniemi T, Berggren M, Adolfsson L: Complete transection of the median and radial nerves during arthroscopic release of post-traumatic elbow contracture. *Arthroscopy* 1999;15(7): 784-787.

26. Hahn M, Grossman JA: Ulnar nerve laceration as a result of elbow arthroscopy. *J Hand Surg Br* 1998;23(1):109.

27. Ruch DS, Poehling GG: Anterior interosseus nerve injury following elbow arthroscopy. *Arthroscopy* 1997;13(6):756-758.

28. Poehling GG, Ekman EF: Arthroscopy of the elbow. *Instr Course Lect* 1995;44:217-223.

29. Kelly EW, Morrey BF, O'Driscoll SW: Complications of elbow arthroscopy. *J Bone Joint Surg Am* 2001;83-A(1):25-34.

Video Reference

15.1: Baker CL: Video. Excerpt: Elbow arthroscopy: Principles, portals and techniques, in Baker CL, ed: *Surgical Techniques in Orthopaedics: Elbow Arthroscopy*. DVD. Rosemont, IL, American Academy of Orthopaedic Surgeons, 2005.

Elbow Arthroscopy: Capitellar Osteochondritis Dissecans and Radiocapitellar Plica

Christopher S. Ahmad, MD
Mark A. Vitale, MD, MPH
Neil S. ElAttrache, MD

Abstract

The combination of excessive radiocapitellar compressive forces and the limited vascularity of the capitellum are responsible for the development of osteochondritis dissecans. Repetitive compressive forces are generated by throwing or racket swinging motions or from constant axial compressive loads on the elbow, which are common in athletes such as gymnasts. Symptoms include activity-associated pain and stiffness. Physical examination findings show tenderness over the radiocapitellar joint and, commonly, loss of extension. Plain radiographs may show flattening and sclerosis of the capitellum, lucencies, and possibly intra-articular loose bodies. MRI can detect bone edema early in the disease process and further delineate the extent of the injury. The management of osteochondritis dissecans lesions is primarily based on the demands of the patient, the size and location of the lesion, and the status and stability of the overlying cartilage. Possible treatments include transarticular drilling; removing detached fragments or loose bodies, followed by drilling; and mosaicplasty.

Radiocapitellar plica can cause chondromalacic changes on the radial head and capitellum, with symptoms including painful clicking and effusions. Arthroscopic plica resection is indicated when nonsurgical treatment fails.

Instr Course Lect 2011;60:181-190.

Dr. Ahmad or an immediate family member has received research or institutional support from Acumed, Arthrex, and Zimmer. Dr. ElAttrache or an immediate family member serves as a board member, owner, officer, or committee member of the American Board of Orthopaedic Surgery and the American Orthopaedic Society for Sports Medicine; has received royalties from Arthrex; is a member of a speakers' bureau or has made paid presentations on behalf of Arthrex; serves as a paid consultant to or is an employee of Acumed and Arthrex; serves as an unpaid consultant to Arthrex; has received research or institutional support from Arthrex; and has received non-income support (such as equipment or services), commercially derived honoraria, or other non–research-related funding (such as paid travel) from Acumed and Arthrex. Neither Dr. Vitale nor any immediate family member has received anything of value from or owns stock in a commercial company or institution related directly or indirectly to the subject of this chapter.

The radiocapitellar compartment of the athlete's elbow is subject to significant stresses during repetitive activities, such as throwing, or upper extremity weight-bearing sports, such as gymnastics.[1] Radiocapitellar compression can lead to Panner disease in preadolescent children or capitellar osteochondritis dissecans (OCD) in adolescents or young adults; it is important to differentiate these two disorders because they have different natural histories and treatments.[2-5] Elbow arthroscopic techniques can be used to treat the OCD lesion with débridement, drilling, and even mosaicplasty and can be used to treat loose bodies that develop secondary to the OCD lesion.

Panner Disease

Panner disease predominantly affects boys younger than 10 years.[6] Patients initially present for treatment with reports of activity-related pain and stiffness in the elbow. Tenderness over the lateral elbow and the capitellum is found on physical examination. Radiographs initially show fissuring, lucencies, fragmentation, and irregularity of the capitellum. Subsequent

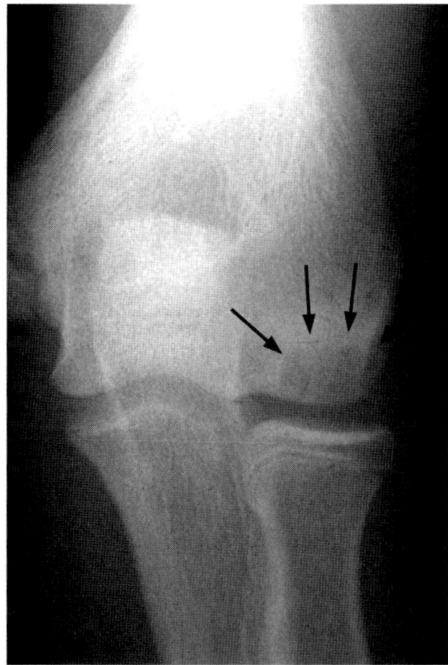

Figure 1 AP radiograph showing an OCD lesion (arrows) in the capitellum of the elbow. (Reproduced with permission from Ahmad CS, ElAttrache NS: Treatment of capitellar osteochondritis dissecans. *Tech Shoulder Elbow Surg* 2006;7: 169-174.)

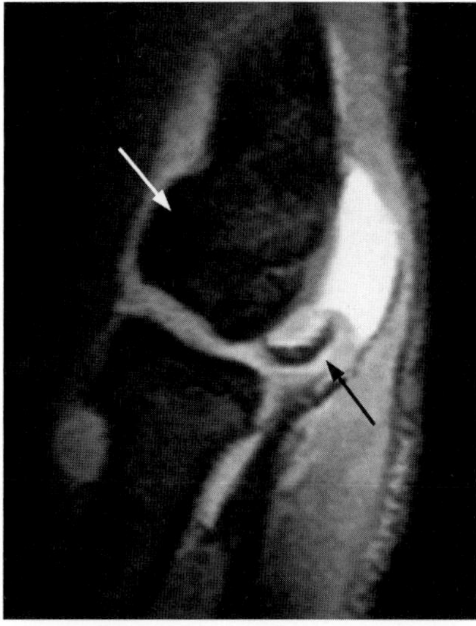

Figure 2 MRI scan showing capitellar OCD lesion (white arrow) with and associated loose body (black arrow). (Adapted with permission from Ahmad CS, ElAttrache NS: Treatment of capitellar osteochondritis dissecans. *Tech Shoulder Elbow Surg* 2006;7:169-174.)

radiographs show larger radiolucent areas followed by reossification, with a corresponding resolution of symptoms. One to 2 years after the initial presentation, the epiphysis regains its normal contour and appearance.[4] MRI scans typically show edema localized to the chondral surface, with less involvement of the subchondral bone in comparison with OCD.

Treatment involves ceasing the activities causing elbow stress, and the use of ice and anti-inflammatory medication. For severe symptoms, the elbow may be immobilized for 3 to 4 weeks. In general, symptoms usually resolve within 6 to 8 weeks, although they occasionally persist for months. Activities are resumed as tolerated. Panner disease has an excellent long-term prognosis, although some patients may experience loss of motion.[4,6]

Osteochondritis Dissecans

OCD of the capitellum is characterized by noninflammatory degeneration of subchondral bone occurring in the context of repetitive loading to the lateral compartment of the elbow. Panner disease and OCD may represent two different stages of the same disorder, but they differ in the patient's age at onset and natural history.[4] Panner disease affects children younger than 10 years, whereas OCD commonly affects older athletes.[7] OCD is not always self-limiting; if untreated it may result in profound destruction of the capitellum.[7]

Etiology

The combination of abnormal radiocapitellar compressive forces and the limited vascularity of the capitellum supplied by end arteries are likely responsible for the development of OCD.[2,5,8,9] Repetitive compressive forces are generated by either large valgus stresses on the elbow during throwing or racket swinging or from constant axial compressive loads on the elbow, such as those experienced by gymnasts.[7,10,11] The capitellum is supplied by two end arteries coursing from posterior to anterior, which are branches of the radial recurrent and interosseous recurrent arteries.[12] Local blood flow to the capitellum may be disrupted by both repetitive microtrauma or a single traumatic event leading to subchondral bone injury.[13,14]

Presentation

Patients with OCD will initially present reporting activity-related pain and stiffness in the elbow. Mechanical symptoms of locking or catching, caused by intra-articular loose bodies, may be present. The physical examination shows tenderness over the radiocapitellar joint. Loss of range of motion with a 15° to 20° flexion contracture is common. The active radiocapitellar compression test suggests an OCD lesion when pain is elicited in the lateral compartment of the elbow and when the patient pronates and supinates the forearm with the arm in extension.

Imaging

Full-extension AP, 45°-flexion AP, and lateral radiographic views of the elbow should be obtained; however, results may be negative early in the disease process (**Figure 1**). As the condition progresses, flattening and sclerosis of the capitellum, typically on its anterolateral aspect, will become apparent. Irregular areas of lucency and intra-articular loose bodies may be seen. It should be noted if the capitellar physis is open or closed. In patients with suspected OCD, an MRI scan of the elbow should always be obtained (**Figure 2**). MRI can detect bone edema early in the disease process.[15] A magnetic resonance arthrogram can further

Table 1
Classification and Treatment of Capitellar Osteochondritis Dissecans Lesions

Stability	Stage	Radiographic Findings	Arthroscopic Findings	Treatment
Stable lesion	I	Normal radiographs T1-weighted MRI: abnormal T2-weighted MRI: normal	Intact articular cartilage Subchondral bone edema but structurally sound	Hinged elbow brace Physical therapy Nonsteroidal anti-inflammatory drugs Follow-up radiograph and/or MRI at 3 to 6 months
Unstable lesion	II	Abnormal radiographs T1- and T2-weighted MRIs: abnormal Contrast shows margin around the lesion	Partially detached fragment Cartilage fracture Subchondral bone collapse Lateral buttress involved; poorer prognosis	Acute: Consider fragment fixation but higher success using treatment for chronic Chronic: (a) < 6 to 7 mm lateral buttress involved/radial head does not engage: fragment removal plus microfracture drilling (b) > 6 to 7 mm lateral buttress involved/head engages: removal plus osteochondral allograft/synthetic graft
	III	Loose bodies	Completely detached loose bodies	Loose body removal Treat as stage II lesion
		Associated radial head deformity	Any of the above	< 30% radial head involvement: treat as stage II lesion > 30% radial head involvement: no osteochondral grafting; microfracture/drilling are OK

(Reproduced with permission from Ahmad CS, ElAttrache NS: Treatment of capitellar osteochondritis dissecans. *Tech Shoulder Elbow Surg* 2006;7: 169-174.)

delineate the extent of the injury because the contrast agent can reveal separation of a detached or partially detached fragment from the subchondral bone.

Management

The management of OCD lesions is based primarily on the demands of the patient and the status and stability of the overlying cartilage. The size and location of the lesion and the status of the capitellar growth plate also influence treatment.[16-18] Several classification systems based on radiographic and arthroscopic findings have been proposed;[16,19,20] however, none has been universally adopted because the systems are cumbersome to use.[21,22] **Table 1** shows a simplified, succinct, three-stage classification system that provides a template for managing capitellar OCD lesions.

Stage I

In stage I lesions, the osteochondral fragment is intact, stable, and nondisplaced. Radiographic findings are often negative. The signal findings on MRI are variable, typically abnormal on T1-weighted MRIs and normal on T2-weighted MRIs, although the T2 signal may also be abnormal. Arthroscopy shows that the articular cartilage is intact, and subchondral stability is generally preserved. Treatment is nonsurgical and includes resting the elbow in a hinged elbow brace for 3 to 6 weeks. Progressive physical therapy should ensue as symptoms abate. Return to sports activities usually can be expected at 3 to 6 months. Follow-up radiographs and MRIs should be obtained at 2- to 3-month intervals to track progress. If symptoms return, an additional rest period is mandated. With persistent refractory symptoms, pitchers may have to change throwing positions, and gymnasts may need to elect a different sport.

Stage II

In stage II OCD of the capitellum, the osteochondral fragment is partially separated as documented both radiographically and arthroscopically. Radiographs will show fissuring, lucencies, and fragmentation. On MRI, both T1- and T2-weighted sequences will show abnormal signals and a margin around the fragment, denoting its instability. CT scans may also show the partially separated fragment. Arthroscopic findings include a broken cartilage surface and unstable and partially displaced subchondral bone. Surgical treatment is needed to return athletes to their sports activity or allow resumption of the activities of daily living as soon as possible.

The size and location of the lesion govern treatment. For smaller lesions, débridement is an option. Patients typically have immediate relief of symptoms; however, early arthritis is associated with the long-term natural history of the disease. Fragment fixation has been advocated by some physicians for stage II lesions, although the healing potential of fixed fragments and the clinical results of the procedure are often unpredictable.[19,20,23,24] Osteochondral autografts or synthetic grafts can be used to treat large defects that engage the radial head and involve the lateral buttress of the capitellum.

This chapter's authors believe that the location of the lesion may be more important than size in guiding treatment. A lesion that extends into the lateral margin of the capitellum, as described by Ruch et al,[25] is associated with a potentially poorer prognosis. The lateral column of the capitellum supports large compressive forces when the elbow is stressed in valgus or with axial loading. Lesions that do not involve a significant portion of the lateral buttress of the capitellum and that do not engage the radial head on arthroscopic examination (pronation and supination with the elbow in extension) have been successfully treated with microfracture or drilling. In this situation, the defect is relatively protected, and healing (predominantly fibrocartilage healing) may occur.

Conversely, lateral column involvement of more than 6 to 7 mm cannot be acceptably treated with microfracture. In this instance, the absence of a lateral buttress allows engagement of the radial head in the defect, which inhibits healing and may lead to accelerated radiocapitellar arthrosis. For these larger, engaging defects or those that extend substantially (more than 6 to 7 mm) into the lateral buttress, this chapter's authors recommend removing the loose fragment and achieving osteochondral restoration by means of mosaicplasty or an osteochondral autograft transfer. If there are partially detached fragments, the detached portion (usually central) should be débrided centrally to laterally. Once stable osteochondral borders have been obtained, the lesion is carefully evaluated arthroscopically to ascertain the extent of the lateral column involvement and determine if the radial head is engaged within the defect. Lesions larger than 1 cm² (mean, 1.32 cm²) with no lateral column involvement were treated successfully with microfracture, whereas those involving the lateral column did well with osteochondral grafting (JD Chappell, MD, and NS ElAttrache, MD, unpublished data presented at the American Orthopaedic Society for Sports Medicine Annual Meeting, Orlando, FL, 2008). Fragment fixation is also an option, but this chapter's authors have had superior and more consistent results with grafting.

Stage III

In stage III capitellar OCD, the fragment is fully displaced and has become a loose body. Patients may present with mechanical symptoms related to loose bodies, such as locking. In this stage of the disease, débridement, drilling, or osteochondral replacement is indicated. If the loose osteochondral fragment is shown to be acutely displaced in a patient with previously documented OCD, fixation to its donor site can be attempted; however, fixation results are inconsistent.[24] Chronic loose bodies (documented by serial radiographs or MRI) should be removed, and the donor bed should be débrided in preparation for one of the previously described treatment options, following the same algorithm.

Radial Head Involvement

Degenerative changes in the radial head, in addition to capitellar pathology, indicate advanced disease and do not generally occur in athletes. If the radial lesion is less than 30% of the size of the radial head, treatment of the capitellar OCD should proceed as previously described. For radial lesions greater than 30% of the size of the radial head, treatment of the capitellar lesion should be limited to débridement, drilling, and microfracture.[6] Severe radiocapitellar degenerative arthritis is a relative contraindication to mosaicplasty.

Surgical Technique

Although alternate surgical patient positioning is possible, the supine position is preferred by the senior author (NSE) because it facilitates general anesthesia, provides an easy conversion to an open procedure if needed, and orients the elbow in an anatomically familiar way. Standard arthroscopic portals are created beginning with the diagnostic arthroscopic procedure in the anterior compartment. The anterior capitellum is inspected and is most often normal, with the pathology residing out of view on the more posterior aspect. In throwing athletes, a valgus stress test with the elbow flexed to 70° can be performed while visualizing the medial ulnohumeral joint. A 1- to 2-mm opening indicates pathologic laxity of the medial collateral ligament, although clinical correlation is mandatory. Diagnostic arthroscopy then proceeds in the posterior compartment, with standard portals to assess for loose bodies and other pathology. Detached OCD fragments are often located in the olecranon fossa.

To visualize the posterior capitellum, a midlateral portal (lateral soft spot) is created in line with the lateral epicondylar ridge and entered with the arthroscope (**Figure 3**). This area often is better suited to a small 2.7-mm arthroscope. The radial head, the capitellum, the trochlear notch, and the trochlear ridge are best seen through this portal. Care should be taken to avoid injury to the posterior antebrachial cutaneous nerve located near this portal. A working portal is created adjacent and slightly ulnar to the midlateral portal. A cadaver study showed that carefully placed, dual, direct lateral portals do not damage lateral ligaments and provide excellent exposure to the capitellum.[26] A thickened radiocapitellar plica is occasionally found in patients with OCD and lateral compartment symptoms; if found, the plica should be resected.

The OCD lesion is then visualized and graded. Grade II and III lesions are treated by removing any loose fragments, shaving loose fragments of cartilage down to subchondral bone, and establishing healthy cartilage borders (**Figure 4**). The size of the lesions is determined using a calibrated probe. The ability of the capitellum to buttress the radial head is determined. At this point, specific procedures are performed as indicated.

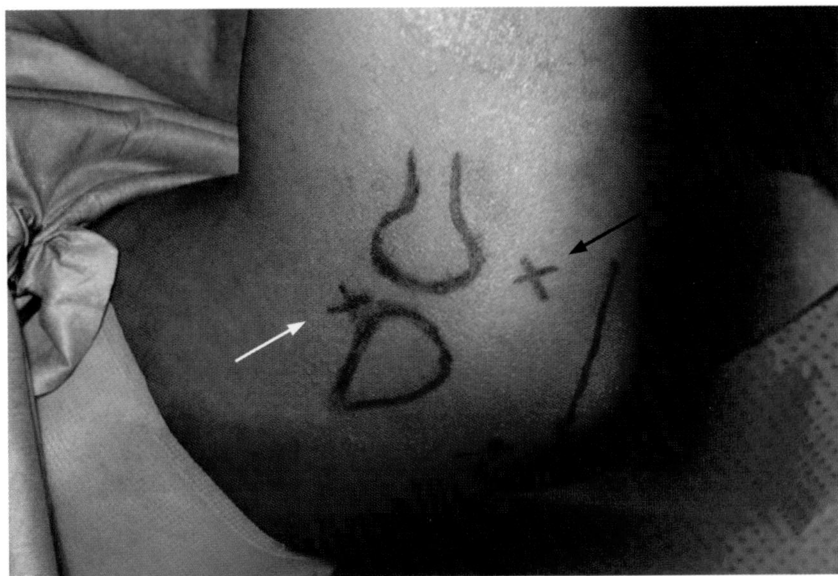

Figure 3 Anterolateral (white arrow) and midlateral (black arrow) portals (soft-spot portals) are outlined. (Reproduced with permission from Ahmad CS, ElAttrache NS: Treatment of capitellar osteochondritis dissecans. *Tech Shoulder Elbow Surg* 2006;7:169-174.)

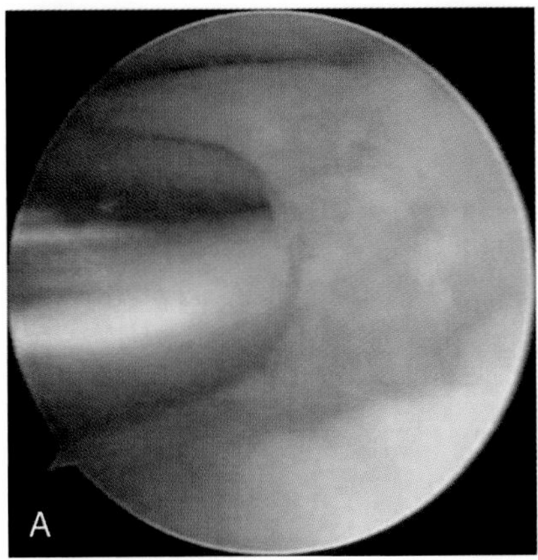

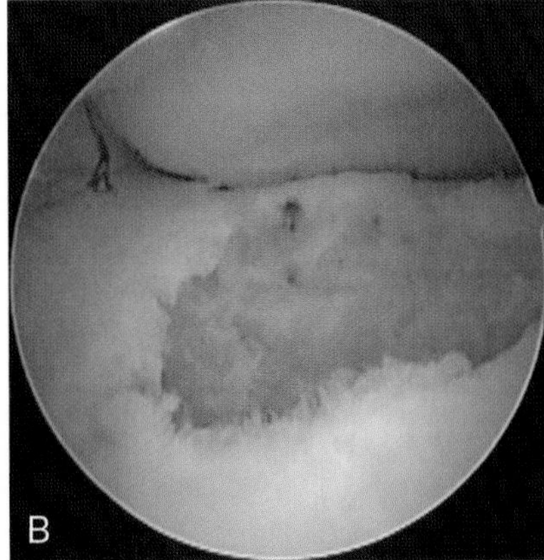

Figure 4 A shaver is used to débride an OCD lesion (**A**) to stable borders (**B**). (Reproduced with permission from Ahmad CS, ElAttrache NS: Treatment of capitellar osteochondritis dissecans. *Tech Shoulder Elbow Surg* 2006;7:169-174.)

Microfracture and Subchondral Drilling

Stage I lesions with cartilage fibrillation and fissuring are treated with transarticular drilling with a small 0.045-inch Kirschner wire. For stage II and III lesions, detached fragments or loose bodies are removed. With the arthroscope in the direct lateral portal, a 0.045-inch or 0.062-inch Kirschner wire is inserted through the accessory lateral portal and used to create vascular channels in the lesion separated by 2 mm (**Figure 5**). Multiple holes are made in the lesion, and efflux of marrow elements is observed to induce a fibrocartilage healing response. Excellent results at 3-year follow-up were obtained in 11 patients treated with this technique; all returned to their previous activity level (JD Chappell, MD, and NS ElAttrache, MD, unpublished data presented at the American Orthopaedic Society for Sports Medicine Annual Meeting, Orlando, FL, 2008). The size of the OCD lesions ranged from 7 × 6 mm to 17 × 15 mm.

Mosaicplasty

In mosaicplasty, small-size osteochondral grafts are obtained arthroscopically from the knee at the lateral periphery or the trochlear edge of the femoral condyles and transplanted into prepared osteochondral defects on the capitellum.[27] Mosaicplasty is indicated when a large capitellar lesion engages the radial head, as observed while rotating the extended arm during arthroscopy, or when there is significant (more than 6 to 7 mm) lateral column involvement. Radial head degeneration and severe deformities of

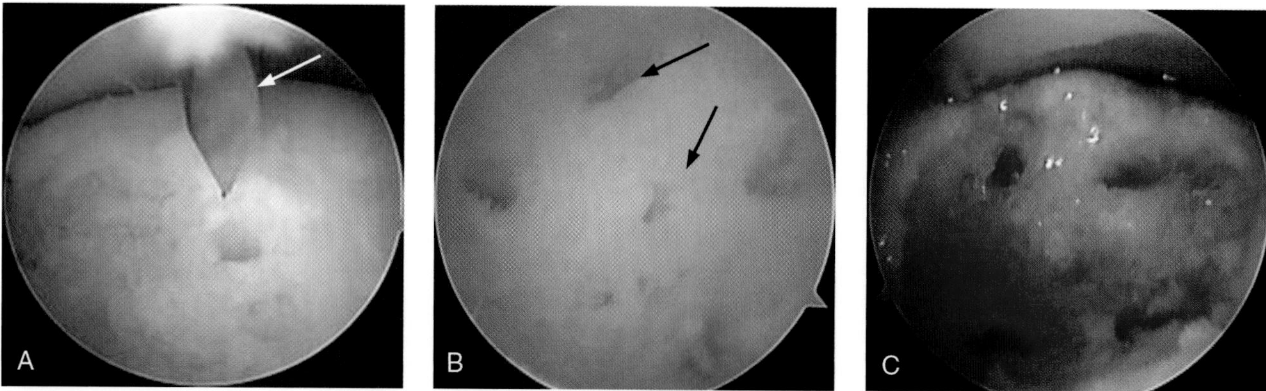

Figure 5 Microfracture technique. **A,** A 0.062-inch Kirschner wire (arrow) is inserted through the accessory midlateral portal and used to perforate the lesion. **B,** Holes (arrows) in the lesion allow marrow elements to produce a fibrocartilage healing response. **C,** The bleeding response from the drilling visualized after the tourniquet is deflated. (Reproduced with permission from Ahmad CS, ElAttrache NS: Treatment of capitellar osteochondritis dissecans. *Tech Shoulder Elbow Surg* 2006;7:169-174.)

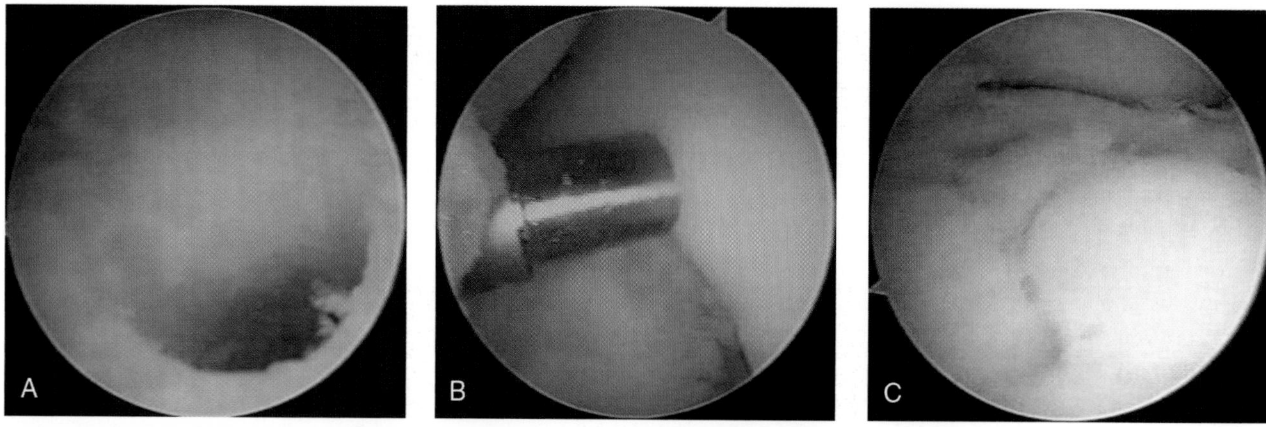

Figure 6 Osteochondral plug reconstruction of a capitellar OCD lesion. **A,** The OCD recipient site is created. **B,** The donor osteochondral graft is harvested from the lateral intercondylar notch. **C,** Final appearance of the capitellum after two osteochondral plugs are placed. (Reproduced with permission from Ahmad CS, ElAttrache NS: Treatment of capitellar osteochondritis dissecans. *Tech Shoulder Elbow Surg* 2006;7:169-174.)

the capitellum are relative contraindications to mosaicplasty.

A midlateral working portal is used to débride the lesion to stable cartilage borders in preparation for drilling. In lesions with a partially detached fragment, the detached region is often located centrally. In this situation, the senior author (NSE) recommends débriding the partially detached portion, beginning centrally and proceeding laterally toward the lateral column. Débridement proceeds until an area of bony integrity, consisting of an osseous connection between the fragment and the subchondral bone, is encountered (if present). The extent of the posterolateral column involvement is then determined, and an arthroscopic evaluation (consisting of supination and pronation of the extended forearm) of radial head engagement in the defect is performed. If more than 6 to 7 mm of the lateral column is involved or the radial head is engaged in the defect, osteochondral grafting proceeds. The goal is to restore a bony buttress to prevent radial head subluxation into the defect; it is not necessary to replace every millimeter of the lesion.

Elbow flexion is increased to 90° to 100°, and a spinal needle is introduced through the anconeus to gauge the feasibility of a perfectly perpendicular approach to the lesion. An incision is created to provide access for a 4- to 6-mm diameter plug. The recipient site is drilled perpendicular to the chondral surface using commercially available osteochondral autograft transfer instrumentation (**Figure 6, A**). The donor osteochondral plug is then arthroscopically harvested from the intercondylar notch (**Figure 6, B**). The arthroscope is placed into an anterolateral portal. Using an anteromedial portal, a donor plug of an appropriate size is then harvested with 1 cm of depth from the medial edge of the lateral femoral condyle toward the notch. The donor plug is introduced into the recipient site and impacted flush with the surrounding cartilage (**Figure 6, C**). The goal is to reconstitute the lateral buttress so that the radial head does not engage into the defect. The process of osteochondral grafting is repeated until lateral column integrity is adequately restored. If some corners of the lesion cannot be fully replaced, they are treated with drilling. If the surgeon does not choose to use autograft, allograft or synthetic scaffolding can be used.

Iwasaki et al[27] reported good or excellent results in seven of eight teenage baseball players with OCD who were treated with osteochondral autograft transplants. Yamamoto et al[28] reported that six of nine adolescents with grade III OCD lesion and eight of nine with grade IV lesions returned to competitive baseball after an osteochondral autograft transplantation procedure. Five baseball players with OCD were treated using an osteochondral autograft transplantation procedure (JD Chappell, MD, and NS ElAttrache, MD, unpublished data presented at the American Orthopaedic Society for Sports Medicine Annual Meeting, Orlando, FL, 2008). All five patients returned to competitive baseball and were still playing 5 years postoperatively. Osteochondral autograft transplantation is particularly recommended when more than 6 to 7 mm of the lateral column is involved, and radial head engagement with the lesion is seen during supination-pronation and flexion-extension of the forearm during a careful arthroscopic examination.

Fragment Fixation

Fragment fixation has been used to treat unstable, partially detached OCD lesions.[23] Kuwahata and Inoue[24] described using cancellous bone grafts and a Herbert screw with an open technique in seven patients. At 32-month follow-up, all patients were free of pain and returned to their sport activities. Takahara et al[19,20] used bone pegs harvested from the lateral olecranon to fix partially detached lesions using an open approach. Newer bioabsorbable implants may facilitate fragment fixation with an arthroscopic approach. Although encouraging results have been reported, the bone quality on the fragment often has limited healing potential. This chapter's authors therefore recommend excision and drilling or grafting for partially detached lesions.

Postoperative Management

Postoperatively, the elbow should be protected for 2 to 3 weeks with a hinged brace. Passive and active assisted motion is performed to avoid postoperative stiffness. Gentle resistance exercises are initiated at 3 months, progressing to greater resistance at 4 months. For throwing athletes, a throwing program is started at 5 months. Return to full participation in sports is usually achieved at 6 months after surgery. Athletes who are treated with simple débridement and drilling or microfracture can usually return to sport activities 1 to 2 months sooner than those treated with open procedures and grafting, depending on the progress of rehabilitation.

Prognosis

Takahara et al[19,20] retrospectively reviewed 106 patients with capitellar OCD with an average follow-up of 7 years. The authors found stable lesions healed completely with nonsurgical treatment when three common characteristics were present: an open capitellar growth plate, localized flattening or radiolucency of the subchondral bone, and good elbow motion. The prognosis for OCD of the capitellum is better for patients with stage I disease compared to those with stage II or III OCD. Early stage OCD responds better to nonsurgical treatment than advanced stages, so identifying the disease promptly can have a significant impact on a patient's prognosis. Matsuura et al[29] reported that 91% of early-stage OCD but only 53% of advanced-stage OCD improved after nonsurgical treatment.

Unfortunately, most capitellar OCD lesions are diagnosed at stage II. Although surgery will usually alleviate symptoms and allow a return to sports, these patients have a less favorable long-term outcome. Longitudinal studies have documented that osteoarthritis will develop in 50% of patients with radiocapitellar OCD.[30] Newer techniques, including osteochondral grafting (mosaicplasty) may change the long-term degenerative process.

Fragment stability also affects the final outcome. If the fragment is stable, Mitsunaga et al[31] reported that less than 50% of those lesions will become unstable in the long term. However, Takahara et al[19] showed that fragments that become unstable have a low rate of healing. Patient age has not been correlated with the likelihood of healing in some studies.[25,32] Mihara et al[18] noted a significant correlation between open capitellar growth plates and healing, reporting that 94% of patients with early-stage OCD with open growth plates healed, whereas only 71% with closed growth plates healed.

Return to Sport Activities

Return to sport activities following treatment of capitellar OCD has varied. Historically, gymnasts have inferior outcomes compared with throwing athletes, perhaps because of the signifi-

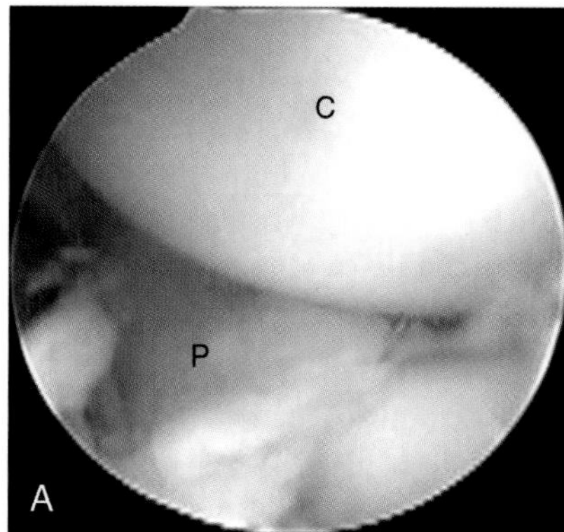

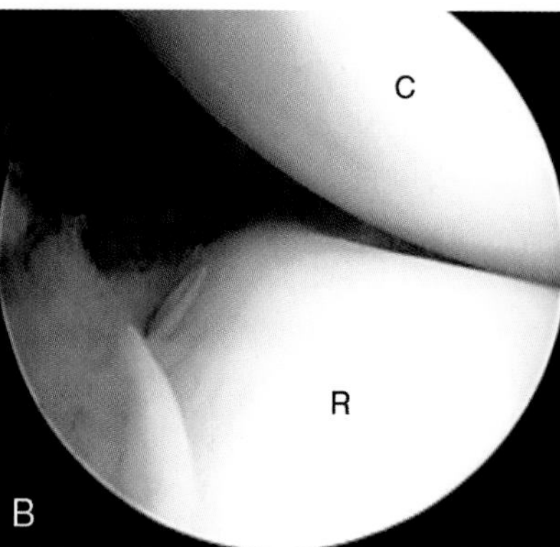

Figure 7 Arthroscopic image of the radiocapitellar plica. **A,** Radiocapitellar plica (P) adjacent to the capitellum (C). **B,** After plica excision of radial head (R) and capitellum (C), the articulation is unobstructed.

cantly increased axial elbow loads. In a study by Jackson et al,[3] 10 female gymnasts were treated with removal of loose bodies and drilling after failed nonsurgical treatment for capitellar OCD; only 1 patient returned to gymnastics. More recently, Bojanić et al[33] reported that all three female gymnasts in their study successfully returned to their previous sports level after loose body removal and microfracture. Byrd et al[34] reported that 4 of 10 adolescent baseball players returned to competitive baseball after arthroscopic débridement, whereas Yamamoto et al[28] reported return to sports in 14 of 18 juvenile baseball players after osteochondral autograft transplantation. One hundred percent (8 of 8) of male baseball players returned to their previous level of sport activities at an average 3-year follow-up after either microfracture or osteochondral autograft transplantation (JD Chappell, MD, and NS ElAttrache, MD, unpublished data presented at the American Orthopaedic Society for Sports Medicine Annual Meeting, Orlando, FL, 2008).

Radiocapitellar Plica

Posterolateral elbow impingement can be caused by a thickened radiocapitellar plica and can occur in combination with capitellar OCD.[35-37] The plica can cause chondromalacic changes on the radial head and capitellum.[35] Symptoms include painful clicking or catching and effusions. If there is snapping, it often occurs with elbow flexion greater than 90° with the forearm in pronation.[35,37] If identified during arthroscopic evaluation, the plica should be resected. Kim et al[36] reported excellent results in throwing athletes and golfers after plica débridement.

A camera is introduced in the proximal anteromedial portal, and a proximal anterolateral working portal is established. Synovitis surrounding the radial neck and the anterior capsule is débrided. The lateral plica is visualized as a fibrous band folding over the radial head. During elbow flexion and extension, the plica will snap back over the radial neck and head. An area of chondromalacia is often present on the anterolateral radial head. A combination of basket resection instruments and shavers are used to resect the plica back to the normal annular ligament (**Figure** 7). The scope is then placed in the posterolateral portal and/or direct midlateral portal, and the plica excision is continued from the midlateral portal (if viewing from the posterolateral portal) or from an accessory midlateral portal (if viewing from the midlateral portal).

Summary

Young male throwing athletes and female gymnasts are at highest risks for the development of capitellar OCD, which must be distinguished from Panner disease. Advanced OCD lesions require surgical treatment. The size and location of the lesion as well as its functional relationship to the radial head should help guide surgical treatment decisions. Factors that influence results include open growth plates, the size and stability of the lesion, and good elbow motion at the initial patient presentation.

References

1. Brown R, Blazina ME, Kerlan RK, Carter VS, Jobe FW, Carlson GJ: Osteochondritis of the capitellum. *J Sports Med* 1974; 2(1): 27-46.
2. Douglas G, Rang M: The role of trauma in the pathogenesis of the osteochondroses. *Clin Orthop Relat Res* 1981;158:28-32.
3. Jackson DW, Silvino N, Reiman P: Osteochondritis in the female gymnast's elbow. *Arthroscopy* 1989;5(2):129-136.
4. Ruch DS, Poehling GG: Arthroscopic treatment of Panner's disease. *Clin Sports Med* 1991; 10(3):629-636.
5. Singer KM, Roy SP: Osteochondrosis of the humeral capitellum. *Am J Sports Med* 1984;12(5): 351-360.
6. Kobayashi K, Burton KJ, Rodner C, Smith B, Caputo AE: Lateral compression injuries in the pediatric elbow: Panner's disease and osteochondritis dissecans of the capitellum. *J Am Acad Orthop Surg* 2004;12(4):246-254.
7. Voloshin I, Schena A: Elbow injuries, in Schepsis AA, Busconi BD, eds: *Sports Medicine*. Philadelphia, PA, Lippincott Williams & Wilkins, 2006.

8. Duthie RB, Houghton GR: Constitutional aspects of the osteochondroses. *Clin Orthop Relat Res* 1981;158:19-27.

9. Yamaguchi K, Sweet FA, Bindra R, Morrey BF, Gelberman RH: The extraosseous and intraosseous arterial anatomy of the adult elbow. *J Bone Joint Surg Am* 1997;79(11):1653-1662.

10. Lord J, Winell JJ: Overuse injuries in pediatric athletes. *Curr Opin Pediatr* 2004;16(1):47-50.

11. Lyman S, Fleisig GS, Waterbor JW, et al: Longitudinal study of elbow and shoulder pain in youth baseball pitchers. *Med Sci Sports Exerc* 2001;33(11): 1803-1810.

12. Haraldsson S: On osteochondrosis deformas juvenilis capituli humeri including investigation of intraosseous vasculature in distal humerus. *Acta Orthop Scand Suppl* 1959;38:1-232.

13. Krappel FA, Bauer E, Harland U: Are bone bruises a possible cause of osteochondritis dissecans of the capitellum? A case report and review of the literature. *Arch Orthop Trauma Surg* 2005;125(8): 545-549.

14. Yang Z, Wang Y, Gilula LA, Yamaguchi K: Microcirculation of the distal humeral epiphyseal cartilage: Implications for posttraumatic growth deformities. *J Hand Surg Am* 1998;23(1): 165-172.

15. Griffith JF, Roebuck DJ, Cheng JC, et al: Acute elbow trauma in children: Spectrum of injury revealed by MR imaging not apparent on radiographs. *AJR Am J Roentgenol* 2001;176(1): 53-60.

16. Baumgarten TE, Andrews JR, Satterwhite YE: The arthroscopic classification and treatment of osteochondritis dissecans of the capitellum. *Am J Sports Med* 1998;26(4):520-523.

17. DiFelice GS, Meunier M, Paletta GJ: Elbow injury in the adolescent athlete, in Altchek DW Andrews JR, eds: *The Athlete's Elbow*. Philadelphia, PA, Lippincott Williams & Wilkins, 2001, pp 231-248.

18. Mihara K, Tsutsui H, Nishinaka N, Yamaguchi K: Nonoperative treatment for osteochondritis dissecans of the capitellum. *Am J Sports Med* 2009;37(2):298-304.

19. Takahara M, Mura N, Sasaki J, Harada M, Ogino T: Classification, treatment, and outcome of osteochondritis dissecans of the humeral capitellum. *J Bone Joint Surg Am* 2007;89(6):1205-1214.

20. Takahara M, Mura N, Sasaki J, Harada M, Ogino T: Classification, treatment, and outcome of osteochondritis dissecans of the humeral capitellum: Surgical technique. *J Bone Joint Surg Am* 2008; 90(Suppl 2, Pt 1):47-62.

21. Petrie RB: Osteochondritis dissecans of the humeral capitellum, in DeLee J, Drez D, Miller D, eds: *Orthopaedic Sports Medicine: Principles and Practice*. Philadelphia, PA, Elsevier Health Science, 2003.

22. Bradley JP, Petrie RS: Osteochondritis dissecans of the humeral capitellum: Diagnosis and treatment. *Clin Sports Med* 2001; 20(3):565-590.

23. Larsen MW, Pietrzak WS, DeLee JC: Fixation of osteochondritis dissecans lesions using poly(l-lactic acid)/poly(glycolic acid) copolymer bioabsorbable screws. *Am J Sports Med* 2005;33(1): 68-76.

24. Kuwahata Y, Inoue G: Osteochondritis dissecans of the elbow managed by Herbert screw fixation. *Orthopedics* 1998;21(4): 449-451.

25. Ruch DS, Cory JW, Poehling GG: The arthroscopic management of osteochondritis dissecans of the adolescent elbow. *Arthroscopy* 1998;14(8):797-803.

26. Davis JT, Idjadi JA, Siskosky MJ, ElAttrache NS: Dual direct lateral portals for treatment of osteochondritis dissecans of the capitellum: An anatomic study. *Arthroscopy* 2007;23(7):723-728.

27. Iwasaki N, Kato H, Ishikawa JS, Saitoh S, Minami A: Autologous osteochondral mosaicplasty for capitellar osteochondritis dissecans in teenaged patients. *Am J Sports Med* 2006;34(8):1233-1239.

28. Yamamoto Y, Ishibashi Y, Tsuda E, Sato H, Toh S: Osteochondral autograft transplantation for osteochondritis dissecans of the elbow in juvenile baseball players: Minimum 2-year follow-up. *Am J Sports Med* 2006;34(5): 714-720.

29. Matsuura T, Kashiwaguchi S, Iwase T, Takeda Y, Yasui N: Conservative treatment for osteochondrosis of the humeral capitellum. *Am J Sports Med* 2008;36(5): 868-872.

30. Bauer M, Jonsson K, Josefsson PO, Lindén B: Osteochondritis dissecans of the elbow: A long-term follow-up study. *Clin Orthop Relat Res* 1992;284:156-160.

31. Mitsunaga MM, Adishian DA, Bianco AJ Jr: Osteochondritis dissecans of the capitellum. *J Trauma* 1982;22(1):53-55.

32. Takahara M, Ogino T, Sasaki I, Kato H, Minami A, Kaneda K: Long term outcome of osteochondritis dissecans of the humeral capitellum. *Clin Orthop Relat Res* 1999;363:108-115.

33. Bojanić I, Ivković A, Borić I: Arthroscopy and microfracture technique in the treatment of osteochondritis dissecans of the humeral capitellum: Report of three adolescent gymnasts. *Knee Surg Sports Traumatol Arthrosc* 2006; 14(5):491-496.

34. Byrd JW, Jones KS: Arthroscopic surgery for isolated capitellar osteochondritis dissecans in adolescent baseball players: Minimum three-year follow-up. *Am J Sports Med* 2002;30(4):474-478.

35. Antuna SA, O'Driscoll SW: Snapping plicae associated with radiocapitellar chondromalacia. *Arthroscopy* 2001;17(5): 491-495.

36. Kim DH, Gambardella RA, El-Attrache NS, Yocum LA, Jobe FW: Arthroscopic treatment of posterolateral elbow impingement from lateral synovial plicae in throwing athletes and golfers. *Am J Sports Med* 2006;34(3):438-444.

37. Steinert AF, Goebel S, Rucker A, Barthel T: Snapping elbow caused by hypertrophic synovial plica in the radiohumeral joint: A report of three cases and review of literature. *Arch Orthop Trauma Surg* 2010;130(3):347-351.

Elbow Arthroscopy: Valgus Extension Overload

Christopher S. Ahmad, MD
John E. Conway, MD

Abstract

Valgus torque combined with deceleration produces high compression and shear forces acting on the posteromedial olecranon and the posteromedial trochlea. This valgus extension overload process may cause posteromedial trochlea chondromalacia, chondral flap formation, osteochondrosis, subchondral erosion, a subchondral insufficiency fracture, and marginal exostosis formation. Olecranon pathologies include proximal stress reaction, a posteromedial tip stress fracture, a transverse proximal process stress fracture, exostosis formation, exostosis fragmentation, and intra-articular loose bodies. Symptoms include posteromedial elbow pain during the deceleration phase of the throwing motion. The extension impingement test reproduces posterior or posteromedial pain similar to that experienced while throwing. Special radiographic techniques and CT scans can show loose bodies and osteophyte fragmentation. Surgical treatment is indicated when symptoms persist despite nonsurgical management. Based on clinical and basic science research, all patients with valgus extension overload should be comprehensively evaluated for medial ulnar collateral ligament insufficiency. Surgical treatment is limited to the resection of osteophytes only; normal olecranon should not be resected.

Instr Course Lect 2011;60:191-197.

In 1959, Bennett[1] described traumatic injury to the tip of the olecranon and the adjacent surface of the condyles of the humerus that resulted from throwing a baseball. He believed the injury caused "exfoliation of cartilage producing loose bodies, synovial thickening, and/or partially detached cartilaginous masses, which obstruct extension of the elbow."[1] This was the first published account that attempted to describe the pathologic process now commonly called valgus extension overload. In 1968, Slocum[2] classified the conditions seen in the thrower's elbow into three groups: medial tension, lateral compression, and extension injuries. He speculated that the extension injuries were caused by the "interplay of torsional, traction, and extension forces" that occur during the follow-through phase of throwing. Slocum later reclassified these three groups as overload conditions, including medial tension, lateral compression, and valgus extension.[2] In 1983, Wilson et al[3] evaluated five baseball pitchers with valgus extension overload and postulated the mechanism as a "wedging effect of the olecranon in the olecranon fossa," occurring during the acceleration phase of throwing.

Etiology

Biomechanical and clinical data currently suggest that the forces leading to the destructive process of valgus extension overload occur during the late acceleration and early follow-through phases of the throwing motion. During the acceleration phase, high tensile loads occur across the medial elbow as a result of valgus torque; the elbow angular velocity may ultimately reach 5,000°/s. The medial ulnar collateral ligament (MUCL) resists more than 50% of this force on the elbow, and dynamic forces and bony geometry resist the remainder. As the throwing motion approaches ball release, the elbow begins to decelerate. During early follow-through, the elbow reaches a deceleration rate measured at more than 500,000°/s^2. Valgus torque combined with deceleration produces high compression and shear forces that act

Dr. Ahmad or an immediate family member has received research or institutional support from Acumed, Arthrex, and Zimmer. Neither Dr. Conway nor any immediate family member has received anything of value from or owns stock in a commercial company or institution related directly or indirectly to the subject of this chapter.

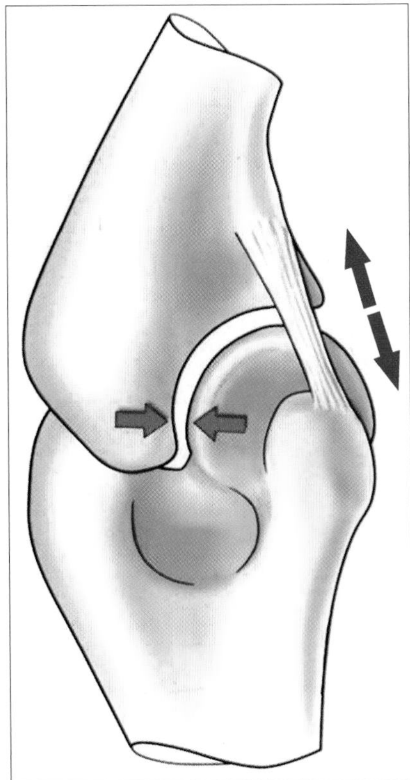

Figure 1 Valgus extension overload results from valgus torque resisted by the MUCL (blue arrows) and shear forces developed in the posteromedial ulnohumeral joint (red arrows).

Table 1
Posteromedial Impingement Describes a Group of Conditions Caused by Valgus Extension Overload

Olecranon	Trochlea
Proximal stress reaction	Chondromalacia
Posterior medial tip stress fracture	Chondral flaps
Transverse proximal process stress fracture	Osteochondral lesions
Marginal osteophytes	Subchondral erosion
Marginal fragmentation	Subchondral insufficiency fracture
Loose bodies	Marginal exostosis

on the posteromedial olecranon and the posteromedial trochlea (**Figure 1**). Chondrocyte damage may occur and disrupt the articular cartilage matrix. Although adjacent viable chondrocytes may proliferate to synthesize new matrix, the injury response is ineffective. Pathologic consequences to the shear and compression forces also induce osteogenesis that results in the formation of osteophytes, which are localized to the posteromedial tip of the olecranon. This valgus extension overload process results in a constellation of findings collectively known as posterior impingement.

There are three types of posterior impingement: posteromedial, posterior, and posterolateral. Although each type has been reported in overhead athletes, posteromedial impingement is directly caused by valgus extension overload and most commonly occurs in throwers. Posteromedial impingement includes the following conditions involving the posteromedial trochlea: chondromalacia, chondral flap formation, osteochondrosis, subchondral erosion, a subchondral insufficiency fracture, and marginal exostosis formation. Conditions involving the olecranon include proximal stress reaction, a posteromedial tip stress fracture, a transverse proximal process stress fracture, exostosis formation, exostosis fragmentation, and intra-articular loose bodies (**Table 1**).

Andrews and Timmerman[4] reported that posterior impingement was the most common diagnosis (78%) requiring surgical treatment in a large group of baseball players. Reedy et al[5] later reported that this condition was the most common diagnosis requiring arthroscopy in a group of athletes participating in a variety of sports. It is important to recognize that valgus extension overload may produce osseous changes suggesting posterior impingement but without clinical symptoms. It has been postulated that symptoms and the loss of performance most commonly develop with exostosis fragmentation, loose body formation, and trochlea chondral injury.[6]

The relationship between posteromedial impingement and valgus stability has been the focus of several clinical and biomechanical studies.[7-9] In an unpublished report of radiographic data from 135 asymptomatic professional pitchers, 32 of the 135 pitchers (24%) had a measurable olecranon tip exostosis formation seen on lateral radiographic views, and 21% had more than 1.0 mm of increased relative valgus laxity on stress radiographs. For those pitchers with exostosis formation, 34% had relative valgus laxity measured at 1.0 mm or more; for those pitchers without exostosis formation, only 16% had relative valgus laxity measured at 1.0 mm or more (J Conway, MD, Las Vegas, NV, unpublished data presented at the American Academy of Orthopaedic Surgeons annual meeting, 2009). If exostosis formation is the result of valgus extension overload, then these unpublished data suggest a possible relationship between posteromedial impingement and valgus laxity; however, many other related factors must be considered, and a clearly accepted relationship has not been established.

Using a cadaver model, Ahmad et al[9] showed that increased MUCL laxity altered contact forces medially between the trochlea and the olecranon. If valgus instability is defined as elbow disability caused by increased valgus laxity, and if posteromedial impingement is assumed to be caused by altered contact forces between the trochlea and the olecranon, then these data suggest that patients with symptomatic valgus extension overload and posteromedial impingement may have underlying valgus instability, even though MUCL pain may not be the presenting symptom. Other studies have suggested that extensive removal of the posteromedial olecranon, as described in the past to treat posteromedial impingement, increases both valgus laxity[8] and MUCL strain, potentially leading to future MUCL compromise.[7]

History

Patients with valgus extension overload have a history of throwing or other repetitive overhead activities. Events preceding the elbow pain may indicate a change in activity level, such as the type or number of pitches thrown. Players often report a decrease in pitching velocity and control, along with difficulty warming up or early fatigue. A history of locking or catching suggests loose bodies or chondral injury. For isolated posteromedial impingement, elbow pain is localized to the posteromedial aspect of the olecranon and usually occurs just after ball release during the deceleration phase of throwing as the elbow approaches full extension. Posterior osteophytes may limit full elbow extension. Sometimes patients have a history of a previous MUCL injury. Pain during the acceleration phase of throwing may indicate a MUCL injury and the presence of posterior osteophytes.

Ulnar neuritis may also occur concomitantly and manifests as pain, local tenderness, and, sometimes, numbness or paresthesias in the fourth and fifth digits when throwing. The ulnar nerve is a critical source of pathology and of potential arthroscopic complications. Stability of the ulnar nerve within the cubital tunnel is important for safe placement of the medial portal during arthroscopy.

Physical Examination

An examination of the elbow begins with an assessment of its carrying angle. An increased carrying angle may indicate adaptation to repetitive valgus stress; angles greater than 15° have been observed in professional pitchers.[10,11] It is important to document the overall range of motion as well as the nature of the end points of extension and flexion. Normal extension terminates in the firm sensation of the posterior bony articulation making contact in the olecranon fossa. Loss of extension is present in up to 50% of professional pitchers.[11] Local tenderness over the posteromedial olecranon is often elicited. The extension impingement test is performed by the examiner, forcing the relaxed patient's flexed elbow into terminal extension. Reproduction of posterior or posteromedial pain similar to the pain felt while throwing is considered a positive test. Simultaneous valgus loading during the maneuver often increases the pain, whereas varus loading diminishes the pain.

In all throwers presenting with medial elbow pain, the MUCL should be evaluated using direct palpation and the moving valgus stress test.[12] The patient's shoulder is placed in 90° of abduction and external rotation, and the forearm is held in the neutral position. The examiner grasps the affected distal forearm and humerus to create a valgus stress across the elbow while the elbow undergoes passive motion from 70° to 120° of flexion. A positive examination reproduces pain, instability, or apprehension during this maneuver. The moving valgus stress test is highly sensitive and specific if the pain produced is medial and localized clearly to the MUCL. Posteromedial, posterior, and posterolateral pain suggests other pathologies. A careful examination of the flexor-pronator muscle mass also should be performed. A patient with injury to the flexor-pronator muscle mass will have pain that is worsened with wrist flexion and/or forearm pronation against resistance and usually has tenderness over the medial epicondyle.

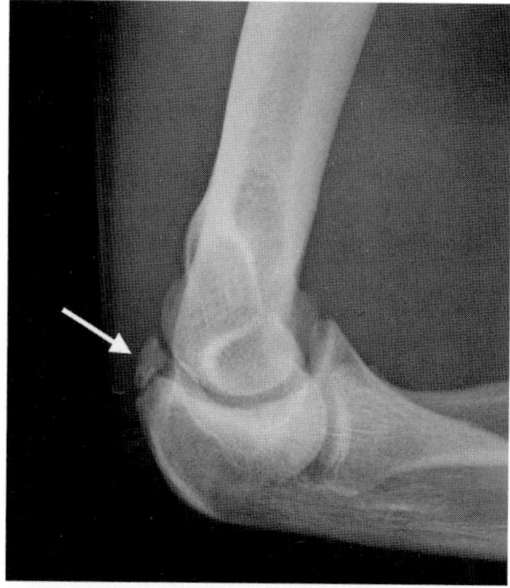

Figure 2 Lateral radiograph shows a fractured osteophyte (arrow) on the olecranon tip.

Imaging Studies

AP, lateral, oblique, and axillary radiographic views of the elbow may reveal posteromedial olecranon osteophytes and/or loose bodies (**Figure 2**). Several views have been described to better visualize the posterior compartment. The cubital tunnel view is an AP view of the elbow with 130° of flexion, the humerus in 15° of external rotation, and the beam directed at 0°. The Andrews-Wilson view is an AP view of the elbow with 110° of flexion, the humerus in 0° of external rotation, and the beam directed 25° proximal. A modified AP radiographic view of the humerus with 140° of elbow flexion and the humerus in 40° of external rotation has been developed to better visualize osteophytes on the posteromedial olecranon in patients with pos-

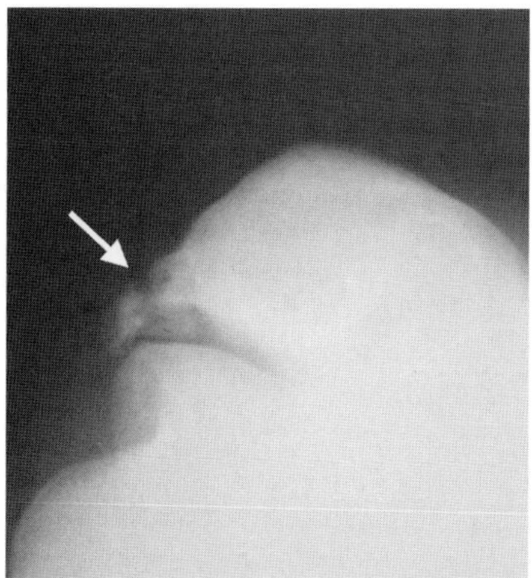

Figure 3 Axial radiographic view shows posteromedial olecranon osteophytes (arrow).

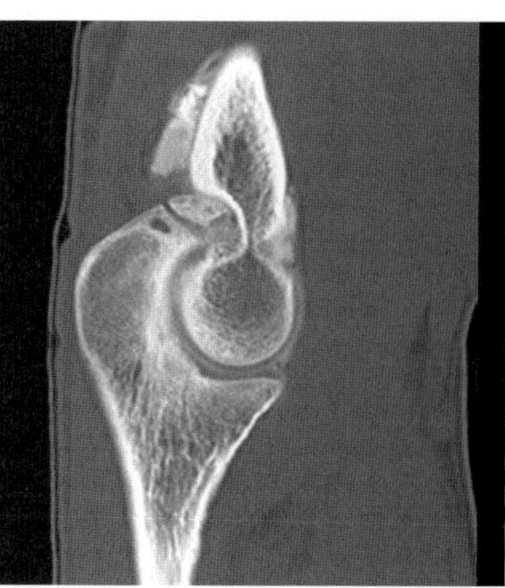

Figure 4 Sagittal CT reconstruction shows a posterior olecranon osteophyte.

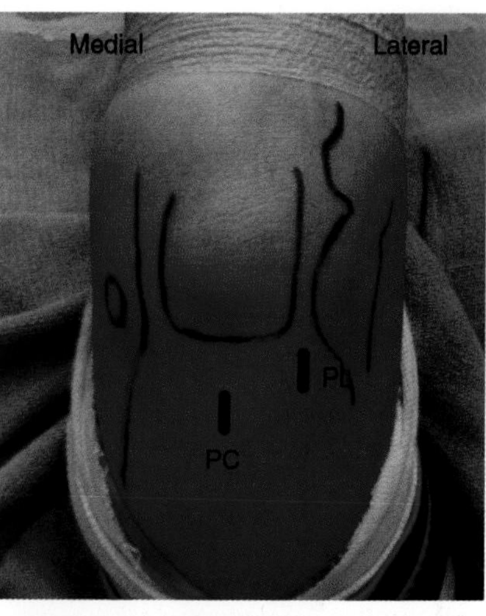

Figure 5 The location of posterior portal placements are marked on the elbow. PL = posterolateral, PC = posterocentral.

teromedial impingement[13] (**Figure 3**).

A CT scan with two-plane (sagittal and coronal), two-dimensional reconstructions may be useful in examining posterior compartments (**Figure 4**). Three-dimensional surface renderings can show the overall morphologic changes, loose bodies, and osteophyte fragmentation. A fractured osteophyte is occasionally observed, particularly in a symptomatic patient. MRI also provides useful information, especially if MUCL pathology is suspected. MRI can show osteochondral damage, synovial plicae, edema, and early stress fractures that can occur in the olecranon. If a stress fracture is not seen on an MRI scan but is clinically suspected, a bone scan should be performed. Stress fractures can involve the olecranon tip, the olecranon process, the posteromedial trochlea, and the sublime tubercle.

Treatment

An initial course of nonsurgical treatment consists of activity modification with a period of rest from throwing, intra-articular cortisone injections, and nonsteroidal anti-inflammatory drugs. Pitching mechanics should be evaluated, and instruction should be given to correct techniques that may be contributing to the injury. After a period of rest, a progressive throwing program is instituted under the supervision of experienced therapists and trainers. Surgical treatment is indicated for those patients who maintain symptoms despite nonsurgical management and desire a return to the same level of competition.

In a report of professional baseball players treated with olecranon débridement for elbow disorders, valgus instability developed in 25% who eventually required MUCL reconstruction.[4] Subsequent basic science studies showed that excessive olecranon resection increases the demands on the MUCL during valgus stress and increases valgus instability.[7,8] Because these studies suggest that MUCL insufficiency may develop following posteromedial decompression, it is currently recommended that olecranon resection be limited to osteophyte removal only, and removal of normal olecranon should be avoided. It has also been shown that existing MUCL insufficiency created in cadaver specimens causes contact alterations in the posteromedial compartment that may cause symptomatic chondrosis and osteophyte formation, which eventually manifests as valgus extension overload.[14] Osteophyte formation may contribute to elbow stability despite a MUCL injury; therefore, removing the bony impingement may convert an asymptomatic MUCL into a painful MUCL. The MUCL should be thoroughly evaluated in patients with posteromedial elbow pain, and overly aggressive resection of posteromedial osteophytes should be avoided.[9]

Surgical Techniques

Anesthesia and patient positioning is performed according to the surgeon's preference. The anatomic landmarks, including the ulnar nerve, are appropriately marked (**Figure 5**). The elbow is then distended using a 60 mL syringe attached to an 18-gauge needle introduced into the soft-spot lateral portal. The joint distention facilitates the introduction of the trocar but more importantly shifts the neurovascular structures further away from the bone, which decreases the risk of nerve injury. Anterior compartment arthroscopy begins with a superficial incision made at the proximal medial portal; the soft tissues are then spread with a blunt clamp to prevent injury to the neurovascular structures. A blunt-

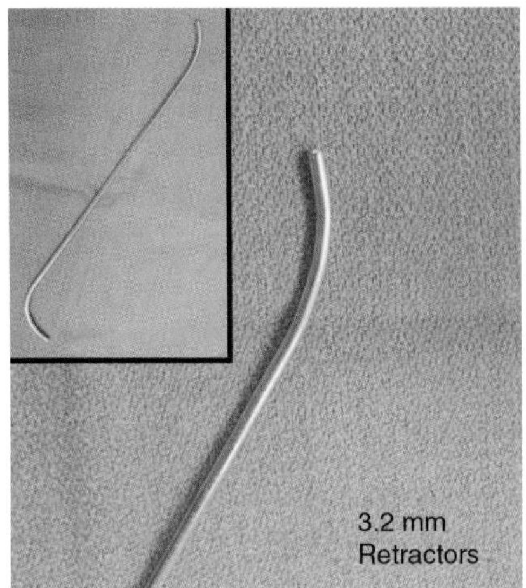

Figure 6 Curved retractor created from a switching stick is used to protect the ulnar nerve and improve visualization during arthroscopy.

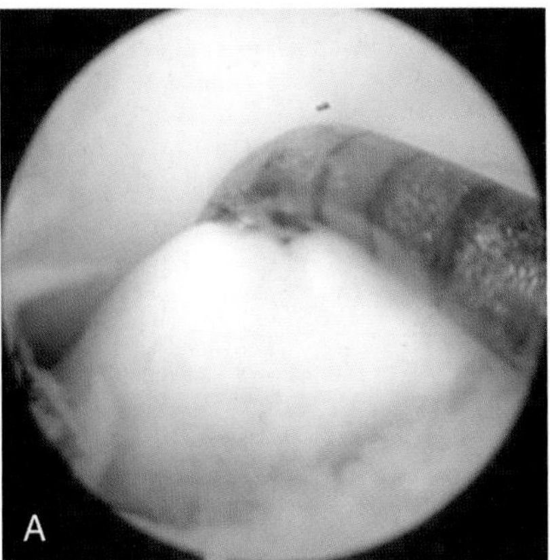

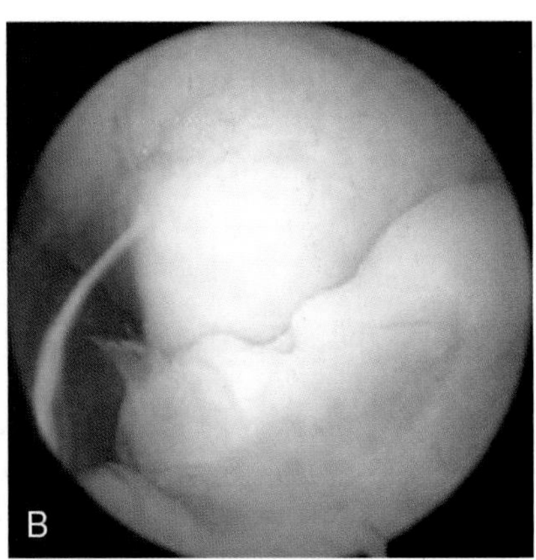

Figure 7 Arthroscopic views of the removal of an olecranon osteophytes and posterior compartment débridement. **A,** The osteophyte is probed. **B,** The osteophyte is removed.

tipped trocar is then introduced into the anterior compartment, hugging the anterior humerus and directed toward the radiocapitellar joint.

Diagnostic arthroscopy is performed anteriorly to look for loose bodies and thoroughly examine the articular cartilage and synovium. The anterior radiocapitellar joint is evaluated for osteochondral lesions of the capitellum and the radial head. The coronoid tip and fossa are then examined for osteophytes, followed by visualization of the trochlea to identify cartilage lesions. The anterior capsule is evaluated for thickening or contracture in the context of loss of passive extension. Because the radial nerve lies in close proximity to the anterolateral capsule, débridement in this area should be done using a retractor (such as a switching stick) introduced through an accessory portal with no suction, with the hood of the shaver to the capsule to prevent iatrogenic injury. To test for valgus laxity, an arthroscopic valgus stress test can be performed; however, valgus laxity is not pathognomonic for MUCL insufficiency. With the arthroscope in the proximal lateral portal visualizing the medial compartment, a valgus stress is applied manually to the elbow. A gap of 3 mm or more seen between the coronoid process and the medial trochlea indicates marked valgus laxity, probable valgus instability, and MUCL insufficiency.[15]

After completing the anterior arthroscopy, a posterolateral viewing portal is established. A direct posterior portal is then established as a working portal. Diagnostic arthroscopy is then performed to evaluate for osteophytes on the posteromedial aspect of the olecranon, loose bodies, and any evidence of chondromalacia. Synovial hypertrophy in the olecranon fossa may be removed using an ablation device or a shaver. The posterior radiocapitellar joint is inspected from the posterolateral portal.

Motorized instruments may cause injury to the ulnar nerve when used in the medial aspect of the posterior compartment. It is imperative to appreciate the position of the ulnar nerve just superficial to the capsule in the posteromedial gutter. The use of cautery and suction when the shaver is near this area of the capsule should be avoided. A curved retractor can be placed through an accessory posterolateral portal to assist in protecting the nerve (**Figure 6**). The pathology of the osteophyte on the posteromedial olecranon is then identified; the osteophyte is often fractured (**Figure 7**). Some osteophytes are encased in soft tissues and may require probing and débridement with a shaver introduced in the direct posterior portal. A small osteotome may be inserted through the direct posterior portal to free the osteophytes. The olecranon can be further contoured with a burr and a shaver if necessary. This chapter's authors prefer removing only the olecranon osteophytes and do not remove any normal bone.[7] When olecranon contouring is complete, radiographic views showing lateral and posterior impingement may be obtained intraoperatively to assess the adequacy of bone removal.

Osteophytes, which are often present in the olecranon fossa, are débrided. The trochlear chondral surfaces are examined for a kissing lesion opposite the olecranon osteophytes. Chondral flaps are débrided; if a well-contained lesion surrounded by normal cartilage can be prepared, microfracture is performed (**Figure 8**).

After arthroscopy is completed, the fluid is evacuated from the posterior cannulas, and the portals are closed with simple, interrupted, 3.0-nylon

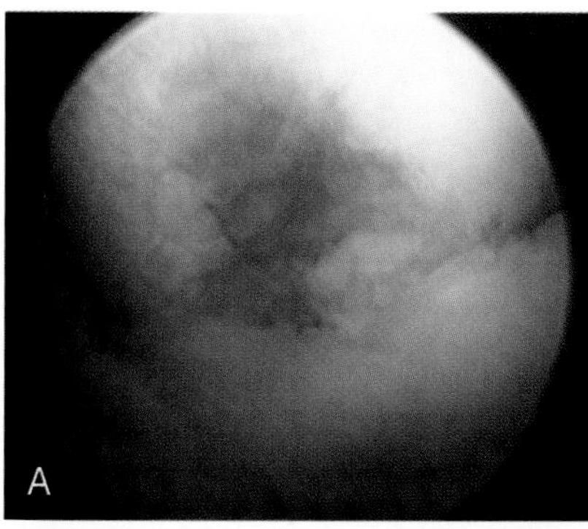

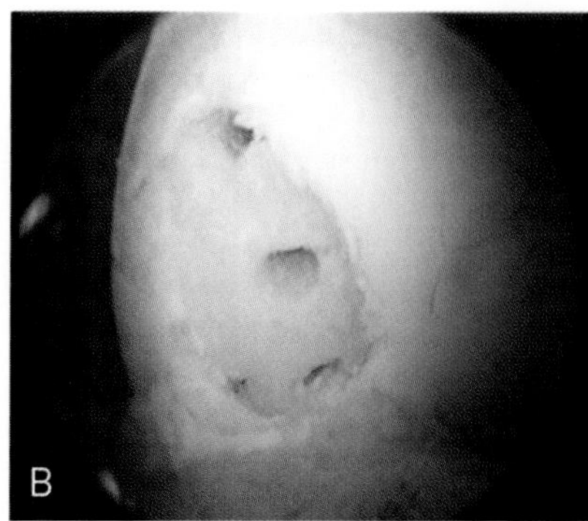

Figure 8 Microfracture performed on the posteromedial trochlea. **A,** Before microfracture. **B,** After microfracture.

sutures. If MUCL reconstruction is required, the patient is placed supine (if arthroscopy was not performed in the supine position), and the patient is reprepped and redraped.

Postoperative Management

After the surgical procedure, the patient is placed in a compressive dressing and simple sling. Some surgeons prefer to use an overnight extension splint to diminish swelling. The dressing may be removed on the first postoperative day. The sling is worn for comfort only and discontinued within 1 week. Active elbow flexion and extension exercises are initiated immediately. The restoration of flexor-pronator strength is also emphasized. Trunk, scapular, and shoulder stabilization exercises are included to avoid shoulder injuries on return to throwing. At 6 weeks, a progressive throwing program is begun, and plyometric exercises and neuromuscular training is enhanced. Return to competition is typically allowed at 3 to 4 months postoperatively after the patient attains full range of motion and full strength and has no pain or tenderness on stress testing and palpation.

Results

With the improvements in arthroscopic equipment and a clear understanding of portal placement and the proximity to neurovascular structures, elbow arthroscopy has become a reliable, safe, and effective way to treat pathology in the thrower's elbow.[15-17] In a study of five pitchers treated with open osteophyte excision, Wilson et al[3] reported that at 8 to 20 months of follow-up, all five patients returned to play for at least one season. One patient required repeat osteophyte excision within two seasons. Andrews and Timmerman[4] reported on 72 professional baseball players treated with either open or arthroscopic elbow surgery. Posteromedial osteophytes were identified in 65% of these patients. The authors reported a 41% reoperation rate in the group treated with olecranon débridement and found that 25% of the patients had underlying MUCL insufficiency and required ulnar collateral ligament reconstruction within 2 years of the initial arthroscopy. They concluded that the incidence of MUCL insufficiency is underestimated, and treatment focused solely on the secondary effects of MUCL insufficiency without treating the underlying MUCL pathology will lead to unsatisfactory results.

Reddy et al[5] reported on 187 arthroscopic elbow procedures. The most common diagnoses were posterior impingement (51%), loose bodies (31%), and degenerative joint disease (22%). The average Figgie score improved from 27.7 points to 45.4 points, with the largest increase occurring in the pain score. Excellent results were achieved in 51% of patients, good results in 36%, fair results in 11%, and poor results in 4%. Forty-seven of 55 baseball players (85%) were able to return to their preoperative level of competition.

Summary

Elbow arthroscopy has evolved to be a safer procedure because the neurovascular structures about the elbow are better understood, and surgeons are able to avoid the structures during portal placement and intra-articular procedures on or near the capsule. However, the real risk of serious nerve injury remains. The use of arthroscopic soft-tissue retractors is extremely helpful when working in the medial gutter to protect the ulnar nerve. Complications specific to olecranon débridement for valgus extension overload include missed MUCL injury and overly aggressive olecranon resection. As previously mentioned, a preexisting MUCL injury may become symptomatic after the patient recovers from the arthroscopic débridement procedure. It is critical to remove the osteophyte only, not normal olecranon. Removing normal olecranon can increase valgus angulation of the elbow and increase MUCL strain during valgus loading, which can contribute to MUCL pathology. Patients who elect arthroscopic posteromedial decompression of the elbow should be counseled on the possibility that future MUCL injury and symptoms may develop.

References

1. Bennett GE: Elbow and shoulder lesions of baseball players. *Am J Surg* 1959;98:484-492.
2. Slocum DB: Classification of elbow injuries from baseball pitching. *Tex Med* 1968;64(3):48-53.

3. Wilson FD, Andrews JR, Blackburn TA, McCluskey G: Valgus extension overload in the pitching elbow. *Am J Sports Med* 1983; 11(2):83-88.
4. Andrews JR, Timmerman LA: Outcome of elbow surgery in professional baseball players. *Am J Sports Med* 1995;23(4):407-413.
5. Reddy AS, Kvitne RS, Yocum LA, ElAttrache NS, Glousman RE, Jobe FW: Arthroscopy of the elbow: A long-term clinical review. *Arthroscopy* 2000;16(6):588-594.
6. O'Driscoll SW: Valgus extension overload and plica, in Levine WN, ed: *The Athlete's Elbow*. Rosemont, IL, American Academy of Orthopaedic Surgeons, 2008, pp 71-83.
7. Kamineni S, ElAttrache NS, O'driscoll SW, et al: Medial collateral ligament strain with partial posteromedial olecranon resection: A biomechanical study. *J Bone Joint Surg Am* 2004; 86-A(11):2424-2430.
8. Kamineni S, Hirahara H, Pomianowski S, et al: Partial posteromedial olecranon resection: A kinematic study. *J Bone Joint Surg Am* 2003;85-A(6):1005-1011.
9. Ahmad CS, Park MC, ElAttrache NS: Elbow medial ulnar collateral ligament insufficiency alters posteromedial olecranon contact. *Am J Sports Med* 2004;32(7): 1607-1612.
10. Cain EL Jr, Dugas JR, Wolf RS, Andrews JR: Elbow injuries in throwing athletes: A current concepts review. *Am J Sports Med* 2003;31(4):621-635.
11. King JW, Brelsford HJ, Tullos HS: Analysis of the pitching arm of the professional baseball pitcher. *Clin Orthop Relat Res* 1969;67:116-123.
12. O'Driscoll SW, Lawton RL, Smith AM: The "moving valgus stress test" for medial collateral ligament tears of the elbow. *Am J Sports Med* 2005;33(2):231-239.
13. David TS: Medial elbow pain in the throwing athlete. *Orthopedics* 2003;26(1):94-105.
14. Park MC, Ahmad CS: Dynamic contributions of the flexor-pronator mass to elbow valgus stability. *J Bone Joint Surg Am* 2004;86-A(10):2268-2274.
15. Field LD, Altchek DW: Evaluation of the arthroscopic valgus instability test of the elbow. *Am J Sports Med* 1996;24(2):177-181.
16. Andrews JR, Carson WG: Arthroscopy of the elbow. *Arthroscopy* 1985;1(2):97-107.
17. O'Driscoll SW, Morrey BF: Arthroscopy of the elbow: Diagnostic and therapeutic benefits and hazards. *J Bone Joint Surg Am* 1992;74(1):84-94.

Fractures and Dislocations of the Elbow: A Return to the Basics

George S. Athwal, MD, FRCSC
Matthew L. Ramsey, MD
Scott P. Steinmann, MD
Jennifer Moriatis Wolf, MD

Abstract

Elbow instability is classified as simple or complex. Complex elbow instability, an elbow dislocation with associated fractures, had historically poor outcomes. Most complex elbow dislocations render the elbow unstable, necessitating surgical treatment. The primary goal of surgery is to restore sufficient stability to the critical anatomy to initiate early range of motion, which has been shown to be a key factor for a successful outcome. Recent literature has improved the understanding of elbow anatomy, biomechanics, and the pathoanatomy of complex instability, thereby allowing the development of systematic approaches for treatment and rehabilitation. These advances in knowledge combined with improved implants and surgical techniques have translated into better outcomes for patients with simple and complex elbow instability.

Instr Course Lect 2011;60:199-214.

The elbow is one of the most commonly dislocated joints in the body, with dislocations occurring with an annual incidence of approximately 6 per 100,000 persons.[1] Dislocations of the elbow can be categorized as simple or complex. Simple elbow dislocations, which are much more common than complex dislocations, are defined as traumatic dislocations, involving only soft-tissue injuries. Complex dislocation or instability, however, involves concomitant fractures. Bony injuries that frequently occur with elbow instability are fractures of the radial head, the coronoid, and the proximal ulna.

The management of complex and simple elbow instability requires an understanding of the normal bony and ligamentous anatomy, the contributions of elbow structures to stability, the natural history of these injuries, the various surgical approaches and techniques used for treatment, and the associated complications. The basics of elbow anatomy and stability will be reviewed, and a principle-based approach to the management of simple and complex elbow instability will be discussed.

Anatomy

The elbow is a trochoid ginglymoid joint, meaning that it has trochoid (rotatory or pivoting) motion through the radiocapitellar and proximal radioulnar joints, and ginglymoid (hingelike) motion through the ulnohumeral joint. An understanding of the com-

Dr. Athwal or an immediate family member is a member of a speaker's bureau or has made paid presentation on behalf of CONMED Livatec and has received research or institutional support from Wright Medical Technology and Tornier. Dr. Ramsey or an immediate family member serves as a board member, owner, officer, or committee member of the Philadelphia Orthopaedic Society; has received royalties from Zimmer and Ascension; is a member of a speakers bureau or has made paid presentations on behalf of DePuy/Mitek; serves as a paid consultant to or is an employee of Zimmer and Ascension; has received research or institutional support from Ortho-McNeil Janssen Scientific Affairs and Biomet; and has stock or stock options held in Johnson & Johnson, Novartis, and Teva. Dr. Steinmann or an immediate family member has received royalties from DePuy; serves as a paid consultant to or is an employee of Arthrex, DePuy, and Wright Medical Technology; and has received research or institutional support from Wright Medical Technology. Dr. Wolf or an immediate family member serves as a board member, owner, officer, or committee member of the American Society for Surgery of the Hand and the Rocky Mountain Hand Surgery Society.

plex bony anatomy of the elbow, the soft-tissue stabilizers, and the neighboring neurovascular structures is imperative when surgically treating elbow fracture-dislocations.

The proximal ulna has two articular zones: the greater sigmoid notch and the lesser sigmoid notch (radial notch). The greater sigmoid notch, with its central guiding ridge, articulates with the trochlea, whereas the lesser notch forms an articulation with the radial head as the proximal radioulnar joint. The greater sigmoid notch is composed of the olecranon and coronoid processes. The coronoid process is composed of a tip, a body, an anteromedial facet, an anterolateral facet, and the sublime tubercle; it is an important anterior and varus stabilizer to the elbow joint. The crista supinatoris, which is the insertion site for the lateral ulnar collateral ligament, is located distal to the lesser sigmoid notch on the lateral aspect of the proximal ulna.

The proximal radius consists of the radial head and neck. The radial head is elliptic and is offset from the neck. The radial head articulates with the capitellum and the lesser sigmoid notch; therefore, articular cartilage covers all of the articular dish and most of the articular margin. With the forearm in neutral rotation, the lateral aspect of the radial head is devoid of hyaline cartilage and is deemed the safe area for hardware because it does not articulate with the lesser sigmoid notch. The radial head is an important secondary stabilizer of the elbow.

There are important ligamentous stabilizers associated with the bony anatomy. The lateral collateral ligament (LCL) complex consists of the lateral ulnar collateral ligament (a primary elbow stabilizer), the radial collateral ligament, and the annular ligament. The lateral ulnar collateral ligament originates at an isometric point on the lateral epicondyle and inserts on the crista supinatoris of the proximal ulna. The LCL complex functions as an important restraint to varus and posterolateral rotatory instability.

The medial collateral ligament (MCL) consists of the anterior bundle, posterior bundle, and transverse ligament. The anterior bundle originates on the anteroinferior aspect of the medial epicondyle and inserts on the sublime tubercle of the coronoid. The anterior bundle of the MCL functions as an important restraint to valgus and posteromedial rotatory instability.

Biomechanics

The bony and soft-tissue components of the elbow that contribute to stability can be classified as primary or secondary stabilizers. The triad of primary stabilizers of the elbow are the anterior bundle of the MCL, the lateral ulnar collateral ligament, and the ulnohumeral joint. These structures are termed primary stabilizers because their integrity is required for the elbow to remain stable.

The ulnohumeral joint is the primary bony stabilizer in the flexion-extension plane. The coronoid process is an important part of the ulnohumeral joint; several biomechanical studies have demonstrated its significance in elbow stability.[2,3] Hull et al[2] examined the role of the coronoid process in elbow stability. In this study, progressive transverse cuts were made in the coronoid process, accounting for 25%, 33%, and 40% of the coronoid. A statistically significant decrease in load resistance to varus displacement occurred only after removal of 50% of the coronoid process. This study suggests that the bony contributions of the coronoid process to elbow stability may not be significant if less than 25% of the coronoid is fractured.

Schneeberger et al[3] examined the role of the radial head and the coronoid process in posterolateral rotatory stability. When 30% of the coronoid was resected along with the entire radial head, complete ulnohumeral dislocation occurred at 60° of elbow flexion. When the radial head was replaced with a metallic implant, stability was restored even though 30% of the coronoid had been removed. A 50% deficiency of the coronoid combined with a resected radial head could not be stabilized by radial head replacement alone. This study emphasized the importance of either repairing or replacing the radial head in the presence of posterolateral rotatory instability. If a small coronoid fracture (less than 30%) is present, ulnohumeral stability may be achieved primarily by focusing the surgical plan on restoring the radial head and repairing the LCL.[4-6]

Simple Elbow Dislocations

The elbow joint is the second most commonly dislocated joint in adults; the shoulder is the most frequently dislocated joint.[1] Associated injuries occur in 10% to 15% of patients with elbow dislocations, including ipsilateral shoulder, humerus, distal radius, ulna, and carpal bone fractures or sprains. Disruption of the interosseous membrane that stabilizes the radial and ulnar shafts can also occur. Many injuries occur during athletic participation, with the most common mechanism being a fall onto an outstretched hand.

The biomechanical forces in an elbow dislocation cause sequential soft-tissue failure. The LCL ruptures first, followed by disruption of the anterior and posterior elbow capsule. If the energy of the dislocation is sufficient, the last soft-tissue structure to fail is the MCL.[7]

Posterior or posterolateral dislocations make up approximately 90% of all elbow dislocations. Lateral, medial, and anterior dislocations are rare. Divergent dislocations, those in which the radius and ulna are separated and widely displaced from each other and the humerus, are extremely rare and generally result from high-energy trauma; these injuries are often associated with a rupture of the forearm interosseous membrane and the annular ligament.[8]

Patient Evaluation

Patients presenting with acute elbow dislocations generally have an obvious deformity and severe elbow pain. The physical examination should include a neurovascular evaluation; radiographic studies should be obtained to determine the direction of the dislocation. A reduction should be performed using sedation or general anesthesia. Gentle traction, manipulation of the olecranon anteriorly, and bringing the elbow into flexion will typically reduce the elbow joint. Once reduced, the elbow should be tested for motion and blocks to rotation and stability. The postreduction stable arc of motion should be documented to assist with rehabilitation.

Nonsurgical Treatment

Nonsurgical treatment of simple elbow dislocations is recommended in most instances when the elbow joint is stable at 45° to 60° of extension.[9] An acute elbow dislocation can be splinted or placed in a sling. Early follow-up is recommended within 5 to 7 days to begin range of motion if the elbow proves stable and repeat radiographs show a concentric joint reduction. If the elbow begins to subluxate beyond 60° of extension, a hinged brace with an extension block can be used to begin rehabilitation within the stable arc of motion. The extension block can be increased 10° to 20° per week to regain motion.

Nonsurgical treatment generally achieves good outcomes, with studies showing that early range of motion leads to less stiffness and extension loss at the final follow-up.[10-12] Typically, some terminal extension is lost, averaging 10° to 20°.[12] Josefsson et al[13] conducted a retrospective comparison of nonsurgical versus surgical treatment of simple elbow dislocations and reported no difference between final outcomes at 2-year follow-up. Maripuri et al,[14] in a retrospective cohort study of patients with acute elbow dislocations treated in a sling or immobilized in a splint, showed that both groups had excellent outcomes; however, the group treated in a sling had significantly better Quick Disabilities of the Arm, Shoulder, and Hand questionnaire results; Mayo Elbow Performance scores; and a faster return to work.

Surgical Treatment

When a simple elbow dislocation shows continued instability, surgical treatment is recommended. Although many authors previously recommended exploration and repair of both the LCL and the MCL, more recent studies in complex elbow dislocations suggest that LCL repair is the most critical factor.[13,15-17] Forthman et al[16] and McKee et al[17] repaired the LCL in complex fracture-dislocations of the elbow in association with the fixation of bony structures and then tested the stability of the elbow. If the elbow proved to be stable through a full range of motion, the MCL was not repaired.

The technique of LCL repair in unstable simple elbow dislocations involves supine positioning of the patient and the use of minifluoroscopy. A posterior midline skin incision or a direct lateral skin incision may be used. The deep lateral approach to the LCL may be conducted through the Kocher interval or via an extensor digitorum communis tendon split.[18] Parts of the common extensor origin along with the lateral ligament are often avulsed from the lateral epicondyle. The ligament can be repaired to the isometric point on the lateral epicondyle using a transosseous technique or with suture anchors. The isometric point on the lateral epicondyle is determined by the center of the radius of curvature of the capitellum (**Figure 1**). Two drill tunnels are made (or a suture anchor is placed) starting at the isometric point (origin of the LCL) and exiting posteriorly, separated by a bone bridge. A high-strength suture is used to grasp the LCL in a running locking fashion. The free ends of the suture used to stitch the LCL are passed through the separate drill tunnels, tensioned, and then tied over a bone bridge. In osteopenic bone, the sutures may be tied over a plate. After repair of the LCL, the extensor origin is repaired. Ligament reconstruction using autograft or allograft is rarely necessary in the acute situation.

The elbow is then examined through a full range of motion and with fluoroscopy. If stability has been achieved, the elbow is rehabilitated in pronation to protect the lateral ligament repair. If the MCL is disrupted, most patients can be effectively managed with an "MCL-off" rehabilitation protocol maintaining forearm supination. Typically, the MCL does not require repair. In rare instances, if instability persists after LCL repair that cannot be managed with supination, the MCL should undergo direct repair. Very rarely, the elbow remains unstable after LCL and MCL repair. In these circumstances, joint reduction can be maintained with a static external fixator, a hinged fixator, or transarticular pinning.

The outcomes of surgical repair of the collateral ligaments in simple elbow dislocations are generally good, although heterotopic ossification is reported more frequently than in nonsurgically treated patients. Micic et al[15]

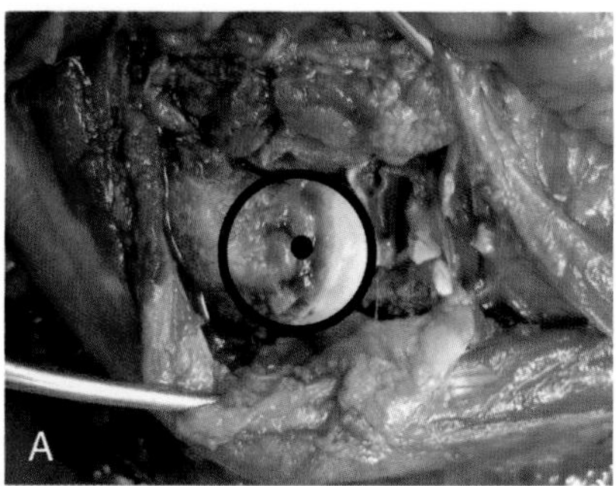

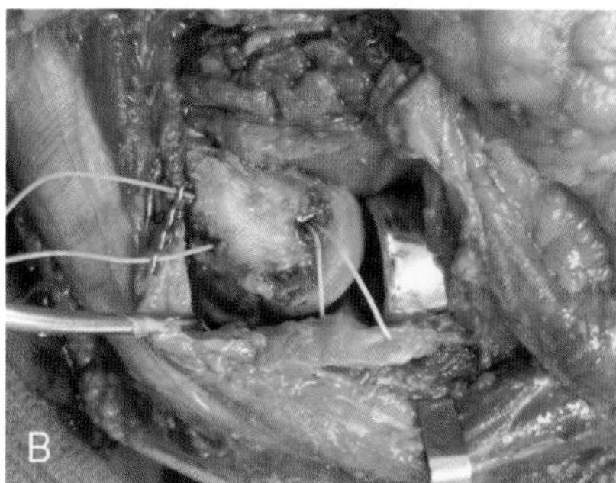

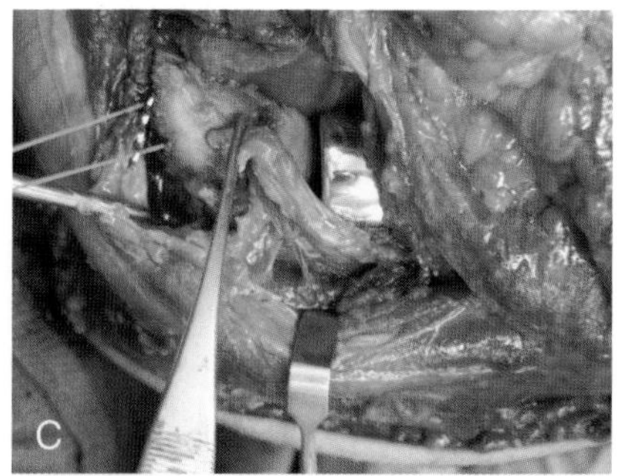

Figure 1 The LCL is repaired to its isometric origin on the lateral epicondyle with suture anchors or transosseous sutures (preferred). **A,** The isometric point is determined by the center (black dot) of the radius of curvature of the capitellum (black circle). **B,** Two drill tunnels are made (or a suture anchor is placed) starting at the isometric point and exiting posteriorly, separated by a bone bridge. **C,** The suture ends used to stitch the LCL are passed through separate drill tunnels, tensioned, and then tied over a bone bridge. In osteopenic bone, the sutures are tied over a plate to prevent the suture from cutting through the bone tunnels.

treated 20 patients with simple elbow dislocations, with LCL injuries in 80% and MCL injuries in 55%. The authors reported good to excellent outcomes in most patients at 2-year follow-up, with a mean extension loss of 14° and heterotopic ossification in 65% of patients. A prospective study by Joseffsson et al[13] compared surgical and nonsurgical outcomes after simple elbow dislocation. The authors reported a higher incidence of pain with use, weather-related symptomatology, weakness, and pain at rest in the surgical group at an average of 2 years after injury.

Complications

Complications of simple elbow dislocation include contracture, heterotopic ossification, nerve and/or artery injury, and residual elbow instability. Elbow contracture, specifically a loss of terminal extension, is very common and averages 10° to 20°.[10,11,13] Elbows requiring surgical treatment generally have more soft-tissue injury and thus greater associated motion loss.[15,19] Similarly, a greater degree of heterotopic ossification is reported in surgically treated elbows,[15] although the overall estimate is that asymptomatic heterotopic ossification develops in 55% of patients with simple dislocations, generally within the collateral ligaments.[9] The study authors recommend heterotopic ossification prophylaxis in patients with surgically treated elbows.

The ulnar nerve is the most commonly injured nerve after a simple elbow dislocation. Symptoms are persistent in fewer than 10% of patients, and few patients require surgical nerve decompression.[10,20,21] Vascular injuries in elbow dislocations, specifically brachial artery injuries, are relatively rare and typically occur with open injuries and fracture-dislocations.[20]

Conclusion

Overall, nonsurgical treatment and early range of motion has been shown to lead to excellent outcomes in most patients with simple elbow dislocations. In patients displaying continued instability after reduction, surgical repair of one or both of the collateral ligaments is indicated and has shown good outcomes.

Complex Elbow Dislocations

Complex elbow dislocations represent some of the most challenging injuries to treat in orthopaedic traumatology. Complex instability can be broadly classified into three injury patterns: (1) dislocation with a radial head fracture with or without a coronoid fracture, (2) varus posteromedial instability with an anteromedial coronoid fracture, and (3) transolecranon or Monteggia-type injuries.

Dislocation With a Radial Head Fracture

Elbow dislocations with an associated fracture of the radial head are common. The mechanism of injury is typically a fall onto an outstretched hand that results in a posterolateral rotatory instability pattern. Dislocation and postreduction radiographs are usually sufficient to diagnose the instability pattern and identify associated radial head fractures. Radiographs, however, may not allow complete characterization of the size, displacement, and comminution of fracture fragments. Radiographs also should be critically examined to rule out associated fractures of the coronoid, capitellum, and trochlea. CT, although not absolutely necessary, is useful in better characterizing radial head fractures and associated bony injuries. CT can be useful in determining the degree of comminution, the amount of fracture displacement, and the size and location of fragments.

Classification

Several classification systems are available to categorize radial head fractures. The Broberg and Morrey[22] modification of the Mason[23] classification system characterizes the size and displacement of fracture fragments. Type I fractures are nondisplaced or minimally displaced (< 2 mm). Type II fractures are displaced more than 2 mm and involve more than 30% of the articulation. Type III fractures are comminuted, and type IV fractures are associated with an elbow dislocation.[24] All radial head fractures associated with complex elbow instability are, by default, type IV. In most instances, classification systems for radial head fractures are descriptive and cannot be used to reliably guide treatment.

Management

The management of an elbow dislocation with an associated radial head fracture follows the principles of obtaining joint stability followed by treating the fracture to maximize the quality of the patient's outcome. If joint reduction cannot be maintained, the principles discussed in the previous section on simple elbow dislocations with continued instability should be followed. In addition, the treatment algorithms should be interpreted in the context of patient factors, such as functional demands, medical comorbidities, and cognitive status.

Nonsurgical treatment is generally used for type I nondisplaced or minimally displaced (< 2 mm) radial head fractures. If the elbow dislocation is reduced and classified as stable, type I fractures are treated nonsurgically with a rehabilitation protocol similar to that of simple elbow dislocations, providing there are no blocks to rotation. In the rare circumstance of an unstable type I radial head elbow fracture, surgery is indicated. The primary goal of the surgical procedure is to repair the lateral ulnar collateral ligament (with or without MCL repair) to obtain stability; however, fixation of the type I radial head fracture also is recommended to prevent delayed fracture displacement during rehabilitation.

The treatment of type II radial head fractures is controversial. Several studies have reported good outcomes with open reduction and internal fixation of fractures displaced more than 2 mm and involving more than 30% of the articular surface,[25-27] whereas other studies have reported equally good results with nonsurgical management.[28,29] Surgical treatment for a type II radial head fracture associated with an elbow dislocation is indicated if stability cannot be maintained nonsurgically or if the surgeon prefers surgical treatment of the fracture. In general, this chapter's authors recommend surgical fixation of type II fractures.

Type III radial head fractures associated with instability are usually surgically managed. The treatment options include open reduction and internal fixation, radial head resection, and radial head arthroplasty. Radial head resection is contraindicated in the setting of complex elbow instability because the radial head is a necessary secondary stabilizer.

The surgical approach may involve a posterior longitudinal or a direct lateral incision. The deep approach may be conducted through the Kocher interval or an extensor digitorum communis split. The advantage of using the Kocher interval is that origin and insertion of the lateral ulnar collateral ligament are easily accessible for repair.

Open Reduction and Internal Fixation

Open reduction and internal fixation of displaced radial head fractures may be accomplished with small-diameter (1.5- to 3.0-mm) standard screws, headless compression screws, or plates. Good results can be achieved when rigid fixation is stable enough to allow early range of motion; however, fractures with comminution of three or more parts have poor results with fixation.[25-27,30-33]

Arthroplasty

Radial head arthroplasty is indicated if there is extensive radial head and/or neck comminution or poor bone quality. Several metallic implant designs are available, and no one implant has shown clinical superiority. A modular system that allows variable head sizes, stem diameters, and stem heights to ensure optimal sizing is recommended. Silastic implants are not recommended because they have inferior biomechanical properties that preclude the restoration of valgus and axial stability. Correct sizing of a radial head implant is critical to decrease complications related to implant overlengthening.[34-40] The excised fragments of the radial head are used as a template for correct sizing. A trial reduction with trial implants is imperative to assess implant sizing, implant tracking, elbow range of motion, and radiocapitellar contact. To ensure the correct implant length, the proximal extent of the implant should be approximately parallel to the proximal edge of the lesser sigmoid notch.[34,39] Recently, radial head arthroplasty in elbows with complex instability has shown reproducible good to excellent outcomes in more than 75% of patients.[17,32,41-45]

Fragment Excision

Excision of a radial head fracture fragment is rarely indicated in the setting of complex elbow instability. Fragment excision is considered only in elbows with small fragments, typically less than 25% of the surface area, which are deemed irreparable.[46]

Once the radial head fracture has been treated with fixation or replacement, the lateral ulnar collateral ligament must be repaired. The technique has been previously described in this chapter. After lateral ligament repair,

Table 1
Rehabilitation Protocol After Surgical Treatment of Elbow Dislocations With Radial Head Fracture With or Without Coronoid Fracture

Scenario	Splint	Rehabilitation	Comments
LCL repair MCL intact	90° resting splint, forearm in neutral or pronation	Unrestricted active flexion Extension in neutral or forearm pronation	If the LCL repair is tenuous (poor tissue), the forearm may be pronated to protect the LCL repair.
LCL repair MCL deficient	90° resting splint, forearm supination	Unrestricted active flexion Extension in forearm supination	If elbow is unstable after LCL repair, which cannot be corrected with supination, the MCL should be repaired (rare).
LCL repair MCL repair	90° resting splint, forearm in neutral	Unrestricted active flexion Extension in neutral rotation	If elbow remains unstable after LCL and MCL repairs, external fixation can be used (very rare).

LCL = lateral collateral ligament, MCL = medial collateral ligament

the elbow must be examined for MCL injury and residual instability. The intraoperative management of continued instability and the postoperative rehabilitation protocols are outlined in **Table 1**.

Dislocation With Radial Head and Coronoid Fractures

Elbow dislocations with associated fractures of the radial head and the coronoid have been termed the terrible triad injury because of historically poor outcomes.[47] By understanding the relevant anatomy and the role of the primary and secondary elbow stabilizers and by using advances in surgical techniques, a systematic algorithm was developed that has led to reproducibly good outcomes.[17,48,49] The mechanism of injury in terrible triad injuries is believed to be in the spectrum of posterolateral rotatory instability. The dislocation and fractures typically occur because of indirect forces transmitted to the elbow as a patient falls onto an outstretched hand.

The patient history and physical examination are important in determining the mechanism of injury, the energy level of the injury (high or low), associated injuries, neurovascular status, and skin integrity. Prereduction and postreduction radiographs should be carefully examined to characterize the fracture and assess the congruency of the ulnohumeral and radiocapitellar joints. This chapter's authors routinely investigate terrible triad injuries with a CT scan to classify the injury and investigate fracture patterns, displacement, and comminution.

A single classification system for terrible triad injuries does not exist; therefore, classification systems that address the individual components of the injury are used. McKee et al[50] classified LCL injuries into six patterns. The most common injury pattern involved proximal avulsion of the LCL from the isometric point on the lateral epicondyle.

Coronoid Fracture Classification Systems

Regan and Morrey[51] classified coronoid fractures into three types based on their appearance on lateral radiographs. Type I is a shear fracture of the tip of the process; type II, a fragment involving less than 50% of the process; and type III, a fragment involving more than 50% of the coronoid process. This classification system predated the use of CT. With the greater use of CT scanning, it is now understood that coronoid fractures may occur not only as transverse fractures but also as fractures in more oblique planes. A recent study updated the Regan and Morrey classification system to include two additional types of fractures: an anterolateral coronoid fracture, in which the fracture plane tilts obliquely toward the radial head, and an anteromedial fracture plane, in which the fracture plane tilts medially toward the sublime tubercle.[52] These latter two fracture types have been described as type IV medial and type IV lateral. This four-part classification system was recently tested for intraobserver and interobserver reliability and was found to demonstrate good reliability in both types of observations.[52]

O'Driscoll et al[53] proposed a seven-part coronoid classification system based on the anatomic location of the fracture (**Table 2**). This classification includes three main types of coronoid fractures: type 1, a transverse fracture of the tip of the coronoid process; type 2, a fracture of the anteromedial facet of the coronoid process; and type 3, a fracture of the coronoid base with or without a fracture of the olecranon process. This is the first classification system that takes into account realistic patterns of coronoid fracture types. As complex elbow instability can broadly be classified into three injury patterns, each with its own unique coronoid fracture type, the O'Driscoll classification system appropriately accounts for these patterns. Although the reliability of this system must be validated, the focus on the tip, the anteromedial facet, and the base may enhance the understanding of coronoid fracture patterns.

Table 2
O'Driscoll Classification of Coronoid Process Fractures

Fracture Type and Location	Subtype	Description
Tip	1	≤ 2 mm of coronoid bony height (flake fracture)
	2	> 2 mm of coronoid body height
Anteromedial	1	Anteromedial rim
	2	Anteromedial rim + tip
	3	Anteromedial rim + sublime tubercle (± tip)
Basal	1	Coronoid body and base
	2	Transolecranon basal coronoid fractures

Management

Most terrible triad injuries require surgical treatment; however, a small subset of these injuries may be managed nonsurgically if strict criteria are present. For nonsurgical management, the elbow must be concentrically reduced, the radial head fracture must not meet surgical indications (minimally displaced without a block to motion), the coronoid fracture must be small, and the elbow must be sufficiently stable to allow early range of motion (extending to at least 30° to 45° before becoming unstable).

Typically, terrible triad injuries are treated surgically. The lateral side of the elbow is approached first because most terrible triad injuries can be surgically stabilized from the lateral side. A systematic surgical algorithm[18] for the treatment of terrible triad injuries is shown in **Figure 2**. A posterior longitudinal skin incision is usually used followed by elevation of a lateral flap, with the deep approach to the lateral elbow conducted through the Kocher interval. A primary technical principle in the surgical management of terrible triad injuries is to survey the damage from outside in and then treat the injury from inside out. This means that the LCL injury is identified first but repaired near the end of the surgical procedure. Once the LCL injury is identified, the radial head is assessed. The radial head-neck fracture is characterized, and the surgeon decides if it is repairable. If the radial head fracture is repairable, it is not fixed until the coronoid injury is characterized and

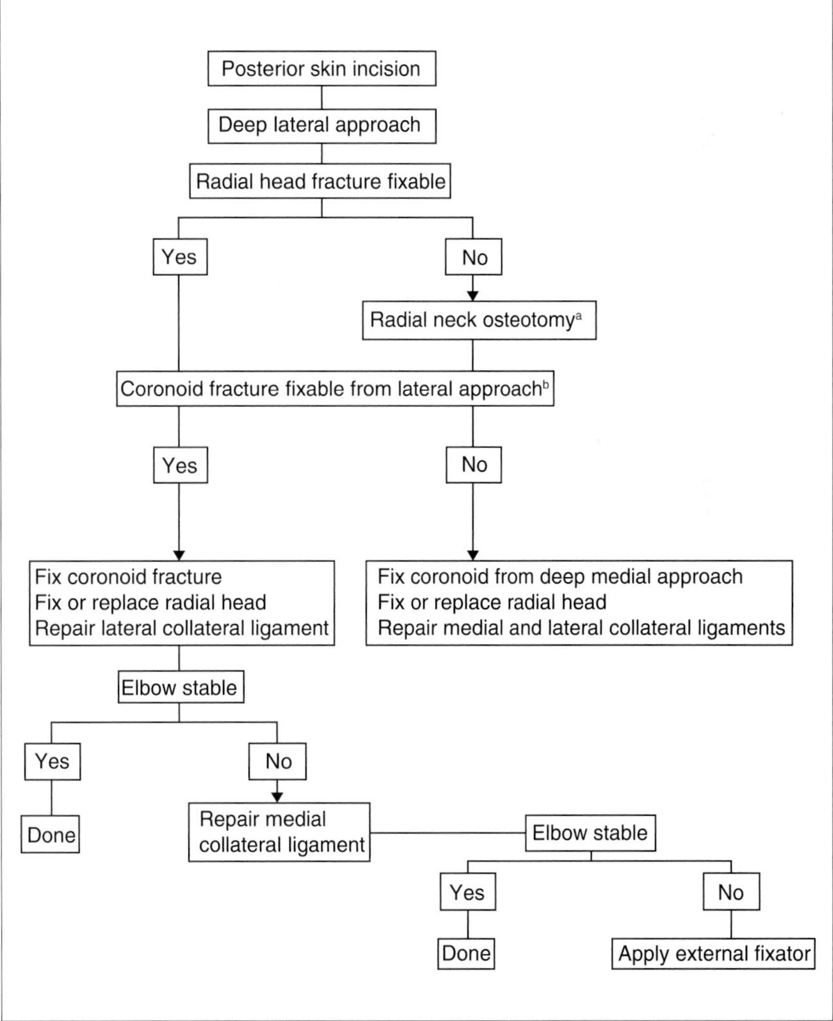

Figure 2 The surgical algorithm for treating terrible triad injuries. [a]Radial neck osteotomy in preparation for radial head replacement. [b]Type I coronoid fractures may not require repair. (Reproduced from Matthew PK, Athwal GS, King GJ: Terrible triad injury of the elbow: Current concepts. *J Am Acad Orthop Surg* 2009;17:137-151.)

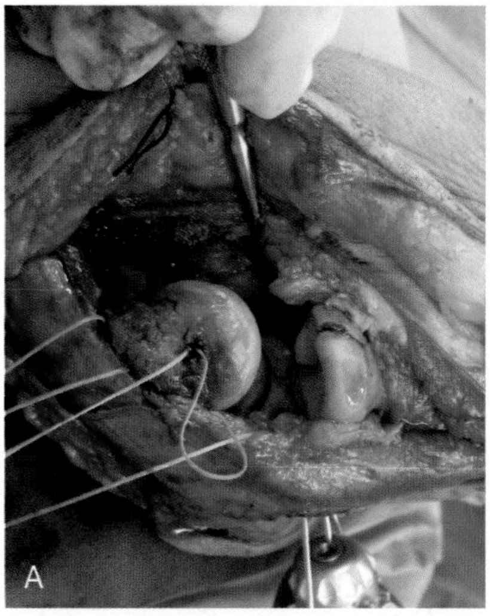

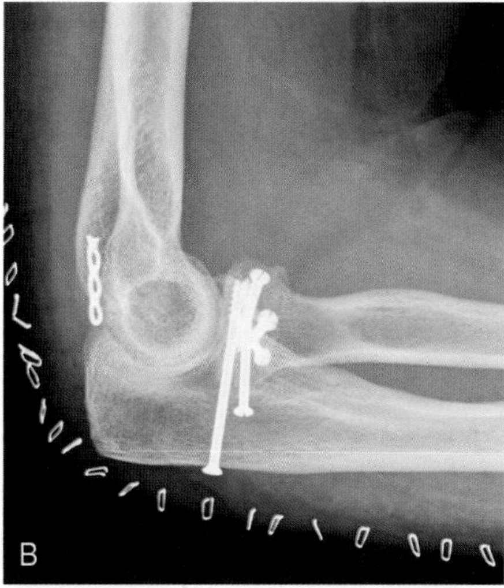

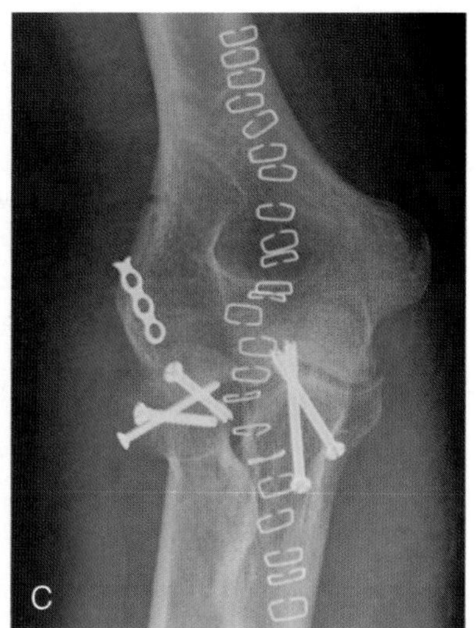

Figure 3 **A,** Intraoperative photograph of retrograde cannulated screw fixation of a Regan and Morrey type II coronoid fracture. The joint is intentionally subluxated to allow access to the coronoid for reduction and fixation from the lateral arthrotomy. The LCL has been sutured, with the free ends passed through drill tunnels at the isometric point in preparation for repair after completion of open reduction and internal fixation of the coronoid and the radial head. Postoperative lateral (**B**) and AP (**C**) radiographs show a reduced joint with fixation of the radial head and the coronoid.

treated. Similarly, if the radial head is irreparable and arthroplasty is planned, a radial neck osteotomy is conducted to improve visualization of the coronoid, but the radial head implant is not inserted until the coronoid injury is treated.

Biomechanical studies have determined that the coronoid is an important elbow stabilizer in response to varus, axial, posterolateral, and posteromedial rotatory forces.[2,3,6] Small tip fractures, involving less than 10% of the coronoid height, have a minimal effect on elbow stability and therefore are not typically repaired.[6] Coronoid fractures associated with terrible triad injuries may be fixed with a retrograde screw technique or with transosseous sutures. If the coronoid fracture fragment is large, a retrograde cannulated screw technique is preferred (**Figure 3**). A targeted guide or a freehand technique is used to pass guidewires from the subcutaneous border of the ulna into the reduced coronoid. The guidewires are then sequentially exchanged for cannulated screws. In smaller comminuted fractures, a high-strength suture is used to reduce fracture fragments via transosseous tunnels made from the subcutaneous border of the ulna to the fractured surface of the coronoid (**Figure 4**). If the coronoid fracture cannot be adequately visualized or fixated from the lateral arthrotomy, a separate medial approach is used.

After open reduction and internal fixation of the coronoid, the radial head is definitively fixed or replaced as described in the preceding section (Dislocation With Radial Head Fracture). The LCL and the extensor origin are then repaired to the isometric point on the lateral epicondyle and the supracondylar ridge, respectively. After lateral ligament repair, the elbow is examined for residual instability, and the algorithm in **Figure 2** is followed. Postoperative rehabilitation follows the protocol outlined in **Table 1**.

Outcomes

Recent literature on the outcomes of terrible triad injuries treated with a systematic protocol has been favorable.[16,17,48,49] Good to excellent outcomes can be expected in approximately 75% to 80% of patients, with a mean arc of motion between 110° to 120°. Risks associated with terrible triad injuries include residual instability, arthritis, heterotopic ossification, stiffness, neuropathy, infection, malunion, and nonunion.

Varus Posteromedial Instability With an Anteromedial Coronoid Fracture

The coronoid helps resist varus stress on the elbow similar to the way the radial head resists valgus forces. The proximal ulna is narrower than the distal humerus but widens to form the coronoid process. The coronoid, therefore, matches the distal articular surface of the trochlea. On average, 60% of the anteromedial facet of the coronoid is unsupported by the proximal ulnar metaphysis, making it prone to fracture from varus stress.[54]

A coronoid fracture can be difficult to visualize on plain AP or lateral radiographs. Often, a coronoid fracture may be mistaken for a fracture of the radial head. It is possible, however, for the coronoid to fracture without a con-

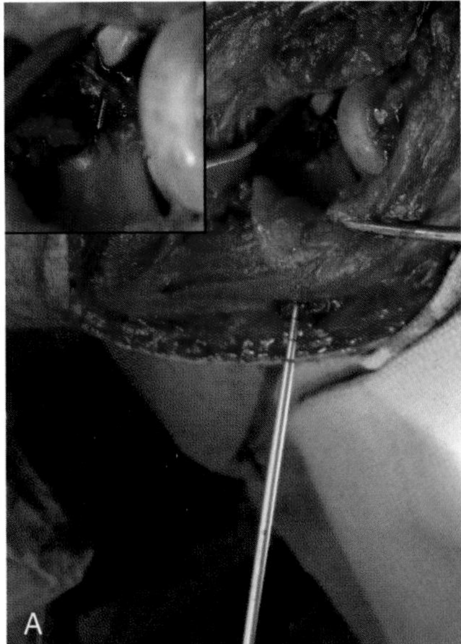

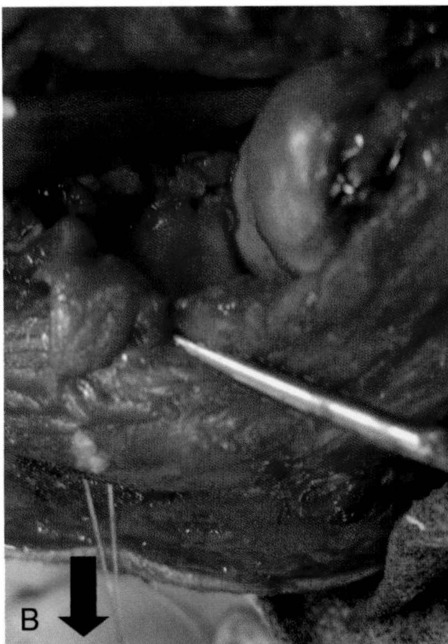

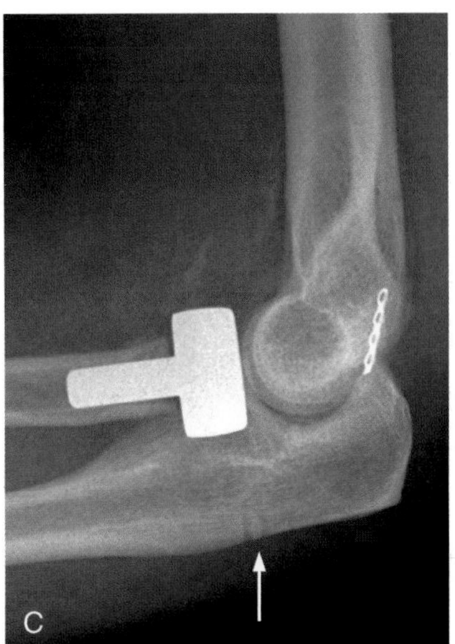

Figure 4 Intraoperative photographs showing suture fixation of a coronoid fracture. **A,** A targeted guide or a freehand technique is used to create two bone tunnels from the subcutaneous border of the ulna into the coronoid fracture site (inset image). The coronoid is sutured with the free ends of suture passed through the bone tunnels. **B,** Traction on the sutures reduces the coronoid fracture (arrow). **C,** Postoperative lateral radiograph showing the transosseous suture tunnels (arrow).

current fracture of the radial head. If a patient is seen with a suspected elbow dislocation and there is no obvious fracture of the radial head, the area of the coronoid on the radiographs must be examined for a potential fracture. A CT scan of the elbow is recommended if a coronoid fracture is suspected because such a fracture can be readily seen with this imaging modality.

Varus posteromedial rotatory instability is hypothesized to occur when an axial load is applied to the extended pronated forearm, resulting in a varus moment and posteromedial rotation of the radius and the ulna. This injury pattern typically results in an anteromedial coronoid fracture in association with ruptures of the LCL and the posterior bundle of the MCL. As the lateral structures of the elbow tear, the coronoid is forced against and under the medial trochlea, resulting in an anteromedial coronoid fracture. The size of the coronoid fracture will depend on the degree of force imparted to the elbow. When the sublime tubercle is involved in the fracture, medial elbow instability usually occurs. Fractures to the radial head are uncommon with this injury pattern.

If a significant anteromedial coronoid fracture with concurrent elbow instability is not discovered and remains untreated, the ulnohumeral joint may subluxate. This malalignment, with the trochlea articulating with the fractured surface of the anteromedial coronoid, will result in greater stress on the cartilage of the medial aspect of the trochlea, leading to early onset posttraumatic arthritis. For this reason, anteromedial coronoid fractures should be identified early in the treatment process to prevent late instability and degenerative changes from occurring.

Management

Because there are few studies in the literature on the management and outcomes of anteromedial coronoid fractures, the surgical indications, approaches, and techniques for this type of fracture are still being developed. The current recommendations for treating varus posteromedial injuries are based on expert opinion and small case series.[53-59]

For an anteromedial coronoid fracture, either a direct medial skin incision or a posterior incision can be used. A posterior incision is preferred because it allows an approach through the watershed area, which avoids injury to branches of the medial or lateral cutaneous sensory nerves. Once the skin flaps have been created, the ulnar nerve is identified in the cubital tunnel, and an in situ release of the ulnar nerve is performed. The nerve is not routinely transposed during coronoid fracture repair but simply released in situ and then retracted posteriorly for exposure (**Figure 5**).

After the ulnar nerve is exposed and retracted posteriorly, the coronoid is approached through the floor of the ulnar nerve on the ulna. The flexor pronator group is carefully elevated off the ulna from a distal to proximal di-

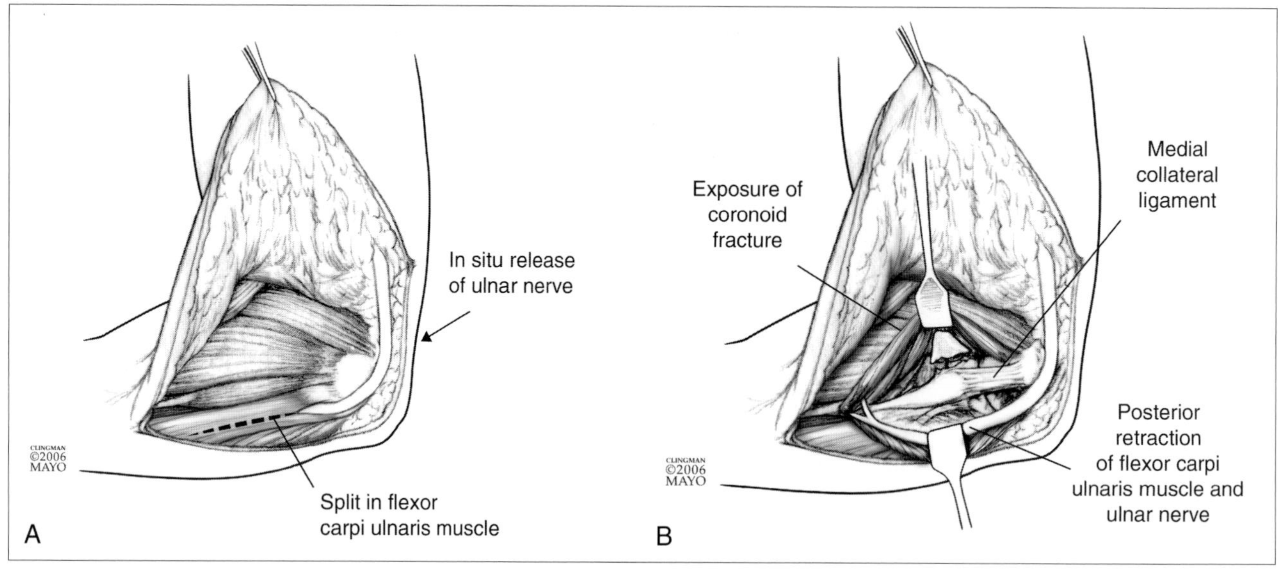

Figure 5 The surgical approach to the medial elbow for fixation of anteromedial coronoid fractures involves an in situ ulnar nerve release (**A**) and exposure of the proximal ulna via an incision that splits the humeral and ulnar heads of the flexor carpi ulnaris muscle (**B**). (Reproduced with permission from the Mayo Foundation for Medical Education and Research, Rochester, MN.)

rection, exposing the sublime tubercle, the coronoid fracture, and the anterior bundle of the MCL. The flexor pronator group itself does not need to be taken down or removed from the medial epicondyle but is simply elevated off the anterior coronoid while preserving the attachments of the MCL.

After the coronoid is exposed, the fracture can be provisionally stabilized with a large reduction clamp or multiple Kirschner wires. Definitive fixation can then be achieved using either a small plate or screws. Precontoured plates specifically made for the coronoid are now available through several manufacturers. The primary role of the plate is to provide a buttress against posterior subluxation of the ulna (**Figure 6**). If screw fixation is used from a posterior to an anterior direction, this can be more accurately done while using an anterior cruciate ligament drill guide. Usually, a minimum of two screws are used for adequate fracture stabilization. After fixation of the coronoid, the LCL should be assessed and repaired to achieve ulnohumeral stability.

If there is severe comminution of the coronoid based on the CT scan, open reduction and rigid fixation of the fragments may be unsuccessful. This type of injury can be approached by reducing the elbow joint in the operating room, repairing the LCL, and applying an external fixator (static or hinged fixator) to maintain stability while the LCL and the comminuted area of the coronoid heal (**Figure 7**). Comminuted fragments of the coronoid also can be reduced and relatively stabilized with small-diameter Kirschner wires, with the elbow joint forces neutralized by the external fixator until healing.

Outcomes

There are few reports in the literature on the outcomes of coronoid process fractures because these fractures rarely occur in isolation. A recent study evaluated 103 coronoid fractures.[60] In this study, most coronoid fractures were associated with other injuries, either bony or ligamentous. Doornberg and Ring[59] examined 18 patients who were treated for anteromedial coronoid facet fractures. Anteromedial plate fixation was used in nine patients, and seven were treated nonsurgically. On follow-up, 6 of the 18 patients had malalignment of the ulnohumeral joint, which resulted in partial varus subluxation and ulnohumeral arthrosis. When the coronoid fracture was secured and healed, good elbow function resulted. This study also emphasized the importance of identifying and treating a significant coronoid fracture discovered during complex elbow trauma.

Monteggia-Type Injuries

Monteggia fractures were initially described by Monteggia[61] in 1814 as an anterior dislocation of the radial head in association with a fracture of the ulnar shaft. Bado[62] coined the term "Monteggia lesions" to describe any fracture of the ulna associated with a dislocation of the radiocapitellar joint and provided a classification for these injuries.

Classification

Bado[62] classified Monteggia fractures as type I, anterior dislocation of the radial head with fracture of the diaphysis of the ulna with anterior angulation of the ulna fracture; type II, posterior or posterolateral dislocation of the radial head with fracture of the ulnar diaphysis with posterior angulation of the ulna fracture; type III, lateral or anterolateral dislocation of the radial head with fracture of the ulnar metaphysis; and type IV, anterior dislocation of the radial head with a fracture of the proximal third of the radius and the ulna at the same level.

In 1991, Jupiter et al[63] further subdivided Bado type II lesions because of their higher prevalence in adults. These fractures were subclassified as type IIA, a fracture at the level of the greater sigmoid notch; type IIB, an ulna fracture at the metaphyseal-diaphyseal junction, distal to the coronoid; type IIC, a diaphyseal ulna fracture; and type IID, comminuted fractures involving more than one region.

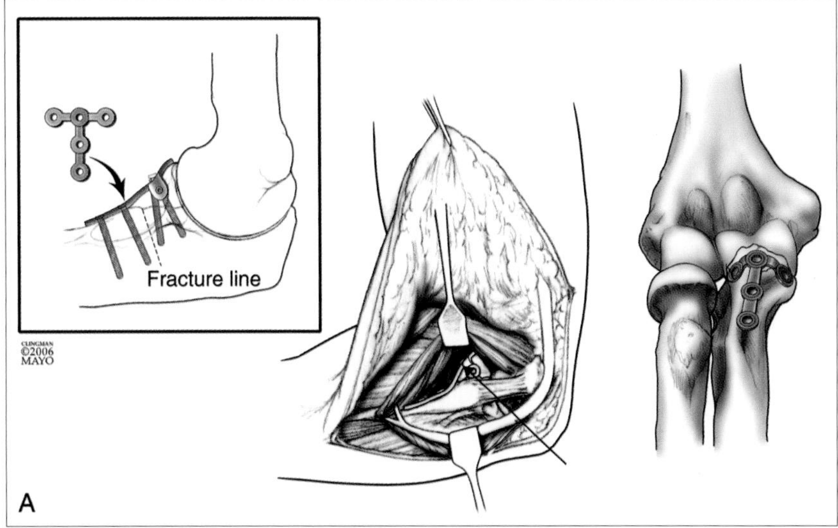

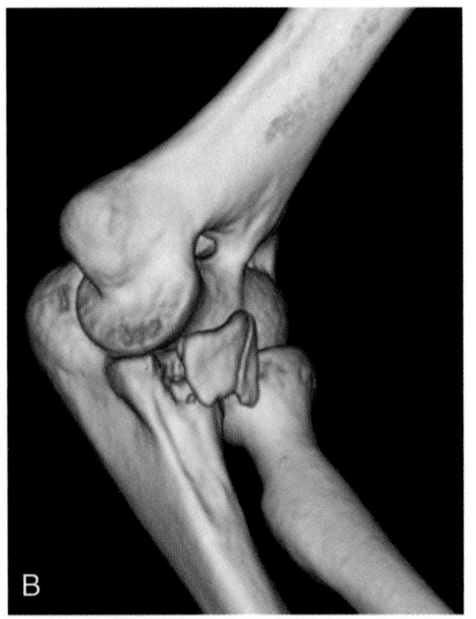

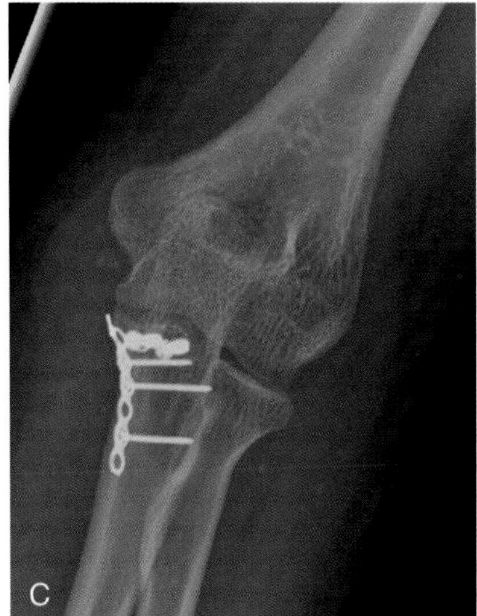

Figure 6 **A,** Illustrations showing plate positioning on the coronoid process. Lateral view of plate fixation (left); plate reduction (arrow) of the coronoid fracture (center); and anterior view of plate fixation (right). (Reproduced with permission from the Mayo Foundation for Medical Education and Research, Rochester, MN.) The fixation of large coronoid fractures may be accomplished with plates and/or cannulated screws. **B,** Three-dimensional CT scan showing a large coronoid fracture. **C,** Postoperative AP radiograph showing combined plate and screw fixation.

Imaging

Orthogonal radiographs of the elbow, forearm, and wrist are mandatory to characterize the injury pattern. Typically, the ulnar fracture is easily identified; however, it can occasionally be difficult to fully appreciate the exact fracture pattern of the ulna on plain radiographs. The radial head fracture or dislocation can be subtle, especially after reduction of the radial head dislocation. CT scans, particularly three-dimensional reconstructions, can be helpful in determining the extent of the bony injury and the location of the fracture fragments. Three-dimensional reconstructions are particularly helpful in identifying fractures involving the coronoid, the olecranon, and the radial head (**Figure 8**).

Management

Monteggia fractures in adults require surgery. The initial management of these patients should define the injury pattern and any associated injuries. The fracture-dislocation should be reduced and stabilized in a long arm posterior splint. The integrity of the skin and the neurovascular status of the extremity should be monitored.

Repeated attempts to reduce the radial head should be avoided. The stability of the radial head is dictated by the ulnar fracture. Comminution of the ulnar fracture affecting the longitu-

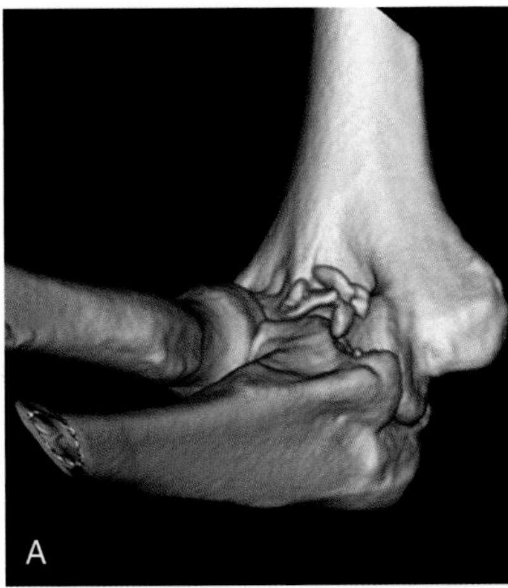

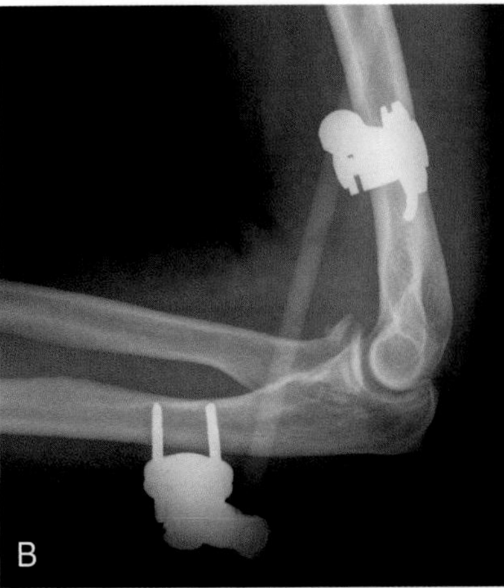

Figure 7 **A,** Three-dimensional CT scan of a severely comminuted anteromedial coronoid fracture treated with LCL repair. **B,** Lateral radiograph showing static external fixation to allow healing of the ligaments and bony comminution.

dinal stability of the ulna will require the radial head to remain dislocated. Repeated attempts to reduce the radial head will further traumatize the soft tissues and theoretically increases the risk of heterotopic ossification.

The timing of surgery depends on the condition of the soft tissues and the availability of necessary equipment and personnel. Potential equipment requirements include small fragment plates and screws or an anatomic plating system, a minifragment fixation system, headless compression screws, threaded Kirschner wires, fluoroscopy, and a radial head replacement system. Bone graft (allograft or autograft) or bone graft substitutes may also be required.

Patients can be placed in the supine or lateral decubitus position. The lateral decubitus position with the arm over a padded arm support is preferred because the deforming effect of gravity is eliminated. A midline posterior skin incision placed lateral to the tip of the olecranon is used, and full-thickness fasciocutaneous flaps are elevated. The interval between the flexor carpi ulnaris and the anconeus is developed along the subcutaneous border of the ulna to expose the fracture site. The amount of dissection required for exposure is dictated by the fracture pattern and the type of fixation to be used. Subperiosteal dissection of the flexor carpi ulnaris along the medial wall of the ulna will typically allow enough exposure to treat an associated fracture of the coronoid and/or medial wall of the ulna. If fixation of the radial head is required, the anconeus can be mobilized more extensively through a Boyd approach. If the ulna fracture permits, the radial head can be fixed through the fracture bed of the ulna before definitive fixation of the ulna. After the ulna is fixed, access to the radial head is not possible.

Fixation Techniques

Because the repaired or replaced radial head can help establish the ulnar length by reestablishing the integrity of the lateral part of the forearm, associated radial head fractures are typically fixed before the ulna fracture. If the lesser sigmoid notch of the ulna is involved, it can be difficult to determine radial length when radial head replacement is required. In this situation, the ulna fracture may need to be fixed before the radius to establish appropriate radial head sizing. A variety of fixation options and a radial head replacement system should be available if a radial head fracture is present.

Plate fixation is required for ulnar fractures associated with Monteggia-type injuries. When ulnar fractures occur distal to the coronoid, the plate can be applied laterally or along the subcutaneous border of the ulna. Lateral plate placement is preferred by some surgeons to prevent hardware prominence; however, this chapter's authors recommend posterior plate placement. Anatomic alignment of the ulna is critical to obtaining reduction of the radial head and a stable joint. Failure to reestablish ulnar geometry can result in persistent subluxation or dislocation of the radial head (**Figure 9**).

Fractures extending proximally to involve the coronoid require that the plate be placed on the subcutaneous border of the ulna to accommodate the complex geometry of this region. If the fracture involves significant comminution, a supplemental medial or lateral plate may be helpful. It is critical to fully appreciate the extent of coronoid involvement.

In general, the ulna fracture is reconstructed from distal to proximal. The fracture is reconstructed by fixing the distal fragments, which may require interfragmentary fixation or subarticular Kirschner wires. As fixation progresses proximally, reconstruction of the coronoid and the greater sigmoid notch is performed. Larger fragments can be fixed with interfragmentary screws from the dorsal aspect of the ulna or can be provisionally fixed with threaded wires and ultimately definitively fixed after the plate is applied to the subcutaneous aspect of the ulna. The final fragment to be fixed is the proximal olecranon fragment. The attached triceps will obscure fracture reduction if reduced before distal reconstruction.

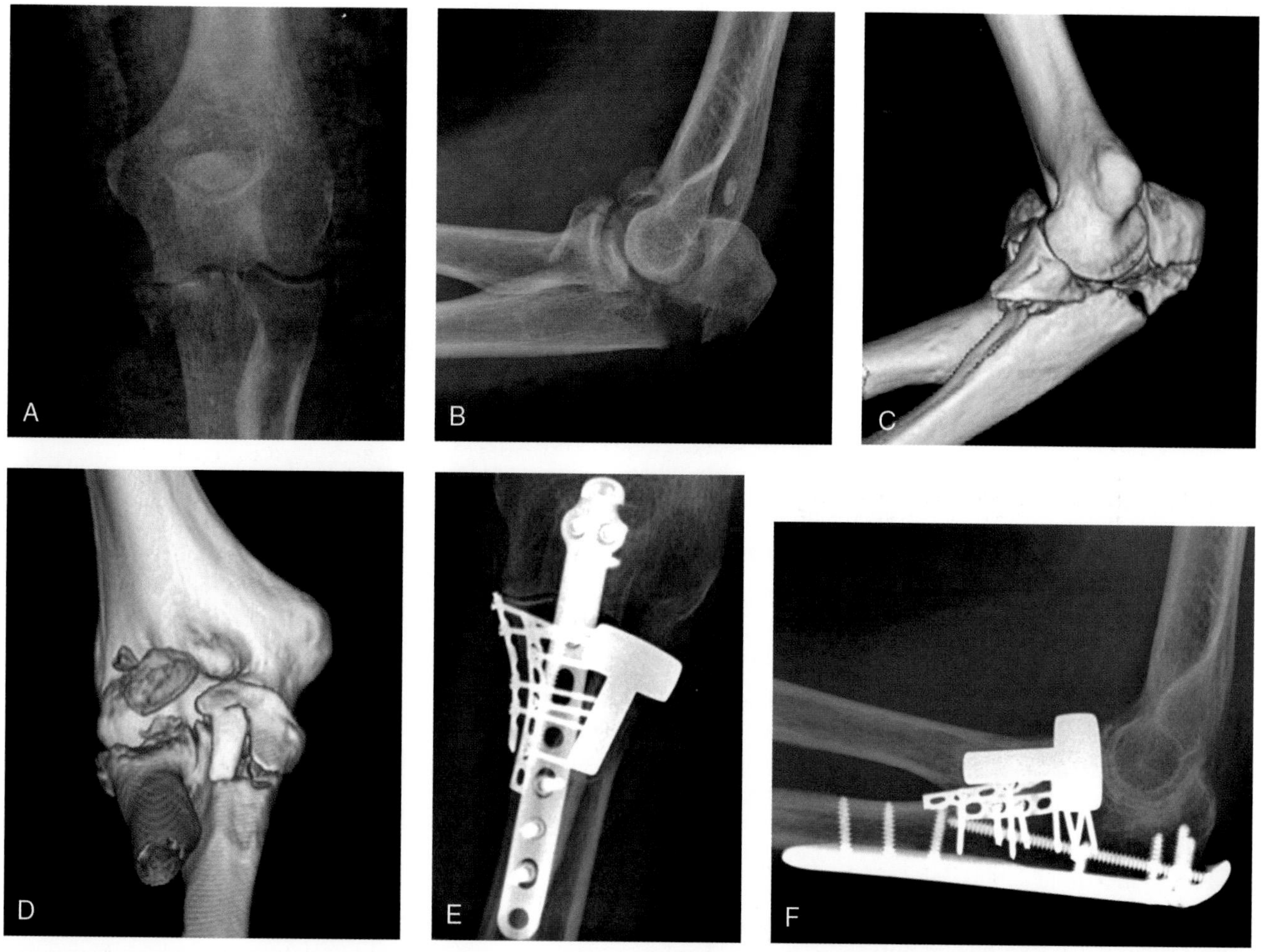

Figure 8 AP (**A**) and lateral (**B**) radiographs of an elbow fracture-dislocation that inadequately characterized the extent of bony injury. Lateral (**C**) and AP (**D**) three-dimensional CT scans show the comminuted radial head fracture and the associated basal coronoid fracture. AP (**E**) and lateral (**F**) radiographs after open reduction and internal fixation of the proximal ulna and coronoid with radial head replacement. A satisfactory outcome with functional range of motion was achieved.

Postoperatively, the arm is splinted in nearly full extension with an anteriorly applied plaster slab to reduce pressure on the posterior soft tissues. Active or active-assisted flexion and gravity-assisted extension exercises are started after the surgical dressings are removed.

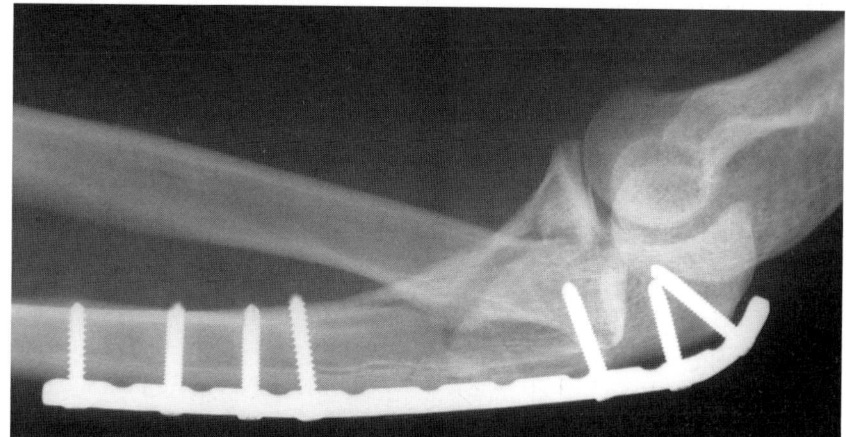

Figure 9 Lateral radiograph showing malunion of the ulna with apex dorsal angulation resulting in dislocation of the radial head.

Outcomes

Historically, the surgical treatment results of Monteggia fracture-dislocations have been unpredictable; however, the advent of rigid internal fixation has improved outcomes.[63-68] Konrad et al[68] found that certain factors, such as a Bado type II injury, a

Jupiter type IIA injury, fracture of the radial head, coronoid fracture, and complications requiring further surgery are associated with poor clinical results.

Complications

Complications following the treatment of Monteggia fracture-dislocations are common. A multicenter study by Reynders et al[69] showed a 43% complication rate, with an unsatisfactory outcome in 46% of the adult patients treated for Monteggia fracture-dislocations.

Nerve injuries associated with Monteggia injuries most commonly involve the posterior interosseous nerve, whereas median and ulnar nerve injuries are much less common. Malreduction or malunion is most commonly associated with type II fractures with anterior comminution that is not appreciated or treated. Malreduction or malunion of the ulna must be considered if radial head subluxation persists. Nonunion is associated with inadequate internal fixation and infection and has a higher incidence with type 2 injuries. These fractures require compression plate fixation. In general, semitubular and reconstruction plates are not recommended because of their insufficient strength.

Heterotopic ossification is common after the surgical treatment of Monteggia injuries and may lead to loss of motion or radioulnar synostosis. Radioulnar synostosis more commonly occurs with high-energy injuries with radial head/neck fracture and ulnar comminution at the same level.

Summary

The treatment of simple and complex elbow instability requires an understanding of the bony and ligamentous anatomy of the elbow, the contributions of elbow structures to stability, the natural history of these injuries, and the various surgical approaches and techniques. Surgeons must critically examine radiographs and advanced imaging modalities to determine the extent of bony and ligamentous injuries. Once classified, a systematic approach should be followed to optimize outcomes and minimize complications. A primary treatment goal is the restoration of the critical anatomy with sufficient stability to initiate early range of motion, which has been shown to be a key factor for a successful outcome.

References

1. Linscheid RL, Wheeler DK: Elbow dislocations. *JAMA* 1965; 194(11):1171-1176.
2. Hull JR, Owen JR, Fern SE, Wayne JS, Boardman ND III: Role of the coronoid process in varus osteoarticular stability of the elbow. *J Shoulder Elbow Surg* 2005;14(4):441-446.
3. Schneeberger AG, Sadowski MM, Jacob HA: Coronoid process and radial head as posterolateral rotatory stabilizers of the elbow. *J Bone Joint Surg Am* 2004; 86-A(5):975-982.
4. Beingessner DM, Dunning CE, Gordon KD, Johnson JA, King GJ: The effect of radial head excision and arthroplasty on elbow kinematics and stability. *J Bone Joint Surg Am* 2004; 86-A(8):1730-1739.
5. Beingessner DM, Dunning CE, Stacpoole RA, Johnson JA, King GJ: The effect of coronoid fractures on elbow kinematics and stability. *Clin Biomech (Bristol, Avon)* 2007;22(2):183-190.
6. Beingessner DM, Stacpoole RA, Dunning CE, Johnson JA, King GJ: The effect of suture fixation of type I coronoid fractures on the kinematics and stability of the elbow with and without medial collateral ligament repair. *J Shoulder Elbow Surg* 2007;16(2): 213-217.
7. O'Driscoll SW, Morrey BF, Korinek S, An KN: Elbow subluxation and dislocation: A spectrum of instability. *Clin Orthop Relat Res* 1992;280:186-197.
8. Kazuki K, Miyamoto T, Ohzono K: A case of traumatic divergent fracture-dislocation of the elbow combined with Essex-Lopresti lesion in an adult. *J Shoulder Elbow Surg* 2005;14(2): 224-226.
9. Hildebrand KA, Patterson SD, King GJ: Acute elbow dislocations: Simple and complex. *Orthop Clin North Am* 1999;30(1): 63-79.
10. Mehlhoff TL, Noble PC, Bennett JB, Tullos HS: Simple dislocation of the elbow in the adult: Results after closed treatment. *J Bone Joint Surg Am* 1988;70(2): 244-249.
11. Protzman RR: Dislocation of the elbow joint. *J Bone Joint Surg Am* 1978;60(4):539-541.
12. Schippinger G, Seibert FJ, Steinböck J, Kucharczyk M: Management of simple elbow dislocations: Does the period of immobilization affect the eventual results? *Langenbecks Arch Surg* 1999;384(3):294-297.
13. Josefsson PO, Gentz CF, Johnell O, Wendeberg B: Surgical versus non-surgical treatment of ligamentous injuries following dislocation of the elbow joint: A prospective randomized study. *J Bone Joint Surg Am* 1987;69(4): 605-608.
14. Maripuri SN, Debnath UK, Rao P, Mohanty K: Simple elbow dislocation among adults: A comparative study of two different methods of treatment. *Injury* 2007;38(11):1254-1258.
15. Micic I, Kim SY, Park IH, Kim PT, Jeon IH: Surgical management of unstable elbow dislocation without intra-articular frac-

ture. *Int Orthop* 2009;33(4): 1141-1147.

16. Forthman C, Henket M, Ring DC: Elbow dislocation with intra-articular fracture: The results of operative treatment without repair of the medial collateral ligament. *J Hand Surg Am* 2007; 32(8): 1200-1209.
17. McKee MD, Pugh DM, Wild LM, Schemitsch EH, King GJ: Standard surgical protocol to treat elbow dislocations with radial head and coronoid fractures: Surgical technique. *J Bone Joint Surg Am* 2005;87 (Pt 1, Suppl 1):22-32.
18. Mathew PK, Athwal GS, King GJ: Terrible triad injury of the elbow: Current concepts. *J Am Acad Orthop Surg* 2009;17(3): 137-151.
19. Duckworth AD, Kulijdian A, McKee MD, Ring D: Residual subluxation of the elbow after dislocation or fracture-dislocation: Treatment with active elbow exercises and avoidance of varus stress. *J Shoulder Elbow Surg* 2008;17(2): 276-280.
20. Martin BD, Johansen JA, Edwards SG: Complications related to simple dislocations of the elbow. *Hand Clin* 2008;24(1):9-25.
21. Ristic S, Strauch RJ, Rosenwasser MP: The assessment and treatment of nerve dysfunction after trauma around the elbow. *Clin Orthop Relat Res* 2000;370: 138-153.
22. Broberg MA, Morrey BF: Results of treatment of fracture-dislocations of the elbow. *Clin Orthop Relat Res* 1987;216: 109-119.
23. Mason ML: Some observations on fractures of the head of the radius with a review of one hundred cases. *Br J Surg* 1954;42(172): 123-132.
24. Johnston GW: A follow-up of one hundred cases of fracture of the head of the radius with a review of the literature. *Ulster Med J* 1962; 31:51-56.
25. King GJ, Evans DC, Kellam JF: Open reduction and internal fixation of radial head fractures. *J Orthop Trauma* 1991;5(1):21-28.
26. Geel CW, Palmer AK, Ruedi T, Leutenegger AF: Internal fixation of proximal radial head fractures. *J Orthop Trauma* 1990;4(3): 270-274.
27. Ring D, Quintero J, Jupiter JB: Open reduction and internal fixation of fractures of the radial head. *J Bone Joint Surg Am* 2002; 84-A(10):1811-1815.
28. Akesson T, Herbertsson P, Josefsson PO, Hasserius R, Besjakov J, Karlsson MK: Primary nonoperative treatment of moderately displaced two-part fractures of the radial head. *J Bone Joint Surg Am* 2006;88(9):1909-1914.
29. Herbertsson P, Josefsson PO, Hasserius R, et al: Uncomplicated Mason type-II and III fractures of the radial head and neck in adults: A long-term follow-up study. *J Bone Joint Surg Am* 2004; 86-A(3):569-574.
30. Hotchkiss RN: Displaced fractures of the radial head: Internal fixation or excision? *J Am Acad Orthop Surg* 1997;5(1):1-10.
31. Lindenhovius AL, Felsch Q, Doornberg JN, Ring D, Kloen P: Open reduction and internal fixation compared with excision for unstable displaced fractures of the radial head. *J Hand Surg Am* 2007;32(5):630-636.
32. Pike JM, Athwal GS, Faber KJ, King GJ: Radial head fractures: An update. *J Hand Surg Am* 2009; 34(3):557-565.
33. Rosenblatt Y, Athwal GS, Faber KJ: Current recommendations for the treatment of radial head fractures. *Orthop Clin North Am* 2008;39(2):173-185.
34. Doornberg JN, Linzel DS, Zurakowski D, Ring D: Reference points for radial head prosthesis size. *J Hand Surg Am* 2006;31(1): 53-57.
35. Frank SG, Grewal R, Johnson J, Faber KJ, King GJ, Athwal GS: Determination of correct implant size in radial head arthroplasty to avoid overlengthening. *J Bone Joint Surg Am* 2009;91(7):1738-1746.
36. Rowland AS, Athwal GS, MacDermid JC, King GJ: Lateral ulnohumeral joint space widening is not diagnostic of radial head arthroplasty overstuffing. *J Hand Surg Am* 2007;32(5):637-641.
37. Shors HC, Gannon C, Miller MC, Schmidt CC, Baratz ME: Plain radiographs are inadequate to identify overlengthening with a radial head prosthesis. *J Hand Surg Am* 2008;33(3): 335-339.
38. Van Glabbeek F, Van Riet RP, Baumfeld JA, et al: Detrimental effects of overstuffing or understuffing with a radial head replacement in the medial collateral-ligament deficient elbow. *J Bone Joint Surg Am* 2004;86-A(12): 2629-2635.
39. van Riet RP, van Glabbeek F, de Weerdt W, Oemar J, Bortier H: Validation of the lesser sigmoid notch of the ulna as a reference point for accurate placement of a prosthesis for the head of the radius: A cadaver study. *J Bone Joint Surg Br* 2007;89(3):413-416.
40. Van Riet RP, Van Glabbeek F, Verborgt O, Gielen J: Capitellar erosion caused by a metal radial head prosthesis: A case report. *J Bone Joint Surg Am* 2004; 86-A(5):1061-1064.
41. Doornberg JN, Parisien R, van Duijn PJ, Ring D: Radial head arthroplasty with a modular metal spacer to treat acute traumatic elbow instability. *J Bone Joint Surg Am* 2007;89(5):1075-1080.
42. Furry KL, Clinkscales CM: Comminuted fractures of the radial head: Arthroplasty versus internal

fixation. *Clin Orthop Relat Res* 1998;353:40-52.

43. Grewal R, MacDermid JC, Faber KJ, Drosdowech DS, King GJ: Comminuted radial head fractures treated with a modular metallic radial head arthroplasty: Study of outcomes. *J Bone Joint Surg Am* 2006;88(10):2192-2200.

44. Harrington IJ, Sekyi-Otu A, Barrington TW, Evans DC, Tuli V: The functional outcome with metallic radial head implants in the treatment of unstable elbow fractures: A long-term review. *J Trauma* 2001;50(1):46-52.

45. Moro JK, Werier J, MacDermid JC, Patterson SD, King GJ: Arthroplasty with a metal radial head for unreconstructible fractures of the radial head. *J Bone Joint Surg Am* 2001;83-A(8): 1201-1211.

46. Beingessner DM, Dunning CE, Gordon KD, Johnson JA, King GJ: The effect of radial head fracture size on elbow kinematics and stability. *J Orthop Res* 2005; 23(1): 210-217.

47. Hotchkiss RN: Fractures and dislocations of the elbow, in Rockwood G, Bucholz RW, Heckman JD, eds: *Rockwood and Green's Fractures in Adults*, ed 4. Philadelphia, PA, Lippincott-Raven, 1996, pp 929-1024.

48. Pugh DM, McKee MD: The "terrible triad" of the elbow. *Tech Hand Up Extrem Surg* 2002;6(1): 21-29.

49. Pugh DM, Wild LM, Schemitsch EH, King GJ, McKee MD: Standard surgical protocol to treat elbow dislocations with radial head and coronoid fractures. *J Bone Joint Surg Am* 2004;86-A(6):1122-1130.

50. McKee MD, Schemitsch EH, Sala MJ, O'Driscoll SW: The pathoanatomy of lateral ligamentous disruption in complex elbow instability. *J Shoulder Elbow Surg* 2003;12(4):391-396.

51. Regan W, Morrey B: Fractures of the coronoid process of the ulna. *J Bone Joint Surg Am* 1989;71(9): 1348-1354.

52. Adams JE, Kallina IV CF, Amrami KK, Steinmann SP: Abstract: Coronoid fracture morphology. *75th Annual Meeting Proceedings.* Rosemont, IL, American Academy of Orthopaedic Surgeons, 2008, p 593.

53. O'Driscoll SW, Jupiter JB, Cohen MS, Ring D, McKee MD: Difficult elbow fractures: Pearls and pitfalls. *Instr Course Lect* 2003;52:113-134.

54. Doornberg JN, de Jong IM, Lindenhovius AL, Ring D: The anteromedial facet of the coronoid process of the ulna. *J Shoulder Elbow Surg* 2007;16(5):667-670.

55. Sanchez-Sotelo J, O'Driscoll SW, Morrey BF: Anteromedial fracture of the coronoid process of the ulna. *J Shoulder Elbow Surg* 2006; 15(5):e5-e8.

56. Sanchez-Sotelo J, O'Driscoll SW, Morrey BF: Medial oblique compression fracture of the coronoid process of the ulna. *J Shoulder Elbow Surg* 2005;14(1):60-64.

57. Cohen MS: Fractures of the coronoid process. *Hand Clin* 2004; 20(4):443-453.

58. Doornberg JN, Ring D: Coronoid fracture patterns. *J Hand Surg Am* 2006;31(1):45-52.

59. Doornberg JN, Ring DC: Fracture of the anteromedial facet of the coronoid process. *J Bone Joint Surg Am* 2006;88(10):2216-2224.

60. Adams JE, Hoskin TL, Morrey BF, Steinmann SP: Management and outcome of 103 acute fractures of the coronoid process of the ulna. *J Bone Joint Surg Br* 2009;91(5):632-635.

61. Monteggia GB: *Instituzioni Chirurgiche*, Milan, Italy, Maspero, 1814.

62. Bado JL: The Monteggia lesion. *Clin Orthop Relat Res* 1967; 50:71-86.

63. Jupiter JB, Leibovic SJ, Ribbans W, Wilk RM: The posterior Monteggia lesion. *J Orthop Trauma* 1991;5(4):395-402.

64. Bruce HE, Harvey JP, Wilson JC Jr: Monteggia fractures. *J Bone Joint Surg Am* 1974; 56(8):1563-1576.

65. Reckling FW: Unstable fracture-dislocations of the forearm (Monteggia and Galeazzi lesions). *J Bone Joint Surg Am* 1982;64(6): 857-863.

66. Reckling FW, Cordell LD: Unstable fracture-dislocations of the forearm: The Monteggia and Galeazzi lesions. *Arch Surg* 1968; 96(6):999-1007.

67. Boyd HB, Boals JC: The Monteggia lesion: A review of 159 cases. *Clin Orthop Relat Res* 1969;66: 94-100.

68. Konrad GG, Kundel K, Kreuz PC, Oberst M, Sudkamp NP: Monteggia fractures in adults: Long-term results and prognostic factors. *J Bone Joint Surg Br* 2007;89(3):354-360.

69. Reynders P, De Groote W, Rondia J, Govaerts K, Stoffelen D, Broos PL: Monteggia lesions in adults: A multicenter Bota study. *Acta Orthop Belg* 1996;62 (Suppl 1):78-83.

19

The Recurrent Unstable Elbow: Diagnosis and Treatment

Anand M. Murthi, MD
Jay D. Keener, MD
April D. Armstrong, MD
Charles L. Getz, MD

Abstract

The elbow is a difficult joint to treat because of the subtle nuances involved in pathology, examination, and treatment. Patients experiencing the sequelae of recurrent elbow instability can lose substantial function in the affected upper extremity. Elbow instability comprises a wide spectrum of diseases, ranging from valgus instability in the throwing athlete to traumatic recurrent rotatory instability to iatrogenic damage. For the orthopaedic surgeon to develop a systematic algorithm for treating elbow instability disorders, it is necessary to understand the basic elbow biomechanics and the alterations that occur in the unstable elbow. A thorough knowledge of the history, physical examination techniques, and imaging studies necessary to diagnose these injury patterns is also needed. Cutting-edge advances in the surgical reconstruction of the unstable elbow will allow those caring for patients with these difficult injuries to make the proper management decisions.

Instr Course Lect 2011;60:215-226.

Biomechanics of Elbow Stability

The elbow joint is a stable articulation comprising the distal humeral, proximal ulnar, and proximal radial articular surfaces. The stabilizers of the elbow are classified as having primary or secondary roles. The primary stabilizers include the conformity of the articular surfaces (both the ulnohumeral and the radiocapitellar articulations), the anterior bundle of the medial ulnar collateral ligament, and the lateral collateral ligament complex. The articular conformity of the ulnohumeral joint arises from the mating of the trochlea of the distal part of the humerus to the greater sigmoid notch of the ulna. This articulation is augmented by the presence of a guiding ridge within the greater sigmoid notch that articulates with the trochlear sulcus. The anterior aspect of the ulnohumeral joint is supported by the coronoid process located at the distal aspect of the greater sigmoid notch. The relative contributions of the articular surfaces and the soft-tissue restraints about the elbow depend on the angle of elbow flexion and the type of force (varus or valgus) applied to the joint.[1] Muscular forces augment osseous stability throughout all arcs of motion by generating joint compressive forces.

The lateral collateral ligament complex comprises the lateral ulnar collateral ligament, the radial collateral ligament, and the annular ligament. The lateral ligaments provide varus stability to the elbow and are the primary restraint to posterolateral rotational forces at the ulnohumeral joint.[2,3] These ligaments are not discrete anatomic and biomechanical structures, and they act in concert to provide stability to the elbow joint. The lateral ulnar collateral ligament and radial collateral ligament originate from the lateral epicondyle near the flexion-extension axis of the elbow. The radial collateral ligament is isometric; however, the lateral ulnar collateral

Dr. Murthi or an immediate family member serves as a paid consultant to or is an employee of Zimmer and Ascension Orthopaedics and has received research or institutional support from Arthrex, DePuy, and Synthes. Dr. Getz or an immediate family member has received research or institutional support from Zimmer, Smith & Nephew, Johnson & Johnson, and Biomet. Neither of the following authors or any immediate family member has received anything of value from or owns stock in a commercial company or institution related directly or indirectly to the subject of this chapter: Dr. Keener and Dr. Armstrong.

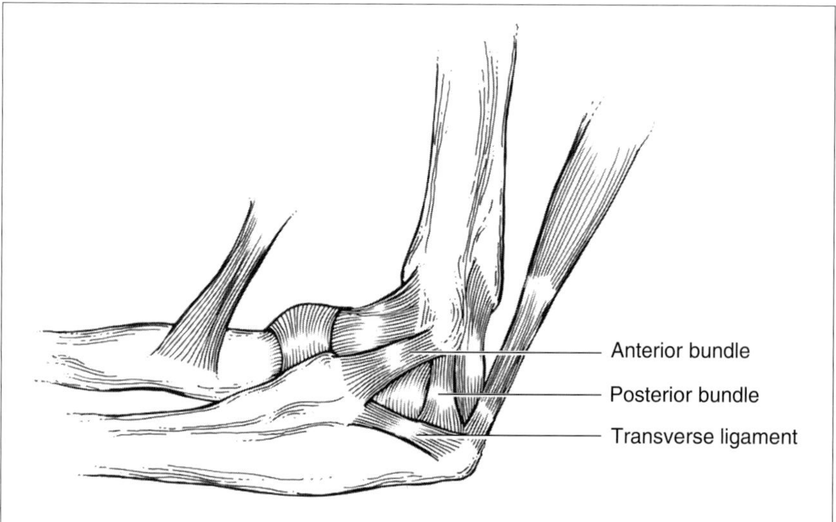

Figure 1 The medial collateral ligament of the elbow. (Reproduced with permission from Bryce CD, Armstrong AD: Anatomy and biomechanics of the elbow. *Orthop Clin North Am* 2008;39(2):141-154.)

capsule, and the muscular forces around the joint. The radial head is an important contributor to elbow stability. In light of the valgus angulation of the elbow, it is estimated that, in full extension, 60% of the joint reactive forces occur at the radiocapitellar articulation.[17] The radial head augments valgus stability of the elbow, particularly in the presence of an incompetent medial ulnar collateral ligament complex.[18] In addition, the radial head provides some restraint to posterolateral rotatory forces at the elbow.[19] The anterior and posterior aspects of the capsule consist of relatively thin, weak tissue and play a smaller but probably important role in elbow stability. The anterior aspect of the capsule makes its greatest contribution to stability in terminal elbow extension; it provides the greatest resistance to distraction forces, and an equal contribution to valgus stability, compared with the roles of the medial ulnar collateral ligament complex and the osseous anatomy.

ligament loosens in elbow extension and becomes more taut with increasing elbow flexion.[4] Biomechanical studies of cadavers have shown that both the lateral ulnar collateral ligament and the radial collateral ligament must be injured to compromise the stability offered by the lateral collateral ligament complex.[5-8]

The primary valgus stabilizer of the elbow is the medial ulnar collateral ligament complex. This ligament complex is divided into the anterior oblique ligament (the anterior bundle of the medial ulnar collateral ligament complex), the posterior oblique ligament, and the transverse ligament[9,10] (**Figure 1**). The anterior bundle of the medial ulnar collateral ligament complex arises from the deep anterior aspect of the medial epicondyle at the flexion-extension axis of the elbow and inserts near the sublime tubercle of the ulna at the base of the medial aspect of the coronoid process. The anterior bundle of the medial ulnar collateral ligament complex is the primary valgus stabilizer of the elbow.[11-14] This ligament is functionally divided into the anterior and posterior bands. The anterior band is taut for the first 60° of elbow flexion, and the posterior band is taut from 60° to 120° of flexion. This provides a reciprocal function of resisting valgus forces at various ranges of flexion and extension motion.[3,13] Although it has been theorized that there is an isometric central band to the anterior bundle of the medial ulnar collateral ligament complex, a recent study showed that there was no true isometric portion of this ligament.[11,15] Injuries to the anterior bundle of the medial ulnar collateral ligament complex are primarily related to attritional stress from repetitive throwing. These stresses are greatest during the early acceleration phase of throwing, producing up to 64 Nm of valgus torque at the elbow,[16] which is believed to exceed the ultimate tensile strength of the medial ulnar collateral ligament complex. These data highlight the importance of other joint stabilizers and dynamic muscular forces in buffering the large valgus moments that occur with throwing.

The secondary stabilizers of the elbow joint include the radial head, the anterior and posterior aspects of the

Muscular forces across the elbow are important augmenters of elbow stability. Forces from the brachialis, biceps, and triceps muscles augment osseous stability through joint compression and increase varus and valgus stability independent of the position of the forearm.[20] The common wrist extensors have imparted substantial stability to the lateral aspect of the elbow in cadaver testing.[2,21] On the medial aspect of the joint, the flexor-pronator muscles, particularly the flexor carpi ulnaris and flexor digitorum superficialis, augment valgus stability at the elbow.[22-25] These muscles are particularly important in throwers; the torque across the medial aspect of the elbow during the throwing motion is estimated to exceed the ultimate strength of the anterior band of the medial collateral ligament. Despite the theoretic benefit of flexor-pronator-mass muscle activity in protecting the medial ulnar collateral ligament complex, some clinical electromyographic studies have failed to show compensatory activity of these muscles in throwing athletes.[26,27]

Injury Mechanisms and Pathomechanics

Substantial trauma is generally necessary to subluxate or dislocate an elbow. Most initial elbow instability injuries are the result of a fall onto an outstretched hand. This mechanism most commonly results in a pattern of injury termed posterolateral instability.[28] Typically, the elbow is slightly flexed, and the forearm is pronated as the hand contacts the ground. The humerus rotates internally around the fixed forearm, imparting a valgus and external rotation (supination) moment to the elbow. If the force is sufficient, the ulna and radius will rotate and displace posterolaterally on the distal part of the humerus. In one report, surgical evaluation of both simple and complex elbow dislocations showed disruption of the lateral collateral ligament complex in all elbows, with proximal avulsion being the most common injury pattern.[29] The common extensor tendons were injured in 66% of the cases, and the anterior bundle of the medial collateral ligament was disrupted in 50% of the cases.

A predictable pattern of capsular and ligamentous injury must occur for the proximal parts of the ulna and radius to subluxate or dislocate.[2,28,30] The soft-tissue injury begins at the lateral collateral ligament complex and the common wrist extensor origin. There are three stages of posterolateral elbow instability. In stage 1, the lateral tissues are disrupted (a proximal avulsion typically occurs off the lateral epicondyle), allowing the ulna and radius to subluxate. In stage 2, the soft-tissue injury propagates to the anterior and posterior aspects of the capsule, allowing the proximal part of the ulna and the coronoid to perch under the distal humeral articular surface. In stage 3, there is a complete posterolateral dislocation of the ulna and the radius. This stage is divided according to the integrity of the anterior band of the medial collateral ligament. In stage 3A injuries, the medial collateral ligament remains intact, and the proximal parts of the ulna and radius dislocate and pivot around the intact medial ligaments. In stage 3B injuries, the anterior band of the medial collateral ligament is disrupted, typically resulting in a fixed dislocation with wide displacement of the articular surfaces. Associated elbow fractures are commonly associated with injuries that produce a dislocation of the elbow.

Residual laxity is more likely when the lateral ligaments are injured than when the medial collateral ligaments are injured. This is possibly caused by chronic tensile gravitational loads on the lateral aspect of the elbow, especially when the arm is abducted with varus force across the elbow. Although it is widely believed that the medial ligaments heal well after simple dislocations, in one study valgus stress testing showed laxity in 24 of 50 elbows after nonsurgical treatment.[31] Up to 15% to 35% of elbow dislocations are followed by recurrence of the instability, which is typically caused by much less energy than that producing the initial trauma.[32,33]

Posterolateral rotatory instability also occurs in association with a variety of predisposing situations. Attritional laxity of the lateral collateral ligaments can occur in elbows with a cubitus varus deformity, such as is seen after malunion of a supracondylar humeral fracture in a child.[34,35] Insufficiency of the lateral collateral ligaments has been reported in patients with lateral epicondylitis, and it is possibly secondary to repetitive corticosteroid injections.[36] Intensive débridement in the surgical treatment of lateral epicondylitis can weaken the lateral ligaments to the extent that the elbow becomes unstable. This complication can also occur after surgical management of a radial head fracture through the Kocher interval, especially if radial head resection is performed.[37-39]

Injuries to the medial collateral ligament are usually attritional and most often occur in overhead throwing athletes. The anterior band of the medial ulnar collateral ligament is the primary restraint to valgus moments. It is supplemented by dynamic muscular support from the flexor-pronator mass. Injuries to the medial ulnar collateral ligament are believed to be the result of cumulative stress from repetitive throwing. Occasionally, the medial collateral ligament ruptures as a result of acute trauma producing a severe valgus moment to the joint.[40] These injuries may or may not produce elbow dislocation and often occur in the context of avulsion of the flexor-pronator muscle mass and acute ulnar nerve symptoms.

History and Physical Examination

Most patients with recurrent posterolateral elbow instability recall a distinct injury that may have produced a complete dislocation. The chief symptom in patients with recurrent posterolateral instability is often subtle, consisting of position-dependent elbow pain or apprehension.[39] Occasionally, clunking, popping, and shifting sensations are felt when the elbow is extended, especially when an axial load is applied to the limb. Provocative activities include those that require forced elbow extension, such as pushing up from a chair or pushing a heavy object with an extended arm. Some patients describe a history consistent with repeated self-reductions.

Patients with symptomatic insufficiency of the medial collateral ligament usually have a gradual onset of symptoms. Some throwers relate the onset of pain to a single throwing event, occasionally accompanied by a painful "pop" in the elbow. More commonly, there is a gradual onset of pain at the medial aspect of the elbow during the acceleration phase of throwing. Frequently, the throwing athlete will have noticed a loss of velocity and control with certain pitches before having symptoms of instability. Typically, patients with medial collateral ligament insufficiency have few or no symptoms with activities of daily living or nonthrowing sports activities.

Most patients with recurrent elbow instability have posterolateral instability. On physical examination, the range of motion of the elbow and forearm is normal, and varus and valgus stress tests are usually not provocative. A variety of special tests have been developed to assess for posterolateral instability of the elbow. The pivot-shift test is designed to replicate the rotatory instability characteristics of this disorder.[41] To perform this test, the examiner stands at the head of the patient, who is supine. The patient's shoulder is flexed as the examiner braces the patient's elbow laterally with one hand and the patient's wrist with the other. The patient's forearm is supinated, and a valgus moment is applied to the patient's elbow. The examiner then slowly moves the patient's elbow from flexion to extension. The test is considered positive when there is subluxation of the elbow at 20° to 30° of extension. A sudden rotatory shift is felt, and the radial head becomes more prominent. Flexion from that point reduces the elbow. Frequently, a patient will not allow subluxation to occur because of pain or apprehension. Alternatively, the clinician can perform this test with the patient sitting. The examiner imparts a posterolateral drawer and supination force to the proximal part of the patient's forearm with the patient's elbow slightly flexed and the humerus stabilized.

Several functional tasks serve as clinical indicators of posterolateral instability. These tests include pushing up from a chair, the tabletop test, and attempting a push-up with the forearm supinated.[42,43] These tasks re-create apprehension or instability symptoms by simulating an axial load on the extending elbow with the forearm supinated. The test results are considered positive if the patient is reluctant to fully extend the loaded elbow. The diagnosis of posterolateral instability is sometimes based only on a clinical impression because the patient cannot tolerate the subluxation of the elbow. An examination performed with the patient under anesthesia will confirm the clinical suspicion of posterolateral instability and may be necessary before definitive treatment is initiated.

A careful physical examination of a throwing athlete with symptomatic insufficiency of the medial collateral ligament is important to facilitate decision making and care. The flexor-pronator mass is examined for tenderness and pain with strength testing. A careful evaluation of the shoulder should be performed, with the examiner focusing on rotator cuff and scapular stabilizer strength, identifying a glenohumeral internal rotation deficit, and analyzing pitching mechanics. The medial aspect of the elbow is examined for localized tenderness directly over the origin of the flexor-pronator mass, the sublime tubercle, the medial aspect of the olecranon, and the cubital tunnel. The range of motion of the elbow is usually preserved. The ulnar nerve should be assessed during elbow motion to rule out subluxation. Pain and tenderness in the posteromedial aspect of the elbow with valgus force into terminal extension can indicate valgus extension overload, which is another common cause of medial elbow pain in throwers.[44,45] Valgus stress testing is conducted with the elbow flexed from 20° to 30° (this unlocks the olecranon from the humerus) and the forearm pronated. Laxity is difficult to appreciate unless fluoroscopic images or stress radiographs are made, but the test is considered positive if the patient has pain with valgus stress. A medial ulnohumeral space opening of 3 mm or more compared with that of the contralateral elbow on valgus stress radiographs indicates medial collateral ligament insufficiency.

Two other tests for medial collateral ligament laxity are the milking maneuver and the moving valgus stress test.[46] The milking maneuver is done by pulling on the patient's thumb with the arm supinated and the elbow flexed beyond 90°, creating a valgus stress. For the moving valgus stress test, the arm is taken to maximal external rotation of the shoulder while the milking maneuver is done (**Figure 2**). The elbow is then flexed and extended with constant valgus torque, and the test is considered positive when the medial elbow pain is reproduced and is maximal between 70° and 120°.

Imaging

Standard radiographic images of patients with recurrent elbow instability include AP, lateral, and internal and external rotation oblique views. By definition, simple dislocations occur without associated elbow fractures. Occasionally, calcification or ossification is seen along the lateral epicondyle and within the substance of the lateral collateral ligaments or, in throwing athletes, the anterior band of the medial collateral ligament, but these are nonspecific findings. After an acute simple elbow dislocation has been reduced, the ulnohumeral joint is carefully inspected to confirm a concentric reduction. The presence of a "drop sign" after acute dislocation indicates an elbow with ligamentous and soft-tissue injury and an increased risk of recurrent instability.[47] A drop sign is a widening of the ulnohumeral joint and represents a subtle resting subluxation of the elbow joint. Radiographs should be inspected for avulsion fractures of the medial collateral ligament at the base of the medial epicondyle or the sublime tubercle. Stress radiographs or fluoroscopy are useful for patients with suspected medial collateral ligament insufficiency. Stress radiographs of patients with posterolateral instability are less reliable because of difficulty in reproducing the positions of instability and because of the onset of pain while the imaging study is conducted. Posterolateral instability can be assessed with fluoroscopy during an examination with the patient under anesthesia.

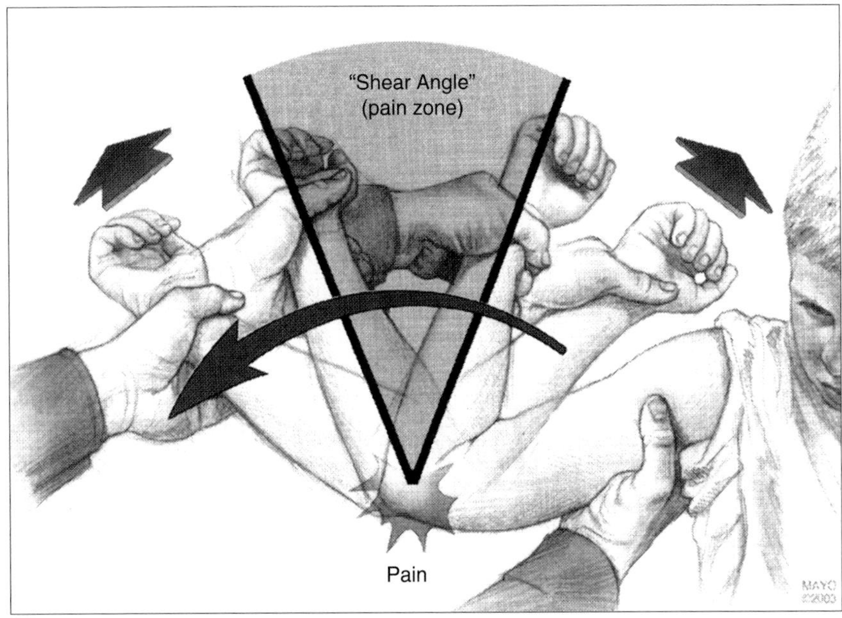

Figure 2 The moving valgus stress test. (Reproduced with permission from the Mayo Foundation of Medical Education and Research, Rochester, MN.)

MRI is indicated after an acute simple dislocation when a nonconcentric reduction is present and no cause for the persistent subluxation can be seen on a plain radiograph. Incarcerated cartilage fragments or soft tissue can be seen on the scan. MRI may also help in the evaluation of a patient who has elbow pain without an obvious cause, but it is not routinely performed in cases of suspected posterolateral instability because the lateral collateral ligament is a poorly defined structure.

MRI may help the clinician diagnose medial collateral ligament injuries. Disruption of the medial collateral ligament can be seen at the origin, at the insertion, or within the midsubstance of the tendon. Intra-articular contrast medium improves the accuracy of detecting partial articular-sided tears of the medial collateral ligament.[48,49] In addition, MRI identifies associated injuries to the radial head, capitellum, and flexor-pronator mass; stress fractures within the olecranon; and the presence of loose bodies and osteophytes. Dynamic ultrasonography is also used to evaluate the medial collateral ligament and can detect increased laxity with valgus instability.[50]

Medial Collateral Ligament Insufficiency of the Elbow

Background and Anatomy

The anterior and posterior bands of the medial ulnar collateral ligament complex tighten in a reciprocal fashion so that the anterior band is lax in extremes of flexion and the posterior band is lax in elbow extension.[11] The existence of a distinct central isometric band remains a point of controversy.[51,52] In one biomechanical study, a single 3-mm central band of the anterior bundle was sufficient to provide elbow stability[53] (**Figure 3**). This band is nearly mechanically isometric, and its origin lies very close to the anatomic axis of rotation of the elbow.[3,15] This concept becomes important clinically when the surgeon is considering single-point tunnel fixation on the ulna and medial epicondyle. To decrease tension in a medial collateral ligament reconstruction, the medial epicondyle drill hole should be located at the anatomic axis of rotation of the elbow.

Long-term studies of chronic elbow instability caused by a traumatic medial collateral ligament injury suggest that symptomatic arthritic changes develop over time in up to 50% of patients, and there is a 15% to 35% prevalence of symptomatic valgus instability.[31-33] Therefore, although it is known that many patients who do not participate in activities that require valgus loading of the elbow can live with an insufficient medial collateral ligament, the sequelae of this injury may not be as benign as was once believed.

Treatment

Initial treatment of chronic medial collateral ligament insufficiency (especially in athletes) focuses first on rest and anti-inflammatory drugs, and then there is gradual progression into an interval throwing program. Early

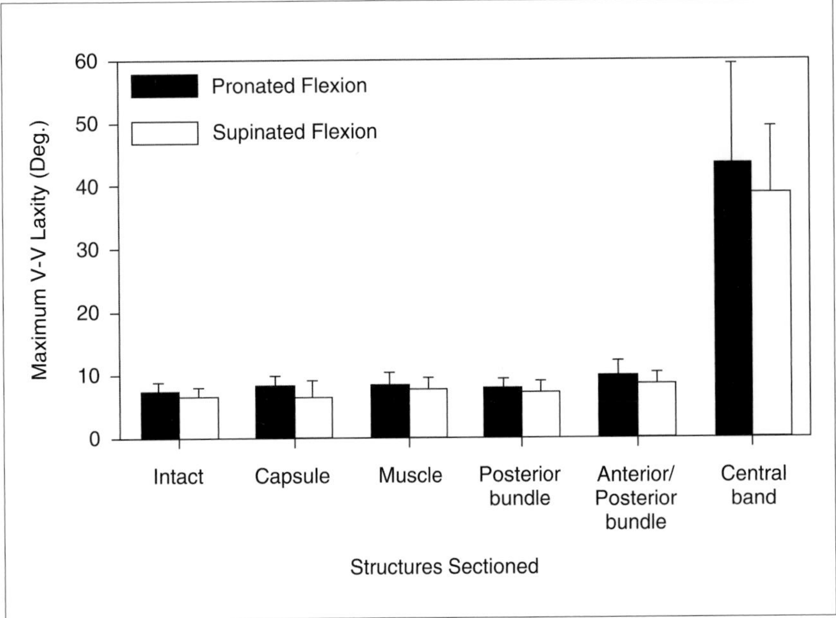

Figure 3 Sequential sectioning of the medial elbow valgus stabilizers does not result in valgus instability until the 3-mm central band of the anterior bundle of the medial collateral ligament has been cut. There was no significant difference between any of the sectioning sequences until the central band was cut ($P < 0.0001$). V-V = varus-valgus. (Reproduced with permission from Armstrong AD, Dunning CE, Faber KJ, Johnson JA, King GJ: Single-strand ligament reconstruction of the medial collateral ligament restores valgus elbow stability. *J Shoulder Elbow Surg* 2002;11(1):65-71.)

acute rehabilitation should focus on stretching and strengthening of the flexor-pronator mass, the rotator cuff, and the scapular stabilizers. Therapy then progresses to a comprehensive program involving normalization of the glenohumeral arc of motion through posterior shoulder stretching. The focus should be on improving strength and endurance of the flexor-pronator muscles and also on addressing core stability and lower-extremity strength and flexibility. Strengthening of the core musculature and the lower extremities plays an important role in transferring energy from the lower extremity to the upper extremity. The athlete then progresses into an interval throwing program. The Youth Baseball Athletes USA Baseball Medical and Safety Advisory Committee provides guidelines for specific pitch counts and rest periods.[54]

Close to 50% of all patients with a medial collateral ligament injury return to their sport within approximately 6 months following the initiation of nonsurgical treatment.[55] It is not possible to predict who will require surgery; therefore, a 3- to 6-month directed rehabilitative program is recommended. If nonsurgical treatment fails to control pain and allow a return to participation in sports, surgical reconstruction of the anterior bundle of the medial collateral ligament is recommended.

Medial collateral ligament reconstruction is either single stranded or two stranded. The first two-strand reconstruction, a figure-of-8 reconstruction, was described in 1986.[56] The exposure required release of the flexor-pronator group with an ulnar nerve transposition. It consisted of three drill holes in the medial epicondyle and two drill holes in the ulna, and the tendon graft was passed in a figure-of-8 fashion and sewn to itself. Approximately two thirds of patients returned to their sport after this procedure, but there was a 21% prevalence of ulnar nerve injury.[57] A late modification split the flexor-pronator mass and transposed the ulnar nerve only if clinically indicated. This modified approach was reported to result in a higher return to sports participation (74% to 81%) than the original method and only a 5% prevalence of ulnar nerve injury.[58,59]

Another flexor-pronator-mass-splitting technique involves use of a single drill hole in the medial epicondyle at the elbow's axis of rotation. Sutures are passed through two separate, smaller exit tunnels superiorly and anteriorly and are tied over an osseous bridge. This is called a "docking" method (**Figure 4**). The two drill holes in the ulna are the same as those originally described. The return-to-sports rate after this procedure has been reported to be 92% to 95%.[60-62]

Single-strand reconstruction has been shown to restore normal kinematics to the elbow.[53] Several fixation techniques have been described for single-strand reconstructions, including the use of interference screws, EndoButtons (Smith & Nephew, Memphis, TN), and no additional hardware. The interference construct provides stability similar to that of a native elbow.[63] A biomechanical study comparing four different reconstruction techniques showed that, with cyclic loading to failure, an EndoButton reconstruction technique was equivalent to the two-strand reconstructions and had a higher load to failure than an interference construct and the traditional figure-of-8 reconstruction.[64] The only other technique reported clinically (for single-strand reconstruction) is the DANE TJ hybrid technique, which involves placing an interference screw in the ulna with a docking procedure at the medial epicondyle. An 85% return-to-sports rate has been reported following that procedure.[65]

Graft choices for any of these reconstructions are at the surgeon's discretion. Palmaris longus, gracilis, plantaris, toe extensor, and Achilles autografts; allografts; and GraftJacket (Wright Medical Technology, Arlington, TN), an acellular dermal allograft, have all been used.

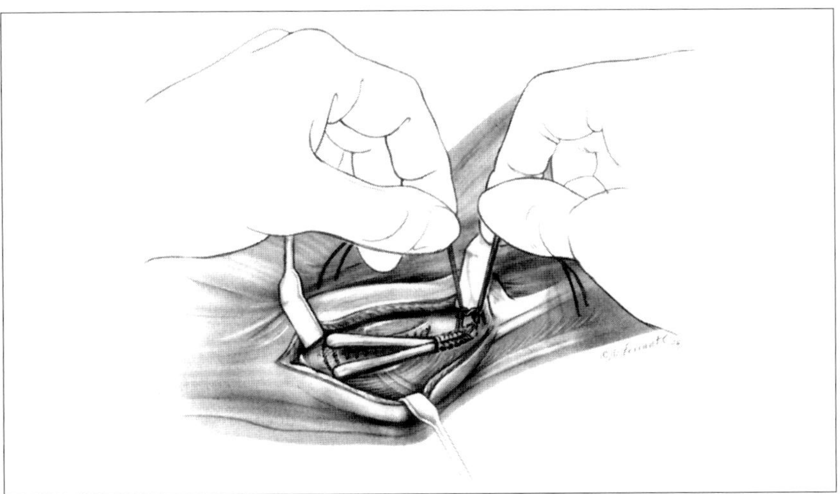

Figure 4 Docking reconstruction technique for treatment of medial collateral ligament insufficiency. (Reproduced with permission from Rohrbough JT, Altchek DW, Hyman J, Williams RJ III, Botts JD: Medial collateral ligament reconstruction of the elbow using the docking technique. *Am J Sports Med* 2002;30(4):541-548.)

Specific Surgical Technique

This chapter's authors recommend the flexor-pronator-mass-splitting approach.[66] In this technique, the flexor-pronator mass is split along its anterior two thirds and posterior one third. There is a palpable raphe that can be used to find the anterior bundle of the medial collateral ligament. An incision slightly posterior to the plane of the medial epicondyle helps to protect the medial cutaneous nerves. The sublime tubercle is identified for placement of the ulnar drill holes. For a two-strand technique, drill holes are placed anterior and posterior to the sublime tubercle with a 1-cm bone bridge. For a single-strand reconstruction, a single drill hole is created directly over the sublime tubercle. The elbow should be kept extended while the 4- or 5-mm holes are drilled into the ulna so that the ulnar nerve falls away from the drill bit. The drill is aimed away from the articular cartilage. The drill hole in the humerus should be at the anteroinferior aspect of the medial epicondyle, close to the trochlea, at the anatomic axis of rotation of the humerus.[15,67] Two smaller drill holes exit the far cortex of the medial epicondyle to create a bone bridge to tie the suture ends of the tendon.

After surgery, the elbow is placed in a soft cast, flexed to 90° with the forearm in supination. At 1 week, the soft cast is removed and the elbow is placed in a static removable splint with the forearm in supination, as forearm supination is the position of stability for the medial collateral ligament. Active motion and muscular contraction provide compressive stability to the elbow.[68] Thus, it is important that the patient actively move the elbow during therapy to provide the least stress on the medial collateral ligament reconstruction. Active-assisted range-of-motion exercises to full flexion and extension with the forearm in supination are begun and continued for 5 weeks. Active forearm pronation and supination are allowed with the elbow at 90°. At 6 weeks, the patient is weaned off the static splint, and a full active range of motion of the elbow is initiated. The patient starts a gradual strengthening program at 3 months and an interval throwing program at 9 to 12 months. With the possibility of the patient returning to competitive throwing, careful emphasis should be placed on body and throwing mechanics.

A systematic review of the treatment of medial collateral ligament injuries identified no prospective cohort or randomized controlled trials comparing reconstruction techniques.[69] The rate of return to sports was 83%, with the time until the return to sports ranging from 9.8 to 26.4 months. The complication rate was 10%, with ulnar nerve injury being the most common postoperative complication, occurring in 6% of cases. The muscle-splitting approaches have a lower complication rate. Compared with previous methods, the docking technique has been shown to result in a higher rate of return to sports and a lower complication rate. In summary, medial collateral ligament reconstruction is an effective treatment for valgus elbow instability in the throwing athlete. Future research and education should emphasize prevention, considering that the incidence in athletes seems to be increasing.[70]

Posterolateral Rotatory Instability of the Elbow

The radial head receives most of the attention in discussions of posterolateral rotatory instability because it is often easier to see malalignment between the radial head and the capitellum than it is to see malalignment of the ulnohumeral joint on plain radiographs. However, the primary cause of the instability is supination of the ulna away from the distal part of the humerus, and the lateral ulnar collateral ligament is the primary stabilizer preventing this instability. Therefore, treatment is aimed at restoring the integrity of the ulnohumeral stabilizers.

The radial head plays a role in rotatory stability, as the lateral ulnar collateral ligament courses around the radial head on its way to the ulna. This results in a mechanical block to the radial head, and the radial head helps to create tension in the lateral ulnar collateral ligament. Posterolateral rotational laxity increases by 145% after radial head excision.[71,72] Hall and McKee[37] identified a series of patients with posterolateral rotatory instability after a radial head resection. It is unclear whether the instability was caused by an unrecognized or iatrogenic lateral collateral ligament injury. In an experimental model, stability after isolated lateral collateral ligament reconstruction was found to be similar to that after lateral collateral ligament reconstruction with radial head replacement.[73]

Nonsurgical Management

Little has been written about the efficacy of nonsurgical treatment of patients with posterolateral rotatory instability. Treatment strategies include educating the patient about avoiding the most unstable positions of the upper extremity. Bracing can be used to stabilize the elbow and possibly limit motion, preventing the position of provocation. Physical therapy can strengthen the dynamic stabilizers and help the patient with coping strategies.

Surgical Techniques

Surgical treatment is focused on restoring rotational stability of the ulnohumeral joint by reconstructing the lateral ulnar collateral ligament. In cases of chronic recurrent posterolateral rotatory instability, grafting of the lateral ulnar collateral ligament has produced more reproducible results than has the use of local tissue. A native palmaris or plantaris graft, or allograft, is used. Novel techniques for arthroscopic imbrication and repair of the lateral collateral ligament complex are being developed.[74]

The patient is positioned supine with the arm on a hand table, and a nonsterile tourniquet is applied. A lateral approach over the lateral epicondyle that is sufficient to provide exposure from the supinator crest to the lateral column of the humerus while sparing the large cutaneous nerves is used. The antebrachial fascia is then incised just posterior to the lateral collateral ligament at the rolled edge of the extensor carpi ulnaris and the anconeus. The lateral collateral ligament is deep and anterior to the thickened rolled edge of the extensor carpi ulnaris. If the lateral collateral ligament has been previously avulsed, scarring might be present in the area. The lateral collateral ligament is incised parallel to the radial head and along the axis of the radial neck to allow visualization of the joint. The anconeus is swept posteriorly to allow placement of the ulnar tunnels. A hole is made with a 4-mm high-speed burr at the proximal portion of the supinator crest, a second hole is made more proximally and posteriorly at the insertion of the anular ligament with a bone bridge of at least 1 cm, and the graft is passed through the ulnar tunnel (**Figure 5**).

The humeral attachment of the lateral collateral ligament is at the isometric point of the lateral epicondyle. Although neither the native nor the reconstructed setting has a true isometric point, this so-called isometric point approximates a best fit.[75] It is at the center of a circle circumscribed along the contour of the capitellum. The other method for locating this point is to place a suture through the ulnar drill holes and apply the suture ends to the lateral epicondyle while moving the elbow through a range of motion (**Figure 6**). The isometric point is found when the sutures maintain the most constant tension through the arc of motion. The humeral drill hole should be placed so that the isometric point is at the distalmost and posteriormost part of the drill hole.

The graft can be attached to the humerus by either a figure-of-8 weave or the docking technique. The figure-of-8 weave requires the creation of diverging 4-mm tunnels from a 5-mm drill hole at the isometric point. The graft should be measured to allow the creation of a yoke with 1 cm of graft to recess into the condyle and a free limb of graft to pass through the humeral tunnel. The suture from the yoke will exit the humeral tunnel opposite the graft limb. The graft exiting the humerus can then be brought back through the opposite humeral tunnel. Before the graft is secured, the capsule should be repaired so that the graft lies extra-articularly. The elbow is reduced and placed in 45° of flexion with the forearm in pronation and with an axial load applied while the graft is secured.

The graft can also be secured to the humerus with a docking technique. The yoke is measured to allow at least 1 cm of tissue to recess into the humerus. Two small humeral tunnels are placed to accommodate the high-strength suture that is sewn to the yoke and brought through the humeral tunnels. The sutures are tied to tension and secure the graft.

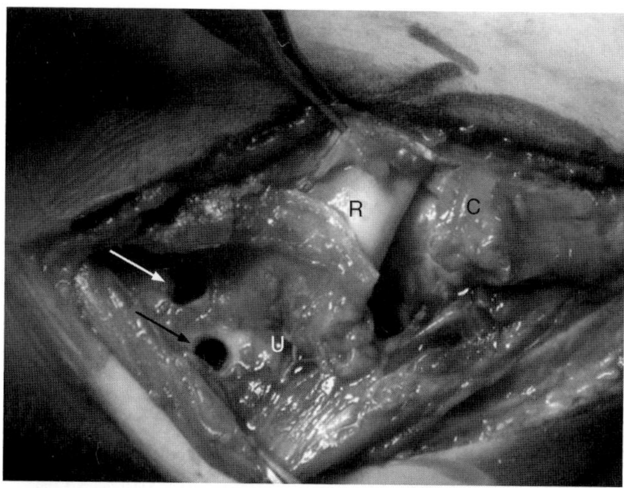

Figure 5 Tunnels (arrows) are placed in the ulna to re-create the broad insertion of the lateral collateral ligament. R = radial head, C = capitellum, U = ulna.

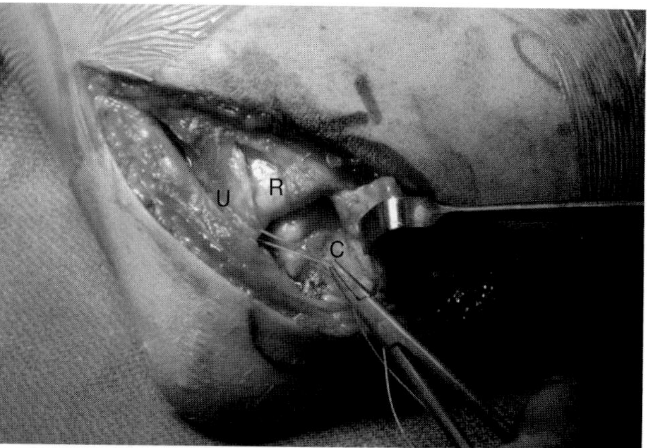

Figure 6 The most isometric point of the lateral epicondyle of the humerus is identified with a suture placed through the ulnar drill holes and by moving the elbow through an arc of motion. R = radial head, C = isometric point on capitellum, U = ulna.

Aftercare

The elbow is splinted at 90° of flexion with the forearm in pronation for 7 to 10 days. At the first postoperative visit, the splint is removed and a hinged elbow brace with a 30° extension block is applied. For the first 6 weeks, the patient performs active-assisted elbow range-of-motion exercises. Flexion and extension range-of-motion exercises are done with the forearm in pronation. Pronation and supination range-of-motion exercises are done with the elbow in 90° of flexion. The patient should not lift anything weighing more than 1 lb (0.45 kg) for 6 weeks.

The hinge on the brace is unlocked 6 weeks after surgery, and the patient continues active-assisted exercises with progression of the range of motion to include flexion and extension with the forearm in neutral and then in supination. Strengthening can be added after 8 weeks. The brace is removed between 8 and 12 weeks after surgery, depending on the compliance of the patient. Unrestricted activity is allowed 4 to 6 months after surgery. Care is taken during the early phase of recovery to avoid varus elbow stresses, including arm abduction.

Results

In one series, 10 of 11 patients with posterolateral rotatory instability who underwent reconstruction had a stable elbow at the time of follow-up,[38] and 7 results were classified as excellent. The authors believed that success required re-creation of a competent lateral ulnar collateral ligament. In another report, 44 patients were surgically treated for posterolateral rotatory instability at the Mayo Clinic.[39] Various techniques were used. At the time of follow-up, 39 patients were deemed to have a stable elbow, with 75% having a good or excellent result. The best outcomes were believed to be in patients with posterolateral rotatory instability caused by trauma and in those who reported instability rather than only pain. The authors believed that using a graft provided better results than did using local tissue.

Summary

The treatment of the unstable elbow requires an understanding of the nuances of the pathologic characteristics. To treat these injuries properly, it is necessary to understand the intricate anatomy and the contributions of both the osseous articulations and the soft tissues to elbow stability.

Acknowledgment

The authors thank senior editor and writer Dori Kelly, MA, University of Maryland School of Medicine, for an outstanding job of manuscript editing.

References

1. An KN, Zobitz ME, Morrey BF: Biomechanics of the elbow, in Morrey BF, Sanchez-Sotelo J, eds: *The Elbow and Its Disorders*, ed 4. Philadelphia, PA, Saunders, 2009, pp 39-63.
2. Cohen MS, Hastings H II: Rotatory instability of the elbow. The anatomy and role of the lateral stabilizers. *J Bone Joint Surg Am* 1997;79(2):225-233.
3. Morrey BF, An KN: Functional anatomy of the ligaments of the elbow. *Clin Orthop Relat Res* 1985;201:84-90.
4. Moritomo H, Murase T, Arimitsu S, Oka K, Yoshikawa H, Sugamoto K: The in vivo isometric point of the lateral ligament of the elbow. *J Bone Joint Surg Am* 2007; 89(9):2011-2017.

5. Dunning CE, Zarzour ZD, Patterson SD, Johnson JA, King GJ: Ligamentous stabilizers against posterolateral rotatory instability of the elbow. *J Bone Joint Surg Am* 2001;83-A(12):1823-1828.
6. McAdams TR, Masters GW, Srivastava S: The effect of arthroscopic sectioning of the lateral ligament complex of the elbow on posterolateral rotatory stability. *J Shoulder Elbow Surg* 2005;14(3): 298-301.
7. Olsen BS, Søjbjerg JO, Nielsen KK, Vaesel MT, Dalstra M, Sneppen O: Posterolateral elbow joint instability: The basic kinematics. *J Shoulder Elbow Surg* 1998;7(1):19-29.
8. Olsen BS, Søjbjerg JO, Dalstra M, Sneppen O: Kinematics of the lateral ligamentous constraints of the elbow joint. *J Shoulder Elbow Surg* 1996;5(5): 333-341.
9. Cohen MS, Bruno RJ: The collateral ligaments of the elbow: Anatomy and clinical correlation. *Clin Orthop Relat Res* 2001;383: 123-130.
10. Bryce CD, Armstrong AD: Anatomy and biomechanics of the elbow. *Orthop Clin North Am* 2008;39(2):141-154, v.
11. Callaway GH, Field LD, Deng XH, et al: Biomechanical evaluation of the medial collateral ligament of the elbow. *J Bone Joint Surg Am* 1997;79(8):1223-1231.
12. Hotchkiss RN, Weiland AJ: Valgus stability of the elbow. *J Orthop Res* 1987;5(3):372-377.
13. Regan WD, Korinek SL, Morrey BF, An KN: Biomechanical study of ligaments around the elbow joint. *Clin Orthop Relat Res* 1991;271:170-179.
14. Morrey BF, An KN: Articular and ligamentous contributions to the stability of the elbow joint. *Am J Sports Med* 1983;11(5):315-319.
15. Armstrong AD, Ferreira LM, Dunning CE, Johnson JA, King GJ: The medial collateral ligament of the elbow is not isometric: An in vitro biomechanical study. *Am J Sports Med* 2004; 32(1):85-90.
16. Fleisig GS, Andrews JR, Dillman CJ, Escamilla RF: Kinetics of baseball pitching with implications about injury mechanisms. *Am J Sports Med* 1995;23(2): 233-239.
17. Halls AA, Travill A: Transmission of pressures across the elbow joint. *Anat Rec* 1964;150:243-247.
18. Morrey BF, Tanaka S, An KN: Valgus stability of the elbow. A definition of primary and secondary constraints. *Clin Orthop Relat Res* 1991;265:187-195.
19. Schneeberger AG, Sadowski MM, Jacob HA: Coronoid process and radial head as posterolateral rotatory stabilizers of the elbow. *J Bone Joint Surg Am* 2004; 86-A(5):975-982.
20. Seiber K, Gupta R, McGarry MH, Safran MR, Lee TQ: The role of the elbow musculature, forearm rotation, and elbow flexion in elbow stability: An in vitro study. *J Shoulder Elbow Surg* 2009;18(2):260-268.
21. Dunning CE, Zarzour ZD, Patterson SD, Johnson JA, King GJ: Muscle forces and pronation stabilize the lateral ligament deficient elbow. *Clin Orthop Relat Res* 2001;388:118-124.
22. Hsu JE, Peng Q, Schafer DA, Koh JL, Nuber GW, Zhang LQ: In vivo three-dimensional mechanical actions of individual. *J Appl Biomech* 2008;24(4): 325-332.
23. Park MC, Ahmad CS: Dynamic contributions of the flexor-pronator mass to elbow valgus stability. *J Bone Joint Surg Am* 2004;86-A(10):2268-2274.
24. Lin F, Kohli N, Perlmutter S, Lim D, Nuber GW, Makhsous M: Muscle contribution to elbow joint valgus stability. *J Shoulder Elbow Surg* 2007;16(6):795-802.
25. Udall JH, Fitzpatrick MJ, McGarry MH, Leba TB, Lee TQ: Effects of flexor-pronator muscle loading on valgus stability of the elbow with an intact, stretched, and resected medial ulnar collateral ligament. *J Shoulder Elbow Surg* 2009;18(5):773-778.
26. Hamilton CD, Glousman RE, Jobe FW, Brault J, Pink M, Perry J: Dynamic stability of the elbow: electromyographic analysis of the flexor pronator group and the extensor group in pitchers with valgus instability. *J Shoulder Elbow Surg* 1996;5(5):347-354.
27. Glousman RE, Barron J, Jobe FW, Perry J, Pink M: An electromyographic analysis of the elbow in normal and injured pitchers with medial collateral ligament insufficiency. *Am J Sports Med* 1992;20(3):311-317.
28. O'Driscoll SW, Morrey BF, Korinek S, An KN: Elbow subluxation and dislocation: A spectrum of instability. *Clin Orthop Relat Res* 1992;280:186-197.
29. McKee MD, Schemitsch EH, Sala MJ, O'driscoll SW: The pathoanatomy of lateral ligamentous disruption in complex elbow instability. *J Shoulder Elbow Surg* 2003;12(4):391-396.
30. O'Driscoll SW, Bell DF, Morrey BF: Posterolateral rotatory instability of the elbow. *J Bone Joint Surg Am* 1991;73(3):440-446.
31. Eygendaal D, Verdegaal SH, Obermann WR, van Vugt AB, Pöll RG, Rozing PM: Posterolateral dislocation of the elbow joint: Relationship to medial instability. *J Bone Joint Surg Am* 2000;82(4): 555-560.
32. Mehlhoff TL, Noble PC, Bennett JB, Tullos HS: Simple dislocation of the elbow in the adult: Results after closed treatment. *J Bone Joint Surg Am* 1988;70(2): 244-249.

33. Josefsson PO, Johnell O, Gentz CF: Long-term sequelae of simple dislocation of the elbow. *J Bone Joint Surg Am* 1984;66(6): 927-930.

34. O'Driscoll SW, Spinner RJ, McKee MD, et al: Tardy posterolateral rotatory instability of the elbow due to cubitus varus. *J Bone Joint Surg Am* 2001;83-A(9): 1358-1369.

35. Abe M, Ishizu T, Morikawa J: Posterolateral rotatory instability of the elbow after posttraumatic cubitus varus. *J Shoulder Elbow Surg* 1997;6(4):405-409.

36. Kalainov DM, Cohen MS: Posterolateral rotatory instability of the elbow in association with lateral epicondylitis. A report of three cases. *J Bone Joint Surg Am* 2005;87(5):1120-1125.

37. Hall JA, McKee MD: Posterolateral rotatory instability of the elbow following radial head resection. *J Bone Joint Surg Am* 2005; 87(7):1571-1579.

38. Nestor BJ, O'Driscoll SW, Morrey BF: Ligamentous reconstruction for posterolateral rotatory instability of the elbow. *J Bone Joint Surg Am* 1992;74(8):1235-1241.

39. Sanchez-Sotelo J, Morrey BF, O'Driscoll SW: Ligamentous repair and reconstruction for posterolateral rotatory instability of the elbow. *J Bone Joint Surg Br* 2005;87(1):54-61.

40. Richard MJ, Aldridge JM III, Wiesler ER, Ruch DS: Traumatic valgus instability of the elbow: Pathoanatomy and results of direct repair. *J Bone Joint Surg Am* 2008;90(11):2416-2422.

41. O'Driscoll SW: Classification and evaluation of recurrent instability of the elbow. *Clin Orthop Relat Res* 2000;370:34-43.

42. Regan W, Lapner PC: Prospective evaluation of two diagnostic apprehension signs for posterolateral instability of the elbow. *J Shoulder Elbow Surg* 2006;15(3):344-346.

43. Arvind CH, Hargreaves DG: Tabletop relocation test: A new clinical test for posterolateral rotatory instability of the elbow. *J Shoulder Elbow Surg* 2006;15(6):707-708.

44. Miller CD, Savoie FH III: Valgus extension injuries of the elbow in the throwing athlete. *J Am Acad Orthop Surg* 1994;2(5):261-269.

45. Wilson FD, Andrews JR, Blackburn TA, McCluskey G: Valgus extension overload in the pitching elbow. *Am J Sports Med* 1983; 11(2):83-88.

46. O'Driscoll SW, Lawton RL, Smith AM: The "moving valgus stress test" for medial collateral ligament tears of the elbow. *Am J Sports Med* 2005;33(2):231-239.

47. Coonrad RW, Roush TF, Major NM, Basamania CJ: The drop sign, a radiographic warning sign of elbow instability. *J Shoulder Elbow Surg* 2005;14(3):312-317.

48. Cotten A, Jacobson J, Brossmann J, et al: Collateral ligaments of the elbow: Conventional MR imaging and MR arthrography with coronal oblique plane and elbow flexion. *Radiology* 1997; 204(3):806-812.

49. Munshi M, Pretterklieber ML, Chung CB, et al: Anterior bundle of ulnar collateral ligament: Evaluation of anatomic relationships by using MR imaging, MR arthrography, and gross anatomic and histologic analysis. *Radiology* 2004;231(3):797-803.

50. Sasaki J, Takahara M, Ogino T, Kashiwa H, Ishigaki D, Kanauchi Y: Ultrasonographic assessment of the ulnar collateral ligament and medial elbow laxity in college baseball players. *J Bone Joint Surg Am* 2002;84-A(4):525-531.

51. Fuss FK: The ulnar collateral ligament of the human elbow joint: Anatomy, function and biomechanics. *J Anat* 1991;175: 203-212.

52. Ochi N, Ogura T, Hashizume H, Shigeyama Y, Senda M, Inoue H: Anatomic relation between the medial collateral ligament of the elbow and the humero-ulnar joint axis. *J Shoulder Elbow Surg* 1999; 8(1):6-10.

53. Armstrong AD, Dunning CE, Faber KJ, Johnson JA, King GJ: Single-strand ligament reconstruction of the medial collateral ligament restores valgus elbow stability. *J Shoulder Elbow Surg* 2002; 11(1):65-71.

54. American Sports Medicine Institute: USA Baseball Medical and Safety Advisory Committee guidelines. May 2006. http://www.asmi.org/asmiweb/usabaseball.htm. Accessed January 15, 2010.

55. Rettig AC, Sherrill C, Snead DS, Mendler JC, Mieling P: Nonoperative treatment of ulnar collateral ligament injuries in throwing athletes. *Am J Sports Med* 2001; 29(1):15-17.

56. Jobe FW, Stark H, Lombardo SJ: Reconstruction of the ulnar collateral ligament in athletes. *J Bone Joint Surg Am* 1986;68(8):1158-1163.

57. Conway JE, Jobe FW, Glousman RE, Pink M: Medial instability of the elbow in throwing athletes: Treatment by repair or reconstruction of the ulnar collateral ligament. *J Bone Joint Surg Am* 1992;74(1):67-83.

58. Azar FM, Andrews JR, Wilk KE, Groh D: Operative treatment of ulnar collateral ligament injuries of the elbow in athletes. *Am J Sports Med* 2000;28(1):16-23.

59. Thompson WH, Jobe FW, Yocum LA, Pink MM: Ulnar collateral ligament reconstruction in athletes: Muscle-splitting approach without transposition of the ulnar nerve. *J Shoulder Elbow Surg* 2001;10(2):152-157.

60. Rohrbough JT, Altchek DW, Hyman J, Williams RJ III, Botts

JD: Medial collateral ligament reconstruction of the elbow using the docking technique. *Am J Sports Med* 2002;30(4):541-548.

61. Koh JL, Schafer MF, Keuter G, Hsu JE: Ulnar collateral ligament reconstruction in elite throwing athletes. *Arthroscopy* 2006;22(11): 1187-1191.

62. Paletta GA Jr, Wright RW: The modified docking procedure for elbow ulnar collateral ligament reconstruction: 2-year follow-up in elite throwers. *Am J Sports Med* 2006;34(10):1594-1598.

63. Ahmad CS, Lee TQ, ElAttrache NS: Biomechanical evaluation of a new ulnar collateral ligament reconstruction technique with interference screw fixation. *Am J Sports Med* 2003;31(3):332-337.

64. Armstrong AD, Dunning CE, Ferreira LM, Faber KJ, Johnson JA, King GJ: A biomechanical comparison of four reconstruction techniques for the medial collateral ligament-deficient elbow. *J Shoulder Elbow Surg* 2005;14(2): 207-215.

65. Dines JS, ElAttrache NS, Conway JE, Smith W, Ahmad CS: Clinical outcomes of the DANE TJ technique to treat ulnar collateral ligament insufficiency of the elbow. *Am J Sports Med* 2007; 35(12):2039-2044.

66. Smith GR, Altchek DW, Pagnani MJ, Keeley JR: A muscle-splitting approach to the ulnar collateral ligament of the elbow: Neuroanatomy and operative technique. *Am J Sports Med* 1996; 24(5):575-580.

67. O'Driscoll SW, Jaloszynski R, Morrey BF, An KN: Origin of the medial ulnar collateral ligament. *J Hand Surg Am* 1992;17(1): 164-168.

68. Armstrong AD, Dunning CE, Faber KJ, Duck TR, Johnson JA, King GJ: Rehabilitation of the medial collateral ligament-deficient elbow: An in vitro biomechanical study. *J Hand Surg Am* 2000;25(6):1051-1057.

69. Vitale MA, Ahmad CS: The outcome of elbow ulnar collateral ligament reconstruction in overhead athletes: A systematic review. *Am J Sports Med* 2008;36(6): 1193-1205.

70. Kerut EK, Kerut DG, Fleisig GS, Andrews JR: Prevention of arm injury in youth baseball pitchers. *J La State Med Soc* 2008;160(2): 95-98.

71. Deutch SR, Olsen BS, Jensen SL, Tyrdal S, Sneppen O: Ligamentous and capsular restraints to experimental posterior elbow joint dislocation. *Scand J Med Sci Sports* 2003;13(5):311-316.

72. Seki A, Olsen BS, Jensen SL, Eygendaal D, Søjbjerg JO: Functional anatomy of the lateral collateral ligament complex of the elbow: Configuration of Y and its role. *J Shoulder Elbow Surg* 2002; 11(1):53-59.

73. Jensen SL, Olsen BS, Tyrdal S, Søjbjerg JO, Sneppen O: Elbow joint laxity after experimental radial head excision and lateral collateral ligament rupture: Efficacy of prosthetic replacement and ligament repair. *J Shoulder Elbow Surg* 2005;14(1):78-84.

74. Savoie FH III, Field LD, Gurley DJ: Arthroscopic and open radial ulnohumeral ligament reconstruction for posterolateral rotatory instability of the elbow. *Hand Clin* 2009;25(3):323-329.

75. Goren D, Budoff JE, Hipp JA: Isometric placement of lateral ulnar collateral ligament reconstructions: A biomechanical study. *Am J Sports Med* 2010;38(1): 153-159.

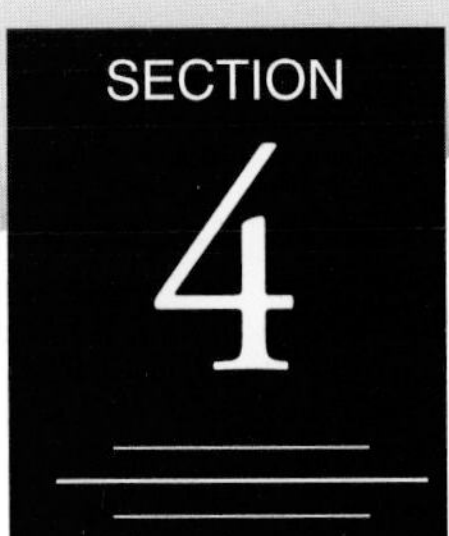

Adult Reconstruction: Hip and Knee

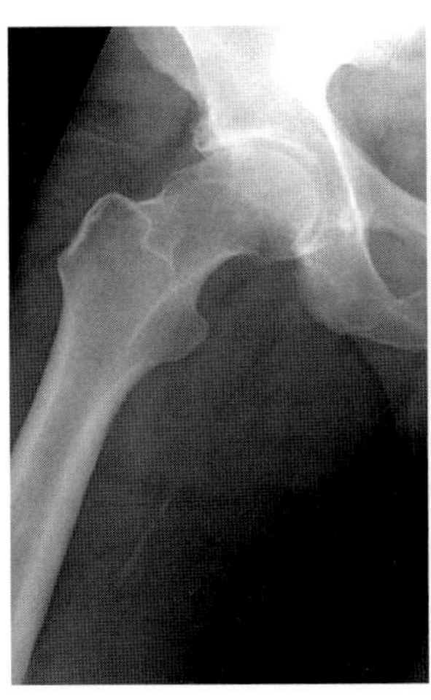
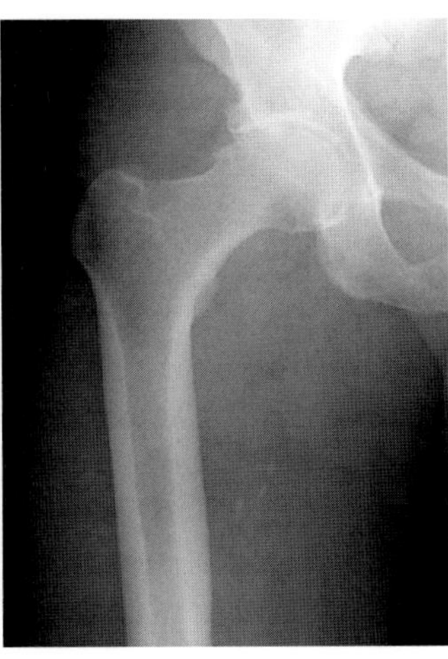

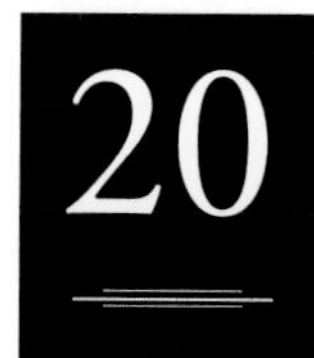

Achieving Stability and Lower Limb Length in Total Hip Arthroplasty

Keith R. Berend, MD
Scott M. Sporer, MD
Rafael J. Sierra, MD
Andrew H. Glassman, MD
Michael J. Morris, MD

Abstract

Total hip arthroplasty is an exceptionally cost-effective and successful surgical procedure. Dislocation, infection, osteolysis, and limb-length inequality are among the most common complications affecting the long-term success of total hip arthroplasty. Instability is a challenging complication to treat. The surgeon frequently must try to achieve a stable hip at the cost of increasing the length of the operated extremity. It is important to understand the factors associated with stability and limb length; the surgical options available; the effect and role of the various surgical approaches; and methods to manage instability, with and without limb-length inequality.

Instr Course Lect 2011;60:229-246.

Total hip arthroplasty is an exceptionally cost-effective and successful surgical intervention.[1,2] Dislocation, infection, osteolysis, and limb-length inequality are among the most common complications affecting the long-term success of total hip arthroplasty.[2-8] Instability with dislocation is a complication that is costly to the patient, surgeon, and hospital.[9] The surgeon is frequently faced with the challenge of obtaining a stable hip at the cost of increasing the length of the lower extremity.[10] This chapter addresses the common issues that surround the achievement of both stability and limb-length equality with total hip arthroplasty. The preoperative patient education and factors associated with stability and limb length, the effect and role of various surgical approaches, the surgical techniques, and the management of instability with and without limb-length inequality are reviewed.

Instability

Dislocation rates are reported to be 0.3% to 10% after primary total hip arthroplasty and up to 28% after revision total hip arthroplasty. The incidence appears to be highest within the first year and rises at a rate of about 1% per 5 years to 7% at 25 years postoperatively.[11-21] A recent national database study reported that instability/dislocation was the most common diagnosis resulting in revision total hip arthroplasty in the United States.[3] There are patient-specific risk factors associated with in-

Dr. Berend or an immediate family member serves as a board member, owner, officer, or committee member of Mount Carmel New Albany Surgical Hospital and the American Association of Hip and Knee Surgeons Education Committee; has received royalties from Biomet; serves as a paid consultant to or is an employee of Biomet, Salient Surgical, and Synvasive; has received research or institutional support from Biomet; and owns stock or stock options in Angiotech. Dr. Sporer or an immediate family member is a member of a speakers' bureau or has made paid presentations on behalf of Zimmer; serves as a paid consultant to or is an employee of Zimmer; and has received research or institutional support from Zimmer. Dr. Sierra or an immediate family member is a member of a speakers' bureau or has made paid presentations on behalf of Biomet; serves as a paid consultant to or is an employee of Biomet; and has received research or institutional support from DePuy, Zimmer, and Stryker. Dr. Glassman or an immediate family member serves as a board member, owner, officer, or committee member of the Hip Society; has received royalties from Zimmer and Innomed; and owns stock or stock options in Stryker. Dr. Morris or an immediate family member has received research or institutional support from Biomet.

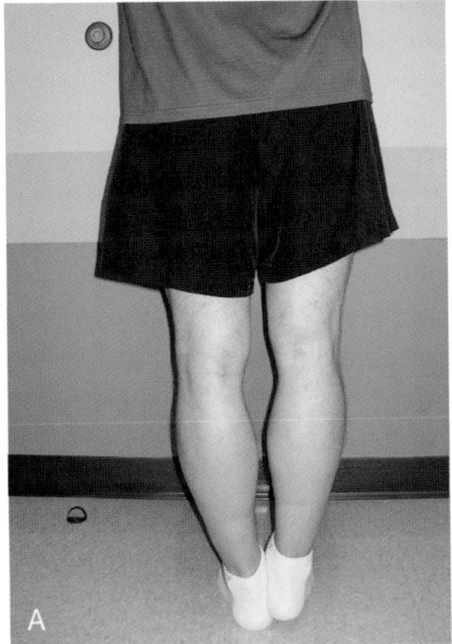

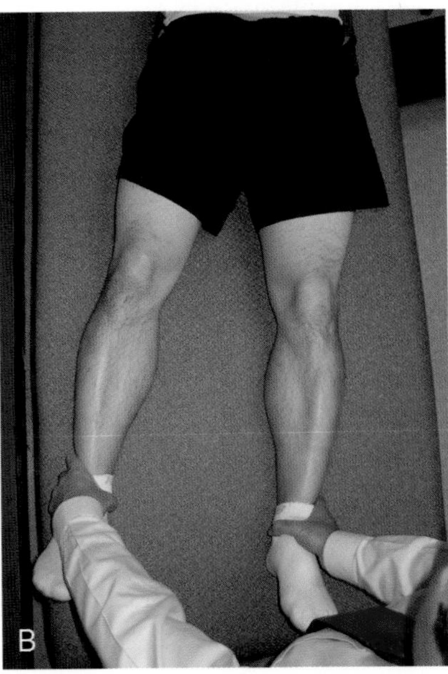

Figure 1 **A,** There is a limb-length discrepancy, with the right lower limb shorter than the left. Note the elevated heel of the right foot. **B,** Adduction contracture is present on the left, leading to the appearance of, but not true, limb-length discrepancy.

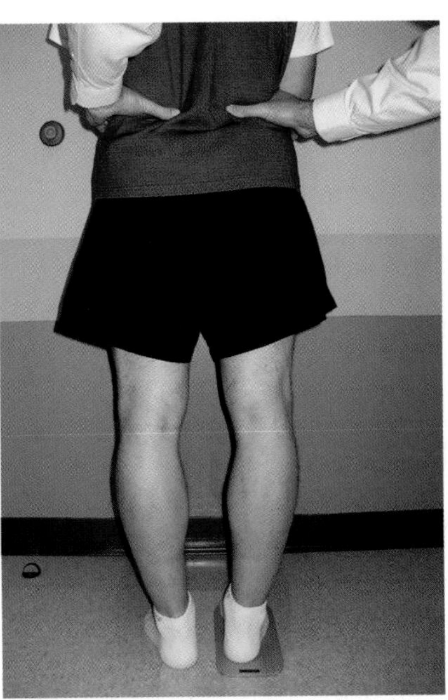

Figure 2 Standing evaluation of clinical limb length is performed by measuring the pelvic obliquity and limb-length difference. The examiner's hands palpate the superior iliac crests, and blocks are added under the short lower limb until the pelvis is level. The block height needed to level the pelvis is the limb-length difference.

stability, including female sex, increasing age, a diagnosis of osteonecrosis or femoral neck fracture, obesity, a high preoperative range of motion, and comorbidities.[5,13,15,22-33] There are variables under the surgeon's direct control, including the surgical approach, component position and orientation, femoral head size, restoration of offset, preservation of soft-tissue integrity, limb lengths, and prosthetic impingement. Surgeon experience is a variable, and the risk of instability is inversely related to the case volume of the operating surgeon.[5,13,15,30-32,34,35]

Preoperative Evaluation

Postoperative limb-length inequality and hip instability are common causes of litigation.[36-38] A thorough preoperative discussion establishes realistic patient expectations. A hierarchy of reconstruction goals should be outlined: first, well-fixed acetabular and femoral components; second, a dynamically stable construct; and third, equalization of limb lengths. The patient must understand and accept that lengthening of the lower limb may be required to achieve the first two goals.

A complete medical and surgical history should be obtained. Previous surgery on either extremity can create limb-length inequality that is not appreciated on a pelvic radiograph alone. Previous fracture, infection, physeal arrest, and various dysplasias may result in limb shortening. Abnormalities of the axial skeleton, such as prior spinal fusion, scoliosis, or neuromuscular disorders, or soft-tissue contractures associated with the hip or knee result in apparent limb-length discrepancy. The combination of "true" and "apparent" limb lengths contribute to the patient's subjective perception of limb-length inequality[39] (**Figure 1**).

Physical Examination

Observation of the patient's gait identifies pelvic obliquity, weak abductors, and dependence on assistive devices. The major muscles around the hip (abductors, adductors, and flexors) as well as the iliotibial band are assessed for contractures. The levels of the iliac crests are compared with the patient standing (**Figure 2**), and the thoracic and lumbar spine is assessed for coronal or sagittal deformity.

True limb length is determined by measuring the actual length of the extremity clinically or radiographically. The apparent limb length is determined by adding the effects of pelvic obliquity and soft-tissue contractures. Clinically, true limb length is measured from the anterior-superior iliac spine to the medial malleolus (**Figure 3**). Accurate identification of the osseous and anatomic landmarks can be difficult, especially in obese patients. A compensatory, flexible scoliosis may develop in the presence of a true limb-length inequality. The flexible deformities are corrected when a block is placed under the shorter extremity or when the patient sits. A

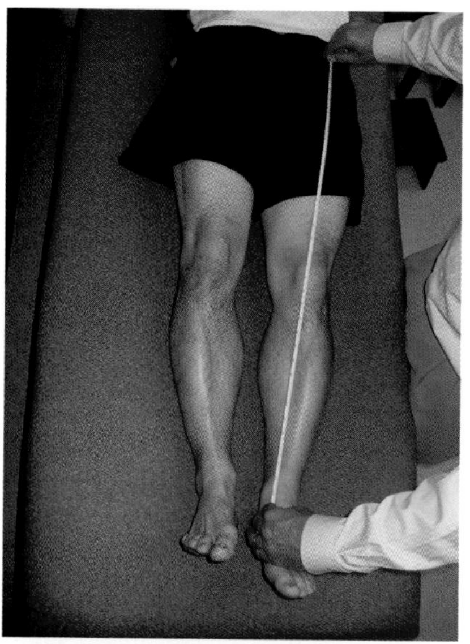

Figure 3 Supine evaluation of limb-length inequality is performed by measuring the distance between the anterior superior iliac spine and the medial malleolus with a tape measure.

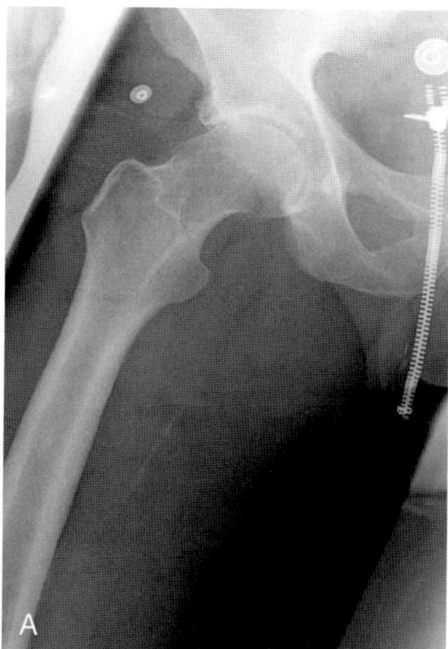

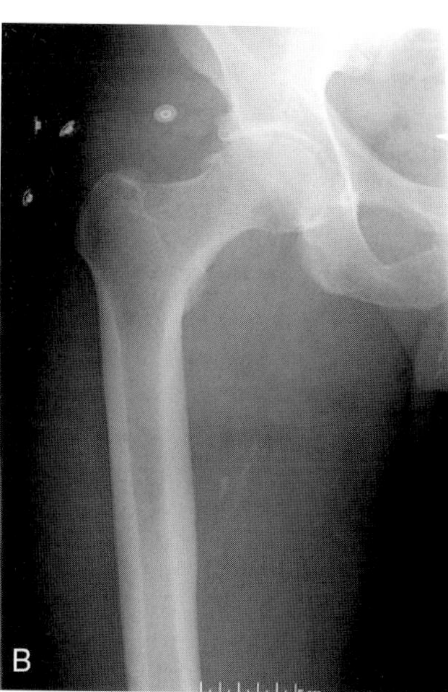

Figure 4 **A,** AP radiograph of a right femur in an externally rotated position. A false femoral offset is seen. **B,** AP radiograph of the same right femur with the hip in 20° of internal rotation. Note the marked femoral offset.

rigid coronal spinal deformity remains unchanged with these maneuvers.

Radiographic Assessment

Standing AP pelvic, AP femoral, and lateral femoral radiographs should be obtained. Because an arthritic hip frequently has an external rotation deformity, the AP pelvic and femoral radiographs should be made with the femur in 20° of internal rotation to avoid underestimation of femoral offset (**Figure 4**).

Preoperative radiographs provide an estimation of true limb-length inequality. A line drawn between the inferior aspects of the obturator foramina, ischia, or radiographic "teardrops" on a supine AP view of the pelvis is used as the pelvic reference. The distance between this line and a fixed point on the femur (the lesser or greater trochanter) can be compared with that of the contralateral hip. The difference between these two distances is the true limb-length inequality (**Figure 5**). This method is valid only if the limb lengths are equal below the chosen reference point and the two lower limbs are held in the same anatomic position.

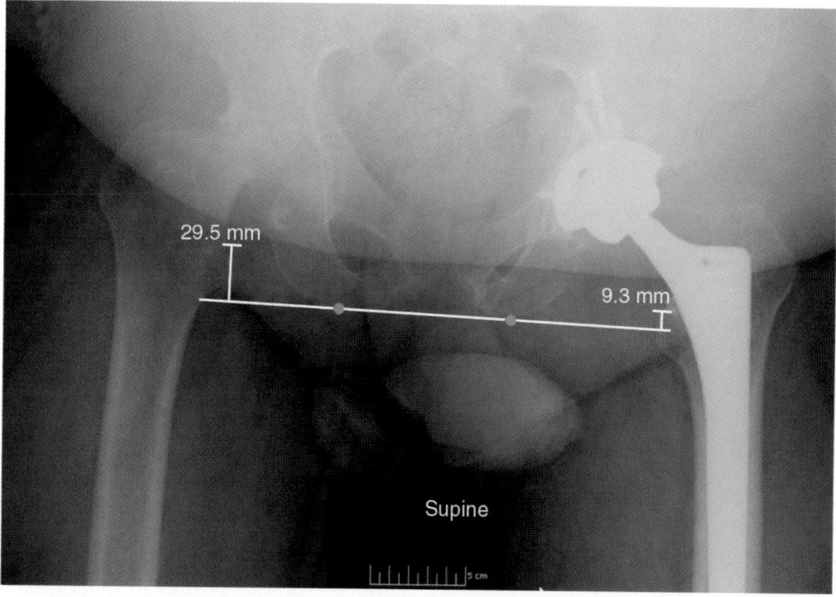

Figure 5 Preoperative AP pelvic radiograph made with the patient supine shows severe erosive arthritis of the right hip. A line is drawn at the most inferior portions of the ischia, providing the pelvic reference line. A perpendicular line is drawn bilaterally from the transischial line to the superior aspect of the lesser trochanter to determine the limb-length difference. The patient has a preoperative limb-length discrepancy of 2.0 cm.

Preoperative templating is essential to minimize limb-length inequality, restore offset, and therefore minimize

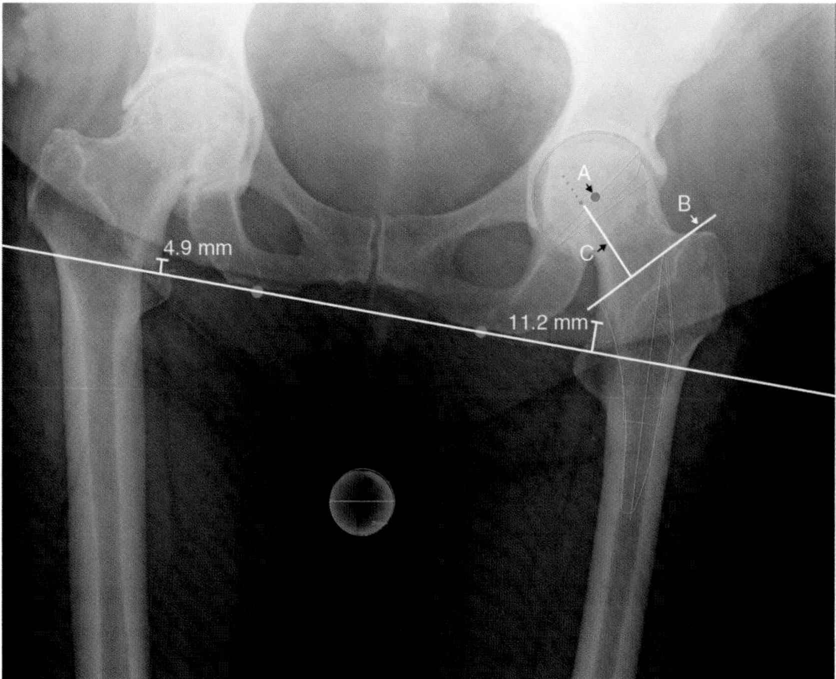

Figure 6 Preoperative templating can be performed with computerized radiology software. The new, anatomic center of rotation is templated (A), and the acetabular implant size is determined using the hip that is not being operated on. The appropriate femoral stem size and position are templated. The corresponding neck cut (B), prosthetic neck length (C), and limb-length difference are noted.

the possibility of instability (**Figure 6**). First, the new center of rotation for the hip is determined by selecting the optimal position of the acetabular component. In general, the inferomedial aspect of the acetabular component is placed in close approximation to the radiographic teardrop such that the inferiormost aspect of the acetabular implant template is aligned with the radiographic teardrop in the vertical plane.

With femoral templating, the examiner should determine (1) the prosthetic size (the fit and fill of the femur needed to achieve axial and rotational stability), (2) the component offset (extended-offset implants or a lateralized acetabular liner may be required to restore offset), and (3) limb length. Limb lengthening (or, rarely, shortening) is planned on the basis of the preoperative radiographic evaluation as well as the clinical assessment of apparent limb-length inequality.

Not all patients with a true limb-length inequality require lengthening. Patients with a fixed adduction contracture or a pelvic obliquity may believe that the limb is excessively long if the true limb length is restored. A common reason for dislocation is the failure to adequately restore offset, which is the distance between the center of hip rotation and the center of the femoral canal.[40] Technically, templating can be performed on the contralateral, normal hip, and changes in limb length or offset can be extrapolated to the hip that is to be operated on. Subsequently, femoral head-neck length and implant offset can be anticipated. Alternatively, templating of the hip that is to be operated on can allow immediate recognition of how much length or offset will be changed by anatomic placement of components, compared with the nonsurgical side.

Patient Expectations

Preoperative discussions about limb-length inequality and the possibility of hip dislocation are critical and should set realistic goals and reiterate the hierarchy of surgical priorities.[36] Patients must be aware that in some situations the lower limb must be lengthened to achieve component stability. Additionally, patients should be told that their lower limb will feel long immediately after the surgery and that this is a normal physiologic response following hip replacement. Patients who have a sense that the lower limb is longer preoperatively but actually have normal limb lengths, or those with a shortened extremity but the perception of equal limb lengths, are particularly at risk for perceiving that they have a discrepancy after surgery and should be appropriately warned preoperatively.[41]

Advantages and Disadvantages of Surgical Approaches in Terms of Limb Length and Stability

Anterior Approaches

The true anterior approaches expose the hip through the interval between the sartorius and tensor fascia femoris muscles, with several variations. The classic approach is the Smith-Petersen approach with either preservation or detachment of the direct head of the rectus femoris tendon. A variation of this approach—the Hueter approach (a fascial incision over the tensor fascia femoris)—has gained interest because of its theoretic ability to provide protection to the lateral femoral cutaneous nerve, which is at risk with the classic Smith-Petersen approach.[42-44]

Limb Length

A major advantage of the direct anterior approach is the ability to directly measure limb lengths because the patient is in the supine position and the true limb length can be measured at the ankle or heel. An intraoperative supine radiograph or fluoroscopy is helpful for measuring limb lengths and component position. Studies have shown an average mean limb-length discrepancy of 3.9 mm with this approach.[43,44] This small amount of lengthening is well tolerated and accepted by the patient, making this approach one of the most accurate in terms of limb-length reconstruction.

Stability

The direct anterior exposure is a true internervous plane between the sartorius (femoral nerve) and tensor fascia femoris (superior gluteal nerve). This approach minimizes soft-tissue damage about the hip and preserves the major abductor attachment. Only the anterior aspect of the capsule is excised. Advocates point out that no muscle detachment is necessary to deliver the femur anteriorly. The dislocation rate after a single-incision anterior approach ranges from 0.6% to 1.3%.[42-44]

Disadvantages

The approach is technically demanding and may or may not require the use of a specialized fracture table. There is a steep learning curve associated with the procedure.[42,45] The lateral femoral cutaneous nerve is always retracted, and the risk of injury to this nerve should be discussed with the patient preoperatively.

Two-Incision Technique

The two-incision technique was described by Light and Keggi[46] and was popularized by Berger.[47,48] It is basically an anterior Smith-Petersen approach with an additional posterior smaller incision for placement of the femoral component.

Limb Length

The advantages of this approach are similar to those of the direct anterior approach.

Stability

Excessive femoral anteversion is a risk because it is difficult to maintain anatomic version while inserting the femoral component through the small posterior incision. The reported dislocation rate after this procedure is relatively low (1.0%).[47-50]

Disadvantages

The two-incision approach is not popular because it is technically difficult, has a steep learning curve, and has a high intraoperative complication rate. In addition, there may be injury to the abductor muscles.[49,51-53]

Anterolateral, Direct Lateral, or Hardinge Approach

Direct lateral approaches include the Hardinge approach, in which the gluteus medius tendon is displaced with the vastus lateralis anteriorly and the hip is dislocated anteriorly.[54] Mallory et al[55] described a modified direct lateral approach in which the anterior portion of the gluteus medius is dissected and displaced anteriorly with the vastus lateralis.

Limb Length

Some surgeons perform this approach with the patient in the supine position, and this position may be advantageous in terms of obtaining equal limb lengths. The approaches that dislocate the hip anteriorly offer some additional protection against dislocation compared with posterolateral approaches.[56] Therefore, slight laxity in the hip to keep the lower limbs of equal length is acceptable.

Stability

The cumulative 10-year rate of dislocation has been reported to be 3.1% after anterolateral approaches but 6.9% after posterolateral approaches.[48,57,58]

Disadvantages

This approach violates the abductor mechanism and is sometimes associated with a postoperative limp. Damage to the superior gluteal nerve can occur and leads to denervation of the muscles that it enervates.[59] Heterotopic ossification is more common than it is with other approaches; this heterotopic bone has required removal in 1% of patients,[58] a rate that is higher than that associated with other approaches.

Posterolateral Approach

The posterolateral approach is the most extensile of all approaches, allowing complete exposure of the femur and acetabulum. It is the most commonly used approach in North America, primarily because it avoids damage to the abductor muscles.[50,60,61] Small-incision techniques have gained favor in recent years.[61] The debate over the clinical benefit and the effect on limb length and stability of this approach is beyond the scope of this chapter.[61,62]

Limb Length

When the posterolateral approach is used, the limb lengths are difficult to accurately measure with physical examination or radiographs, so some other means of determining limb length is necessary. Because of concerns about postoperative dislocation, it is not uncommon for the extremity to be overlengthened during the hip arthroplasty with this approach.[63]

Stability

The risk of dislocation associated with the posterior approach is higher than that found with transtrochanteric, anterolateral, and anterior-based approaches.[13,16,21,64] In a study of

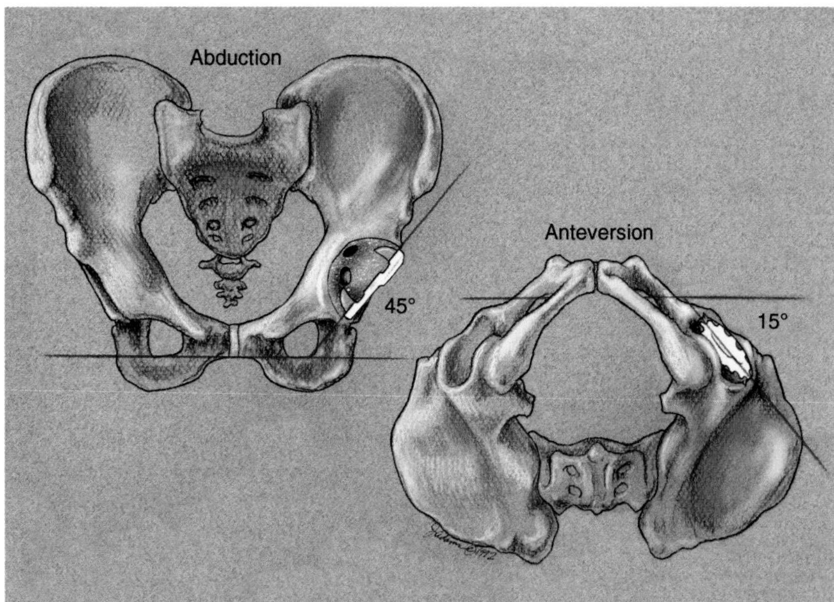

Figure 7 The so-called safe zone for orientation of the acetabular component. (Reproduced with permission of Joint Implant Surgeons, Inc, New Albany, Ohio.)

more than 21,000 primary total hip arthroplasties, Berry et al[13] reported dislocation rates at the time of a 10-year follow-up of 3.1%, 3.4%, and 6.9% for the anterolateral, transtrochanteric, and posterolateral approaches, respectively. A meta-analysis by Masonis and Bourne[64] suggested that the dislocation rate associated with the posterior approach is sixfold higher than that observed with a direct lateral approach. Proper repair of the capsule and short external rotators after a posterior approach reduces the incidence of dislocation.[60,64-69] Furthermore, Kim et al[70] advocated preserving the external rotators during the posterior approach, a technique that resulted in no dislocations.

Disadvantages

The risk of injury to the sciatic nerve with the posterior approach is reported to be 0.6%.[71,72] However, as a result of the proximity of the nerve with this approach, the risk of sciatic nerve injury is higher than that associated with all other surgical approaches.[59,70,73]

Surgical Technique

Implant Positioning: Acetabular Component

Implant malposition is a major contributor to instability and dislocation. Correct implant position decreases wear and reduces the risk of dislocation, but other factors play a role in hip stability.[74,75] Multiple investigators have attempted to define a safe zone of acetabular component anteversion and inclination, or abduction. It is widely believed that the acetabular component should be placed in approximately 45° (40° to 60°) of abduction and should be anteverted 15° to 20°[18] (**Figure** 7). The safe zone is 15° ± 10° of anteversion and 40° ± 10° of abduction.[18] Total hip arthroplasty components that dislocate anteriorly have mean anteversion and abduction angles that are greater than the safe zone, whereas those that dislocate posteriorly have mean anteversion and abduction angles that are less than the safe zone.[76] The position of the acetabular cup is not the only factor affecting instability and dislocation. Hassan et al[77] reported that 42% of total hip prostheses in which the acetabular cup was positioned outside the safe zone did not dislocate. Rittmeister and Callitsis[78] noted that although nearly 20% of acetabular cups were positioned outside the safe zone in their study, there was no increase in dislocations in that group.

Implant Positioning: Reference Landmarks

Landmarks are useful in assisting with positioning of the acetabular component. McCollum and Gray[79] investigated multiple external reference points for acetabular component positioning and found that significant changes in pelvic position and orientation occur when the patient is in the lateral decubitus position. Care must be taken to evaluate the effects of body position when using external cues for orientation of the acetabular component during surgery.

Fixed anatomic landmarks, in contrast to external aiming devices, are independent of patient positioning. Useful landmarks include the transverse acetabular ligament, the acetabular sulcus on the ischium, the most lateral prominence of the superior pubic rami (pubis), and the most superior aspect of the acetabulum.[80,81] These landmarks define a plane of orientation for acetabular component positioning that provides stability within a safe arc of motion.[81] An average cup position of 44° of abduction and 13° of anteversion can be achieved with use of these landmarks.[81]

Computer navigation, or computer-assisted orthopaedic surgery, has been proposed as a method for accurately determining correct acetabular component positioning. Computer-assisted orthopaedic surgery reduces outliers but is not totally reliable.[82-84] The cost and technical aspects of computer-assisted orthopaedic surgery currently prohibit its widespread use.

Implant Positioning: Femoral Component

The positioning of the femoral component affects limb length, offset, abductor tension, and stability. All other factors being equal, a distally placed femoral stem will result in a limb that is shorter than that resulting from a more proximally placed stem. The level of the femoral component has an equally important, albeit less obvious, effect on femoral offset. Femoral offset is defined as the distance from the center of rotation of the femoral head to a line bisecting the long axis of the femur. Reconstruction of the femoral offset is important for restoring the biomechanics of the hip and specifically the abductor lever arm. Proper restoration of offset enhances hip motion and reduces the risk of dislocation.[85] A high femoral neck resection can be combined with a short neck length to yield the same limb length as provided by a low femoral neck resection combined with a long modular head. However, the first combination yields less femoral offset and may be appropriate in the presence of coxa valga. The second combination yields greater offset and is better for hips with coxa vara. Varus or valgus malpositioning of the stem will increase or decrease offset and should be avoided. Rotational alignment of the stem to the appropriate femoral anteversion influences the amount of hip motion that is possible before impingement occurs as well as abductor tension. Herrlin et al[86] reported that femoral anteversion was significantly reduced in hips that dislocated after total hip arthroplasty. The ideal femoral anteversion is 15° to 20° in an osteoarthritic hip with otherwise normal anatomy. Acetabular deformity or deficiency may dictate less than ideal orientation of the acetabular component. To compensate for this, the femoral component may need to be placed in greater or less anteversion. In recognition of this possibility, the concept of combined acetabular and femoral component anteversion has been introduced. Using a mathematical model, Widmer and Zurfluh[87] determined that the acetabular component should be in 40° to 45° of inclination (abduction) and 20° to 28° of anteversion (forward flexion). This is combined with femoral anteversion such that the femoral anteversion multiplied by 0.7, plus the cup anteversion, should equal 37° to provide the greatest range of motion without impingement. Modular femoral components of various designs that allow adjustments in offset and anteversion without limb lengthening are now available from various manufacturers.[4,88]

There are some general rules of thumb for placing a femoral stem in the correct position. The proximal-distal position of the femoral stem is assessed in relation to the greater and lesser trochanters. Alternatively, the center of the femoral head in relation to the tip of the greater trochanter is noted. Additionally, the piriformis fossa can serve as a landmark for femoral neck resection. When the posterior approach is used, the templated neck resection can be easily reproduced by measuring the level of resection from the top of the lesser trochanter. This landmark is easily visualized on preoperative radiographs and intraoperatively, even through limited exposures. Woolson et al[89] described using the templated femoral neck and head segment as a guide for placing the femoral stem. By placing the femoral stem at that osteotomy level, they achieved an appropriate limb length in 97% of cases.

Soft-Tissue Balancing

By restoring femoral offset and limb length, proper balancing of the soft tissues around the hip minimizes postoperative instability, pain, and limp.[90,91] Inadequate restoration of femoral offset increases the risk of dislocation by decreasing soft-tissue tension.[91] Excessive limb lengthening can result when intraoperative instability caused by inadequate offset is inappropriately treated by increasing the neck length in an attempt to restore soft-tissue tension.[38] As mentioned previously, the combination of these factors is critical for understanding prosthetic hip stability.[19]

Better wear performance of the implants has been observed after femoral head medialization and femoral shaft lateralization. In addition, restoration of offset is associated with better functional and clinical results.[85,92,93] Bourne and Rorabeck[90] reviewed the available methods to restore offset. The most common approach is the use of a lateralized (high-offset) femoral stem (**Figure 8**). Another option is to use a lateralized acetabular liner. However, such liners decrease the abductor moment arm, increase the joint reactive force, and result in accelerated polyethylene wear.[90] A lower-level neck resection and more distal femoral stem placement combined with a longer neck segment can lateralize the femoral shaft without lengthening the limb. However, longer heads with skirts should be avoided because they decrease motion as a result of impingement.

Concerns have been raised that excessive femoral lateralization may increase the incidence of thigh pain and trochanteric bursitis or place undue strains on the bone-cement or biologic interfaces, leading to loosening. This latter concern has been refuted, and data show that, when indicated, a lateralized stem improves the accuracy of

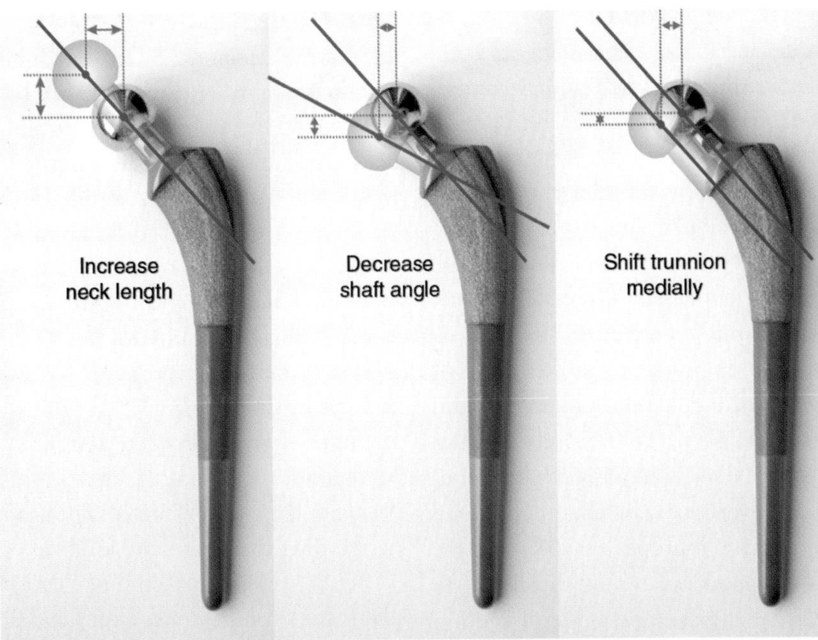

Figure 8 Various methods of restoring offset with use of the femoral stem. (Reproduced with permission of Joint Implant Surgeons, Inc, New Albany, Ohio.)

hip soft-tissue reconstruction and does not increase thigh pain, trochanteric pain, or loosening.[56] In fact, proper soft-tissue balancing, obtained with a lateralized stem, is associated with less thigh and trochanteric pain.[94] However, overlateralization should be avoided. Incavo et al[95] showed that excessive lateralization led to a 15% incidence of trochanteric pain. The value of intraoperative tests of soft-tissue balance, such as the shuck test or drop-kick test, is highly dependent on the surgical approach, the anesthetic technique, and surgeon experience.[90] These tests, however, can provide the surgeon with an assessment of the overall tightness of the reconstructed hip. The shuck test is performed by attempting to distract the total hip prosthesis in an inferior direction to assess soft-tissue tension. The drop-kick test is performed by placing the hip in extension, flexing the knee to 90°, and releasing the lower limb to assess the amount of recoil as the knee springs back toward extension. In addition, intraoperative motion of the hip is important to evaluate for potential bone or prosthetic impingement and prosthetic stability. These intraoperative assessments coupled with proper preoperative templating should allow the surgeon to restore proper hip offset and limb length.

Measuring Limb Length

Substantial limb-length discrepancy occurs after up to 3% of total hip arthroplasties, but the clinical relevance is not known.[69] The definition of clinically relevant limb-length discrepancy is not universally agreed on, with a range between 6 and 35 mm having been reported.[96-99] Most authors have agreed that discrepancies of less than 1 cm are well tolerated.[97] Edwards et al[71] reported average lengthening of 2.7 cm and 4.4 cm in 23 total hip arthroplasties complicated by peroneal and sciatic nerve palsy, respectively. White and Dougall[99] reported that lengthening of up to 35 mm does not affect clinical results. Edeen et al[37] reported that 32% of patients who had a total hip arthroplasty were aware of a limb-length inequality. Relevant limb-length discrepancy results in a limp, low back pain, and functional impairment and is a major cause of litigation.[38,100] There are several methods for the intraoperative assessment of limb length, with varied degrees of accuracy, technical difficulty, and expense. Many of the methods involve an intraoperative measuring device, which may also enable the measurement of offset.[41,63,101-103] These instruments measure from a fixed point on the pelvis to a fixed point on the femur and are used before femoral head dislocation and after total hip arthroplasty reconstruction. They are accurate if the position of the limb before the dislocation is correctly reproduced for the postarthroplasty measurement.[104] There is a learning curve with these devices as well as the need for additional expense and time for surgery. An average limb lengthening of 3.4 mm was observed with the use of one specific device; limb lengthening of more than 12 mm was observed in 5% of cases, and 7% had symptomatic lengthening requiring a heel lift.[103]

Alternatively, preoperative templating and intraoperative "well-leg" referencing for limb length is as accurate as other methods, with few radiographic outliers.[56] Preoperative templating is performed. The center of the acetabulum on the normal, contralateral side is identified with acetabular templates (**Figure 6**). The femoral component size and osteotomy level are determined, and the neck length is selected. The level of the femoral neck osteotomy is referenced intraoperatively with regard to the greater trochanter, the lesser trochanter, the piriformis fossa, or the distance from the center of the resected head. Direct measurement of limb length with the patient supine is performed before positioning for the total hip arthroplasty and preparation of the extremity. This measurement is correlated with the preoperative templating. The patient is positioned in the lateral decubitus position, and the uninvolved lower limb is used as a reference, with the relative difference felt at the patellar tendon (**Figure 9**). The relative difference is reassessed after trial components have been placed. In one series of 410 patients treated with a primary total hip arthroplasty, an average lengthening of 3.9 mm was seen and only 2 patients perceived a limb-length discrepancy.[56]

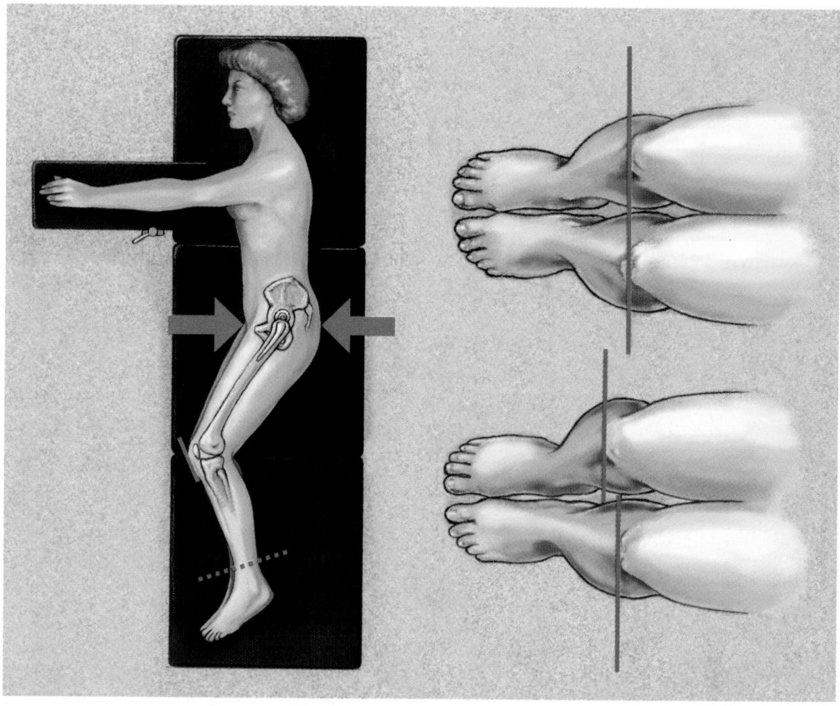

Figure 9 With the patient in a lateral position, the uninvolved lower limb is used to reference limb lengths intraoperatively. The pelvis needs to be perpendicular to the floor. With the feet symmetrically positioned, the patellar tendons are palpated, and the limb-length difference is assessed. The goal is to have symmetric positioning of the patellar tendons with the pelvis and feet. (Reproduced with permission of Joint Implant Surgeons, Inc., New Albany, Ohio.)

Implant-Related Factors

Femoral head size affects hip stability after a total hip arthroplasty.[13,105-107] Dislocation rates for all approaches decrease as femoral head size increases from 22 mm to 32 mm.[13] Smith et al[108] reported no dislocations when a 38-mm head had been used. Cuckler et al[109] also reported no dislocations with 38-mm heads, but 2.5% of the total hip prostheses with a 28-mm head dislocated. Peters et al[110] found no dislocations with 38-mm heads, a 0.4% rate with 38 to 56-mm heads, and a 2.5% rate with 28-mm heads. Smit[111] studied anatomically sized femoral heads (femoral heads with a size that was 6 mm less than the acetabular size) in primary total hip arthroplasties and reported no dislocations at 1-year follow-up. Others believe that a good capsular repair as well as a larger femoral head protects against a dislocation. Lachiewicz and Soileau[112] found that when a formal posterior capsular repair had been used, there was no change in the dislocation risk associated with 36- and 40-mm metal femoral heads compared with that for historic controls with standard-sized heads. Despite the overall impressive reduction in the dislocation rate associated with large femoral heads in these studies, Amstutz et al[113] reported a dislocation rate of 3.5% with large femoral heads in primary total hip arthroplasty. However, Amstutz et al[113] reported an advantage of using larger heads in revision total hip arthroplasties. In addition, the use of large heads increases volumetric wear, and a thinner polyethylene acetabular liner is needed to accommodate the larger head. To avoid the adverse mechanical and fatigue properties associated with thin liners, implant companies commonly offer offset liners to increase polyethylene thickness.[114] Offset liners may increase femoral offset, which affects the joint mechanics as previously discussed.

Management of Instability

An accurate and complete patient history is critical for defining the cause of hip instability. Surgical records are reviewed to determine the surgical approach, type of soft-tissue repair, and specific implant used, including the manufacturer's implant stickers if possible. The mechanism of the dislocation may be evaluated according to the direction of dislocation and the position of instability. Limb length, associated skeletal conditions such as scoliosis and contractures, neurologic function of both the affected limb and the abductors, and the overall neurologic function of the patient should be assessed. A thorough evaluation for infection is necessary.[115]

Radiographic studies are essential. AP and true lateral views of the hip and an AP view of the pelvis are the minimal imaging studies needed for these patients. Limb-length differences, femoral offset, the status of the greater trochanter, and the component orientation are noted. A preoperative CT scan to evaluate the position of the acetabular cup can provide important information regarding acetabular version.[116-119] Following evaluation and definition of the etiology of the dislocation, a treatment algorithm is established.[120,121]

The treatment options include closed reduction of the dislocated hip with or without bracing, total hip arthroplasty component revision, exchange of modular parts, cementing a liner into a well-fixed acetabular shell, bipolar or tripolar arthroplasty, use of a large femoral head, use of a constrained liner, advancement of the greater trochanter, and soft-tissue augmentation.[122-129] An understanding of the risk factors, the causes of dislocation, and management options enables the surgeon to effectively minimize the incidence of dislocation after total hip arthroplasty as well as to establish a strategy for treating a patient with an unstable total hip prosthesis.

Treatment Indications

Selection of the appropriate treatment option is guided by the cause and timing of the dislocation. Early dislocations occur within the first 3 to 6 months after the operation, and in most patients a single episode of dislocation can be adequately treated with closed reduction.[130] The role of cast-bracing or casting is controversial, and there are data supporting and refuting the use of this treatment after reduction of the hip.[123,126,129] Late dislocations are those that occur 5 years or more after the index procedure. Patients with a first-time late dislocation are at high risk for recurrent instability.[131] Late dislocations have multiple possible causes, including polyethylene wear, trauma, decline in neurologic function, increased soft-tissue laxity, or malposition of a total hip arthroplasty component.[132] Dislocations termed "intermediate" occur between 6 months and 5 years after the total hip arthroplasty. Patients in whom this is the first dislocation can usually be managed with closed reduction. Surgical management should be considered for patients with recurrent instability following the initial closed reduction.[73,132] Successful surgical management is critically dependent on accurate identification of the cause(s) of instability.[133]

Techniques and Results of Revision Total Hip Arthroplasty for Instability

Component revision is indicated when implants are seen to be malpositioned on radiographs, CT scans, or intraoperative evaluation.[118,119] Malpositioning of acetabular and femoral implants, limb-length inequality, and improper femoral offset can be corrected and restored in a reasonably predictable fashion with component revision.[11,58,120,134] Perhaps the easiest and most attractive option for managing recurrent instability in the presence of implants that appear to be in an appropriate position and alignment is modular component exchange, or so-called dry revision.[135] This option is indicated, however, only if the components are reasonably well positioned.[135] Increasing the head size and/or neck length and changing the acetabular liner are among the simplest solutions. Varying degrees of success with this approach have been reported in multiple small series. Toomey et al[135] successfully prevented recurrent dislocation with modular component exchange in 12 of 13 hips, although 3 hips dislocated once during the follow-up period. Importantly, these modular revisions also included excision of soft tissue and bone causing impingement in 10 hips. Nine of the hips were converted to either a lipped-bearing implant or an implant with a higher degree of lipped bearing. In another study, liner exchange was successful in 82% of cases of late instability associated with polyethylene wear.[136] In contrast, Barrack et al[88] reported multiple complications with modular component exchange, including liner dissociation and impingement, instability, and femoral head dislodgement from the stem trunnion. In cases of polyethylene wear-related instability, cementing a new liner into a well-fixed shell may provide an alternative to complete revision if the components are oriented correctly.[137,138]

High-walled liners can be valuable for treating or preventing dislocation of well-positioned components, as reported by Cobb et al[139] Similarly, in revision total hip arthroplasty, an augmentation device can act as an elevated-rim liner. McConway et al[140] reported a 1.6% dislocation rate in 307 patients treated with revision total hip arthroplasty with a posterior lip-augmentation device. Adding an augmentation device to the existing liner or socket has also been described and is effective in certain cases.[141-143] Currently, high-wall or lipped liners are used more sparingly because of concerns regarding impingement, wear, and limited hip motion.

Large femoral heads increase the head-neck ratio, thereby increasing the range of motion before impingement occurs, and increase the jump distance required for the head to dislocate.[107] In a series in which large femoral heads (36 mm and larger) were used, Beaulé et al[144] reported that more than 90% of the hips had no more instability after an average duration of follow-up of 6.5 years and only one had recurrent instability. Amstutz et al[113] reported that the dislocation rate after revisions for recurrent instability was higher than that after revisions for other etiologies. More troubling results were reported by Skeels et al,[145] who observed a 17% rate of recurrent dislocation in patients who had undergone revision surgery with a femoral head that was 36 mm or larger.

Another, less commonly used strategy to manage instability involves soft-tissue augmentation, or reinforcement of the hip abductor muscles and/or the posterior aspect of the hip capsule.[19] Reconstructions with an Achilles tendon allograft and a bone block, fascia lata, or a synthetic ligament have all been reported.[146-148] Indications for these procedures are unclear but may include deficiency of the hip abductor muscles or posterior aspect of the hip capsule in the setting of well-positioned, well-fixed total hip arthroplasty components.

Trochanteric advancement has been advocated for patients with well-positioned, well-fixed total hip arthroplasty implants.[124,149,150] Nonunion of the greater trochanter is a major concern, and trochanter-related hip pain is common. Ekelund[124] and Kaplan et al[150] independently reported 80% success rates with this approach in 21 patients each with recurrent dislocation and properly oriented components. Similarly, trochanteric osteotomy and advancement can be used for complex primary total hip arthroplasty to enhance stability.[151]

Bipolar arthroplasty is based on the principle of increasing the overall range of motion with articulation at two different bearing surfaces.[133,152,153] This provides a greater safe arc of motion before dislocation occurs and optimizes head-neck ratios while providing a larger jump distance. Parvizi and Morrey[133] reported the elimination of recurrent dislocation in 22 of 27 hips (81%). Attarian[152] and Ries and Wiedel[154] achieved 100% success using this technique. Medial and/or superior migration of the prosthesis, with resultant groin pain, is a concern if this technique is used.

Unconstrained tripolar hip arthroplasty uses a bipolar head to articulate with an acetabular shell and liner; this combination increases the head-neck ratio and the jump distance.[154-156] Grigoris et al[155] and Beaulé et al[154] used an unconstrained tripolar implant to successfully treat instability without compromising acetabular fixation in 95% of their patients. Levine et al[156] reported a 93% success rate in a series of 31 patients in whom an unstable total hip prosthesis had been treated with an unconstrained tripolar construct.

The final salvage option involves the use of a constrained acetabular liner.[19,157-169] Indications for this technique include hip abductor deficiency, neurologic impairment, low-demand patients with well-fixed components, instability for which the cause cannot be determined, and persistent intraoperative instability.[19,122,127,157,166,167] Constrained acetabular liners reduce the hip motion before impingement and therefore increase the risk of impingement and the acetabular shear stresses, which could lead to accelerated wear, loosening, or failure of fixation. These implants can be cemented into a well-fixed acetabular shell to reduce the morbidity of revision total hip arthroplasty.[137] Callaghan et al[162] reported no dislocations and two liner failures (a 94% success rate) with this technique in patients with a well-fixed, well-positioned, cementless acetabular shell. This procedure is considered a low-morbidity treatment option in the setting of a well-fixed, properly oriented acetabular component, especially in older, low-demand patients.[162]

Favorable results with the use of constrained devices have been reported in several studies, but these components should be considered only if no other treatment options are available.[170] At an average of 10.2 years after the use of 56 constrained tripolar devices, Goetz et al[163,164] reported a 7% failure rate secondary to recurrent dislocation, osteolysis, or aseptic loosening. Bremner et al[160] reported similar results, with a 6% failure rate secondary to recurrent dislocation or liner failure at 10.2 years. There is concern about the stability of fixation of constrained devices. Shrader et al[168] noted that, while no dislocations were seen, there were acetabular cup radiolucencies in 14% of their cases. Su and Pellicci[169] reported a 98% rate of success in terms of preventing instability in 85 hips with a constrained tripolar implant. There are modes of failure specific to tripolar constrained devices.[171-173] Guyen et al[172] reported 43 failures of tripolar constrained devices, with four types of failure: the bone-implant interface, the mechanism holding the constrained acetabular liner to the metal shell, the locking mechanism of the bipolar component, and dislocation of the head at the inner bearing. Methods for closed reduction of a constrained component have been described, but long-term outcomes have not yet been reported.[174]

Berend et al[158] reported on 755 alternatively designed constrained total hip arthroplasty components with a capture mechanism and locking ring design. The dislocation rate for the 667 hips followed for 10 years was 17.5%, and aseptic loosening of the cup and stem were also major long-term causes of failure that required a reoperation.[158] Newer designs allowing greater hip motion before impingement have been introduced. In another study, Berend et al[159] reported a 99% rate of success in terms of preventing recurrent dislocation in a group of 81 total hip arthroplasty revisions performed with a novel constrained device.

Summary

The intraoperative challenge of achieving stability and limb-length equality after total hip arthroplasty starts with preoperative planning, including physical examination, radiographic evaluation, templating, and aligning patient and surgeon expectations. Each surgical approach has advantages and disadvantages in terms of stability and limb length. It is the responsibility of the surgeon to be familiar with the benefits and drawbacks of each approach and use a method that most easily accomplishes the goals of a stable prosthetic construct, hip stability, and restoration of limb-length equality. Familiarity and experience with a total hip arthroplasty technique reduce the risk of dislocation and limb-length inequality. Intraoperatively, the prosthetic design, including the femoral head size and femoral offset, component orientation, and reconstruction of the hip soft tissues, are the critical variables for achieving success. Preoperative radiographic templating is paramount, and intraoperative maneuvers to determine limb length are important for obtaining the best result. Dislocation continues to be a major mode of failure of total hip arthroplasty. Obtaining a stable hip at the time of the initial total hip arthroplasty reduces the risk of this complication.

References

1. Bourne RB, Maloney WJ, Wright JG: An AOA critical issue: The outcome of the outcomes movement. *J Bone Joint Surg Am* 2004;86-A(3):633-640.
2. Chang RW, Pellisier JM, Hazen GB: A cost-effectiveness analysis of total hip arthroplasty for osteoarthritis of the hip. *JAMA* 1996;275(11):858-865.
3. Bozic KJ, Kurtz SM, Lau E, Ong K, Vail TP, Berry DJ: The epidemiology of revision total hip arthroplasty in the United States. *J Bone Joint Surg Am* 2009;91(1): 128-133.
4. Goldstein WM, Gordon A, Branson JJ: Leg length inequality in total hip arthroplasty. *Orthopedics* 2005;28(9, Suppl):S1037-S1040.
5. Khatod M, Barber T, Paxton E, Namba R, Fithian D: An analysis of the risk of hip dislocation with a contemporary total joint registry. *Clin Orthop Relat Res* 2006; 447:19-23.
6. Kurtz S, Ong K, Lau E, Mowat F, Halpern M: Projections of primary and revision hip and knee arthroplasty in the United States from 2005 to 2030. *J Bone Joint Surg Am* 2007;89(4):780-785.
7. Levy RN, Levy CM, Snyder J, Digiovanni J: Outcome and long-term results following total hip replacement in elderly patients. *Clin Orthop Relat Res* 1995;316: 25-30.
8. Phillips CB, Barrett JA, Losina E, et al: Incidence rates of dislocation, pulmonary embolism, and deep infection during the first six months after elective total hip replacement. *J Bone Joint Surg Am* 2003;85-A(1):20-26.
9. Sanchez-Sotelo J, Haidukewych GJ, Boberg CJ: Hospital cost of dislocation after primary total hip arthroplasty. *J Bone Joint Surg Am* 2006;88(2):290-294.
10. Abraham WD, Dimon JH III: Leg length discrepancy in total hip arthroplasty. *Orthop Clin North Am* 1992;23(2):201-209.
11. Alberton GM, High WA, Morrey BF: Dislocation after revision total hip arthroplasty: An analysis of risk factors and treatment options. *J Bone Joint Surg Am* 2002; 84-A(10):1788-1792.
12. Berry DJ, von Knoch M, Schleck CD, Harmsen WS: The cumulative long-term risk of dislocation after primary Charnley total hip arthroplasty. *J Bone Joint Surg Am* 2004;86-A(1):9-14.
13. Berry DJ, von Knoch M, Schleck CD, Harmsen WS: Effect of femoral head diameter and operative approach on risk of dislocation after primary total hip arthroplasty. *J Bone Joint Surg Am* 2005;87(11):2456-2463.
14. Callaghan JJ, Templeton JE, Liu SS, et al: Results of Charnley total hip arthroplasty at a minimum of thirty years: A concise follow-up of a previous report. *J Bone Joint Surg Am* 2004;86-A(4):690-695.
15. Conroy JL, Whitehouse SL, Graves SE, Pratt NL, Ryan P, Crawford RW: Risk factors for revision for early dislocation in total hip arthroplasty. *J Arthroplasty* 2008;23(6):867-872.
16. Eftekhar NS: Dislocation and instability complicating low friction arthroplasty of the hip joint. *Clin Orthop Relat Res* 1976;121: 120-125.
17. Heithoff BE, Callaghan JJ, Goetz DD, Sullivan PM, Pedersen DR, Johnston RC: Dislocation after total hip arthroplasty: A single surgeon's experience. *Orthop Clin North Am* 2001;32(4):587-591, viii.
18. Lewinnek GE, Lewis JL, Tarr R, Compere CL, Zimmerman JR: Dislocations after total hip-replacement arthroplasties. *J Bone Joint Surg Am* 1978;60(2): 217-220.
19. Parvizi J, Picinic E, Sharkey PF: Revision total hip arthroplasty for instability: Surgical techniques and principles. *J Bone Joint Surg Am* 2008;90(5):1134-1142.
20. Ritter MA: Dislocation and subluxation of the total hip replacement. *Clin Orthop Relat Res* 1976; 121:92-94.
21. Woo RY, Morrey BF: Dislocations after total hip arthroplasty. *J Bone Joint Surg Am* 1982;64(9):1295-1306.
22. Sadr Azodi O, Adami J, Lindström D, Eriksson KO, Wladis A,

Bellocco R: High body mass index is associated with increased risk of implant dislocation following primary total hip replacement: 2,106 patients followed for up to 8 years. *Acta Orthop* 2008;79(1): 141-147.

23. Ekelund A, Rydell N, Nilsson OS: Total hip arthroplasty in patients 80 years of age and older. *Clin Orthop Relat Res* 1992;281:101-106.
24. Jibodh SR, Gurkan I, Wenz JF: In-hospital outcome and resource use in hip arthroplasty: Influence of body mass. *Orthopedics* 2004; 27(6):594-601.
25. Jolles BM, Zangger P, Leyvraz PF: Factors predisposing to dislocation after primary total hip arthroplasty: A multivariate analysis. *J Arthroplasty* 2002;17(3): 282-288.
26. Kim Y, Morshed S, Joseph T, Bozic K, Ries MD: Clinical impact of obesity on stability following revision total hip arthroplasty. *Clin Orthop Relat Res* 2006;453: 142-146.
27. Krenzel BA, Berend ME, Malinzak RA, et al: High preoperative range of motion is a significant risk factor for dislocation in primary total hip arthroplasty. *J Arthroplasty* 2010;25(6, Suppl): 31-35.
28. Lachiewicz PF, Soileau ES: Stability of total hip arthroplasty in patients 75 years or older. *Clin Orthop Relat Res* 2002;405:65-69.
29. Lee BP, Berry DJ, Harmsen WS, Sim FH: Total hip arthroplasty for the treatment of an acute fracture of the femoral neck: Long-term results. *J Bone Joint Surg Am* 1998;80(1):70-75.
30. Meek RM, Allan DB, McPhillips G, Kerr L, Howie CR: Epidemiology of dislocation after total hip arthroplasty. *Clin Orthop Relat Res* 2006;447:9-18.
31. Morrey BF: Instability after total hip arthroplasty. *Orthop Clin North Am* 1992;23(2):237-248.
32. Morrey BF: Difficult complications after hip joint replacement: Dislocation. *Clin Orthop Relat Res* 1997;344:179-187.
33. Zwartelé RE, Brand R, Doets HC: Increased risk of dislocation after primary total hip arthroplasty in inflammatory arthritis: A prospective observational study of 410 hips. *Acta Orthop Scand* 2004;75(6):684-690.
34. Battaglia TC, Mulhall KJ, Brown TE, Saleh KJ: Increased surgical volume is associated with lower THA dislocation rates. *Clin Orthop Relat Res* 2006;447:28-33.
35. Katz JN, Losina E, Barrett J, et al: Association between hospital and surgeon procedure volume and outcomes of total hip replacement in the United States medicare population. *J Bone Joint Surg Am* 2001;83-A(11):1622-1629.
36. Austin MS, Hozack WJ, Sharkey PF, Rothman RH: Stability and leg length equality in total hip arthroplasty. *J Arthroplasty* 2003; 18(3, Suppl 1):88-90.
37. Edeen J, Sharkey PF, Alexander AH: Clinical significance of leg-length inequality after total hip arthroplasty. *Am J Orthop (Belle Mead NJ)* 1995;24(4): 347-351.
38. Parvizi J, Sharkey PF, Bissett GA, Rothman RH, Hozack WJ: Surgical treatment of limb-length discrepancy following total hip arthroplasty. *J Bone Joint Surg Am* 2003;85-A(12):2310-2317.
39. Ranawat CS, Rodriguez JA: Functional leg-length inequality following total hip arthroplasty. *J Arthroplasty* 1997;12(4):359-364.
40. Charles MN, Bourne RB, Davey JR, Greenwald AS, Morrey BF, Rorabeck CH: Soft-tissue balancing of the hip: The role of femoral offset restoration. *Instr Course Lect* 2005;54:131-141.
41. Itokazu M, Masuda K, Ohno T, Itoh Y, Takatsu T, Wenyi Y: A simple method of intraoperative limb length measurement in total hip arthroplasty. *Bull Hosp Jt Dis* 1997;56(4):204-205.
42. Berend KR, Lombardi AV Jr, Seng BE, Adams JB: Enhanced early outcomes with the anterior supine intermuscular approach in primary total hip arthroplasty. *J Bone Joint Surg Am* 2009; 91(Suppl 6):107-120.
43. Kennon RE, Keggi JM, Wetmore RS, Zatorski LE, Huo MH, Keggi KJ: Total hip arthroplasty through a minimally invasive anterior surgical approach. *J Bone Joint Surg Am* 2003;85-A(Suppl 4):39-48.
44. Matta JM, Shahrdar C, Ferguson T: Single-incision anterior approach for total hip arthroplasty on an orthopaedic table. *Clin Orthop Relat Res* 2005;441:115-124.
45. Seng BE, Berend KR, Ajluni AF, Lombardi AV Jr: Anterior-supine minimally invasive total hip arthroplasty: Defining the learning curve. *Orthop Clin North Am* 2009;40(3):343-350.
46. Light TR, Keggi KJ: Anterior approach to hip arthroplasty. *Clin Orthop Relat Res* 1980;152: 255-260.
47. Berger RA: Total hip arthroplasty using the minimally invasive two-incision approach. *Clin Orthop Relat Res* 2003;417:232-241.
48. Berger RA: Mini-incision total hip replacement using an anterolateral approach: Technique and results. *Orthop Clin North Am* 2004; 35(2):143-151.
49. Archibeck MJ, White RE Jr: Learning curve for the two-incision total hip replacement. *Clin Orthop Relat Res* 2004;429: 232-238.
50. Berry DJ, Berger RA, Callaghan JJ, et al: Minimally invasive total hip arthroplasty: Development, early results, and a critical analysis. Presented at the Annual Meeting of the American Orthopaedic Association, Charleston,

South Carolina, USA, June 14, 2003. *J Bone Joint Surg Am* 2003; 85-A(11):2235-2246.

51. Bal BS, Haltom D, Aleto T, Barrett M: Early complications of primary total hip replacement performed with a two-incision minimally invasive technique. *J Bone Joint Surg Am* 2005; 87(11):2432-2438.

52. Mardones R, Pagnano MW, Nemanich JP, Trousdale RT: The Frank Stinchfield Award: Muscle damage after total hip arthroplasty done with the two-incision and mini-posterior techniques. *Clin Orthop Relat Res* 2005;441:63-67.

53. Pagnano MW, Leone J, Lewallen DG, Hanssen AD: Two-incision THA had modest outcomes and some substantial complications. *Clin Orthop Relat Res* 2005;441:86-90.

54. Hardinge K: The direct lateral approach to the hip. *J Bone Joint Surg Br* 1982;64(1):17-19.

55. Mallory TH, Lombardi AV Jr, Fada RA, Herrington SM, Eberle RW: Dislocation after total hip arthroplasty using the anterolateral abductor split approach. *Clin Orthop Relat Res* 1999;358:166-172.

56. Iagulli ND, Mallory TH, Berend KR, et al: A simple and accurate method for determining leg length in primary total hip arthroplasty. *Am J Orthop (Belle Mead NJ)* 2006;35(10):455-457.

57. Demos HA, Rorabeck CH, Bourne RB, MacDonald SJ, McCalden RW: Instability in primary total hip arthroplasty with the direct lateral approach. *Clin Orthop Relat Res* 2001;393:168-180.

58. Ritter MA, Harty LD, Keating ME, Faris PM, Meding JB: A clinical comparison of the anterolateral and posterolateral approaches to the hip. *Clin Orthop Relat Res* 2001;385:95-99.

59. Kenny P, O'Brien CP, Synnott K, Walsh MG: Damage to the superior gluteal nerve after two different approaches to the hip. *J Bone Joint Surg Br* 1999;81(6): 979-981.

60. Goldstein WM, Gleason TF, Kopplin M, Branson JJ: Prevalence of dislocation after total hip arthroplasty through a posterolateral approach with partial capsulotomy and capsulorrhaphy. *J Bone Joint Surg Am* 2001;83-A(Pt 1, Suppl 2):2-7.

61. Woolson ST, Mow CS, Syquia JF, Lannin JV, Schurman DJ: Comparison of primary total hip replacements performed with a standard incision or a mini-incision. *J Bone Joint Surg Am* 2004;86-A(7):1353-1358.

62. Ogonda L, Wilson R, Archbold P, et al: A minimal-incision technique in total hip arthroplasty does not improve early postoperative outcomes: A prospective, randomized, controlled trial. *J Bone Joint Surg Am* 2005;87(4): 701-710.

63. Huddleston HD: An accurate method for measuring leg length and hip offset in hip arthroplasty. *Orthopedics* 1997;20(4):331-332.

64. Masonis JL, Bourne RB: Surgical approach, abductor function, and total hip arthroplasty dislocation. *Clin Orthop Relat Res* 2002;405: 46-53.

65. Chiu FY, Chen CM, Chung TY, Lo WH, Chen TH: The effect of posterior capsulorrhaphy in primary total hip arthroplasty: A prospective randomized study. *J Arthroplasty* 2000;15(2): 194-199.

66. Pellicci PM, Bostrom M, Poss R: Posterior approach to total hip replacement using enhanced posterior soft tissue repair. *Clin Orthop Relat Res* 1998;355:224-228.

67. Sierra RJ, Raposo JM, Trousdale RT, Cabanela ME: Dislocation of primary THA done through a posterolateral approach in the elderly. *Clin Orthop Relat Res* 2005;441:262-267.

68. Suh KT, Park BG, Choi YJ: A posterior approach to primary total hip arthroplasty with soft tissue repair. *Clin Orthop Relat Res* 2004;418:162-167.

69. Weeden SH, Paprosky WG, Bowling JW: The early dislocation rate in primary total hip arthroplasty following the posterior approach with posterior soft-tissue repair. *J Arthroplasty* 2003;18(6): 709-713.

70. Kim YS, Kwon SY, Sun DH, Han SK, Maloney WJ: Modified posterior approach to total hip arthroplasty to enhance joint stability. *Clin Orthop Relat Res* 2008; 466(2):294-299.

71. Edwards BN, Tullos HS, Noble PC: Contributory factors and etiology of sciatic nerve palsy in total hip arthroplasty. *Clin Orthop Relat Res* 1987;218:136-141.

72. Navarro RA, Schmalzried TP, Amstutz HC, Dorey FJ: Surgical approach and nerve palsy in total hip arthroplasty. *J Arthroplasty* 1995;10(1):1-5.

73. Lachiewicz PF: Dislocation, in Hozack WJ, Parvizi J, Bender B, eds: *Surgical Treatment of Hip Arthritis: Reconstruction, Replacement, and Revision*. Philadelphia, PA, Saunders Elsevier, 2010, pp 429-436.

74. Kadakia NR, Noble PC, Sugano N, Paravic V: Posterior dislocation of the artificial hip joint: Effect of cup anteversion. *Orthop Trans* 1998-1999;22: 905-906.

75. Paterno SA, Lachiewicz PF, Kelley SS: The influence of patient-related factors and the position of the acetabular component on the rate of dislocation after total hip replacement. *J Bone Joint Surg Am* 1997;79(8):1202-1210.

76. Biedermann R, Tonin A, Krismer M, Rachbauer F, Eibl G, Stöckl B: Reducing the risk of dislocation after total hip arthroplasty: The effect of orientation of

the acetabular component. *J Bone Joint Surg Br* 2005;87(6):762-769.

77. Hassan DM, Johnston GH, Dust WN, Watson G, Dolovich AT: Accuracy of intraoperative assessment of acetabular prosthesis placement. *J Arthroplasty* 1998; 13(1):80-84.

78. Rittmeister M, Callitsis C: Factors influencing cup orientation in 500 consecutive total hip replacements. *Clin Orthop Relat Res* 2006;445:192-196.

79. McCollum DE, Gray WJ: Dislocation after total hip arthroplasty: Causes and prevention. *Clin Orthop Relat Res* 1990;261:159-170.

80. Archbold HA, Mockford B, Molloy D, McConway J, Ogonda L, Beverland D: The transverse acetabular ligament: An aid to orientation of the acetabular component during primary total hip replacement. A preliminary study of 1000 cases investigating post-operative stability. *J Bone Joint Surg Br* 2006;88(7):883-886.

81. Sotereanos NG, Miller MC, Smith B, Hube R, Sewecke JJ, Wohlrab D: Using intraoperative pelvic landmarks for acetabular component placement in total hip arthroplasty. *J Arthroplasty* 2006; 21(6):832-840.

82. Honl M, Schwieger K, Salineros M, Jacobs J, Morlock M, Wimmer M: Orientation of the acetabular component: A comparison of five navigation systems with conventional surgical technique. *J Bone Joint Surg Br* 2006; 88(10):1401-1405.

83. Jaramaz B, DiGioia AM III, Blackwell M, Nikou C: Computer assisted measurement of cup placement in total hip replacement. *Clin Orthop Relat Res* 1998; 354:70-81.

84. Spencer JM, Day RE, Sloan KE, Beaver RJ: Computer navigation of the acetabular component: A cadaver reliability study. *J Bone Joint Surg Br* 2006;88(7): 972-975.

85. McGrory BJ, Morrey BF, Cahalan TD, An KN, Cabanela ME: Effect of femoral offset on range of motion and abductor muscle strength after total hip arthroplasty. *J Bone Joint Surg Br* 1995; 77(6):865-869.

86. Herrlin K, Selvik G, Pettersson H, Kesek P, Onnerfält R, Ohlin A: Position, orientation and component interaction in dislocation of the total hip prosthesis. *Acta Radiol* 1988;29(4):441-444.

87. Widmer KH, Zurfluh B: Compliant positioning of total hip components for optimal range of motion. *J Orthop Res* 2004;22(4): 815-821.

88. Barrack RL, Burke DW, Cook SD, Skinner HB, Harris WH: Complications related to modularity of total hip components. *J Bone Joint Surg Br* 1993; 75(5):688-692.

89. Woolson ST, Hartford JM, Sawyer A: Results of a method of leg-length equalization for patients undergoing primary total hip replacement. *J Arthroplasty* 1999; 14(2):159-164.

90. Bourne RB, Rorabeck CH: Soft tissue balancing: the hip. *J Arthroplasty* 2002;17(4, Suppl 1):17-22.

91. Longjohn D, Dorr LD: Soft tissue balance of the hip. *J Arthroplasty* 1998;13(1):97-100.

92. Asayama I, Naito M, Fujisawa M, Kambe T: Relationship between radiographic measurements of reconstructed hip joint position and the Trendelenburg sign. *J Arthroplasty* 2002;17(6):747-751.

93. Sakalkale DP, Sharkey PF, Eng K, Hozack WJ, Rothman RH: Effect of femoral component offset on polyethylene wear in total hip arthroplasty. *Clin Orthop Relat Res* 2001;388:125-134.

94. Mineo R, Berend KR, Mallory TH, Lombardi AV Jr: A lateralized tapered titanium cementless femoral component does not increase thigh or trochanteric pain. *Surg Technol Int* 2007;16: 210-214.

95. Incavo SJ, Havener T, Benson E, McGrory BJ, Coughlin KM, Beynnon BD: Efforts to improve cementless femoral stems in THR: 2- to 5-year follow-up of a high-offset femoral stem with distal stem modification (Secur-Fit Plus). *J Arthroplasty* 2004;19(1): 61-67.

96. Bhave A, Paley D, Herzenberg JE: Improvement in gait parameters after lengthening for the treatment of limb-length discrepancy. *J Bone Joint Surg Am* 1999;81(4): 529-534.

97. Gurney B, Mermier C, Robergs R, Gibson A, Rivero D: Effects of limb-length discrepancy on gait economy and lower-extremity muscle activity in older adults. *J Bone Joint Surg Am* 2001; 83-A(6):907-915.

98. Maloney WJ, Keeney JA: Leg length discrepancy after total hip arthroplasty. *J Arthroplasty* 2004; 19(4, Suppl 1):108-110.

99. White TO, Dougall TW: Arthroplasty of the hip: Leg length is not important. *J Bone Joint Surg Br* 2002;84(3):335-338.

100. Ranawat CS, Rao RR, Rodriguez JA, Bhende HS: Correction of limb-length inequality during total hip arthroplasty. *J Arthroplasty* 2001;16(6):715-720.

101. Jasty M, Webster W, Harris W: Management of limb length inequality during total hip replacement. *Clin Orthop Relat Res* 1996; 333:165-171.

102. Matsuda K, Nakamura S, Matsushita T: A simple method to minimize limb-length discrepancy after hip arthroplasty. *Acta Orthop* 2006;77(3):375-379.

103. Shiramizu K, Naito M, Shitama T, Nakamura Y, Shitama H: L-shaped caliper for limb length measurement during total hip

arthroplasty. *J Bone Joint Surg Br* 2004;86(7):966-969.

104. Sarin VK, Pratt WR, Bradley GW: Accurate femur repositioning is critical during intraoperative total hip arthroplasty length and offset assessment. *J Arthroplasty* 2005;20(7):887-891.

105. Bartz RL, Nobel PC, Kadakia NR, Tullos HS: The effect of femoral component head size on posterior dislocation of the artificial hip joint. *J Bone Joint Surg Am* 2000;82(9):1300-1307.

106. Kung PL, Ries MD: Effect of femoral head size and abductors on dislocation after revision THA. *Clin Orthop Relat Res* 2007;465: 170-174.

107. Sariali E, Lazennec JY, Khiami F, Catonné Y: Mathematical evaluation of jumping distance in total hip arthroplasty: Influence of abduction angle, femoral head offset, and head diameter. *Acta Orthop* 2009;80(3):277-282.

108. Smith TM, Berend KR, Lombardi AV Jr, Emerson RH Jr, Mallory TH: Metal-on-metal total hip arthroplasty with large heads may prevent early dislocation. *Clin Orthop Relat Res* 2005;441: 137-142.

109. Cuckler JM, Moore KD, Lombardi AV Jr, McPherson E, Emerson R: Large versus small femoral heads in metal-on-metal total hip arthroplasty. *J Arthroplasty* 2004; 19(8, Suppl 3):41-44.

110. Peters CL, McPherson E, Jackson JD, Erickson JA: Reduction in early dislocation rate with large-diameter femoral heads in primary total hip arthroplasty. *J Arthroplasty* 2007;22(6, Suppl 2): 140-144.

111. Smit MJ: Hip stability in primary total hip arthroplasty using an anatomically sized femoral head. *Orthopedics* 2009;32(7):489.

112. Lachiewicz PF, Soileau ES: Dislocation of primary total hip arthroplasty with 36 and 40-mm femoral heads. *Clin Orthop Relat Res* 2006;453:153-155.

113. Amstutz HC, Le Duff MJ, Beaulé PE: Prevention and treatment of dislocation after total hip replacement using large diameter balls. *Clin Orthop Relat Res* 2004; 429:108-116.

114. Halley D, Glassman A, Crowninshield RD: Recurrent dislocation after revision total hip replacement with a large prosthetic femoral head: A case report. *J Bone Joint Surg Am* 2004;86-A(4): 827-830.

115. Spangehl MJ, Masri BA, O'Connell JX, Duncan CP: Prospective analysis of preoperative and intraoperative investigations for the diagnosis of infection at the sites of two hundred and two revision total hip arthroplasties. *J Bone Joint Surg Am* 1999;81(5):672-683.

116. Barmeir E, Dubowitz B, Roffman M: Computed tomography in the assessment and planning of complicated total hip replacement. *Acta Orthop Scand* 1982;53(4): 597-604.

117. Lasda NA, Levinsohn EM, Yuan HA, Bunnell WP: Computerized tomography in disorders of the hip. *J Bone Joint Surg Am* 1978;60(8):1099-1102.

118. Mian SW, Truchly G, Pflum FA: Computed tomography measurement of acetabular cup anteversion and retroversion in total hip arthroplasty. *Clin Orthop Relat Res* 1992;276:206-209.

119. Pierchon F, Pasquier G, Cotten A, Fontaine C, Clarisse J, Duquennoy A: Causes of dislocation of total hip arthroplasty: CT study of component alignment. *J Bone Joint Surg Br* 1994;76(1):45-48.

120. Dorr LD, Wan Z: Causes of and treatment protocol for instability of total hip replacement. *Clin Orthop Relat Res* 1998;355: 144-151.

121. Ritter MA: A treatment plan for the dislocated total hip arthroplasty. *Clin Orthop Relat Res* 1980; 153:153-155.

122. Cameron HU: Use of a constrained acetabular component in revision hip surgery. *Contemp Orthop* 1991;23:481-484.

123. Clayton ML, Thirupathi RG: Dislocation following total hip arthroplasty: Management by special brace in selected patients. *Clin Orthop Relat Res* 1983;177: 154-159.

124. Ekelund A: Trochanteric osteotomy for recurrent dislocation of total hip arthroplasty. *J Arthroplasty* 1993;8(6):629-632.

125. LaPorte DM, Mont MA, Pierre-Jacques H, Peyton RS, Hungerford DS: Technique for acetabular liner revision in a nonmodular metal-backed component. *J Arthroplasty* 1998;13(3):348-350.

126. Mallory TH, Vaughn BK, Lombardi AV Jr, Kraus TJ: Prophylactic use of a hip cast-brace following primary and revision total hip arthroplasty. *Orthop Rev* 1988; 17(2):178-183.

127. Russin LA, Sonni A: Indications for the use of a constrained THR prosthesis. *Orthop Rev* 1981;10: 81-84.

128. Sioen W, Simon JP, Labey L, Van Audekercke R: Posterior transosseous capsulotendinous repair in total hip arthroplasty: A cadaver study. *J Bone Joint Surg Am* 2002; 84-A(10):1793-1798.

129. Williams JF, Gottesman MJ, Mallory TH: Dislocation after total hip arthroplasty: Treatment with an above-knee hip spica cast. *Clin Orthop Relat Res* 1982;171:53-58.

130. Woolson ST, Rahimtoola ZO: Risk factors for dislocation during the first 3 months after primary total hip replacement. *J Arthroplasty* 1999;14(6):662-668.

131. von Knoch M, Berry DJ, Harmsen WS, Morrey BF: Late dislocation after total hip arthroplasty. *J Bone Joint Surg Am* 2002; 84-A(11):1949-1953.

132. Joshi A, Lee CM, Markovic L, Vlatis G, Murphy JC: Prognosis of dislocation after total hip arthroplasty. *J Arthroplasty* 1998; 13(1):17-21.

133. Parvizi J, Morrey BF: Bipolar hip arthroplasty as a salvage treatment for instability of the hip. *J Bone Joint Surg Am* 2000;82-A(8): 1132-1139.

134. Olerud S, Karlström G: Recurrent dislocation after total hip replacement: Treatment by fixing an additional sector to the acetabular component. *J Bone Joint Surg Br* 1985;67(3):402-405.

135. Toomey SD, Hopper RH Jr, McAuley JP, Engh CA: Modular component exchange for treatment of recurrent dislocation of a total hip replacement in selected patients. *J Bone Joint Surg Am* 2001;83-A(10):1529-1533.

136. Parvizi J, Wade FA, Rapuri V, Springer BD, Berry DJ, Hozack WJ: Revision hip arthroplasty for late instability secondary to polyethylene wear. *Clin Orthop Relat Res* 2006;447:66-69.

137. Beaulé PE, Ebramzadeh E, LeDuff M, Prasad R, Amstutz HC: Cementing a liner into a stable cementless acetabular shell: The double-socket technique. *J Bone Joint Surg Am* 2004; 86-A(5):929-934.

138. Heck DA, Murray DG: In vivo construction of a metal-backed, high-molecular-weight polyethylene cup during McKee-Farrar revision total joint arthroplasty: A case report. *J Arthroplasty* 1986; 1(3):203-206.

139. Cobb TK, Morrey BF, Ilstrup DM: The elevated-rim acetabular liner in total hip arthroplasty: Relationship to postoperative dislocation. *J Bone Joint Surg Am* 1996;78(1):80-86.

140. McConway J, O'Brien S, Doran E, Archbold P, Beverland D: The use of a posterior lip augmentation device for a revision of recurrent dislocation after primary cemented Charnley/Charnley Elite total hip replacement: Results at a mean follow-up of six years and nine months. *J Bone Joint Surg Br* 2007;89(12): 1581-1585.

141. Mogensen B, Arnason H, Jónsson GT: Socket wall addition for dislocating total hip: Report of two cases. *Acta Orthop Scand* 1986;57(4):373-374.

142. Rogers M, Blom AW, Barnett A, Karantana A, Bannister GC: Revision for recurrent dislocation of total hip replacement. *Hip Int* 2009;19(2):109-113.

143. Williamson JB, Galasko CS, Rowley DI: Failure of acetabular augmentation for recurrent dislocation after hip arthroplasty: Report of 3 cases. *Acta Orthop Scand* 1989;60(6):676-677.

144. Beaulé PE, Schmalzried TP, Udomkiat P, Amstutz HC: Jumbo femoral head for the treatment of recurrent dislocation following total hip replacement. *J Bone Joint Surg Am* 2002;84-A(2):256-263.

145. Skeels MD, Berend KR, Lombardi AV Jr: The dislocator, early and late: The role of large heads. *Orthopedics* 2009;32(9).

146. Barbosa JK, Khan AM, Andrew JG: Treatment of recurrent dislocation of total hip arthroplasty using a ligament prosthesis. *J Arthroplasty* 2004;19(3): 318-321.

147. Lavigne MJ, Sanchez AA, Coutts RD: Recurrent dislocation after total hip arthroplasty: Treatment with an Achilles tendon allograft. *J Arthroplasty* 2001;16(8, Suppl 1):13-18.

148. Strømsøe K, Eikvar K: Fascia lata plasty in recurrent posterior dislocation after total hip arthroplasty. *Arch Orthop Trauma Surg* 1995; 114(5):292-294.

149. Dennis DA, Lynch CB: Trochanteric osteotomy and advancement: A technique for abductor related hip instability. *Orthopedics* 2004; 27(9):959-961.

150. Kaplan SJ, Thomas WH, Poss R: Trochanteric advancement for recurrent dislocation after total hip arthroplasty. *J Arthroplasty* 1987;2(2):119-124.

151. Della Valle CJ, Berger RA, Rosenberg AG, Jacobs JJ, Sheinkop MB, Paprosky WG: Extended trochanteric osteotomy in complex primary total hip arthroplasty: A brief note. *J Bone Joint Surg Am* 2003;85-A(12):2385-2390.

152. Attarian DE: Bipolar arthroplasty for recurrent total hip instability. *J South Orthop Assoc* 1999;8(4): 249-253.

153. Ries MD, Wiedel JD: Bipolar hip arthroplasty for recurrent dislocation after total hip arthroplasty: A report of three cases. *Clin Orthop Relat Res* 1992;278:121-127.

154. Beaulé PE, Roussignol X, Schmalzried TP, Udomkiat P, Amstutz HC, Dujardin FH: Tripolar arthroplasty for recurrent total hip prosthesis dislocation. *Rev Chir Orthop Reparatrice Appar Mot* 2003;89(3):242-249.

155. Grigoris P, Grecula MJ, Amstutz HC: Tripolar hip replacement for recurrent prosthetic dislocation. *Clin Orthop Relat Res* 1994;304:148-155.

156. Levine BR, Della Valle CJ, Deirmengian CA, et al: The use of a tripolar articulation in revision total hip arthroplasty: A minimum of 24 months' follow-up. *J Arthroplasty* 2008;23(8):1182-1188.

157. Anderson MJ, Murray WR, Skinner HB: Constrained acetabular components. *J Arthroplasty* 1994; 9(1):17-23.

158. Berend KR, Lombardi AV Jr, Mallory TH, Adams JB, Russell JH, Groseth KL: The long-term outcome of 755 consecutive constrained acetabular components in total hip arthroplasty examining the successes and fail-

ures. *J Arthroplasty* 2005;20(7, Suppl 3):93-102.

159. Berend KR, Lombardi AV Jr, Welch M, Adams JB: A constrained device with increased range of motion prevents early dislocation. *Clin Orthop Relat Res* 2006;447:70-75.

160. Bremner BR, Goetz DD, Callaghan JJ, Capello WN, Johnston RC: Use of constrained acetabular components for hip instability: An average 10-year follow-up study. *J Arthroplasty* 2003;18(7, Suppl 1):131-137.

161. Callaghan JJ, O'Rourke MR, Goetz DD, Lewallen DG, Johnston RC, Capello WN: Use of a constrained tripolar acetabular liner to treat intraoperative instability and postoperative dislocation after total hip arthroplasty: A review of our experience. *Clin Orthop Relat Res* 2004;429: 117-123.

162. Callaghan JJ, Parvizi J, Novak CC, et al: A constrained liner cemented into a secure cementless acetabular shell. *J Bone Joint Surg Am* 2004;86-A(10): 2206-2211.

163. Goetz DD, Bremner BR, Callaghan JJ, Capello WN, Johnston RC: Salvage of a recurrently dislocating total hip prosthesis with use of a constrained acetabular component: A concise follow-up of a previous report. *J Bone Joint Surg Am* 2004;86-A(11):2419-2423.

164. Goetz DD, Capello WN, Callaghan JJ, Brown TD, Johnston RC: Salvage of a recurrently dislocating total hip prosthesis with use of a constrained acetabular component: A retrospective analysis of fifty-six cases. *J Bone Joint Surg Am* 1998;80(4): 502-509.

165. Goetz DD, Capello WN, Callaghan JJ, Brown TD, Johnston RC: Salvage of total hip instability with a constrained acetabular component. *Clin Orthop Relat Res* 1998;355:171-181.

166. Lombardi AV Jr, Mallory TH, Kraus TJ, Vaughn BK: Preliminary report on the S-ROM constraining acetabular insert: A retrospective clinical experience. *Orthopedics* 1991;14(3):297-303.

167. Padgett DE, Warashina H: The unstable total hip replacement. *Clin Orthop Relat Res* 2004;420: 72-79.

168. Shrader MW, Parvizi J, Lewallen DG: The use of a constrained acetabular component to treat instability after total hip arthroplasty. *J Bone Joint Surg Am* 2003; 85-A(11):2179-2183.

169. Su EP, Pellicci PM: The role of constrained liners in total hip arthroplasty. *Clin Orthop Relat Res* 2004;420:122-129.

170. Kaper BP, Bernini PM: Failure of a constrained acetabular prosthesis of a total hip arthroplasty: A report of four cases. *J Bone Joint Surg Am* 1998;80(4):561-565.

171. Fisher DA, Kiley K: Constrained acetabular cup disassembly. *J Arthroplasty* 1994;9(3):325-329.

172. Guyen O, Lewallen DG, Cabanela ME: Modes of failure of Osteonics constrained tripolar implants: A retrospective analysis of forty-three failed implants. *J Bone Joint Surg Am* 2008;90(7): 1553-1560.

173. Robertson WJ, Mattern CJ, Hur J, Su EP, Pellicci PM: Failure mechanisms and closed reduction of a constrained tripolar acetabular liner. *J Arthroplasty* 2009; 24(2):322, e5-e11.

174. McPherson EJ, Costigan WM, Gerhardt MB, Norris LR: Closed reduction of dislocated total hip with S-ROM constrained acetabular component. *J Arthroplasty* 1999;14(7):882-885.

The Evolution and Modern Use of Metal-on-Metal Bearings in Total Hip Arthroplasty

Mark H. Gonzalez, MD, MEng
Ryan Carr, MD
Sharon Walton, MD
William M. Mihalko, MD, PhD

Abstract

Metal-on-metal bearings have been used in total hip arthroplasty for decades. Because younger patients with higher physical demands are now being treated with hip arthroplasty, the popularity and use of metal-on-metal bearings has increased over the past 10 years. New concerns, however, have emerged regarding the percentage of patients with a hypersensitivity reaction or pseudotumor formation after arthroplasty with these bearings. These concerns have raised questions concerning long-term outcomes for patients treated with metal-on-metal bearings. It is important for orthopaedic surgeons to review these issues so that better educated decisions can be made in treating their patients.

Instr Course Lect 2011;60:247-255.

First-generation metal-on-metal hip implants were introduced in the late 1930s. Despite long-term survival, many implants showed significant radiographic loosening.[1] Poor manufacturing techniques, crude designs, and the lack of adequate fixation were some of the problems encountered with the early designs.[1-4] Additional concerns over metal sensitivity and the early success of the metal-on-polyethylene Charnley prosthesis eventually led to a decline in the use of metal-on-metal hip implants.[2] In 1984, there was renewed interest in the metal-on-metal hip prosthesis because of evolving evidence of very low volumetric wear rates and a lack of periprosthetic inflammatory changes, unlike those seen in the polyethylene designs. The growing interest in metal-on-metal bearings used in implants for total hip arthroplasty (THA) has heightened concerns over the effects of the metal ions released from the degradation of these implants. This fact, coupled with recent Australian and US experience of increased revision rates with the ASR Hip System (DePuy, Warsaw, IN; device recently recalled in the United States) and the British medical alert concerning hip resurfacing devices has made surgeons aware of the possible reaction to particulate metal debris that patients may experience and that may increase the risk for an early revision.[5,6] Monitoring recommendations from the British medical device alert for patients with metal-on-metal bearings are summarized in **Table 1**.[5] This chapter will discuss the literature regarding the local and systemic effects of metal-on-metal implants as well as hypersensitivity and carcinogenic effects.

Dr. Gonzalez or an immediate family member has received royalties from Johnson & Johnson; serves as a paid consultant to or is an employee of Smith & Nephew and owns stock or stock options in Ortho Sensing Technology. Dr. Mihalko or an immediate family member has received royalties from Aesculap/B. Braun; is a member of a speakers' bureau or has made paid presentations on behalf of Aesculap/B. Braun; serves as a paid consultant to or is an employee of Aesculap/B. Braun; has received research or institutional support from Aesculap/B. Braun, Smith & Nephew, Stryker, and Corin USA; and has received nonincome support (such as equipment or services), commercially derived honoraria, nor other non–research-related funding (such as paid travel) from Aesculap/B. Braun. Neither of the following authors or any immediate family member has received anything of value from or owns stock in a commercial company or institution related directly or indirectly to the subject of this chapter: Dr. Carr and Dr. Walton.

Table 1
Monitoring Recommendation From the British Medical Device Alert for Patients With Metal-on-Metal Bearings

Patient follow-up should be done at least annually for 5 years postoperatively and more frequently in the presence of symptoms. Beyond 5 years, follow up in accordance with locally agreed protocols.
Evaluate patients with painful metal-on-metal hip replacements. Specific tests should include an evaluation of cobalt and chromium ion levels in the patient's blood and cross-sectional imaging, including MRI or ultrasound scanning.
Consider measuring cobalt and chromium ion levels in the blood and/or cross-sectional imaging for the following patient groups:
Patients with radiologic features associated with adverse outcomes, including component position
Patients with small component size (hip resurfacing arthroplasty only)
If the patient or surgeon is concerned about a metal-on-metal hip replacement
Cohorts of patients in which there is concern about higher than expected rates of failure
If either cobalt or chromium ion levels are elevated above seven parts per billion, a second test should be performed 3 months after the first to identify patients who require closer surveillance, which may include cross-sectional imaging.
If imaging shows soft-tissue reactions, fluid collections, or tissue masses, revision surgery should be considered

Wear Characteristics of Metal, Polyethylene, and Ceramic Prostheses

An analysis of second-generation metal-on-metal hip prostheses showed a biphasic wear distribution comparable to first-generation prostheses. The initial volumetric run-in wear rate is threefold to fivefold that of the steady-state wear rate.[4] This is believed to result from the opposing surface asperities that are polished away during initial use. Steady-state wear is believed to occur after one million cycles (mc) and produces a volumetric wear rate of 0.43 mm^3/y (range, 0.02 to 1.63 mm^3/y) for the low carbon Sikomet prosthesis (Endoprothetik AG, Modling, Austria) and 1.0 ± 1.64 mm^3/mc for the high carbon Metasul prosthesis (Zimmer, Warsaw, IN).[7,8] Particle analysis demonstrates mean particle size in the range of 25 to 36 nm and generates 4×10^{12} to 6×10^{13} particles per million cycles as shown in high and low carbon pairings.[9]

This pattern differs from polyethylene prostheses that produce a monophasic wear pattern and a volumetric wear rate of 16.6 ± 0.4 mm^3/mc to 20.0 ± 2.6 mm^3/mc.[10] Particle analysis showed particles in the range of 0.1 to 10 μm and generation of 5×10^{11} particles per million cycles.[9] Polyethylene prostheses produce larger particles and greater volumetric wear than metallic prostheses.

Ceramic prostheses also have a monophasic wear pattern. The volumetric wear rates are 0.05 to 1.6 mm^3/mc.[11,12] Particle analysis demonstrates mean particle size of 0.39 μm (range, 0.13 to 78.4 μm).[3] Ceramic prostheses produce lower volumetric wear rates compared to metallic and polyethylene prostheses.

Volumetric wear is now understood to comprise tribology (the science related to the mechanisms of friction, lubrication, and wear of surfaces that are in relative motion with each other), as well as the composition of the prostheses. Low carbon pairings of a femoral head and an acetabular cup were shown to have significantly higher bedding-in and steady-state wear rates than mixed and high carbon pairings.[9] Mixed evidence also has led to the belief that larger femoral heads (of approximately 36 mm) produce fluid film lubrication conditions that allow more of the load to be carried by the fluid film as opposed to asperity contact seen in smaller femoral heads and in those with mixed lubrication conditions. Lubrication films within the bearing are important because the thicker the film, the lower the number of wear particles produced by the bearing. Analysis showed that 16- and 22.25-mm femoral heads produce no surface separation, and volumetric wear rates of 4.85 mm^3/mc and 6.3 mm^3/mc, respectively.[13] Larger femoral heads of 28 mm and 36 mm produce mixed and fluid film lubrications and volumetric wear rates of 0.54 mm^3/mc and 0.07mm^3/mc, respectively.[13]

Clearance is also clinically significant. The clearance of a bearing relates to the difference between the convex and concave curvatures of the opposite sides of the bearing. In the metal-on-metal hip, if the ball is slightly smaller (for example, 30 μm), then the bearing allows fluid film to form and decreases bearing wear. Evidence reveals that an increase in clearance results in greater volumetric wear,[14] whereas a decrease in clearance results in increased fluid film thickness and decreased contact pressure. However, there is a fine balance between having a low clearance, which optimizes the fluid film condition, and a clearance that is too low and increases the contact pressure. Critically low clearance rates cause concern for the reemergence of locking, increased friction, and increased wear rates.[15] Equatorial contact resulting from decreased clearance has shown greater wear rates and a higher release of particulate debris.

Metal-on-Polyethylene Versus Metal-on-Metal

It is now widely accepted that the larger polyethylene particles seen in metal-on-polyethylene bearing surfaces stimulate the activation of multinucleated giant cells, causing bone reabsorption and aseptic loosening. An examination of tissue adjacent to the prostheses during revisions has revealed inflamed periarticular tissue.[16] Histologic examination of the joint capsule showed polyethylene particles within macrophages.[16] Aseptic loosening is now understood to result from a biologically induced reaction stimulated by polyethylene particles. Twenty-year survival rates in metal-on-polyethylene THA prostheses with no reoperation were 81.3%, and 89.4% with no component removal or revision for aseptic loosening; however, implant survivorship has been reported as low as 73%.[17] Because of the high incidence of aseptic failure, alternate materials (including metal-on-metal prostheses) are being studied.

Although metallic particles seen in metal-on-metal hip prostheses did not produce the aseptic loosening response of polyethylene particles, there is convincing evidence that the greater number of metallic particles stimulates an immunologic reaction similar to type IV hypersensitivity,[8] which is discussed in greater detail later in this chapter. Histologic examination reveals diffuse and perivascular lymphocytic aggregates in the presence of moderate metallic wear debris.[8] Further evaluation shows persistently high levels of chromium and cobalt in serum and urine. The deleterious effects of metallic particles on levels of CD4 and CD8 T lymphocytes also have been reported.[18] Although the clinical significance has not yet been determined, there are concerns regarding the carcinogenic and mutagenic effects of metal particles. Despite a lower incidence of osteolysis in metal-on-metal THAs, aseptic loosening remained the dominant feature at the time of revision.[8]

Nickel, cobalt, and chromium are the most common metal allergens. Currently, it is unclear if early osteolysis seen in metal-on-metal hip implants is caused by preexisting metal sensitivity or if patients later develop sensitivity as a result of the failed THA and exposure to a large amount of particulate metal debris. In a study by Park et al,[19] 165 patients treated with metal-on-metal hip implants were evaluated. Within 24 months of surgery, nine patients had radiographic evidence of osteolysis. Skin-patch testing determined that eight of the nine patients had a higher sensitivity to cobalt chloride in comparison with a control group. The authors concluded that patients who had radiographic findings of osteolysis had significantly higher rates of sensitivity to metals in comparison to control groups.[19] Willert et al[20] evaluated the first 19 consecutive revisions of metal-on-metal hip implants performed at a single institution for patients with hip pain and osteolysis. At 1- to 7-year follow-ups, three of five patients treated with revision to a metal-on-metal hip prosthesis had persistent pain in the hip and thigh. The 14 patients treated with revision to alumina-on-polyethylene or metal-on-polyethylene prostheses had symptom relief. It was believed that the patients treated with revision to metal-on-metal hip implants had become sensitized to the metal particles, and an immunologic reaction led to the persistent painful symptoms.[20] However, the overall incidence of tissue reaction to metal-on-metal hip implants remains low. Engh et al[21] evaluated 828 patients (945 hips) treated with large head (36 mm) metal-on-metal hip prostheses and determined that 3 patients had a local tissue reaction that was likely attributed to the metal-on-metal implant (0.3%). The authors continued to use metal-on-metal implants but considered a sensitivity reaction to the metal as a possible factor in all failed implants.[21]

The incidence of hypersensitivity is markedly increased in metal-on-metal hip prostheses compared with metal-on-polyethylene prostheses. Although metallic ions induce an immunologic reaction, it is not clear if this response contributes to the development of osteolysis.

A recent analysis of surface engineered metal-on-metal prostheses containing titanium niobium, chromium nitrogen, chromium-carbon-nitrogen, and diamond-like carbon produced a volumetric wear rate 36 times lower and a metallic ion concentration rate 20 times lower than traditional metal-on-metal prostheses.[22] In prosthetic designs using metals, the possibility remains for producing extremely low volumetric wear rates and low metallic ion concentrations, which has the potential to reduce the incidence of hypersensitivity, minimize osteolysis, and prolong prostheses survival rates.

Metal-on-metal implants remain a viable alternative, especially in younger and more active patients in whom implant longevity is an issue, although the problem of hypersensitivity must be considered. An alternative to traditional THA is hip resurfacing with metal-on-metal designs, but this approach has recently been questioned by the British National Health Service.[6]

Hip Resurfacing

Several different metal-on-metal hip resurfacing designs exist, including the Conserve Plus (Wright Medical Technology, Arlington, TN), the McMinn prosthesis (Corin Medical, Cirencester, England), the Cormet (Corin, Tampa, FL), and the Birmingham (Smith & Nephew, Memphis, TN). Each design consists of a high carbon chromium-cobalt alloy with a press-fit acetabular cup and cemented femoral stem. The differences among the prostheses result from the manufacturing process of the alloy. Wrought alloy is harder than cast alloy and can be highly polished, thus producing more wear resistance and decreased surface roughness compared with cast alloy.[23] Additional processing can include postcast heat treatments, such as solution heat treatment or hot isostatic processing. This process can cause depletion of surface carbides, which are a mix of carbon and the surrounding metal.[23] These carbides are significantly harder than the surrounding metal and provide a higher resistance to wear. Although processing was originally believed to produce different wear characteristics, recent analysis has not shown a significant difference.[24,25] Instead, wear is considered to be a function of radial clearance, lubrication conditions, carbon content, and surface roughness.[23,26]

McKellop et al[27] reported similar wear rates between hip resurfacing and THA. The development of pseudotumors is a unique characteristic of the metallic wear particles in hip resurfacing.[28] Although the etiology of pseudotumors is likely multifactorial, it is believed that toxic levels of metallic ions contribute to their development.[28] Among 1,300 metal-on-metal hip resurfacing prostheses, 12 were found to contain a soft-tissue mass.[28] Histologic examination showed metallic wear particles within necrotic connective tissue surrounded by macrophages and lymphocytes.[28] Although rare occurrences of cysts with lymphocytic infiltration have been seen in THA, this response is considered to be more extensive and suggestive of a new complication unique to hip resurfacing. The predilection to women is not well understood but may suggest a prior sensitivity to metallic ions.[28] Recently, reports have linked smaller size femoral heads with a higher likelihood of metal reactivity about these implants.[29] The smaller femoral head seems to be susceptible to higher wear rates because of the smaller contact area in an acetabular component that is aligned with greater inclination and or anteversion.[29,30] The higher wear rate of a smaller femoral head needs to be considered when an orthopaedic surgeon is weighing the pros and cons of a metal-on-metal bearing. If templating suggests the need for small head and acetabular component sizes, then hard-on-hard bearings, such as ceramic bearings, should be considered.

Radiographic analysis of resurfaced hips has shown a 77% incidence of femoral neck narrowing.[31] Hing et al[31] identified narrowing greater than 10% in 28% of patients, although there has been no indication that this finding is of clinical significance.[32] The etiology of femoral neck narrowing is largely unknown but may be related to stress shielding or a decreased blood supply to the femoral head and neck, as seen in the posterior approach to hip resurfacing.

Femoral neck fracture is identified as the most common and significant complication associated with hip resurfacing, with an overall incidence ranging from 1.46% to 7.2%. A learning curve for surgeons is also related to the hip resurfacing procedure.[32-35] In a study by Shimmin and Back,[32] femoral neck notching and varus placement of more than 5° was seen in 46.6% and 71.1% of patients, respectively. No case of femoral neck fracture was identified in prostheses placed in valgus position in relationship to the preoperative neck-shaft angle;[32] however, prostheses placed in excessive valgus position were associated with notching along the superior lateral border of the femoral neck.[34] Marker et al[33] reported that 12 of 14 femoral neck fractures (86%) occurred in the first 69 hip resurfacing procedures performed by a single surgeon, after which time the incidence decreased to 0.4%, thereby suggesting a learning curve. However, Shimmin and Back[32] did not find any association between the surgeon's experience and the incidence of femoral neck fractures. To help identify patients at risk for this complication, Beaulé and Antoniades[26] developed the surface arthroplasty risk index. Evidence shows that resurfaced hips with higher surface arthroplasty risk index numbers were more likely to fail. When surgeons implemented stricter patient selection criteria (body mass index < 35, no osteopenia, no femoral cysts > 1 cm), the overall complication rate decreased from 13.4% to 2.1%, and femoral neck fractures decreased from 7.2% to 0.8%.[35]

Early analyses of hip resurfacing procedures seemed to indicate higher rates of revision among females when compared with males. This difference is now attributed to the smaller femoral heads used in female patients and the decreased area of contact that can result from excessive inclination and/or anteversion of the acetabulum.[29,30,36] McBryde et al[36] reported a similar risk of revision in both sexes when the same size component was used. It was concluded that revision rates were more significantly related to femoral head size than to sex.

Resurfacing Versus Total Hip Arthroplasty

Although THA has traditionally produced excellent results in older patients, significantly higher failure rates have occurred in younger patients.[37-39] Although the transition to cementless prostheses did not show any early significant differences in implant survival rates compared with cemented prostheses, a recent analysis by Lombardi et al[40] showed excellent long-term survival rates for uncemented proximal porous-coated titanium tapered stems. Kaplan-Meier analysis showed a 95.5% cumulative survival rate for any stem revision at 20 years.[40] Although uncemented prostheses have excellent long-term survival rates, hip resurfacing helps maintain bone stock and offers a relatively easy transition to THA. Recent studies indicate similar survival rates in patients younger than 55 years treated with hip resurfacing compared with THA.[41] The larger femoral heads used in hip resurfacing are believed to provide greater stability, fewer dislocations, and greater range of motion. Proponents also believe that hip resurfacing produces a more physiologic load transfer than stemmed prostheses, thereby minimizing stress shielding, bone remodeling, and bone loss.[42] Although some surgeons believe this load transfer enables patients to resume higher levels of activity, gait studies do not indicate superiority. Gait characteristics between patients treated with hip resurfacing and large femoral head THAs were not found to be statistically different; however, Lavigne et al[43] reported significant differences in gait characteristics in patients treated with THAs with smaller femoral heads. Although hip resurfacing offers several advantages to THA, hip resurfacing remains more technically challenging. For this reason, some orthopaedic surgeons believe that hip resurfacing should not replace THA but should serve as a viable alternative.

Wear Particle Consideration in Metal-on-Metal Prostheses

Local Toxicity

Tissue samples obtained from hips with metal-on-metal prostheses were markedly more ulcerated than those obtained from hips with metal-on-polyethylene implants, particularly in the area adjacent to areas of perivascular lymphocytic infiltration.[44] This type of reaction is consistent with an aseptic lymphocytic vasculitis-associated lesion (type IV hypersensitivity reaction) because there was no histologic evidence of acute infection.[44,45] The characteristic histologic features of tissue from patients with metal-on-metal implants were perivascular infiltrates of T and B lymphocytes, plasma cells, high endothelial venules, massive fibrin exudation, the accumulation of macrophages, and infiltrates of eosinophilic granulocytes and necrosis. There was no such immune response in the tissues of patients with nonmetal implants.[44]

Mikhael et al[45] described two patients with metal-on-metal implant failure who presented with signs that mimicked a hip infection. The etiology of symptoms differed between the two patients. The first patient had a local hypersensitivity type IV reaction to the metal-on-metal implant. Previously reported clinical presentations have included pain within 10 months to 5 years following THA surgery or early radiographic signs of loosening. In this study, the patient also had constitutional symptoms and elevated serum levels of inflammatory biomarkers. Tissue specimens from the patient showed perivascular lymphocytic infiltrates and was positive for B and T lymphocytes, similar to the results in studies by Hallab et al[46,47] involving human lymphocytes and metal alloy degradation. The second patient had a mismatch between the sizes of the femoral head and the acetabular socket that led to a rapid increase in the production of local metal debris and tissue hyperreactivity to the metal. In contrast to the chronic inflammation identified in the first patient, the samples from the second patient revealed acellular necrotic tissue. The large amount of metal debris caused an inflammatory reaction leading to elevated inflammatory markers, which were probably exacerbated by some form of metal hypersensitivity. The inappropriate pairing of the acetabular and femoral components also may have caused elevated inflammatory markers. Both patients had complete resolution of symptoms following exchange of the metal liner for a polyethylene component.[45]

Systemic Toxicity

Multiple studies have shown elevated metal ions in the serum and urine of patients with metal-on-metal implants (particularly in those with long-term implants).[48-51] In a 4-year prospective study assessing serum levels of metal ions in patients with THAs, cobalt levels were shown to steadily decrease over a 4-year period compared with chromium levels.[52] Furthermore, metal-on-metal bearings with a large diameter resulted in a greater systemic exposure of metal ions than bearings with a small diameter.[53]

The number of chromosomal aberrations found in patients with metal-on-metal bearings was greater than those in a control group. Structural aberrations were not seen in the control group, and this difference was highly significant (P = 0.003).[54] Also, the number of chromosomal aberrations in the metal-on-metal group was greater than in patients who had revision surgery from metal-on-metal to metal-on-polyethylene implants.[54,55] The clinical consequences of the chromosomal changes seen in this study are unknown, and it is unknown if the changes are present in other cells in the body. Decreased levels of CD8(+) T cells and an increase in the number of debris particles in the liver and spleen were found in patients with metal-on-metal THAs compared with a control group.[56,57] In one rare instance, granulomas had formed in the liver, spleen, and abdominal lymph nodes in response to the heavy accumulation of wear debris from a hip prosthesis.[57] Cobalt and chromium have also been shown to cross the placenta in women with metal-on-metal THAs.[58] Although the pathologic importance of these results have not been elucidated, they emphasize the need for additional investigations into the effect of chronic exposure to elevated levels of metal ions produced by orthopaedic implants.

Hypersensitivity Responses

Components of metal alloys, such as benzoyl peroxide, have been shown to be potential allergens in patients treated with THAs.[45] It is clear that some patients have excessive immune reactions directly associated with implanted metallic materials leading to an aseptic lymphocytic vasculitis-associated lesion.[44,45] However, these reactions are rare, with reported estimated prevalences of 1% to 2% and up to 5% for certain alloys such as cobalt and chromium.[59] In one study, blood samples were taken from patients with no known prior metal allergies or exposures having a primary THA. Repeat blood samples were taken 3 months to 1 year later. Sensitivity to at least one of the antigens developed in 32% of the patients, but a severe reaction developed in only 5%.[59] In a histologic analysis of patients with metal-on-metal THAs at a mean follow-up of 77 months postoperatively, it was concluded that periprosthetic osteolysis and aseptic loosening in the hips were possibly associated with hypersensitivity to metal debris.[20] The lymphocyte response to serum protein complexed with metal from implant degradation was investigated using human lymphocytes from healthy volunteers. Even in healthy patients, there is a lymphocyte proliferative response to both cobalt-chromium-molybdenum and titanium alloy metalloprotein degradation products. Histologic samples were taken from patients who had hip revision surgery with ceramic, metal-on-polyethylene, or metal-on-metal implants. The induction of T cell activation by metal particles suggests that lymphocytes may contribute to the inflammation that mediates osteolysis in patients with particle debris.[60]

Carcinogenic Effects

Animal studies have documented the carcinogenic potential of orthopaedic implant materials. Small increases in rat sarcoma rates were correlated with metal implants; however, lymphomas were more common in rats with metallic implants.[61] The occurrence of tumor-like reactions at the site of metallic implants in humans also has been reported.[62] The most common lesion was a malignant fibrous histiocytoma.[63] Slight increases in the risk of lymphoma and leukemia were observed in patients with metal-on-metal THAs.[64] In contrast, studies have shown a decreased incidence of certain tumors, including breast carcinoma, sarcoma, and stomach cancer in patients with metal-on-metal THAs. In a 1988 Swedish study of 154 patients treated with THA and followed for 20 years, the overall relative risk of cancer increased by 3%, with most cancers originating from connective tissue.[64] A 1996 Finnish study evaluated the incidence of cancer in patients with metal-on-metal THAs compared with patients with polyethylene implants. There was a 4% and 4.5% increase in the incidence of cancer in the metal-on-metal and polyethylene groups, respectively. Also, there was a threefold to fourfold risk for tumors of the lymphatic and hematopoietic systems after THA compared with a control group.[65] Neither study separated patients with degenerative and inflammatory joint disease, suggesting that there could be factors other than THA that play a major role in the origin of cancer.

Practice Recommendations

This chapter's authors avoid the use of metal-on-metal endbearing hip replacements in patients requiring a cup size smaller than 50 to 52 mm. A full radius (180°) cup should be used with high carbon content. Surgical technique is paramount, especially in properly placing the acetabular cup. Excessive anteversion or lateral opening can produce end loading and increased metallic wear.

Patients are followed with an examination and radiographic evaluation every 12 months. Patients with pain or radiologic signs of early implant failure are evaluated for cobalt-chromium ion levels and with MRI. Patients with elevated ion levels alone are reevaluated in 3 to 6 months with repeat ion level testing and imaging. Revision is advised if there is a soft-tissue reaction or abnormal fluid collection noted on imaging studies.

Summary

Clearly, there seems to be a subset of patients that may be more susceptible to complications caused by metallic debris from metal-on-metal bearing articulations. Whether this susceptibility is related to implant size, implant contact area, a combination of patient genetic factors, or patient predisposition is not yet clear. Long-term epidemiologic studies are needed to fully address the issues of metal implant-associated local and remote toxicity, as well as hypersensitivity reactions and carcinogenesis. Advances in science and patient screening procedures will increase the understanding of host compatibility to metal implants. However, it should be remembered that modern metal-on-metal bearings have achieved good results in most patients.

References

1. Dumbleton JH, Manley MT: Metal-on-metal total hip replace-

ment: What does the literature say? *J Arthroplasty* 2005;20(2): 174-188.

2. Amstutz HC, Grigoris P: Metal on metal bearings in hip arthroplasty. *Clin Orthop Relat Res* 1996; 329(Suppl):S11-S34.
3. Santavirta S, Böhler M, Harris WH, et al: Alternative materials to improve total hip replacement tribology. *Acta Orthop Scand* 2003;74(4):380-388.
4. Amstutz HC, Campbell P, McKellop H, et al: Metal on metal total hip replacement workshop consensus document. *Clin Orthop Relat Res* 1996;329(Suppl): S297-S303.
5. Meier B: With warning, a hip device is withdrawn. *New York Times*, March 9, 2010.
6. Medical Device Alert: All metal-on-metal (MoM) hip replacements. Ref: MDA/2010/033. Issued: April 22, 2010. http://www.mhra.gov.uk/Publications/Safetywarnings/MedicalDeviceAlerts/CON079157. Accessed September 3, 2010.
7. Anissian HL, Stark A, Good V, Dahlstrand H, Clarke IC: The wear pattern in metal-on-metal hip prostheses. *J Biomed Mater Res* 2001;58(6):673-678.
8. Milosev I, Trebse R, Kovac S, Cör A, Pisot V: Survivorship and retrieval analysis of Sikomet metal-on-metal total hip replacements at a mean of seven years. *J Bone Joint Surg Am* 2006;88(6): 1173-1182.
9. Firkins PJ, Tipper JL, Saadatzadeh MR, et al: Quantitative analysis of wear and wear debris from metal-on-metal hip prostheses tested in a physiological hip joint simulator. *Biomed Mater Eng* 2001;11(2):143-157.
10. St John KR, Zardiackas LD, Poggie RA: Wear evaluation of cobalt-chromium alloy for use in a metal-on-metal hip prosthesis. *J Biomed Mater Res B Appl Biomater* 2004;68(1):1-14.
11. Fisher J, Jin ZM, Tipper JL, Stone MH, Ingham E: Tribology of alternative bearings. *Clin Orthop Relat Res* 2006;453:25-34.
12. Stewart T, Tipper J, Streicher R, Ingham E, Fisher J: Long-term wear of HIPed alumina on alumina bearings for THR under microseparation conditions. *J Mater Sci Mater Med* 2001; 12(10-12):1053-1056.
13. Smith SL, Dowson D, Goldsmith AA: The effect of femoral head diameter upon lubrication and wear of metal-on-metal total hip replacements. *Proc Inst Mech Eng H* 2001;215(2):161-170.
14. Udoifa IJ, Yew A, Jin ZM: Contact mechanics analysis of metal-on-metal hip resurfacing prostheses. *Proc Inst Mech Eng H* 2004; 218(5):293-305.
15. Goldsmith AA, Dowson D, Isaac GH, Lancaster JG: A comparative joint simulator study of the wear of metal-on-metal and alternative material combinations in hip replacements. *Proc Inst Mech Eng H* 2000;214(1):39-47.
16. Müller ME: The benefits of metal-on-metal total hip replacements. *Clin Orthop Relat Res* 1995;311:54-59.
17. Berry DJ, Harmsen WS, Cabanela ME, Morrey BF: Twenty-five-year survivorship of two thousand consecutive primary Charnley total hip replacements: Factors affecting survivorship of acetabular and femoral components. *J Bone Joint Surg Am* 2002;84-A(2):171-177.
18. Hart AJ, Skinner JA, Winship P, et al: Circulating levels of cobalt and chromium from metal-on-metal hip replacement are associated with CD8+ T-cell lymphopenia. *J Bone Joint Surg Br* 2009; 91(6):835-842.
19. Park YS, Moon YW, Lim SJ, Yang JM, Ahn G, Choi YL: Early osteolysis following second-generation metal-on-metal hip replacement. *J Bone Joint Surg Am* 2005;87(7):1515-1521.
20. Willert HG, Buchhorn GH, Fayyazi A, et al: Metal-on-metal bearings and hypersensitivity in patients with artificial hip joints: A clinical and histomorphological study. *J Bone Joint Surg Am* 2005; 87(1):28-36.
21. Engh CA Jr, Ho H, Engh CA: Metal-on-metal hip arthroplasty: Does early clinical outcome justify the chance of an adverse local tissue reaction? *Clin Orthop Relat Res* 2010;468(2):406-412.
22. Fisher J, Hu XQ, Stewart TD, et al: Wear of surface engineered metal-on-metal hip prostheses. *J Mater Sci Mater Med* 2004; 15(3):225-235.
23. Grigoris P, Roberts P, Panousis K, Bosch H: The evolution of hip resurfacing arthroplasty. *Orthop Clin North Am* 2005;36(2): 125-134.
24. Nevelos J, Shelton JC, Fisher J: Metallurgical considerations in the wear of metal-on-metal hip bearings. *Hip Int* 2004;14(1): 1-10.
25. Dowson D, Hardaker C, Flett M, Isaac GH: A hip joint simulator study of the performance of metal-on-metal joints: Part I. The role of materials. *J Arthroplasty* 2004;19(8, Suppl 3):118-123.
26. Beaulé PE, Antoniades J: Patient selection and surgical technique for surface arthroplasty of the hip. *Orthop Clin North Am* 2005; 36(2):177-185.
27. McKellop H, Amstutz H, Lu B, Timmerman I,Carroll M: A hip simulator study of the wear of large diameter, metal-on-metal hip surface replacements, in *Society for Biomaterials 27th Annual Meeting Transactions.* Mt Laurel, NJ, Society for Biomaterials, 2001, p 339.

28. Pandit H, Glyn-Jones S, McLardy-Smith P, et al: Pseudotumours associated with metal-on-metal hip resurfacings. *J Bone Joint Surg Br* 2008;90(7): 847-851.
29. Langton DJ, Jameson SS, Joyce TJ, Hallab NJ, Natu S, Nargol AV: Early failure of metal-on-metal bearings in hip resurfacing and large-diameter total hip replacement: A consequence of excess wear. *J Bone Joint Surg Br* 2010;92(1):38-46.
30. Langton DJ, Jameson SS, Joyce TJ, Webb J, Nargol AV: The effect of component size and orientation on the concentrations of metal ions after resurfacing arthroplasty of the hip. *J Bone Joint Surg Br* 2008;90(9): 1143-1151.
31. Hing CB, Young DA, Dalziel RE, Bailey M, Back DL, Shimmin AJ: Narrowing of the neck in resurfacing arthroplasty of the hip: A radiological study. *J Bone Joint Surg Br* 2007;89(8):1019-1024.
32. Shimmin AJ, Back D: Femoral neck fractures following Birmingham hip resurfacing: A national review of 50 cases. *J Bone Joint Surg Br* 2005;87(4):463-464.
33. Marker DR, Seyler TM, Jinnah RH, Delanois RE, Ulrich SD, Mont MA: Femoral neck fractures after metal-on-metal total hip resurfacing: A prospective cohort study. *J Arthroplasty* 2007;22 (7, Suppl 3):66-71.
34. Mont MA, Schmalzried TP: Modern metal-on-metal hip resurfacing: Important observations from the first ten years. *J Bone Joint Surg Am* 2008;90(Suppl 3): 3-11.
35. Mont MA, Seyler TM, Ulrich SD, et al: Effect of changing indications and techniques on total hip resurfacing. *Clin Orthop Relat Res* 2007;465:63-70.
36. McBryde CW, Theivendran K, Thomas AM, Treacy RB, Pynsent PB: The influence of head size and sex on the outcome of Birmingham hip resurfacing. *J Bone Joint Surg Am* 2010;92(1): 105-112.
37. Beaulé PE, Dorey FJ, LeDuff M, Gruen T, Amstutz HC: Risk factors affecting outcome of metal-on-metal surface arthroplasty of the hip. *Clin Orthop Relat Res* 2004;418:87-93.
38. Duffy GP, Berry DJ, Rowland C, Cabanela ME: Primary uncemented total hip arthroplasty in patients < 40 years old: 10- to 14-year results using first-generation proximally porous-coated implants. *J Arthroplasty* 2001;16(8, Suppl 1):140-144.
39. Ortiguera CJ, Pulliam IT, Cabanela ME: Total hip arthroplasty for osteonecrosis: Matched-pair analysis of 188 hips with long-term follow-up. *J Arthroplasty* 1999;14(1):21-28.
40. Lombardi AV Jr, Berend KR, Mallory TH, Skeels MD, Adams JB: Survivorship of 2000 tapered titanium porous plasma-sprayed femoral components. *Clin Orthop Relat Res* 2009;467(1): 146-154.
41. Buergi ML, Walter WL: Hip resurfacing arthroplasty: The Australian experience. *J Arthroplasty* 2007;22(7 Suppl 3):61-65.
42. Daniel J, Pynsent PB, McMinn DJ: Metal-on-metal resurfacing of the hip in patients under the age of 55 years with osteoarthritis. *J Bone Joint Surg Br* 2004; 86(2):177-184.
43. Lavigne M, Vendittoli P-A, Nantel J, Prince F: Abstract: Gait analysis in three types of hip replacement. *75th Annual Meeting Procedings*. Rosemont, IL, American Academy of Orthopaedic Surgeons, 2008, p 431.
44. Davies AP, Willert HG, Campbell PA, Learmonth ID, Case CP: An unusual lymphocytic perivascular infiltration in tissues around contemporary metal-on-metal joint replacements. *J Bone Joint Surg Am* 2005;87(1):18-27.
45. Mikhael MM, Hanssen AD, Sierra RJ: Failure of metal-on-metal total hip arthroplasty mimicking hip infection: A report of two cases. *J Bone Joint Surg Am* 2009; 91(2):443-446.
46. Hallab NJ, Anderson S, Stafford T, Glant T, Jacobs JJ: Lymphocyte responses in patients with total hip arthroplasty. *J Orthop Res* 2005;23(2):384-391.
47. Hallab NJ, Mikecz K, Vermes C, Skipor A, Jacobs JJ: Orthopaedic implant related metal toxicity in terms of human lymphocyte reactivity to metal-protein complexes produced from cobalt-base and titanium-base implant alloy degradation. *Mol Cell Biochem* 2001; 222(1-2):127-136.
48. Back DL, Young DA, Shimmin AJ: How do serum cobalt and chromium levels change after metal-on-metal hip resurfacing? *Clin Orthop Relat Res* 2005;438: 177-181.
49. Brodner W, Bitzan P, Meisinger V, Kaider A, Gottsauner-Wolf F, Kotz R: Serum cobalt levels after metal-on-metal total hip arthroplasty. *J Bone Joint Surg Am* 2003;85-A(11):2168-2173.
50. Schaffer AW, Pilger A, Engelhardt C, Zweymueller K, Ruediger HW: Increased blood cobalt and chromium after total hip replacement. *J Toxicol Clin Toxicol* 1999;37(7):839-844.
51. Sauvé P, Mountney J, Khan T, De Beer J, Higgins B, Grover M: Metal ion levels after metal-on-metal ring total hip replacement: A 30-year follow-up study. *J Bone Joint Surg Br* 2007;89(5): 586-590.
52. Daniel J, Ziaee H, Pradhan C, Pynsent PB, McMinn DJ: Blood and urine metal ion levels in young and active patients after Birmingham hip resurfacing ar-

throplasty: Four-year results of a prospective longitudinal study. *J Bone Joint Surg Br* 2007;89(2): 169-173.

53. Clarke MT, Lee PT, Arora A, Villar RN: Levels of metal ions after small- and large-diameter metal-on-metal hip arthroplasty. *J Bone Joint Surg Br* 2003;85(6): 913-917.

54. Dunstan E, Ladon D, Whittingham-Jones P, Carrington R, Briggs TW: Chromosomal aberrations in the peripheral blood of patients with metal-on-metal hip bearings. *J Bone Joint Surg Am* 2008;90(3):517-522.

55. Ladon D, Doherty A, Newson R, Turner J, Bhamra M, Case CP: Changes in metal levels and chromosome aberrations in the peripheral blood of patients after metal-on-metal hip arthroplasty. *J Arthroplasty* 2004;19(8, Suppl 3):78-83.

56. Hart AJ, Hester T, Sinclair K, et al: The association between metal ions from hip resurfacing and reduced T-cell counts. *J Bone Joint Surg Br* 2006;88(4): 449-454.

57. Urban RM, Jacobs JJ, Tomlinson MJ, Gavrilovic J, Black J, Peoc'h M: Dissemination of wear particles to the liver, spleen, and abdominal lymph nodes of patients with hip or knee replacement. *J Bone Joint Surg Am* 2000; 82(4):457-476.

58. Ziaee H, Daniel J, Datta AK, Blunt S, McMinn DJ: Transplacental transfer of cobalt and chromium in patients with metal-on-metal hip arthroplasty: A controlled study. *J Bone Joint Surg Br* 2007;89(3):301-305.

59. Merritt K, Rodrigo JJ: Immune response to synthetic materials: Sensitization of patients receiving orthopaedic implants. *Clin Orthop Relat Res* 1996;326:71-79.

60. Hallab NJ, Mikecz K, Vermes C, Skipor A, Jacobs JJ: Differential lymphocyte reactivity to serum-derived metal-protein complexes produced from cobalt-based and titanium-based implant alloy degradation. *J Biomed Mater Res* 2001;56(3):427-436.

61. Memoli VA, Urban RM, Alroy J, Galante JO: Malignant neoplasms associated with orthopedic implant materials in rats. *J Orthop Res* 1986;4(3):346-355.

62. Jacobs JJ, Urban RM, Wall J, Black J, Reid JD, Veneman L: Unusual foreign-body reaction to a failed total knee replacement: Simulation of a sarcoma clinically and a sarcoid histologically. A case report. *J Bone Joint Surg Am* 1995;77(3):444-451.

63. Tait NP, Hacking PM, Malcolm AJ: Malignant fibrous histiocytoma occurring at the site of a previous total hip replacement. *Br J Radiol* 1988;61(721):73-76.

64. Visuri T, Pukkala E, Paavolainen P, Pulkkinen P, Riska EB: Cancer risk after metal on metal and polyethylene on metal total hip arthroplasty. *Clin Orthop Relat Res* 1996;329(Suppl):S280-S289.

65. Paavolainen P, Pukkala E, Pulkkinen P, Visuri T: Cancer incidence in Finnish hip replacement patients from 1980 to 1995: A nationwide cohort study involving 31,651 patients. *J Arthroplasty* 1999;14(3):272-280.

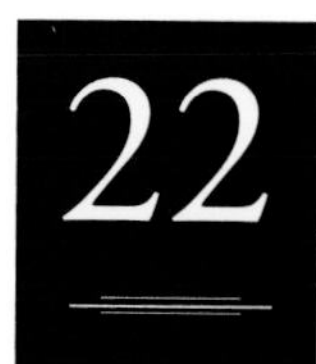

Alternative Bearing Surface Options for Revision Total Hip Arthroplasty

Deepan Patel, MD
Javad Parvizi, MD, FRCS
Peter F. Sharkey, MD

Abstract

Despite the overall success of total hip arthroplasty (THA), there has been an increase in the rate of revision hip surgeries performed each year in the United States. These revision surgeries result in several billion dollars in health care costs. Bearing surface wear can result in the need for revision surgery through a variety of mechanisms. Many implant failures necessitating the need for revision surgeries occur secondary to dislocations, which are often related to prothesis wear and eventual loosening of the components. Wear also can lead to osteolysis and may play a role in aseptic loosening. Specific concerns regarding the wear rates of metal-on-polyethylene (the most common bearing surface) have encouraged the manufacture of newer polyethylene implants with improved wear properties, as well as alternative bearing surfaces. The goal is to improve the durability of revision implants and/or reduce the incidence of revision THAs. Revision arthroplasty involves using alternative surfaces, such as replacing the metal femoral head with a ceramic component or changing the entire prosthesis to a metal-on-metal or ceramic-on-ceramic articulation. It is important to review the characteristics of these alternative bearing surface options and their contributions to improved THA tribology and prolonged prosthesis longevity.

The choice of a bearing surface for a revision THA should consider factors such as the patient's age and activity level, the cost of the implant, and both the surgeons' and patients' preferences. Although laboratory studies and small clinical trials have generated optimistic results for these alternative implants in vitro and in vivo, much still needs to be learned about the long-term performance of these materials in patients after total hip revision surgery.

Instr Course Lect 2011;60:257-267.

Total hip arthroplasty (THA) is a treatment option for patients with advanced stages of degenerative joint disease. For these patients, joint surgery improves the quality of life and provides relief from the chronic, persistent pain that interferes with daily activities and is refractory to conservative therapy. More than 200,000 artificial hips were implanted last year in the United States. The success of this surgery is attributed to advances in prosthetic devices and surgical techniques, which have ultimately led to reduced risks and an increase in immediate and long-term benefits. However, despite the success of THA, there has been an annual increase in the rate (approximately 7% to 8%) of revision hip surgeries performed in the United States, which translates to several billion dollars in health care costs.[1,2]

Many implant failures requiring revision surgery occur secondary to dislocations that are often related to wear of the prostheses. Bearing surface wear can cause osteolysis and eventual loosening of the components.[1,3,4] Other less common causes of failure include joint infection, limb-length inequality, and gradual bone loss around the implant. Specific concerns exist over the wear rates of the most common bearing surface—the metal-on-polyethylene implant—in younger, more active patients who are at an increased risk for prosthesis wear and future revision surgery. The relative motion between the two bearing surfaces contributes to the generation of most of the in vivo, wear-related, particulate debris.[4] This debris leads to macrophage accumulation and a subsequent inflammatory response. The presence of lytic enzymes, proinflammatory cytokines, and bone-resorbing mediators in the area of the prosthesis have been documented.[4] This process results in osteolysis that can cause aseptic loosening and fixation failure.[5,6]

Revision THA is considered by many surgeons to be a more technically complicated procedure with inferior outcomes compared with primary THA. Problems arise because of the diminished quality of bone and the inability to adequately secure the components of the revision hip replacement. In addition, removing the original hip implant can necessitate more extensive surgery and bone loss. These factors, coupled with the discovery of periprosthetic wear debris, has encouraged the development and manufacture of newer polyethylene implants with improved wear properties as well as alternative bearing surfaces. The ultimate goals are to improve the durability of revision implants and reduce the incidence of re-revision THAs. Revision surgery may include replacing the metal femoral head with a ceramic component or changing the entire prosthesis to a metal-on-metal or ceramic-on-ceramic articulation. The characteristics of these alternative bearing surface options and their contribution to improved THA tribology and component longevity are discussed in this chapter.

Tribology

Before any formal discussion of alternative bearing surfaces, it is important to first review the principles of tribology and how it relates to implant design. Tribology refers to the science of surfaces (for example, bearings) interacting under an applied load and in relative motion. Broadly defined, tribology encompasses three aspects of science and technology—wear, lubrication, and friction.

Wear refers to the removal of material and the resultant generation of particles caused by the relative motion between two opposing surfaces under loading. There are three known mechanisms of wear: adhesion, abrasion, and fatigue.[7] Adhesive wear is caused by the bonding between two surfaces in close contact and the matter that is subsequently pulled off the weaker surface.[8] Abrasive wear involves the removal of material from the softer surface secondary to microcutting from hard surface asperities that have rooted themselves into the opposing soft surface.[8] Fatigue refers to the progressive and localized structural damage that occurs when a material is subjected to repetitive loading cycles, such as exists in an artificial hip joint.[8]

Lubrication occurs when two opposing surfaces are separated by a lubricant film that carries the force of the applied load as a fluid pressure and removes the load from the opposing surface materials.[9] Boundary lubrication arises when the two bodies are not completely separated; thus, occasional abrasion from hard surface asperities will occur.[7,9] The gamma (λ) ratio compares fluid-film thickness to surface roughness. A higher λ value translates into reduced friction and wear.[7] A λ value greater than 3 indicates fluid-film or hydrodynamic lubrication in which complete separation of the bearing surfaces is achieved, and abrasive wear is minimal (if present at all).[7]

Friction is the force that opposes the relative motion or tendency toward such motion of two surfaces in contact.[10] Ideally, when prostheses are designed, bearing surfaces are manufactured to be smoother to reduce the coefficient of friction and yield lower frictional forces across the joint. The coefficient of friction of a normal hip joint is 0.008 to 0.02; most artificial hip joints are designed with a coefficient at or below those values.[11]

Metal-on-Polyethylene Prostheses

Much of the current success of THA is attributed to the work of Charnley, whose implant design became the foremost model for arthroplasty by the 1970s. Charnley's design consisted of three parts: the stainless steel femoral component, a polyethylene acetabular component, and cement to fix the component to bone. The Charnley implant used a small 22-mm femoral head to decrease the wear rate of the joint; however, it was later recognized that smaller femoral heads could increase the rate of hip dislocation.[7]

Currently, the most common bearing surface used in hip replacement is a cobalt alloy femoral head that

Dr. Parvizi or an immediate family member serves as a board member, owner, officer, or committee member of the American Association of Hip and Knee Surgeons, the American Board of Orthopaedic Surgery, the British Orthopaedic Association, the Hip Society, the Orthopaedic Research and Education Foundation, the Orthopaedic Research Society, and SmartTech; serves as a paid consultant to or is an employee of Stryker; and has received research or institutional support from 3M, the Musculoskeletal Transplant Foundation, Smith & Nephew, and Stryker. Dr. Sharkey or an immediate family member serves as a board member, owner, officer, or committee member of Physician Recommended Nutriceuticals and the American Association of Hip and Knee Surgeons; has received royalties from Stryker and Stelkast; serves as a paid consultant to or is an employee of Stryker; has received research or institutional support from Stryker and Stelkast; and owns stock or stock options in Cross Current, Physician Recommended Nutriceuticals, CardoMedical, and Knee Creations. Neither Dr. Patel nor any immediate family member has received anything of value from or owns stock in a commercial company or institution related directly or indirectly to the subject of this chapter.

articulates with an ultra-high molecular weight polyethylene (UHMWPE) acetabular cup. The advantages of this design are that it is a proven product, which has demonstrated excellent results in clinical studies; is nontoxic to patients; is cost effective; and allows the surgeon some flexibility with implantation because of multiple polyethylene liner options.[6] However, one major disadvantage of this bearing couple is that the longevity of this prosthesis can be compromised by eventual wearing of the UHMWPE cup, resulting in subsequent osteolysis and failure of the joint.[3,12] Given these concerns, when revising a THA, this chapter's authors prefer to reserve the use of metal-on-polyethylene implants for elderly and/or less active patients who have a reduced risk for component wear. Nonetheless, if a well-fixed, cemented, all-polyethylene socket or a nonmodular liner with minimal wear is present, the risk-to-benefit ratio of removing this device must be carefully considered.

UHMWPE is manufactured by either extrusion, bulk compression molding, or net-shape molding, and its wear properties can be enhanced by irradiating the material to induce cross-linking.[13] Cross-linked UHMWPE has more than 95% improved wear resistance compared with non–cross-linked polyethylene.[14] Non–cross-linked polyethylene can generate approximately 0.1 mm/y microparticulate debris, with a mean particle size of 0.4 µm.[11] Oxidative degradation secondary to sterilization of polyethylene by gamma radiation has been cited as an important cause of polyethylene deformation, accelerated wear, and, ultimately, liner fracture.[6] Additionally, laboratory studies have shown a tradeoff, with gamma radiation resulting in increased wear resistance at the cost of lower yield strength, ultimate tensile strength, and percentage of strain on the polyethylene before it fails.[14] To counter these detrimental effects, the manufacturing process has been modified and improved to incorporate sterilization in an inert atmosphere, such as nitrogen or argon gas, to prevent oxidation of free radicals, which reduce the mechanical properties of components.[14] When planning for a revision THA, the surgeon should try to determine the type of polyethylene currently implanted and should assess the risk for future failure if the component is not revised.

In an effort to further improve the wear properties of the polyethylene cup, highly cross-linked UHMWPE was developed in the late 1990s.[15,16] The theory behind this new composite material suggests that cross-linking improves wear resistance by decreasing adhesive and abrasive wear.[17] However, radiation alone generates free radicals only, and these free radicals can couple with other free radicals and cross-link only if the polymeric chains are given mobility. This can be achieved through annealing or remelting the polyethylene. In the annealing process, the polyethylene is heated to a temperature below its melting point.[18] Annealing preserves mechanical and fatigue properties of the material, but it still contains free radicals because there is not enough mobility for all free radicals to cross-link.[18] In the remelting process, the polyethylene is heated to a temperature beyond its melting point, which results in lower mechanical and fatigue properties; however, there are no detectable residual free radicals after the process.[18]

In vitro studies have reported that highly cross-linked UHMWPE offers the additional advantage of having wear properties that are independent of the femoral head size.[3,15,19] This is a major advantage compared with conventional UHMWPE components, which exhibits increased wear in proportion to an increasing femoral head size. Using larger femoral heads is particularly important in revision surgery where the risk of postoperative dislocation is increased. Using larger heads translates into increased hip range of motion, reduced dislocation rates, and a lack of component-to-component impingement.[19-21] In a study by Muratoglu et al,[22] significant improvements in the wear resistance characteristics of UHMWPE were reported with up to 10 Mrads of gamma radiation. With more than 10 mrads of gamma radiation, the mechanical properties of the polyethylene exponentially decline, and the rate of improved wear resistance begins to drastically diminish. Caution must be taken when introducing more cross-linking into the polyethylene because studies have reported an indirect relationship of more cross-linking with loss of material fatigue strength, ultimate strength, and the percentage of ultimate elongation, leading to polyethylene fracture and long-term component failure.[14,22-24]

Metallic alloys used for hip implants should have a high level of corrosion resistance as well as mechanical properties that can withstand the demanding requirements of the replaced hip. The three materials used for artificial femoral heads are titanium, stainless steel, and cobalt-chromium alloys. All three metallic alloys have a modulus of elasticity significantly higher than that of bone, which causes the implant to be stiffer than natural bone.[25] Titanium femoral heads have great biocompatibility and low levels of corrosion in vivo, along with the lowest modulus of elasticity compared to cobalt-based alloys or surgical stainless steel.[25] However, because titanium has significant vulnerability to abrasion, it is no longer used as a femoral head bearing.[13] Concerns have been expressed about in vivo corrosion in surgical stainless steel alloys used for hip implants.[16] The low carbon in 316 L stainless steel reduces corrosion rates and is still used for some hip replacements, predominantly outside the United States.[16] Cast or forged cobalt-chromium components offer more resistance to corrosion compared with stainless steel. Forged components have a smaller grain size and greater hardness compared with cast alloys.[13] Currently, cobalt-chromium, which is well suited for long-term weight bearing, is the most common metallic surface used for femoral head replacements. Although surgeons are unlikely to encounter a titanium or stainless steel femoral head during revision THA, this contingency should be considered if the primary surgery was done before the early 1990s or outside the United States.

Ceramic-on-Polyethylene Implants

An alternative bearing option available for revision THA is the replacement of metallic femoral heads with ceramic components, mainly alumina or zirconium. Both materials offer improved biocompatibility and durability compared with their metallic counterparts. Alumina bearings have high hardness, wettability (lower friction), lower surface roughness, and high tensile strength.[26] These properties may translate to a fivefold to tenfold reduction in polyethylene wear and a higher resistance to femoral head surface abrasion.[26,27] The zirconium femoral head has even higher hardness and burst strength compared with the alumina head; however, in vivo studies have shown that it is not as thermostable as alumina.[28] Practically speaking, this makes it dangerous to sterilize zirconium components in an autoclave. In a case study by Haraguchi et al,[28] deterioration and an increase in the surface roughness of two zirconia ceramic femoral head implants was associated with in vivo phase transformation of the ceramics after implantation. Therefore, despite its high mechanical durability, many surgeons and implant designers believe that zirconia is not stable enough to be considered an optimal bearing surface for femoral head replacement. Nonetheless, the product is still available and is an option for revision THA.

Oxidized zirconium alloy implants, made from a zirconium base that is heated and infused with oxygen so that the outer coating of the metal transforms into a ceramic shell, have recently been introduced. These implants retain the light yet strong characteristics of the zirconium metal while also adopting the smooth, tough properties inherent in ceramic implants. Specifically, the ceramic coating reduces friction between the oxidized zirconium femoral head and the polyethylene cup leading to potentially diminished wear compared with standard metal-on-polyethylene devices.[29,30] Oxidized zirconium also is harder and more than 4,900 times more resistant to scratching compared with cobalt-chromium and has a minimum fatigue load equivalent to its metal counterparts.[29] However, with oxidized zirconium, the ceramic coating is thin and can be easily scratched, greatly diminishing its wear properties. When revising an oxidized zirconium head, it should be carefully inspected and revised if scratched. Interestingly, oxidized zirconium contains no detectable level of nickel, which some investigators suspect causes allergic reactions in patients following the implantation of metal bearings.[29] It is hoped that clinical trials will confirm the superior qualities of oxidized zirconium. Replacing a metal head with a ceramic head during revision surgery is generally discouraged. If any damage of the femoral trunion is present, the risk of catastrophic head fracture is increased. An oxidized zirconium head could potentially provide enhanced wear protection without the risk of fracture.

Metal-on-Metal Implants

Metal-on-metal hip implants were first introduced in the 1950s with limited success.[31] Many surgeons and implant manufacturers believed that the initial problems associated with metal-on-metal components resulted from poor manufacturing practices for the first generation of this type of prosthesis (specifically, poor alloy quality and mismatched articulating surfaces) rather than from design flaws.[32] However, despite poor manufacturing practices, some first-generation metal-on-metal implants lasted more than 20 years in vivo.[33,34] This fact, combined with the potential for 100 times less wear debris versus polyethylene components (because of increased hardness) and resistance to dislocation, has led to a renewed interest in second-generation metal-on-metal implants.[27,35,36] The particles generated by metal-on-metal implants are smaller than those generated by polyethylene and are less likely to result in macrophage stimulation.[27] Also, it is now understood that there is an early spike in the level of metal debris during the "breaking in" period; after this period, there is a large decrease in the number of particles produced.[37] Hip simulator studies and laboratory measurements of friction and wear in metal-on-metal joints have identified wear rates of approximately 0.01 mm/y with a mean particle debris size of 0.05 µm.[11,38] Metal-on-metal implants also allow for a larger femoral head, which leads to increases in sliding velocity and pulls more fluid into the articulation.[7,38] This ultimately results in greater joint stability and fewer postoperative dislocations.[7] When performing revision THA for chronic instability, the use of a metal-on-metal articulation should be considered.

Second-generation metal-on-metal designs developed in the late 1980s, such as the Metasul Hip (Zimmer Orthopaedics, Warsaw, IN) featured lower steady-state wear rates, optimal clearance, and improved tribology versus earlier devices. The conventional plastic polyethylene insert in the Metasul Hip implant has a cobalt-chromium metal inlay that articulates with the cobalt-chromium-molybdenum metallic alloy of the femoral head.[39] In a 5-year follow-up study of 78 patients with metal-on-metal uncemented THAs, Wagner and Wagner[39] reported no metallosis at the time of revision, a reduction in wear properties, and no evidence that the metal-on-metal articulation led to additional complications in vivo. Newer cobalt-chromium-molybdenum bearings also have an intrinsic capacity to smooth surface scratches caused by third-body particles.[40] In a small, randomized controlled study, Pabinger et al[41] reported that the metal-on-metal implants showed lower migration rates at 6 and 12 months (0.13 mm and 0.27 mm, respectively) compared with ceramic-on-polyethylene prostheses (0.63 mm and 0.82 mm, respectively). There were no significant differences reported between the two surfaces in terms of radiolucency, activity limitations, degree of pain, or range of motion.[41] A prospective, randomized, clinical trial of 171 patients, which compared 95 patients with a metal-on-metal prosthesis with a control group of 76 patients with a metal-on-polyethylene prosthesis, reported no statistically significant differences in the average Harris hip scores, degree of pain, presence of a limp, range of motion, and radiolucencies.[42] A 7-year follow-up study on the clinical performance of 161 THAs with Metasul metal-on-metal hip prostheses reported no complications from failed cup fixation, no evidence of large amounts of particulate debris, and no other unusual complications.[43]

Despite the advantages of metal-on-metal prostheses, concerns exist over the long-term biologic effect of metal particulate wear debris released into body tissues and fluids. Studies have reported an association between wear and metal sensitivity in patients. Metallosis results in the potential for mutagenic and carcinogenic effects, as well as a possible delayed-type hypersensitivity response to the metal ions.[7,44,45] The term "metallosis" has been used to describe the intraoperative findings of gross metallic debris and blackening of periprosthetic tissue.[45] The quantity of metal debris generated annually from a metal-on-metal prosthesis can be up to 500 times the number of polyethylene particles produced from a traditional metal-on-polyethylene implant.[46] Many studies have reported the release of cytokines and inflammatory mediators secondary to low to moderate doses of metallic particulate debris, which in theory may lead to cell destruction and subsequent periprosthetic osteolysis and aseptic loosening.[44,47-50] In contrast, other studies have suggested that metallic debris is too small to induce an inflammatory cascade and is not associated with loosening of the prosthesis.[51,52] Various clinical trials and laboratory studies have shown higher levels (up to 50 to 100 times higher) of cobalt and chromium in the blood and urine of patients with metal-on-metal implants compared with normal human levels.[7,44,53,54] Consequently, the use of metal-on-metal bearings is precluded in patients with chronic renal failure because of the risk of reduced urine clearance of metallic ions and in women of childbearing age because of the possibility of metal particles crossing the placenta.[55,56] A Finnish study compared the incidence of cancer after metal-on-metal total THA versus metal-on-polyethylene implantation.[57] Results showed an increased ratio for all cancers in the metal-on-metal group (0.95) over the polyethylene group (0.76), which translated into an overall risk of cancer in the metal-on-metal group of 1.23-fold compared with the risk in patients who had metal-on-polyethylene THAs.[57] Despite the suggestion that metallic implants may lead to carcinogenic and other adverse effects, other factors may also be contributing to the overall risks; therefore, more studies are needed to fully explore this issue.[57] Revising a metal-on-metal THA creates numerous issues. Metal-on-metal acetabular components are often nonmodular. If a surgeon decides not to use a metal-on-metal articulation, equipment should be available to revise the entire acetabular component. Alternatively, a dual mobility polyethylene insert (for example, Mobile Bearing Hip; Stryker Orthopaedics, Mahwah, NJ) can be inserted into the existing acetabular shell.

Ceramic-on-Ceramic Implants

The appeal of a ceramic-on-ceramic hip implant is the inherent properties of improved hardness and durability compared with a metal implant, as well as its biologic inertness in the body. Ceramic is regarded as the hardest bearing material used in THA, and it is the bearing surface that is most resistant to wear.[58] In vivo, ceramic implant debris usually produces no inflammatory response or osteolysis. Ceramic implants are often used in a younger, more active patient who is at risk of wearing out the bearing in his or her lifetime.[58] Hip simulator studies and laboratory measurements of friction and wear in ceramic-on-ceramic joint implants have identified wear rates of approximately 0.0001 mm/y with a mean particle debris size of 0.02 μm.[59] As was the case with first-generation metal-on-metal total hip prostheses, early ceramic prostheses had design flaws and material inequalities that commonly led to catastrophic fractures, impingement, implant loosening, and higher than predicted wear rates.[60-62] Improvements in implant design and the material grain structure of ceramic devices have produced a bearing surface with improved hardness, fracture toughness, and burst strength compared with early designs.[7] These properties are attributed to smaller average grain size and lower porosity of the ceramic material and its higher density and purity.[63] In a study comparing the results of ceramic-on-ceramic with metal-on-polyethylene bearings, D'Antonio et al[64] reported that revisions were necessary in 2.7% of patients with ceramic (alumina) bearings compared with 7.5% of the control group with metal-on-polyethylene bearings. Osteolysis was reported in 1.4% of the patients with an alumina bearing compared with 14.0% of the control group.[64]

Ceramics also are hydrophilic, which allows for improved wettability of the joint articulation.[7] This attribute, combined with the ability to polish a ceramic bearing to a low surface roughness, allows for a higher λ ratio compared with its metal counterpart and less friction and overall wear.[7,65] Because laboratory trials have demonstrated no ion release from the wear of ceramic bearings, in theory these bearings are more biologically compatible; however, these same studies have reported some ceramic particle-induced inflammatory reaction, but it is much less than seen with metal debris.[66] In the revision setting, even with copious irrigation, residual debris (such as bone, metal, and polymethylmethacrylate cement) may be present. Because ceramic-on-ceramic bearings are highly resistant to third body wear caused by debris, a ceramic-on-ceramic bearing should be considered for a young patient undergoing revision of all hip components.

Ceramic-on-ceramic implants also have disadvantages. Early alumina-on-alumina models, plagued with faulty designs and poor manufacturing, experienced excessive wear rates of 5 to 9 μm/y to 90 μm over 3 years.[67] The most common concerns surrounding ceramic bearings are the heightened fracture risk because of brittleness, the potential for acetabular liner chipping over time, the limited availability in femoral neck lengths, and postoperative squeaking with joint movement. The fracture rate of newer ceramic models is reported at 0.012%, and the incidence of acetabular liner chipping occurs in approximately 1% to 2% of all implants.[68] Squeaking has been reported in metal-on-metal bearings but is more common with ceramic articulations. In metal-on-polyethylene implants, squeaking may be attributed to femoral head wear through the polyethylene liner and the resulting articulation with the metal cup underneath.[69] Squeaking of a metal-on-polyethylene bearing requires urgent evaluation and treatment. In ceramic-on-ceramic implants, malpositioning of the cup can lead to component impingement and squeaking.[70] A relatively low incidence of squeaking (1 in 700 patients) has been reported with newer models of ceramic-on-ceramic implants.[69] Revision surgeries secondary to the failure of ceramic implants, most notably ceramic fracture, is complicated by the presence of highly abrasive ceramic particulate debris.[71] Nevertheless, an approach using total synovectomy, cup exchange, and the insertion of a new ceramic femoral ball minimizes the chance of accelerated bearing wear and the need for additional revision surgeries.[72] The limited choices of head, neck, and liner sizes available with ceramic components creates an added challenge when they are used in revision surgery.

Despite concerns, the outlook for ceramic implants appears positive. In a 5-year minimum follow-up study of alumina-on-alumina THAs in 79 patients younger than 65 years (93 hips), postoperative imaging and examination results showed no hip dislocations, component loosening, wear, or osteolysis.[73] In addition, ceramic fractures did not occur in any of the patients under ordinary circumstances.[73] A prospective, randomized, multicenter study with 495 patients and 514 hips compared patients with an alumina-on-alumina ceramic bearing to a control group with cobalt chromium-on-polyethylene bearings.[74] No significant differences in clinical outcomes were observed after a mean follow-up of 4 years.[74] No fractures of the ceramic head or liner were reported nor were any revisions needed because of liner-related complications.[74] These encouraging results with newer ceramic bearings may provide a safe option for younger and more active patients in need of primary or revision THAs.

Ceramic-on-Metal Implants

The most recent combination of bearing surfaces introduced for joint reconstruction is the ceramic-on-metal implant. Early studies reported lower friction, wear, and ion levels (specifically, cobalt and chromium) in ceramic-on-metal bearings compared with metal-on-metal implants and nearly equivalent tribologic properties as ceramic-on-ceramic implants.[75,76] These results are further supported by in vitro studies that evaluated the tribology of various bearing surfaces. The differential hardness of ceramic-on-metal bearings and ceramic-like coatings on metal reduce wear and metallic ion levels by up to 50% compared with metal-on-metal articulations.[77] In a study by Firkins et al,[78] the differential hardness of the ceramic-on-metal bearings contributed to the approximately 100-fold lower wear rates of these implants compared with metal-on-metal implants. Although early investigative clinical trials have reported optimistic results for ceramic-on-metal hip replacements, further long-term studies are needed before surgeons can confidently choose these bearing surfaces for treating their patients.

Discussion of Bearing Surface Options

Each of the previously discussed bearing surface options may be suitable for patients undergoing revision THA because of their favorable wear rates and low incidence of osteolysis (**Table 1**). A metal-on-polyethylene hip bearing is the workhorse of revision THA because of its very good wear resistance, multiple liner options, and lower cost versus other bearing surfaces. Polyethylene is not associated with in vivo toxicity, and osteolysis usually occurs only with significant wear. However, these benefits come at the cost of increased wear rates compared with other bearing surfaces. Metal-on-metal implants offer higher wear resistance and long-term in vivo durability and easily support larger diameter femoral heads, which reduce the risk of dislocation. However, concerns about the biotoxicity of wear particles should be considered before making this type of bearing a routine choice in THA. Because ceramic-on-ceramic implants have the highest wear resistance, have good long-term in vivo results, and show minimal evidence of particle toxicity, these implants are often used in younger, more active patients. The disadvantages of ceramic-on-ceramic implants include the risk of acetabular liner chipping, catastrophic fracturing of the implant, and squeaking. However, these concerns may be subjugated when considering ceramic bearings for younger patients because of the need to avoid future revision surgery that may occur secondary to implant wear (**Table 2**).

Table 1
Comparison of Hip Implant Materials

Properties	Metal-on-Polyethylene	Metal-on-Metal	Ceramic-on-Ceramic
Hardness (MPa)	Low	350	2,300
Fracture risk	Yes	No	Yes
Run-in wear	100 µm	25 µm	1 µm
Steady-state wear	10-20 µm	5 µm	0-3 µm
Metal ion level in body fluids	N/A	Yes	N/A
Cell toxicity	N/A	Yes	N/A
Allergic component	Yes, minor	Yes, major	No
Squeaking	No	Yes	Yes
Clicking	No	Yes	Yes

N/A = not available

Table 2
Advantages and Disadvantages of Hip Implant Materials

	Metal-on-Polyethylene	Metal-on-Metal	Ceramic-on-Ceramic
Advantages	High wear resistance No toxicity Low cost Multiple liner options Proven product	Very high wear resistance Larger head diameters Long in vivo experience	Highest wear resistance Bioinert Long in vivo experience Wettability Decreased surface roughness Resistant to oxidative wear
Disadvantages	Reduced material properties Material failure Increased bioactivity Particles/osteolysis	Increased ion levels Delayed-type hypersensitivity response Carcinogenic Corrosion at metal junctions Precise machining required	Acetabular liner chipping Fracture risk Squeaking Increased cost Limited neck lengths

Summary

Over the years, impressive advances in the design and durability of bearing surfaces for THA have occurred. The choice of a bearing surface for revision THA should take into account factors such as the patient's age and activity level, the cost of the implant, and both the surgeon's and patient's preference and experience with various bearing options. Currently, most revision THAs are performed using a metal-on-polyethylene articulation. However, as the revision burden increases and the average age of patients undergoing revision surgery decreases, the use of more durable bearing surfaces should be considered. Although laboratory studies and small clinical trials have reported optimistic in vivo results for alternative bearing surface options, much has to be learned about the long-term performance of these materials in patients treated with revision THA. Although long-term clinical studies confirming the better wear performance of newer bearing surfaces are needed, a decline in the incidence of wear-induced osteolysis and loosening with these new bearing surface options for revision THA is likely based on optimistic and extensive in vitro evaluation.

References

1. Furnes O, Havelin LI, Espehaug B, Engesaeter LB, Lie SA, Vollset SE: The Norwegian registry of joint prostheses: 15 beneficial years for both the patients and the health care. *Tidsskr Nor Laegeforen* 2003;123(10): 1367-1369.
2. Kurtz S, Mowat F, Ong K, Chan N, Lau E, Halpern M: Prevalence of primary and revision total hip and knee arthroplasty in the United States from 1990 through 2002. *J Bone Joint Surg Am* 2005;87(7):1487-1497.
3. Harris WH: The problem is osteolysis. *Clin Orthop Relat Res* 1995;311:46-53.
4. Jazrawi LM, Kummer FJ, Di-Cesare PE: Alternative bearing surfaces for total joint arthroplasty. *J Am Acad Orthop Surg* 1998;6(4):198-203.
5. Schmalzried TP, Kwong LM, Jasty M, et al: The mechanism of loosening of cemented acetabular components in total hip arthroplasty: Analysis of specimens retrieved at autopsy. *Clin Orthop Relat Res* 1992;274:60-78.
6. Harris WH, Muratoglu OK: A review of current cross-linked polyethylenes used in total joint arthroplasty. *Clin Orthop Relat Res* 2005;430:46-52.
7. Heisel C, Silva M, Schmalzried TP: Bearing surface options for total hip replacement in young patients. *Instr Course Lect* 2004; 53:49-65.
8. Garvey R: Wear rates impact maintenance priorities. Machinery Lubrication Website. 2003. http://www.machinerylubrication.com/Read/468/wear-rate-maintenance. Accessed November 16, 2010.
9. Jacobson B: Thin film lubrication of real surfaces. *Tribology Intl* 2000;33:205-210.
10. Czichos H: *Tribology: A Systems Approach to the Science and Technology of Friction, Lubrication, and Wear.* Amsterdam, The Netherlands, Elsevier Scientific Publishing, 1978, p 414.
11. Dumbleton JH, Manley MT, Edidin AA: A literature review of the association between wear rate and osteolysis in total hip arthroplasty. *J Arthroplasty* 2002;17(5): 649-661.
12. Sochart DH: Relationship of acetabular wear to osteolysis and loosening in total hip arthroplasty. *Clin Orthop Relat Res* 1999;363: 135-150.
13. McKellop HA: Bearing surfaces in total hip replacements: State of the art and future developments. *Instr Course Lect* 2001;50: 165-179.
14. McKellop H, Shen FW, Lu B, Campbell P, Salovey R: Effect of sterilization method and other modifications on the wear resistance of acetabular cups made of ultra-high molecular weight polyethylene: A hip-simulator study. *J Bone Joint Surg Am* 2000; 82-A(12):1708-1725.
15. Muratoglu OK, Bragdon CR, O'Connor DO, Jasty M, Harris WH: A novel method of cross-linking ultra-high-molecular-weight polyethylene to improve wear, reduce oxidation, and retain mechanical properties: Recipient of the 1999 HAP Paul Award. *J Arthroplasty* 2001;16(2): 149-160.
16. Sharkey PF, Hozack WJ, Dorr LD, Maloney WJ, Berry D: The bearing surface in total hip arthroplasty: Evolution or revolution. *Instr Course Lect* 2000; 49:41-56.
17. Kurtz SM, Manley M, Wang A, Taylor S, Dumbleton J: Comparison of the properties of annealed crosslinked (Crossfire) and conventional polyethylene as hip bearing materials. *Bull Hosp Jt Dis* 2002-2003;61(1-2):17-26.
18. Wannomae KK, Christensen SD, Freiberg AA, Bhattacharyya S, Harris WH, Muratoglu OK: The effect of real-time aging on the oxidation and wear of highly cross-linked UHMWPE acetabular liners. *Biomaterials* 2006;27(9): 1980-1987.
19. Burroughs BR, Rubash HE, Harris WH: Femoral head sizes larger than 32 mm against highly cross-linked polyethylene. *Clin Orthop Relat Res* 2002;405:150-157.
20. Livermore J, Ilstrup D, Morrey B: Effect of femoral head size on wear of the polyethylene acetabu-

lar component. *J Bone Joint Surg Am* 1990;72(4):518-528.

21. Burroughs BR, Golladay GJ, Hallstrom B, Harris WH: A novel constrained acetabular liner design with increased range of motion. *J Arthroplasty* 2001;16(8, Suppl 1):31-36.
22. Muratoglu OK, Bragdon CR, O'Connor DO, et al: Unified wear model for highly crosslinked ultra-high molecular weight polyethylenes (UHMWPE). *Biomaterials* 1999;20(16):1463-1470.
23. McKellop HA, Shen FW, Campbell P, Ota T: Effect of molecular weight, calcium stearate, and sterilization methods on the wear of ultra high molecular weight polyethylene acetabular cups in a hip joint simulator. *J Orthop Res* 1999;17(3):329-339.
24. Colwell CW, et al: Effect of head size and crosslinking on wear in polyethylene acetabular components. *Trans AAHKS* 2001;11:46.
25. Leventhal GS: Titanium: A metal for surgery. *J Bone Joint Surg Am* 1951;33-A(2):473-474.
26. Clarke IC, Manaka M, Green DD, et al: Current status of zirconia used in total hip implants. *J Bone Joint Surg Am* 2003; 85-A(Suppl 4):73-84.
27. Manley MT, Dumbleton J: Bearing surfaces, in Barrack RL, Booth RE Jr, Lonner JH, eds: *Orthopaedic Knowledge Update: Hip and Knee Reconstruction*, ed 3. Rosemont, IL, American Academy of Orthopaedic Surgeons, 2006, pp 333-344.
28. Haraguchi K, Sugano N, Nishii T, Miki H, Oka K, Yoshikawa H: Phase transformation of a zirconia ceramic head after total hip arthroplasty. *J Bone Joint Surg Br* 2001;83(7): 996-1000.
29. Smith & Nephew: Welcome to Oxinium Hip and Knee Placements. 2003-2005. http://www.oxinium.co.uk/index.php. Accessed September 22, 2010.
30. Bourne RB, Barrack R, Rorabeck CH, Salehi A, Good V: Arthroplasty options for the young patient: Oxinium on cross-linked polyethylene. *Clin Orthop Relat Res* 2005;441:159-167.
31. Amstutz HC, Le Duff MJ: Background of metal-on-metal resurfacing. *Proc Inst Mech Eng H* 2006;220(2):85-94.
32. Willert HG, Buchhorn GH, Göbel D, et al: Wear behavior and histopathology of classic cemented metal on metal hip endoprostheses. *Clin Orthop Relat Res* 1996; 329(Suppl):S160-S186.
33. Jacobsson SA, Djerf K, Wahlström O: Twenty-year results of McKee-Farrar versus Charnley prosthesis. *Clin Orthop Relat Res* 1996;329(Suppl):S60-S68.
34. Jacobsson SA, Djerf K, Wahlström O: A comparative study between McKee-Farrar and Charnley arthroplasty with long-term follow-up periods. *J Arthroplasty* 1990;5(1):9-14.
35. MacDonald SJ, McCalden RW, Chess DG, et al: Metal-on-metal versus polyethylene in hip arthroplasty: A randomized clinical trial. *Clin Orthop Relat Res* 2003;406: 282-296.
36. Dorr LD, Wan Z, Longjohn DB, Dubois B, Murken R: Total hip arthroplasty with the use of the Metasul metal-on-metal articulation: Four to seven-year results. *J Bone Joint Surg Am* 2000;82(6): 789-798.
37. Archibeck MJ, Jacobs JJ, Black J: Alternate bearing surfaces in total joint arthroplasty: Biologic considerations. *Clin Orthop Relat Res* 2000;379:12-21.
38. Dowson D, Jin ZM: Metal-on-metal hip joint tribology. *Proc Inst Mech Eng H* 2006;220(2): 107-118.
39. Wagner M, Wagner H: Medium-term results of a modern metal-on-metal system in total hip replacement. *Clin Orthop Relat Res* 2000;379:123-133.
40. McKellop H, Park SH, Chiesa R, et al: In vivo wear of three types of metal on metal hip prostheses during two decades of use. *Clin Orthop Relat Res* 1996;329 (Suppl):S128-S140.
41. Pabinger C, Biedermann R, Stöckl B, Fischer M, Krismer M: Migration of metal-on-metal versus ceramic-on-polyethylene hip prostheses. *Clin Orthop Relat Res* 2003;412:103-110.
42. Jacobs M, Gorab R, Mattingly D, Trick L, Southworth C: Three- to six-year results with the Ultima metal-on-metal hip articulation for primary total hip arthroplasty. *J Arthroplasty* 2004;19(7, Suppl 2):48-53.
43. Long WT, Dorr LD, Gendelman V: An American experience with metal-on-metal total hip arthroplasties: A 7-year follow-up study. *J Arthroplasty* 2004;19 (8, Suppl 3):29-34.
44. Lhotka C, Szekeres T, Steffan I, Zhuber K, Zweymüller K: Four-year study of cobalt and chromium blood levels in patients managed with two different metal-on-metal total hip replacements. *J Orthop Res* 2003;21(2): 189-195.
45. McGovern TF, Moskal JT: Radiographic evaluation of periprosthetic metallosis after total knee arthroplasty. *J South Orthop Assoc* 2002;11(1):18-24.
46. Silva M, Heisel C, Schmalzried TP: Metal-on-metal total hip replacement. *Clin Orthop Relat Res* 2005;430:53-61.
47. Lee SH, Brennan FR, Jacobs JJ, Urban RM, Ragasa DR, Glant TT: Human monocyte/macrophage response to cobalt-chromium corrosion products and titanium particles in patients with total joint replacements. *J Orthop Res* 1997;15(1):40-49.

48. Shanbhag AS, Jacobs JJ, Black J, Galante JO, Glant TT: Human monocyte response to particulate biomaterials generated in vivo and in vitro. *J Orthop Res* 1995;13(5): 792-801.

49. Korovessis P, Petsinis G, Repanti M: Zweymueller with metal-on-metal articulation: Clinical, radiological and histological analysis of short-term results. *Arch Orthop Trauma Surg* 2003; 123(1):5-11.

50. Park YS, Moon YW, Lim SJ, Yang JM, Ahn G, Choi YL: Early osteolysis following second-generation metal-on-metal hip replacement. *J Bone Joint Surg Am* 2005;87(7):1515-1521.

51. Green TR, Fisher J, Stone M, Wroblewski BM, Ingham E: Polyethylene particles of a "critical size" are necessary for the induction of cytokines by macrophages in vitro. *Biomaterials* 1998; 19(24):2297-2302.

52. Willert HG, Semlitsch M: Tissue reactions to plastic and metallic wear products of joint endoprostheses. *Clin Orthop Relat Res* 1996;333:4-14.

53. Grübl A, Weissinger M, Brodner W, et al: Serum aluminium and cobalt levels after ceramic-on-ceramic and metal-on-metal total hip replacement. *J Bone Joint Surg Br* 2006;88(8):1003-1005.

54. Savarino L, Greco M, Cenni E, et al: Differences in ion release after ceramic-on-ceramic and metal-on-metal total hip replacement: Medium-term follow-up. *J Bone Joint Surg Br* 2006;88(4): 472-476.

55. Santavirta S, Böhler M, Harris WH, et al: Alternative materials to improve total hip replacement tribology. *Acta Orthop Scand* 2003;74(4):380-388.

56. Jacobs JJ, Skipor AK, Doorn PF, et al: Cobalt and chromium concentrations in patients with metal on metal total hip replacements. *Clin Orthop Relat Res* 1996;329 (Suppl):S256-S263.

57. Visuri T, Pukkala E, Paavolainen P, Pulkkinen P, Riska EB: Cancer risk after metal on metal and polyethylene on metal total hip arthroplasty. *Clin Orthop Relat Res* 1996;329(Suppl):S280-S289.

58. Hannouche D, Hamadouche M, Nizard R, Bizot P, Meunier A, Sedel L: Ceramics in total hip replacement. *Clin Orthop Relat Res* 2005;430:62-71.

59. Tipper JL, Hatton A, Nevelos JE, et al: Alumina-alumina artificial hip joints: Part II. Characterisation of the wear debris from in vitro hip joint simulations. *Biomaterials* 2002;23(16):3441-3448.

60. Mittelmeier H, Heisel J: Sixteen-years' experience with ceramic hip prostheses. *Clin Orthop Relat Res* 1992;282:64-72.

61. Walter A: On the material and the tribology of alumina-alumina couplings for hip joint prostheses. *Clin Orthop Relat Res* 1992;282: 31-46.

62. Mahoney OM, Dimon JH III: Unsatisfactory results with a ceramic total hip prosthesis. *J Bone Joint Surg Am* 1990;72(5): 663-671.

63. D'Antonio J, Capello W, Manley M: Alumina ceramic bearings for total hip arthroplasty. *Orthopedics* 2003;26(1):39-46.

64. D'Antonio J, Capello W, Manley M, Naughton M, Sutton K: Alumina ceramic bearings for total hip arthroplasty: Five-year results of a prospective randomized study. *Clin Orthop Relat Res* 2005;436:164-171.

65. Prudhommeaux F, Hamadouche M, Nevelos J, Doyle C, Meunier A, Sedel L: Wear of alumina-on-alumina total hip arthroplasties at a mean 11-year followup. *Clin Orthop Relat Res* 2000;379:113-122.

66. Germain MA, Hatton A, Williams S, et al: Comparison of the cytotoxicity of clinically relevant cobalt-chromium and alumina ceramic wear particles in vitro. *Biomaterials* 2003;24(3):469-479.

67. Boutin P, Christel P, Dorlot JM, et al: The use of dense alumina-alumina ceramic combination in total hip replacement. *J Biomed Mater Res* 1988;22(12):1203-1232.

68. Garino JP: Ceramic component fracture: Trends and recommendations with modern components based on improved reporting methods, in D'Antonio JA, Dietrich M, eds: *Bioceramics and Alternative Bearings in Joint Arthroplasty: 10th Biolox Symposium Proceedings*. Darmstadt, Germany, Steinkopff Verlag, 2005, pp 157-168.

69. Walter WL, Insley GM, Walter WK, Tuke MA: Edge loading in third generation alumina ceramic-on-ceramic bearings: Stripe wear. *J Arthroplasty* 2004; 19(4):402-413.

70. Eickmann T, Masakazu M, et al: Squeaking and neck-socket impingement in a ceramic total hip arthroplasty. *Key Eng Mater* 2003; 240-242:849-852.

71. Barrack RL, Burak C, Skinner HB: Concerns about ceramics in THA. *Clin Orthop Relat Res* 2004;429:73-79.

72. Allain J, Roudot-Thoraval F, Delecrin J, Anract P, Migaud H, Goutallier D: Revision total hip arthroplasty performed after fracture of a ceramic femoral head: A multicenter survivorship study. *J Bone Joint Surg Am* 2003; 85-A(5):825-830.

73. Yoo JJ, Kim YM, Yoon KS, Koo KH, Song WS, Kim HJ: Alumina-on-alumina total hip arthroplasty: A five-year minimum follow-up study. *J Bone Joint Surg Am* 2005;87(3):530-535.

74. Capello WN, Dantonio JA, Feinberg JR, Manley MT: Alternative bearing surfaces: Alumina ceramic

bearings for total hip arthroplasty. *Instr Course Lect* 2005;54: 171-176.

75. Williams S, Schepers A, Isaac G, et al: Ceramic-on-metal hip arthroplasties: A comparative in vitro and in vivo study. *Clin Orthop Relat Res* 2007;465:23-32.

76. Brockett C, Williams S, Jin Z, Isaac G, Fisher J: Friction of total hip replacements with different bearings and loading conditions. *J Biomed Mater Res B Appl Biomater* 2007;81(2):508-515.

77. Fisher J, Jin Z, Tipper J, Stone M, Ingham E: Tribology of alternative bearings. *Clin Orthop Relat Res* 2006;453:25-34.

78. Firkins PJ, Tipper JL, Ingham E, Stone MH, Farrar R, Fisher J: A novel low wearing differential hardness, ceramic-on-metal hip joint prosthesis. *J Biomech* 2001; 34(10):1291-1298.

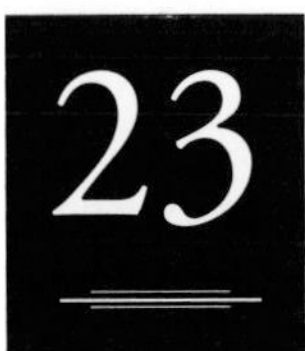

Revision Total Knee Arthroplasty: What the Practicing Orthopaedic Surgeon Needs to Know

David J. Jacofsky, MD
Craig J. Della Valle, MD
R. Michael Meneghini, MD
Scott M. Sporer, MD
Robert M. Cercek, MD

Abstract

The number of revision total knee arthroplasties (TKAs) continues to steadily increase. The evaluation of painful and revision TKAs may be challenging for the general orthopaedic surgeon, but a standardized, systematic approach to each patient will allow predictable surgical outcomes. This approach begins with a consistent and thorough preoperative patient evaluation. Revision surgery should not be performed until the etiology of failure of the index arthroplasty is known. The possibility of infection in the revision setting also must be considered because this complication will drastically alter the treatment algorithm.

Adjunctive techniques, including the quadriceps snip, the medial collateral ligament slide, and the tibial tubercle osteotomy, can greatly enhance surgical exposure and the efficient removal of components in revision TKAs. A thorough knowledge of the reconstructive options for replacing bone loss is crucial, and the availability of appropriate revision instrumentation is required for surgical efficiency. A concise diagnostic algorithm coupled with clear reconstructive principles will allow more efficient and confident management of a patient with a failed TKA.

Instr Course Lect 2011;60:269-281.

Total knee arthroplasties (TKAs) are very common, and the overall results are excellent, with 95% of the implants surviving for at least 15 years.[1,2] The 5% that fail represent a substantial number, and orthopaedic surgeons are seeing an increasing number of patients who initially had a successful total knee replacement but then had pain, radiographic evidence of failure, and/or dysfunction caused by failure of the arthroplasty. Extensive bone loss, instability, infection, dysfunction of the extensor mechanism, and periarticular arthrofibrosis are frequent challenges encountered during revision surgery. A systematic approach to the evaluation of patients requiring revision TKA can help identify the correct diagnosis and guide the surgical intervention, thereby optimizing success.

Before doing a revision, the surgeon should know the cause of the pain in a patient with a prior TKA. A revision TKA done for unexplained pain has a very low probability of success.[3] The surgeon should identify the current implants by reviewing previous surgical records. Medical comorbidities should be appropriately managed so that the patient can be in the best health before a revision is done. Sometimes revision surgery is contraindicated, such as in a patient with Charcot arthropathy or neuromuscular disease. Wound healing after revision TKA is critical to success and is often more difficult to achieve than after a primary TKA. If there is doubt about soft-tissue coverage and/or viability, the use of a rotational muscle flap or consultation with a plastic surgeon should be considered.

Dr. Jacofsky or an immediate family member has received royalties from Stryker and Smith & Nephew; serves as a paid consultant for or is an employee of Stryker; owns stock or stock options in Bacterin; and has received research or institutional support from Biomet, Stryker, Smith & Nephew, and Arthrex. Dr. Della Valle or an immediate family member serves as a paid consultant for or is an employee of Angiotech, Biomet, Kinamed, and Smith & Nephew; has received research or institutional support from Pacira and Zimmer; and serves as a board member, owner, officer, or committee member for the American Association of Hip and Knee Surgeons and the Arthritis Foundation. Dr. Sporer or an immediate family member serves as a paid consultant for or is an employee of Smith & Nephew and Zimmer and has received research or institutional support from Coolsystems. Dr. Meneghini or an immediate family member is a member of a speakers' bureau or has made paid presentations on behalf of Stryker; serves as a paid consultant to or is an employee of Stryker; and has received research or institutional support from Stryker. Neither Dr. Cercek nor any immediate family member has received anything of value from or owns stock in a commercial company or institution related directly or indirectly to the subject of this chapter.

Preoperative Evaluation

The causes of dysfunction and pain after TKA are numerous.[4-6] There are two broad categories to consider: extrinsic (extra-articular) and intrinsic (intra-articular). Extrinsic sources of pain include the ipsilateral hip, the lumbar spine (stenosis or radiculopathy), soft-tissue inflammation (pes anserinus bursitis or iliotibial, patellar, or quadriceps tendinitis), complex regional pain syndrome, neuroma, vascular claudication, fracture (tibial stress fracture, patellar stress fracture, femoral stress fracture, or traumatic fracture), and rarely an intrapelvic lesion compressing the medial or lateral femoral cutaneous nerve. Intrinsic sources include aseptic loosening, polyethylene wear, osteolysis, malalignment, instability (coronal instability, flexion instability, or global instability), infection, implant fracture, arthrofibrosis, soft-tissue impingement, component overhang, and dysfunction of the extensor mechanism (instability, fracture, maltracking, lateral patellar facet impingement, excessive component construct thickness, patella baja, and patellar or quadriceps tendon rupture). A working and complete knowledge of these causes will improve the surgeon's ability to correctly determine the reason or reasons for the failed TKA.

History and Physical Examination

The history and physical examination are critical first steps in the evaluation of patients with pain after a TKA, and often they alone allow identification and/or elimination of most pathologic etiologies. The primary symptom should be clearly defined (pain, swelling, instability, or stiffness), as should the time of onset, the duration, and the frequency of the symptoms as well as any activities that are associated with them. Pain that was present before the surgery and has persisted without change suggests an extrinsic etiology. Pain that began within the first year after the surgery suggests infection, malrotation, or soft-tissue impingement. Pain that began after 1 year suggests wear, osteolysis, loosening, or infection (acute hematogenous or late chronic). Comorbid conditions, such as diabetes, peripheral vascular disease, and lumbar stenosis, should be considered. The physical examination should include visual inspection; careful palpation (for swelling or point tenderness); stability testing in extension, midflexion, and 90° of flexion;[7,8] and evaluation of patellofemoral stability, including palpation of the patella and its retinaculum. The surgeon should (1) watch the patient walk; (2) measure the active and passive ranges of knee motion; (3) evaluate patellar tracking (patellar clunk refers to impingement of scar tissue on the undersurface of the quadriceps tendon as the knee extends from a flexed position; this is less common with modern trochlear and femoral box designs);[9] (4) perform a thorough neurovascular examination with careful assessment of quadriceps and vastus medialis obliquus strength and the quality and symmetry of peripheral pulses; and (5) examine adjacent joints, including the hip, lumbar spine, foot, and ankle (a planovalgus foot deformity can lead to the failure of a cruciate-retaining arthroplasty).[10]

Radiographic Evaluation

Examining plain radiographs can reveal many of the intrinsic causes of pain in a patient treated with TKA, and examining a series of radiographs made over time, including preoperatively, can be particularly useful. Hip-to-ankle weight-bearing AP, lateral, and Merchant views of the knee and radiographs of the ipsilateral hip should be evaluated. The AP radiograph should be scrutinized for evidence of polyethylene wear; osteolysis; radiolucent lines; and overhang, subsidence, or a change in the position of the tibial component. The lateral radiograph should be assessed for femoral component size, posterior femoral offset, patellar height and thickness, and tibial component slope and subsidence. The Merchant radiograph should be evaluated for patellar tilt, malalignment, femoral overhang, lateral patellofemoral impingement, and patellar composite thickness. Serial radiographs are invaluable for determining subtle signs of loosening, such as late progression of radiolucent lines, changes or fractures in the cement mantle, progression of osteolysis, or a subtle change in component position.

Fluoroscopic examination may be useful for evaluating the interface in cementless arthroplasty designs. The extent of osteolytic lesions is best seen on CT or MRI scans with metal artifact suppression, but these modalities are not universally available.[11] CT and MRI can also be used to accurately assess the rotation of the femoral and tibial components; the femoral component is compared with the transepicondylar axis, and the tibial component is compared with the medial third of the tibial tubercle. Excessive internal rotation of either component can be associated with patellar instability and lateral flexion laxity, leading to poorer clinical function.[12,13] Radionuclide scans may help in diagnosing aseptic loosening, infection, complex regional pain syndrome, and periprosthetic stress fractures. These scans are nonspecific and may be falsely positive in the first few postoperative years; a technetium bone scan demonstrates increased uptake in approximately 90% of tibial and 65% of femoral components at 1 year after TKA.[14] The value of radionuclide scans in the diagnosis of infection has been explored with mixed results.[15-17] Technetium bone scans are sensitive but are unable to differentiate septic from aseptic failure. Indium 111-labeled white blood cell scans have value for the exclusion of infection when they are negative, and their specificity is optimal when they are combined with sulfur colloid bone marrow scans to correct for marrow packing in the vicinity of prosthetic components. Positron emission tomography and MRI may be useful for diagnosing infection; however, their utility has not yet been determined. Given the ease, accuracy, and low cost of knee joint aspiration and synovial fluid analysis and culture, advanced imaging should be used only for second-line testing (if no fluid can be obtained with an aspiration or if repeated aspirations lead to equivocal findings).

Preoperative Laboratory Testing

Every patient who presents with a failed TKA or pain following a TKA must be evaluated for a deep periprosthetic infection. Even if the cause of failure seems obvious, concomitant infection may be present; the treatment of an infection-related failure of a TKA is fundamentally different from the treatment of aseptic failure. The patient's medical history and the history surrounding the index arthroplasty may suggest an infection. Patient-related risk factors include diabetes mellitus, inflammatory arthritis, obesity, a history of septic arthritis of the native knee, skin disorders, prior ipsilateral knee surgery, revision as opposed to a primary procedure, malnourishment, renal insufficiency (especially when it requires dialysis), and any immunocompromised state. The patient should be specifically questioned regarding the presence of wound-healing complications immediately following the surgery, the extended use of antibiotics, or a return to the operating room, as the patient may not understand the importance of such events with regard to the present pain symptoms. A lack of pain relief since the TKA, particularly if the character of the pain is different from that experienced preoperatively, increases the clinical suspicion of infection, as does a recent systemic illness (particularly if it was associated with bacteremia), which may indicate hematogenous infection. Early loosening of a prosthetic component (within the first 2 to 5 years postoperatively) should be considered suspicious for infection.

Basic laboratory testing includes an evaluation of the erythrocyte sedimentation rate and C-reactive protein level. These are sensitive tests for identifying infection, and it is unlikely both will yield normal results if there is an infection;[18] thus, they are ideal screening tools for the identification of patients who require additional testing. If either test is abnormal or clinical suspicion remains high, the joint should be aspirated, and the aspirated fluid should be sent for Gram stain, culture, and a synovial fluid white blood cell count and differential. The patient should not receive antibiotics for a minimum of 2 weeks before the aspiration to optimize the culture results.[19] The aspiration should be repeated if clinical suspicion remains high. A synovial fluid white blood cell count of between 1,100 and 3,000 cells/mm^3 from the site of a total joint arthroplasty is strongly suggestive of an infection.[20-22] This is much lower than the 50,000 to 100,000 cells/mm^3 range that suggests an infection in a native knee. The percentage of neutrophils in the aspirated fluid is also an accurate predictor of infection. If the percentage of neutrophils is between 60% and 80%, infection is likely. When the white blood cell count is less than 1,100 cells/mm^3 and the percentage of neutrophils is less than 64%, the negative predictive value is 98.2%; in contrast, when both are greater than these values, the positive predictive value for infection is 98.6%.[23] Determining the white blood cell count in aspirated fluid has a low cost, is objective, can be performed preoperatively or intraoperatively, and is available to surgeons worldwide.

Intraoperative Laboratory Testing

Both intraoperative appearance and intraoperative Gram stains have been shown to have low sensitivity and should not be relied on for diagnosing periprosthetic joint infection.[24] Histopathologic examination of periprosthetic tissues has been shown to be useful for diagnosing infection;[25] however, for this examination to be accurate, a skilled pathologist must be available. The histologic criteria for diagnosing infection are controversial, but in general an average of more than 10 polymorphonuclear cells per high-power field is diagnostic for infection. The most suspicious-appearing areas should be sampled, and the leukocytes must be in tissue (and not fibrin) to be counted. The possibility of an occult infection should be discussed with the pathologist so that the synovial tissue can be prepared and interpreted properly.

Preoperative Planning

The surgeon should thoroughly review the radiographs, while remembering that the degree of bone loss surrounding the components is underestimated on the basis of plain radiographs.[26] The function of the extensor mechanism should be ascertained before surgery. A preoperative extension lag may be caused by relative shortening of the lower extremity secondary to component loosening or catastrophic bearing failure and a subsequent loss of resting tension. This type of extension lag can improve with revision surgery. Conversely, chronic quadriceps or patellar tendon dysfunction may require augmentation with an extensor mechanism or an Achilles tendon allograft at the time of the surgery. The appropriate height of the joint line should be assessed to improve the kinematics of the knee. Radiographs available from before the index arthroplasty or radiographs of the native contralateral knee help to determine the anatomic location of the joint line and the amount of posterior femoral offset in a given patient. Patella baja is frequently encountered during revision surgery and may be a result of an intrinsic contracture of the patellar tendon. Frequently, distal femoral augmentation is required in revision surgery to avoid excessive elevation of the joint line. The joint line can be approximated on the basis of the fibular head, the femoral epicondyles, or the superior pole of the patella in relation to the superior aspect of the trochlear groove.

Isolated patellar revision or tibial polyethylene exchange is rarely indicated as they do not usually address the underlying failure mechanism, which is often component malposition.[27,28] The indications for arthroscopy for a patient with pain related to a TKA are also very limited. Some authors have reported successful arthroscopic lysis of adhesions for the treatment of arthrofibrosis, and others have reported successful arthroscopic débridement in cases of soft-tissue impingement, such as patellar clunk or popliteus tendon impingement.[29-31]

Surgical Technique

Exposure

Adequate exposure is essential for a successful surgical reconstruction. The exposure must allow complete exposure of the implant, a thorough débridement of osteolysis, visualization of the remaining bone stock, and reimplantation of the components. Exposure can be quite challenging in the presence of arthrofibrosis, osteoporotic or osteolytic bone, patella baja, and/or obesity.

The medial parapatellar arthrotomy is the workhorse of revision TKA;[32] however, a previous lateral arthrotomy may dictate a repeat lateral approach to avoid patellar osteonecrosis. Often, only a single incision was used previously, and this incision can generally be used for the revision surgery. The incision may be straight and anterior, medialized, or curvilinear. If a transverse or oblique incision was used, it should be crossed at the most obtuse angle possible to minimize wound-healing complications at the corners created by this intersection. If multiple longitudinal incisions were used, the more lateral incision should generally be used because the blood supply travels from the medial to the lateral side of the knee.[33] However, if all incisions were made more than 2 years previously and did not involve a surrounding soft-tissue flap, the surgeon should choose the incision that is most advantageous for the revision surgery. A minimum 6-cm skin bridge should be maintained if previous incisions cannot be used. When there is excessive tension on the skin edges, making the incision longer is advisable, full-thickness flaps should be made, and undermining of tissue should be avoided.

During the exposure, previously placed sutures should be removed as part of the débridement whenever possible. The medial and lateral gutters are re-created, and the suprapatellar pouch is freed of fibrotic tissue to assist with mobilization of the extensor mechanism. In cases of arthrofibrosis and stiffness, a quadricepsplasty is beneficial to free the extensor mechanism from the anterior aspect of the femur.[34] A release of the soft-tissue adhesions between the anterior aspect of the tibia and the patellar tendon proximal to the level of the tubercle insertion will also improve patellar mobilization. Patellar subluxation (as opposed to eversion) is generally sufficient to allow adequate exposure of the knee. The extensor mechanism must be protected throughout the procedure, as fibrosis, osteolysis in the region of the tibial tubercle, and multiple prior surgical procedures place the extensor mechanism at risk for iatrogenic avulsion. A copious medial release to the posteromedial corner of the tibia should then be performed if component revision is required; this allows tibial external rotation and anterior subluxation for removal of the polyethylene liner. This step is often referred to as a "medial collateral ligament (MCL) slide." The polyethylene insert is then removed to improve the surgeon's ability to mobilize the soft tissues, and in many cases this provides sufficient exposure for revision surgery.[35]

A more extensile approach should be considered if patellar subluxation persists and/or visualization of the components remains difficult. The quadriceps snip is the first option for improving exposure. It is particularly helpful in patients with patella baja. It consists of an oblique apical extension of the arthrotomy from the superomedial capsulotomy, and it continues proximally and laterally, exiting the quadriceps tendon laterally and splitting the fibers of the vastus lateralis obliquus. This improves patellar eversion, knee flexion, and lateralization of the extensor mechanism. The quadriceps snip should exit the quadriceps tendon distal to the musculotendinous junction of the rectus femoris muscle (**Figure 1**). Proximal extension of the arthrotomy beyond the tendon before the oblique snip will lead to transection of a portion of the rectus femoris fibers and should be avoided. Because the closure is nearly identical to a normal capsular closure and there is no change in postoperative rehabilitation or outcome, the quadriceps snip may be used liberally to improve exposure.[36]

If exposure is still inadequate, an extended tibial tubercle osteotomy can be performed. It is most useful in the presence of patella baja, for the removal of a cemented tibial stem, and in cases of extensor mechanism maltracking and tibial tubercle malposition that require correction.[37] The tibial tubercle osteotomy is a long osteotomy of at least 8 cm in length. Ideally, a proximal shelf of bone is left to prevent proximal migration of the osteotomy fragment (**Figure 2**); in practice, however, extensive osteolysis, or the need to move the tibial tubercle proximally, often obviates the surgeon's ability to leave a structurally sound proximal shelf. The osteotomy is made along the proximal and medial aspect of the tubercle and is hinged about the lateral side with osteotomes. The soft-tissue sleeve is left intact laterally, and the osteotomy is repaired with cerclage wires at the time of closure. Holes for these wires can be predrilled before the osteotomy is hinged open. When the patient has reasonable bone stock, no alteration in postoperative rehabilitation is necessary. Although there may be symptoms related to the hardware, nonunion is extremely rare unless the prosthetic site is infected.[38]

If improved exposure of the components is still required, a medial femoral peel may be performed. This provides outstanding exposure of both the femoral component and the posterior aspect of the femoral condyles. It is often necessary when contraction of the medial side is found, such as during reimplantation following an infection and the use of static spacers. The medial femoral peel can be performed with cautery, achieving a subperiosteal removal of the origin of the MCL and the soft tissues around the medial side of the knee. It is imperative to keep the entire medial sleeve intact, from the region of the extensor mechanism proximally to the superficial MCL distally, because this is critical for maintaining medial-sided stability. No alteration of postoperative rehabilitation is required.[39] A medial epicondylar osteotomy can be performed in more severe cases, but generally it is not required unless a malunion is present. Should an epicondylar osteotomy be required, the surgeon must be certain that osteolysis of the medial femoral condyle is minimal, as extensive osteolysis may result in a large uncontained femoral bone defect.

In general, the most useful approach for most revision procedures is a generous MCL release to the posterior aspect of the tibia, in conjunction with a quadriceps snip. A tibial tubercle osteotomy is a useful extensile approach for removing a cemented tibial stem or correcting patella baja, and in cases of severe arthrofibrosis, such as during reimplantation TKA, a medial femoral peel may be required. In rare cases, a traditional V-Y turndown of the quadriceps may be indicated; however, this is now generally reserved for severe quadriceps tendon contracture. The turndown should never be used in a knee with multiple previous surgeries, a history of quadriceps fibrosis, or a previous infection (for example, during reimplantation).[40] A fibrotic extensor mechanism may fail at the closure of the V-Y turndown, and quadriceps necrosis has been reported after this exposure. Additionally, postoperative extension lag is frequently a result even in patients in whom an initially contracted extensor mechanism required lengthening to achieve adequate range of motion.

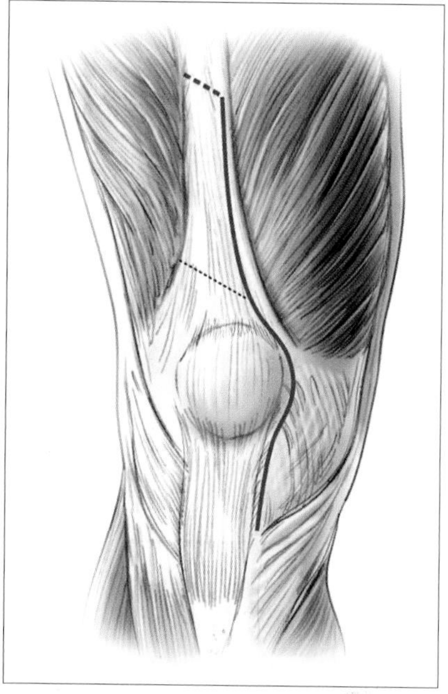

Figure 1 Illustration showing a medial parapatellar arthrotomy (blue solid line) and quadriceps snip modification (blue dashed line). It is important to keep the longitudinal incision in the tendon and to extend it proximally to the top of the tendon before creating an oblique incision (quadriceps snip) at the proximal extent of the tendon. A transverse or oblique incision across the quadriceps tendon closer to the patella (black dashed line) must be avoided because this may be associated with postoperative extensor mechanism disruption. (Reproduced with permission from Nelson CL, Kim J, Lotke PA: Stiffness after total knee arthroplasty: Surgical technique. *J Bone Joint Surg Am* 2005;87 [suppl 1]:264-270.)

Component Removal

Once adequate exposure has been obtained, the bone-cement or bone-implant interfaces of all three components should be fully exposed with a needle-nose rongeur. The components should be evaluated for loosening, malposition, or impingement. The determination of which components to revise depends on these findings and the preoperative diagnosis. The components can be removed with

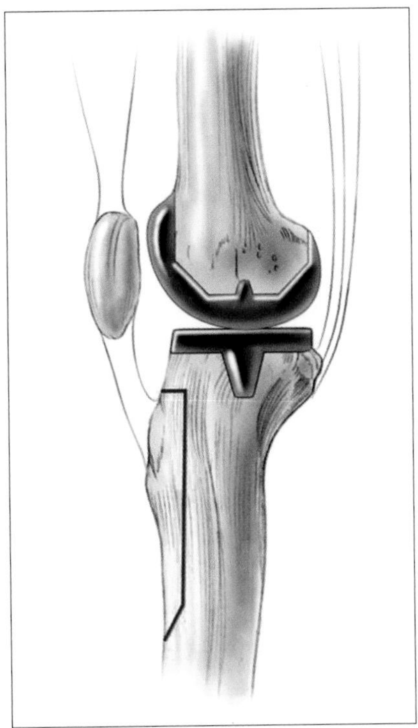

Figure 2 Illustration showing a tibial tubercle osteotomy site from the lateral view, emphasizing the transverse nature of the proximal extent of the osteotomy and the oblique nature of the distal extent of the osteotomy. (Reproduced with permission from Nelson CL, Kim J, Lotke PA: Stiffness after total knee arthroplasty: Surgical technique. *J Bone Joint Surg Am* 2005;87 [suppl 1]:264-270.)

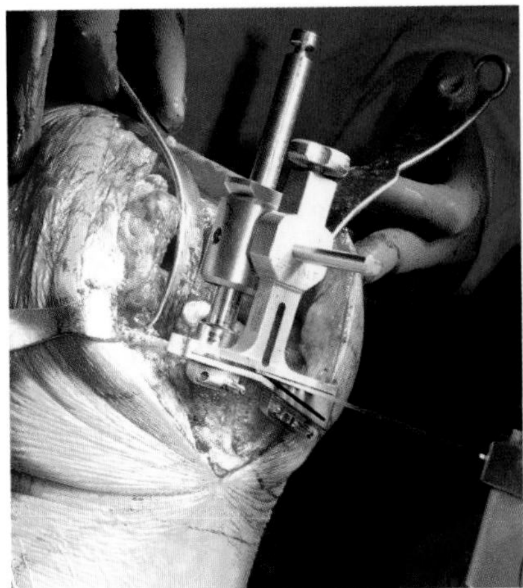

Figure 3 A trial tibial stem can be used to hold the tibial cutting block. A minimal tibial resection that still provides a stable platform on which to rest the tibial component should be performed. The use of a 0° cutting block allows unlimited positioning of the saw capture without affecting the tibial cut.

osteotomes, a Gigli saw, or a small oscillating saw. A thin, narrow blade should be used for precise steering and to minimize inadvertent soft-tissue damage.

The interface beneath the tibial tray is disrupted with use of the saw from the medial and anterior sides. A small, thin osteotome is then used to reach the far lateral side; placing the knee in extension can also improve access. Extensive damage to the bone may occur if the interface between the implant and the host bone is not fully developed. Even if the components appear grossly loose radiographically, the soft-tissue attachments and fibrous tissue must be released from the implant before implant removal. The area between the tibial tray and the proximal tibial tubercle often contains fibrotic tissue. It should be exposed and débrided with a curved osteotome or cautery. In the case of a nonstemmed total knee prosthesis, a slap hammer or stepped impactor can then be used to remove the tibial tray. Osteotomes should not be used to lever the implant off the tibia, as even a relatively loose tibial component may be stronger than the surrounding osteoporotic bone, leading to a tibial fracture or unnecessary bone damage. If there is a cemented stem, a tibial tubercle osteotomy, as described previously, can be performed if necessary; however, axial impaction of the tibial tray often allows removal of the stemmed component, leaving the cement mantle behind. Cement removal is then performed; this may require using ultrasonic equipment or specialized osteotomes.

The femoral component is treated in a similar fashion. The interface is disrupted with a small oscillating saw. A slap hammer can be placed distally, or a stepped impactor can be placed on the anterior flange, but it must be driven in a collinear manner to avoid a flexion moment and condylar fracture. A Gigli saw is quite popular for removing components; however, caution must be used because the saw will generally follow the path of least resistance and can often inadvertently remove excessive portions of bone from the anterior aspect of the femur. After the femoral component is removed, additional soft tissue along the posterior aspect of the tibia can be released to allow further anterior tibial subluxation.

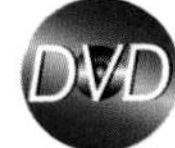

Video 23.1: Revision Total Knee Arthroplasty With Flexion Instability: Component Removal. David G. Lewallen, MD (7 min)

Should a long, well-fixed cemented stem be present on the femoral or tibial side, windows can be created in the tibial or femoral diaphysis to assist with dislodging the implant. Rarely, a metal cutting tool, such as a high-speed diamond wheel, is needed to separate the articular tibial or femoral component from the stem while leaving the stem in place for later removal. Trephines that approximate the size of the stem should be available to assist with stem removal. Subsequent cement removal is done as previously described.

Tibial Reconstruction

Once the components have been successfully removed, surgical reconstruction should begin with the tibia, as the platform created will equally affect both the flexion and the extension gap.[41] A reverse hook and reamers should be used to remove any remaining fibrous membrane from the tibial canal. An intramedullary stem can then be used as a cutting guide if tibial deformity is not severe. Extramedullary guides may be preferred, especially if tibial bowing is excessive. Most systems include revision instrumentation that allows the proximal part of the tibia to be cut with use of a 0° guide (**Figure 3**); this allows the bone resection to be performed independent of the rotational position of the cutting guide. Bone loss may be managed with cement, cancellous allograft, structural cortical allograft, metal wedges and augments, or custom implants.[42] In general, surgical options that minimize the removal of additional bone should be used. The Anderson Orthopaedic Research Institute Bone Defect Classification helps in defining the severity of bone loss intraoperatively. Type 1 is minor femoral or tibial defects with intact metaphyseal bone not compromising the stability of a revision implant. Type 2 is damaged metaphyseal bone requiring femoral or tibial bone reconstruction (with cement, augments, or bone graft); type 2A is involvement of one femoral or tibial condyle, and type 2B is involvement of both condyles. Type 3 is a deficient metaphyseal segment compromising a major portion of either the femoral condyle or the tibial plateau.

Custom implants are now rarely used because of their expense and the inability to modify them intraoperatively. Most patients treated with revision surgery have some degree of cavitary bone loss within the proximal part of the tibia. This defect can generally be filled with cement, if a stemmed tibial implant is used.[43] Impaction bone grafting provides support for the tibial baseplate if a peripheral cortical rim is present and may be preferable in younger patients.[44] Bulk allograft or metal augments should be considered when larger structural defects are present. Bulk allograft can be used if a segmental defect is present that involves a large portion of the tibial plateau,[45] whereas metal augmentation has gained popularity as a result of its ease of insertion, lack of resorption, and ability to be easily customized intraoperatively.[46] In general, the metal augment has become the workhorse of revision knee arthroplasty. A tumor prosthesis is generally reserved for severe bone loss in elderly, low-demand patients.

A stem extension can be used during both the tibial and the femoral reconstruction. Stem extensions transfer stress from the deficient proximal part of the tibia more distally to the intact diaphyseal bone.[47] These extensions also provide additional surface area for fixation and can assist with component orientation. The optimal length of a tibial or femoral stem extension remains controversial. In general, uncemented stems should engage diaphyseal bone and should bypass any metaphyseal-diaphyseal defects. Stems can be fully cemented, or a hybrid fixation technique can be used, whereby the tibial baseplate and the metaphyseal region are cemented and the stem extension is press-fit into the canal.[48] Undersized uncemented diaphyseal stems and metaphyseal engaging stems have a higher rate of loosening and should be avoided.[49] The main advantage of uncemented stems is easier removal in the future. The disadvantages of uncemented stems include the difficulty of their use in deformed tibial bone, occasional malalignment if excessive tibial bowing is present, the potential for pain at the stem tip, and their inability to fully offload the tibial plateau. Cemented stems allow improved surface area for cement interdigitation, but they are much more difficult to remove. Although cemented stems do not assist with alignment because they do not fill the medullary canal, they can permit the use of an extramedullary cutting guide and a "perfect" proximal tibial cut without concern for the ability to seat an uncemented canal-filling stem in the presence of tibial bowing. Offset stem extensions offer the additional advantage of improved tibial coverage but are generally needed only if an uncemented stem is used. An offset tibial stem allows the implant to be placed anteriorly and laterally in relationship to the tibial canal. The optimal tibial component design is dependent on the degree of bone loss and associated ligamentous stability. Full block augments allow easier reconstruction of tibial defects than is possible with hemiblocks or wedges and may be preferred unless their use results in excessive bone resection. After reconstruction of the tibial side, the joint line should be within the midrange of polyethylene inserts available, and the final position is based on gap balancing and the femoral reconstruction.

Femoral Reconstruction

Femoral reconstruction begins once secure tibial fixation has been established. The surgeon should start with a thorough posterior capsular release before treating any osseous defects. Tight posterior capsular structures result in an apparently loose flexion gap and a tight extension gap; the removal of more distal femoral bone, which is usually the method for correcting this problem, can lead to inadvertent elevation of the joint line. Most femoral revisions require the use of a femoral stem extension. The degree of component valgus is generally between 5° and 6°. The femoral stem extension can be used to determine the coronal orientation. Most femoral revisions require augmentation of the distal part of the femur to lower the joint line.[50] Many revisions also require the use of a posterolateral augment to avoid inadvertent internal rotation of the femoral component. The transepicondylar axis remains a useful landmark to ensure appropriate component rotation. Additionally, more anterolateral than anteromedial bone should be exposed if femoral rotation is appropriate, although bone loss in this area often makes this guideline impossible to use. Severe femoral bone loss can be treated with bulk structural allografts or the use of metal augmentation. Although allografts have been used successfully in the past, metal augmentation is now common because of its relative ease of use and the avoidance of graft resorption. Type 3 femoral defects are typically associated with damaged or absent collateral ligaments, necessitating the use of a hinged component.

Undersizing of the femoral component, which is the tendency when there is femoral bone loss, should be avoided. Using an undersized femoral component will result in a larger flexion gap and poor posterior femoral offset, leading to flexion instability and limited range of motion. Once appropriate bone preparation has been completed, the long stem can be converted to a shorter, thicker stem. An offset stem can be used on the femur to not only improve coverage of the distal part of the femur but also allow adjustment of the implant posteriorly, which improves stability in flexion, or laterally, which improves patellar tracking. If a total hip prosthesis is present on the ipsilateral side, a femoral stem that allows a minimum of three cortical diameters between implants should be used to avoid creating a stress riser and the potential for an interprosthetic fracture.

The joint line should be re-created as close to the anatomic state as possible to optimize knee kinematics and stability.[51] The landmarks frequently used to assess the joint line may be absent during revision surgery because of bone loss and soft-tissue damage. Landmarks from which to choose include the previous meniscal scar, the fibular head (1 cm above), the inferior pole of the patella (1 cm below), and the medial femoral epicondyle (25 to 32 mm below). The contralateral extremity should be examined because the height above the fibular head may be variable, and the height of the patella may be altered by patella baja. The flexion gap generally opens more than the extension gap with a revision TKA; therefore, slight elevation of the joint line may be required to appropriately balance the flexion and extension gaps. Although restoration of the joint line is desirable, its importance is trumped by the need to balance the flexion and extension gaps because there is a limit to how large an implant can be reasonably used to tighten the gap in flexion.

Patellar Reconstruction

The patellar component should be exposed and assessed during all knee revision surgeries. The patellar component should be retained if it is well fixed, well positioned, and reasonably compatible with the revision femoral component. Removal of a well-fixed implant may result in bone loss and thereby preclude resurfacing and/or may result in subsequent patellar fracture. If the implant is loose, is incompatible with the femoral component, or shows severe wear, it should be removed. A sagittal saw is used to remove the articular portion of the implant, and a high-speed burr is used to remove the posts and cement. In some situations, the patellar remnant is less than 10 mm thick and will not accept an implant. A patelloplasty may be performed, or a so-called gull-wing osteotomy can be undertaken.[52]

Stability Assessment

Once the trial femoral and tibial components have been inserted, the knee is brought through a range of motion and its stability is assessed. The knee must have full extension, and the patella must track centrally throughout the range of motion. The stability of the knee should be assessed in full extension, midrange flexion, and deep flexion. Obtaining stability in both the coronal and sagittal planes is crucial, but most instability patterns can be treated without the need for excessive constraint. A higher tibial post is generally sufficient in situations of unidirectional instability or a slight flexion-extension mismatch. The least constrained insert possible should be used to avoid increased stresses on the cement mantle. Longer stem extensions should be considered as the degree of constraint increases. A more constrained, hinge-type implant is reserved for patients with a marked flexion-extension mismatch, global instability caused by collateral ligament insufficiency, or uncontrolled recurvatum.[53]

Component Insertion

The technique of component insertion depends on the mode of stem fixation. If a fully cemented stem is chosen, a canal restrictor should be used to allow cement pressurization and limit distal extravasation. Cement should be applied to the undersurface of the tibial and femoral components as well as along the metaphyseal regions of the bone; small holes should be made in sclerotic cortical bone to improve cement interdigitation and fixation. It is crucial to examine the rotation of the tibial component during insertion because inadvertent internal rotation is common.

Management of Infection at the Site of a TKA

Treating an infection at the site of a TKA is most easily understood when using the classification described by Segawa et al.[54] This system describes four different clinical presentations of prosthesis-related infections.

Positive Intraoperative Cultures

Patients with positive intraoperative cultures include those in whom the cause of failure was believed to be aseptic but two or more of the intraoperative cultures are positive. Recent work has verified that a single positive culture does not necessarily indicate a need for treatment.[55] It is advisable to have an infectious disease specialist review such cases and help make the decision about whether further treatment is appropriate. Because of the potential for this scenario, the routine use of antibiotic-loaded cement is recommended for all revision TKAs. Recent work has shown a decreased risk of subsequent infection if antibiotic-impregnated cement is used.[56] Furthermore, prophylactic antibiotic therapy should be continued for 3 days postoperatively or until the final culture results are known.

Acute Postoperative Infections

The treatment of an acute postoperative infection (a deep joint infection identified within the first 4 to 6 weeks after the arthroplasty) has become more controversial. The most commonly accepted treatment includes surgical débridement and exchange of the polyethylene liner, followed by 6 weeks of intravenous antibiotics and, at most centers, an additional course of oral antibiotics.[57] However, recent studies have shown that the rate of success of this regimen, particularly in patients who are infected with resistant and/or biofilm-producing organisms (such as *Staphylococcus*), is less than 20%.[58] On the basis of these reports, patients should be counseled regarding the success of this approach, and serious consideration should be given to component removal if the infecting organism is *Staphylococcus* and is resistant to methicillin.

Late Chronic Infections

In North America, late chronic infections are most commonly treated with a two-stage exchange protocol. This is based on the results of multiple studies that showed a cure rate of approximately 90%.[59-61] Attempts at débridement with retention of the components are associated with an unacceptable rate of failure, and this approach should not be used.[62] The first stage of the two-stage exchange protocol includes the removal of all prosthetic components, all associated cement, and all infected-appearing tissues, followed by insertion of an antibiotic-loaded spacer that contains a minimum of 4 g of antibiotics per 40 g of bone cement (although the use of higher concentrations has been reported).[63,64] The medullary canals of the femur and tibia should be opened, débrided, and lavaged, and intramedullary dowels of antibiotic-loaded cement should be inserted. The most commonly used antibiotics in the cement spacer are a combination of vancomycin and an aminoglycoside, as the combination of the two improves overall elution.[65]

The spacer can be either static or articulating, and there is controversy concerning which approach is best. Studies suggest that the cure rates for the two are similar; however, a static spacer may be associated with more bone loss between stages, whereas an articulating spacer may allow limited weight bearing and joint motion, resulting in a greater final range of motion and higher knee scores.[66] Regardless of the type of spacer used, the cement should extend into the metaphysis, and antibiotic-loaded dowels should be placed into the medullary canals (**Figure 4**).

Following removal of the implants, the patient is treated with a 6-week course of organism-specific antibiotics. The erythrocyte sedimentation rate and C-reactive protein level are used to monitor treatment response. Although these values typically decrease with successful treatment, they often do not return to normal even after the infection has been eradicated; they are not as reliable in identifying persistent infection as they are as an initial screening test, as outlined previously.[67] The knee is then aspirated, and the aspirate is sent for a cell count and culture at a minimum of 2 weeks following cessation of the antibiotic therapy, although there is controversy regarding the value of cultures in this setting.[68,69] If all data indicate that the infection has been eradicated, it is appropriate to proceed with reimplantation. Otherwise, a repeat débridement should be

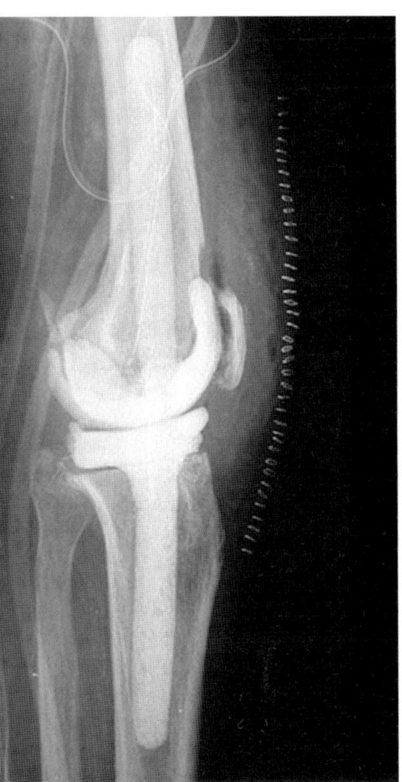

Figure 4 Postoperative lateral radiograph showing an all-cement articulating spacer constructed from plastic molds. Note the antibiotic-loaded cement dowels in the femur and tibia. The tibial dowel is incorporated into the tibial component to prevent it from dislodging.

performed. At the time of surgery, specimens should be obtained for frozen-section analysis. Further débridement and lavage is performed, followed by the insertion of components with the use of standard-dose premixed antibiotic-impregnated cement. Intravenous administration of the antibiotics is once again continued postoperatively until negative results are obtained for all cultures. Antibiotic therapy may then be discontinued, although many surgeons prescribe oral antibiotics for an extended period of time (often for life).

Acute Hematogenous Infections

A patient is considered to have an acute hematogenous infection when a bacteremic event occurs at the site of a TKA that had previously been functioning well. Patients typically present with fever, acute severe pain, and the inability to bear weight on the extremity. Although only limited data on this subject are available, with most reports describing relatively small series of patients,[70,71] it seems that many of these infections are associated with sensitive microorganisms; therefore, the recommended treatment is surgical débridement, modular polyethylene liner exchange, and component retention, followed by a 6-week course of intravenous antibiotics (and potentially additional oral antibiotic treatment), particularly if the duration of symptoms has been short.[72] In practice, however, it is often difficult to determine exactly when the knee became infected, leading to an unclear distinction between an acute hematogenous and a late chronic infection. Failure is often associated with infection with a resistant staphylococcal organism, similar to the situation with early postoperative infection, and should be treated with a two-stage exchange.

Summary

The management of a failed TKA can seem quite challenging to the general orthopaedic surgeon, but with a systematic evaluation that includes a thorough history and physical examination, radiographs, and appropriate serologic testing, the etiology of the failure can be identified in most cases. Infection must always be considered and ruled out. The etiology of failure then dictates the appropriate surgical intervention. Useful adjuncts to the standard surgical exposure for TKA include a copious posteromedial release, the quadriceps snip, the tibial tubercle osteotomy, and the medial femoral peel. Care must be taken to minimize bone loss during component removal. Modular metal augments have proved to be very useful in the management of bone defects, and constraint should be minimized to the least amount necessary for a stable outcome. Finally, with the ever-increasing prevalence of drug-resistant organisms, strong consideration should always be given to a two-stage revision in the management of infection at the site of a THA.

References

1. Ranawat CS, Flynn WF Jr, Saddler S, Hansraj KK, Maynard MJ: Long-term results of the total condylar knee arthroplasty: A 15-year survivorship study. *Clin Orthop Relat Res* 1993;286:94-102.
2. Ritter MA, Berend ME, Meding JB, Keating EM, Faris PM, Crites BM: Long-term followup of anatomic graduated components posterior cruciate-retaining total knee replacement. *Clin Orthop Relat Res* 2001;388:51-57.
3. Mont MA, Serna FK, Krackow KA, Hungerford DS: Exploration of radiographically normal total knee replacements for unexplained pain. *Clin Orthop Relat Res* 1996;331:216-220.
4. Fehring TK, Odum S, Griffin WL, Mason JB, Nadaud M: Early failures in total knee arthroplasty. *Clin Orthop Relat Res* 2001; 392:315-318.
5. Mulhall KJ, Ghomrawi HM, Scully S, Callaghan JJ, Saleh KJ: Current etiologies and modes of failure in total knee arthroplasty revision. *Clin Orthop Relat Res* 2006;446:45-50.
6. Sharkey PF, Hozack WJ, Rothman RH, Shastri S, Jacoby SM: Why are total knee arthroplasties failing today? *Clin Orthop Relat Res* 2002;404:7-13.
7. Pagnano MW, Hanssen AD, Lewallen DG, Stuart MJ: Flexion instability after primary posterior cruciate retaining total knee arthroplasty. *Clin Orthop Relat Res* 1998;356:39-46.
8. Schwab JH, Haidukewych GJ, Hanssen AD, Jacofsky DJ, Pagnano MW: Flexion instability without dislocation after posterior stabilized total knees. *Clin Orthop Relat Res* 2005;440:96-100.
9. Clarke HD, Fuchs R, Scuderi GR, Mills EL, Scott WN, Insall JN: The influence of femoral component design in the elimination of patellar clunk in posterior-stabilized total knee arthroplasty. *J Arthroplasty* 2006;21(2): 167-171.
10. Meding JB, Keating EM, Ritter MA, Faris PM, Berend ME, Malinzak RA: The planovalgus foot: A harbinger of failure of posterior cruciate-retaining total knee replacement. *J Bone Joint Surg Am* 2005;87(Suppl 2):59-62.
11. Vessely MB, Frick MA, Oakes D, Wenger DE, Berry DJ: Magnetic resonance imaging with metal suppression for evaluation of periprosthetic osteolysis after total knee arthroplasty. *J Arthroplasty* 2006;21(6):826-831.
12. Berger RA, Crossett LS, Jacobs JJ, Rubash HE: Malrotation causing patellofemoral complications after

total knee arthroplasty. *Clin Orthop Relat Res* 1998;356:144-153.

13. Romero J, Stähelin T, Binkert C, Pfirrmann C, Hodler J, Kessler O: The clinical consequences of flexion gap asymmetry in total knee arthroplasty. *J Arthroplasty* 2007; 22(2):235-240.
14. Hofmann AA, Wyatt RW, Daniels AU, Armstrong L, Alazraki N, Taylor A Jr: Bone scans after total knee arthroplasty in asymptomatic patients: Cemented versus cementless. *Clin Orthop Relat Res* 1990;251:183-188.
15. Joseph TN, Mujtaba M, Chen AL, et al: Efficacy of combined technetium-99m sulfur colloid/indium-111 leukocyte scans to detect infected total hip and knee arthroplasties. *J Arthroplasty* 2001;16(6):753-758.
16. Kraemer WJ, Saplys R, Waddell JP, Morton J: Bone scan, gallium scan, and hip aspiration in the diagnosis of infected total hip arthroplasty. *J Arthroplasty* 1993; 8(6):611-616.
17. Scher DM, Pak K, Lonner JH, Finkel JE, Zuckerman JD, Di Cesare PE: The predictive value of indium-111 leukocyte scans in the diagnosis of infected total hip, knee, or resection arthroplasties. *J Arthroplasty* 2000;15(3): 295-300.
18. Schinsky MF, Della Valle CJ, Sporer SM, Paprosky WG: Perioperative testing for joint infection in patients undergoing revision total hip arthroplasty. *J Bone Joint Surg Am* 2008;90(9):1869-1875.
19. Lachiewicz PF, Rogers GD, Thomason HC: Aspiration of the hip joint before revision total hip arthroplasty: Clinical and laboratory factors influencing attainment of a positive culture. *J Bone Joint Surg Am* 1996;78(5): 749-754.
20. Barrack RL, Jennings RW, Wolfe MW, Bertot AJ: The value of preoperative aspiration before total knee revision. *Clin Orthop Relat Res* 1997;345:8-16.
21. Mason JB, Fehring TK, Odum SM, Griffin WL, Nussman DS: The value of white blood cell counts before revision total knee arthroplasty. *J Arthroplasty* 2003; 18(8):1038-1043.
22. Della Valle CJ, Sporer SM, Jacobs JJ, Berger RA, Rosenberg AG, Paprosky WG: Preoperative testing for sepsis before revision total knee arthroplasty. *J Arthroplasty* 2007;22(6, Suppl 2):90-93.
23. Ghanem E, Parvizi J, Burnett RS, et al: Cell count and differential of aspirated fluid in the diagnosis of infection at the site of total knee arthroplasty. *J Bone Joint Surg Am* 2008;90(8):1637-1643.
24. Morgan PM, Sharkey P, Ghanem E, et al: The value of intraoperative Gram stain in revision total knee arthroplasty. *J Bone Joint Surg Am* 2009;91(9):2124-2129.
25. Lonner JH, Desai P, Dicesare PE, Steiner G, Zuckerman JD: The reliability of analysis of intraoperative frozen sections for identifying active infection during revision hip or knee arthroplasty. *J Bone Joint Surg Am* 1996; 78(10):1553-1558.
26. Nadaud MC, Fehring TK, Fehring K: Underestimation of osteolysis in posterior stabilized total knee arthroplasty. *J Arthroplasty* 2004;19(1):110-115.
27. Leopold SS, Silverton CD, Barden RM, Rosenberg AG: Isolated revision of the patellar component in total knee arthroplasty. *J Bone Joint Surg Am* 2003;85-A(1): 41-47.
28. Babis GC, Trousdale RT, Pagnano MW, Morrey BF: Poor outcomes of isolated tibial insert exchange and arthrolysis for the management of stiffness following total knee arthroplasty. *J Bone Joint Surg Am* 2001;83-A(10): 1534-1536.
29. Parisien JS: The role of arthroscopy in the treatment of postoperative fibroarthrosis of the knee joint. *Clin Orthop Relat Res* 1988; 229:185-192.
30. Lucas TS, DeLuca PF, Nazarian DG, Bartolozzi AR, Booth RE Jr: Arthroscopic treatment of patellar clunk. *Clin Orthop Relat Res* 1999;367:226-229.
31. Allardyce TJ, Scuderi GR, Insall JN: Arthroscopic treatment of popliteus tendon dysfunction following total knee arthroplasty. *J Arthroplasty* 1997;12(3): 353-355.
32. Barrack RL, Smith P, Munn B, Engh G, Rorabeck C: Comparison of surgical approaches in total knee arthroplasty. *Clin Orthop Relat Res* 1998;356:16-21.
33. Colombel M, Mariz Y, Dahhan P, Kénési C: Arterial and lymphatic supply of the knee integuments. *Surg Radiol Anat* 1998;20(1): 35-40.
34. Aglietti P, Windsor RE, Buzzi R, Insall JN: Arthroplasty for the stiff or ankylosed knee. *J Arthroplasty* 1989;4(1):1-5.
35. Della Valle CJ, Berger RA, Rosenberg AG: Surgical exposures in revision total knee arthroplasty. *Clin Orthop Relat Res* 2006;446: 59-68.
36. Meek RM, Greidanus NV, McGraw RW, Masri BA: The extensile rectus snip exposure in revision of total knee arthroplasty. *J Bone Joint Surg Br* 2003;85(8): 1120-1122.
37. Whiteside LA: Exposure in difficult total knee arthroplasty using tibial tubercle osteotomy. *Clin Orthop Relat Res* 1995;321:32-35.
38. Mendes MW, Caldwell P, Jiranek WA: The results of tibial tubercle osteotomy for revision total knee arthroplasty. *J Arthroplasty* 2004;19(2):167-174.

39. Younger AS, Duncan CP, Masri BA: Surgical exposures in revision total knee arthroplasty. *J Am Acad Orthop Surg* 1998;6(1): 55-64.
40. Scott RD, Siliski JM: The use of a modified V-Y quadricepsplasty during total knee replacement to gain exposure and improve flexion in the ankylosed knee. *Orthopedics* 1985;8(1):45-48.
41. Dennis DA, Berry DJ, Engh G, et al: Revision total knee arthroplasty. *J Am Acad Orthop Surg* 2008;16(8):442-454.
42. Whittaker JP, Dharmarajan R, Toms AD: The management of bone loss in revision total knee replacement. *J Bone Joint Surg Br* 2008;90(8):981-987.
43. Bush JL, Wilson JB, Vail TP: Management of bone loss in revision total knee arthroplasty. *Clin Orthop Relat Res* 2006;452: 186-192.
44. Lonner JH, Lotke PA, Kim J, Nelson C: Impaction grafting and wire mesh for uncontained defects in revision knee arthroplasty. *Clin Orthop Relat Res* 2002;404: 145-151.
45. Engh GA, Ammeen DJ: Use of structural allograft in revision total knee arthroplasty in knees with severe tibial bone loss. *J Bone Joint Surg Am* 2007;89(12):2640-2647.
46. Long WJ, Scuderi GR: Porous tantalum cones for large metaphyseal tibial defects in revision total knee arthroplasty: A minimum 2-year follow-up. *J Arthroplasty* 2009;24(7):1086-1092.
47. Bourne RB, Finlay JB: The influence of tibial component intramedullary stems and implant-cortex contact on the strain distribution of the proximal tibia following total knee arthroplasty: An in vitro study. *Clin Orthop Relat Res* 1986;208:95-99.
48. Peters CL, Erickson J, Kloepper RG, Mohr RA: Revision total knee arthroplasty with modular components inserted with metaphyseal cement and stems without cement. *J Arthroplasty* 2005;20(3): 302-308.
49. Fehring TK, Odum S, Olekson C, Griffin WL, Mason JB, McCoy TH: Stem fixation in revision total knee arthroplasty: A comparative analysis. *Clin Orthop Relat Res* 2003;416:217-224.
50. Mahoney OM, Kinsey TL: Modular femoral offset stems facilitate joint line restoration in revision knee arthroplasty. *Clin Orthop Relat Res* 2006;446:93-98.
51. Porteous AJ, Hassaballa MA, Newman JH: Does the joint line matter in revision total knee replacement? *J Bone Joint Surg Br* 2008;90(7):879-884.
52. Rorabeck CH, Mehin R, Barrack RL: Patellar options in revision total knee arthroplasty. *Clin Orthop Relat Res* 2003;416:84-92.
53. Ries MD, Haas SB, Windsor RE: Soft-tissue balance in revision total knee arthroplasty: Surgical technique. *J Bone Joint Surg Am* 2004;86-A(Suppl 1):81-86.
54. Segawa H, Tsukayama DT, Kyle RF, Becker DA, Gustilo RB: Infection after total knee arthroplasty: A retrospective study of the treatment of eighty-one infections. *J Bone Joint Surg Am* 1999; 81(10):1434-1445.
55. Barrack RL, Aggarwal A, Burnett RS, et al: The fate of the unexpected positive intraoperative cultures after revision total knee arthroplasty. *J Arthroplasty* 2007; 22(6, Suppl 2)94-99.
56. Chiu FY, Lin CF: Antibiotic-impregnated cement in revision total knee arthroplasty: A prospective cohort study of one hundred and eighty-three knees. *J Bone Joint Surg Am* 2009;91(3): 628-633.
57. Moyad TF, Thornhill T, Estok D: Evaluation and management of the infected total hip and knee. *Orthopedics* 2008;31(6):581-590.
58. Bradbury T, Fehring TK, Taunton M, et al: The fate of acute methicillin-resistant Staphylococcus aureus periprosthetic knee infections treated by open debridement and retention of components. *J Arthroplasty* 2009;24 (6, Suppl):101-104.
59. Insall JN, Thompson FM, Brause BD: Two-stage reimplantation for the salvage of infected total knee arthroplasty. *J Bone Joint Surg Am* 1983;65(8): 1087-1098.
60. Goldman RT, Scuderi GR, Insall JN: 2-stage reimplantation for infected total knee replacement. *Clin Orthop Relat Res* 1996; 331:118-124.
61. Mittal Y, Fehring TK, Hanssen A, Marculescu C, Odum SM, Osmon D: Two-stage reimplantation for periprosthetic knee infection involving resistant organisms. *J Bone Joint Surg Am* 2007;89(6): 1227-1231.
62. Chiu FY, Chen CM: Surgical débridement and parenteral antibiotics in infected revision total knee arthroplasty. *Clin Orthop Relat Res* 2007;461:130-135.
63. Jacobs C, Christensen CP, Berend ME: Static and mobile antibiotic-impregnated cement spacers for the management of prosthetic joint infection. *J Am Acad Orthop Surg* 2009;17(6): 356-368.
64. Springer BD, Lee GC, Osmon D, Haidukewych GJ, Hanssen AD, Jacofsky DJ: Systemic safety of high-dose antibiotic-loaded cement spacers after resection of an infected total knee arthroplasty. *Clin Orthop Relat Res* 2004; 427:47-51.
65. Penner MJ, Masri BA, Duncan CP: Elution characteristics of vancomycin and tobramycin combined in acrylic bone-cement.

J Arthroplasty 1996;11(8): 939-944.

66. Freeman MG, Fehring TK, Odum SM, Fehring K, Griffin WL, Mason JB: Functional advantage of articulating versus static spacers in 2-stage revision for total knee arthroplasty infection. *J Arthroplasty* 2007;22(8): 1116-1121.
67. Ghanem E, Azzam K, Seeley M, Joshi A, Parvizi J: Staged revision for knee arthroplasty infection: What is the role of serologic tests before reimplantation? *Clin Orthop Relat Res* 2009;467(7):1699-1705.
68. Lonner JH, Siliski JM, Della Valle C, DiCesare P, Lotke PA: Role of knee aspiration after resection of the infected total knee arthroplasty. *Am J Orthop (Belle Mead NJ)* 2001;30(4):305-309.
69. Mont MA, Waldman BJ, Hungerford DS: Evaluation of preoperative cultures before second-stage reimplantation of a total knee prosthesis complicated by infection: A comparison-group study. *J Bone Joint Surg Am* 2000; 82-A(11):1552-1557.
70. Deirmengian C, Greenbaum J, Stern J, et al: Open debridement of acute gram-positive infections after total knee arthroplasty. *Clin Orthop Relat Res* 2003;416: 129-134.
71. Fulkerson E, Della Valle CJ, Wise B, Walsh M, Preston C, Di Cesare PE: Antibiotic susceptibility of bacteria infecting total joint arthroplasty sites. *J Bone Joint Surg Am* 2006;88(6):1231-1237.
72. Cook JL, Scott RD, Long WJ: Late hematogenous infections after total knee arthroplasty: Experience with 3013 consecutive total knees. *J Knee Surg* 2007; 20(1):27-33.

Video Reference

23.1: Lewallen DG: Video. Excerpt. Revision total knee arthroplasty with flexion instability, in Stiehl J, Ayers DC, eds: *Surgical Techniques in Orthopaedics: Ligament Balancing for Total Knee Arthroplasty.* DVD. Rosemont, IL, American Academy of Orthopaedic Surgeons, 2010.

What Is the State of the Art in Orthopaedic Thromboprophylaxis in Lower Extremity Reconstruction?

Clifford W. Colwell Jr, MD

Abstract

Venous thromboembolic events, including deep venous thromboses and pulmonary embolisms, have a high risk of occurrence in patients treated with lower extremity arthroplasty and hip fracture surgery. Although the prevalence of these complications has been lowered with the use of venous thromboembolic prophylaxis, the current rate is still troublesome because of the possibility of death or the need for lifetime treatment of postthrombotic syndrome and/or pulmonary hypertension. Prophylactic methods currently include mechanical devices and pharmacologic agents. Mechanical devices are difficult to compare because they are not standardized, the devices are often used in multimodal prophylactic regimens, and the devices cannot be used when the patient is ambulating or at home. A new portable compression device allows use during ambulation and can be used by the patient at home. A recent study of this portable device in patients treated with total hip arthroplasty showed an efficacy similar to that of low-molecular-weight heparin, with fewer major bleeding complications. Pharmacologic prophylaxis includes low-molecular-weight heparin, synthetic pentasaccharide, warfarin, and aspirin. All of these agents have different degrees of efficacy and safety. New oral agents for thromboprophylaxis are on the horizon but are not yet approved by the Food and Drug Administration.

Instr Course Lect 2011;60:283-290.

The 1986 Consensus Conference convened by the National Institutes of Health emphasized the unacceptably high rates of venous thromboembolism (VTE), including proximal and distal deep venous thrombosis (DVT), pulmonary embolism (PE), and death in orthopaedic patients treated with lower extremity surgery without prophylaxis.[1] In the more than 25 years since that conference, the interest in the use of prophylaxis has increased, along with the number of total joint arthroplasties, which currently number approximately 1 million per year in the United States.[2] The number of total joint arthroplasties and the number of hip fractures is expected to increase to almost 4 million yearly over the next 20 years as the US population ages.[2]

The argument for thromboprophylaxis for all patients treated with total joint arthroplasty is based on the overall risk in this patient population for VTE, including DVT and PE (**Table 1**).[3] The goals of thromboprophylaxis are to prevent death from PE, proximal and distal DVT, chronic pulmonary hypertension, and the possibility of postthrombosis syndrome in patients with a venous thromboembolic event. Such events may necessitate a lifetime of treatment for these patients. Any patient with VTE is always at higher risk of recurrent VTE with any future surgery.

The ideal prophylactic regimen would be clinically proven as effective, have a low risk of adverse side effects, be practical to use (easy to administer and monitor), and would be cost effective. Currently, no single modality meets all these requirements or is appropriate for every patient. Orthopaedic surgeons have many

Dr. Colwell serves as a paid consultant to or is an employee of Stryker and has received research or institutional support from Stryker and Medical Compression Systems.

Table 1
VTE Prevalence After TKA, THA, and Hip Fracture Surgery Based on Mandatory Venography in Patients Who Received Placebo or No Prophylaxis

Type of Surgery	DVT Prevalence	Proximal DVT Prevalence	PE Prevalence	Fatal PE Prevalence
TKA	41% to 85%	5% to 22%	1.5% to 10%	0.1% to 1.7%
THA	42% to 57%	18% to 36%	0.9% to 28%	0.1% to 2.0%
Hip Fracture	46% to 60%	23% to 30%	3% to 11%	0.3% to 7.5%

VTE = venous thromboembolism, TKA = total knee arthroplasty, THA = total hip arthroplasty, DVT = deep venous thrombosis, PE = pulmonary embolism

prophylactic protocols to choose from, including single and/or additive mechanical and pharmacologic agents with varying time frames of patient exposure. Some clinicians continue to rely on clinical signs and symptoms as the initial presentation of DVT or PE; however, the accuracy of diagnosis based on signs and symptoms is considered to be low.[3,4] Objective testing has determined that many symptomatic patients are negative for venous thrombosis, and asymptomatic patients are often positive for venous thrombosis.

Prophylactic Modalities

Two major types of modalities exist for thromboprophylaxis: mechanical techniques and pharmacologic techniques. Both of these modalities have elicited positive and negative responses from clinicians and patients.

Mechanical Prophylaxis

Mechanical prophylactic methods, including graduated compression stockings, intermittent pneumatic compression of the calf or calf and thigh, and venous foot pumps are reported effective in combination with early ambulation;[5-7] in many protocols, pharmacologic prophylaxis is included while the patient is ambulating or after discharge from the hospital. Compression devices can be applied preoperatively and used during the surgical procedure. These devices have no clinically significant adverse side effects, and bleeding is similar to that experienced with placebo. Until recently, these devices could not be worn by the patient while ambulating or after discharge from the hospital.

Mechanical devices appear to be effective when used properly; however, few data are available for these devices compared with antithrombotic pharmacologic agents. It is difficult to quantify the effectiveness of these devices because of the lack of standardization. The results from a study of one device cannot be applied to another device.[8] Two key concerns of mechanical devices are proper fit and the percentage of time of daily use. Some patients find the devices too warm or uncomfortable to wear, and many devices require a large motorized pump, which can be noisy and cumbersome. Although early ambulation is encouraged, many devices must be disconnected when the patient is ambulating, which makes compliance an issue for both the patient and staff. Shorter hospital stays of 3 to 5 days also present a problem because traditional devices are not designed for use outside the hospital. Home use of VTE prophylaxis is important because VTE is reported to develop an average of 8 days after total knee arthroplasty (TKA) and an average of 21 days after total hip arthroplasty (THA).[9]

The scant data available on graduated compression stockings indicate that they provide little or no protection from DVT. A study evaluating above-knee and below-knee graduated compression stockings found no reduction in DVT rates with either type of stocking compared with a control group that received no form of prophylaxis.[10] In another study, 98% of graduated compression stockings failed to produce the "ideal" pressure gradient from the ankle to the knee.[11]

Of the various types of compression devices available, a portable device has recently been studied.[12] In a multicenter study comparing the mobile compression device (Continuous Enhanced Circulation Therapy plus Synchronized Flow Technology; Medical Compression Systems, Akiva, Israel) with enoxaparin (a low-molecular-weight heparin [LMWH]) after THA, the rate of VTE was similar, but the rate of major bleeding was significantly different (**Table 2**). The mobile compression device was applied preoperatively, and the LMWH was started the morning after surgery. Both treatments were continued for 10 days after surgery, with a duplex ultrasound performed on days 10 through 12 after surgery. Clinical follow-up on patients continued for 3 months.

The portability of the mobile compression device allows use of the device at home. In the hospital, the device can be used when the patient is out of his or her bed without disconnecting the device, which may increase com-

Table 2
Studies of a Mobile Compression Device (the CECT) Showing the Incidence of VTE and Major Bleeding

Authors	Patient Compliance	VTE Incidence With CECT	LMWH	*P*	Major Bleeding
Edwards et al[13]	85%	+ enoxaparin: TKA: VTE = 5/141 (3.5%) THA: VTE = 1/65 (1.5%)	TKA: VTE = 15/77 (9.5%) THA: VTE = 2/59 (3.4%)	0.018 NS	No difference
Gelfer et al[14]	Not reported	TJA: VTE = 4/61 (6.6%)	TJA: VTE = 17/60 (28%)	0.049	Not reported
Froimson et al[15]	83% CECT 49% other non-mobile compression device	TJA: VTE = 3/223 (1.3%)	+ Other compression device TJA: VTE = 55/1,354 (4.3%)	< 0.05	Not reported
Colwell et al[12]	83%	THA: VTE = 10/197 (5.1%)	THA: VTE = 10/192 (5.2%)	NS	CECT 0/199 LMWH 11/196 (5.6%) $P < 0.0007$

CECT = Continuous Enhanced Circulation Therapy system, VTE = venous thromboembolism, LMWH = low-molecular-weight heparin, TKA = total knee arthroplasty, THA = total hip arthroplasty, TJA = total joint arthroplasty, NS = not significant

pliance. The portable pump, which weighs 1.6 lb, is small enough to be worn with a shoulder strap and can run on battery power for 6 hours before recharging. The disposable limb sleeves are placed over the patient's calves in a form-fitting manner and are secured with hook and loop fasteners. The device also contains a sensor (synchronized flow technology) that monitors respiratory-related venous phasic flow and times the compression during the expiratory phase when the thoracic pressure is low and filling of the right side of the heart is maximal. The compliance rate during the 10-day usage period was 83%, or 20 hours per day.[12] Other studies have shown that in patients with total joint arthroplasty treated with this mobile device, the incidence of DVT ranged from 1.3% to 8%, whereas DVT in those treated with enoxaparin ranged from 3.6% to 23% (**Table 2**).[13-15]

Pharmacologic Prophylaxis

Pharmacologic methods of prophylaxis include LMWH, synthetic pentasaccharide, vitamin K antagonists, unfractionated heparin, and aspirin. Worldwide, LMWH is the most commonly used category of drug for VTE prophylaxis. The LMWHs are administered subcutaneously in different doses with different timing depending on the particular drug; they do not require laboratory monitoring or dose adjustment. Extensive data have shown that this category of drugs is safe and effective, although concerns exist about related bleeding. Fondaparinux, a subcutaneously administered synthetic pentasaccharide, is also used for prophylaxis. Although the pentasaccharide provides excellent prophylaxis for VTE, many surgeons are concerned with the risk of increased bleeding. Warfarin, a vitamin K antagonist, is administered orally. The dosage of warfarin is adjusted by checking the prothrombin time using the international normalized ratio. Aspirin is prescribed in varying dosages and is often used as part of a multimodal prophylactic approach with mechanical devices. Low-dose unfractionated heparin or aspirin prophylaxis has been shown to be more effective than no prophylaxis in meta-analyses, but both agents are less effective than other prophylactic regimens in high-risk patients treated with total joint arthroplasty.[3] Unwanted bleeding is a potential adverse side effect of each drug. **Table 3** provides information on the efficacy and bleeding events reported with each of these agents.[5,16-25]

Low-Molecular-Weight Heparin

LMWH consists of fragments of unfractionated heparin produced by either chemical or enzymatic depolymerization. The shorter chains in LMWH bind less to proteins and endothelial cells, resulting in a more predictable dose response, a dose-independent mechanism of clearance, and a longer plasma half-life. LMWH has highly predictable pharmacokinetic properties and high bioavailability with a half-life of 4.5 hours. The effects of LMWH can be reversed by protamine sulfate, but no laboratory monitoring or dose adjustment is necessary. There is a small risk of heparin-induced thrombocytopenia (an immunologic response to heparin).

Pentasaccharide

Fondaparinux, a synthetic pentasaccharide, provides anticoagulation through inhibition of factor Xa. Effective prophylaxis can be achieved

Table 3
The Incidence of VTE and Bleeding That Occurs in TKA, THA, and Hip Fracture Surgery With Pharmacologic Prophylaxis

Data From	Surgery Type	Agent	Total DVT	Proximal DVT	PE	Bleeding
Brookenthal et al[16]	TKA	LMWH	31.7% (568/1,793)	6.2% (88/1,422)	0.2% (4/1,805)	2.4% (43/1,765)
Bauer et al[18]	TKA	Pentasaccharide	12.4% (45/361)	2.4% (9/368)	0.2% (1/517)	1.9% (10/517)
Mismetti et al[24]	TKA	Vitamin K antagonist	37.2% (148/298)	8.8% (35/398)	0.2% (1/398)	1.3% (5/398)
Westrich et al[5] Geerts et al[25]	TKA	Aspirin	53% (1,701/3,214)	8.9% (39/443)	1.3% (23/1,800)	Not available
Freedman et al[17]	THA	LMWH	16.6% (918/5,512)	6.2% (342/5,512)	0.36% (19/5,238)	2.2% (120/5,412)
Turpie et al[19] Lassen et al[20]	THA	Pentasaccharide	4.1% (80/1,962)	1.1% (20/1,738)	0.3% (7/2,555)	2.9% (67/2,268)
Freedman et al[17]	THA	Vitamin K antagonist	21.6% (590/2,731)	5.4%(149/2,731)	0.16% (2/1,232)	1.7% (23/1,381)
Freedman et al[17]	THA	Aspirin	31.1% (214/687)	11.9% (82/687)	1.3% (8/625)	0.7% (5/687)
Eriksson et al[21]	Hip fracture	LMWH	19.1% (117/623)	4.3% (28/646)	0.3% (3/840)	2.2% (19/842)
Eriksson et al[21]	Hip fracture	Pentasaccharide	7.9% (49/624)	0.9% (6/650)	0.4% (3/831)	2.2% (18/831)
Mismetti et al[24]	Hip fracture	Vitamin K antagonist	22.2% (93/418)	12.6% (13/103)	1.2% (3/240)	5.7% (14/244)
Powers et al[22] Gent et al[23]	Hip fracture	Aspirin	43% (66/153)	12.6% (19/150)	1.0% (2/192)	2.6% (5/192)

VTE = venous thromboembolism, TKA = total knee arthroplasty, THA = total hip arthroplasty, DVT = deep venous thrombosis, PE = pulmonary embolism, LMWH = low-molecular-weight heparin

with once-daily dosing for total joint arthroplasty and hip fracture surgery, with no laboratory monitoring or dose adjustment. Pentasaccharide is administered subcutaneously and has a half-life of 18 hours with no known antidote.

Vitamin K Antagonist

Adjusted-dose warfarin sodium is the most common vitamin K antagonist and is used for prophylactic protocols by approximately 50% of orthopaedic surgeons in North America. Warfarin oral anticoagulation should be administered in a dose sufficient to prolong the international normalized ratio to a target of 2.5 (range 2 to 3). Adjusted-dose warfarin has the potential advantage of allowing continued prophylaxis after hospital discharge, provided that there is supporting infrastructure available to continue home therapy effectively and safely. The half-life of warfarin is 36 to 42 hours and can be reversed with the administration of vitamin K. Even with early initiation of warfarin therapy, the international normalized ratio does not usually reach the target range until the third postoperative day. Many factors interact with warfarin, including medications, smoking, alcohol, foods, and changes in activity. Patients discharged with warfarin prophylaxis must be aware of these interactions and monitor themselves for any symptoms of overanticoagulation.

Unfractionated Heparin

Unfractionated heparin is seldom used for prophylaxis because of the need for continued dosing adjustments and the adverse side effect of bleeding. Unfractionated heparin has been used intraoperatively with success as part of a multimodal prophylactic regimen.[26]

Aspirin

Aspirin (acetylsalicylic acid) is a nonsteroidal anti-inflammatory agent used to inhibit platelet aggregation and vasoconstriction and is effective as an antithrombotic agent in heart disease and arterial thrombosis. However, the clots that form on the venous circulatory side are seldom platelet based but rather are formed from clotting proteins and erythrocytes, which are not affected by aspirin alone. A study comparing aspirin with aspirin and a mechanical device in TKA showed that aspirin alone was less effective (67% DVT) than aspirin and a mechanical device (27% DVT).[27] The Pulmonary Embolism Prevention Trial, a major study of aspirin prophylaxis, compared the efficacy of 160 mg of aspirin with a placebo for symptomatic VTE in 17,444 patients worldwide treated for hip fractures or with elective arthroplasties.[28] Because the trial allowed the use of other anticoagulants in many of the patients, the reported reduction of VTE disease from 2.3% with placebo to 1.6% with aspirin is questionable. Aspirin is often used in a multimodal prophylactic regimen along with mechanical devices.

New Oral Agents

Three new oral anticoagulant drugs are in clinical trials with Food and Drug Administration oversight before possible approval. Included are two factor Xa inhibitory drugs, Apixaban (Bristol-Myers Squibb, New York, NY) and Rivaroxaban (Bayer HealthCare, Wuppertal, Germany), and Dabigatran (Boehringer Ingleheim, Ridgefield, CT), an oral direct thrombin inhibitor. Potential advantages of these drugs are oral administration, no needed monitoring of blood levels, and no dosing adjustments. Trials of these medications in patients treated with total joint arthroplasty have been reported in the literature.[29-34]

Other Considerations

Inferior Vena Cava Filters

Inferior vena cava filters may be used in patients with an increased risk of bleeding or a prior history of VTE disease to minimize bleeding and PE events after total joint arthroplasty. Both permanent and retrievable inferior vena cava filters are available. Substantially more data are available on permanent filters, with reports on patients at follow-up periods up to 8 years. Follow-up data on retrievable filters are mostly short term and involve only a small number of patients.[35] These filters are not always retrievable, with reports of successful recovery ranging from 77% to 98%.[36] Retrievable filters were originally intended to be removed after 14 days, but reports are available of retrieval of filters up to 100 days after placement. Although complications for both permanent and retrievable filters are reported to be minor, there have been case reports of filter fracture or migration with serious complications.[35,36]

In a retrospective examination of a cohort of 95 patients treated with total joint arthroplasty who received inferior vena cava filters either preoperatively or perioperatively, two recurrent nonfatal PE events were reported.[37] Although 11 patients died, no deaths were related to VTE or inferior vena cava filter failures. At a minimum 2-year follow-up, 15 patients reported a persistent and painful swollen lower extremity, and 5 patients had new or extension of existing DVT. In another retrospective study that evaluated 58 orthopaedic patients who were treated with retrievable inferior vena cava filters, no patient had a PE, and 64% of the filters were removed without complications.[38] The remaining filters were retained for ongoing prevention of PE (20%), for clots on the filter (8%), and for incorporation of the filter into the vena cava (8%). Few complications have been reported with inferior vena cava filters, although one study reported a 36% recurrence of DVT in nonfilter-treated patients at 8-year follow-up but no increase in mortality.[39]

Surgery and Anesthesia

A decrease in VTE has been reported with regional anesthesia;[40,41] however, regional anesthesia does not decrease the rate of VTE disease sufficiently to be used as the only method of prophylaxis. Combined with other methods, such as pharmacologic or mechanical prophylaxis, regional anesthesia can further decrease the rate of VTE.[42] Some surgeons believe that decreased surgical time also reduces the incidence of VTE disease. Theoretically, this belief makes sense, although no studies have reported reduced rates of VTE with shorter surgical times.

Genetic and Clotting Factors

Genetic factors, including mutations of factor V Leiden and prothrombin gene *G20210A*, have been reported to increase the risk of VTE in the general population.[43] A study of patients treated with TKA or THA indicated that the prothrombin gene mutation, *G20210A*, was significantly represented in groups of patients with symptomatic VTE (P = 0.0002). A tendency toward an increased risk of VTE was found with factor V Leiden mutation (P = 0.09).[43] General preoperative genotype screening is of questionable value because 90% of the general population who have these genetic risk factors have not developed VTE disease.

Clotting factors associated with VTE disease are increased levels of factor VIII and fibronectin.[44,45] Also implicated is a low level of high-density lipoprotein.[46] These factors have not been examined in relationship to orthopaedic surgery patients and VTE.

A relationship between two genetic variants of the enzyme that metabolizes warfarin, cytochrome P-450 2C9 (CYP2C9) and vitamin K epoxide reductase (VKORC1), has been reported to be responsible for patient differences in the response to warfarin dosages.[47] In a study of 92 TKA and THA patients,[48] a proposed algorithm for warfarin dosing after orthopaedic surgery considered genetic types, clinical variables, current medications, and preoperative and postoperative laboratory values. If this algorithm is validated, a safer, more effective process for initiating warfarin therapy may be provided. Individual patients at the extremes of dosing requirements are more likely to benefit from genotype anticoagulant therapy than the entire patient population.[49]

Guidelines

The strength of any guideline depends on the risk-benefit ratio of the prophylaxis and the strength of the methodology leading to the estimated prophylactic effect. Thromboprophylaxis guidelines are available to assist in practicing evidence-based medicine.

The American College of Chest Physicians released the eighth edition of their antithrombotic and thrombotic therapy guidelines in 2008.[3] These guidelines are based on current literature that reports on the effectiveness and safety of various types of thromboprophylaxis in preventing VTE. The American Academy of Orthopaedic Surgeons released a guideline in 2007 for the prevention of symptomatic and fatal PE in patients treated with total joint arthroplasty.[50] Because most studies with symptomatic PE as the end point were underpowered to evaluate the benefit of prophylaxis, these recommendations allow for multiple as well as additive protocols. The evidence available regarding the prevention of PE does not indicate that any one protocol is more or less effective. More information on both of these guidelines is available in chapter 26.

In the United States, the prevention of thrombosis after total joint arthroplasty has been mandated by several regulatory agencies, including the Surgical Care Improvement Project, the National Quality Forum, and The Joint Commission. The Surgical Care Improvement Project recommends VTE prophylaxis for every surgery patient, and prophylaxis should be started within 24 hours of surgery or hospital admission.[51] More information on the Surgical Care Improvement Project guidelines is available in chapter 26. In 2008, the National Quality Forum released six measures to prevent VTE disease directed at all hospital patients, not just surgery patients. The measures include appropriately documenting the risk of VTE, documenting prescribed and received VTE prophylaxis, and providing instructions on VTE to patients at hospital discharge.[52] In late 2009, The Joint Commission approved six VTE core measures available for data collection and reporting. These measures include (1) VTE prophylaxis, (2) intensive care unit VTE prophylaxis, (3) VTE patients with anticoagulation overlap therapy, (4) VTE patients receiving unfractionated heparin with dosages and platelet count monitoring by protocol or nomogram, (5) VTE discharge instructions, and (6) the incidence of potentially preventable VTE.[53]

Summary

Overall, the risks of VTE disease have decreased significantly for patients treated with orthopaedic lower extremity reconstruction since the 1986 Consensus Conference by the National Institutes of Health because of a multitude of factors. The lower rates of VTE achieved with many varying prophylactic protocols, both mechanical and pharmacologic, have made it difficult to judge improvements made by changes in protocols and the introduction of new prophylactic agents.

References

1. Prevention of venous thrombosis and pulmonary embolism: NIH Consensus Development. *JAMA* 1986;256(6):744-749.
2. Kurtz S, Ong K, Lau E, Mowat F, Halpern M: Projections of primary and revision hip and knee arthroplasty in the United States from 2005 to 2030. *J Bone Joint Surg Am* 2007;89(4):780-785.
3. Geerts WH, Bergqvist D, Pineo GF, et al; American College of Chest Physicians: Prevention of venous thromboembolism: American College of Chest Physicians evidence-based clinical practice guidelines (8th edition). *Chest* 2008;133(6, Suppl):381S-453S.
4. Anderson DR, Gross M, Robinson KS, et al: Ultrasonographic screening for deep vein thrombosis following arthroplasty fails to reduce posthospital thromboembolic complications: The Postarthroplasty Screening Study (PASS). *Chest* 1998;114(2, Suppl Evidence)119S-122S.
5. Westrich GH, Haas SB, Mosca P, Peterson M: Meta-analysis of thromboembolic prophylaxis after total knee arthroplasty. *J Bone Joint Surg Br* 2000;82(6): 795-800.
6. Amaragiri SV, Lees TA: Elastic compression stockings for prevention of deep vein thrombosis. *Cochrane Database Syst Rev* 2000; 3(3):CD001484.
7. Pitto RP, Young S: Foot pumps without graduated compression stockings for prevention of deep-vein thrombosis in total joint replacement: Efficacy, safety and patient compliance. A comparative, prospective clinical trial. *Int Orthop* 2008;32(3):331-336.
8. Morris RJ, Woodcock JP: Evidence-based compression: Prevention of stasis and deep vein thrombosis. *Ann Surg* 2004; 239(2):162-171.
9. Warwick D, Friedman RJ, Agnelli G, et al: Insufficient duration of venous thromboembolism prophylaxis after total hip or knee replacement when compared with the time course of thromboembolic events: Findings from the Global Orthopaedic Registry. *J Bone Joint Surg Br* 2007;89(6): 799-807.
10. Sajid MS, Tai NR, Goli G, Morris RW, Baker DM, Hamilton G: Knee versus thigh length

graduated compression stockings for prevention of deep venous thrombosis: A systematic review. *Eur J Vasc Endovasc Surg* 2006; 32(6):730-736.

11. Best AJ, Williams S, Crozier A, Bhatt R, Gregg PJ, Hui AC: Graded compression stockings in elective orthopaedic surgery: An assessment of the in vivo performance of commercially available stockings in patients having hip and knee arthroplasty. *J Bone Joint Surg Br* 2000;82(1):116-118.
12. Colwell CW Jr, Froimson MI, Mont MA, et al: Thrombosis prevention after total hip arthroplasty: A prospective, randomized trial comparing a mobile compression device with low-molecular-weight heparin. *J Bone Joint Surg Am* 2010;92(3):527-535.
13. Edwards JZ, Pulido PA, Ezzet KA, Copp SN, Walker RH, Colwell CW Jr: Portable compression device and low-molecular-weight heparin compared with low-molecular-weight heparin for thromboprophylaxis after total joint arthroplasty. *J Arthroplasty* 2008;23(8):1122-1127.
14. Gelfer Y, Tavor H, Oron A, Peer A, Halperin N, Robinson D: Deep vein thrombosis prevention in joint arthroplasties: Continuous enhanced circulation therapy vs low molecular weight heparin. *J Arthroplasty* 2006;21(2): 206-214.
15. Froimson MI, Murray TG, Fazekas AF: Venous thromboembolic disease reduction with a portable pneumatic compression device. *J Arthroplasty* 2009;24(2): 310-316.
16. Brookenthal KR, Freedman KB, Lotke PA, Fitzgerald RH, Lonner JH: A meta-analysis of thromboembolic prophylaxis in total knee arthroplasty. *J Arthroplasty* 2001;16(3):293-300.
17. Freedman KB, Brookenthal KR, Fitzgerald RH Jr, Williams S, Lonner JH: A meta-analysis of thromboembolic prophylaxis following elective total hip arthroplasty. *J Bone Joint Surg Am* 2000; 82-A(7):929-938.
18. Bauer KA, Eriksson BI, Lassen MR, Turpie AG; Steering Committee of the Pentasaccharide in Major Knee Surgery Study: Fondaparinux compared with enoxaparin for the prevention of venous thromboembolism after elective major knee surgery. *N Engl J Med* 2001;345(18): 1305-1310.
19. Turpie AG, Bauer KA, Eriksson BI, Lassen MR; Pentathalon 2000 Study Steering Committee: Postoperative fondaparinux versus postoperative enoxaparin for prevention of venous thromboembolism after elective hip-replacement surgery: A randomised double-blind trial. *Lancet* 2002; 359(9319):1721-1726.
20. Lassen MR, Bauer KA, Eriksson BI, Turpie AG; European Pentasaccharide Elective Surgery Study (EPHESUS) Steering Committee: Postoperative fondaparinux versus preoperative enoxaparin for prevention of venous thromboembolism in elective hip-replacement surgery: A randomised double-blind comparison. *Lancet* 2002;359(9319): 1715-1720.
21. Eriksson BI, Bauer KA, Lassen MR, Turpie AG; Steering Committee of the Pentasaccharide in Hip-Fracture Surgery Study: Fondaparinux compared with enoxaparin for the prevention of venous thromboembolism after hip-fracture surgery. *N Engl J Med* 2001;345(18):1298-1304.
22. Powers PJ, Gent M, Jay RM, et al: A randomized trial of less intense postoperative warfarin or aspirin therapy in the prevention of venous thromboembolism after surgery for fractured hip. *Arch Intern Med* 1989;149(4):771-774.
23. Gent M, Hirsh J, Ginsberg JS, et al: Low-molecular-weight heparinoid orgaran is more effective than aspirin in the prevention of venous thromboembolism after surgery for hip fracture. *Circulation* 1996;93(1):80-84.
24. Mismetti P, Laporte S, Zufferey P, Epinat M, Decousus H, Cucherat M: Prevention of venous thromboembolism in orthopedic surgery with vitamin K antagonists: A meta-analysis. *J Thromb Haemost* 2004;2(7): 1058-1070.
25. Geerts WH, Heit JA, Clagett GP, et al: Prevention of venous thromboembolism. *Chest* 2001;119(1, Suppl):132S-175S.
26. Westrich GH, Salvati EA, Sharrock N, Potter HG, Sánchez PM, Sculco TP: The effect of intraoperative heparin administered during total hip arthroplasty on the incidence of proximal deep vein thrombosis assessed by magnetic resonance venography. *J Arthroplasty* 2005;20(1):42-50.
27. Westrich GH, Sculco TP: Prophylaxis against deep venous thrombosis after total knee arthroplasty: Pneumatic plantar compression and aspirin compared with aspirin alone. *J Bone Joint Surg Am* 1996; 78(6):826-834.
28. Prevention of pulmonary embolism and deep vein thrombosis with low dose aspirin: Pulmonary Embolism Prevention (PEP) trial. *Lancet* 2000;355(9212):1295-1302.
29. Kakkar AK, Brenner B, Dahl OE, et al; RECORD2 Investigators: Extended duration rivaroxaban versus short-term enoxaparin for the prevention of venous thromboembolism after total hip arthroplasty: A double-blind, randomised controlled trial. *Lancet* 2008;372(9632):31-39.
30. Eriksson BI, Borris LC, Friedman RJ, et al; Record1 Study Group: Rivaroxaban versus enoxaparin for thromboprophylaxis after hip arthroplasty. *N Engl J Med* 2008;358(26):2765-2775.

31. Lassen MR, Ageno W, Borris LC, et al; Record3 Investigators: Rivaroxaban versus enoxaparin for thromboprophylaxis after total knee arthroplasty. *N Engl J Med* 2008;358(26):2776-2786.

32. Lassen MR, Davidson BL, Gallus A, Pineo G, Ansell J, Deitchman D: The efficacy and safety of apixaban, an oral, direct factor Xa inhibitor, as thromboprophylaxis in patients following total knee replacement. *J Thromb Haemost* 2007;5(12):2368-2375.

33. Wolowacz SE, Roskell NS, Plumb JM, Caprini JA, Eriksson BI: Efficacy and safety of dabigatran etexilate for the prevention of venous thromboembolism following total hip or knee arthroplasty: A meta-analysis. *Thromb Haemost* 2009;101(1):77-85.

34. Eriksson BI, Dahl OE, Rosencher N, et al; Re-model Study Group: Oral dabigatran etexilate vs. subcutaneous enoxaparin for the prevention of venous thromboembolism after total knee replacement: the RE-MODEL randomized trial. *J Thromb Haemost* 2007;5(11):2178-2185.

35. Berczi V, Bottomley JR, Thomas SM, Taneja S, Gaines PA, Cleveland TJ: Long-term retrievability of IVC filters: should we abandon permanent devices? *Cardiovasc Intervent Radiol* 2007; 30(5):820-827.

36. Chung J, Owen RJ: Using inferior vena cava filters to prevent pulmonary embolism. *Can Fam Physician* 2008;54(1):49-55.

37. Austin MS, Parvizi J, Grossman S, Restrepo C, Klein GR, Rothman RH: The inferior vena cava filter is effective in preventing fatal pulmonary embolus after hip and knee arthroplasties. *J Arthroplasty* 2007;22(3):343-348.

38. Strauss EJ, Egol KA, Alaia M, Hansen D, Bashar M, Steiger D: The use of retrievable inferior vena cava filters in orthopaedic patients. *J Bone Joint Surg Br* 2008;90(5):662-667.

39. PREPIC Study Group: Eight-year follow-up of patients with permanent vena cava filters in the prevention of pulmonary embolism: The PREPIC (Prevention du Risque d'Embolie Pulmonaire par Interruption Cave) randomized study. *Circulation* 2005;112(3): 416-422.

40. Prins MH, Hirsh J: A comparison of general anesthesia and regional anesthesia as a risk factor for deep vein thrombosis following hip surgery: A critical review. *Thromb Haemost* 1990;64(4):497-500.

41. Bottner F, Sculco TP: Nonpharmacologic thromboembolic prophylaxis in total knee arthroplasty. *Clin Orthop Relat Res* 2001;392: 249-256.

42. Pellegrini VD Jr, Sharrock NE, Paiement GD, Morris R, Warwick DJ: Venous thromboembolic disease after total hip and knee arthroplasty: Current perspectives in a regulated environment. *Instr Course Lect* 2008;57:637-661.

43. Wåhlander K, Larson G, Lindahl TL, et al: Factor V Leiden (G1691A) and prothrombin gene G20210A mutations as potential risk factors for venous thromboembolism after total hip or total knee replacement surgery. *Thromb Haemost* 2002;87(4):580-585.

44. Kyrle PA, Minar E, Hirschl M, et al: High plasma levels of factor VIII and the risk of recurrent venous thromboembolism. *N Engl J Med* 2000;343(7):457-462.

45. Pecheniuk NM, Elias DJ, Deguchi H, Averell PM, Griffin JH: Elevated plasma fibronectin levels associated with venous thromboembolism. *Thromb Haemost* 2008; 100(2):224-228.

46. Eichinger S, Pecheniuk NM, Hron G, et al: High-density lipoprotein and the risk of recurrent venous thromboembolism. *Circulation* 2007;115(12):1609-1614.

47. Schwarz UI, Ritchie MD, Bradford Y, et al: Genetic determinants of response to warfarin during initial anticoagulation. *N Engl J Med* 2008;358(10):999-1008.

48. Millican EA, Lenzini PA, Milligan PE, et al: Genetic-based dosing in orthopedic patients beginning warfarin therapy. *Blood* 2007;110(5):1511-1515.

49. Stehle S, Kirchheiner J, Lazar A, Fuhr U: Pharmacogenetics of oral anticoagulants: A basis for dose individualization. *Clin Pharmacokinet* 2008;47(9):565-594.

50. Johanson NA, Lachiewicz PF, Lieberman JR, et al: Prevention of symptomatic pulmonary embolism in patients undergoing total hip or knee arthroplasty. *J Am Acad Orthop Surg* 2009;17(3): 183-196.

51. Venous thromboembolism: Includes deep vein thrombosis and pulmonary embolism. Premier Website. http://premierinc.com/all/safety/topics/Venous-Thromboembolism/venous-thromboembolism.jsp. Accessed August 24, 2009.

52. The National Quality Forum Website. http://www.qualityforum.org/news/releases/051508-endorsed-measures.asp. Accessed December 1, 2008.

53. The Joint Commission Website. http://www.jointcommission.org/. Accessed December 1, 2008.

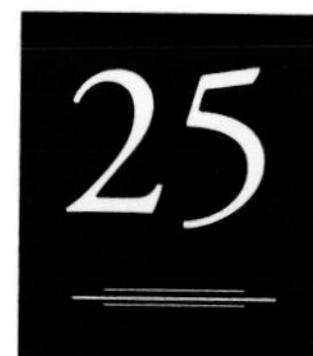

New Oral Anticoagulants for Venous Thromboembolism Prophylaxis in Orthopaedic Surgery

Richard J. Friedman, MD, FRCSC

Abstract

Anticoagulant drugs reduce the risk of venous thromboembolic events after total hip and knee arthroplasty. However, the use of current drugs, such as low-molecular-weight heparins, is hampered by their subcutaneous administration. The use of a vitamin K antagonist, such as warfarin, is hampered by the required routine coagulation monitoring and dose titration to provide effective anticoagulation without an increased risk of bleeding. Numerous possible food and drug interactions must also be considered. New classes of oral anticoagulant agents have been developed that have a fixed dose, do not require coagulation monitoring, do not have food and drug interactions, and demonstrate similar or better efficacy and safety profiles when compared with current agents.

Instr Course Lect 2011;60:291-300.

In the United States, in 2007, the number of total hip arthroplasties (THAs) and total knee arthroplasties (TKAs) performed was approximately 300,000 and 500,000, respectively.[1] The number of THAs is expected to increase to 572,000 and the number of TKAs to 3.48 million by 2030. As has been well documented, patients treated with THA or TKA are at significant risk of developing venous thromboembolism (VTE), comprising deep venous thrombosis and (DVT) and pulmonary embolism (PE).[2] Without thromboprophylaxis, 42% to 57% of patients treated with THA have venographically confirmed total (proximal or distal) DVT. In patients treated with TKA without thromboprophylaxis, 41% to 85% have venographically confirmed total DVT.

The appropriate use of antithrombotic agents has been shown to reduce the risk of VTE after THA and TKA; guidelines by several organizations, such as the American College of Chest Physicians (ACCP) and the American Academy of Orthopaedic Surgeons (AAOS), recommend their routine use after this type of surgery. More information on the guideline recommendations is available in chapter 26. However, symptomatic clinical events still occur in approximately 2% to 4% of patients and occur at a mean of 9.7 days after TKA and 21.5 days after THA[3] (**Figure 1**). With the current trend toward shorter hospital stays, which average fewer than 3 days for THA and TKA, VTE prophylaxis has become essentially an outpatient issue.

Pharmacologic Prophylaxis

Options and Limitations

Recommended pharmacologic options for thromboprophylaxis after THA or TKA include vitamin K antagonists (such as warfarin), low-molecular-weight heparins (such as enoxaparin and dalteparin), and an indirect factor Xa inhibitor (fondaparinux). The limitations of warfarin include the requirement for regular coagulation monitoring, the potential for food and drug interactions, and a delayed onset of action.[3,4] Parenteral anticoagulants, such as enoxaparin and fondaparinux, may be less convenient than those administered orally. There is also a risk of heparin-induced thrombocytopenia with low-molecular-weight heparins.[5]

Although warfarin offers the convenience of oral administration, its use in

Dr. Friedman or an immediate family member serves as a board member, owner, officer, or committee member of the AAOS, the American Shoulder and Elbow Surgeons, and the BOS; has received royalties from DJ Orthopaedics and CRC Press; serves as a paid consultant to or is an employee of Johnson & Johnson, Astellas US, Boehringer Ingelheim, and DJO Surgical; and has received research or institutional support from Astellas US.

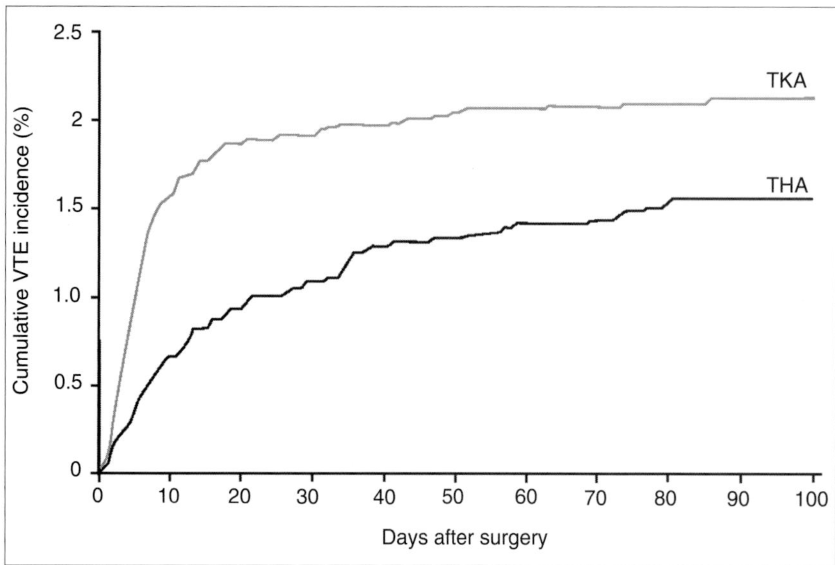

Figure 1 Graph showing the cumulative incidence of VTE, with the mean time to a symptomatic event after TKA being 9.7 days and 20.5 days after THA. (Reproduced with permission from Warwick D, Friedman W, Agnelli G, et al: Insufficient duration of venous thromboembolism prophylaxis after total hip or knee replacement when compared with the time course of thromboembolic events. *J Bone Joint Surg Br* 2007;89:799-807.)

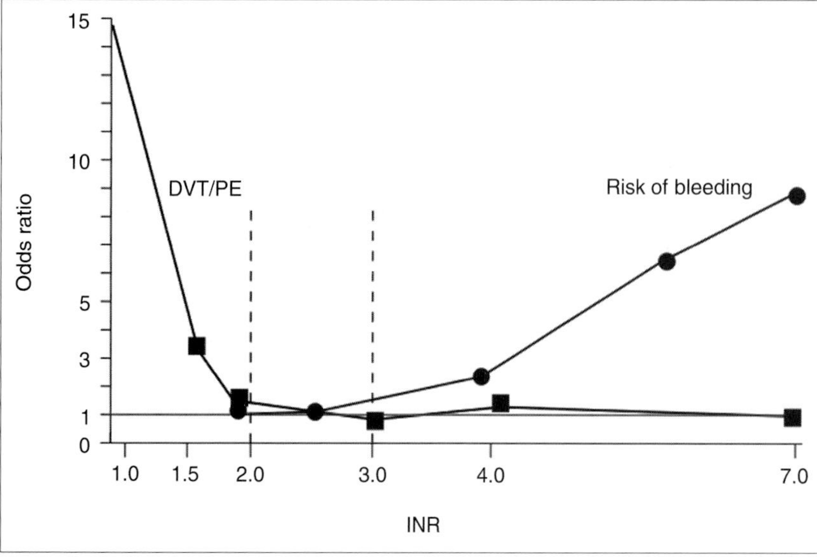

Figure 2 Graph showing the narrow therapeutic range of warfarin. (Adapted with permission from Friedman RJ: Prevention of thrombophlebitis in total knee arthroplasty, in Scott WN: *Surgery of the Knee*, ed 4. Philadelphia, PA, Churchill-Livingstone, 2006, vol 2, pp 1837-1847.)

clinical practice can be complicated. It has a narrow therapeutic window and shows considerable individual variability in its dose-response relationship[6] (**Figure 2**). With a narrow therapeutic window, an international normalized ratio (INR) of less than 2.0 is associated with a low risk of bleeding but reduced efficacy and therefore an increased risk for DVT and PE. If the INR rises above 3.0, the risk for thromboembolic complications is low, but the risk of surgical site and remote bleeding rises exponentially. Warfarin is subject to numerous dietary and drug interactions, and the need for regular dose adjustments to achieve and maintain a target INR can lead to additional problems, such as nonadherence to the medication regimen or communication difficulties between the physician and the patient.[6] These factors make it difficult for the patient to achieve and maintain adherence to the narrow therapeutic window of efficacy and safety.

New Oral Anticoagulant Agents

To overcome these limitations, new oral anticoagulants that do not require regular coagulation monitoring, are unlikely to interact with food and drugs, and have a fast onset and offset of action are being developed. Because patients often need to self-administer injectable thromboprophylaxis at home, an ideal anticoagulant would allow easier administration. Oral anticoagulants have a clear advantage over parenteral agents.

Several new oral anticoagulants in development have shown promising benefit-risk profiles in clinical trials with similar or better efficacy and safety profiles compared with current agents.[7-10] Clinical studies have focused on the use of oral, direct factor Xa inhibitors (such as apixaban and rivaroxaban) and a direct thrombin inhibitor (dabigatran etexilate) for thromboprophylaxis following THA and TKA. At the time of this writing, these agents are classified by the Food and Drug Administration as investigational and have not been cleared for clinical use in the United States.

Because currently available anticoagulant drugs are administered subcutaneously or require monitoring and dose adjustment to provide effective anticoagulation without increasing bleeding risk, their use presents a clinical challenge for orthopaedic surgeons. It is hoped that new drugs will meet the needs of orthopaedic surgeons in providing improved VTE prophylaxis for their patients.

An ideal anticoagulant should be efficacious without increasing bleeding risk, safe, convenient to use, and administered orally once daily with fixed dosing—factors that could potentially improve patient compliance. The most promising new oral anticoagulants are the direct thrombin inhibitors and the direct factor Xa inhibitors. These agents directly target a single coagulation factor in the coagulation cascade (**Figure 3**). Dabigatran is approved for use in Europe, Canada, and other countries. It is dosed at 110 mg within 1 to 4 hours of surgery and then 220 mg once daily for 28 to 35 days after THA and 10 days after TKA, for VTE prophylaxis after elective THA and TKA.[11] Rivaroxaban is also approved in Europe, Canada, and numerous other countries for the prevention of VTE in patients after elective THA or TKA at a dose of 10 mg 6 to 10 hours after surgery and then once daily for 35 days after THA and 14 days after TKA.[12] These two drugs represent the first new oral agents for VTE prophylaxis in THA and TKA in more than 50 years.

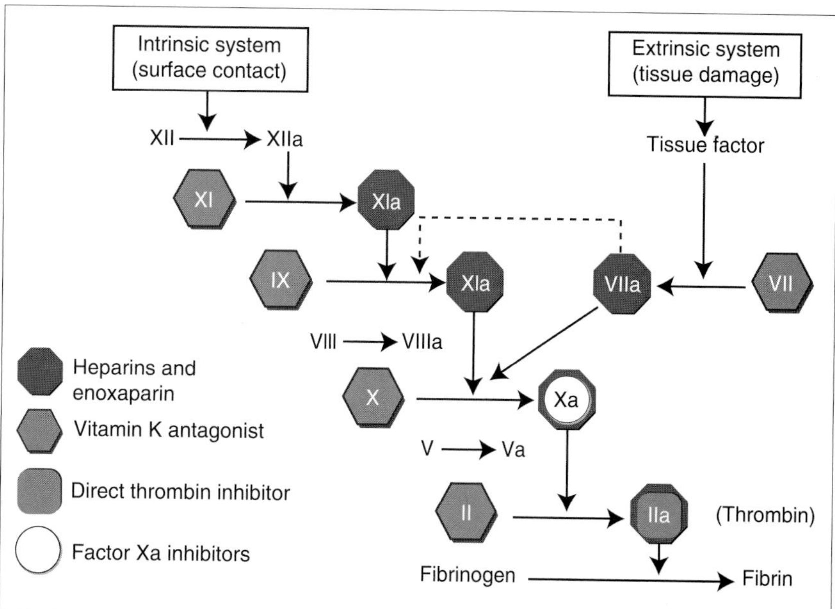

Figure 3 Schematic diagram of the simplified coagulation cascade showing sites of action of anticoagulant drugs used in thromboprophylaxis. (Adapted with permission from Friedman RJ: Prevention of thrombophlebitis in total knee arthroplasty, in Scott WN: *Surgery of the Knee*, ed 4. Philadelphia, PA, Churchill-Livingstone, 2006, vol 2, pp 1837-1847.)

Direct Thrombin Inhibitors

Mode of Action

Thrombin is an enzyme that catalyzes the conversion of fibrinogen to fibrin, which leads to thrombus formation. Direct thrombin inhibitors bind to thrombin and block the interaction of thrombin with its substrate, thereby preventing the conversion of fibrinogen to fibrin.[4] Direct thrombin inhibitors offer some potential advantages over indirect thrombin inhibitors. Because of low levels of plasma protein binding, direct inhibitors offer a more predictable anticoagulant effect than indirect inhibitors and also are effective against both circulating and clot-bound thrombin (whereas heparins are ineffective against clot-bound thrombin, which remains biologically active). An important advantage of direct thrombin inhibitors is their oral administration, which (as with the oral direct factor Xa inhibitors) provides added convenience and may encourage patient compliance.

Dabigatran Etexilate

Dabigatran etexilate is rapidly absorbed and converted to its active form, dabigatran.[13] The bioavailability of dabigatran after oral administration is low (6% to 7%). After oral administration of a 200-mg dose of dabigatran, the half-life is approximately 9 hours. The predominant elimination pathway is renal excretion, through which more than 80% of the systemically available dabigatran is eliminated. Because renal function declines with increasing age, dabigatran elimination would be expected to be prolonged in elderly patients with compromised renal function. In a pharmacokinetic study of healthy individuals age 65 years or older, dabigatran dosed at 150 mg twice daily for 6 days and once on day 7 resulted in a half-life of 12 to 14 hours.[14]

The sex of the patient has not been shown to have any clinically important effects on dabigatran pharmacokinetics, and there is limited clinical experience in patients with extreme body weight.[14] Food consumption delays the time to peak plasma concentration by 2 hours but does not affect the extent of absorption.[15] Comedications (such as diuretics, drugs that accelerate the gastrointestinal transit time, acetaminophen, and CYP3A4 inhibitors), demographics, and standard laboratory parameters had no relevant effect on standard coagulation tests in a population pharmacodynamic analysis in patients treated with THA.[16] The

CYP450 system does not appear to play an important role in the pharmacodynamics of dabigatran; therefore, drugs that are metabolized by this system are unlikely to interact with therapeutic doses of dabigatran.[3] Dabigatran does not require regular coagulation monitoring.[17]

Three phase III studies have been completed for dabigatran.[18-20] The RE-NOVATE study was conducted in patients treated with THA, and the RE-MODEL and RE-MOBILIZE studies in patients treated with TKA. All three studies were prospective, randomized, double-blind, double-dummy, controlled trials. The primary efficacy end point in the three studies was the composite of total VTE (venographic or symptomatic DVT or symptomatic PE) and death.

In the RE-NOVATE THA study of 3,494 patients, dabigatran (150 mg or 220 mg once daily) was compared with enoxaparin (40 mg once daily), with both drugs administered for 28 to 35 days.[18] The primary efficacy end point occurred in 8.6% of the 150-mg group (absolute risk difference versus enoxaparin, 1.9%), 6.0% of the 220-mg group (absolute risk difference versus enoxaparin, –0.7%), and 6.7% of the enoxaparin group. Both doses of dabigatran were noninferior to enoxaparin ($P < 0.0001$ for noninferiority for both doses). Symptomatic DVT occurred in 0.8% of the 150-mg group, 0.5% of the 220-mg group, and 0.1% of the enoxaparin group. Rates of major bleeding were 1.3% for the 150-mg group ($P = 0.60$), 2.0% for the 220-mg group ($P = 0.44$), and 1.6% for the enoxaparin group. Clinically relevant, nonmajor bleeding occurred in 4.7%, 4.2%, and 3.5% of the dabigatran 150 mg, dabigatran 220 mg, and enoxaparin groups, respectively. The rate of wound complications was 3% in each of the dabigatran groups and 4% in the enoxaparin group. Bleeding events leading to reoperation occurred in 0.3% of patients receiving dabigatran 150 mg, 0.2% of patients receiving dabigatran 220 mg, and 0.3% of patients receiving enoxaparin.

In the RE-MODEL TKA study of 2,101 patients, dabigatran (150 mg and 220 mg once daily) was compared with enoxaparin (40 mg once daily; n = 699).[19] The primary efficacy end point occurred in 40.5% of patients in the 150-mg group (absolute risk difference versus enoxaparin, 2.8%; $P = 0.017$ for noninferiority), 36.4% of the dabigatran 220 mg group (absolute risk difference versus enoxaparin, –1.3%; $P = 0.0003$ for noninferiority), and 37.7% of the enoxaparin group. Rates of major bleeding were 1.3% for the 150-mg group ($P = 1.0$), 1.5% for the 220-mg group ($P = 0.82$), and 1.3% for the enoxaparin group. Symptomatic DVT occurred in 0.4% of patients in the 150-mg group, 0.1% of patients the 220-mg group, and 1.2% of patients in the enoxaparin group. Clinically relevant, nonmajor bleeding occurred in 6.8% of the dabigatran 150-mg group, 5.9% of the dabigatran 220-mg group, and 5.3% of the enoxaparin group. Bleeding leading to reoperation occurred in 0.1% of patients receiving dabigatran 150 mg, 0.4% of patients receiving dabigatran 220 mg, and 0.1% of patients receiving enoxaparin.

In the RE-MOBILIZE TKA study of 2,615 patients, dabigatran (150 mg and 220 mg once daily) was compared with enoxaparin (30 mg twice daily).[20] Dabigatran did not meet the noninferiority criteria for either dose. The primary efficacy outcome occurred in 33.7% of the 150-mg group, 31.1% of the 220-mg group, and 25.3% of the enoxaparin group. For the 150-mg group, the risk difference was 8.4% ($P = 0.0009$), and for the 220-mg group, the risk difference was 5.8% ($P = 0.0234$) compared with enoxaparin. Major bleeding occurred in 0.6% of the 150-mg group, 0.6% of the 220-mg group, and 1.4% of the enoxaparin group. Clinically relevant, nonmajor bleeding occurred in 2.5%, 2.7%, and 2.4% of the dabigatran 150 mg, dabigatran 220 mg, and enoxaparin groups, respectively. No patients in the dabigatran arm experienced bleeding that led to reoperation, but one patient in the enoxaparin group required reoperation because of bleeding.

Dabigatran showed noninferiority to the enoxaparin 40-mg once-daily regimen after THA and TKA but failed to meet the noninferiority criteria compared with the North American enoxaparin 30-mg twice-daily regimen after TKA. In all three studies, the incidence of liver enzyme elevations (alanine aminotransferase > 3 times the upper limit of the normal range) and acute coronary events was similar between the three groups.

A meta-analysis of the three trials has been completed.[10] A meta-analysis of the dabigatran 220-mg dose showed no significant differences between dabigatran 220 mg and enoxaparin in any of the end points when all three trials were included in the analysis. Major bleeding rates did not differ significantly when the RE-MODEL and RE-NOVATE studies were analyzed ($P = 0.41$ for random effect and fixed effect analyses) or when RE-MOBILIZE was included in the analysis ($P = 0.85$ for random effects and $P = 0.95$ for fixed effects). Clinically relevant, nonmajor bleeding also did not differ significantly in the two-trial analysis ($P = 0.34$ for random effects and $P = 0.33$ for fixed effects) or when all three trials were analyzed together ($P = 0.31$ for both random effect and fixed effect analyses). These findings support the conclusions of RE-MODEL and RE-NOVATE that dabigatran 220 mg is noninferior to enoxaparin 40 mg once daily, with a similar safety profile.

Based on this information, 2,055 patients treated with THA were entered in the RE-NOVATE II study, a double-blind, noninferiority trial, in which patients were randomized to treatment for 28 to 35 days with oral dabigatran, 220 mg once daily, starting with a half dose 1 to 4 hours after surgery; or subcutaneous enoxaparin 40 mg once daily.[21] The primary efficacy outcome was a composite of total VTE (venographic or symptomatic) and death from all causes. The main secondary composite outcome was major VTE (proximal DVT or nonfatal PE) plus VTE-related death. The main safety outcome was major bleeding during treatment. The primary efficacy outcome occurred in 61 of 792 patients (7.7%) in the dabigatran group versus 69 of 785 patients (8.8%) in the enoxaparin group (absolute risk difference –1.1%, 95% confidence interval [CI], –3.8% to 1.6%; $P < 0.0001$) for the prespecified noninferiority margin. The main secondary efficacy outcome occurred in 18 of 805 patients (2.2%) in the dabigatran group versus 33 of 794 patients (4.2%) in the enoxaparin group (absolute risk difference –1.9%; 95% CI, –3.6% to –0.2%; $P = 0.03$). Major bleeding occurred in 1.4% of the dabigatran group and 0.9% of the enoxaparin group ($P = 0.40$). The incidence of adverse events, including liver and cardiac events, did not differ significantly between the groups. Extended prophylaxis with oral dabigatran 220 mg once daily was as effective as subcutaneous enoxaparin 40 mg once daily in reducing the risk of VTE after THA. The risk of bleeding and the safety profiles were similar.

Direct Factor Xa Inhibitors

Mode of Action

The enzyme factor X is an attractive target for inhibition because it occupies a critical junction between the intrinsic and extrinsic coagulation cascade pathways and is essential for the conversion of prothrombin to thrombin, which leads to thrombus formation[22,23] (**Figure 3**). In response to vascular injury, factor X is activated to factor Xa by either the contact (intrinsic pathway) or by the tissue factor/factor VIIa (extrinsic pathway). Factor Xa combines with its cofactor, factor Va, on phospholipid membranes to form the prothrombinase complex. This complex converts prothrombin to thrombin, which leads to the amplified generation of thrombin.

The indirect factor Xa inhibitors, such as subcutaneous fondaparinux, showed that factor Xa is an effective target for anticoagulation. Direct factor Xa inhibitors have some advantages over indirect factor Xa inhibitors. Unlike indirect factor Xa inhibitors, which catalyze factor Xa inhibition by antithrombin, direct factor Xa inhibitors bind directly to factor Xa, thus preventing the subsequent reactions leading to thrombin generation.[22,23] In addition, they inhibit both free and platelet-bound factor Xa and factor Xa bound to the prothrombinase complex. Some direct factor Xa inhibitors in development are administered parenterally (for example, DX-9065a), whereas others (for example, apixaban and rivaroxaban) are orally active.

Apixaban

Apixaban is an oral, direct factor Xa inhibitor that has no food and relatively few drug interactions. Peak concentrations occur 3 to 4 hours after oral administration, and the terminal half-life is 9 to 12 hours. Bioavailability is 50%, and there is a dual mode of excretion, with 25% excreted renally. A phase II study of apixaban was used to establish the dose to be used for the phase III clinical development program.[24] In this study, 1,238 patients were randomized to one of six double-blind apixaban doses (5, 10, or 20 mg once daily or 2.5, 5, or 10 mg twice daily), enoxaparin (30 mg twice daily subcutaneously), or open-label warfarin (titrated to an INR of 1.8 to 3.0) for 10 to 14 days. The primary efficacy outcome (the composite of VTE and all cause mortality) decreased with an increasing apixaban dose ($P = 0.09$ with once- or twice-daily regimens combined; $P = 0.19$ for once-daily and $P = 0.13$ for twice-daily dosing). There was a significant dose-related increase of total adjudicated bleeding events for the once-daily ($P = 0.01$) and twice-daily ($P = 0.02$) regimens. The authors concluded that apixaban administered at 2.5 mg twice daily and 5 mg once daily might have a promising risk–benefit profile compared with enoxaparin 30 mg twice daily and warfarin.

The ADVANCE-1 phase III study of 3,195 patients compared apixaban 2.5 mg twice daily with the enoxaparin regimen commonly used in North America of 30 mg twice daily for the prevention of VTE after TKA.[8] The primary efficacy outcome (composite of venographic DVT; symptomatic, objectively confirmed DVT; nonfatal PE; or death from any cause) occurred in 9.0% of patients receiving apixaban and 8.9% of patients receiving enoxaparin (relative risk, 1.02; 95% CI, 0.78 to 1.32; $P = 0.06$ for noninferiority; absolute risk difference, 0.1%; 95% CI, –2.2 to 2.44; $P < 0.001$ for noninferiority) during the treatment period. The rates of PE were 1.0% in the apixaban group and 0.4% in the enoxaparin group; two PEs were fatal in the apixaban group, and none were fatal in the enoxaparin group. Major or clinically relevant nonmajor bleeding occurred in 2.9% and 4.3% of patients receiving apixaban and enoxaparin, respectively ($P = 0.03$). Major bleeding occurred in 0.7% and 1.4% of patients receiving apixaban and enoxaparin, respectively ($P = 0.05$). One patient in the enoxaparin group died from bleeding; no patients in the apixaban group died from bleeding.

In the ADVANCE-2 study, which compared apixaban 2.5 mg twice daily with enoxaparin 40 mg once daily in 3,057 patients treated with TKA, it was hypothesized that apixaban would be noninferior to enoxaparin based on a prespecified margin for the primary efficacy outcome in which the upper limit of the two-sided 95% CI is less than 1.25 for relative risk and less than 0.056 for the absolute risk difference.[7] The primary efficacy end point (the same as in ADVANCE-1 study) occurred in 15.1% of the apixaban group and 24.4% of the enoxaparin group (relative risk 0.62; 95% CI, 0.51 to 0.74; $P < 0.001$; absolute risk difference, −9.3%; 95% CI, −12.7 to −5.8; $P < 0.001$). Major VTE, the composite of proximal DVT, PE, and VTE death, was also significantly less in the apixaban group (1.1%) versus the enoxaparin group (2.2%) (relative risk, 0.50; 95% CI, 0.26 to 0.97; $P = 0.019$). The rates of PE were 0.26% in the apixaban group and 0.0% in the enoxaparin group; one PE was fatal in the apixaban group, and none was fatal in the enoxaparin group. Major or clinically relevant, nonmajor bleeding occurred in 3.5% and 4.8% of patients receiving apixaban and enoxaparin, respectively ($P = 0.09$). Major bleeding occurred in 0.6% and 0.9% of patients receiving apixaban and enoxaparin, respectively ($P = 0.3$).

In the ADVANCE-3 THA study, 5,407 patients were randomized to receive either apixaban 2.5 mg twice daily or enoxaparin 40 mg for 35 days.[25] The same primary and secondary efficacy outcomes were used as in the previous two studies. Total VTE occurred in 1.4% of the apixaban patients compared with 3.9% of the enoxaparin patients (relative risk 0.36; 95% CI, 0.22 to 0.54; $P < 0.0001$; absolute risk difference, 2.5; 95% CI, 1.5 to 3.5; $P < 0.0001$). The secondary efficacy endpoint, major VTE, occurred in 0.5% of the apixaban patients and 1.1% in the enoxaparin patients (relative risk, 0.40; 95% CI, 0.15 to 0.80; $P < 0.0001$; absolute risk difference, 0.7; 95% CI, 0.2 to 1.3; $P < 0.0001$). Major or clinically relevant, nonmajor bleeding occurred in 4.8% and 5.0% of patients receiving apixaban and enoxaparin, respectively ($P = 0.72$). Major bleeding occurred in 0.8% and 0.7% of patients receiving apixaban and enoxaparin, respectively ($P = 0.54$). After THA, one major VTE is prevented for each of the 146 patients treated with apixaban compared with enoxaparin, without an increased risk of bleeding. Symptomatic rates were extremely low for both groups, 0.15% for apixaban versus 0.37% for enoxaparin.

In all three studies, there were no differences in the occurrence of liver function enzyme elevations, thrombocytopenia, or cardiac events (stroke or myocardial infarction). The findings of these studies suggest that apixaban 2.5 mg daily is superior to the 40-mg once-daily enoxaparin regimen at reducing the composite of DVT, PE, and death by any cause and similar to the 30-mg twice-daily dosing, with a trend toward decreased bleeding.

Rivaroxaban

Rivaroxaban is an oral, direct factor Xa inhibitor, which is rapidly absorbed and has a mean terminal half-life of 7 to 11 hours.[12] It exhibits a predictable pharmacokinetic and pharmacodynamic profile and does not require dose adjustment for age, sex, or weight.[26,27] Rivaroxaban and its metabolites have a dual route of elimination: one third of the administered drug is cleared as unchanged active drug by the kidneys, one third is metabolized to inactive metabolites and then excreted by the kidneys, and one third is metabolized to inactive metabolites and then excreted by the fecal route.[28]

Rivaroxaban has a low propensity for drug-drug interaction with frequently used concomitant medications such as naproxen, aspirin, or clopidogrel, and no interaction with the cardiac glycoside digoxin.[29-32] Dietary restrictions are not necessary, and rivaroxaban was given with or without food in the phase III VTE prevention studies (RECORD studies 1 to 4). Phase II studies showed that all investigated rivaroxaban dose regimens had similar efficacy to enoxaparin, and the incidence of major bleeding was not significantly different compared with enoxaparin across a fourfold dose range (5 to 20 mg total daily rivaroxaban dose).[33-36]

The RECORD program consisted of four phase III studies investigating the efficacy and safety of rivaroxaban in 12,500 patients treated with THA and TKA.[37-40] All patients received rivaroxaban 10 mg once daily 6 to 8 hours after surgery, and there was no upper age or weight limit for participation. The primary efficacy end point was the composite of DVT (as detected by mandatory bilateral venography) nonfatal PE, and all-cause mortality up to days 30 to 42 after surgery for RECORD1 and RECORD2, up to days 13 to 17 for RECORD3, and up to day 17 for RECORD4. The secondary efficacy end points were the incidence of major VTE (composite of proximal DVT, nonfatal PE, or death from VTE). Any DVT, symptomatic VTE during treatment and follow-up, and death during follow-up were also evaluated.

The main safety end point was the incidence of treatment-emergent (observed no later than 2 days after the last dose of the study drug) major bleeding events, which were defined as fatal events, bleeding into a critical organ (for example, retroperitoneal, intracranial, intraocular, and intraspinal bleeding) requiring reoperation, clinically overt extra surgical-site bleeding associated with a fall in hemoglobin of at least 2 g/dL, or needing transfusion of two or more units of whole blood or packed cells. Clinically relevant, nonmajor bleeding events (defined as multiple-source bleeding, excessive wound hematomas, nose bleeding for more than 5 minutes, gingival bleeding for more than 5 minutes, macroscopic hematuria, rectal bleeding, coughing of blood, hematemesis, vaginal bleeding, intra-articular bleeding with trauma, surgical-site bleeding, unexpected hematoma or blood in semen), hemorrhagic wound complications, and postoperative wound infection were among the other outcomes reported.[37-40]

RECORD1 showed that 5 weeks of extended-duration rivaroxaban (10 mg once daily for 31 to 39 days after surgery) was significantly more effective than enoxaparin (40 mg once daily for 31 to 39 days) for extended-duration prophylaxis in patients treated with THA (1.1% versus 3.7% for the primary efficacy end point, $P < 0.001$).[37] Major bleeding events did not differ significantly between the groups (0.3% for the rivaroxaban group versus 0.1% for the enoxaparin group, $P = 0.18$). Clinically relevant nonmajor bleeding occurred in 2.9% of the rivaroxaban group versus 2.4% of the enoxaparin group; hemorrhagic wound complications in 1.5% versus 1.7% of patients; and postoperative wound infections in 0.4% of patients in both groups. The incidence of symptomatic VTE during treatment was not significantly different between the groups (0.3% for the rivaroxaban group versus 0.5% for the enoxaparin group, $P = 0.22$).

RECORD2 showed that extended-duration rivaroxaban prophylaxis (10 mg once daily for 31 to 39 days after surgery) was significantly more effective than short-duration prophylaxis with enoxaparin (40 mg once daily for 10 to 14 days) followed by placebo in patients treated with THA (2.0% for the rivaroxaban group versus 9.3% for the enoxaparin group for the primary efficacy end point, $P < 0.0001$).[38] The incidence of bleeding was comparable between extended-regimen rivaroxaban and short-duration enoxaparin. Major bleeding events occurred in fewer than 0.1% of patients in both groups. Clinically relevant nonmajor bleeding was recorded in 3.3% of the rivaroxaban group versus 2.7% of the enoxaparin group; hemorrhagic wound complications in 1.6% versus 1.7% of patients; and postoperative wound infections in 0.7% versus 0.5% of patients, respectively. Significantly fewer patients in the rivaroxaban group had symptomatic VTE (0.2%) than in the enoxaparin group (1.2%, $P = 0.004$) during the active study period.

In RECORD3, rivaroxaban prophylaxis (10 mg once daily for 10 to 14 days) was significantly more effective than the European enoxaparin regimen for prophylaxis (40 mg once daily) in patients treated with TKA (9.6% versus 18.9% for the primary efficacy end point, $P < 0.001$), with a similar safety profile.[39] Rates of major bleeding were similar in the rivaroxaban and enoxaparin groups (0.6% versus 0.5%, $P = 0.77$). Clinically relevant, nonmajor bleeding occurred in 2.7% of rivaroxaban versus 2.3% of enoxaparin patients, hemorrhagic wound complications in 2.0% versus 1.9%, and postoperative wound infections in 0.6% versus 0.9%, respectively. There was a significant reduction in the number of symptomatic VTE events in the rivaroxaban group (0.7% versus 2.0%, $P = 0.005$).

In RECORD4, rivaroxaban showed significantly better efficacy than the enoxaparin regimen (30 mg every 12 hours) commonly used in North America for short-term prophylaxis after TKA (6.9% versus 10.1%, respectively for the primary efficacy end point, $P = 0.0118$).[40] The rates of major bleeding were 0.7% versus 0.3% ($P = 0.1096$) respectively, and major and clinically relevant nonmajor bleeding 3.0% versus 2.3% ($P = 0.179$), respectively. The observed incidences of symptomatic VTE in those receiving rivaroxaban or enoxaparin were 0.7% versus 1.2% ($P = 0.187$), respectively.

In the four studies comparing rivaroxaban with enoxaparin, rivaroxaban demonstrated superior efficacy compared with enoxaparin. In addition, extended thromboprophylaxis with rivaroxaban was significantly more effective than short-term enoxaparin plus placebo in the prevention of total, major, and symptomatic VTE after THA. The incidence of treatment-emergent major and clinically relevant nonmajor bleeding was low for rivaroxaban and enoxaparin ($P = 0.21$ for RECORD1, P value not reported for RECORD2, $P = 0.44$ for RECORD3, and $P = 0.18$ for RECORD4). There was no evidence of compromised liver function or rebound cardiovascular events associated with rivaroxaban.

In a pooled analysis of the RECORD1, 2, and 3 studies (which compared rivaroxaban with enoxaparin 40 mg once daily after THA and TKA), the prespecified primary efficacy outcome (the composite of symptomatic VTE [DVT or PE] and all-cause mortality at 2 weeks) was 0.4% and 0.8%, respectively ($P = 0.005$).[41] The rates were 0.5% and 1.3%, respectively, at the end of the planned medication period ($P < 0.001$). Rates of on-treatment major bleeding were 0.2% for both drugs at 2 weeks ($P = 0.662$), and 0.3% for rivaroxaban and 0.2% for enoxaparin at the end of the planned medication period (*P* = 0.305). Rates of clinically relevant, nonmajor bleeding were 2.6% for rivaroxaban and 2.3% for enoxaparin at 2 weeks, and 3.0% and 2.5%, respectively, at the end of the planned medication period.

In a pooled analysis of the four RECORD studies, the primary efficacy end point (the composite of symptomatic VTE [DVT or PE] and death) was significantly reduced for the rivaroxaban regimens compared with enoxaparin regimens at day 12 ± 2 (0.5% versus 1.0%, *P* = 0.001) and in the planned treatment period (0.6% versus 1.3%, *P* < 0.001).[9] Rates of treatment-emergent major bleeding were not significantly different between the groups at any of the time points analyzed. The composite of major and clinically relevant, nonmajor bleeding for the rivaroxaban and enoxaparin regimens were 2.9% versus 2.5% (*P* = 0.186) at day 12 ± 2 and 3.2% versus 2.6% (*P* = 0.039), respectively, in the planned treatment period. Rates of the composite of PE and death were lower for rivaroxaban compared with enoxaparin in the planned treatment period and at follow-up (0.5% versus 0.8%, *P* = 0.039).[42]

Summary

It is difficult to achieve a good balance between efficacy and safety when administering prophylaxis for orthopaedic surgical procedures. With insufficient anticoagulation prophylaxis, the patient is at increased risk of VTE, whereas too much anticoagulation prophylaxis places the patient at increased risk for a bleeding event. Although guidelines (such as the ACCP and AAOS) for thromboprophylaxis are available, a substantial proportion of orthopaedic patients still do not receive adequate prophylaxis.[43] The discovery of new oral anticoagulants with promising benefit-risk profiles for VTE prevention after THA and TKA could be an important advance for orthopaedic surgeons and patients. Research has focused on oral direct factor Xa inhibitors and direct thrombin inhibitors, which have several advantages over conventional agents. Phase III studies have shown that some of these new agents can improve the benefit-risk ratio. With the convenience of oral dosing and the potential for simplified postoperative management of patients, it is possible that these new agents will replace the more conventional anticoagulants currently in clinical practice.

References

1. Kurtz S, Ong K, Lau E, Mowat F, Halpern M: Projections of primary and revision hip and knee arthroplasty in the United States from 2005 to 2030. *J Bone Joint Surg Am* 2007;89(4):780-785.
2. Geerts WH, Bergqvist D, Pineo GF, et al: Prevention of venous thromboembolism: American College of Chest Physicians Evidence-Based Clinical Practice Guidelines (8th edition). *Chest* 2008;133(6, Suppl):381S-453S.
3. Warwick D, Friedman RJ, Agnelli G, et al: Insufficient duration of venous thromboembolism prophylaxis after total hip or knee replacement when compared with the time course of thromboembolic events: Findings from the Global Orthopaedic Registry. *J Bone Joint Surg Br* 2007;89 (6):799-807.
4. Weitz JI, Hirsh J, Samama MM; American College of Chest Physicians: New antithrombotic drugs: American College of Chest Physicians Evidence-Based Clinical Practice Guidelines (8th Edition). *Chest* 2008;133(6, Suppl):234S-256S.
5. Hirsh J, Bauer KA, Donati MB, et al: Parenteral anticoagulants: American College of Chest Physicians Evidence-Based Clinical Practice Guidelines (8th edition). *Chest* 2008;133(6, Suppl):141S-159S.
6. Ansell J, Hirsh J, Hylek E, et al: Pharmacology and management of the vitamin K antagonists: American College of Chest Physicians Evidence-Based Clinical Practice Guidelines (8th edition). *Chest* 2008;133(6, Suppl):S160-S198.
7. Lassen MR, Raskob GE, Gallus AS, et al: Apixaban versus enoxaparin for thromboprophylaxis after knee replacement (ADVANCE-2): A randomised double-blind trial. *Lancet* 2010; 375(9717):807-815.
8. Lassen MR, Raskob GE, Gallus A, Pineo G, Chen D, Portman RJ: Apixaban or enoxaparin for thromboprophylaxis after knee replacement. *N Engl J Med* 2009; 361(6):594-604.
9. Turpie AGG, Lassen MR, Kakkar AK et al: A pooled analysis of four pivotal studies of rivaroxaban for the prevention of venous thromboembolism after orthopaedic surgery: Effect on symptomatic venous thromboembolism and death, and bleeding. *Haematologica* 2009;94(Suppl 2):439.
10. Wolowacz SE, Roskell NS, Plumb JM, Caprini JA, Eriksson BI: Efficacy and safety of dabigatran etexilate for the prevention of venous thromboembolism following total hip or knee arthroplasty: A meta-analysis. *Thromb Haemost* 2009;101(1):77-85.
11. Summary of Product Characteristics. Pradaxa Website. http://www.pradaxa.com/Include/media/pdf/Pradaxa_SPC_EMEA.pdf. Accessed May 10, 2010.
12. Summary of Product Characteristics. Xarelto Website. http://www.xarelto.com/html/

downloads/Xarelto_Summary_of_Product_ Characteristics_May2009.pdf. Accessed May 10, 2010.

13. Blech S, Ebner T, Ludwig-Schwellinger E, Stangier J, Roth W: The metabolism and disposition of the oral direct thrombin inhibitor, dabigatran, in humans. *Drug Metab Dispos* 2008;36(2):386-399.
14. Stangier J, Stähle H, Rathgen K, Fuhr R: Pharmacokinetics and pharmacodynamics of the direct oral thrombin inhibitor dabigatran in healthy elderly subjects. *Clin Pharmacokinet* 2008;47(1): 47-59.
15. Stangier J, Eriksson BI, Dahl OE, et al: Pharmacokinetic profile of the oral direct thrombin inhibitor dabigatran etexilate in healthy volunteers and patients undergoing total hip replacement. *J Clin Pharmacol* 2005;45(5):555-563.
16. Eriksson BI, Quinlan DJ, Weitz JI: Comparative pharmacodynamics and pharmacokinetics of oral direct thrombin and factor Xa inhibitors in development. *Clin Pharmacokinet* 2009;48(1): 1-22.
17. Stangier J: Clinical pharmacokinetics and pharmacodynamics of the oral direct thrombin inhibitor dabigatran etexilate. *Clin Pharmacokinet* 2008;47(5):285-295.
18. Eriksson BI, Dahl OE, Rosencher N, et al: Dabigatran etexilate versus enoxaparin for prevention of venous thromboembolism after total hip replacement: A randomised, double-blind, non-inferiority trial. *Lancet* 2007; 370(9591):949-956.
19. Eriksson BI, Dahl OE, Rosencher N, et al: Oral dabigatran etexilate vs. subcutaneous enoxaparin for the prevention of venous thromboembolism after total knee replacement: The RE-MODEL randomized trial. *J Thromb Haemost* 2007;5(11): 2178-2185.
20. RE-MOBILIZE Writing Committee; Ginsberg JS, Davidson BL, et al: Oral thrombin inhibitor dabigatran etexilate vs the North American enoxaparin regimen for the prevention of venous thromboembolism after knee arthroplasty surgery. *J Arthroplasty* 2009; 24(1):1-9.
21. Eriksson B, Dahl OE, Kurth AA, et al: Oral dabigatran versus enoxaparin for thromboprophylaxis after primary total hip arthroplasty: The RE-NOVATE II randomised trial (Abstract OC645). *Pathophysiol Haemost Thromb* 2010;37(Suppl 1):A20.
22. Leadley RJ Jr: Coagulation factor Xa inhibition: Biological background and rationale. *Curr Top Med Chem* 2001;1(2):151-159.
23. Mann KG, Butenas S, Brummel K: The dynamics of thrombin formation. *Arterioscler Thromb Vasc Biol* 2003;23(1):17-25.
24. Lassen MR, Davidson BL, Gallus A, Pineo G, Ansell J, Deitchman D: The efficacy and safety of apixaban, an oral, direct factor Xa inhibitor, as thromboprophylaxis in patients following total knee replacement. *J Thromb Haemost* 2007;5(12):2368-2375.
25. Lassen MR, Gallus A, Raskob GE, Pineo G, Chen D, Ramirez LM: ADVANCE-3 Investigators: Randomized double blind comparison of apixaban and enoxaparin for thromboprophylaxis after hip replacement. The ADVANCE-3 trial (Abstract #OC356). *Pathophysiol Haemost Thromb* 2010; 37(Suppl 1):A20.
26. Kubitza D, Becka M, Mueck W, Zuehlsdorf M: The effect of extreme age, and gender, on the pharmacology and tolerability of rivaroxaban, an oral, direct factor Xa inhibitor. *Blood* 2006;108(11): 905.
27. Kubitza D, Becka M, Zuehlsdorf M, Mueck W: Body weight has limited influence on the safety, tolerability, pharmacokinetics, or pharmacodynamics of rivaroxaban (BAY 59-7939) in healthy subjects. *J Clin Pharmacol* 2007; 47(2):218-226.
28. Weinz C, Schwarz T, Kubitza D, Mueck W, Lang D: Metabolism and excretion of rivaroxaban, an oral, direct factor Xa inhibitor, in rats, dogs, and humans. *Drug Metab Dispos* 2009;37(5):1056-1064.
29. Kubitza D, Becka M, Mueck W, Zuehlsdorf M: Rivaroxaban (BAY 59-7939), an oral direct factor Xa inhibitor, has no clinically relevant interaction with naproxen. *Br J Clin Pharmacol* 2007;63(4): 469-476.
30. Kubitza D, Becka M, Mueck W, Zuehlsdorf M: Safety, tolerability, pharmacodynamics, and pharmacokinetics of rivaroxaban, an oral direct factor Xa inhibitor, are not affected by aspirin. *J Clin Pharmacol* 2006;46(9):981-990.
31. Kubitza D, Becka M, Mueck W, Zuehlsdorf M: Co-administration of rivaroxaban, a novel, oral, direct factor Xa inhibitor, and clopidogrel in healthy subjects. *Eur Heart J* 2007;28:1272.
32. Kubitza D, Becka M, Zuehlsdorf M: No interaction between the novel, oral direct factor Xa inhibitor BAY 59-7939 and digoxin. *J Clin Pharmacol* 2006; 46:702.
33. Eriksson BI, Borris LC, Dahl OE, et al: Dose-escalation study of rivaroxaban (BAY 59-7939), an oral, direct Factor Xa inhibitor, for the prevention of venous thromboembolism in patients undergoing total hip replacement. *Thromb Res* 2007;120(5): 685-693.
34. Eriksson BI, Borris LC, Dahl OE, et al: Oral, direct factor Xa inhibition with BAY 59-7939 for the prevention of venous thromboembolism after total hip replacement. *J Thromb Haemost* 2006;4(1): 121-128.

35. Eriksson BI, Borris LC, Dahl OE, et al: A once-daily, oral, direct factor Xa inhibitor, rivaroxaban (BAY 59-7939), for thromboprophylaxis after total hip replacement. *Circulation* 2006;114(22): 2374-2381.

36. Turpie AG, Fisher WD, Bauer KA, et al: BAY 59-7939: An oral, direct factor Xa inhibitor for the prevention of venous thromboembolism in patients after total knee replacement. A phase II dose-ranging study. *J Thromb Haemost* 2005;3(11): 2479-2486.

37. Eriksson BI, Borris LC, Friedman RJ, et al: Rivaroxaban versus enoxaparin for thromboprophylaxis after hip arthroplasty. *N Engl J Med* 2008;358(26):2765-2775.

38. Kakkar AK, Brenner B, Dahl OE, et al: Extended duration rivaroxaban versus short-term enoxaparin for the prevention of venous thromboembolism after total hip arthroplasty: A double-blind, randomised controlled trial. *Lancet* 2008;372(9632):31-39.

39. Lassen MR, Ageno W, Borris LC, et al: Rivaroxaban versus enoxaparin for thromboprophylaxis after total knee arthroplasty. *N Engl J Med* 2008;358(26): 2776-2786.

40. Turpie AG, Lassen MR, Davidson BL, et al: Rivaroxaban versus enoxaparin for thromboprophylaxis after total knee arthroplasty (RECORD4): A randomised trial. *Lancet* 2009;373(9676):1673-1680.

41. Eriksson BI, Kakkar AK, Turpie AG, et al: Oral rivaroxaban for the prevention of symptomatic venous thromboembolism after elective hip and knee replacement. *J Bone Joint Surg Br* 2009;91(5): 636-644.

42. Friedman RJ, Turpie AG, Lassen MR, et al: A pooled analysis of four pivotal studies of rivaroxaban for the prevention of venous thromboembolism after hip or knee arthroplasty. *122nd Annual Meeting of the American Orthopaedic Association Proceedings*. Rosemont, IL, American Orthopaedic Association, 2009, p 62.

43. Friedman RJ, Gallus AS, Cushner FD, Fitzgerald G, Anderson FA Jr; Global Orthopaedic Registry Investigators: Physician compliance with guidelines for deep-vein thrombosis prevention in total hip and knee arthroplasty. *Curr Med Res Opin* 2008;24(1): 87-97.

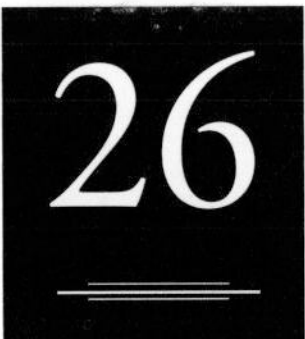

Comparing and Contrasting Current Guidelines for Venous Thromboembolism Prophylaxis After Total Hip and Total Knee Arthroplasty

Paul F. Lachiewicz, MD

Abstract

Orthopaedic surgeons may be impacted by three different clinical venous thromboembolism guidelines: the American College of Chest Physicians guidelines, the Surgical Care Improvement Project guidelines, and, most recently, the American Academy of Orthopaedic Surgeons (AAOS) guideline. The American College of Chest Physicians guidelines use deep venous thrombosis detected by venography or ultrasonography as their primary outcome measure. High-grade recommendations are based on prospective randomized studies only, usually comparing one pharmacologic agent to another. The Surgical Care Improvement Project guidelines are essentially based on the 2004 American College of Chest Physicians guidelines and seek to determine if surgeons prescribe venous thromboembolism prophylaxis within 24 hours of admission. Compliance with these guidelines may affect the quality rating of a particular hospital. The AAOS guideline was designed with the clinical outcome measures of symptomatic pulmonary embolism, fatal pulmonary embolism, major bleeding, and all-cause mortality. This guideline recommends that surgeons preoperatively evaluate the patient's risks (standard or elevated) for pulmonary embolism and serious bleeding and individualize pharmacologic prophylaxis based on a risk-benefit ratio. The three guidelines all have advantages and disadvantages.

Instr Course Lect 2011;60:301-307.

Clinical guidelines in medical specialties and orthopaedic surgery have been devised to standardize and improve patient care for a variety of disorders. A clinical guideline addresses an important clinical problem, has a defined evidence base, and strength of recommendations. These recommendations are reached by both a review of available published medical literature and, when no data exist, through a consensus process of experts in the field. A clinical guideline should also encourage and guide future clinical research in the field. It is important to remember that a clinical guideline is not a predefined protocol or dogmatic statement that is incapable of changing and is not a substitute for sound clinical judgment. Clinical guidelines in orthopaedic surgery have recently addressed the nonsurgical treatment of osteoarthritis of the knee and the treatment of pediatric fractures of the femur. There are currently three clinical guidelines dealing with thromboembolism prophylaxis after total hip and total knee arthroplasty. These are the guidelines of the American College of Chest Physicians (ACCP), the Surgical Care Improvement Project (SCIP), and, most recently, the American Academy of Orthopaedic Surgeons (AAOS). This chapter will compare and contrast the ACCP clinical practice guidelines on the prevention of venous thromboembolism, the SCIP guidelines, and the AAOS clinical guideline: "Prevention of Sympto-

Dr. Lachiewicz or an immediate family member serves as a board member, owner, officer, or committee member of the Hip Society, Southern Orthopaedic Association, and Orthopaedic Surgery and Trauma Society; has received royalties from Innomed; is a member of a speakers' bureau or has made paid presentations on behalf of Zimmer, DJO Global, and Covidien; serves a paid consultant to or is an employee of GlaxoSmithKline; and has received research or institutional support from Zimmer.

matic Pulmonary Embolism in Patients Undergoing Total Hip or Knee Arthroplasty."

ACCP Guidelines

The ACCP is an organization of more than 16,500 members who provide clinical respiratory, sleep, critical care, and cardiothoracic patient care. The venous thromboembolism guidelines proposed by this organization first appeared in 1986, and the most recent eighth edition of the guidelines was published in June 2008.[1] The SCIP guidelines are essentially based on the 2004 ACCP guidelines. Deep venous thrombosis, detected by venography or ultrasonography, was the primary outcome measure in the development of these guidelines. The strongest recommendations (grade 1A) are based on a review of prospective randomized studies only, with most of these studies comparing the efficacy of one pharmacologic agent to another or to a placebo. Few studies were related to mechanical or multimodal (combined) prophylaxis. Surgical patients are grouped as low, medium, or high risk; however, all total hip and knee arthroplasty patients are considered high risk regardless of the patient's age, activity level, and comorbidities.

The 2008 ACCP guidelines contain general recommendations, warnings, and specific recommendations for elective hip and knee arthroplasty.[1] Included in the general recommendations is a grade 1A recommendation that every hospital should develop a formal active strategy for the prevention of venous thromboembolism. Strategies to increase thromboprophylaxis adherence include computer decision support systems (grade 1A) and preprinted orders (grade 1B; these recommendations are less strong than grade 1A recommendations because of the absence of high-quality prospective randomized studies or lesser grades of evidence in published studies on the topic of interest). The warnings include the use of appropriate caution when using anticoagulants in patients undergoing neuraxial anesthesia, analgesia, or deep peripheral nerve blocks (grade 1A).

For elective hip replacement procedures, the guidelines provide a grade 1A recommendation for the routine use of one of the following regimens: low-molecular-weight heparin (LMWH) with the usual high-risk dose (30 mg twice daily) started 12 hours preoperatively or 12 to 24 hours postoperatively, or alternatively, one half the high-risk dose started 4 to 6 hours postoperatively; fondaparinux (2.5 mg) started 6 to 24 hours postoperatively; or warfarin with a target international normalized ratio (INR) of 2.5 (range, 2 to 3). However, for patients with a high risk of bleeding (not specified) treated with hip arthroplasty, the optimal use of mechanical thromboprophylaxis with intermittent pneumatic compression (IPC) is recommended (grade 1A). This last recommendation is a major change from the 2004 ACCP guidelines.

For elective knee replacement procedures, routine thromboprophylaxis with the same anticoagulants listed above was recommended (grade 1A). However, the use of IPC was recommended (grade 1B) as an acceptable alternative to anticoagulants. For knee patients with a high risk of bleeding (not specified), the optimal use of mechanical prophylaxis with IPC (grade 1A) or venous foot pumps (grade 1B) was recommended. For patients treated with hip or knee arthroplasty, the recommended duration of prophylaxis was at least 10 days (grade 1A), with an extension up to 35 days for hip patients (grade 1A). Recommended prophylactic agents for patients treated with hip arthroplasty were LMWH (grade 1A), warfarin (grade 1B), or fondaparinux (grade 1C). For knee patients, extending prophylaxis up to 35 days was not as highly recommended (grade 2B), with grade 1C recommendations for the prophylactic agents of LMWH, warfarin, and fondaparinux.

Orthopaedic Surgeons' Concerns With the ACCP Guidelines

Several orthopaedic surgeons have expressed serious concerns with the ACCP guidelines, which emphasize prophylaxis with strong pharmacologic agents.[2] Asymptomatic thrombi, detected by venography or ultrasonography, are considered as important an outcome as symptomatic thromboembolism. Only data from prospective randomized studies were used to obtain a grade 1A recommendation. Thus, the data from even large (> 1,000 patients) cohort studies of one prophylactic method or multimodal prophylaxis cannot obtain a grade 1A recommendation. Because prospective randomized studies of the efficacy of pharmaceutical agents include only carefully selected patients with few comorbidities, these guidelines may not be applicable to the wide spectrum of patients treated with total hip or total knee arthroplasty. The ACCP guidelines appear to underestimate the risks of bleeding complications and other adverse outcomes, including prolonged wound drainage, hematoma, or deep infection, related to the use of pharmacologic anticoagulants.[2]

The risk of serious bleeding complications has been described in a nonselected group of total hip and knee arthroplasty patients treated with the ACCP grade 1A level recommended 10-day course of LMWH.[3] In this study of 290 patients, major bleeding occurred in 9% of patients, with 4.7% requiring hospital readmission. The efficacy of this protocol was also questioned because symptomatic deep venous thrombosis occurred in 3.8% of patients and nonfatal, symptomatic pulmonary embolism occurred in 1.3%. Another study showed that patients who require surgical treatment for evacuation of a postoperative hematoma within 30 days after total knee arthroplasty are at a significantly increased risk for the development of deep infection or other major surgery.[4]

SCIP Guidelines

SCIP guidelines are voluntary consensus standards, endorsed by the National Quality Forum, for the inpatient hospital care of surgical patients. Hospitals are rated on compliance with a variety of performance measures (standards), including the timing and duration of perioperative antibiotic prophylaxis and thromboembolism prophylaxis for all types of inpatient surgical patients. The thromboembolism guidelines are based on selected surgical procedures from the 2004 ACCP guidelines. The documentation of initiation of prophylaxis 24 hours before surgery to 24 hours after surgery is recommended by a consensus of the SCIP technical expert panel. For elective total hip arthroplasty, any of the following are recommended to be started within 24 hours of surgery: a LMWH (dose not specified), a factor Xa inhibitor (for example, fondaparinux), or warfarin (INR level not specified). Patients who receive neuraxial anesthesia (epidural catheter) or have a documented contraindication to pharmacologic prophylaxis may be considered to have passed the SCIP hospital performance measure if mechanical prophylaxis (with either IPC or a venous foot pump) is ordered.

For elective total knee arthroplasty, any of the following are recommended to be started within 24 hours of surgery: a LMWH (dose not specified), a factor Xa inhibitor, warfarin (target INR not specified), IPC, or a venous foot pump. Patients who receive neuraxial anesthesia or have a documented contraindication to pharmacologic prophylaxis may be considered to have passed the performance measure if either appropriate pharmacologic or mechanical prophylaxis is ordered.

Orthopaedic Surgeons' Concerns With the SCIP Guidelines

There is great concern that the SCIP guidelines are based on the 2004 ACCP guidelines rather than the 2008 ACCP guidelines. The 2004 ACCP guidelines were devised by an expert panel that did not review any references published after 2004. Compliance with these guidelines will apparently be used by regulatory agencies, such as the Joint Commission and the Centers for Medicare and Medicaid Services, to gauge inpatient hospital quality. There has been some mention of considering symptomatic venous thromboembolism as a "pay for performance" event; however, it is not possible to eliminate all symptomatic thromboembolic complications, even if appropriate prophylaxis has been ordered. The SCIP guidelines permit a physician's clinical judgement to withhold pharmacologic prophylaxis if there is a risk of bleeding or when there is a contraindication to pharmacologic prophylaxis.

AAOS Guideline

Symptomatic pulmonary embolism is relatively rare after total hip or total knee arthroplasty. The 90-day rate of fatal pulmonary embolism was 0.22% after 44,785 total hip arthroplasties and 0.15% after 27,000 total knee arthroplasties in the Scottish Registry.[5] In a review of more than 200,000 total knee arthroplasties in a California database, the 90-day rate of symptomatic pulmonary embolism was 0.41%.[6]

In 2006, the AAOS formed a working group to develop a consensus guideline for the prevention of symptomatic pulmonary embolism after total hip and total knee arthroplasty.[7-9] This working group was composed of eight members of the AAOS with known expertise in the field. The group consulted an evidence review team from the Center for Clinical Evidence Synthesis at Tufts-New England Medical Center. The key goals or questions were to determine the rates of fatal and symptomatic pulmonary embolism after total hip and knee arthroplasty with several interventions (aspirin, warfarin, LMWHs, pentasaccharides, and mechanical methods) and the rates of adverse events (bleeding or death) associated with these interventions. The evidence base, determined by a consensus of the working group, was a review of the literature that met certain strict criteria. The selected criteria were as follows: a prospective study of hip or knee arthroplasty procedures performed since 1996; a cohort study with at least 100 patients per group; or a randomized, controlled trial with at least 10 patients per treatment group.[9] There were no recent studies of the natural history (pulmonary embolism without prophylaxis) that included at least 1,000 patients. Studies that included surgical procedures performed before 1996 were excluded because the consensus of the working group was that techniques and postoperative rehabilitation had greatly changed since that time.

The literature review included 2,713 citations from search engines and 10 other articles known to the working group that had not been retrieved by the search engines.[7-9] Only 42 of the 2,723 citations met the pre-

Table 1
AAOS Guideline Recommendations for the Prevention of Symptomatic Pulmonary Embolism After Total Hip and Total Knee Arthroplasty

Recommendation	Level of Evidence/Strength of the Recommendation
Every patient should be evaluated preoperatively by the orthopaedic surgeon for the risk (standard or elevated) of pulmonary embolism.	III/B
Every patient should be evaluated preoperatively (and postoperatively, if necessary) for the risk of bleeding complications (standard or elevated).	III/C
The surgeon should consider placement of an inferior vena cava filter for patients who have contraindications for anticoagulation and an elevated risk for pulmonary embolism.	V/C
The surgeon should consider using mechanical prophylaxis intraoperatively or immediately postoperatively.	III/B
The patient and surgeon should consider (in consultation with the anesthesiologist) the use of regional anesthesia.	IV/C
The surgeon should consider the use of mechanical prophylaxis postoperatively.	IV/C
The patient should be mobilized rapidly.	V/C
Postoperative screening for asymptomatic deep venous thrombosis (with ultrasonography) or pulmonary embolism is not recommended.	III/B
There should be appropriate patient education, before discharge, regarding the early symptoms of venous thromboembolism.	V/B

viously specified criteria of the working group. Of the 42 articles, 26 articles with cohorts totaling 16,304 total hip arthroplasties and 16 articles with cohorts totaling 11,665 total knee arthroplasties were reviewed by the evidence review team. There were numerous limitations in the literature review. No study had pulmonary embolism as the primary outcome measure, and the reporting of pulmonary embolism was often vague. There was great clinical heterogenicity in these studies. Pooled averages were used to estimate event rates because of inadequate sample sizes in many studies. Because of the limitations of the published literature, most of the recommendations have a level of evidence grade of III or IV and a strength of recommendation of B or C.

Conclusions from the literature review of both total hip and total knee arthroplasty studies were described together. The rate of fatal pulmonary embolism was approximately 1 per 1,700 arthroplasties, and there was no difference among prophylactic methods. With any prophylactic method, the rate of nonfatal pulmonary embolism was approximately 1 per 300 arthroplasties. The rate of death from bleeding was approximately 1 per 3,000 arthroplasties. Major bleeding complications were more common in patients treated with systemic pharmacologic prophylaxis (random effects model summary estimate, 1.8%; 95% confidence interval [CI], 1.4% to 2.5%) than in patients treated with mechanical prophylaxis and aspirin (random effects model summary estimate, 0.14%; 95% CI, 0.03% to 0.8%).

The AAOS guideline recommendations were derived from the working group consensus process and the literature review and analysis process.[9] All aspects of the guideline are to be followed, rather than using selective implementation. The working group consensus process established nine recommendations with a level of evidence and strength of the recommendation (**Table 1**).

From the literature review and analysis, the AAOS guideline recommendations for medication are stratified into four groups based on the risk of pulmonary embolism and risk of major bleeding. For patients with a standard risk of pulmonary embolism and a standard risk of major bleeding, either aspirin, a LMWH, a pentasaccharide, or warfarin (INR ≤ 2) is recommended (grade III/B; grade C for dosing and timing). For patients with an elevated risk of pulmonary embolism but a standard risk of major bleeding, a LMWH, a pentasaccharide, or warfarin (INR ≤ 2) is recommended (grade III/B; grade C for dosing and timing). For patients with a standard risk of pulmonary embolism and an elevated risk of major bleeding, aspirin, warfarin (INR ≤ 2), or no medication is recommended (grade III/C). For patients with both an elevated risk of pulmonary embolism and major bleeding, either aspirin, warfarin (INR ≤ 2), or no medication is recommended (grade III/C). The AAOS Board of Directors approved these guideline recommendations in May 2007; the guideline has been published in many formats.[7-9]

Controversy exists as to which patients have an elevated risk for pulmonary embolism. This category would include patients with a prior documented history of symptomatic venous thromboembolism, patients with a history of thrombophilia (for example, factor V Leiden or protein S or C deficiency), patients kept at bed rest or unable to be mobilized rapidly, and patients with other risk factors based on the surgeon's judgment. Patients with an elevated risk for major bleeding include those undergoing complex primary or revision arthroplasties with extensive dissections, or patients with other remote potential bleeding sites.

Several studies support preoperative risk assessment and multimodal thromboprophylaxis, which are the cornerstones of the AAOS guideline.[10-14] Dorr et al[10] reported preoperative assessment and the use of calf compression and aspirin in 1,179 patients treated with total hip or knee arthroplasty, with no fatal pulmonary embolisms and 0.25% nonfatal pulmonary embolisms. In two studies using multimodal prophylaxis, including mechanical prophylaxis (IPC) and aspirin, Westrich et al[11] reported 0.04% fatal and 1% nonfatal pulmonary embolisms in 2,592 total hip arthroplasties and Lachiewicz and Soileau[12] reported 0.09% fatal and 0.7% nonfatal pulmonary embolisms. Lotke and Lonner[13] reported the results of 3,473 total knee arthroplasties treated with foot pumps and aspirin. Preoperatively identified high-risk patients were excluded and given warfarin prophylaxis. With multimodal prophylaxis, the rate of nonfatal pulmonary embolism was 0.26%, and the rate of fatal pulmonary embolism was 0.06% to 0.14%. Lachiewicz and Soileau[14] reported a 0.5% rate of nonfatal pulmonary embolism in 856 total knee arthroplasties in patients treated with calf mechanical compression and aspirin.

Concerns With the AAOS Guideline and ACCP Guidelines

The AAOS guideline has encountered some negative comments and criticisms. Eikelboom et al[15] support the continued use of the ACCP guidelines for hip and knee arthroplasty patients and believe that the use of asymptomatic deep venous thrombosis is a valid surrogate outcome measure for pulmonary embolism. There are some nonarthroplasty studies that show a parallel reduction of deep venous thrombosis and pulmonary embolism when antithrombotic agents are compared to placebo or untreated control groups. However, the position of the AAOS is that there is insufficient evidence to conclude that, in patients treated with total hip or knee arthroplasty, asymptomatic deep venous thrombosis meets the criterion of a valid surrogate marker. The impact of the harm of treatment, especially bleeding, was not addressed in the Eikelboom et al[15] commentary.

There are other criticisms of the AAOS guidelines. Although the studies dealing with total hip and total knee arthroplasty patients were analyzed separately in the AAOS guideline, these two groups of patients are considered as one group for the risk assessment analysis and the recommendations for medication. Because of the lack of prospective randomized studies of symptomatic pulmonary embolism after total hip and knee arthroplasty, most of the recommendations in the AAOS guideline have only a level of evidence of III or IV, rather than level I, as do the strongest recommendations of the ACCP guidelines. The AAOS guideline does not offer any recommendations concerning prophylaxis of asymptomatic deep venous thrombosis other than recommending against routine postoperative screening with ultrasonography. The AAOS guideline is a relatively new document, having been approved by the Board of Directors in May 2007, whereas the ACCP guidelines have been in existence since 1986. The AAOS guideline has, to date, had limited influence on governmental and other agencies that propose regulations and requirements on hospitals that impact reimbursement for the inpatient care of those treated with total hip or knee arthroplasty.

The ACCP guidelines have also encountered some recent criticism regarding methodology. Brown[16] stated that there were four methodological flaws incorporated in the ACCP guidelines. These include (1) exclusion of randomized controlled trials without venographic outcome assessment; (2) lack of measurement of the outcome measures of symptomatic deep venous thrombosis, pulmonary embolism, fatal pulmonary embolism, major surgical site bleeding, and major nonsurgical site bleeding complications; (3) the absence of a meta-analysis or pooled analysis of randomized controlled trials to estimate the incidence of the previously listed outcome measures; and (4) the potential conflicts of interest for several members of the guideline drafting committee. Brown[16] also performed a pooled analysis of the 14 randomized controlled trials cited by the ACCP and included two other randomized controlled trials mentioned but excluded from the ACCP guidelines because the studies did not include venography. There were no statistically significant differences in the rates of symptomatic deep venous thrombosis, pulmonary embolism, and fatal pulmonary embolism with aspirin, vitamin K antagonists, LMWHs, and pentasaccharides.

However, the relative risks of surgical site bleeding with vitamin K antagonists, LMWH, and pentasaccharides were 4.9, 6.4, and 4.2, respectively, compared with aspirin prophylaxis. Sharrock et al[17] also performed a meta-analysis of venous thromboembolism prophylactic studies using 3-month all-cause mortality as the end point. Group A included patients treated with LMWH, ximelagatran, fondaparinux, or rivaroxiban. Group B included patients treated with multimodal prophylaxis (regional anesthesia, pneumatic compression, and aspirin). Group C included patients treated with warfarin. The random effects meta-analysis found that the relative risk of 3-month all-cause mortality in comparing group A with group B was 2.48 (95% CI, 1.28 to 4.32; $P < 0.01$) and in comparing group C with group B was 2.29 (95% CI, 1.06-4.96; $P = 0.03$). Another criticism of the ACCP guidelines is the hypothesized correlation between asymptomatic deep venous thrombosis (detected by venography or ultrasonography) and postphlebitic syndrome with its associated morbidity. At present, there are no level 1 data nor clinical evidence that postphlebitic syndrome is a major complication after total hip or total knee arthroplasty.

Summary

The ACCP, SCIP, and AAOS guidelines dealing with venous thromboembolism prophylaxis differ greatly in their rationale, methodology, and end point analysis. The ACCP guidelines focus on the prevention of asymptomatic deep venous thrombosis, with the strongest recommendations based on randomized controlled trials only. The SCIP guidelines are based on the ACCP guidelines, but meeting a performance measure (prescription of thromboembolism prophylaxis) in the hospital within 24 hours of surgery is the only outcome. The AAOS guideline focuses predominantly on the clinical outcomes of symptomatic pulmonary embolism, fatal pulmonary embolism, and major bleeding. There are advantages and criticisms of all three guidelines. The orthopaedic surgeon must consider the individual patient's risk-benefit ratio in the decision for strong pharmacologic intervention.

References

1. Geerts WH, Bergqvist D, Pineo GF, et al; American College of Chest Physicians: Prevention of venous thromboembolism: American College of Chest Physicians Evidence-Based Clinical Practice Guidelines (8th Edition). *Chest* 2008;133(6, suppl):381S-453S.
2. Callaghan JJ, Dorr LD, Engh GA, et al; American College of Chest Physicians: Prophylaxis for thromboembolic disease: Recommendations from the American College of Chest Physicians. Are they appropriate for orthopaedic surgery? *J Arthroplasty* 2005;20(3): 273-274.
3. Burnett RS, Clohisy JC, Wright RW, et al: Failure of the American College of Chest Physicians-1A protocol for lovenox in clinical outcomes for thromboembolic prophylaxis. *J Arthroplasty* 2007;22(3):317-324.
4. Galat DD, McGovern SC, Hanssen AD, Larson DR, Harrington JR, Clarke HD: Early return to surgery for evacuation of a postoperative hematoma after primary total knee arthroplasty. *J Bone Joint Surg Am* 2008; 90(11):2331-2336.
5. Howie C, Hughes H, Watts AC: Venous thromboembolism associated with hip and knee replacement over a ten-year period: A population-based study. *J Bone Joint Surg Br* 2005;87(12):1675-1680.
6. SooHoo NF, Lieberman JR, Ko CY, Zingmond DS: Factors predicting complication rates following total knee replacement. *J Bone Joint Surg Am* 2006;88(3): 480-485.
7. Haas SB, Barrack RL, Westrich G, Lachiewicz PF: Venous thromboembolic disease after total hip and knee arthroplasty. *J Bone Joint Surg Am* 2008;90(12):2764-2780.
8. Johanson NA, Lachiewicz PF, Lieberman JR, et al: Prevention of symptomatic pulmonary embolism in patients undergoing total hip or knee arthroplasty. *J Am Acad Orthop Surg* 2009;17(3): 183-196.
9. Lachiewicz PF: Prevention of symptomatic pulmonary embolism in patients undergoing total hip and knee arthroplasty: Clinical guideline of the American Academy of Orthopaedic Surgeons. *Instr Course Lect* 2009;58: 795-804.
10. Dorr LD, Gendelman V, Maheshwari AV, Boutary M, Wan Z, Long WT: Multimodal thromboprophylaxis for total hip and knee arthroplasty based on risk assessment. *J Bone Joint Surg Am* 2007; 89(12):2648-2657.
11. Westrich GH, Farrell C, Bono JV, Ranawat CS, Salvati EA, Sculco TP: The incidence of venous thromboembolism after total hip arthroplasty: A specific hypotensive epidural anesthesia protocol. *J Arthroplasty* 1999;14(4): 456-463.
12. Lachiewicz PF, Soileau ES: Multimodal prophylaxis for THA with mechanical compression. *Clin Orthop Relat Res* 2006;453: 225-230.
13. Lotke PA, Lonner JH: The benefit of aspirin chemoprophylaxis for thromboembolism after total knee arthroplasty. *Clin Orthop Relat Res* 2006;452:175-180.
14. Lachiewicz PF, Soileau ES: Mechanical calf compression and

aspirin prophylaxis for total knee arthroplasty. *Clin Orthop Relat Res* 2007;464:61-64.

15. Eikelboom JW, Karthikeyan G, Fagel N, Hirsh J: American Association of Orthopedic Surgeons and American College of Chest Physicians guidelines for venous thromboembolism prevention in hip and knee arthroplasty differ: What are the implications for clinicians and patients? *Chest* 2009;135(2):513-520.

16. Brown GA: Venous thromboembolism prophylaxis after major orthopaedic surgery: A pooled analysis of randomized controlled trials. *J Arthroplasty* 2009;24(6, Suppl):77-83.

17. Sharrock NE, Gonzalez Della Valle A, Go G, Lyman S, Salvati EA: Potent anticoagulants are associated with a higher all-cause mortality rate after hip and knee arthroplasty. *Clin Orthop Relat Res* 2008;466(3):714-721.

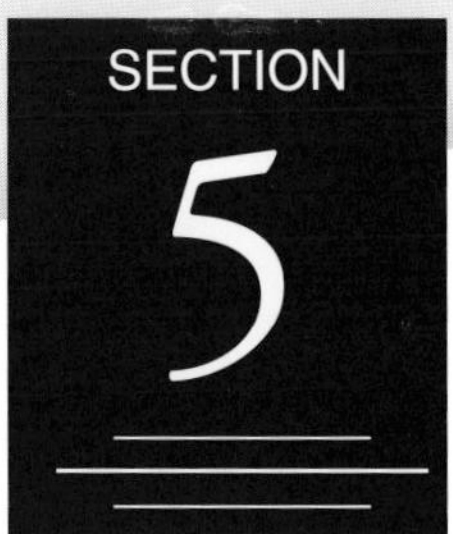

Foot and Ankle

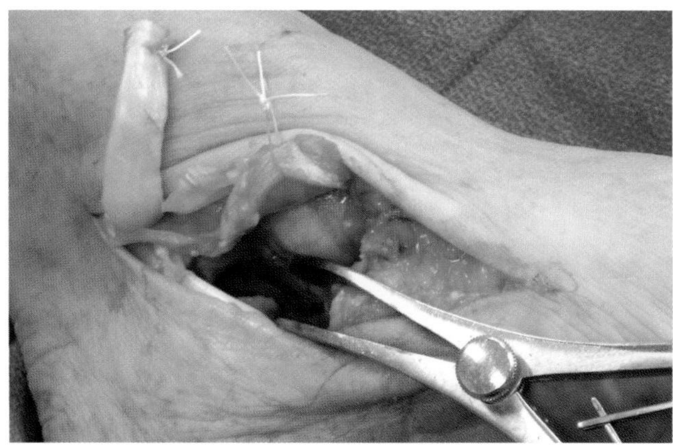

The Use of Arthrodesis to Correct Rigid Flatfoot Deformity

J. Kent Ellington, MD
Mark S. Myerson, MD

Abstract

Rigid adult flatfoot deformity ranges in severity and is caused by a variety of conditions. Treatment is based on the etiology, the severity of symptoms, the stage of the deformity, and patient goals. Posterior tibial tendon pathology, osteoarthritis, posttraumatic arthritis/deformity, inflammatory arthropathy, and neuropathic arthropathy are all known causes of adult flatfoot deformity. Regardless of the cause, treatment goals are the same—restore a plantigrade foot, decrease symptoms, and increase function. When nonsurgical modalities have failed, many surgical reconstructive options are available to restore anatomy and function.

Instr Course Lect 2011;60:311-320.

Anatomy and Pathophysiology

Rigid adult flatfoot deformity (AFD) can evolve over time from a flexible flatfoot deformity, beginning either in childhood or acquired later in adult life, commonly from a rupture of the posterior tibial tendon (PTT). Rigid hindfoot deformity in the adult can also be the result of trauma, osteoarthritis, inflammatory arthropathy, neuromuscular imbalance, or neuroarthropathy. In the child, this deformity results from various types of tarsal coalition or a congenital oblique or vertical talus. It has been shown that the triceps surae has the most significant arch flattening effect in the sagittal plane and also contributes largely to the abduction of the forefoot in the transverse plane.[1,2] As the anatomy of the foot changes, the weight-bearing axis is shifted medially as the hindfoot progresses into more valgus. The cumulative increase of force of the tight triceps results in an increased force across the arch, which weakens, leading to stretching or tearing of the spring ligament, the PTT, and the midfoot joint capsules.[3]

As the arch flattens, the talus plantar flexes and the calcaneus subluxates posteriorly. Consequently, the anterior process of the calcaneus does not support the talar head, and the forefoot and midfoot rotate dorsally and laterally around the talus, leading to a lack of coverage of the talus by the navicular. Continued dorsolateral peritalar subluxation leads to increased stress on the PTT. Whether a weak PTT leads to a deformity or is caused by a deformity is unclear, although it is known that the PTT weakens and may rupture through a degenerative process.[4] However, flatfoot deformity is not solely caused by a weak or ruptured PTT. As the talus assumes a more plantar-flexed position, the spring ligament attenuates or ruptures, leading to a nonlinear talar-first metatarsal axis. Although this deformity occurs predominantly at the talonavicular joint, similar subluxation may occur at either the naviculocuneiform or the tarsometatarsal joints. The plantar-flexed talus pushes the calcaneus further laterally and posteriorly, and the cuboid

Dr. Ellington or an immediate family member has received nonincome support (such as equipment or services), commercially derived honoraria, or other non–research-related funding (such as paid travel) from Smith & Nephew and Wright Medical Technology. Dr. Myerson or an immediate family member has received royalties from DePuy and Biomet; is a member of a speakers' bureau or has made paid presentations on behalf of DePuy, Medtronic, and Orthohelix; serves as a paid consultant to or is an employee of DePuy, Biomet, Orthohelix, Tornier, and Medtronic; serves as an unpaid consultant to DePuy; has received research or institutional support from Biomet and Synthes; and has received nonincome support (such as equipment or services), commercially derived honoraria, or other non–research-related funding (such as paid travel) from Elsevier.

slides with the calcaneus, bringing with it the forefoot and therefore increasing abduction. As the deformity progresses, the calcaneus impinges against the fibula, which leads to another source of stress and lateral foot and ankle pain.[5] Combined with all these described changes, the added deformity leads to deltoid ligament attenuation, causing the ankle to tilt into valgus.[3] It is not clear why a rupture of the deltoid ligament develops in some ankles but not in others. Based on the experience of the senior author (MSM), when the talonavicular joint is severely subluxated, the stress on the ankle (and hence the deltoid ligament) may be minimized because most of the force on the medial ankle is directed across the talonavicular joint. With more rigid deformities, the valgus load on the ankle is greater, and the deltoid is subjected to greater stress and may be more prone to attenuation or rupture.

A rigid deformity implies that the hindfoot cannot be reduced into a neutral position with manual manipulation. The degree of rigidity varies; in some instances, there is absolutely no movement of the subtalar or transverse tarsal joint; in others, some flexibility remains at one of the joints. Also, when manually correcting the heel into neutral position from valgus, there is a very fixed supination deformity of the forefoot. This adaptive forefoot supination compensates for the fixed hindfoot valgus because the forefoot has to progressively supinate to maintain a plantigrade position.[6,7] This forefoot supination deformity may be associated with arthritis or instability of the first tarsometatarsal or the naviculocuneiform joint or with a fixed elevation of the first metatarsal or the entire medial column.

Flatfoot rigidity associated with tarsal coalition, trauma, and arthritides is easy to explain mechanically. The transition from a flexible deformity into a rigid deformity is poorly understood but is likely to represent a gradual mechanical change resulting from increased tension on the triceps surae that leads to flattening of the arch.[1-3] In 1939, Todd[8] suggested that the change from a flexible to a rigid deformity was caused by habitual overstrain in patients who are developmentally weak. In 1948, Lapidus[9] stated the transition was caused by injury to the interosseous ligament of the subtalar joint. The long-lasting incongruity of the affected joints leads to arthrosis, soft-tissue contractures, and, finally, a rigid deformity. It is likely that the gradual attenuation of the medial soft-tissue structures, including the PTT, the spring ligament, and the talonavicular capsule, is followed by contraction of the lateral soft tissues, including the peroneal muscles and the interosseous ligament. This is followed by adaptive changes in the periarticular capsuloligamentous structures, ultimately leading to the rigid deformity.

Patient Evaluation

It is useful to examine the patient while he or she is standing and walking. The entire lower extremity should be visible, and the foot should be inspected from the front, above, and behind the patient. With the patient standing and the examiner viewing from behind the patient, the patient should be asked to stand up on the toes of both feet and then one foot (a double- and single-limb heel rise). Patients with a rigid deformity are unable to perform a single-limb heel rise, and even a double-limb heel rise may be impossible because of weakness or pain. Regardless of the magnitude of the deformity, if the hindfoot is flexible, during the heel rise the hindfoot will transition into varus and the arch will reconstitute. The strength of the PTT is not relevant in the management of a rigid deformity, but the location of pain and tenderness is important. The range of motion of the ankle and the subtalar, transverse tarsal, and first tarsometatarsal joints must be evaluated because each component of the deformity, stiffness, and compensatory motion must be addressed surgically. Additional associated features of a rigid valgus deformity are subfibular impingement between the tip of the fibula and the lateral margin of the calcaneus and varying degrees of fixed lateral subluxation or abduction of the talonavicular joint, referred to as uncovering of the talar head. In a longstanding deformity, this may lead to callus formation under the plantar medial head of the talus as well as the navicular. These fixed articular deformities are in addition to the contracture of the peroneal tendons and the Achilles or the gastrocnemius muscle. With repetitive subfibular impingement, the fibula is compressed; this, in addition to the fixed valgus deformity of the hindfoot, can lead to a stress fracture of the fibula, which is generally approximately 6 cm proximal to the tip. The fibula usually heals in slight valgus, further perpetuating the valgus deformity of the hindfoot but now also potentially causing a valgus deformity of the ankle joint. Additional medial ankle pain can result from stretching the tibial nerve and tarsal tunnel syndrome.

In these patients, it is important to evaluate ankle stability in the coronal plane for both medial and lateral instability. The medial instability is straightforward and is associated with attenuation or rupture of the deltoid ligament. With chronic, rigid, hindfoot valgus deformity, the lateral aspect is compressed against the fibula, which can lead to erosion of the calcaneofibular ligament and ultimately to multiplanar coronal plane instability. The texture of the skin is important because patients with chronic, fixed, hindfoot valgus deformity, particularly those with any rheumatologic disease and any venous stasis, have taut lateral skin. When the foot is corrected from fixed valgus to a neutral position of the hindfoot, there is marked stretching of the lateral skin, which can lead to wound dehiscence and infection. If the skin is very taut laterally, it is preferable to use a medial approach to correct the hindfoot deformity, avoiding any lateral incision.

Weight-bearing radiographs are required, including AP and lateral views of the foot, a hindfoot alignment view, and an AP view of the ankle.[10] On the AP radiograph of the foot, the talonavicular coverage, the extent of forefoot abduction, and any secondary changes in the midfoot, including arthritis and/or deformity of the tarsometatarsal and naviculocuneiform joints, are evaluated. On the lateral foot radiograph, the talometatarsal angle (normal angle, 0° to 10°) and the distance of the medial cuneiform from the floor should be measured (normal distance, 15 to 25 mm), along with careful inspection for a subtalar coalition and any changes of the talonavicular joint, such as talar beaking. The oblique foot radiograph also should be inspected for a calcaneonavicular coalition, which can lead to a rigid deformity. The ankle series should be evaluated for any valgus tilt in the tibiotalar joint. Fluoroscopic examination is useful to evaluate the mobility and stability of the ankle joint, particularly in a patient with a valgus deformity of the ankle with or without associated arthritis. It is important to determine if the ankle valgus deformity is passively correctable because this may determine the type of surgery needed; ideally, this examination should be performed fluoroscopically. MRI has no value in preoperative planning, unless severe osteonecrosis of the talus is present and associated with a rigid ankle and hindfoot deformity. A CT scan may be useful to determine the alignment of the calcaneus relative to the talus and confirm the extent of peritalar subluxation as well as fracture of the sustentaculum, which occurs in severe cases of peritalar subluxation. These scans are rarely taken with any weight or pressure on the subtalar joint and should be carefully interpreted.[11]

Classification

In 1989, Johnson and Strom[12] described three clinical stages of PTT dysfunction. This classification was modified in 1997 by Myerson[13] by adding a fourth stage, which is defined as the presence of ankle valgus caused by a rupture of the deltoid ligament with or without arthritis of the ankle joint. The classification of flatfoot deformity was further refined by Bluman et al[14] in 2007. In the Myerson classification, although stage III is still characterized by rigid hindfoot valgus, it is further defined by the presence of forefoot abduction. In stage IIIA, the deformity is corrected by a triple arthrodesis. In stage IIIB, the forefoot abduction is so severe that to correct the deformity, the triple arthrodesis is combined with bone graft lengthening of the calcaneocuboid joint. Additional procedures, such as Achilles lengthening, medial cuneiform osteotomy, medial column arthrodesis, and lengthening or transfer of the peroneal or anterior tibial tendons, are performed as necessary.

Treatment

Nonsurgical treatment can be successful despite the rigidity of the deformity. Although an orthotic arch support cannot correct the fixed deformity, a soft, multilayered, arch support may provide relief of the bone prominence of the head of the talus. If more support is required, a custom, molded, leather, ankle gauntlet referred to as a Baldwin or Arizona brace should be considered. The brace fits into a comfortable shoe and stabilizes the ankle area and the talocalcaneal, midtarsal, and subtalar joints. It provides medial and lateral stability to minimize sinus tarsi impingement and reduce forefoot motion. The brace improves the function of the limb for most patients but does not correct the deformity, which can progress if the brace is not worn.

Most patients eventually stop wearing the brace and elect surgery to correct the deformity. The goal of surgery is to provide a plantigrade foot, decrease pain, and increase function. Because there are many surgical options available, choosing the procedure(s) to correct the deformity is dependent on the stage of deformity and the patient's goals, age, weight considerations (such as obesity), and the presence of arthritis. Usually, a rigid flatfoot deformity must be treated with an arthrodesis of some type, supplemented with osteotomy and tendon transfer as required. It is important to recognize the characteristics of a deformity that is too stiff or "not flexible enough" to correct with tendon transfer or osteotomy, the latter of which is always preferable to maximize and maintain motion in the hindfoot. If the hindfoot is stiff, adequate deformity correction is unlikely without arthrodesis, and the option of tendon transfer should not be advocated. The hindfoot can often be manually reduced to neutral; however, this is accompanied by severe forefoot supination deformity. In some instances, the "feel" of this examination may help the examiner determine that arthrodesis is preferable, has a greater degree of predictability, and will adequately meet the patient's needs. Although arthrodesis is generally used to correct a rigid deformity, under certain circumstances it may also be indicated in a patient with a flexible flatfoot. For example, in an obese patient, a tendon transfer and hindfoot osteotomies have a higher chance of failure. In some patients with severe laxity of the hindfoot (whether associated with generalized ligamentous laxity, hypermobility, or a rupture of the spring ligament), a talonavicular arthrodesis may be a more predictable procedure.

Several procedures are available for treating a rigid flatfoot, and should be added in sequence in a systematic approach commencing with reduction of the subtalar joint and then moving distally depending on the presence of additional deformity. The heel should be reduced to a more physiologic valgus, the subfibular impingement should be corrected, and the medial arch pain and deformity eliminated. The surgical options listed in this chapter include the type of procedure along with a description of the technique and indications. In all cases, equinus should be evaluated, and an Achilles lengthening procedure should be performed (gastrocnemius recession versus tendon Achilles lengthening if appropriate).

Triple Arthrodesis

Triple arthrodesis is a very common procedure for correcting a rigid flatfoot deformity. The phrase "triple arthrodesis" was first used by Ryerson[15] in 1923. This procedure was traditionally performed with joint preparation without any internal fixation and with a long-leg plaster cast. By the early 1980s, there was less reliance on cast immobilization and various types of more rigid internal fixation became more commonly used for correction. With these changes in fixation methods, there was a marked increase in the rate of union, but there were also potential disadvantages, including an increase in varus malunion from overcorrecting the talonavicular joint.[16] Although the surgical goal is to create a functional plantigrade foot, preserving motion is also important. In some instances, a modification of the triple arthrodesis procedure is used on the hindfoot joints, such as a talonavicular and subtalar arthrodesis or a subtalar and calcaneocuboid arthrodesis. This approach must be carefully considered because a single or double arthrodesis cannot correct deformity as reliably as a triple arthrodesis. Although the approach to the procedure may have changed over the decades, triple arthrodesis has remained a standard for correcting severe deformity regardless of the etiology.

Surgical Approaches

Single-Incision Lateral Approach

The traditional triple arthrodesis was originally performed through a single-incision lateral approach through the sinus tarsi, but the incidence of complications, including persistent deformity and nonunion, was common with this approach because of limited visualization of the talonavicular joint. A cadaver model evaluating preparation of the three joints using the single lateral approach showed that the cartilage can be successfully removed in 90% of the calcaneocuboid joint, 80% of the subtalar joint, but only 38% of the talonavicular joint. Additional reported complications included obliteration of the talonavicular joint, inadvertent division of the talar neck or talar head, removal of excess bone, medial skin punctures, and an iatrogenic cut through the talar dome.[17] Over the past two decades, the two-incision technique has become far more popular because it allows the surgeon to better visualize the adequate preparation, reduction, and alignment of the joints.

Two-Incision Approach

With the patient supine, a lateral incision is made, extending from the tip of the fibula to the base of the fourth metatarsal. The sural nerve is retracted plantarly, the peroneal tendons are protected, and the extensor digitorum brevis is elevated dorsally and preserved. The sinus tarsi is opened, débrided, and distracted with a laminar spreader to visualize the subtalar joint. Care must be taken to remove all the cartilage from the entire posterior, middle, and anterior facets, followed by perforation of the subchondral plate with systematic drilling of both the talus and the calcaneus with a 2.0-mm drill bit at 2-mm intervals, generating abundant bone slurry. A 5-mm, curved osteotome is then used to shingle the joint surfaces to further generate a good cancellous bed of bone. The calcaneocuboid joint is prepared in a similar manner. Next, a dorsomedial incision just medial to the anterior tibial tendon is made. This joint is much more difficult to visualize, and although a laminar spreader can be used to try to twist open the joint for distraction, the talar bone quality may be poor, causing the head of the talus to be crushed by the spreader. It may be easier to use a pin distractor to open the joint, which is then prepared as previously described, along with drill holes, which are particularly important if the navicular is sclerotic. It is essential to preserve the bone on both joint surfaces, maintaining the contour of the talonavicular joint. If bone is inadvertently removed, the medial column of the foot will shorten, followed by a varus malunion.

The sequence of fixation is subjective, but this chapter's authors believe that the talonavicular joint should be fixed first because this joint functions as the hinge to the hindfoot. If the deformity is mild to moderate, the talonavicular joint is always corrected first, followed by the subtalar joint, which "falls into place." With the talonavicular joint held reduced, the first ray is plantar flexed by dorsiflexing the hallux, which further corrects the forefoot relative to the hindfoot. If there is a complete peritalar dislocation, the subtalar joint is reduced first because it is difficult to translate the subtalar joint medially and simultaneously correct heel valgus in these very severe deformities. In contrast, if the subtalar joint is reduced first, it is easy to overcorrect the talonavicular joint; this overcorrection must be avoided to prevent a varus or adductus malunion. Two points of fixation of the talonavicular joint are recommended. This chapter's authors use one 5.0-mm screw from distal to proximal in compression mode along with a two-hole locking compression plate placed more dorsolaterally. The subtalar joint is fixed next with one 7-mm screw, followed by fixation of the calcaneocuboid joint. It is useful to notch the side of the calcaneus for insertion of the 5-mm screw into the calcaneocuboid joint to prevent splitting the distal calcaneus. Alternatively, a plate or staples can be used quite effectively to compress the calcaneocuboid joint. If a gap is present in the calcaneocuboid joint following correction of pronounced forefoot abduction, it may be necessary to lengthen the lateral column through the calcaneocuboid joint using a structural bone block graft. The results of simultaneous triple arthrodesis and lateral column lengthening are favorable.[18]

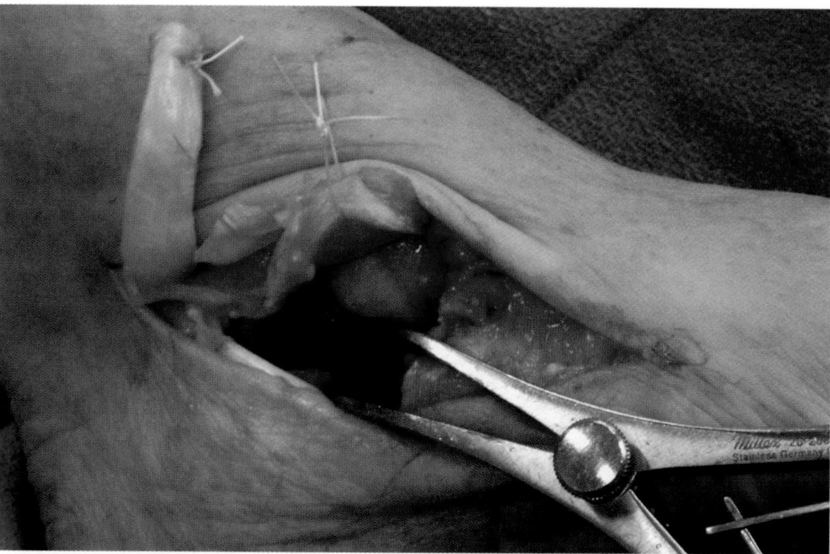

Figure 1 Intraoperative photograph of the medial approach for a triple arthrodesis to correct a hindfoot deformity.

Single-Incision Medial Approach

Variations of standard triple arthrodesis have been described for correcting rigid hindfoot deformity, including more limited fusions of either the talonavicular and the subtalar joints or the subtalar and the calcaneocuboid joints. A single-incision medial approach also has been used with a predictable outcome to perform triple arthrodesis in patients who are at risk for wound healing complications associated with correcting a hindfoot valgus deformity.[19] This approach can be accomplished through a rather small incision (**Figure 1**). Jeng et al[19] treated 17 patients with a rigid hindfoot valgus deformity using triple arthrodesis with a single medial incision. The indication for surgery was refractory pain associated with hindfoot valgus deformities in patients with taut lateral skin and poor skin conditions laterally because of contracture. The severity of the hindfoot deformity itself was not the indication for this procedure. A subtalar and talonavicular arthrodesis was achieved in all patients and an asymptomatic nonunion of the calcaneocuboid arthrodesis was reported in 2 of 17 patients. In a cadaver study, Jeng et al[20] showed that through the single medial incision, 91% of the subtalar, 91% of the talonavicular, and 90% calcaneocuboid joints could be prepared. The medial approach to either a triple or a hindfoot double arthrodesis is a reliable procedure that can be used in patients with poor-quality lateral skin and a fixed hindfoot valgus deformity and in those in whom correction with a two-incision approach could lead to a lateral wound complication. Brilhault[21] performed a subtalar and talonavicular arthrodesis procedure in 11 patients and reported the occurrence of wound healing and arthrodesis as well as an asymptomatic calcaneocuboid joint in all patients. More importantly, significant radiographic improvements were reported in the AP talonavicular coverage angle (from 38.5° to 7°), the lateral talonavicular–first metatarsal angle (from 21° to 0°), and the hindfoot-frontal alignment angle (from 18° to 7.5°).

As this chapter's authors gained more experience with the medial approach to correct deformity, it became apparent that the calcaneocuboid joint does not always need to be included in the arthrodesis. More recently, this chapter's authors have attempted to treat most rigid AFDs with a single medial incision, either including the calcaneocuboid joint or not including that joint, depending on the ability to completely correct the deformity. The isolated subtalar and talonavicular arthrodesis must be performed with caution because inferior subluxation of the cuboid relative to the calcaneus

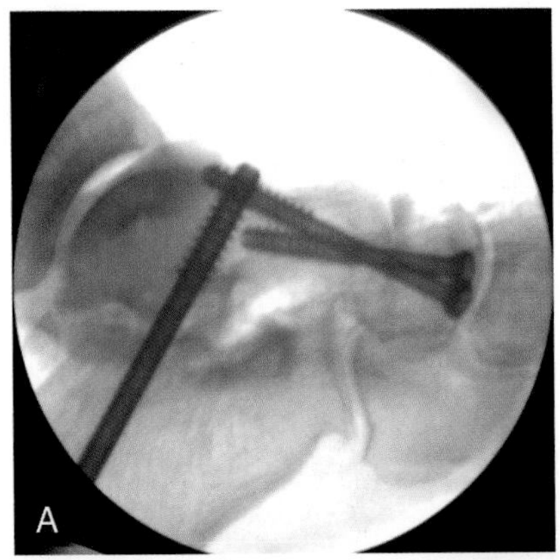

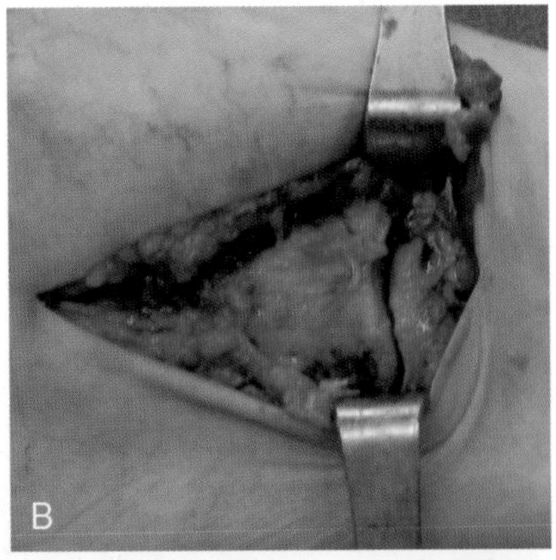

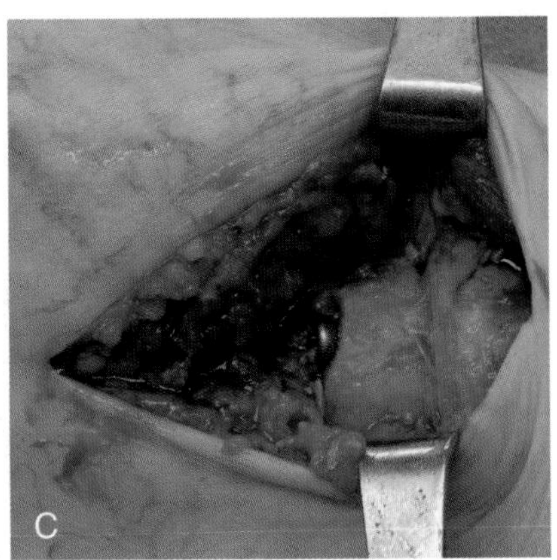

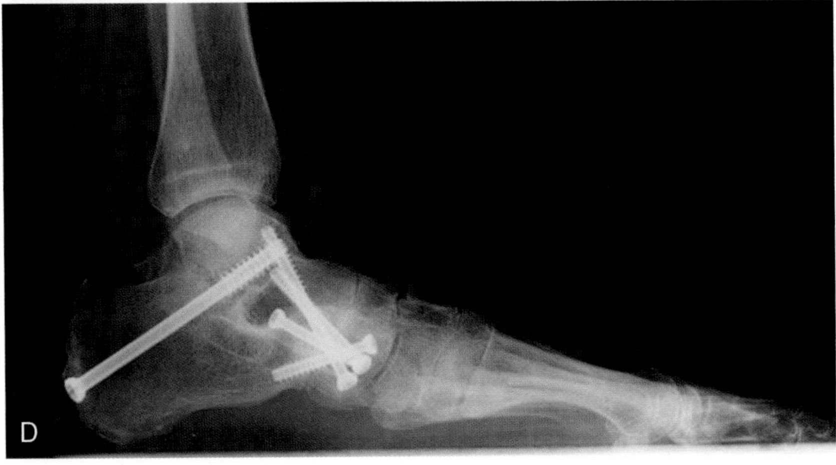

Figure 2 **A,** Lateral radiograph of the foot after a double arthrodesis showing subluxation of the calcaneocuboid joint. **B,** Photograph of the foot after a double arthrodesis showing subluxation of the calcaneocuboid joint. **C,** Photograph of the foot after reduction and fixation of the subluxated calcaneocuboid joint. **D,** Lateral radiograph of the foot after reduction and fixation of the subluxated calcaneocuboid joint.

may occur, resulting in a fixed rotation of the transverse tarsal joint, which will then lead to pain under the cuboid and the base of the fifth metatarsal (**Figure 2**).

Adjunctive Procedures

Following any hindfoot arthrodesis, adjunctive procedures are frequently necessary to achieve the desired correction of a plantigrade foot. To some extent, these procedures must be planned ahead of the triple arthrodesis because the incisions may vary slightly as these additional osteotomies and tendon transfers are performed. With a severe abduction deformity, correction may be difficult because of peroneal tendon contracture; the tendons can be lengthened or cut or the peroneus brevis can be transferred to the peroneus longus. The latter procedure has a twofold purpose—to lengthen the lateral contracted tendon and improve the plantar-flexion strength of the first metatarsal. With very severe inferior subluxation of the talus under the navicular, there is a contracture of the anterior tibial tendon, which then elevates the first ray even further and adds to the deformity. In some instances, correction of the sagittal alignment of the first ray cannot be attained without lengthening or a lateral transfer of the anterior tibial tendon. The elevation and/or the anterior tibial tendon may need to be released if the desired correction cannot be obtained. Correcting the medial column alignment in the sagittal plane is essential to the success of a triple arthrodesis because loss of medial column support will lead to insufficient weight bearing, which forces the hindfoot into valgus and creates further deformity. As the medial column support fails, even if the talonavicular joint is fused, the subtalar joint must evert to maintain a plantigrade foot. Naviculocuneiform arthrodesis, first tarsometatarsal arthrodesis, or a medial cuneiform opening wedge osteotomy are correction options determined by the location of the deformity and the instability. If fixed forefoot supination is present following the triple arthrodesis, and no arthritis at either the naviculocuneiform or first tarsometatarsal joints is present, it is preferable to maintain as much motion in these joints as possible, performing the realignment at the level of the medial cuneiform. Although the addition of a medial column arthrodesis to the triple arthrodesis adds to the stiffness of the foot and the potential for arthritis at the remaining open medial joint, these deformities cannot be ignored. Restoring the medial column alignment after naviculocuneiform arthrodesis may

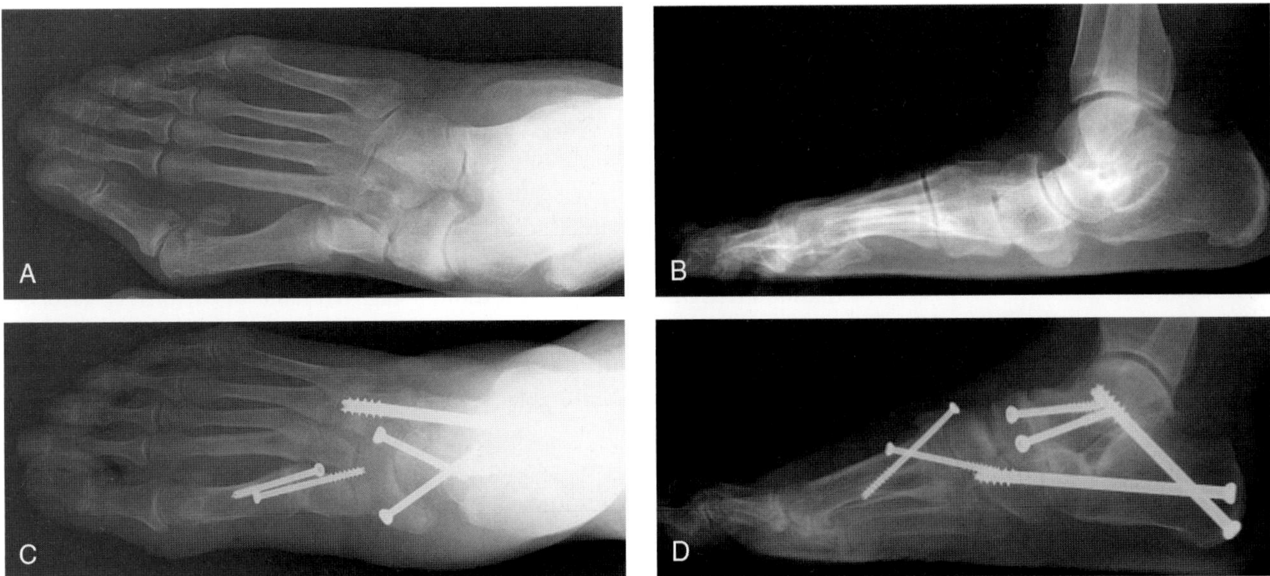

Figure 3 **A,** AP preoperative radiograph of a rigid flatfoot with hallux valgus and instability of the first tarsometatarsal joint. **B,** Lateral radiograph of a rigid flatfoot with hallux valgus and instability of the first tarsometatarsal joint. **C,** Postoperative AP radiograph after a triple arthrodesis and first tarsometatarsal arthrodesis. **D,** Postoperative lateral radiograph of the foot after a triple arthrodesis and first tarsometatarsal arthrodesis.

provide a link between stability of the midfoot and alignment of the hindfoot.[22]

First tarsometatarsal joint arthrodesis is a reliable technique to stabilize the medial column and correct forefoot supination following a triple arthrodesis, especially in the presence of arthritis, instability, metatarsus elevatus, or hallux valgus. It is important to note that this joint is very deep, measuring up to 30 mm, and failure to prepare the plantar aspect of the joint will result in an undesirable dorsal malunion. Fixation is ideally performed with two axial compression screws, although staples or a plate have been successfully used for fixation of this joint (**Figure 3**). In 182 patients treated with a first tarsometatarsal joint arthrodesis as a part of an AFD reconstruction or correction of hallux valgus, no nonunions of the first tarsometatarsal joint were reported when the procedure was performed as part of the AFD correction.[23]

When the hindfoot is fixed in severe valgus, the medial shift of the subtalar joint in conjunction with the triple arthrodesis may not be sufficient. There may be erosion of the lateral subtalar joint, and correction cannot adequately be obtained without an additional medial translational osteotomy of the calcaneus. This procedure must be planned ahead because the incision may vary if the osteotomy is performed simultaneously, by either extending the sinus tarsi incision posteriorly or using a second oblique incision directly inferior to the peroneal tendons over the calcaneus. Following exposure, débridement, and joint preparation of the subtalar joint, the osteotomy is performed and provisionally fixed with Kirschner wires or guide pins. The screws can extend into the talus, simultaneously correcting and fixing both the calcaneus osteotomy and the subtalar joint (**Figure 4**).

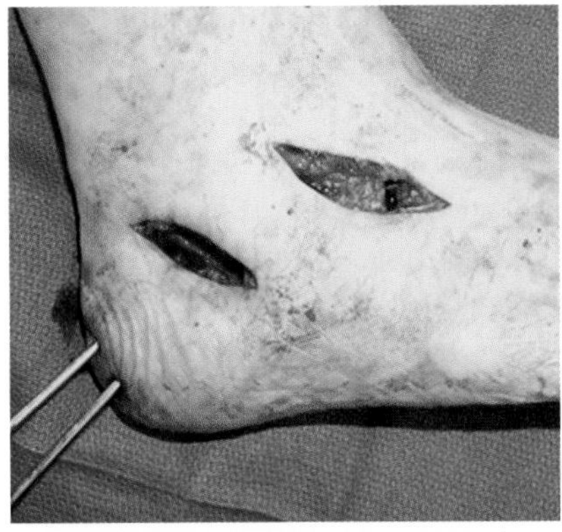

Figure 4 Photograph showing the ability to achieve fixation of both a medial displacement calcaneal osteotomy and subtalar arthrodesis.

Management of the Unstable Ankle

The stability of the ankle should be checked following fixation of the triple arthrodesis, not only for attenuation or rupture of the deltoid ligament but also for lateral ankle instability (particularly for those procedures that are performed for a severe valgus deformity). Chronic valgus impingement between the calcaneus and the fibula may lead to erosion of the calcaneofibular ligament and subsequent ankle instability. If lateral ankle instability is present, it must be stabilized to prevent subsequent ankle arthritis. There is

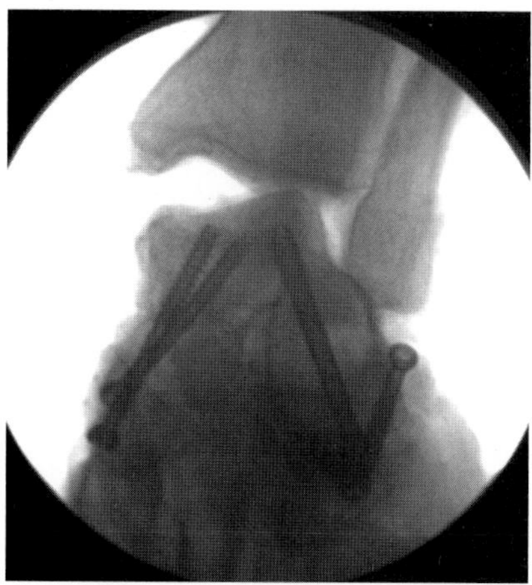

Figure 5 Fluoroscopic image showing an incompetent deltoid after a triple arthrodesis.

never sufficient tissue present to perform a simple reconstruction using a Broström-type procedure; therefore, some reconstruction using the peroneal tendon is preferable. This chapter's authors use a modified Chrisman-Snook procedure.[24] A rupture of the deltoid (stage IV deformity) can be corrected in a variety of ways. The ankle must be examined to determine if the deformity is passively correctable (stage IV-A) or if it is rigid (stage IV-B). Fluoroscopic examination at the time of the triple arthrodesis is helpful, but it is preferable to perform it ahead of time to anticipate the planned procedure (**Figure 5**). In stage IV-B deformity or if the ankle deformity is flexible but associated with arthritis, it should be corrected with either a tibiotalocalcaneal arthrodesis or a pantalar arthrodesis. Total ankle replacement in this setting is highly unreliable, and a fixed valgus deformity of the ankle is best treated with arthrodesis. The use of an intramedullary rod is preferred for primary and revision arthrodesis, especially in revision surgeries for correcting a stage IV deformity. Although tibiotalocalcaneal and pantalar fusions are successful in obtaining a plantigrade foot, there can be associated morbidity. Even after successful fusion, the energy expenditure of ambulation is increased, and functionality and patient satisfaction are decreased.[25] For managing a stage IV-A deformity, the ankle joint can be preserved with a variety of ligament reconstruction techniques performed following the necessary hindfoot and midfoot realignment. The correction of the hindfoot and midfoot alignment must be obtained, with particular attention to ensuring good, stable alignment of the medial column; a first tarsometatarsal arthrodesis should be performed if necessary. Studies have shown that a medial translational osteotomy of the calcaneus is also beneficial because it decreases the valgus force on the deltoid ligament.[26] If the stage IV deformity is associated with malunion of a previously performed hindfoot arthrodesis, then either the correction should be made at the ankle joint in stage IV-B deformities or a revision arthrodesis should be followed by a deltoid reconstruction.

Deltoid reconstruction falls into three categories: repair of the ligament, advancement of the ligament, or the use of a tendon graft (either an autograft or an allograft).[27-30] The local remnant of the deltoid ligament, PTT, and capsule are not sufficient to maintain long-term correction, and failure of these approaches has been reported.[26] This chapter's authors recommend a technique that uses a forked semitendinosus allograft tendon in conjunction with soft-tissue interference screws to reconstruct the deep tibiotalar ligaments and the superficial calcaneofibular fibers. The graft is anchored in a tibial tunnel that is created parallel to the joint at the level of the physeal scar. After a Krackow suture is placed in the distal end of the tendon, it is then passed subcutaneously over the medial malleolus. A talar tunnel is created, and the tendon is passed, manually tensioned, then secured. Next, a calcaneal tunnel is created, and the tendon is passed, tensioned, then secured.[26]

Results

The results of triple arthrodesis for AFD have been studied extensively. A series of 32 triple arthrodeses for stage III and IV deformity (average follow-up, 4.3 years) showed improvement in American Orthopaedic Foot and Ankle Society scores by 36 points, with all but one patient reporting satisfaction with the procedure. There was one nonunion and two malunions.[31] Similarly, in a series of 44 feet (9 with AFD), 34 had good results.[32] In a study of the results of triple arthrodesis in 132 feet (average follow-up, 5.7 years), Pell et al[33] reported an overall patient satisfaction score of 8.3 of 10. Interestingly, 60% of the patients had clear radiographic progression of ankle arthritis, but this did not correlate with patient satisfaction. The longest outcome data available in the literature on triple arthrodesis shows a 95% patient satisfaction rate at 40-year follow-up.[34]

Limited Hindfoot Arthrodesis Procedures

As previously discussed, an isolated talonavicular arthrodesis cannot correct excessive hindfoot valgus or instability of the midfoot joints. It has been shown in a cadaver model that isolated talonavicular fusion was as powerful as both the triple and double arthrodesis; however, it reduced hindfoot motion by 80%.[35] An isolated talonavicular arthrodesis is occasionally indicated for managing rigid flatfoot deformity, but it may be better indicated for severe hypermobility associated with a rupture of the spring ligament and a flexible flatfoot deformity. The talonavicular joint is the apex of the deformity in AFD,[35] and certainly most of the transverse tarsal joint deformity and abduction of the midfoot can be corrected with an isolated talonavicular arthrodesis. Residual hindfoot valgus remains a concern with this technique, and a medial displacement calcaneal osteotomy can be added if necessary to correct the heel deformity. At 27-month follow-up, 26 patients with AFD treated with an isolated talonavicular arthrodesis had favorable outcomes with no pain or pain only after heavy use. Although the procedure was performed for patients with AFD, it was not reported if the deformity was flexible or rigid. A successful fusion was achieved in all the patients and no loss of correction was reported. Mild asymptomatic adjacent joint arthritis was reported in five patients, and ankle plantarflexion was decreased by 10°.[36,37]

A double arthrodesis (talonavicular and calcaneocuboid joints) has been described with an overall satisfaction rate of 83% with the procedure.[38,39] Progressive degeneration of the surrounding joints was common, and the most frequent complication was nonunion at the talonavicular joint. The authors stressed that this procedure was indicated only in rigid flatfeet in which the principle deformity was at the transverse tarsal joints, with no subtalar arthritis present.[39]

Isolated subtalar arthrodesis is an effective procedure for stage II and some stage III deformities.[40] This approach is recommended only when most of the deformity originates from the subtalar joint, less than 30% of the talonavicular joint is uncovered, pain is isolated to the lateral foot and sinus tarsi, and arthritis is present in the subtalar joint; it can also be used as a salvage procedure for a failed prior reconstruction. A subtalar arthrodesis may be performed in conjunction with a flexor digitorum longus transfer and supplemented by a medial column procedure as necessary to correct forefoot supination and instability. In patients with a somewhat flexible deformity that could be treated with tendon transfer and osteotomy, this approach may provide more durable results, particularly if associated with inflammatory arthropathy or obesity. The benefit of isolated subtalar fusion is joint preservation of the transverse tarsal joint. A cadaver study showed a 39% loss of eversion and a 41% loss of inversion with subtalar arthrodesis, with minimal affect on dorsiflexion and plantarflexion.[41] Extending the fusion to a triple arthrodesis showed a 16% reduction in plantarflexion and a 13% decrease in dorsiflexion. The triple arthrodesis also resulted in an additional 20% loss of eversion and 22% loss of inversion. Studies evaluating isolated subtalar arthrodesis for AFD in conjunction with flexor digitorum longus transfer have reported good results.[42,43]

Summary

The surgical management of rigid AFD requires a systematic approach. A careful patient history, a thorough examination, and a detailed review of weight-bearing radiographs are paramount in determining the etiology and the stage of the deformity. After this is achieved, a well-planned surgery can be devised. Many options exist for surgical correction. Careful patient selection and meticulous technique are required for successful outcomes. Regardless of the surgical reconstruction, the goal is a long-lasting plantigrade foot.

References

1. Thordarson DB, Schmotzer H, Chon J, Peters J: Dynamic support of the human longitudinal arch: A biomechanical evaluation. *Clin Orthop Relat Res* 1995;316: 165-172.
2. Pedowitz WJ, Kovatis P: Flatfoot in the adult. *J Am Acad Orthop Surg* 1995;3(5):293-302.
3. Harris RI, Beath T: Hypermobile flat-foot with short tendo achillis. *J Bone Joint Surg Am* 1948; 30A(1):116-140.
4. Mosier SM, Pomeroy G, Manoli A II: Pathoanatomy and etiology of posterior tibial tendon dysfunction. *Clin Orthop Relat Res* 1999;365:12-22.
5. Malicky ES, Crary JL, Houghton MJ, Agel J, Hansen ST Jr, Sangeorzan BJ: Talocalcaneal and subfibular impingement in symptomatic flatfoot in adults. *J Bone Joint Surg Am* 2002;84-A(11): 2005-2009.
6. Hansen ST: Progressive symptomatic flat foot (lateral peritalar subluxation), in Hansen ST, ed: *Functional Reconstruction of the Foot and Ankle.* Philadelphia, PA, Lippincott Willams & Wilkins, 2000, pp 195-207.
7. Mann RA: Flatfoot in adults, in Coughlin MJ, Mann RA, eds: *Surgery of the Foot and Ankle,* ed 7. St Louis, MO, Mosby, 1999, pp 733-767.
8. Todd AH: The treatment of pes cavus. *Proc R Soc Med* 1934;28(2): 117-128.
9. Lapidus PW: The so-called longitudinal arch: Some new thoughts. *Am J Phys Anthropol* 1948; 6(2): 241.
10. Saltzman CL, el-Khoury GY: The hindfoot alignment view. *Foot Ankle Int* 1995;16(9):572-576.
11. Ananthakrisnan D, Ching R, Tencer A, Hansen ST Jr, Sangeorzan BJ: Subluxation of the talocalcaneal joint in adults who have symptomatic flatfoot. *J Bone Joint Surg Am* 1999;81(8):1147-1154.
12. Johnson KA, Strom DE: Tibialis posterior tendon dysfunction. *Clin Orthop Relat Res* 1989;239: 196-206.
13. Myerson MS: Adult acquired flatfoot deformity: Treatment and

dysfunction of the posterior tibial tendon. *Instr Course Lect* 1997;46: 393-405.

14. Bluman EM, Title CI, Myerson MS: Posterior tibial tendon rupture: A refined classification system. *Foot Ankle Clin* 2007; 12(2): 233-249.
15. Ryerson EW: Arthrodesing operations on the feet. *J Bone Joint Surg Am* 1923;5:453-471.
16. Bednarz PA, Monroe MT, Manoli A II: Triple arthrodesis in adults using rigid internal fixation: An assessment of outcome. *Foot Ankle Int* 1999;20(6):356-363.
17. Bono JV, Jacobs RL: Triple arthrodesis through a single lateral approach: A cadaveric experiment. *Foot Ankle* 1992;13(7):408-412.
18. Horton GA, Olney BW: Triple arthrodesis with lateral column lengthening for treatment of severe planovalgus deformity. *Foot Ankle Int* 1995;16(7):395-400.
19. Jeng CL, Vora AM, Myerson MS: The medial approach to triple arthrodesis: Indications and technique for management of rigid valgus deformities in high-risk patients. *Foot Ankle Clin* 2005; 10(3):515-521.
20. Jeng CL, Tankson CJ, Myerson MS: The single medial approach to triple arthrodesis: A cadaveric study. *Foot Ankle Int* 2006;27(12): 1122-1125.
21. Brilhault J: Single medial approach to modified double arthrodesis in rigid flatfoot with lateral deficient skin. *Foot Ankle Int* 2009;30(1):21-26.
22. Greisberg J, Assal M, Hansen ST Jr, Sangeorzan BJ: Isolated medial column stabilization improves alignment in adult-acquired flatfoot. *Clin Orthop Relat Res* 2005;435:197-202.
23. Thompson IM, Bohay DR, Anderson JG: Fusion rate of first tarsometatarsal arthrodesis in the modified Lapidus procedure and flatfoot reconstruction. *Foot Ankle Int* 2005;26(9):698-703.
24. Acevedo JI, Myerson MS: Modification of the Chrisman-Snook technique. *Foot Ankle Int* 2000; 21(2):154-155.
25. Papa JA, Myerson MS: Pantalar and tibiotalocalcaneal arthrodesis for post-traumatic osteoarthrosis of the ankle and hindfoot. *J Bone Joint Surg Am* 1992;74(7):1042-1049.
26. Bluman EM, Myerson MS: Stage IV posterior tibial tendon rupture. *Foot Ankle Clin* 2007; 12(2):341-362.
27. Haddad SL, Myerson MS, Pell RF IV, Schon LC: Clinical and radiographic outcome of revision surgery for failed triple arthrodesis. *Foot Ankle Int* 1997; 18(8):489-499.
28. Raikin SM, Myerson MS: Surgical repair of ankle injuries to the deltoid ligament. *Foot Ankle Clin* 1999;4(7):745-753.
29. Hintermann B, Valderrabano V, Boss A, Trouillier HH, Dick W: Medial ankle instability: An exploratory, prospective study of fifty-two cases. *Am J Sports Med* 2004;32(1):183-190.
30. Deland JT, de Asla RJ, Segal A: Reconstruction of the chronically failed deltoid ligament: A new technique. *Foot Ankle Int* 2004; 25(11):795-799.
31. Fortin PT, Walling AK: Triple arthrodesis. *Clin Orthop Relat Res* 1999;365:91-99.
32. Sangeorzan BJ, Smith D, Veith R, Hansen ST Jr: Triple arthrodesis using internal fixation in treatment of adult foot disorders. *Clin Orthop Relat Res* 1993;294:299-307.
33. Pell RF IV, Myerson MS, Schon LC: Clinical outcome after primary triple arthrodesis. *J Bone Joint Surg Am* 2000;82(1):47-57.
34. Saltzman CL, Fehrle MJ, Cooper RR, Spencer EC, Ponseti IV: Triple arthrodesis: Twenty-five and forty-four-year average follow-up of the same patients. *J Bone Joint Surg Am* 1999; 81(10):1391-1402.
35. O'Malley MJ, Deland JT, Lee KT: Selective hindfoot arthrodesis for the treatment of adult acquired flatfoot deformity: An in vitro study. *Foot Ankle Int* 1995; 16(7):411-417.
36. Harper MC, Tisdel CL: Talonavicular arthrodesis for the painful adult acquired flatfoot. *Foot Ankle Int* 1996;17(11):658-661.
37. Harper MC: Talonavicular arthrodesis for the acquired flatfoot in the adult. *Clin Orthop Relat Res* 1999;365:65-68.
38. Clain MR, Baxter DE: Simultaneous calcaneocuboid and talonavicular fusion: Long-term follow-up study. *J Bone Joint Surg Br* 1994; 76(1):133-136.
39. Mann RA, Beaman DN: Double arthrodesis in the adult. *Clin Orthop Relat Res* 1999;365:74-80.
40. Cohen BE, Johnson JE: Subtalar arthrodesis for treatment of posterior tibial tendon insufficiency. *Foot Ankle Clin* 2001;6(1): 121-128.
41. Gellman H, Lenihan M, Halikis N, Botte MJ, Giordani M, Perry J: Selective tarsal arthrodesis: An in vitro analysis of the effect on foot motion. *Foot Ankle* 1987;8(3):127-133.
42. Stephens HM, Walling AK, Solmen JD, Tankson CJ: Subtalar repositional arthrodesis for adult acquired flatfoot. *Clin Orthop Relat Res* 1999;365:69-73.
43. Johnson JE, Cohen BE, DiGiovanni BF, Lamdan R: Subtalar arthrodesis with flexor digitorum longus transfer and spring ligament repair for treatment of posterior tibial tendon insufficiency. *Foot Ankle Int* 2000;21(9): 722-729.

The Management of Complications Following the Treatment of Flatfoot Deformity

Jason S. Lin, MD
Mark S. Myerson, MD

Abstract

Adult acquired flatfoot deformity encompasses a wide spectrum of clinical conditions. Current management approaches have emerged from a growing understanding of its manifestations, which have been learned from decades of clinical trial and error. Although surgical trends continue to evolve, many basic principles and practices have endured. Adult flatfoot deformity can arise from multiple causes, the most common of which remains posterior tibial tendon rupture with subsequent elongation of secondary supportive structures. Regardless of the cause, the fundamental goals of surgical management include correcting peritalar subluxation, restoring hindfoot-midfoot-forefoot relationships and muscle balance, attaining a plantigrade foot, and preserving motion when possible. Surgical correction may be associated with a variety of potential problems, including errors in decision making, undertreatment, overcorrection, and technical mistakes. These complications can lead to adjacent joint arthritis, recurrent deformity, rigidity, nonunion, and persistent pain.

Instr Course Lect 2011;60:321-334.

Adult acquired flatfoot deformity (AAFD) encompasses a wide spectrum of clinical conditions and exemplifies the complexity of many common foot and ankle disorders and their associated treatments. Current approaches have emerged from a growing understanding of the manifestations of AAFD that have been learned from decades of clinical trial and error. Although surgical trends continue to evolve, many basic treatment principles and practices have endured.

A flatfoot deformity can arise in an adult as a result of ligamentous or plantar fascia rupture, inflammatory processes, osteoarthritis, Charcot arthropathy, or trauma.[1-3] However, the most common cause remains posterior tibial tendon (PTT) rupture with subsequent elongation of the secondary supportive structures. Regardless of the cause of the deformity, the fundamental goals of surgical management for AAFD include correction of peritalar subluxation, restoration of hindfoot-midfoot-forefoot relationships and muscle balance, attainment of a plantigrade foot, and preservation of motion when possible. The surgical correction of AAFD may be associated with a variety of potential problems, including decision-making and technical errors and undertreatment and overcorrection of the condition. These errors can lead to complications such as adjacent joint arthritis, recurrent deformity, rigidity, nonunion, and persistent pain. This chapter presents an overview of the more common treatment choices for AAFD and options for managing its most common complications.

Errors in Decision Making

Proper decision making is essential in treating patients with AAFD. The surgeon evaluates the extent of the

Dr. Myerson or an immediate family member has received royalties from DePuy and Biomet; is a member of a speakers' bureau or has made paid presentations on behalf of DePuy, Biomet, Medtronic, and Orthohelix; serves as a paid consultant for or is an employee of DePuy, Biomet, Orthohelix, Tornier, and Medtronic; serves as an unpaid consultant for DePuy; and has received research or institutional support from Biomet and Synthes. Neither Dr. Lin nor any immediate family member has received anything of value from or owns stock in a commercial company or institution related directly or indirectly to the subject of this chapter.

deformity with respect to its various components—ankle and hindfoot valgus, forefoot supination, midfoot abduction, medial column stability, and foot flexibility (flexible or rigid). In patients with supple hindfoot deformity, it should be determined if there is any fixed forefoot supination or significant abduction deformity. The apex of the deformity should be located. As one component of the deformity is addressed, it is necessary to determine the consequent effect on other parts of the foot and ankle, the presence of instability, ankle involvement, and if a supramalleolar osteotomy or a deltoid ligament reconstruction is needed to correct tibiotalar valgus. The three-stage description of PTT dysfunction by Johnson and Strom[4] along with the stage IV modification by Myerson[5] still serves as a useful organizational scheme for diagnosing and treating AAFD. However, the simplicity of that classification system may inadequately convey the intricacies of a particular flatfoot deformity. Failing to recognize such subtleties preoperatively or intraoperatively may lead to compromised corrective procedures and potential complications. The classification system for PTT was further refined in 2007 by Bluman et al[6] to address this issue.

Undertreatment

Failing to appreciate the magnitude of a flatfoot deformity will lead to undertreatment and recurrent deformity. A common error is treating a rigid foot as if it were flexible; no tendon transfer or osteotomy will overcome the forces of a rigid hindfoot. With AAFD, a flexor digitorum longus (FDL) transfer alone may not provide sufficient power to substitute for the torn PTT and overcome the force of the peroneal muscles. Technical errors, such as performing a simple side-to-side tenodesis of the FDL to the PTT or performing a tendon transfer with insufficient tension, may explain the failure of some corrective procedures. Correction of a flexible deformity may fail in an obese patient, whereas the same procedure would be successful in a nonobese patient. Failing to correct additional components of the deformity, including forefoot supination, midfoot abduction, medial column instability, and persistent gastrocnemius contracture, will ultimately lead to inferior results.

An isolated PTT procedure is generally not successful except in patients with only underlying tenosynovitis (stage I disease) with normal hindfoot anatomy.[4] Tenosynovectomy and débridement alone have achieved good short-term results in appropriately selected patients.[7-9] Long-term failure may occur because of progressive degeneration of the PTT or an error in the initial patient selection process. The success of tenosynovectomy and débridement presupposes that the PTT is inflamed but not torn and there is no hindfoot deformity, which is common in patients with a seronegative spondyloarthropathy.[10] Patients with seronegative arthritis respond well to tenosynovectomy, but those with rheumatoid arthritis or other inflammatory conditions have less successful outcomes with isolated tendon procedures because hindfoot deformity is usually present (particularly at the talonavicular joint), and failure occurs as a result of increasing deformity.

The basic approach to managing AAFD involves a tendon transfer to replace the torn PTT, with additional osteotomies as required to correct the deformity. In patients with an early stage of the disease, with preserved subtalar motion and minor hindfoot valgus, a medial displacement calcaneal osteotomy may be a useful adjunct to soft-tissue correction.[6,11] Biomechanical analysis has shown that this osteotomy helps to normalize talonavicular joint forces in the flatfoot,[12] thereby alleviating medial hindfoot stresses and potentially decelerating further PTT degeneration. The biomechanical rationale behind tendon transfer is best understood in reference to flatfoot-hindfoot imbalance. The tendon transfer acts as a substitute for the dysfunctional PTT to help counter the lateral eversion forces. As hindfoot valgus progresses, the peroneus brevis in conjunction with the lateralized Achilles tendon exacerbate lateral ground reaction forces exerted on the subtalar joint.[1,13] Additionally, the medial and plantar ligaments attenuate and fail to oppose these forces.[14] Because FDL transfer may only partially balance the deforming forces, the addition of a calcaneal osteotomy has been recommended by some authors.[1,5] The effect of combining medial displacement calcaneal osteotomy with FDL transfer is to realign the valgus heel under the mechanical axis of the leg. The goal of this surgery is not necessarily to establish a normal arch, which the tendon transfer and osteotomy procedures cannot accomplish, but rather to relieve pain, improve function, and prevent deformity progression.

Tendon transfer for flexible AAFD correction is always preferable to tenodesis; however, tendon transfer in itself does not effect a change in the overall appearance of the foot.[7,15-18] Tenodesis of the torn PTT to an adjacent tendon, such as the FDL, has a limited role in treating AAFD. Despite earlier reports that FDL tenodesis to the diseased PTT would sufficiently support the flatfoot deformity and alleviate pain, survivorship analysis showed that 50% of procedures had failed at 2-year follow-up.[19] Over time, the medial longitudinal arch collapsed, and radiographic measurements returned to preoperative values.[20] This outcome is not unexpected because of the inherently nonphysiologic nature of the procedure. Tenodesis requires normal muscle function and adequate tendon excursion. When the healthy FDL is sutured to a scarred and immobile PTT, the diseased PTT will restrict FDL function. This form of tenodesis should be avoided. It is unclear if the torn PTT should be left behind after the FDL transfer is performed. Leaving the PTT behind may increase the power of inversion and improve muscle balance, but the torn and pathologic PTT may contain potential pain generators.

An alternative is to cut and excise the torn PTT at the level of the medial malleolus and, if the tendon has normal excursion, to perform a tenodesis to the FDL proximal to the ankle. This technique has the advantage of improving the power of the weaker FDL transfer but can be performed only if the PTT has normal, more proximal excursion. Otherwise, problems may occur as previously discussed, and the diseased PTT will restrict FDL function.

Wacker et al[21] studied the MRI morphometry of the posterior tibial and the FDL muscles in AAFD. In patients with a diseased but intact PTT, there was no fatty infiltration, and the muscle volume was at least 83% of normal. The authors suggested that, in the presence of an intact PTT, the posterior tibial muscle belly may provide some useful function if used to augment the FDL transfer when the diseased tendon is excised. In contrast, Rosenfeld et al[22] reported continued posterior tibial muscle atrophy and complete fatty replacement if the tendon was excised after FDL transfer and a calcaneal osteotomy. The outcome was the same whether the PTT was sacrificed or left intact.[22] The argument for leaving the repaired PTT behind was presented in a study by Valderrabano et al,[23] who evaluated 14 patients at 47 months after surgical reconstruction of a complete PTT rupture with end-to-end repair of the torn PTT and side-to-side augmentation with the FDL in combination with distal calcaneal lateral column lengthening. The authors concluded that the posterior tibial muscle had significant recovery potential even after delayed repair of its ruptured tendon.

Subtalar arthroereisis has been recommended as an alternative to a medial translational osteotomy of the calcaneus to correct hindfoot valgus deformity. By blocking calcaneal eversion at the sinus tarsi, the implant may improve the talonavicular coverage angle and the medial cuneiform height.[24] This procedure is generally performed in conjunction with other hindfoot procedures in adults, although its isolated use has been described.[25] It can also be used as a supplementary procedure in patients with persistent heel valgus despite treatment with a medial displacement calcaneal osteotomy and an FDL transfer.[26] Complications of subtalar arthroereisis include sinus tarsi pain, foreign body reaction, implant failure, osteonecrosis of the talus, and the need for implant removal.[25,27,28] Perhaps the major complication of subtalar arthroereisis is hindfoot stiffness and pain in the sinus tarsi necessitating removal of the implant. Because the goal of the implant is to block calcaneal eversion, it is important not to overdistract the joint with too large an implant, which always causes stiffness and pain. In the experience of this chapter's authors, the use of this implant in the adult population is associated with painful sequelae necessitating removal in approximately 50% of patients. If pain is present following surgery, it is important to determine if the forefoot is plantigrade. If the heel is corrected to a neutral position following surgery and a fixed forefoot supination deformity is present during the foot-flat phase of gait, maintaining a plantigrade forefoot will force the heel into eversion, causing sinus tarsi compression and pain. A corticosteroid injection can relieve pain if the foot is plantigrade, but removal of the implant may be necessary. Deformity may recur with premature implant removal; however, this does not seem to be a problem for most patients if the implant has been left in place for more than 6 months (**Figure 1**).

Occasionally, FDL transfer may fail even when appropriately combined with a calcaneal osteotomy for stage II deformity.[29] Guyton et al[30] reported a middle-term failure rate as high as 7% after combined FDL transfer with medial displacement calcaneal osteotomy. Early failures resulted from the tendon pullout from the navicular, and later deterioration occurred as the hindfoot drifted back into valgus and flatfoot deformity recurred. This recurrence of deformity may arise from undertensioning the transferred FDL. This chapter's authors advocate a tight repair, with FDL tensioning at near maximal excursion. However, the FDL muscle cannot contract if the transfer is overtightened.

Failure of the initial tendon transfer can also occur secondary to adjacent ligamentous attenuation. When PTT rupture occurs, the added stress is redistributed among the remaining medial capsuloligamentous structures. Elongation, attenuation, or tearing of the spring ligament, the talonavicular capsule, and the deltoid ligament in AAFD has been reported.[31,32] Patients with a torn or lax spring ligament in addition to a ruptured PTT may have more severe hindfoot abnormalities than those with only a ruptured tendon.[32] Gazdag and Cracchiolo[32] reported that 18 of 22 patients treated with tendon transfer because of a PTT rupture had evidence of spring ligament injury. For tendon transfer repair

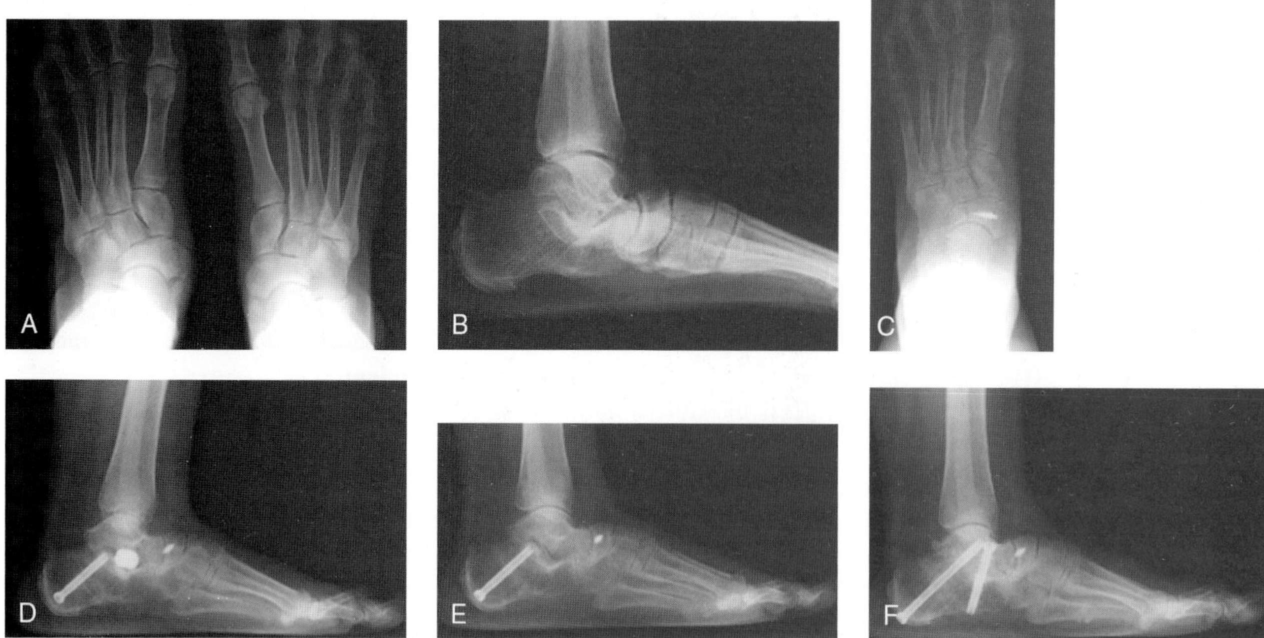

Figure 1 Radiographs of the foot of a 53-year-old patient who presented with painful left flexible flatfoot deformity and accessory navicular. Preoperative AP (**A**) and lateral (**B**) radiographs show hindfoot valgus and talonavicular undercoverage. The deformity was corrected with excision of the accessory navicular with advancement of the PTT and a medial displacement calcaneal osteotomy. **C** and **D,** Persistent heel valgus was treated with the addition of a subtalar arthroereisis implant. **E,** The patient continued to report sinus tarsi pain at 6 months postoperatively despite corticosteroid injection, and the implant was removed at 8 months postoperatively. **F,** The patient required subtalar arthrodesis to treat subtalar arthritis and offload the lateral column. That procedure also was unsuccessful and was complicated by a fifth metatarsal stress fracture. Ultimately a triple arthrodesis was performed.

to succeed, associated soft-tissue lesions must be addressed concurrently. Various spring ligament repair techniques have been proposed, including elliptical tissue excision, ligament advancement, free tissue and tendon grafts, and direct repair of the bone suture anchor.[33] A cadaver study described flatfoot deformity correction using the peroneus longus to anatomically reconstruct the spring ligament.[33] When a rupture of the spring ligament is identified, this chapter's authors use a No. 2 nonresorbable suture on a bone suture anchor into the navicular bone to make the repair.

Recurrent deformity is the reason for most revision surgeries in patients with AAFD. The surgeon must determine the magnitude of the deformity, and the individual components of the recurrence must be accounted for and corrected. In revision surgery, however, additional variables must be taken into consideration. What is the condition of the skin and soft tissues? Will previous incisions aid or compromise any planned surgical approaches? Was the correct procedure initially performed? Has a flexible deformity now become rigid? If tendon transfer repair fails, correction depends on whether the deformity is flexible or fixed and on the type of procedure previously performed because local tissue may not be available for reconstruction.

One of the more challenging problems occurs in revision procedures after failed surgery involving an FDL transfer. Generally, there is significant scarring along the medial foot and ankle, which is associated with pain and/or deformity. When the foot remains flexible, this chapter's authors prefer to excise most of the scar tissue, determine whether any functional excursion remains in the PTT or FDL tendon, and then perform a modified anterior tibial tendon transfer.[34] The use of the flexor hallucis longus (FHL) has been described for primary as well as revision surgeries; if the foot is still flexible and FDL transfer has already been done, the FHL may be used.[35] Toe flexion weakness is not commonly reported by patients following an FDL transfer because most patients have cross connections between the FDL and the FHL just distal to the master knot of Henry. If the FHL is used following an FDL transfer, the flexion strength of the toes will significantly decrease; therefore, the FHL should be used with caution. This chapter's authors use a modification of the Young[34] suspension procedure in anterior tibial tendon transfers in which a prior FDL procedure has failed and the hindfoot remains flexible. The retinaculum of the anterior tibial tendon is opened, and the tendon is left attached distally but passed under the navicular by creating a trough to support the tendon. The tendon functions to elevate the medial column without a loss of dorsiflexion strength (**Figure 2**). Although it does not increase inversion strength, a peroneus brevis transfer can be used to augment a small FDL without causing significant eversion weakness; a peroneus brevis to peroneus longus transfer may also be considered for recurrent deformity. Mizel et al[36] reported that hindfoot valgus associated with PTT deficiency did not occur when peroneus brevis function was absent. Peroneus brevis transfer effectively weakens hindfoot eversion forces while supplementing first-ray plantar-flexion strength derived from the peroneus longus. The addition of a peroneus brevis tendon transfer to maintain sufficient tendon and muscle mass to rebalance the foot has also been described by Song and Deland.[37] The peroneus brevis is passed behind the tibia medially and down the PTT sheath into the same navicular bony tunnel as the FDL transfer. This technique effectively increases inversion strength while simultaneously weakening the eversion force on the hindfoot.

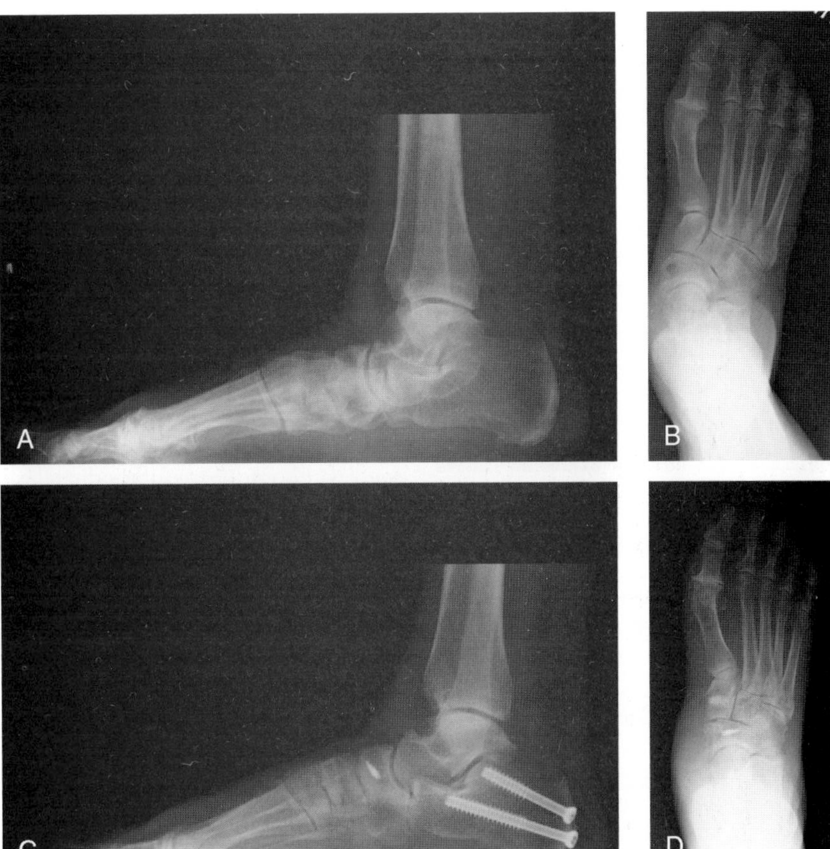

Figure 2 Radiographs of the foot of an adult who was previously treated with isolated FDL tendon transfer for PTT rupture. **A,** Lateral radiograph of the foot after the patient presented with persistent pain and failed deformity correction 1.5 years postoperatively. **B,** AP radiograph showing the previous drill hole in the medial navicular from the prior tendon transfer. Lateral (**C**) and AP (**D**) radiographs after revision surgery was accomplished with a modified Young suspension anterior tibial tendon transfer, a medial displacement calcaneal osteotomy, and a medial cuneiform dorsal opening wedge osteotomy.

Forefoot Supination

The hindfoot-forefoot relationship in AAFD must be assessed. As hindfoot valgus worsens, a progressive and potentially fixed forefoot supination may result. If this condition is not recognized preoperatively or intraoperatively, then correction of hindfoot alignment may lead to problems with forefoot rotation and lateral column overload. The surgeon must determine if the forefoot can adapt and correct on its own. It is important to establish the strength of the peroneus longus if the medial ray plantar-flexion strength is sufficient to pull down the first metatarsal. Assessing forefoot varus after hindfoot correction may help avoid such complications. In patients with a flexible forefoot deformity, the forefoot varus may correct to neutral by applying balanced pressure underneath the first and fifth rays to simulate weight bearing. If the deformity corrects without plantar flexion, then no further surgical treatment is required. If the deformity corrects only with ankle plantar flexion to relax the gastrocnemius, then a gastrocnemius recession or a percutaneous Achilles tendon lengthening may be needed.[38]

The positioning of the forefoot following FDL transfer and a calcaneal osteotomy is the subject of debate. With this procedure, the forefoot is intentionally left quite supinated, with the assumption that it will correct to a plantigrade position over time. Some authors have recommended that any fixed forefoot supination greater than 15° requires bony realignment for adequate correction.[39] Mann and Beaman[39] suggested that double arthrodesis was indicated with this degree of

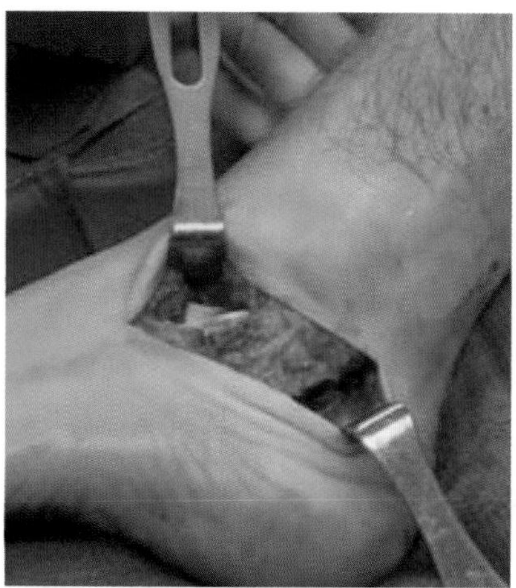

Figure 3 Intraoperative photograph of a double calcaneal osteotomy used for correcting both midfoot abduction and hindfoot valgus associated with flatfoot deformity. A medial displacement calcaneal osteotomy was added to treat residual heel valgus noted after lateral column lengthening through the calcaneal neck. Both procedures were performed through the same lateral incision.

varus, provided that the subtalar joint remained supple and free from arthrosis. Alternatively, a dorsal opening wedge medial cuneiform (Cotton) osteotomy[40] or some form of medial column plantar-flexion realignment procedure, such as first tarsometatarsal or naviculocuneiform joint arthrodesis, can be used to correct fixed forefoot supination after calcaneal osteotomy and FDL transfer.[41] Procedure selection should be based on the degree of medial ray instability and the presence of first tarsometatarsal arthritis.[6]

Although a medial translational osteotomy corrects heel valgus and a lateral column lengthening corrects forefoot abduction, neither procedure reliably corrects medial sagittal plane deformity. The foot becomes more rigid as it moves toward supination, resulting in lateral forefoot overload.[42,43] A Cotton osteotomy or medial column arthrodesis in slight plantar flexion will resolve this secondary problem. This chapter's authors recommend an arthrodesis of the first tarsometatarsal joint only if there is a notable gap on the plantar surface of the joint indicating instability. For most cases with a fixed supination deformity greater than 20° following a lateral column lengthening, a cuneiform osteotomy is recommended.

A plantar-flexion procedure of the medial column may not always be needed in the surgical treatment of stage II AAFD. In a 2008 review, 28 patients with some degree of residual flexible forefoot varus after FDL tendon transfer, medial displacement calcaneal osteotomy, and gastrocnemius recession were evaluated (R Vander Griend, MD, Denver, CO, unpublished data presented at the American Orthopaedic Foot and Ankle Society Meeting, 2008). The patients were treated with cast immobilization of the forefoot-midfoot in valgus (pronation) for 5 to 6 weeks. At 6 months postoperatively, 20 of the patients had normal forefoot rotational alignment based on clinical examinations. The remaining eight patients had asymptomatic residual forefoot varus of less than 10°. These findings suggest that flexible forefoot varus of less than 20° is a compensatory deformity that corrects or improves without direct surgical treatment. If this is true, then forefoot supination deformity may be an overtreated condition.

Midfoot Abduction

Talar head uncovering measured on AP foot radiographs suggests deformity at the level of the transverse tarsal joint. Lengthening of the lateral column should be considered if there is a forefoot abduction deformity with a lack of coverage of the talar head greater than 40%.[6] The procedure addresses the relatively short lateral column associated with moderate flatfoot by restoring the normal parallel transverse tarsal joint relationship. It may be performed proximal to or through the calcaneocuboid joint and in combination with a medial displacement calcaneal osteotomy.[44-46] Typically, lateral column lengthening is not very effective in correcting hindfoot valgus.[47] If heel valgus is present after lateral column lengthening, an additional medial displacement calcaneal osteotomy can be performed[46] (**Figure 3**).

The potential morbidity associated with a lateral column lengthening osteotomy must be considered. A 1-cm calcaneal lengthening results in an eightfold increase in the calcaneocuboid joint compressive force.[48] Although development of calcaneocuboid arthritis has been recognized after calcaneal lengthening,[49-51] this has not presented a major clinical problem based on the experience of this chapter's authors. Bolt et al[52] reported a lower reoperation rate after lateral column lengthening despite a higher incidence of nonunion and adjacent arthritis when compared with a medial translational calcaneal osteotomy. Persistent lateral hindfoot or sinus tarsi pain may be present following an apparently well-performed lateral column lengthening for flatfoot correction. Outcomes are closely associated with the location of the osteotomy, which this chapter's authors recommend be located at approximately 10 mm proximal to the calcaneocuboid joint. This recommendation is in contradistinction to the osteotomy described by Hintermann et al[49] that crosses the calcaneus between the posterior and middle calcaneal facet. The ability to correct midfoot abduction is increased by lengthening the lateral column closer to the calcaneocuboid joint, near the apex of deformity, which offers a more powerful correction by increasing talonavicular coverage. More importantly, it is essential to recognize that when a laminar spreader is inserted into the

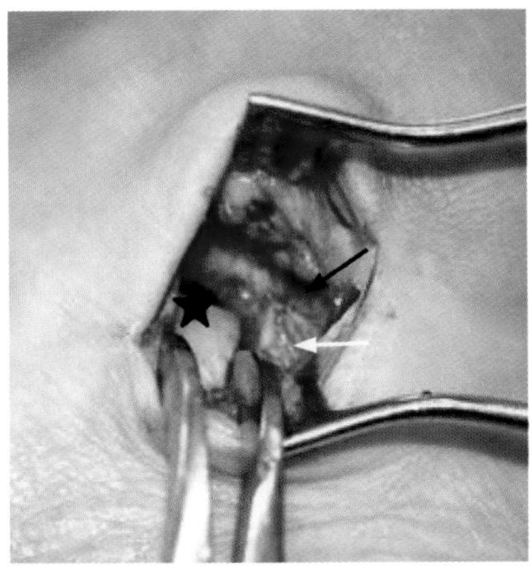

Figure 4 Intraoperative photograph of a lateral column lengthening through the calcaneal neck using cortical allograft (star). When the laminar spreader is inserted into the calcaneus for lengthening, the forefoot adducts and rotates around the talonavicular joint. However, the calcaneal tuberosity also subluxates posteriorly and can cause impingement of the calcaneal neck (white arrow) against the posterior facet (black arrow). This may result in persistent sinus tarsi pain. The neck of the calcaneus was shaved with a saw intraoperatively to prevent impingement.

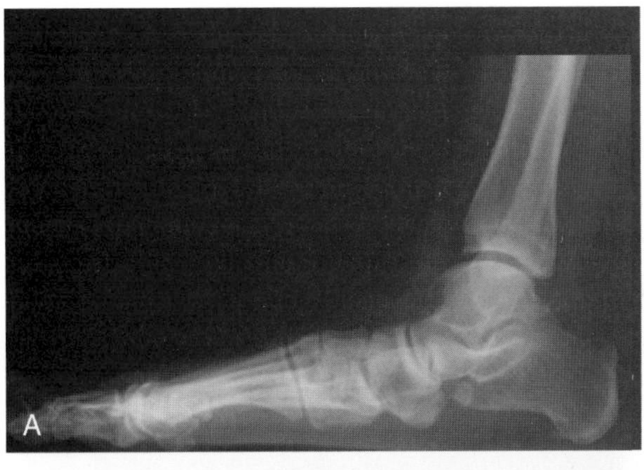

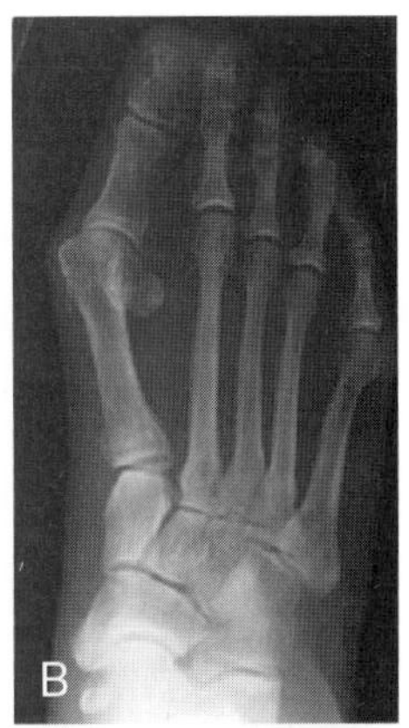

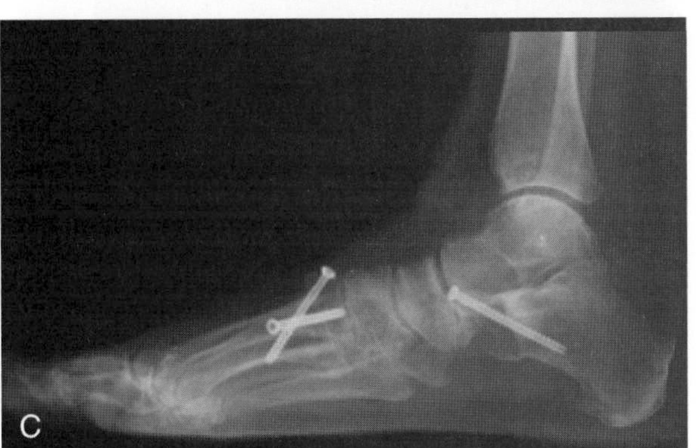

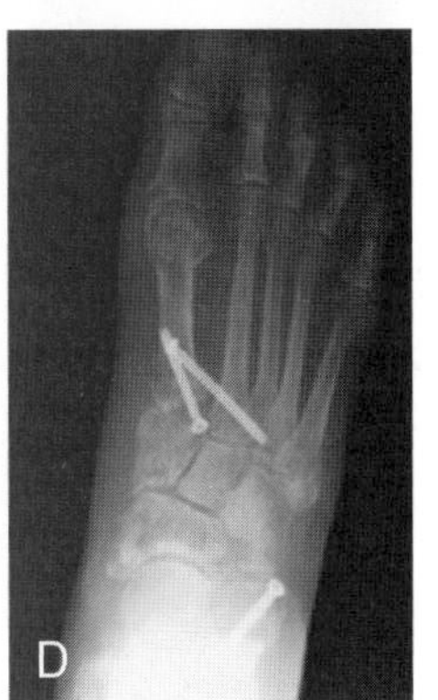

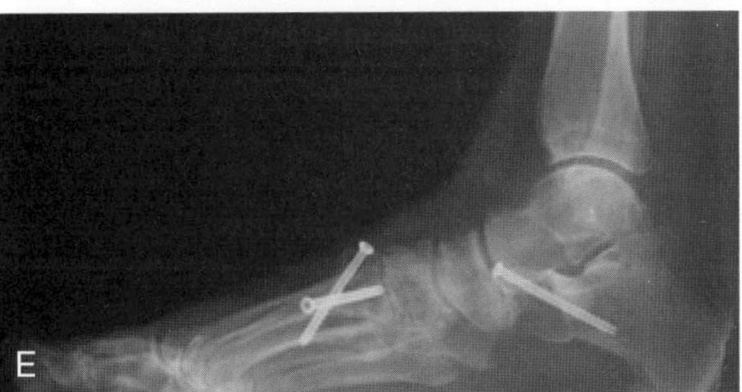

Figure 5 Lateral (**A**) and AP (**B**) radiographs of the foot of a 56-year-old patient who presented with a painful flexible AAFD, hallux valgus, and first tarsometatarsal joint instability. Lateral (**C**) and AP (**D**) radiographs after correction using FDL tendon transfer, the Lapidus procedure, and lateral column lengthening through the calcaneal neck. Note that the osteotomy of the calcaneus had been made too far posterior to the calcaneocuboid joint. **E,** The development of symptomatic sinus tarsi impingement required excavation of the allograft and calcaneal neck to decrease contact with the posterior facet.

calcaneus for lengthening, the forefoot adducts and rotates around the talonavicular joint, but the calcaneal tuberosity also shifts slightly posteriorly. This posterior shift causes calcaneal neck impingement against the posterior facet; the osteotomy will fail because of postoperative sinus tarsi pain (N Espinosa, MD, and MS Myerson, MD, Carden Park, England, unpublished data presented at the British Orthopaedic Foot and Ankle Society Meeting, 2007) (**Figure 4**). These findings were confirmed by Malicky et al[53] who examined CT scans of 19 adult patients with persistent symptoms following lateral column lengthening and found calcaneal neck impingement present in most of the patients.

If a patient presents with pain in the sinus tarsi postoperatively at a routine radiographic evaluation, CT should be used to confirm adequate healing and alignment of the hindfoot. Impingement of the graft in the neck of the calcaneus against the posterior facet is easily diagnosed with CT. A corticosteroid injection is useful to diminish inflammation from the impingement but may not be long lasting. If pain persists, the graft and the neck of the calcaneus should be excavated to decrease the contact between the neck of the calcaneus and the anterior aspect of the lateral process of the talus, which is present particularly with the foot in dorsiflexion and eversion (**Figure 5**).

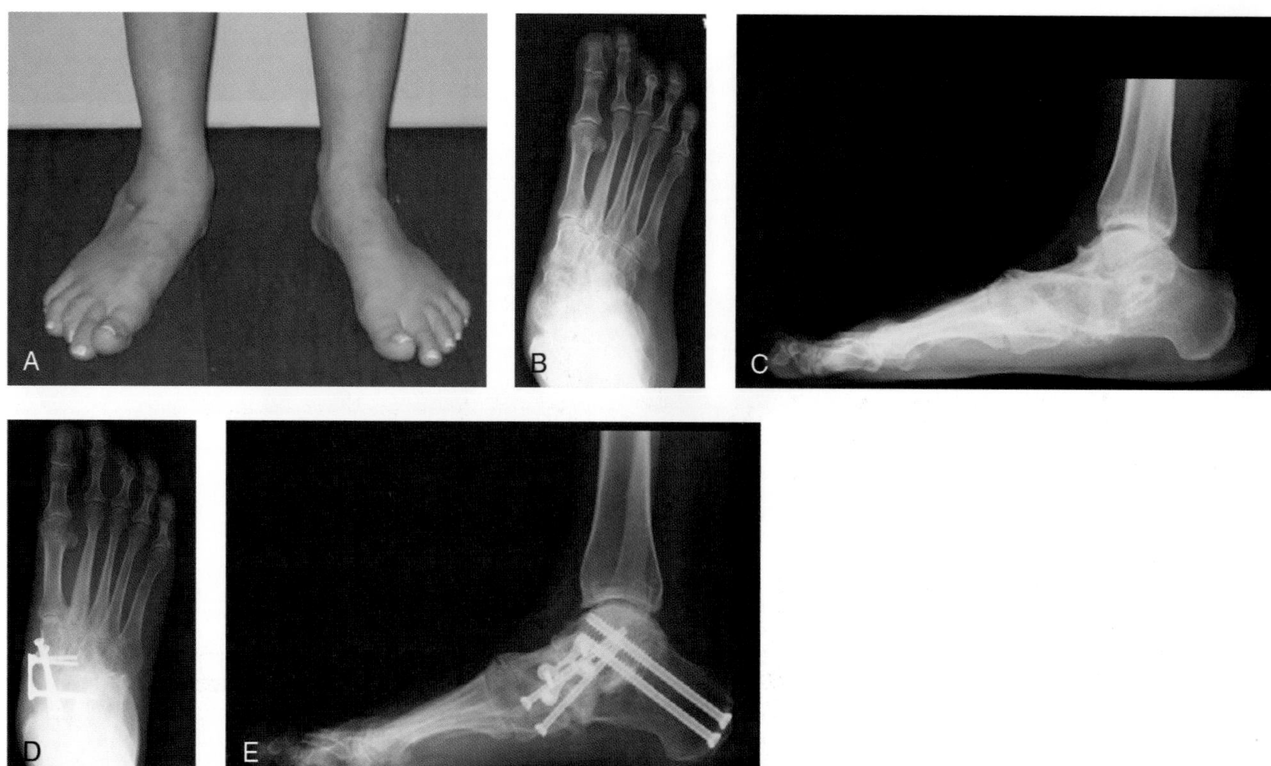

Figure 6 Clinical photograph (**A**) and AP (**B**) and lateral (**C**) radiographs of the foot of a 47-year-old woman who presented with unilateral rigid flatfoot deformity and subfibular impingement after five previous reconstructive procedures, including triple arthrodesis. AP (**D**) and lateral (**E**) radiographs after the marked hindfoot valgus was revised using a medial closing wedge calcaneal osteotomy through a lateral approach; the midfoot abduction deformity was corrected at its apex using a medial biplanar closing wedge osteotomy through the talonavicular joint.

Lengthening of the lateral column with a calcaneocuboid arthrodesis has an unusually high risk of nonunion requiring revision.[41] Toolan et al[54] reported a 20% nonunion rate with this procedure, whereas Conti and Wong[55] reported a 50% nonunion rate. Currently, this technique is less popular, and, under most circumstances, if lengthening of the lateral column is necessary, it is performed with an osteotomy at the neck of the calcaneus. A symptomatic nonunion of the calcaneocuboid joint requires revision bone grafting and more rigid fixation using a variety of plates available for this purpose.

Overcorrection

Overcorrection of AAFD can result in postoperative morbidity and the potential need for revision surgery. Excessive medialization of the osteotomized calcaneal tuberosity or calcaneal inversion through the subtalar joint caused by lateral column overdistraction will create hindfoot varus. Varus hindfoot malalignment has been associated with painful lateral column overload and overuse peroneal tendinitis. Subtalar varus also restricts transverse tarsal joint motion, resulting in a rigid foot and increased ligamentous stress along the lateral ankle. This overcorrection may be reversed with lateral calcaneal repositioning or a lateral closing wedge (Dwyer) osteotomy.[56]

Lateral column overlengthening can also have detrimental effects on the lateral midfoot. Increased compressive forces at the metatarsocuboid articulation may ultimately lead to arthritis or dislocation at that joint.[38] This condition may be salvaged with metatarsocuboid resection arthroplasty or extended lateral column arthrodesis. Alternatively, resection of a laterally based wedge from the arthrodesis site can reverse the overlengthening and preserve mobility. Toolan et al[54] successfully revised an overlengthened distraction arthrodesis of the calcaneocuboid joint with a dorsiflexion-abduction closing wedge osteotomy through the healed tricortical graft. Subtalar arthrodesis should be avoided to preserve accommodative hindfoot motion. If circumstances necessitate a fusion, care must be taken to reposition the subtalar joint into physiologic valgus.

Managing Rigid Deformity

Rigid or severe flatfoot deformity (stage III disease) is characterized by rigid hindfoot valgus; a triple arthro-

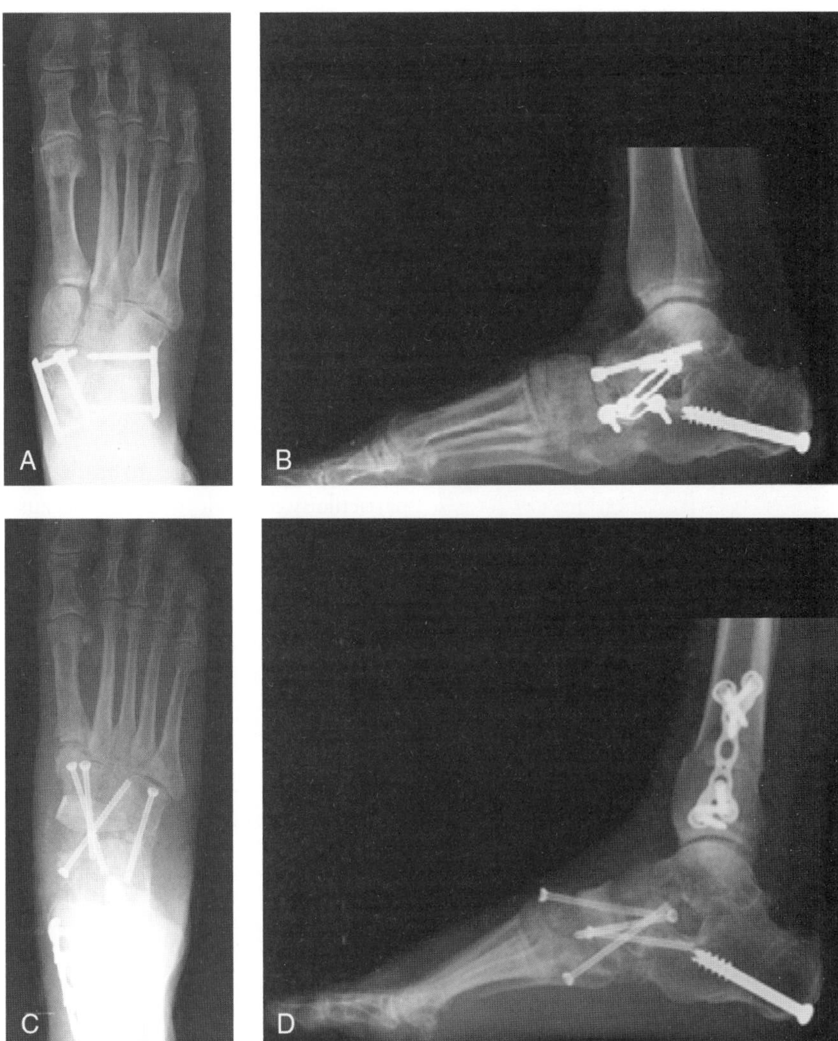

Figure 7 A 58-year-old woman presented with ankle and lateral foot pain after three previous attempts at AAFD correction. AP (**A**) and lateral (**B**) radiographs of the foot after fixed forefoot supination developed secondary to a short medial column and mild varus of the distal tibia. Note the elevated first metatarsal and the prominent plantar lateral bone. AP (**C**) and lateral (**D**) radiographs of the foot after corrective procedures involving an opening wedge supramalleolar osteotomy and revision triple arthrodesis with medial column lengthening and derotational transverse tarsal osteotomy to elevate the lateral column.

desis is needed to achieve adequate correction. Because the condition requires both deformity correction and joint fusion, it is a more challenging than in situ procedures for the well-aligned arthritic foot. Judicious use of a calcaneal osteotomy, lateral column lengthening with a bone block arthrodesis of the calcaneocuboid joint, and medial column plantar-flexion osteotomy or arthrodesis may be necessary in addition to the triple arthrodesis to achieve a stable, plantigrade foot. Additional soft-tissue procedures, such as tendon lengthening and tendon transfers to treat ankle equinus and balance force couples around the foot, may be necessary. Although bone wedges can be removed to correct deformity and facilitate joint reduction, doing so may cause significant complications, including loss of hindfoot height, pseudarthrosis, deformity recurrence, and talar osteonecrosis.[57] In an early review of long-term follow-up after triple arthrodeses, nonunion was reported in more than 20% of patients.[57] In contrast, a nonunion rate of less than 2% was reported in the largest reported series of triple arthrodesis using rigid internal fixation techniques, minimal bone resection, and rotation without resection of bone wedges.[58]

A malpositioned or malunited triple arthrodesis presents a challenging problem that requires systematic management. The use of rigid internal fixation for arthrodesis may increase the incidence of symptomatic malunion because of the marked sensitivity of the talonavicular joint to hindfoot malpositioning. Flatfoot undercorrection can result in residual valgus deformity. Conversely, overpronation or adduction of the talonavicular joint can lead to hindfoot varus. Haddad et al[59] reported results for malunion correction after triple arthrodesis and presented a management algorithm to highlight revision principles in the presence of hindfoot malalignment or rocker-bottom deformity. In general, deformity correction involves various translational and rotational hindfoot osteotomies performed through the apex of the deformity. In more complex cases, multiple apices often must be considered. Correction most often begins with the hindfoot, followed by the midfoot and the forefoot.[59,60]

In patients with valgus malunion, medial displacement calcaneal osteotomy performed in combination with a triple arthrodesis reduces forces on the spring and deltoid ligaments, thereby improving tibiotalar joint mechanics.[61-63] Medial calcaneal translation shifts the Achilles tendon medially and reduces hindfoot valgus forces and lateral ankle joint pres-

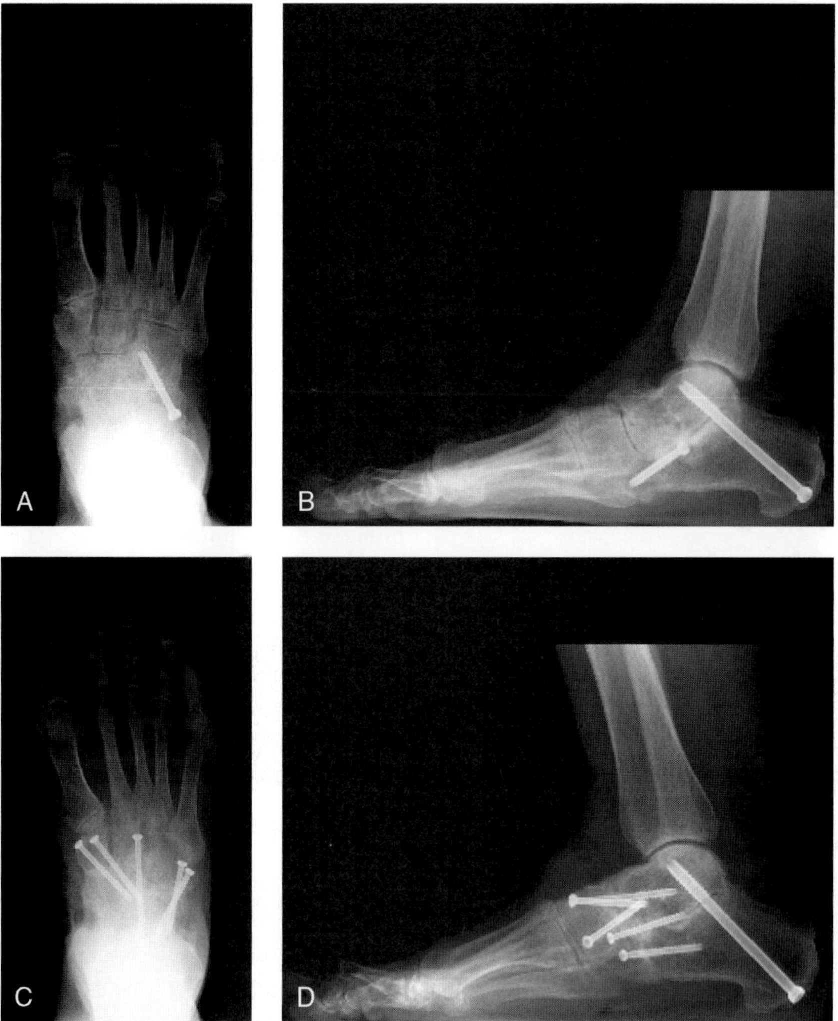

Figure 8 AP (**A**) and lateral (**B**) radiographs of the foot of an adult woman who presented with persistent pain after a previous triple arthrodesis for flatfoot deformity. Although the patient had arthritis of the naviculocuneiform joint and marked shortening of the medial column, a medial approach with opening wedge osteotomy at the talonavicular joint was contraindicated because of poor medial skin on the foot. AP (**C**) and lateral (**D**) radiographs of the foot after treatment with a lateral biplanar closing wedge osteotomy through the calcaneocuboid joint with arthrodesis of the talonavicular cuneiform complex.

sures.[64,65] It is difficult to perform a medially based closing wedge osteotomy at the level of the subtalar joint to correct persistent valgus; a medial displacement calcaneal osteotomy is preferable and can sometimes be combined effectively with a medial closing wedge transverse tarsal osteotomy to correct any residual midfoot abduction.[59] It may be preferable to lengthen the transverse tarsal joint with bone graft laterally, but the success of this procedure will depend on the tolerance of the lateral skin. It is generally safer to perform a medially based closing wedge osteotomy, even though this will result in slight shortening of the foot (**Figure 6**).

Varus malunion can originate from the heel (in patients with subtalar malalignment), the calcaneocuboid joint, or both. Correction of varus malunion is based on similar but opposite principles as valgus malunion, with lateral translational or closing wedge calcaneus osteotomy and lateral closing wedge and/or rotational transverse tarsal osteotomies. Sometimes, there may be an adductus component to the deformity in addition to the varus. In these complex scenarios, the surgeon may need to consider biplanar correction to treat the multiple apices of deformity (**Figures** 7 and **8**).

A rocker-bottom deformity following a malunited triple arthrodesis is particularly difficult to correct because of marked contractures of the Achilles and anterior tibial tendons. It is not possible to restore a plantigrade foot without tendon lengthening and multiplanar osteotomy of the calcaneus and transverse tarsal joint (**Figure 9**).

Long-term follow-up studies have shown that increased stresses on adjacent joints commonly result in degenerative midfoot changes after a triple arthrodesis.[20,58,66] Because triple arthrodesis limits foot dorsiflexion through arthrodesis of the talonavicular and calcaneocuboid joints, more stress is placed on the midfoot joints during gait. A comparison of radiographs preoperatively and at a minimum of 3 years postoperatively showed a progression of midfoot arthritis in 50% of patients, although most patients were asymptomatic or minimally symptomatic.[66]

Stage IV Deformity and Ankle Arthritis

Stage IV PTT rupture involves valgus tilting of the talus within the ankle mortise in association with hindfoot valgus. It is important to preoperatively document the presence of any ankle deformity and/or arthritis because triple arthrodesis causes increased tibiotalar strain that may exacerbate any existing pathology over time.[20,58,65-67] Ankle arthritis and val-

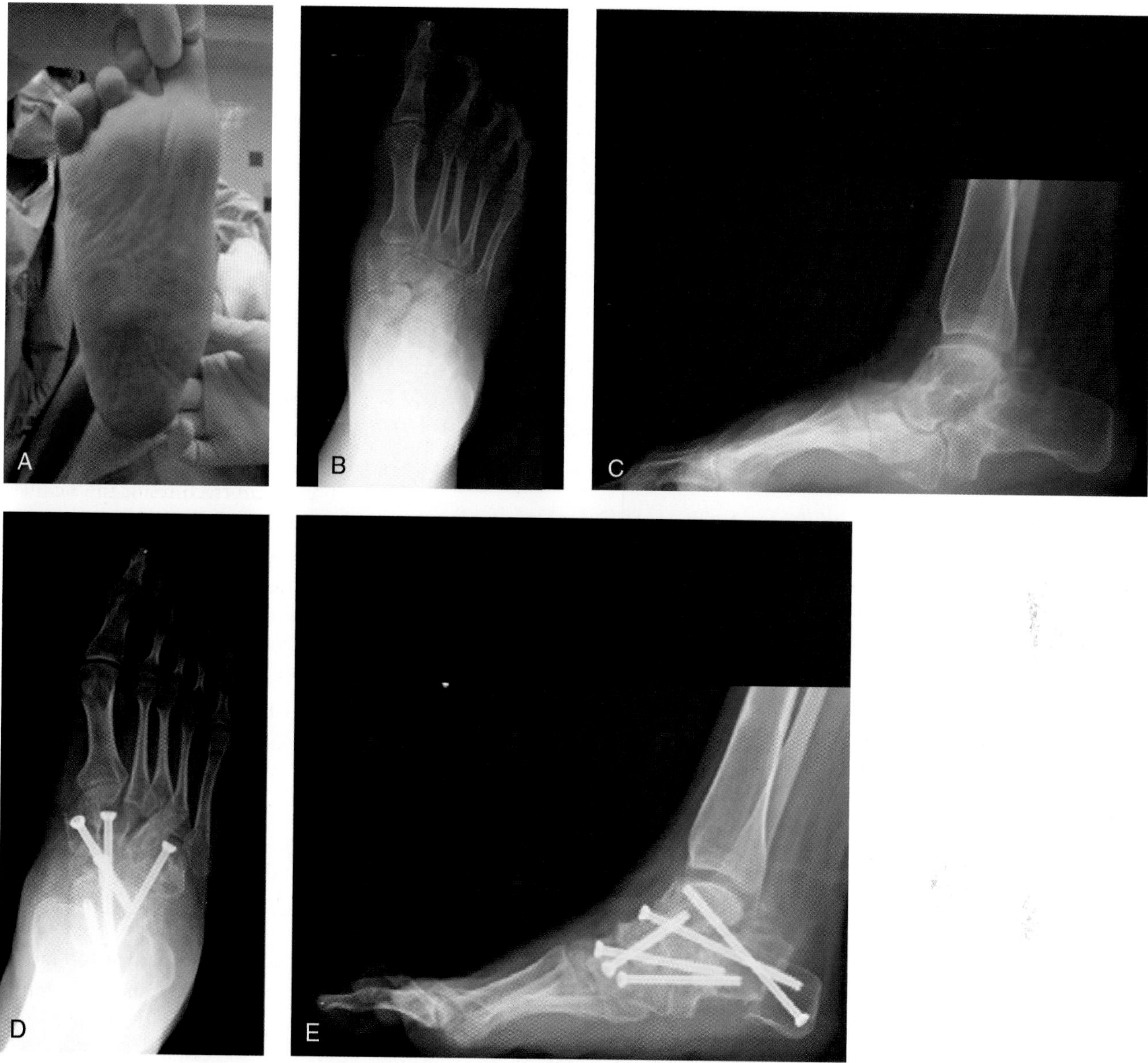

Figure 9 Clinical photograph (**A**) and AP (**B**) and lateral (**C**) radiographs of the foot of a 17-year-old woman who presented with plantar foot pain, an oblique talus, and a rocker-bottom deformity after a previous failed correction of flatfoot deformity that included lateral column lengthening. AP (**D**) and lateral (**E**) radiographs of the foot after the deformity was revised using an open Achilles tendon lengthening, a multiplanar calcaneal osteotomy, and plantar flexion transverse tarsal arthrodesis. Intraoperatively, the calcaneal osteotomy was temporarily held with pins as the calcaneocuboid and subtalar joints were corrected and then fused, and the reduction of the talonavicular joint was approached medially to complete the triple arthrodesis.

gus deformity of the ankle resulting from a deltoid rupture can develop as a consequence of triple arthrodesis malalignment.[6,59]

It is difficult to correct an ankle deformity after triple arthrodesis. The surgeon should recognize that when valgus tilting of the tibiotalar joint occurs, an attempt should be made to minimize compression on the lateral ankle joint surface and tension on the deltoid ligament. Jahss[68] first introduced the concept that a medial displacement calcaneal osteotomy can normalize the hindfoot weight-bearing surface and improve the distribution of weight-bearing forces across the ankle. This concept is important because ankle arthritis after triple arthrodesis is often progressive, particularly when associated with tibiotalar valgus. A study by Southwell et al[69] showed a 58% prevalence of ankle arthritis after triple arthrodesis, and another long-term follow-up study of 132 patients showed 60% had progressive ankle arthritis.[58] Tibiotalar joint deformity may be rigid. Although rigid deformities are best treated with ankle arthrodesis, supple tibiotalar deformity can be treated with joint-sparing procedures involving reconstruction of the deltoid ligament.[70]

Summary

Numerous surgical procedures have been proposed for reconstructing and correcting AAFD. Most procedures include Achilles lengthening and FDL tendon transfer to substitute for a dysfunctional PTT. Soft-tissue procedures are commonly combined with bony procedures to stabilize the correction and treat the pathologic anatomy. Rigid or severe flatfoot deformities require arthrodesis procedures to correct the deformity. All of these procedures can have a range of potential complications, many of which are serious and difficult to salvage. In general, the physician should perform the least invasive procedure that decreases pain and improves function. The effects of each procedure and the associated morbidity and risks must be carefully considered.

References

1. Anderson RB, Davis WH: Management of the adult flatfoot deformity, in Myerson MS, ed: *Foot and Ankle Disorders*. Philadelphia, PA, WB Saunders, 2000, p 1017.
2. Cracchiolo A III: Evaluation of spring ligament pathology in patients with posterior tibial tendon rupture, tendon transfer, and ligament repair. *Foot Ankle Clin* 1997;2:297-307.
3. Pedowitz WJ, Kovatis P: Flatfoot in the adult. *J Am Acad Orthop Surg* 1995;3(5):293-302.
4. Johnson KA, Strom DE: Tibialis posterior tendon dysfunction. *Clin Orthop Relat Res* 1989;239: 196-206.
5. Myerson MS: Adult acquired flatfoot deformity: Treatment of dysfunction of the posterior tibial tendon. *Instr Course Lect* 1997;46: 393-405.
6. Bluman EM, Title CI, Myerson MS: Posterior tibial tendon rupture: A refined classification system. *Foot Ankle Clin* 2007; 12(2):233-249, v.
7. Funk DA, Cass JR, Johnson KA: Acquired adult flat foot secondary to posterior tibial-tendon pathology. *J Bone Joint Surg Am* 1986; 68(1):95-102.
8. Teasdall RD, Johnson KA: Surgical treatment of stage I posterior tibial tendon dysfunction. *Foot Ankle Int* 1994;15(12):646-648.
9. McCormack AP, Varner KE, Marymont JV: Surgical treatment for posterior tibial tendonitis in young competitive athletes. *Foot Ankle Int* 2003;24(7):535-538.
10. Myerson M, Solomon G, Shereff M: Posterior tibial tendon dysfunction: Its association with seronegative inflammatory disease. *Foot Ankle* 1989;9(5):219-225.
11. Koutsogiannis E: Treatment of mobile flat foot by displacement osteotomy of the calcaneus. *J Bone Joint Surg Br* 1971;53(1):96-100.
12. Arangio GA, Chopra V, Voloshin A, Salathe EP: A biomechanical analysis of the effect of lateral column lengthening calcaneal osteotomy on the flat foot. *Clin Biomech (Bristol, Avon)* 2007; 22(4):472-477.
13. Trnka HJ, Easley ME, Myerson MS: The role of calcaneal osteotomies for correction of adult flatfoot. *Clin Orthop Relat Res* 1999;365:50-64.
14. Goldner JL, Keats PK, Bassett FH III, Clippinger FW: Progressive talipes equinovalgus due to trauma or degeneration of the posterior tibial tendon and medial plantar ligaments. *Orthop Clin North Am* 1974;5(1):39-51.
15. Kettelkamp DB, Alexander HH: Spontaneous rupture of the posterior tibial tendon. *J Bone Joint Surg Am* 1969;51(4):759-764.
16. Mann RA: Flatfoot in adults, in Mann RA, Coughlin MJ, eds: *Surgery of the Foot and Ankle*, ed 6. St Louis, Mosby-Year Book, 1993, p 757.
17. Mann RA, Thompson FM: Rupture of the posterior tibial tendon causing flat foot: Surgical treatment. *J Bone Joint Surg Am* 1985; 67(4):556-561.
18. Shereff MJ: Treatment of ruptured posterior tibial tendon with direct repair and FDL tenodesis. *Foot Ankle Clin* 1997;2:281-296.
19. Michelson J, Conti S, Jahss M: Survivorship analysis of tendon transfer surgery for posterior tibial tendon rupture. *Clin Orthop Relat Res* 1992;16:30.
20. Myerson MS, Corrigan J, Thompson F, Schon LC: Tendon transfer combined with calcaneal osteotomy for treatment of posterior tibial tendon insufficiency: A radiological investigation. *Foot Ankle Int* 1995;16(11):712-718.
21. Wacker J, Calder JD, Engstrom CM, Saxby TS: MR morphometry of posterior tibialis muscle in adult acquired flat foot. *Foot Ankle Int* 2003;24(4):354-357.
22. Rosenfeld PF, Dick J, Saxby TS: The response of the flexor digitorum longus and posterior tibial muscles to tendon transfer and calcaneal osteotomy for stage II posterior tibial tendon dysfunction. *Foot Ankle Int* 2005;26(9): 671-674.
23. Valderrabano V, Hintermann B, Wischer T, Fuhr P, Dick W: Recovery of the posterior tibial muscle after late reconstruction following tendon rupture. *Foot Ankle Int* 2004;25(2):85-95.
24. Vora AM, Tien TR, Parks BG, Schon LC: Correction of moderate and severe acquired flexible

flatfoot with medializing calcaneal osteotomy and flexor digitorum longus transfer. *J Bone Joint Surg Am* 2006;88(8):1726-1734.

25. Needleman RL: A surgical approach for flexible flatfeet in adults including a subtalar arthroereisis with the MBA sinus tarsi implant. *Foot Ankle Int* 2006; 27(1):9-18.
26. Zaret DI, Myerson MS: Arthroerisis of the subtalar joint. *Foot Ankle Clin* 2003;8(3):605-617.
27. Siff TE, Granberry WM: Avascular necrosis of the talus following subtalar arthrorisis with a polyethylene endoprosthesis: A case report. *Foot Ankle Int* 2000;21(3): 247-249.
28. Smith SD, Millar EA: Arthrorisis by means of a subtalar polyethylene peg implant for correction of hindfoot pronation in children. *Clin Orthop Relat Res* 1983;181: 15-23.
29. Myerson MS, Corrigan J: Treatment of posterior tibial tendon dysfunction with flexor digitorum longus tendon transfer and calcaneal osteotomy. *Orthopedics* 1996; 19(5):383-388.
30. Guyton GP, Jeng C, Krieger LE, Mann RA: Flexor digitorum longus transfer and medial displacement calcaneal osteotomy for posterior tibial tendon dysfunction: A middle-term clinical follow-up. *Foot Ankle Int* 2001;22(8): 627-632.
31. Johnson JE, Cohen BE, DiGiovanni BF, Lamdan R: Subtalar arthrodesis with flexor digitorum longus transfer and spring ligament repair for treatment of posterior tibial tendon insufficiency. *Foot Ankle Int* 2000;21(9): 722-729.
32. Gazdag AR, Cracchiolo A III: Rupture of the posterior tibial tendon: Evaluation of injury of the spring ligament and clinical assessment of tendon transfer and ligament repair. *J Bone Joint Surg Am* 1997;79(5):675-681.
33. Choi K, Lee S, Otis JC, Deland JT: Anatomical reconstruction of the spring ligament using peroneus longus tendon graft. *Foot Ankle Int* 2003;24(5):430-436.
34. Young CS: Operative treatment of pes planus. *Surg Gynecol Obstet* 1939;68:1099-1101.
35. Sammarco GJ, Hockenbury RT: Treatment of stage II posterior tibial tendon dysfunction with flexor hallucis longus transfer and medial displacement calcaneal osteotomy. *Foot Ankle Int* 2001; 22(4):305-312.
36. Mizel MS, Temple HT, Scranton PE Jr, et al: Role of the peroneal tendons in the production of the deformed foot with posterior tibial tendon deficiency. *Foot Ankle Int* 1999;20(5):285-289.
37. Song SJ, Deland JT: Outcome following addition of peroneus brevis tendon transfer to treatment of acquired posterior tibial tendon insufficiency. *Foot Ankle Int* 2001;22(4):301-304.
38. Neufeld SK, Myerson MS: Complications of surgical treatments for adult flatfoot deformities. *Foot Ankle Clin* 2001;6(1):179-191.
39. Mann RA, Beaman DN: Double arthrodesis in the adult. *Clin Orthop Relat Res* 1999;365:74-80.
40. Cotton FJ: Foot statics and surgery. *N Engl J Med* 1936;214: 353-362.
41. van der Krans A, Louwerens JW, Anderson P: Adult acquired flexible flatfoot, treated by calcaneocuboid distraction arthrodesis, posterior tibial tendon augmentation, and percutaneous Achilles tendon lengthening: A prospective outcome study of 20 patients. *Acta Orthop* 2006;77(1):156-163.
42. Logel KJ, Parks BG, Schon LC: Calcaneocuboid distraction arthrodesis and first metatarsocuneiform arthrodesis for correction of acquired flatfoot deformity in a cadaver model. *Foot Ankle Int* 2007;28(4):435-440.
43. Benthien RA, Parks BG, Guyton GP, Schon LC: Lateral column calcaneal lengthening, flexor digitorum longus transfer, and opening wedge medial cuneiform osteotomy for flexible flatfoot: A biomechanical study. *Foot Ankle Int* 2007;28(1):70-77.
44. Anderson RB, Davis WH: Calcaneocuboid distraction arthrodesis for the treatment of the adult-acquired flatfoot: The modified Evans procedure. *Foot Ankle Clin* 1996;1:279-294.
45. Evans D: Calcaneo-valgus deformity. *J Bone Joint Surg Br* 1975; 57(3):270-278.
46. Pomeroy GC, Manoli A II: A new operative approach for flatfoot secondary to posterior tibial tendon insufficiency: A preliminary report. *Foot Ankle Int* 1997;18(4): 206-212.
47. Sangeorzan BJ, Mosca V, Hansen ST Jr: Effect of calcaneal lengthening on relationships among the hindfoot, midfoot, and forefoot. *Foot Ankle* 1993;14(3): 136-141.
48. Cooper PS, Nowak MD, Shaer J: Calcaneocuboid joint pressures with lateral column lengthening (Evans) procedure. *Foot Ankle Int* 1997;18(4):199-205.
49. Hintermann B, Valderrabano V, Kundert HP: Lengthening of the lateral column and reconstruction of the medial soft tissue for treatment of acquired flatfoot deformity associated with insufficiency of the posterior tibial tendon. *Foot Ankle Int* 1999;20(10):622-629.
50. Phillips GE: A review of elongation of os calcis for flat feet. *J Bone Joint Surg Br* 1983;65(1): 15-18.
51. Moseir-LaClair S, Pomeroy G, Manoli A II: Intermediate follow-up on the double osteotomy and tendon transfer procedure for stage II posterior tibial tendon insufficiency. *Foot Ankle Int* 2001;22(4):283-291.

52. Bolt PM, Coy S, Toolan BC: A comparison of lateral column lengthening and medial translational osteotomy of the calcaneus for the reconstruction of adult acquired flatfoot. *Foot Ankle Int* 2007;28(11):1115-1123.

53. Malicky ES, Crary JL, Houghton MJ, Agel J, Hansen ST Jr, Sangeorzan BJ: Talocalcaneal and subfibular impingement in symptomatic flatfoot in adults. *J Bone Joint Surg Am* 2002;84-A(11):2005-2009.

54. Toolan BC, Sangeorzan BJ, Hansen ST Jr: Complex reconstruction for the treatment of dorsolateral peritalar subluxation of the foot: Early results after distraction arthrodesis of the calcaneocuboid joint in conjunction with stabilization of, and transfer of the flexor digitorum longus tendon to, the midfoot to treat acquired pes planovalgus in adults. *J Bone Joint Surg Am* 1999;81(11):1545-1560.

55. Conti SF, Wong YS: Osteolysis of structural autograft after calcaneocuboid distraction arthrodesis for stage II posterior tibial tendon dysfunction. *Foot Ankle Int* 2002;23(6):521-529.

56. Dwyer FC: Osteotomy of the calcaneum for pes cavus. *J Bone Joint Surg Br* 1959;41-B(1):80-86.

57. Angus PD, Cowell HR: Triple arthrodesis: A critical long-term review. *J Bone Joint Surg Br* 1986;68(2):260-265.

58. Pell RF IV, Myerson MS, Schon LC: Clinical outcome after primary triple arthrodesis. *J Bone Joint Surg Am* 2000;82(1):47-57.

59. Haddad SL, Myerson MS, Pell RF IV, Schon LC: Clinical and radiographic outcome of revision surgery for failed triple arthrodesis. *Foot Ankle Int* 1997;18(8):489-499.

60. Joseph TN, Myerson MS: Correction of multiplanar hindfoot deformity with osteotomy, arthrodesis, and internal fixation. *Instr Course Lect* 2005;54:269-276.

61. Otis JC, Deland JT, Kenneally S: Medial arch strain after lateral column lengthening: An in vitro study. *Foot Ankle Int* 1999;20(12):797-802.

62. Resnick RB, Jahss MH, Choueka J, Kummer F, Hersch JC, Okereke E: Deltoid ligament forces after tibialis posterior tendon rupture: Effects of triple arthrodesis and calcaneal displacement osteotomies. *Foot Ankle Int* 1995;16(1):14-20.

63. Song SJ, Lee S, O'Malley MJ, Otis JC, Sung IH, Deland JT: Deltoid ligament strain after correction of acquired flatfoot deformity by triple arthrodesis. *Foot Ankle Int* 2000;21(7):573-577.

64. Steffensmeier SJ, Saltzman CL, Berbaum KS, Brown TD: Effects of medial and lateral displacement calcaneal osteotomies on tibiotalar joint contact stresses. *J Orthop Res* 1996;14(6):980-985.

65. Fairbank A, Myerson MS, Fortin P, Yu-Yahiro J: The effect of calcaneal osteotomy on contact characteristics of the tibiotalar joint. *Foot* 1995;5:137-142.

66. Bennett GL, Graham CE, Mauldin DM: Triple arthrodesis in adults. *Foot Ankle* 1991;12(3):138-143.

67. Welton EA, Rose GK: Posterior tibial tendon pathology: The foot at risk and its treatment by os calcis osteotomy. *Foot* 1993;3:168-174.

68. Jahss MH: Spontaneous rupture of the tibialis posterior tendon: Clinical findings, tenographic studies, and a new technique of repair. *Foot Ankle* 1982;3(3):158-166.

69. Southwell RB, Sherman FC: Triple arthrodesis: A long-term study with force plate analysis. *Foot Ankle* 1981;2(1):15-24.

70. Bluman EM, Myerson MS: Stage IV posterior tibial tendon rupture. *Foot Ankle Clin* 2007;12(2):341-362.

Diagnosis and Treatment of Chronic Ankle Pain

Dane K. Wukich, MD
Dominick A. Tuason, MD

Abstract

The differential diagnosis for chronic ankle pain is quite broad. Ankle pain can be caused by intra-articular or extra-articular pathology and may be a result of a traumatic or nontraumatic event. A detailed patient history and physical examination, coupled with judicious selection of the appropriate imaging modalities, are vital in making an accurate diagnosis and providing effective treatment. Chronic ankle pain can affect all age groups, ranging from young athletes to elderly patients with degenerative joint and soft-tissue disorders. It has been estimated that 23,000 ankle sprains occur each day in the United States, representing approximately 1 sprain per 10,000 people per day. Because nearly one in five ankle injuries result in chronic symptoms, orthopaedic surgeons are likely to see patients with chronic ankle pain. Many patients with chronic ankle pain do not recall any history of trauma. Reviewing the management of the various disorders that can cause chronic ankle pain will help orthopaedic surgeons provide the best treatment for their patients.

Instr Course Lect 2011;60:335-350.

Chronic ankle pain is common. The causes are numerous, and all ages are affected. Trauma is not necessary but is often the initiating event, so an efficient method for evaluation is beneficial. A detailed history, careful physical examination, and judicious selection of the appropriate imaging modalities are all vital to making an accurate diagnosis and providing effective treatment.

Tarsal Tunnel Syndrome

The tarsal tunnel is bordered by the distal part of the tibia anteriorly and the posterior border of the talus and calcaneus posteriorly. The roof of the tunnel is formed by the flexor retinaculum, which begins 10 cm proximal to the medial malleolus. The contents of the tarsal tunnel include the posterior tibial artery and vein, the posterior tibial tendon, the flexor hallucis and flexor digitorum longus tendons, and the posterior tibial nerve. The posterior tibial nerve has three terminal branches: the medial plantar, lateral plantar, and medial calcaneal nerves. The three terminal nerve branches typically arise in the tarsal tunnel, although variations may occur. Recent evidence has identified separate fascial tunnels distal to the flexor retinaculum for the medial plantar nerve, the lateral plantar nerve, and the medial calcaneal nerve.[1] Tarsal tunnel syndrome is defined as the symptomatic entrapment of the tibial nerve and/or its branches within the confines of the tarsal tunnel or distally. Space-occupying lesions such as ganglion cysts, lipomas, varicose veins, nerve-sheath tumors, and synovitis can result in nerve compression. Similarly, a hypertrophic tarsal coalition or a nonunion of a sustentaculum tali fracture can cause compression of the neural structures within the tunnel. Pathologic hindfoot valgus can produce tension on the posterior tibial nerve and can cause symptoms of nerve irritation. Intraoperative pressure measurements have shown that pronation and plantar flexion increase the pressures in the medial and lateral plantar tunnels.[2] Patients usually report a burning or tingling sensation along the plantar aspect of the foot or

Dr. Wukich or an immediate family member has received royalties from Arthrex; serves as a paid consultant to or is an employee of SBI; and has received research or institutional support from Smith & Nephew. Neither Dr. Tuason nor any immediate family member has received anything of value from or owns stock in a commercial company or institution related directly or indirectly to the subject of this chapter.

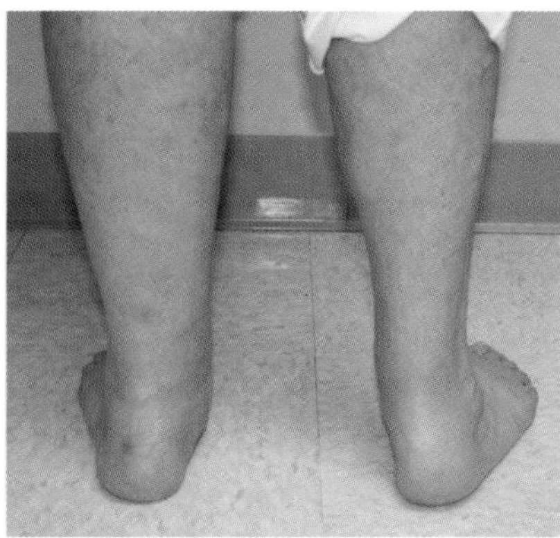

Figure 1 Photograph showing the "too many toes" sign on the right foot, as is seen with posterior tibial tendon degeneration or rupture.

pain radiating proximally into the distal part of the medial aspect of the leg. Symptoms are usually exacerbated by activity such as walking or prolonged standing.

The hallmark of the physical examination is the reproduction of paresthesias with percussion over the posterior tibial nerve (Tinel sign). On physical examination, it is important to inspect for soft-tissue masses on the medial aspect of the ankle and to note any varicosities as well as the presence of any hindfoot malalignment. Positioning the ankle and foot in dorsiflexion and eversion may reproduce the symptoms, analogous to the Phalen sign in the hands.[3] Evaluation of the lumbosacral spine is important because radiculopathy can present in a similar fashion. The patient should also be questioned about other causes of neuropathy, such as diabetes and alcoholism. Electrodiagnostic studies are useful for confirming the site of nerve compression and can eliminate more proximal nerve compression as a source of symptoms. Electrodiagnostic studies are accurate approximately 80% to 90% of the time, and sensory nerve conduction velocity studies are more likely to be abnormal than motor nerve conduction velocity studies. Needle electromyography is of uncertain value in the diagnosis of tarsal tunnel syndrome.[4] MRI is used to exclude a mass within the tunnel.

If there is a mass within the tarsal tunnel, removal is usually recommended, but otherwise the initial treatment is resting the foot and ankle in a removable walking boot. A local injection of a corticosteroid may be used but is associated with a risk of an injury to the posterior tibial tendon. Physical therapy modalities, such as ice, heat, and ultrasound, may be helpful for providing symptomatic relief. Orthotics should be prescribed for patients with biomechanical abnormalities, especially if hyperpronation is present.

The indications for surgical decompression include a failure of nonsurgical treatment as previously described and objective evidence of nerve compression within the tarsal tunnel. The best results of surgery are achieved in patients with positive electrodiagnostic tests, a positive Tinel sign, a space-occupying lesion, and paresthesias in the distribution of the posterior tibial nerve. The results of surgery have been reported to be successful in 50% to 90% of patients. The use of a tourniquet is optional; however, if a tourniquet is used, it should be deflated before closure to ensure that a hematoma does not form. Some authors have recommended distal decompression of the medial and lateral plantar tunnels.[1] Unsatisfactory outcomes are associated with postoperative wound complications such as infection, dehiscence, hematoma formation, incomplete release of the tarsal tunnel, and complex regional pain syndrome.

Posterior Tibial Tendon Dysfunction (Adult-Acquired Flatfoot Deformity)

Adult-acquired flatfoot deformity begins with tenosynovitis or injury to the posterior tibial tendon, eventually resulting in tendon elongation and dysfunction. Originally, this condition was known as posterior tibial dysfunction because tendon failure occurred as a result of tendon degeneration. As the posterior tibial tendon elongates and becomes dysfunctional, unopposed peroneus brevis contraction results in hindfoot eversion, causing stretching of the unsupported medial ankle ligaments and soft tissues. The spring ligament fails, the talus plantar flexes, and the medial longitudinal arch collapses. As the forefoot abducts at the talonavicular joint, the Achilles tendon falls lateral to the midline and contributes further to hindfoot valgus.

A hypovascular zone begins 2 to 4 cm proximal to the insertion of the posterior tibial tendon, rendering this area susceptible to tenosynovitis and/or injury, with overuse being a possible cause. Patients present with posteromedial ankle pain and swelling over the posterior tibial tendon and have difficulty with stair climbing and walking on uneven ground. In later stages, lateral pain predominates because of fibular impingement. Approximately 25% of patients have a history of a previous medial ankle sprain. On clinical examination, a pes planovalgus deformity develops as the tendon elongates; soft-tissue swelling is often observed along the course of the posterior tibial tendon. Observation of the standing patient from the rear demonstrates the "too many toes" sign (**Figure 1**). The patient should be asked to do a single-leg heel rise. With the contralateral foot off the ground, a normal patient will stand on tiptoe, and, in the process, the heel inverts. If the heel does not invert or if the patient is unable to raise the heel off the ground, there is likely dysfunction of the posterior tibial tendon.

Weight-bearing AP and lateral ankle and foot radiographs as well as an

Table 1
Four Stages of Adult-Acquired Flatfoot Deformity

Stage	Deformity	Surgical Treatment
I	No deformity from adult-acquired flatfoot deformity (may have preexisting flatfoot)	Tenosynovectomy, possible tendon transfer, and/or medial slide osteotomy
IIa	Mild/moderate flexible deformity (minimal abduction through talonavicular joint, < 30% talonavicular uncoverage)	Tendon transfer, medial slide osteotomy, possible Cotton procedure
IIb	Severe flexible deformity (abduction deformity through talonavicular joint, > 30% talonavicular uncoverage)	Tendon transfer, medial slide osteotomy, and possible lateral column lengthening or hindfoot fusion (subtalar or talonavicular and calcaneocuboid fusion) Cotton procedure or metatarsal-tarsal fusion performed as needed for elevation of the first ray
III	Fixed deformity (involving the triple-joint complex)	Hindfoot fusion, most commonly triple arthrodesis; correction requires fusion of all three joints
IV	Foot deformity and ankle deformity (lateral talar tilt)	Complete correction of foot deformity, possible deltoid reconstruction For severe arthritis, perform ankle fusion or total ankle arthroplasty, including correction of foot deformity
IVa	Flexible foot deformity	Foot deformity corrected as with stage IIb
IVb	Fixed foot deformity	Foot deformity corrected as with stage III

(Adapted from Deland JT: Adult-acquired flatfoot deformity. *J Am Acad Orthop Surg* 2008;16:399-406.)

axial calcaneal radiograph should be obtained. Particular attention should be paid to the presence of disruption of the normal talar-first metatarsal angle on both the AP and lateral radiographs. Although not necessary for diagnosis, MRI can be a useful adjunct. Axial MRIs have been reported to be 96% accurate for identifying tendon pathology.

Johnson and Strom[5] described three stages of posterior tibial tendon dysfunction, and Myerson[6] added a fourth (**Table 1**). Stage I is characterized by tenosynovitis, no deformity, and preservation of posterior tibial tendon strength. Often, patients report a long history of flatfoot deformity. Stage II is characterized by tendon dysfunction and weakness in the presence of a correctable deformity. Stage II has been further subdivided on the basis of the amount of abduction that is present at the midfoot.[7] Stage IIa disease is characterized by minimal abduction (< 30% peritalar subluxation on a standing AP foot radiograph), whereas stage IIb disease is characterized by uncoverage of more than 30% of the talar head. Stage III deformity is characterized by a rigid deformity with lateral pain caused by fibular impingement. Passive inversion of the triple joint complex is not possible past the neutral position. Stage IV disease is characterized by ankle involvement secondary to deltoid ligament incompetence, although the foot deformity may be either flexible or rigid.

Nonsurgical treatment consists of treatment in a boot, cast, or customized brace such as the Arizona brace, supplemented with nonsteroidal anti-inflammatory drugs or oral steroids. Steroid injections are not recommended because of the risk of tendon rupture. Physical therapy modalities, begun once the initial inflammation subsides, include ultrasound, iontophoresis with dexamethasone, cryotherapy, strengthening with progressive resistance of all muscle groups about the foot and ankle, and stretching of the Achilles tendon with the subtalar joint in a neutral position. Twenty-two of 32 patients with stage II posterior tibial tendon dysfunction who were managed temporarily with a double upright ankle-foot orthosis and were followed for an average of 8.6 years were able to avoid surgical treatment.[8] Five patients continued use of the brace, and an additional five patients had surgery. Alvarez et al[9] reported that 42 of 47 patients with stage I and II posterior tibial tendon dysfunction were effectively managed with an orthosis and structured exercises. A customized brace, such as an articulating ankle-foot orthosis or Arizona brace, is also effective for providing long-term symptomatic relief. Currently, it is unknown if these devices alter the progression of the disease.

Patients should be managed nonsurgically for at least 3 months. Surgical treatment of stage I adult-acquired flatfoot deformity includes tenosynovectomy as well as possible tendon repair or flexor digitorum longus tendon transfer. If tendon transfer is performed, a medializing calcaneal osteotomy should be done concomitantly in patients with a flatfoot deformity.

The surgical treatment of stage IIa deformity involves a transfer of the flexor digitorum longus to the midfoot

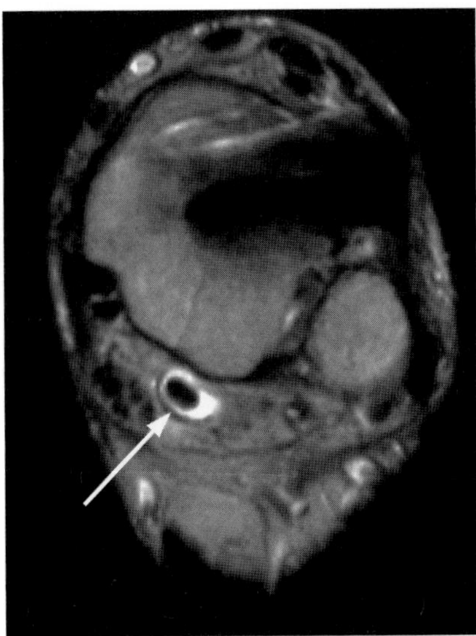

Figure 2 T1-weighted axial MRI scan of the ankle illustrating fluid surrounding the flexor hallucis longus tendon (arrow), consistent with flexor hallucis longus tenosynovitis. (Adapted from Recht MP, Donley BG: Magnetic resonance imaging of the foot and ankle. *J Am Acad Orthop Surg* 2001;9:187-199.)

and a medial displacement osteotomy of the calcaneus. An Achilles tendon lengthening or a Strayer procedure is usually necessary because of the development of an equinus contracture. In a series of 129 surgically managed patients, Myerson et al[10] reported that 97% had pain relief, 94% had improved function, and 84% were able to wear shoes without shoe modifications or orthotics. A medial column fusion or Cotton osteotomy may be performed to treat forefoot varus. In patients with stage IIb deformity, a lateral column lengthening calcaneal osteotomy may be necessary to treat forefoot abduction.

The surgical treatment of stage III deformity involves a triple arthrodesis to correct the plantar flexed talus and the subluxated talonavicular joint. If excessive heel valgus remains after triple arthrodesis, a medial slide osteotomy of the calcaneus is recommended. An Achilles tendon lengthening or a Strayer procedure is usually necessary. Isolated subtalar fusion is not recommended if a rigid forefoot varus deformity is present because correction of the forefoot varus deformity can only be accomplished by including the transverse tarsal joints in the fusion. Surgical treatment of stage IV deformity involves deltoid ligament repair or reconstruction (with use of tendon graft) to correct talar tilt. If the deformities in the hindfoot and ankle are flexible, then the same procedures used for a stage II deformity can be combined with deltoid reconstruction. For rigid deformities, triple arthrodesis with reconstruction of the deltoid ligament is recommended. End-stage posterior tibial tendon dysfunction with associated ankle joint arthrosis requires either a pantalar fusion or a triple arthrodesis and a total ankle replacement.

Patients with seronegative arthropathy (ankylosing spondylitis, psoriasis, and Reiter syndrome) are also at increased risk for the development of a flatfoot deformity. These patients present with enthesopathy, or inflammation and maximum tenderness at the tendon insertion. Planovalgus deformity secondary to tenosynovitis and destruction of the subtalar and talonavicular joints may also develop in patients with rheumatoid arthritis. If these patients have persistent tenosynovitis, early surgical treatment is needed to prevent tendon rupture.

Flexor Hallucis Longus Tendinitis

Flexor hallucis longus tendinitis is differentiated from posterior ankle impingement by the presence of posteromedial pain and soft-tissue swelling along the posteromedial aspect of the ankle. The flexor hallucis longus tendon descends from the leg into the foot through a sulcus, which is bordered by the posteromedial and posterolateral tubercles of the talus. The pain may be aggravated by passive toe motion. Gymnasts, dancers, runners, and tennis players are prone to the development of this condition as a result of activities that require repetitive push-off. On physical examination, crepitus over the flexor hallucis longus may be present. The Thomason test demonstrates that, in the presence of functional hallux rigidus, the patient has normal motion of the metatarsophalangeal joint with the ankle in plantar flexion, but with the ankle in dorsiflexion, passive dorsiflexion of the metatarsophalangeal joint is reduced.[11] In chronic cases, triggering may be present if nodules are present within the substance of the flexor hallucis longus. Radiographs may show a symptomatic os trigonum or fractures. MRI may show fluid within the tendon sheath (**Figure 2**).

Nonsurgical treatment begins with rest and modified training. A removable walking boot should be used as necessary. Ice, cryotherapy, ultrasound, and stretching are done next, before surgery is considered. Local steroid injections are not recommended for the treatment of flexor hallucis longus tendinitis but may be useful to exclude posterior ankle impingement caused by an os trigonum. Surgery, if needed, involves a release of the flexor hallucis longus sheath through a posteromedial approach. After surgery, the foot is placed in a splint for 3 weeks, after which motion and strengthening exercises are begun.

Posterior Ankle Impingement

The posterior process of the talus includes the posteromedial and posterolateral tubercles. The flexor hallucis longus runs between these tubercles and has a discrete osseous tunnel. In 10% of the population, an unfused posterolateral process, or os trigonum, is present.[12] An enlarged posterolateral tubercle is known as a Stieda process. Any of these structures can cause posterior ankle pain with the ankle in plantar flexion. Most commonly, an acute plantar flexion injury will damage the os trigonum or the synchondrosis (**Figure 3**). A symptomatic Stieda process or synovitis in the flexor hallucis longus also can cause these symptoms.

The patient with posterior ankle impingement who does not have flexor hallucis longus tenosynovitis reports posterolateral ankle pain. Activities that require repetitive plantar flexion, such as ballet dancing, downhill running, and soccer, are often associated with this impingement. The patient has posterolateral tenderness and pain on the forced plantar flexion test. The patient frequently sprains the ankle because the foot is placed in an inverted position to avoid impingement. The patient also reports pain with motion of the great toe when flexor hallucis longus tendinitis is present. In addition to standard foot radiographs, a neutral weight-bearing lateral foot and ankle radiograph and a plantar flexion lateral foot and ankle radiograph are beneficial. A plantar flexion lateral radiograph may show an acute or old fracture of the trigonal process, the presence of an os trigonum, or dynamic impingement (**Figure 4**). CT is a useful adjunct to rule out an occult fracture of the posterior process. A normal bone scan eliminates the trigonal process as a source of pathology. MRI is the study of choice to assess for bone edema and possible changes in the soft tissues, such as the flexor hallucis longus.

Nonsteroidal anti-inflammatory drugs, icing, activity modification, and strapping of the foot to minimize ankle dorsiflexion are often successful. Immobilization in a removable boot limits plantar flexion to avoid the foot position that causes pain. Injection with lidocaine and steroid may be used posterolaterally for both diagnostic and therapeutic purposes. After 4 to 6 weeks of this therapy, physiotherapy with stretching and strengthening exercises is prescribed.

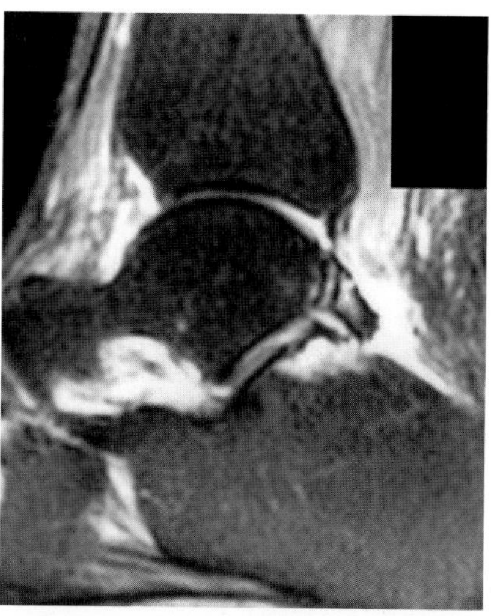

Figure 3 T2-weighted sagittal MRI scan of the ankle, showing an os trigonum. (Adapted from Berkowitz MJ, Kim DH: Process and tubercle fractures of the hindfoot. *J Am Acad Orthop Surg* 2005;13:492-502.)

If nonsurgical treatment fails, surgical excision of the os trigonum and redundant capsule is recommended. For isolated posterior ankle impingement, a posterolateral approach is used. The patient is placed in the prone position, the sural nerve is identified and protected, and a more direct approach to the trigonal process is provided. The limiting factor in this approach is that dissection medial to the flexor hallucis longus is not advisable because of potential damage to the neurovascular structures in the vicinity. For patients with concomitant flexor hallucis longus tenosynovitis and posterior impingement, a posteromedial approach is recommended.

Arthroscopic techniques have been described for the treatment of posterior impingement. Procedures that have been performed have included excision of an os trigonum, decompression of a prominent posterior talar process, tenolysis of the flexor hallucis longus, the removal of loose bodies, and débridement of posterior osteochondritis dissecans lesions. Uncontrolled case series have reported earlier return to activities, less morbidity, and outcomes that compared favorably with open lateral approaches.[13]

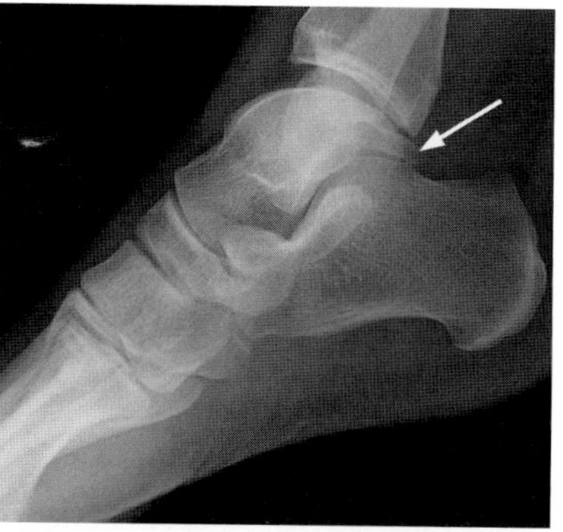

Figure 4 Plantar flexion lateral ankle radiograph showing posterior ankle impingement (arrow) caused by a Stieda process.

Achilles Tendinitis and Retrocalcaneal Bursitis

Disorders of the Achilles tendon and retrocalcaneal bursa are the most common causes of posterior ankle pain. Runners are frequently affected, as are those who participate in jumping sports. The Achilles tendon arises from the gastrocnemius and soleus muscles and broadly inserts onto the calcaneal tuberosity. The tendon receives its vascular supply from proximal muscular branches and distal calcaneal branches. The tendon is protected by an external sheath, the paratenon, and has an avascular zone approximately 2 to 6 cm proximal to its calcaneal insertion due to a watershed zone of its blood supply. A retrocalcaneal bursa, located anterior to the Achilles tendon, lubricates the anterior aspect of the distal part of the Achilles tendon. Pathology of the Achilles tendon can be caused by inflammation limited to the paratenon

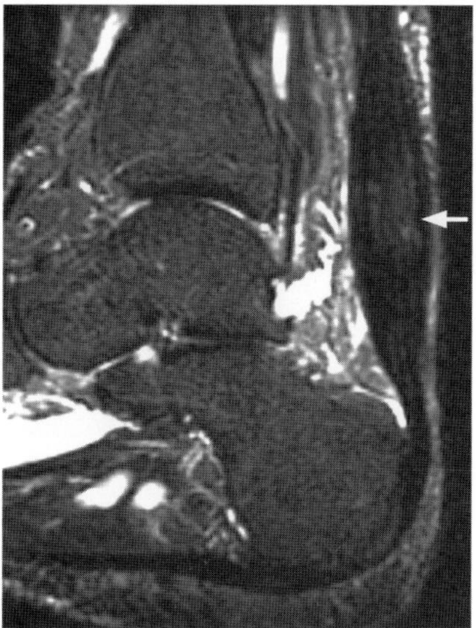

Figure 5 T2-weighted sagittal MRI scan showing thickening of the Achilles tendon and intrasubstance degeneration (arrow), consistent with chronic tendinosis. (Reproduced from Reddy SS, Pedowitz DI, Parekh SG, Omar IM, Wapner KL: Surgical treatment for chronic disease and disorders of the Achilles tendon. *J Am Acad Orthop Surg* 2009;17:3-14.)

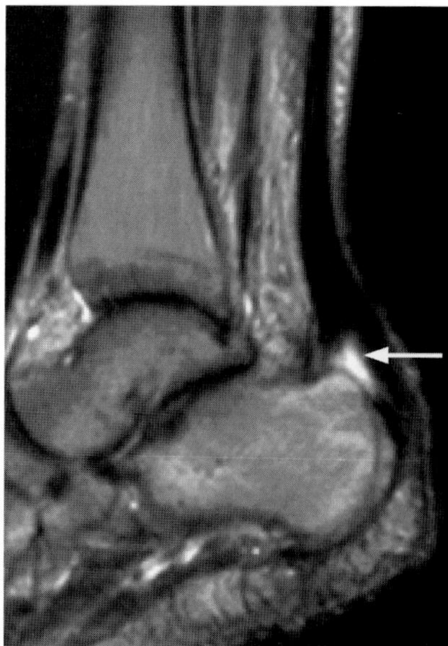

Figure 6 T1-weighted sagittal MRI scan showing insertional Achilles tendinitis and impingement secondary to a Haglund deformity. Area of high signal intensity (arrow) represents a partial tear. (Reproduced from Recht MP, Donley BG: Magnetic resonance imaging of the foot and ankle. *J Am Acad Orthop Surg* 2001;9:187-199.)

(paratenonitis), intrasubstance mucoid degeneration and tendon thickening (tendinosis), or insertional Achilles tendinosis with retrocalcaneal bursitis.

Noninsertional Achilles tendon pathology causes pain in the avascular zone (**Figure 5**). Predisposing factors for noninsertional Achilles tendinitis include increased age, male sex, excessive hindfoot varus or valgus, and overuse. Patients with insertional Achilles tendinosis and retrocalcaneal bursitis present with posterosuperior heel pain that is aggravated by shoe wear and activity. Insertional Achilles tendinitis can be a presenting symptom of seronegative arthritis. Swelling, crepitus, and tenderness are characteristically present in patients with paratenonitis. Tenderness can be elicited by squeezing the tendon proximal to its insertion. Fusiform swelling is typical of degenerative tendinosis. Patients with insertional Achilles tendinitis and retrocalcaneal bursitis have tenderness at the calcaneal insertion (**Figure 6**).

Medial and lateral fullness of the retrocalcaneal space is typical of retrocalcaneal bursitis. In patients with tendinitis and concomitant bursitis, tenderness is present anterior to the Achilles tendon, and an enlargement of the posterior superior calcaneal process (a Haglund deformity) may be present. Standing AP and lateral radiographs of the foot and ankle should be made. Haglund deformity, if present, is seen on the lateral radiograph. Ultrasound has been reported to be sensitive and specific for confirming noninsertional Achilles tendinosis.[14] MRI is useful for evaluating both noninsertional and insertional Achilles tendinitis as well as paratenonitis.

Nonsurgical treatment of noninsertional and insertional Achilles tendinitis is nonsteroidal anti-inflammatory drugs for pain relief, heel lifts, Achilles tendon stretching, shoes that do not put pressure on the back of the heel, and activity modification. Ice, massage, ultrasound, and iontophoresis can be used. Temporary immobilization in a removable boot or night splint or even a short leg cast can be used if the patient has severe pain. Corticosteroid injections are not recommended because of the risk of tendon rupture. Eccentric strengthening of the calf muscle has been recommended as an effective treatment of both insertional and noninsertional tendinopathy.[15,16] Prospective randomized studies have shown that repetitive low-energy shock-wave therapy was superior to eccentric muscle training for patients with insertional and noninsertional tendinopathy.[17,18] In one study, kinematic evaluation of runners with noninsertional tendinopathy showed an increase in eversion of the subtalar joint.[19] Consequently, orthotic devices that control subtalar eversion may help this group of patients. Another study evaluated the effectiveness of platelet-rich plasma in patients with noninsertional tendinopathy.[20] This randomized controlled trial evaluated patients who were managed with eccentric exercises and either saline solution injections (control) or platelet-rich plasma. The authors reported that platelet-rich plasma did not result in significant improvements in terms of pain or function compared with the findings in the group managed with saline solution. Nonsurgical treatment of acute paratenonitis is usually successful, but patients with chronic symptoms are more likely to require surgery.

Surgical treatment of Achilles tendinitis or paratenonitis is indicated for patients in whom symptoms persist despite supervised nonsurgical management for 6 months.

Tenolysis of the paratenon and débridement of the degenerative tendon is used to treat patients with noninsertional disease. If more than 50% of the tendon is involved, augmentation with an autogenous graft is recommended. Excision of a Haglund deformity (if present) and débridement of diseased tendon is done for patients with insertional disease. If more than 50% of the tendon insertion is débrided, augmentation with a flexor hallucis longus transfer is recommended.

A compression dressing is applied after surgery and is kept on for 1 week; the patient is then managed with a cast or a boot for 6 to 8 weeks. The patient should use a heel lift for 6 more weeks and should begin to resume normal activities at 3 months. Maximum medical improvement may take 6 to 12 months, especially in patients with insertional Achilles tendinitis. Following the surgical treatment of chronic Achilles tendinopathy, 86% to 100% of patients have satisfactory results.[21-24]

Chronic Lateral Instability

Nine million people sustain ankle sprains each year in the United States. Most are caused by a plantar-flexed inversion injury that leads to compromise of the anterior talofibular ligament and/or the calcaneofibular ligament. These injuries typically heal uneventfully after short-term immobilization, ice, compression, and elevation, and early range of motion. However, chronic lateral ankle instability and residual symptoms develop in a subset of patients who sustain an injury of these ligaments. These patients have subjective reports of instability without radiographic abnormalities but have functional instability, reporting the ankle "giving way." Some have measurable hypermobility and objective findings of mechanical instability.

Patients reporting "giving way" typically have a history of a severe ankle sprain or recurrent ankle inversion injuries. Pain usually is not a predominant symptom, and, when pain is present, an associated injury should be suspected.[25-27] Commonly associated abnormalities are loose bodies, synovitis, osteochondral injuries, osteophytes, peroneal tendon pathology, and chondromalacia. The evaluation should include an examination for malalignment, particularly hindfoot varus, first-ray plantar flexion, and cavus deformities, which predispose to recurrent inversion injuries. Manual anterior drawer and talar tilt tests are critical for evaluating the integrity of the anterior talofibular ligament and the calcaneofibular ligament, respectively. The involved ankle should be compared with the contralateral ankle to assess for asymmetric laxity. The involved ankle should also be evaluated for peroneal tendon tenderness and subluxation.

In addition to standard radiographs, stress views can be used when the clinical examination is equivocal. The anterior drawer stress radiograph is the most useful. Radiographic signs of instability include more than 10 mm of subluxation, or 3 mm more than the contralateral side. On the talar tilt stress radiograph, more than 10° of varus talar tilt or a side-to-side difference of more than 3° raises the possibility of instability. MRI is not necessary to make the diagnosis of instability; however, it helps to identify associated intra-articular or periarticular sources of pain. Strengthening and proprioceptive training are the mainstays of physical therapy programs and can decrease the episodes of instability. Bracing and orthotics can be used, especially for patients with varus ankle malalignment.

Surgical treatment is reserved for those in whom nonsurgical therapy has failed. More than 80 surgical techniques have been described for the treatment of chronic lateral ankle instability. Anatomic repairs that restore normal anatomy and joint kinematics are preferred. The modified Broström repair, using the extensor retinaculum to reinforce the ligament repair, has a high rate of patient satisfaction[28-30] (**Figure 7**). Patients with generalized ligamentous laxity do not do as well with the modified Broström technique, and nonanatomic repair techniques (for example, the Evans tenodesis and the Chrisman-Snook procedure) are better for these patients. Nonanatomic repair procedures restore stability but sacrifice normal joint kinematics and subtalar motion in the process. Anatomic reconstruction procedures using autogenous tissue (such as hamstring tendons) or allografts are also potential treatment options and do not alter normal ankle kinematics. A split peroneus brevis tendon that is anchored distally at its insertion; routed through bone tunnels in the calcaneus, fibula, and talus; and then sutured back onto itself can also be used for patients with generalized laxity. Case series have indicated

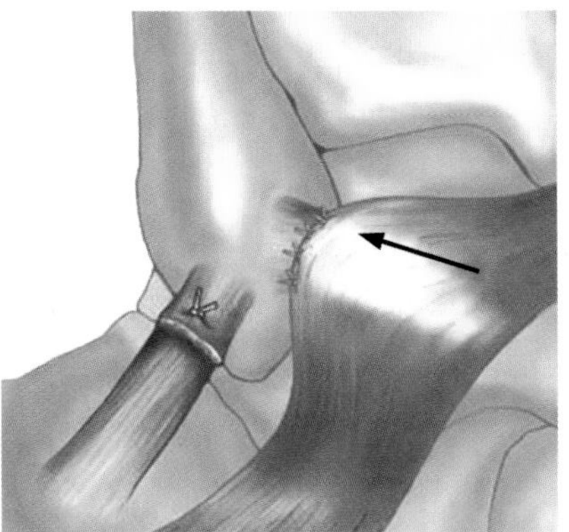

Figure 7 Gould modification of the Broström procedure for lateral ankle instability, with the inferior extensor retinaculum being used to reinforce the ligament repair (arrow). (Reproduced from Maffulli N, Ferran NA: Management of acute and chronic ankle instability. *J Am Acad Orthop Surg* 2008;16:608-615.)

that 83% to 100% of patients managed with anatomic tenodesis report good or excellent outcomes.[31]

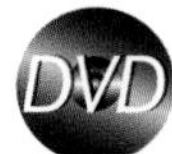

Video 29.1: The Anatomic Reconstruction of Chronic Lateral Ankle Instability: A Modified Broström-Gould Technique. Sameh A. Labib, MD; William S. Kimmerly, MD; Spero G. Karas, MD (6 min)

Peroneal Tendon Pathology

The peroneus longus muscle originates from the lateral condyle of the tibia and the head of the fibula. The tendon travels behind the lateral malleolus through a tunnel known as the retromalleolar groove. This groove is bordered by the fibula anteriorly and by a fibrous band known as the superior peroneal retinaculum posterolaterally. The peroneus longus tendon turns medially at the cuboid groove and inserts into the lateral part of the plantar aspect of the first metatarsal and the medial cuneiform. The function of the peroneus longus is to evert the foot and plantar flex the ankle, but it also plantar flexes the first ray and thus serves as an antagonist to the tibialis anterior muscle.

The peroneus brevis originates from the fibula in the middle third of the leg. It is located anterior and medial to the peroneus longus at the level of the ankle and inserts into the tuberosity of the fifth metatarsal and functions to evert and plantar flex the foot. Occasionally, there is a low-lying brevis muscle belly, which may become symptomatic. In most cases, however, the musculotendinous junctions of both tendons are located proximal to the superior peroneal retinaculum. The os peroneum is present in 20% of the population. It is an ossified sesamoid bone, which is found at the level of the calcaneocuboid joint, and can become symptomatic. A peroneus quartus muscle, found in the lateral compartment in about 20% of the population, originates from the brevis muscle belly and inserts into the peroneal tubercle of the calcaneus. Patients with this muscle have a higher risk of peroneal tubercle hypertrophy and stenosing tenosynovitis.

Patients with peroneal tendon pathology have persistent swelling along the peroneal tendon sheath. Retromalleolar pain or ankle instability is the usual complaint. When the tendons are subluxating or dislocating, the patient may have a snapping sensation. In patients who have a history of an acute injury, tendon rupture should be suspected. The alignment of the hindfoot should be evaluated because a varus heel position is associated with an increased rate of peroneal tendon disorders. Eversion strength should be tested. It should be remembered that the peroneus tertius, extensor digitorum longus, and extensor hallucis longus also provide some eversion of the foot. Peroneal tendon dislocation or subluxation can be identified by rotating the ankle to see if the tendons subluxate anterior to the lateral malleolus.

Weight-bearing AP and lateral radiographs of the symptomatic ankle should be made. In addition, an axial heel radiograph will help show the peroneal tubercle and the retromalleolar groove. CT scans are a valuable adjunct for evaluating osseous abnormalities, such as peroneal tubercle hypertrophy, os peroneum fractures, or an avulsion of the lateral malleolus. MRI has emerged as the imaging modality of choice for this condition because heterogeneity or discontinuity of the tendon, a fluid-filled tendon sheath, marrow edema along the lateral calcaneal wall, a hypertrophied peroneal tubercle, the shape of the posterior part of the fibula, and the integrity of the superior peroneal retinaculum can all be evaluated.

Nonsurgical treatment of peroneal tendinitis involves nonsteroidal anti-inflammatory medications, rest, and activity modification. Mild cases of tendinitis can be treated with a lateral heel wedge. In refractory cases, a short leg cast or controlled ankle motion walker can be used for 6 weeks. If nonsurgical treatment is ineffective, an open tenosynovectomy and débridement of any region of the tendon that appears to be degenerated is recommended. The remaining portion of the tendon is subsequently repaired in a tubelike fashion with a running 4-0 nylon suture (**Figure 8**). If the remaining portion of the tendon is of insufficient size or poor quality, a tenodesis of the diseased tendon to the adjacent peroneal tendon (for example, peroneus brevis to longus tenodesis) should be done.

Peroneal tendon tears or ruptures are treated surgically, unless the patient is not a candidate for surgical treatment because of medical comorbidities. In such cases, the patient can be managed with a lateral heel wedge. If possible, an acute tendon rupture is treated with an end-to-end repair. If this is not possible, a transfer of the flexor digitorum longus to the peroneus brevis is a viable option. Surgical treatment of peroneal tendon tears is based on the amount of remaining viable tendon. Primary repair and tubularization is indicated for tears involving less than 50% of the tendon, and tenodesis is indicated for tears involving more than 50% of the tendon.[32] If both tendons are intact, the torn tissue is débrided and tubularized. If one tendon is torn and irreparable and the other is functional, a tenodesis can be performed with use of the myotendinous junctions of the tendons. If one tendon is torn and irreparable and the other is nonfunctional, flexor digito-

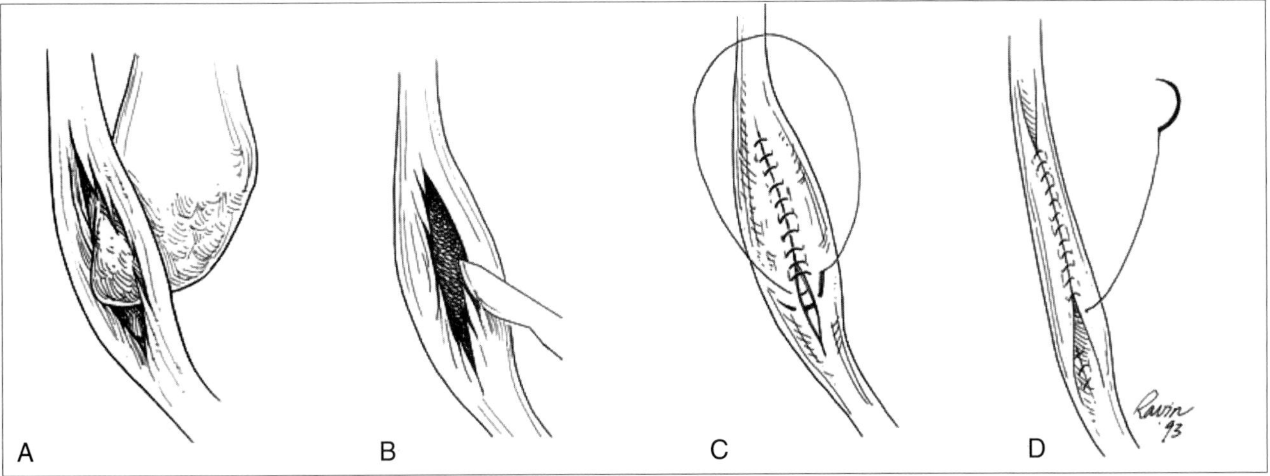

Figure 8 Illustration depicting a peroneal tendon tear (**A**) and repair. Steps may include débridement (**B**), repair (**C**), and tubularization (**D**). (Reproduced from Chiodo CP: Acute and chronic tendon injury, in Richardson EG, ed: *Orthopaedic Knowledge Update: Foot and Ankle 3.* Rosemont, IL, American Academy of Orthopaedic Surgeons, 2003, pp 81-89.)

rum longus transfer as previously described should be considered. Hindfoot varus, ankle instability, and osteophyte formation, which contribute to peroneal tendon tearing, should also be corrected. In one report, residual symptoms were reported to be present in more than 50% of patients and less than 50% of patients returned to sports activities after surgical repair.[33]

Peroneal tendon subluxation occurs following disruption of the superior peroneal retinaculum. Eckert and Davis[34] described three grades of injuries to the superior peroneal retinaculum. In grade I, the superior peroneal retinaculum is elevated from the fibula; in grade II, a fibrocartilaginous ridge is elevated from the fibula; and in grade III, a cortical fragment is avulsed with the superior peroneal retinaculum. Nonsurgical treatment can be attempted for acute grade I and III injuries with use of a short leg cast for 6 weeks. If this treatment fails, the superior peroneal retinaculum is reattached surgically after the creation of an osseous trough along the posterolateral aspect of the fibula. For patients with chronic peroneal subluxation, a fibular groove-deepening procedure is indicated. This procedure involves raising an osseous flap from the posterolateral corner of the fibula and using a burr to remove the cancellous bone beneath the flap. The flap is then reduced and is tamped into place. The superior peroneal retinaculum is then repaired over the tendons, which are located in the newly deepened groove. In a similar fashion, a bone block procedure can be performed, with a sagittal cut of the fibula, translating the more lateral portion posteriorly, and holding the displaced fibula with screws.[35]

Occult Fractures of the Hindfoot

Process and tubercle fractures of the hindfoot can be difficult to diagnose and treat. These injuries are often misdiagnosed as a sprain of the ankle or foot, leading to a delay in diagnosis and suboptimal outcomes.[36] Prompt diagnosis requires a high index of suspicion and a thorough knowledge of the anatomy of the hindfoot. Specialized radiographs as well as CT and MRI may be needed to confirm the diagnosis. Fractures of the anterior process of the calcaneus occur with inversion of the plantar-flexed ankle and are the result of an avulsion injury of the bifurcate ligament. Tenderness is usually reproduced in an area 2 cm anterior and 1 cm inferior to the anterior talofibular ligament. This fracture is typically not visualized on standard AP radiographs of the foot and ankle. An oblique radiograph of the foot with the x-ray beam directed 10° to 25° superior and posterior to the midfoot is necessary. This projects the anterior process away from the talar neck and enables optimal visualization of the fracture. As an adjunct, multiplanar CT imaging with fine 1-mm cuts can be done to provide a more accurate delineation of displacement and fragment size, which influence treatment decisions.

For fracture fragments that are larger than 1 cm in size and are displaced by more than 2 mm, a below-knee, non–weight-bearing cast can be applied for a period of 6 weeks, followed by transition to a removable walking boot and progressive weight bearing. Open reduction and internal fixation is recommended for fractures that are larger than 1 cm in size and are

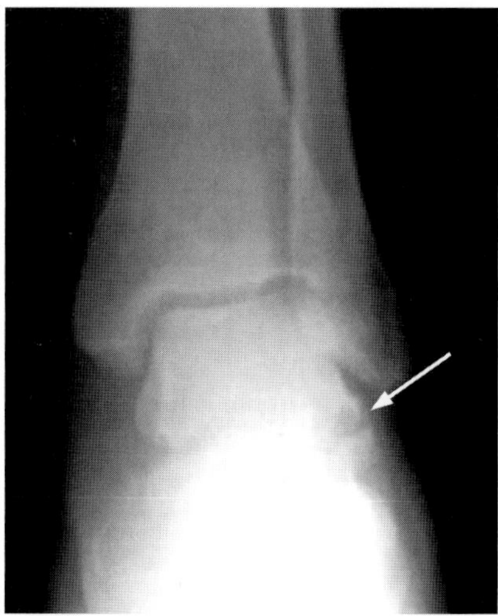

Figure 9 AP ankle radiograph showing a fracture of the lateral talar process (arrow). (Reproduced from Berkowitz MJ, Kim DH: Process and tubercle fractures of the hindfoot. *J Am Acad Orthop Surg* 2005;13:492-502.)

displaced by more than 2 mm with intra-articular involvement.[37]

Lateral talar process fractures typically occur after a fall or motor vehicle crash, but they also occur in association with snowboarding injuries. Approximately 2,000 lateral talar process fractures occur annually in these athletes.[38] The lateral talar process is avulsed by the lateral talocalcaneal ligament with an inversion injury. Another mechanism is an eversion moment that is applied to a dorsiflexed, axially loaded foot, causing compression and fracture of the lateral talar process. Careful palpation just anterior and inferior to the lateral malleolus can elicit pain, which should raise suspicion for this injury. Lateral talar process fractures usually can be visualized on routine radiographs, although subtle fragments just distal to the lateral malleolus may be difficult to appreciate (**Figure 9**). The amount of displacement and the extent of articular involvement of the posterior facet of the subtalar joint are seen on a thin-cut CT scan.[39]

Fracture fragments that are less than 1 cm in size and displaced by more than 2 mm are treated nonsurgically. Displaced fractures are best treated with open reduction and internal fixation or primary excision, with excision favored in scenarios in which the fracture is comminuted. If open reduction and internal fixation is feasible, fixation is typically done with minifragment screws or Kirschner wires.[38]

Sinus Tarsi Syndrome

Sinus tarsi syndrome is associated with persistent lateral ankle pain directly over the sinus tarsi. It is usually a result of an inversion injury, and the patient may report a feeling of instability. Several theories have been advocated to explain the source of pain, including interosseous ligament injury; hypertrophy of the synovium; or hypertrophy of the fat, resulting in impingement of the neural plexus. The diagnosis is one of exclusion and is confirmed on the basis of pain relief after an injection of local anesthetic into the sinus tarsi. Radiographs show normal findings and serve to eliminate other causes of pain, such as occult fractures or subtalar arthritis. MRI scans may show nonspecific inflammation in the sinus tarsi, sinus tarsi fat alterations, chronic synovitis and synovial thickening, interosseous talocalcaneal ligament tears, cervical ligament tears, or a ganglion cyst.[40] Nonsurgical treatment is similar to that for chronic lateral ankle instability. Injections, diagnostic and therapeutic, have been reported to be successful in approximately two thirds of patients. Open and arthroscopic débridement of the contents of the sinus tarsi have been described.[41]

Osteochondral Lesions of the Talar Dome

Osteochondral lesions involving the talar dome were originally believed to be secondary to ischemia; however, most authors currently believe that they are caused by trauma. Various names have been used to describe osteochondral lesions involving the talar dome, including osteochondritis dissecans, transchondral fracture, and osteochondral fracture. The talus has a decreased capacity for repair because of its limited blood supply, and the sequelae of osteochondral talar injury include joint degeneration and limited range of motion at the ankle.

Osteochondral lesions of the talus are frequently associated with more obvious traumatic injuries of the foot and ankle. Diagnosis of talar dome injury is often delayed. In some series, as many as 28% of osteochondral injuries of the talus were associated with other fractures involving the foot and ankle, most frequently the malleoli. Osteochondral lesions of the talus can occur as the result of a single traumatic episode or as the result of repetitive microtrauma, such as recurrent lateral ankle sprains.

Several schemes exist for the classifying osteochondral lesions of the talus on the basis of radiographs, CT, MRI, and arthroscopic findings[42-44] (**Table 2**). In patients with chronic ankle pain and a history of injury, clinical suspicion for an osteochondral lesion should be high. Radiographic evaluation is the initial imaging modality of choice; however, false-negative radiographs are common. Any osteochondral lesions that are identified with standard radiographs should be further evaluated with CT, which provides a more complete delineation of the integrity of the subchondral bone. MRI is a useful adjunct for patients without any radiographic abnormality (**Figure 10**). The superiority of MRI for visualizing the surface of the articular cartilage and edema of the talus makes it the study of choice for the evaluation of suspected stage I osteochondral lesions. The treatment of osteochondral lesions of the talus is based on the stage of the lesion. Cast immobilization for 12 to 16 weeks with progressive weight bearing to full weight bearing at the end of immobilization is recommended for stage I or II lesions. Patients with a stage I or II lesion that remains painful for 1 year and those with a stage III or IV lesion are candidates for surgery. Surgery can involve débridement and lavage, marrow-stimulating procedures, or restorative techniques. Arthroscopic débridement of the lesion and techniques that induce healing by stimulating the underlying marrow are successful in approximately 80% of patients.[43] Lesions measuring more than 1.5 cm^2 do not respond well to these techniques. Restoration of the articular surface with osteochondral autografts has been successful for the treatment of lesions measuring less than 1 cm^2 (**Figure 11**).[45] The major disadvantage of using an autograft is donor-site morbidity. Osteochondral allografts have been used for larger lesions; however, the long-term outcomes remain uncertain.

Autologous chondrocyte implantation is a promising technique and has been used for patients who remain symptomatic after previous surgery.[46] The location of the lesion dictates the appropriate surgical approach and may require the use of osteotomies to optimize visualization. Indications for performing these procedures include a lesion with a diameter of more than 1 cm and a depth of at least 5 mm that cannot be repaired primarily. Autologous chondrocyte implantation into the talus has shown some encouraging results in preliminary studies.[46]

Table 2
Classifications of Osteochondral Lesions of the Talus

Radiographic classification[42]
Stage I: small area of compression of the subchondral bone
Stage II: osteochondral fracture that is partially detached
Stage III: complete detachment from the underlying bed without displacement
Stage IV: complete detachment with displacement resulting in a loose body
CT classification[43]
Stage I: cystic lesion within talar dome with intact roof on all views
Stage IIA: cystic lesion with communication to talar dome surface
Stage IIB: open articular surface lesion with overlying nondisplaced fragment
Stage III: nondisplaced lesion with lucency
Stage IV: displaced fragment
MRI classification[44]
Stage I: subchondral compression with marrow edema; normal radiographs and positive uptake on bone scintigraphy
Stage IIA: subchondral cyst
Stage IIB: incomplete fragment separation
Stage III: unattached, nondisplaced fragment with synovial fluid around the fragment
Stage IV: displaced fragment

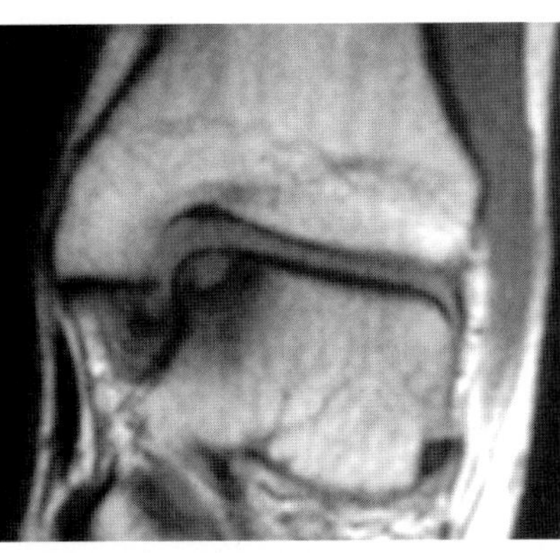

Figure 10 T1-weighted coronal MRI scan of the ankle showing an osteochondral lesion of the medial part of the talus. (Reproduced from Schachter AK, Chen AL, Reddy PD, Tejwani NC: Osteochondral lesions of the talus. *J Am Acad Orthop Surg* 2005;13:152-158.)

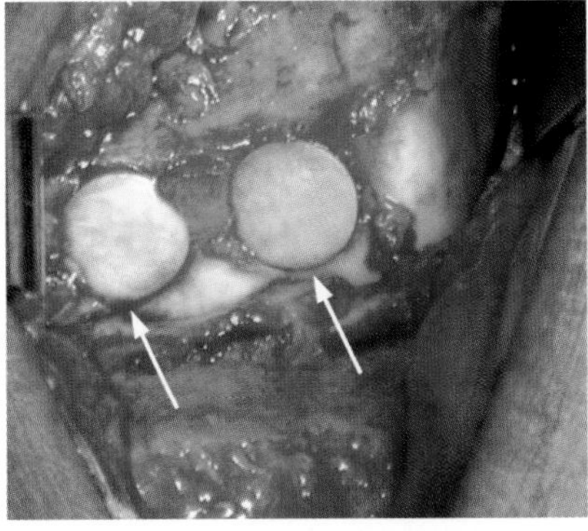

Figure 11 Autologous osteochondral transplant for the treatment of an osteochondral lesion of the talus. Osteochondral autografts are seen (arrows). (Reproduced from Schachter AK, Chen AL, Reddy PD, Tejwani NC: Osteochondral lesions of the talus. *J Am Acad Orthop Surg* 2005;13:152-158.)

Anterior Ankle Impingement

Anterior ankle impingement can be caused by soft-tissue or osseous lesions and typically is related to the superior portion of the anterior talofibular ligament or the distal portion of the anteroinferior tibiofibular ligament.[47] Redundant injured synovial or ligamentous tissue causes joint irritation. Repetitive exaggerated ankle dorsiflexion can lead to soft-tissue impingement, and soccer and basketball players are particularly prone to the development of anterior tibiotalar bone spurs, which result in osseous impingement. Patients report anterior pain, stiffness, and swelling. Walking uphill is painful, whereas downhill walking is more comfortable. The hallmark of the physical examination is

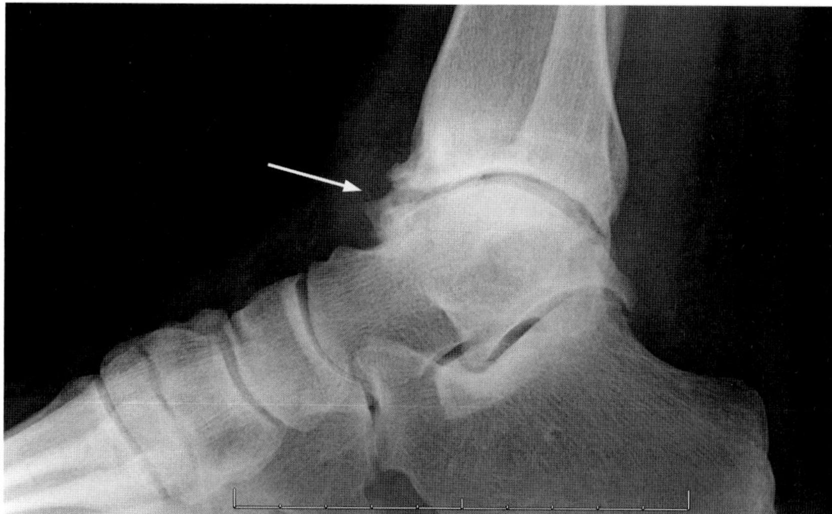

Figure 12 Lateral radiograph of the ankle showing anterior osseous ankle impingement (arrow).

painful limitation of passive dorsiflexion and anterior ankle tenderness. The osseous bone spurs are seen on a lateral ankle radiograph, whereas MRI is useful for seeing the soft-tissue lesions (**Figure 12**). Nonsurgical treatment includes rest, ice, anti-inflammatory medications, and physiotherapy. An intra-articular injection of a local anesthetic and steroid can be diagnostic and therapeutic. Patients often experience symptomatic relief with a small heel lift. Patients who fail to respond to conservative treatment benefit from arthroscopic débridement of soft-tissue lesions. Osseous lesions can be treated with arthroscopic or open methods, depending on the size and location of the lesion as well as the skill of the surgeon.[48]

Nerve Entrapment at the Level of the Ankle

The deep peroneal nerve and the anterior tibial artery are deep to the extensor hallucis longus and the extensor digitorum brevis. Approximately 1 cm proximal to the ankle joint, the nerve branches into a medial motor branch and a lateral sensory branch. The nerve can be compressed by the superior extensor retinaculum, the inferior extensor retinaculum, and the extensor hallucis brevis muscle.[49] Proximal compression by the superior retinaculum causes sensory changes and clawing of the toes. Distal compression by the inferior retinaculum or the extensor hallucis brevis muscle causes isolated sensory deficits.

Patients report burning anterior ankle and dorsal foot pain and may have a history of trauma or recurrent ankle sprains. Paresthesias in the first dorsal web space may be present. An injection of local anesthetic 1 cm proximal to the site of nerve compression should improve or alleviate symptoms. The site of nerve compression is determined by the presence of a positive Tinel sign, which reproduces the symptoms and distal paresthesias in the distribution of the nerve. If the injection does not relieve the symptoms, nerve compression is unlikely. Radiographs may show osteophytes as the source of entrapment, and space-occupying lesions, such as ganglion cysts, can be seen best on MRI scans. Electrodiagnostic testing can determine the location of the lesion, including compression more proximally in the leg or in the lumbar spine.

The superficial peroneal nerve is a pure sensory nerve that becomes superficial in the distal third of the leg, approximately 10 cm proximal to the tip of the fibula. It then continues in the subcutaneous layer and branches into the medial dorsal cutaneous nerve and the intermediate dorsal cutaneous nerve, 6 to 7 cm proximal to the malleolus. Entrapment typically occurs where the nerve becomes subcutaneous, and symptoms rarely radiate proximal to the site of nerve compression. Nerve injury or entrapment can occur in patients with inversion injury as the nerve gets tethered where its exits the fascia.[50] Iatrogenic entrapment can occur after open reduction and internal fixation of fibular fractures and placement of lateral ankle arthroscopic portals.[51,52] Occasionally, space-occupying masses, such as ganglion cysts or fracture callus, will entrap the nerve. Patients present with pain radiating across the ankle and the dorsum of the foot. Tenderness or a Tinel sign is typically present 10 cm proximal to the tip of the distal part of the fibula. Pain is reproduced with several provocative maneuvers, such as foot plantar flexion and inversion, which places the nerve under compression and tightens the fascia. When the foot is dorsiflexed and everted, the nerve is under tension and becomes more sensitive to percussion. The motor and reflex examination reveals normal findings. Ankle stability should be assessed, as instability can place intermittent tension on the superficial peroneal nerve. Proximal causes of nerve irritation, including compression at the fibular neck and lumbar pathology, must be considered. The differential diagnosis should also include exertional compartment syndrome, especially if the patient describes exacerbation of symptoms with activity. A diagnostic injection of local anesthetic just proximal to the site of entrapment helps to confirm the diagnosis.

The lateral sural nerve originates from the common peroneal branch of the sciatic nerve. It innervates the lateral part of the proximal third of the leg. The medial sural nerve originates from the posterior tibial branch of the sciatic nerve and is subfascial. It innervates the posterolateral part of the proximal half of the calf. These two branches meet in the lower third of the calf to form the common sural nerve, which runs along the lateral border of the Achilles tendon, next to the short saphenous vein. It then travels subcutaneously, inferior to the peroneal tendon sheath at the ankle, toward the fifth metatarsal tuberosity, and provides sensation to the lateral aspect of the fifth toe and the fourth web space. Entrapment can occur after closed and surgical treatment of fractures, which cause subsequent scarring in the region of the fifth metatarsal or ankle. Space-occupying lesions can also lead to compression of the nerve.

Patients present with paresthesias in the cutaneous distribution of the sural nerve and have a history of trauma or recurrent ankle sprains. Examination of the entire course of the nerve is necessary, and local tenderness with percussion can identify any areas of impingement. More proximal causes of nerve irritation should be considered. Specifically, S1 nerve-root irritation can cause paresthesias in the lateral aspect of the foot. However, if the S1 nerve root is involved, gastrocnemius-soleus weakness and an abnormal ankle reflex are typical accompanying findings. In patients with isolated sural nerve entrapment, neither of these findings should be seen.

Entrapment of the saphenous nerve over the medial aspect of the anterior part of the ankle is another source of chronic pain. Patients report numbness along the medial border of the foot and pain exacerbated by tight-fitting shoes, particularly with ankle straps. Iatrogenic injury can occur during placement of a medial arthroscopic portal or during open reduction and internal fixation of a medial malleolar fracture.

Radiographs reveal normal findings. MRI is useful for identifying a space-occupying lesion. Electromyography and nerve conduction velocity studies help to assess for a more proximal cause of nerve compression.

Nonsurgical treatment of all nerve entrapments involves the avoidance of tight-fitting shoes, the administration of anti-inflammatory medications, and physical therapy modalities to help to modulate the pain. Supportive ankle bracing and a lateral heel wedge help to prevent inversion of the ankle. Occasionally, medications such as gabapentin or tricyclic antidepressants help to alleviate symptoms.

Surgery, consisting of neurolysis, removal of osteophytes, and excision of any soft-tissue masses, is considered if nonsurgical treatment fails. The decompression should start proximally at a point where the normal anatomy of the nerve can be visualized. The release should be performed distal to the site of the positive Tinel sign. Meticulous hemostasis should be achieved before closure to prevent hematoma formation and additional nerve entrapment. In recurrent cases, excision of the nerve and burying of the stump can help. The saphenous, lateral sural, medial sural, and superficial peroneal nerves do not provide sensation to the plantar aspect of the foot and can be sacrificed if necessary.

Complex Regional Pain Syndrome

A full discourse on the diagnosis and treatment of complex regional pain syndrome is beyond the scope of this chapter. This diagnosis should be considered for patients with chronic ankle pain that is not consistent with the conditions described. Type I complex regional pain syndrome develops after a noxious stimulating event, such as a crush injury, fracture, or sprain. The symptoms typically do not follow the distribution of a single, specific nerve. Type II complex regional pain syndrome develops after injury to a specific nerve, such as a laceration.

Complex regional pain syndrome is more common in females and patients who smoke, and it has been reported to occur in 1% of fractures and up to 5% of patients with peripheral nerve injuries. The stages of complex regional pain syndrome include an acute phase (0 to 3 months), a dystrophic phase (3 to 6 months), and an atrophic stage. Early recognition and treatment are paramount to achieve successful treatment. Burning pain, cold intolerance, temperature changes, swelling, allodynia (pain from a stimulus that does not normally cause pain), and dysesthesias (unpleasant abnormal sensations) are common. Characteristic physical findings include discoloration of the skin (redness, cyanosis, mottling), altered skin temperature (hot or cold), edema, decreased range of motion, atrophy (late), abnormal sweating patterns, loss of hair, and abnormal nail growth.

The kick-off sign has recently been described.[53] Thirty-nine patients with complex regional pain syndrome, while sitting on the examination table, held the affected extremity with the knee extended against gravity. When the leg was pushed back to a relaxed and suspended position, the 39 patients eventually involuntarily resumed the extended position. The position in which the patients held the legs was termed the "kick-off" position sign.

Synovial thickening and equinovarus contractures characterize the late stage of complex regional pain syndrome. Osteopenia secondary to disuse and increased blood flow is a common radiographic finding. Diffuse uptake on the delayed images of a technetium bone scan is characteristically seen, with a specificity of 75% to 98% for the diagnosis of complex regional pain syndrome.[54] A referral to a comprehensive pain management team that uses a combination of medication and physical therapy is recommended. Recalcitrant cases may benefit from sympathetic blockade and spinal cord stimulation. In patients with complex regional pain syndrome who require surgery, preoperative consultation with a pain service is recommended. These patients may benefit from regional anesthesia with indwelling catheters to minimize postoperative pain.

Summary

Chronic ankle pain is a common presenting symptom in orthopaedic surgery. A careful history and physical examination are paramount to arrive at the correct diagnosis. Ancillary imaging may help confirm the diagnosis. The clinician should recognize that both intra-articular and extra-articular pain generators can be responsible for subjective complaints.

References

1. Dellon AL: The four medial ankle tunnels: A critical review of perceptions of tarsal tunnel syndrome and neuropathy. *Neurosurg Clin N Am* 2008;19(4):629-648, vii.
2. Rosson GD, Larson AR, Williams EH, Dellon AL: Tibial nerve decompression in patients with tarsal tunnel syndrome: Pressures in the tarsal, medial plantar, and lateral plantar tunnels. *Plast Reconstr Surg* 2009; 124(4):1202-1210.
3. Kinoshita M, Okuda R, Morikawa J, Jotoku T, Abe M: The dorsiflexion-eversion test for diagnosis of tarsal tunnel syndrome. *J Bone Joint Surg Am* 2001;83-A(12):1835-1839.
4. Patel AT, Gaines K, Malamut R, Park TA, Toro DR, Holland N; American Association of Neuromuscular and Electrodiagnostic Medicine: Usefulness of electrodiagnostic techniques in the evaluation of suspected tarsal tunnel syndrome: An evidence-based review. *Muscle Nerve* 2005;32(2): 236-240.
5. Johnson KA, Strom DE: Tibialis posterior tendon dysfunction. *Clin Orthop Relat Res* 1989;239: 196-206.
6. Myerson MS: Adult acquired flatfoot deformity: Treatment of dysfunction of the posterior tibial tendon. *Instr Course Lect* 1997;46: 393-405.
7. Deland JT: Adult-acquired flatfoot deformity. *J Am Acad Orthop Surg* 2008;16(7):399-406.
8. Lin JL, Balbas J, Richardson EG: Results of non-surgical treatment of stage II posterior tibial tendon dysfunction: A 7- to 10-year followup. *Foot Ankle Int* 2008;29(8): 781-786.
9. Alvarez RG, Marini A, Schmitt C, Saltzman CL: Stage I and II posterior tibial tendon dysfunction treated by a structured nonoperative management protocol: An orthosis and exercise program. *Foot Ankle Int* 2006;27(1):2-8.
10. Myerson MS, Badekas A, Schon LC: Treatment of stage II posterior tibial tendon deficiency with flexor digitorum longus tendon transfer and calcaneal osteotomy. *Foot Ankle Int* 2004; 25(7):445-450.
11. Hamilton WG, Geppert MJ, Thompson FM: Pain in the posterior aspect of the ankle in dancers: Differential diagnosis and operative treatment. *J Bone Joint Surg Am* 1996;78(10):1491-1500.
12. Chao W: Os trigonum. *Foot Ankle Clin* 2004;9(4):787-796, vii.
13. Scholten PE, Sierevelt IN, van Dijk CN: Hindfoot endoscopy for posterior ankle impingement. *J Bone Joint Surg Am* 2008; 90(12):2665-2672.
14. Mitchell AW, Lee JC, Healy JC: The use of ultrasound in the assessment and treatment of Achilles tendinosis. *J Bone Joint Surg Br* 2009;91(11):1405-1409.
15. Fahlström M, Jonsson P, Lorentzon R, Alfredson H: Chronic Achilles tendon pain treated with eccentric calf-muscle training. *Knee Surg Sports Traumatol Arthrosc* 2003;11(5):327-333.
16. Ohberg L, Lorentzon R, Alfredson H: Eccentric training in patients with chronic Achilles tendinosis: Normalised tendon structure and decreased thickness at follow up. *Br J Sports Med* 2004;38(1):8-11.
17. Rompe JD, Furia J, Maffulli N: Eccentric loading compared with shock wave treatment for chronic insertional achilles tendinopathy: A randomized, controlled trial. *J Bone Joint Surg Am* 2008;90(1): 52-61.
18. Rompe JD, Furia J, Maffulli N: Eccentric loading versus eccentric loading plus shock-wave treatment for midportion achilles tendinopathy: A randomized controlled trial. *Am J Sports Med* 2009;37(3):463-470.
19. Ryan M, Grau S, Krauss I, Maiwald C, Taunton J, Horstmann T: Kinematic analysis of runners with achilles mid-portion tendinopathy. *Foot Ankle Int* 2009; 30(12):1190-1195.
20. de Vos RJ, Weir A, van Schie HT, et al: Platelet-rich plasma injection for chronic Achilles tendinopathy: A randomized controlled trial. *JAMA* 2010;303(2):144-149.
21. Den Hartog BD: Flexor hallucis longus transfer for chronic Achilles tendonosis. *Foot Ankle Int* 2003;24(3):233-237.
22. Martin RL, Manning CM, Carcia CR, Conti SF: An outcome study of chronic Achilles tendinosis after excision of the Achilles

tendon and flexor hallucis longus tendon transfer. *Foot Ankle Int* 2005;26(9):691-697.

23. Will RE, Galey SM: Outcome of single incision flexor hallucis longus transfer for chronic achilles tendinopathy. *Foot Ankle Int* 2009;30(4):315-317.

24. Saxena A: Results of chronic Achilles tendinopathy surgery on elite and nonelite track athletes. *Foot Ankle Int* 2003;24(9): 712-720.

25. DIGiovanni BF, Fraga CJ, Cohen BE, Shereff MJ: Associated injuries found in chronic lateral ankle instability. *Foot Ankle Int* 2000;21(10):809-815.

26. Komenda GA, Ferkel RD: Arthroscopic findings associated with the unstable ankle. *Foot Ankle Int* 1999;20(11):708-713.

27. Sugimoto K, Takakura Y, Okahashi K, Samoto N, Kawate K, Iwai M: Chondral injuries of the ankle with recurrent lateral instability: An arthroscopic study. *J Bone Joint Surg Am* 2009;91(1): 99-106.

28. Krips R, Brandsson S, Swensson C, van Dijk CN, Karlsson J: Anatomical reconstruction and Evans tenodesis of the lateral ligaments of the ankle: Clinical and radiological findings after follow-up for 15 to 30 years. *J Bone Joint Surg Br* 2002;84(2):232-236.

29. Li X, Killie H, Guerrero P, Busconi BD: Anatomical reconstruction for chronic lateral ankle instability in the high-demand athlete: Functional outcomes after the modified Broström repair using suture anchors. *Am J Sports Med* 2009;37(3):488-494.

30. Messer TM, Cummins CA, Ahn J, Kelikian AS: Outcome of the modified Broström procedure for chronic lateral ankle instability using suture anchors. *Foot Ankle Int* 2000;21(12):996-1003.

31. DiGiovanni CW, Brodsky A: Current concepts: Lateral ankle instability. *Foot Ankle Int* 2006; 27(10):854-866.

32. Heckman DS, Reddy S, Pedowitz D, Wapner KL, Parekh SG: Operative treatment for peroneal tendon disorders. *J Bone Joint Surg Am* 2008;90(2):404-418.

33. Steel MW, DeOrio JK: Peroneal tendon tears: Return to sports after operative treatment. *Foot Ankle Int* 2007;28(1):49-54.

34. Eckert WR, Davis EA Jr: Acute rupture of the peroneal retinaculum. *J Bone Joint Surg Am* 1976; 58(5):670-672.

35. Selmani E, Gjata V, Gjika E: Current concepts review: Peroneal tendon disorders. *Foot Ankle Int* 2006;27(3):221-228.

36. Chan GM, Yoshida D: Fracture of the lateral process of the talus associated with snowboarding. *Ann Emerg Med* 2003;41(6):854-858.

37. Sanders RW, Clare MP: Fractures of the calcaneus, in Coughlin MJ, Mann RA, Saltzman CL, eds: *Surgery of the Foot and Ankle*, ed 8. Philadelphia, PA, Elsevier, 2007, vol 2, pp 2058-2060.

38. von Knoch F, Reckord U, von Knoch M, Sommer C: Fracture of the lateral process of the talus in snowboarders. *J Bone Joint Surg Br* 2007;89(6):772-777.

39. Bonvin F, Montet X, Copercini M, Martinoli C, Bianchi S: Imaging of fractures of the lateral process of the talus, a frequently missed diagnosis. *Eur J Radiol* 2003;47(1):64-70.

40. Lee KB, Bai LB, Park JG, Song EK, Lee JJ: Efficacy of MRI versus arthroscopy for evaluation of sinus tarsi syndrome. *Foot Ankle Int* 2008;29(11):1111-1116.

41. Frey C, Feder KS, DiGiovanni C: Arthroscopic evaluation of the subtalar joint: Does sinus tarsi syndrome exist? *Foot Ankle Int* 1999;20(3):185-191.

42. Berndt AL, Harty M: Transchondral fractures (osteochondritis dissecans) of the talus. *J Bone Joint Surg Am* 1959;41-A:988-1020.

43. Ferkel RD, Hommen JP: Arthroscopy of the ankle and foot, in Coughlin MJ, Mann RA, Saltzman CL, eds: *Surgery of the Foot and Ankle*, ed 8. Philadelphia, PA, Elsevier, 2007, vol 2, pp 1641-1726.

44. Anderson IF, Crichton KJ, Grattan-Smith T, Cooper RA, Brazier D: Osteochondral fractures of the dome of the talus. *J Bone Joint Surg Am* 1989;71(8): 1143-1152.

45. Valderrabano V, Leumann A, Rasch H, Egelhof T, Hintermann B, Pagenstert G: Knee-to-ankle mosaicplasty for the treatment of osteochondral lesions of the ankle joint. *Am J Sports Med* 2009;37(Suppl 1):105S-111S.

46. Whittaker JP, Smith G, Makwana N, et al: Early results of autologous chondrocyte implantation in the talus. *J Bone Joint Surg Br* 2005;87(2):179-183.

47. Stetson WB, Ferkel RD: Ankle arthroscopy: II. Indications and results. *J Am Acad Orthop Surg* 1996;4(1):24-34.

48. Urgüden M, Söyüncü Y, Ozdemir H, Sekban H, Akyildiz FF, Aydin AT: Arthroscopic treatment of anterolateral soft tissue impingement of the ankle: Evaluation of factors affecting outcome. *Arthroscopy* 2005;21(3):317-322.

49. Liu Z, Zhou J, Zhao L: Anterior tarsal tunnel syndrome. *J Bone Joint Surg Br* 1991;73(3): 470-473.

50. O'Neill PJ, Parks BG, Walsh R, Simmons LM, Miller SD: Excursion and strain of the superficial peroneal nerve during inversion ankle sprain. *J Bone Joint Surg Am* 2007;89(5):979-986.

51. Ucerler H, Ikiz AA: The variations of the sensory branches of the superficial peroneal nerve course and its clinical importance. *Foot Ankle Int* 2005;26(11): 942-946.

52. Ferkel RD, Small HN, Gittins JE: Complications in foot and ankle arthroscopy. *Clin Orthop Relat Res* 2001;391:89-104.

53. Trevino SG, Panchbhavi VK, Castro-Aragon O, Rowell M, Jo J: The “kick-off” position: A new sign for early diagnosis of complex regional pain syndrome in the leg. *Foot Ankle Int* 2007;28(1):92-95.

54. Hogan CJ, Hurwitz SR: Treatment of complex regional pain syndrome of the lower extremity. *J Am Acad Orthop Surg* 2002; 10(4):281-289.

Video Reference

29.1: Labib SA, Kimmerly WS, Karas SG: Video. Excerpt. *The Anatomic Reconstruction of Chronic Lateral Ankle Instability: A Modified Broström-Gould Technique.* Atlanta, GA, 2006.

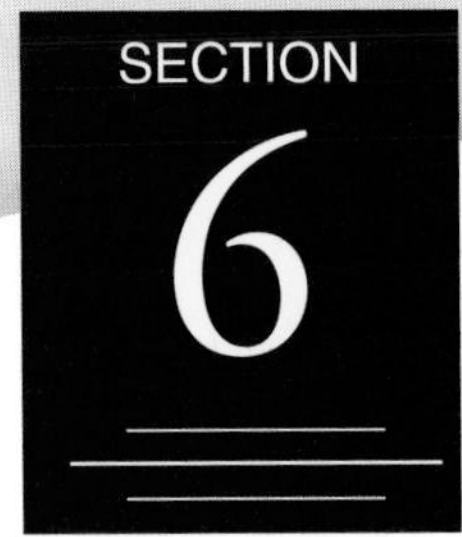

Spine

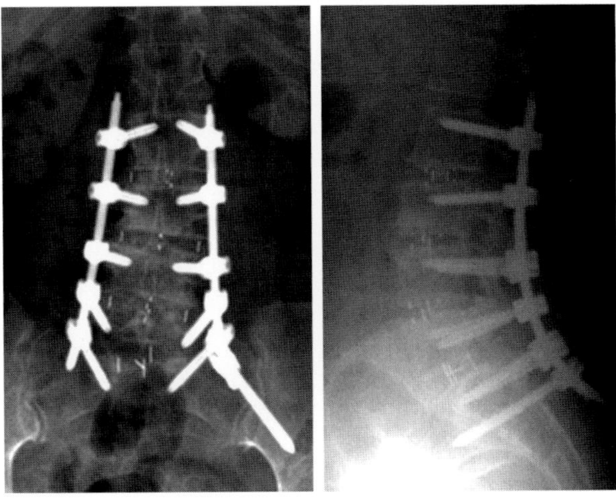

The Current State of Minimally Invasive Spine Surgery

Choll W. Kim, MD, PhD
Krzysztof Siemionow, MD
D. Greg Anderson, MD
Frank M. Phillips, MD

Abstract

Minimally invasive surgery for spinal disorders is predicated on the following basic principles: (1) avoid muscle crush injury by self-retaining retractors; (2) do not disrupt tendon attachment sites of key muscles, particularly the origin of the multifidus muscle at the spinous process; (3) use known anatomic neurovascular and muscle compartment planes; and (4) minimize collateral soft-tissue injury by limiting the width of the surgical corridor. The traditional midline posterior approach for lumbar decompression and fusion violates these key principles of minimally invasive surgery. The tendon origin of the multifidus muscle is detached, the surgical corridor is exceedingly wide, and significant muscle crush injury occurs with the use of powerful self-retaining retractors. The combination of these factors leads to well-described changes in muscle physiology and function. Minimally invasive posterior lumbar surgery is performed with table-mounted tubular retractors that focus the surgical dissection to a narrow corridor directly over the surgical target site. The path of the surgical corridor is chosen based on anatomic planes, specifically avoiding injury to the musculotendinous complex and the neurovascular bundle. With these relatively simple modifications in the minimally invasive surgical technique, significant improvements have been achieved in intraoperative blood loss, postoperative pain, and surgical morbidity. However, minimally invasive surgical techniques remains technically demanding, and a significant complication rate has been reported during a surgeon's initial learning curve for the procedures. Improvements in surgeon training along with long-term prospective studies will be needed for advancements in this area of spine surgery.

Instr Course Lect 2011;60:353-370.

The past decade has seen an evolution of minimally invasive spine surgery with new technologic developments. Minimally invasive spine surgery is believed to decrease postoperative pain and allow quicker recovery by limiting soft-tissue retraction and dissection. Advances in microscopy, tissue retractors, and specialized instruments have enabled surgeons to perform procedures through small incisions. As with the open approach, the goals of the minimally invasive approach are to adequately decompress the involved neural elements, stabilize the motion segment, and/or realign the spinal column according to the needs of the individual patient. This chapter presents an overview of the current state of minimally invasive spine surgery and a discussion of the key biologic concepts of posterior lumbar decompression as well as posterior and lateral fusion techniques.

Key Concepts

Minimally invasive posterior lumbar surgery is based on the following key concepts: (1) avoid muscle crush injury by self-retaining retractors; (2) do not disrupt tendon attachment sites of key muscles, particularly the origin of the multifidus muscle at the spinous process; (3) use known anatomic neurovascular and muscle compartment planes; and (4) minimize collateral soft-tissue injury by limiting the width of the surgical corridor.

One of the main goals of minimally invasive spine surgery is to reduce trauma to the two posterior paraspinal muscle groups: (1) the deep paramedian transversospinalis muscle group, including the multifidus, inter-

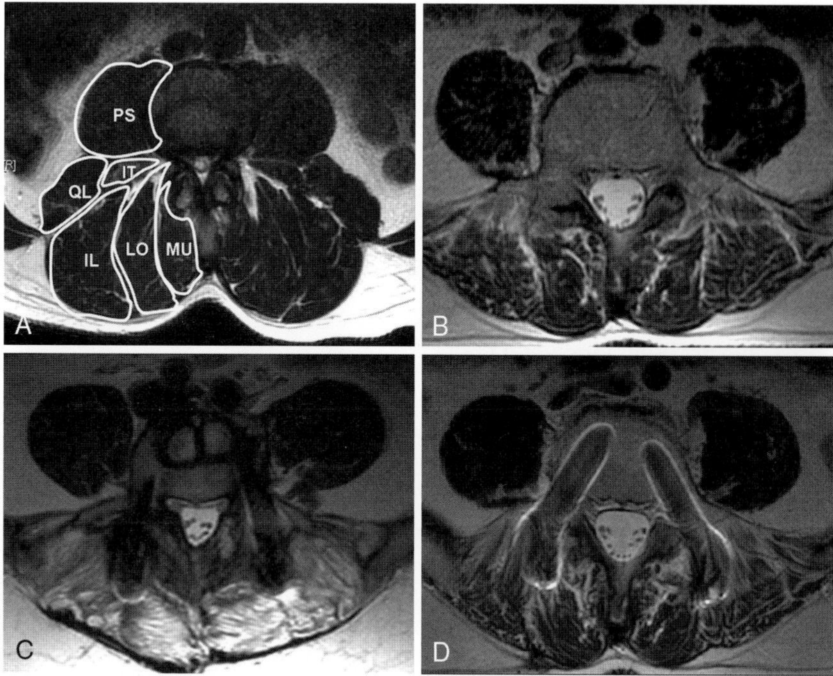

Figure 1 **A,** Axial T2-weighted MRI scan through the L4-L5 disk showing the multifidus (MU), iliocostalis (IL), longissimus (LO), quadratus lumborum (QL), intertransversarii (IT), and psoas (PS) muscles. **B,** Axial T2-weighted MRI scan at the L5 pedicle level in a 57-year-old man with L5-S1 spondylolisthesis before surgery. **C,** Axial T2-weighted MRI scan at the L5 pedicle level in a 45-year-old woman after midline open transforaminal lumbar interbody fusion at L4-L5, showing fatty replacement of the paraspinal muscles. **D,** Axial T2-weighted MRI scan of the same patient in panel B after minimally invasive transforaminal lumbar interbody fusion at L5-S1, showing preservation of the paraspinal muscle architecture.

spinales, intertransversarii, and short rotators; and (2) the more superficial and lateral erector spinae muscles, including the longissimus and iliocostalis (**Figure 1**). These muscles run along the thoracolumbar spine and attach caudally. The multifidus muscle in particular is important for dynamic stability of the spine (**Figure 2**).

The traditional midline posterior approach for lumbar decompression and fusion traumatizes some paraspinous tissue. The tendon origin of the multifidus muscle is detached, the surgical site is wide, and muscle crush injury may occur with the use of self-retaining retractors, all of which may result in muscle atrophy.[1-9] Atrophy, in turn, leads to decreased force-production capacity of the muscle.[10,11] Kim et al[12] compared trunk muscle strength between patients treated with open posterior spinal instrumentation and those managed with percutaneous instrumentation. Patients who had been treated with percutaneous instrumentation had more than 50% improvement in lumbar extension strength, whereas those treated with open surgery had no improvement.

Muscle biopsy specimens from patients undergoing revision spine surgery have shown selective type II fiber atrophy, widespread fiber-type grouping (a sign of reinnervation), and a moth-eaten appearance of muscle fibers.[13] Although there may be several causes, the most important factor responsible for muscle injury is the use of forceful self-retaining retractors. Kawaguchi et al[6,14-17] proposed that injury is induced by a crush mechanism similar to that caused by a pneumatic tourniquet during surgery on the extremities. During the application of self-retaining retractors, elevated pressures lead to decreased intramuscular perfusion.[18,19] The severity of the muscle injury is affected by the degree of intramuscular pressure and the length of the retraction time. Using MRI, Stevens et al[20] assessed the postoperative appearance of the multifidus muscle. Patients treated with a traditional open posterior transforaminal lumbar interbody fusion technique showed marked intramuscular edema on postoperative MRI 6 months after

Dr. Kim or an immediate family member serves as a board member, owner, officer, or committee member of the Society for Minimally Invasive Spine Surgery; has received royalties from Hydrocision; is a member of a speakers' bureau or has made paid presentations on behalf of Medtronic Sofamor Danek, Biomet, DePuy, Synthes, and Globus Medical; serves as a paid consultant to or is an employee of Medtronic Sofamor Danek, Synthes, and Globus Medical; has received research or institutional support from Medtronic Sofamor Danek, DePuy, Biomet, EBI, and Synthes; and owns stock or stock options in Hydrocision and Spinal Elements. Dr. Siemionow or an immediate family member serves as a board member, owner, officer, or committee member of Tolera Therapeutics; has received royalties from Tolera Therapeutics; serves as a paid consultant to or is an employee of Tolera Therapeutics; serves as an unpaid consultant to MAZOR Surgical Technologies and AxioMed; and owns stock or stock options in Tolera Therapeutics. Dr. Anderson or an immediate family member has received royalties from DePuy and Medtronic Sofamor Danek; is a member of a speakers' bureau or has made paid presentations on behalf of DePuy and Medtronic Sofamor Danek; serves as a paid consultant to or is an employee of DePuy, Medtronic Sofamor Danek, the Musculoskeletal Transplant Foundation, Seaspine, and Synthes; and has received research or institutional support from DePuy and Medtronic Sofamor Danek. Dr. Phillips or an immediate family member has received royalties from DePuy and Nuvasive; serves as a paid consultant to or is an employee of DePuy, Nuvasive, Kyphon, AxioMed, Flexuspine, Spinal Kinetics, and CrossTrees; has received research or institutional support from Cervitech, Nuvasive, and Stryker; and owns stock or stock options in AxioMed, Nuvasive, Archus, Spinal Motion, Spinal Kinetics, TissueLink, Flexuspine, K2M, and CrossTrees.

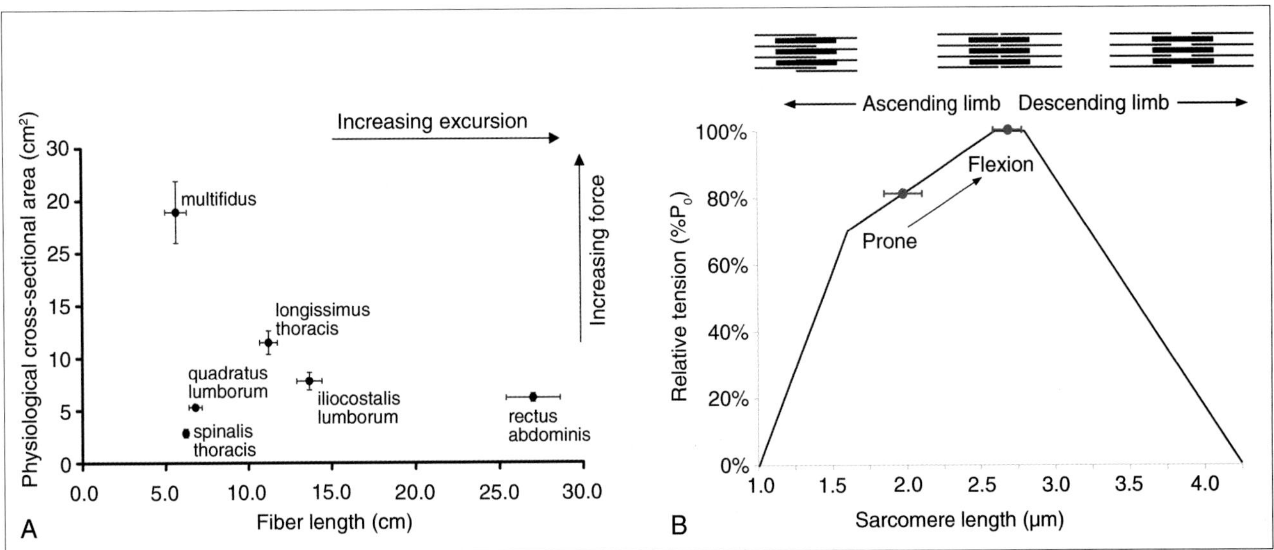

Figure 2 **A,** This scatterplot of physiologic cross-sectional area versus fiber length illustrates the functional design of a muscle because the physiologic cross-sectional area is proportional to muscle force, and the fiber length is proportional to muscle excursion. These data illustrate that the multifidus has the largest force-generating capacity in the lumbar spine and is designed for stability. The bars represent the standard deviation. **B,** Sarcomere length operating range of the multifidus plotted on the human skeletal muscle sarcomere length-tension curve (black line). These data show that the multifidus muscle operates on the ascending limb of the length-tension curve and becomes intrinsically stronger as the spine is flexed (lower arrow). Schematic sarcomeres are shown on the ascending and descending limbs to scale, on the basis of the quantification of actin and myosin filament lengths. (Reproduced with permission from Ward SR, Kim CW, Eng CM, et al: Architectural analysis and intraoperative measurements demonstrate the unique design of the multifidus muscle for lumbar spine stability. *J Bone Joint Surg Am* 2009;91:176-85.)

the surgery, whereas patients treated with a mini-open transforaminal lumbar interbody fusion had nearly normal findings on MRI. Tsutsumimoto et al[21] used MRI to assess the multifidus muscle in patients treated with a posterior lumbar interbody fusion. They compared two groups of patients: those who had been treated with a traditional midline approach and those who had been treated with a mini-open Wiltse approach. The degree of multifidus atrophy and the increase in T2 signal intensity in the multifidus muscle after the mini-open posterior lumbar interbody fusion were significantly lower than those measurements following open posterior lumbar interbody fusion.

Another mechanism leading to degeneration and atrophy following traditional open surgery is muscle denervation. The nerve supply to the multifidus is monosegmental, making it especially vulnerable to injury.[22,23] Damage to the neuromuscular junction following prolonged retraction can also lead to muscle denervation. Muscle biopsies in patients with failed back surgery syndrome showed signs of advanced chronic denervation.[24]

Soft-tissue trauma can have widespread regional and systemic effects. Kim et al[25] compared levels of circulating markers of tissue injury in patients who had been treated with open spinal fusion with those in patients treated with minimally invasive spine surgery. The levels of creatinine kinase, aldolase, proinflammatory cytokines (interleukin [IL]-6 and IL-8), and anti-inflammatory cytokines (IL-10 and IL-1 receptor antagonist) in the patients treated with open surgery were altered several-fold compared with those in the patients treated with minimally invasive surgery. Most markers returned to baseline levels by 3 days after the minimally invasive surgery, whereas they required 7 days to return to baseline levels after the open surgery. Glycerol is an important component of glycerophospholipid, the basic structure of the cell plasma membrane. When the integrity of a cell membrane is destroyed, glycerol is released into the interstitial fluid. Ren et al[26] reported that the glycerol concentrations in the paraspinal muscles of patients who had been treated with posterolateral lumbar fusion with instrumentation were higher than the concentrations in the deltoid muscles of the same patients.

Another goal of minimally invasive spine surgery is to limit the amount of osseous resection to minimize postoperative spinal instability.[27,28] The disruption of facet joint integrity combined with the loss of the midline interspinous ligament-tendon complex associated with traditional laminectomy can contribute to flexion instability.[29-31] Efforts to limit such potentially destabilizing surgery have been pursued via unilateral laminotomies in which the spinous processes and corresponding tendinous attachments of the multifidus muscle and the supraspinous and interspinous ligaments are preserved. A finite element analysis demonstrated that minimizing bone and ligament removal resulted in greater preservation of normal motion of the lumbar spine after surgery.[32]

Minimally Invasive Lumbar Decompression

Minimally Invasive Tubular Microdiskectomy

The treatment of herniated disks via minimally invasive tubular microdiskectomy is the most common minimally invasive spine technique currently used in the United States. This system, developed by Foley and Smith, consists of a series of concentric dilators and thin-walled tubular retractors of variable length.[33-35] The tube, typically 18 mm in diameter, circumferentially defines a surgical corridor. Surgery is typically performed using an operating microscope. Several recent studies have compared minimally invasive lumbar diskectomy with the traditional open approach and have shown that the minimally invasive approach resulted in less intraoperative tissue damage, nerve irritation, blood loss, and immediate postoperative pain as well as a shorter period of hospitalization and a faster recovery and return to work.[36-40] Randomized controlled trials comparing traditional open microdiskectomy with minimally invasive tubular microdiskectomy[41-43] all showed that tubular microdiskectomy is safe and efficacious.

The surgical corridor is defined by the specific pathologic entity. Minimally invasive lumbar decompression can adequately decompress the central, lateral, and foraminal zones of the spinal canal and can be used to remove disk material from the extraforaminal region. However, the access strategy for decompression of each region of the spine should be planned preoperatively. Extraforaminal neural compression may be approached from outside the spinal canal by inserting the tubular retractor over the intertransverse membrane between the transverse processes. The intertransverse membrane is identified and released to expose the exiting nerve root. Once the root is identified, the disk material in the extraforaminal zone can be accessed deep to the nerve root.

Minimally Invasive Lumbar Hemilaminectomy

The key principle in minimally invasive spine decompression is maintaining the multifidus tendon attachment to the spinous process. During a traditional laminectomy, the spinous process is removed, and the multifidus muscle is retracted laterally. On wound closure, the multifidus origin cannot be repaired to the spinous process. However, a thorough decompression can be achieved through a unilateral portal via a hemilaminectomy technique.[44] The central canal and the contralateral recess can be decompressed by angling the tubular retractor dorsally to view the undersurface of the spinous process and the contralateral lamina (**Figure 3**). The dural tube can be gently pushed down, and the ligamentum flavum and the contralateral superior articular process are resected to achieve a bilateral decompression. The upper lumbar spine anatomy differs from the lower lumbar spine anatomy. At L3 and above, the lamina between the spinous process and the facet joint can be narrow (**Figure 3**). With a unilateral approach, it may be difficult to reach the ipsilateral recess without removing an excessive amount of the ipsilateral inferior articular process. An option is to use a bilateral crossover technique to reach the right lateral recess from a left-sided hemilaminectomy and vice versa. In a small preliminary study of four patients and seven levels of decompression performed with this technique, the total operating time averaged 32 minutes per level, and the estimated blood loss averaged 75 mL (G Regev, MD, et al, Henderson, NV, unpublished data presented at the Annual Meeting of the Society for Minimally Invasive Spine Surgery, 2008). The average postoperative stay was 1.2 days. All patients had resolution of neurogenic claudication, and there were no complications.

The efficacy and safety of minimally invasive posterior lumbar decompression have been assessed.[44-54] The learning curve for minimally invasive spine surgery is a concern because patients who had been treated during the initial phases of some studies had higher complication rates.[52,54] In a study of their experience with a minimally invasive unilateral approach to bilateral lumbar decompression for treatment of lumbar stenosis, Ikuta et al[52] reported good short-term results in 38 of 44 patients. The mean improvement in the Japanese Orthopaedic Association score was 72%. Postoperative morbidity was relatively low and, compared with a control group treated with open surgery, the patients had decreased intraoperative blood loss, decreased pain medication requirements, and shorter hospital stays. The authors reported a 25% complication rate, including four dural tears, three fractures of the inferior facet on the approach side, one postoperative cauda equina syndrome requiring a reoperation, and one postoperative epidural hematoma requiring a reoperation.

In a prospective study, Yagi et al[55] randomly assigned 41 patients with lumbar stenosis to treatment with either a minimally invasive microendoscopic decompression (20 patients) or a conventional laminectomy (21 patients). The duration of follow-up averaged 18 months. The patients treated with the minimally invasive decompression had a shorter mean hospital stay, less blood loss, a lower mean creatine phosphokinase muscle isoenzyme level, a lower visual analog scale score for back pain at 1 year postoperatively, and a faster recovery rate. Satisfactory neurologic decompression and symptom relief were achieved in 90% of the patients, and no patient had spinal instability. Castro-Menéndez et al[56] treated 50 patients with lumbar spinal stenosis with a microendoscopic decompression using an 18-mm tubular retractor. The authors reported good or excellent results in 72% of the patients, with 68% expressing good subjective satisfaction, at a mean of 4 years. The mean decrease in the Oswestry Disability Index was 30.23, and the mean decrease in the visual analog scale score for leg pain was 6.02.

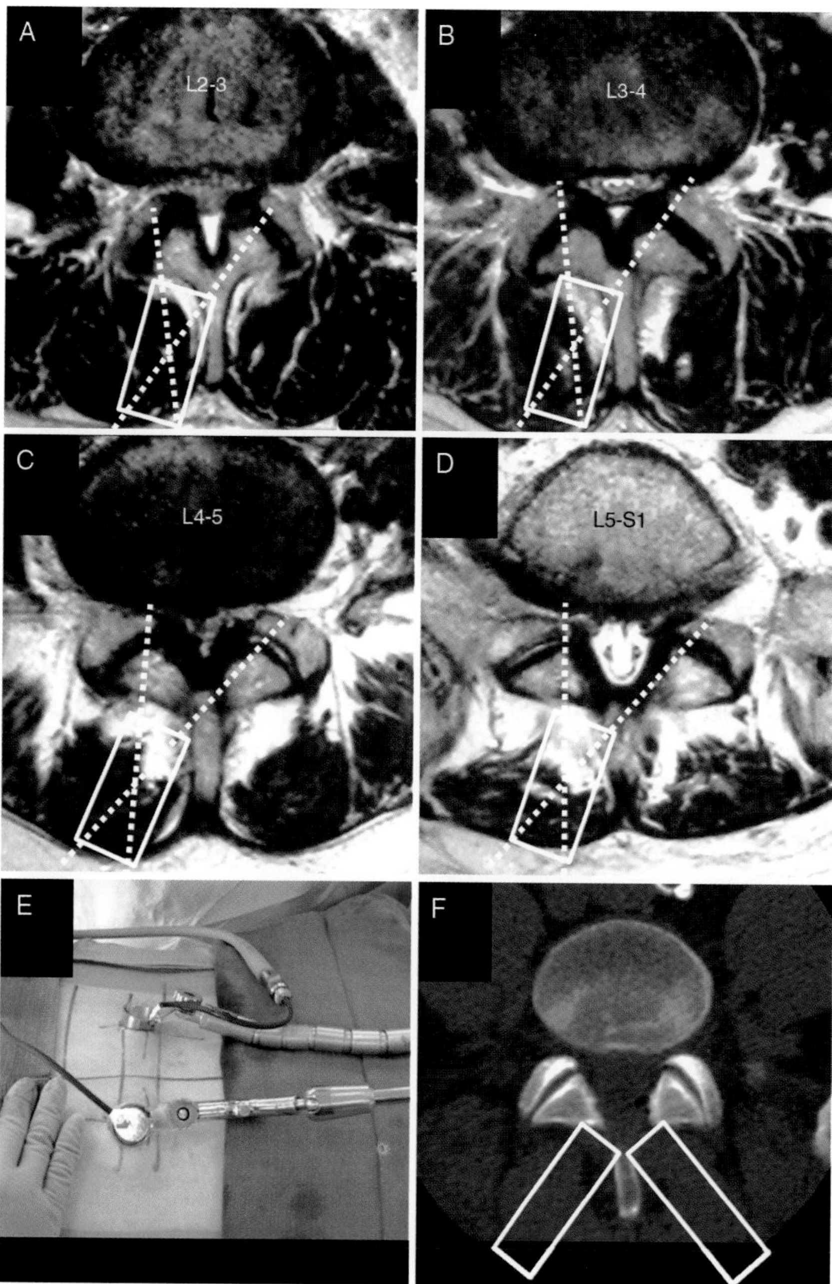

Figure 3 Axial T2-weighted MRI scan through the disk space at L2-L3 (**A**), L3-L4 (**B**), L4-L5 (**C**), and L5-S1 (**D**). The outline of the tubular retractor is overlaid on each image, and the trajectory of the surgical target site is indicated by the dashed lines. Note the proximity of the ipsilateral facet joint at the higher lumbar levels. At L3-L4 and above, care must be exercised to avoid inadvertent injury to the ipsilateral facet joint. A bilateral approach can be used (**E**) to decompress the lateral recess from the contralateral sides (**F**).

Asgarzadie and Khoo[57] reported on 48 patients who had been treated with minimally invasive lumbar decompression for lumbar stenosis. Twenty-eight patients had a one-level decompression, and 20 patients had a two-level decompression. Compared with a control group treated with a traditional open laminectomy, the minimally invasive surgery group had, on average, less intraoperative blood loss (25 versus 193 mL) and a shorter hospital stay (36 versus 94 hours). Four-year clinical outcomes were available for 32 of the 48 patients. All patients reported improvement in walking endurance at 6 months following surgery, and 80% of the patients had maintained improvement in walking endurance at a mean of 38 months. Improvements in both the Oswestry Disability Index and the Medical Outcomes Study 36-Item Short Form score had been sustained during the follow-up period. There were no neurologic complications.

Minimally invasive techniques for spine surgery may be advantageous in patients who are elderly, medically frail, or obese.[40,58-60] In a retrospective case study, Tomasino et al[61] compared

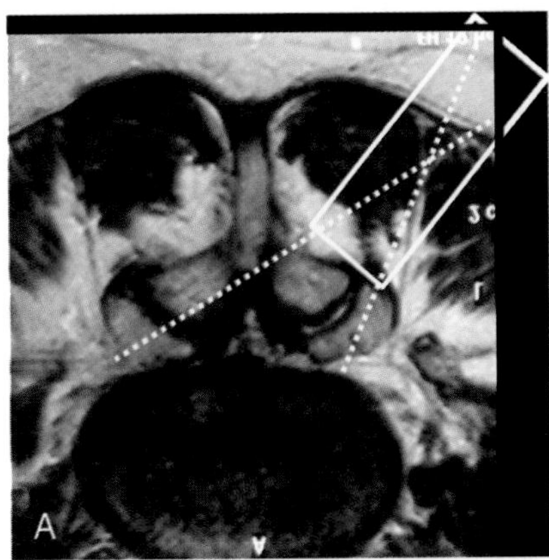
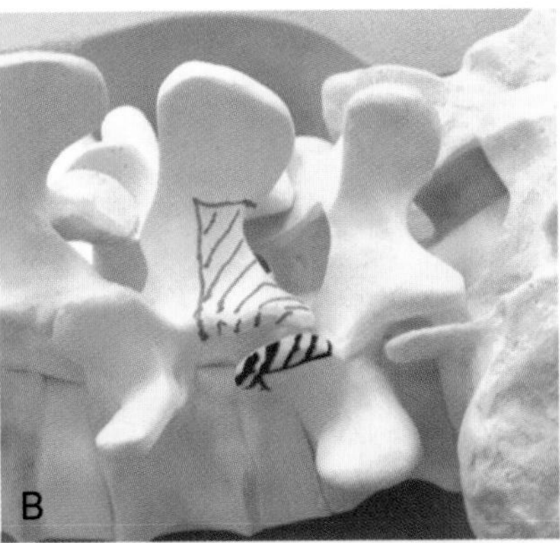
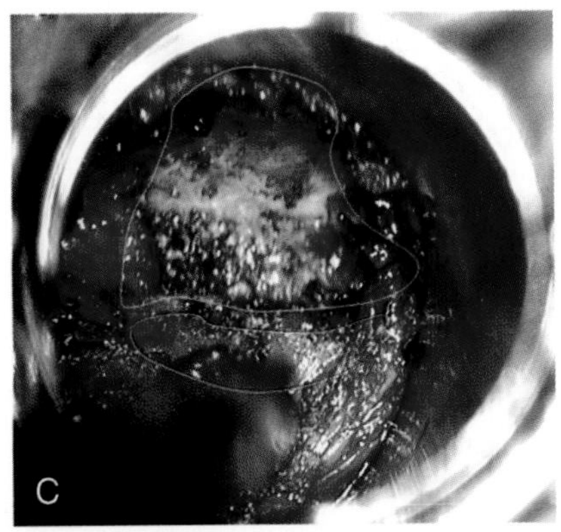

Figure 4 **A,** Axial T2-weighted MRI scan at the L4-L5 level showing the surgical corridor made with a tubular retractor (solid white lines) and the trajectory of the surgical target site (dashed lines). **B,** Synthetic model of the L4-L5 surgical target site with the base of the L4 spinous process and the inferior articular process marked in red and the overhang of the L5 superior articular process marked in black. **C,** Intraoperative microphotograph through a tubular retractor showing the surgical target site analogous to that shown in panel B, with the L4 spinous process and the inferior articular process outlined in orange and the overhang of the L5 superior articular process outlined in blue.

surgical results and patient outcomes among obese and nonobese patients who had been treated with a one-level lumbar microdiskectomy or a laminectomy with the use of tubular retractors. Of 115 patients, 31% were obese. No significant differences were seen among obese and nonobese patients in terms of incision length, surgical time, blood loss, or complications.

Minimally invasive decompression without fusion may be efficacious in patients with degenerative spondylolisthesis. Pao et al[62] performed a microdecompression on 13 patients with stenosis from a grade I spondylolisthesis. There was no progression of vertebral slippage, and all patients reported a good outcome. Sasai et al[63] performed a unilateral approach with bilateral decompression in 23 patients with degenerative spondylolisthesis and 25 patients with degenerative spinal stenosis. At 2 years, the Neurogenic Claudication Outcome Scores and Oswestry Disability Indices were similar between the two groups, although the patients with spondylolisthesis had a somewhat worse outcome. A progression of vertebral slippage of 5% or greater was found in 3 of the 23 patients with degenerative spondylolisthesis. Kleeman et al[64] performed a spinous process and interspinous ligament-preserving decompression to treat spinal stenosis in 15 patients who had an average degenerative spondylolisthesis of 6.7 mm. After an average follow-up of 4 years, 2 patients had progression of slippage, with associated worsening of their symptoms, whereas 12 patients reported good to excellent results.

Transforaminal Lumbar Interbody Fusion

Transforaminal lumbar interbody fusion, originally described by Blume and Rojas[65] and later popularized by Harms and Jeszensky,[66] is an adaptation of the posterior lumbar interbody fusion technique first described by Cloward.[67] In contrast to posterior lumbar interbody fusion, which requires a wide decompression and bilateral nerve root retraction to access the disk space, transforaminal lumbar interbody fusion is done via a unilateral approach to the disk space through the intervertebral foramen (**Figure 4**). Compared with bilateral posterior lumbar interbody fusion, transforaminal lumbar interbody fusion requires less neural retraction.[68-70] One of its main advantages is that the approach allows pathologic conditions such as spinal stenosis to be treated concurrently with an anterior interbody fusion through a single posterior incision (**Figure 5**).

Video 30.1: Minimally Invasive Transforaminal Lumbar Interbody Fusion: Preoperative Planning, Patient Positioning, and Exposure. Choll W. Kim, MD, PhD (10 min)

Peng et al[71] compared the clinical and radiographic outcomes of minimally invasive transforaminal lumbar interbody fusion with those of traditional open transforaminal lumbar interbody fusion. At 2 years, the outcomes were similar, but the patients who had been treated with minimally invasive surgery had the additional benefits of less initial postoperative pain, early rehabilitation, shorter hospitalization, and fewer complications. Dhall et al[72] retrospectively compared the outcomes of 21 patients treated with a mini-open transforaminal lumbar interbody fusion with those of 21 patients treated with a traditional open transforaminal lumbar interbody fusion and reported that there was significantly more blood loss and a longer hospital stay after the open transforaminal lumbar interbody fusion, although there was no difference in the clinical outcomes at 2 years. Selznick et al[73] reported that minimally invasive transforaminal lumbar interbody fusion is technically feasible in revision cases and is not associated with more blood loss or neurologic morbidity than found with primary procedures. However, there was a higher rate of incidental durotomy. Minimally invasive transforaminal lumbar interbody fusions in the revision setting are challenging procedures and should be performed by surgeons with experience using minimally invasive techniques.

In a prospective study, Kasis et al[74] found that limited-exposure posterior lumbar interbody fusion provided better clinical outcomes and shorter hospital stays when compared with a traditional open approach. The authors noted that the following factors were responsible for the improved outcomes: (1) preservation of posterior elements, (2) avoidance of far lateral dissection over the transverse processes, (3) a bilateral total facetectomy, (4) fewer neurologic complications, and (5) an avoidance of iliac crest autograft.

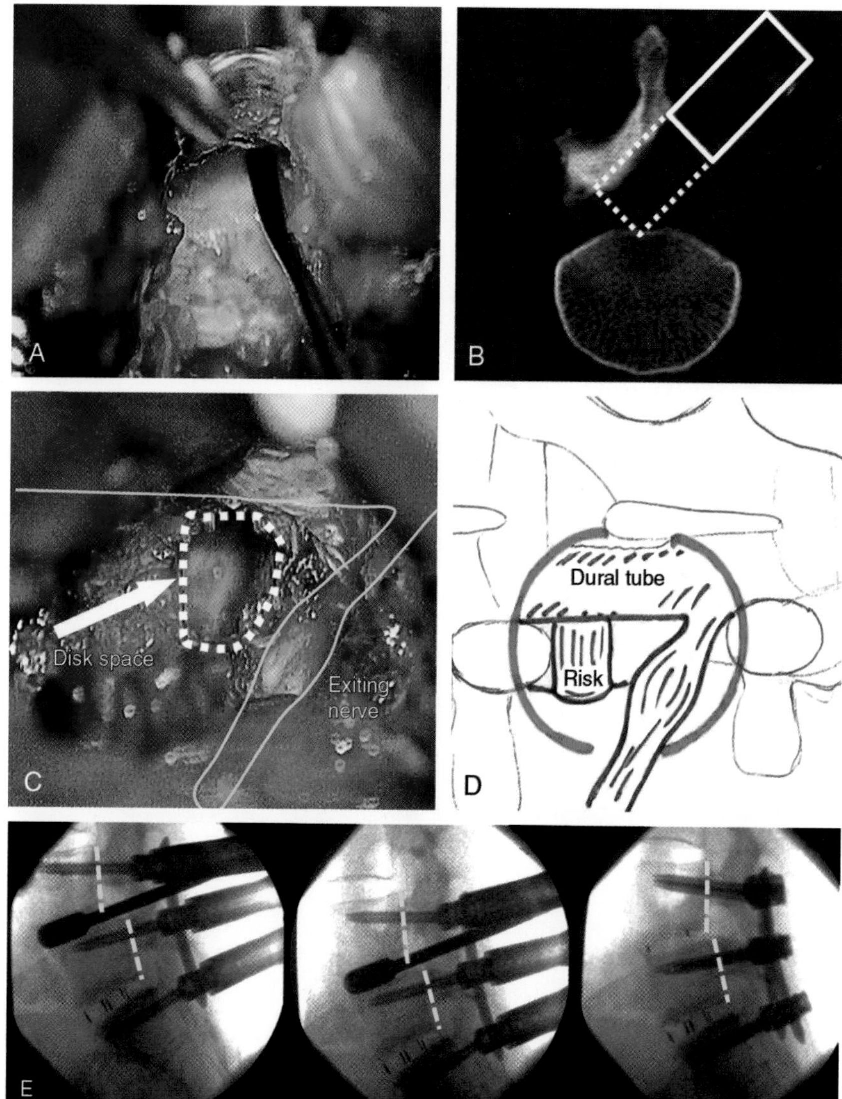

Figure 5 The minimally invasive transforaminal lumbar interbody fusion and decompression is shown. **A,** Intraoperative photograph showing the dural tube. A probe is reaching to the contralateral side. **B,** Axial CT scan showing the surgical corridor. **C,** Intraoperative photograph showing the surgical target site after diskectomy. The dural tube and exiting nerve root are outlined in yellow, and the anulotomy window for posterior interbody fusion is outlined by the dashed white line. **D,** Corresponding drawing of the surgical target site. **E,** Sequential intraoperative lateral images of a spondylolisthesis reduction maneuver with the use of a paddle distractor to mobilize the disk space and a rod reducer to pull the L4 vertebral body posteriorly. The posterior vertebral body line is shown by the yellow dashed lines.

Direct Lateral Interbody Fusion

Interbody lumbar fusion is a popular technique with touted benefits that include eliminating the disk as a potential pain generator, high rates of fusion, and restoration of intervertebral disk height and lumbar lordosis.[75-77] These benefits can be achieved with anterior lumbar interbody fusion, posterior or transforaminal lumbar interbody fusion, or an endoscopic lateral retroperitoneal approach.[78] A minimally invasive retroperitoneal direct lateral transpsoas approach to interbody arthrodesis has been described.[79,80] This technique involves a minimally invasive approach through the retroperitoneal space and the psoas muscle, with reliance on neural monitoring and fluoroscopy to provide the ability to achieve an interbody fusion (**Figures 6** and 7).

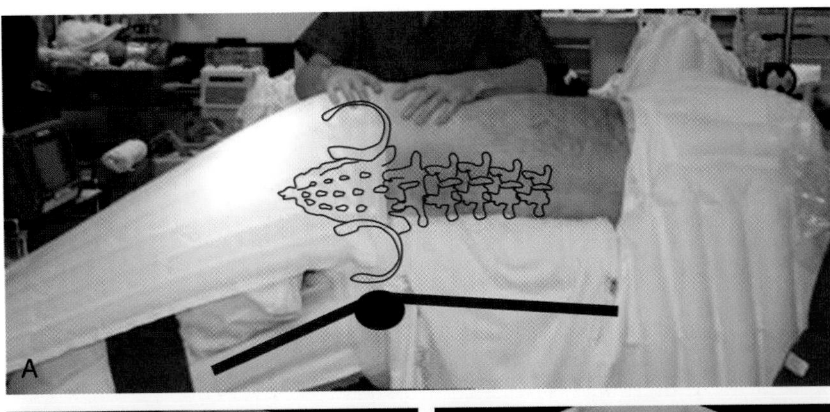

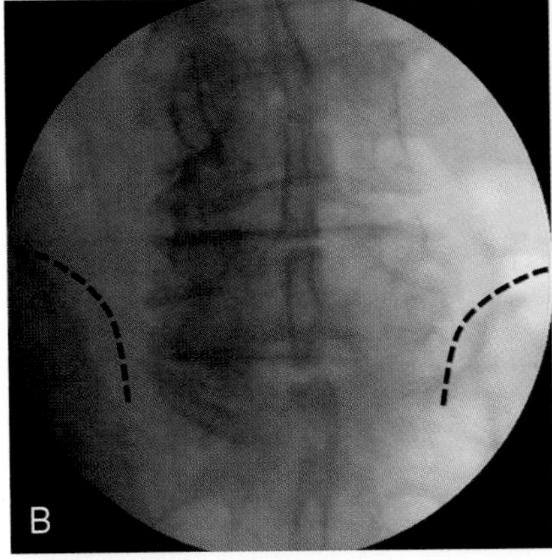

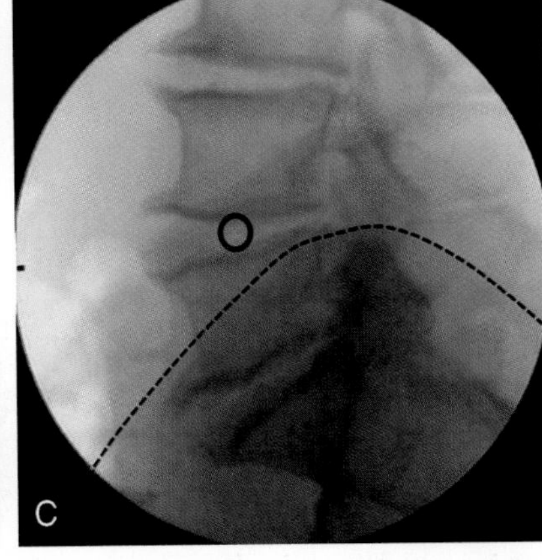

Figure 6 **A,** Intraoperative photograph showing proper positioning for a direct lateral transpsoas approach. The spine and pelvis are outlined in black, and the table break is indicated by a black oval. **B,** Intraoperative AP image with the iliac crests outlined by black dashed lines. **C,** Intraoperative lateral image with the iliac crests outlined by black dashed lines. The surgical target site at the disk center is shown by a black circle.

The iliac wing blocks minimally invasive lateral exposure below L4-L5 (**Figure 6**). Limiting the dissection to the anterior third to anterior half of the psoas muscle reduces the risk of neural injury because the lumbar plexus is in the posterior half of the psoas muscle.[79,81,82] The use of intraoperative electromyographic monitoring helps reduce the risk of neural injury (**Figure 7**).[83] While preparing the disk space for interbody fusion and inserting the interbody device, the end plates should not be violated, and the orientation should be confirmed with both anteroposterior and lateral imaging (**Figure 8**). Indirect foraminal decompression is possible by restoring the neuroforaminal height and sagittal alignment during interbody fusion. The decision whether to include a posterior spinal fusion or decompression is individualized based on the needs of the patient (**Figure 9**).

Knight et al[84] reported on the early complications in 43 female and 15 male patients who had been treated with minimally invasive direct lateral interbody fusion. Six patients had postoperative meralgia paresthetica, and two patients had L4 nerve-root injuries.

Ozgur et al[79] reported on 13 patients treated with a single or multilevel extreme lateral interbody fusion. The patients had significant pain relief and improvement in functional scores without any complications. Anand et al[85] reported on 12 patients treated with direct lateral interbody fusion in combination with a transsacral interbody fusion technique at L5-S1. The patients had an average of 3.6 levels fused, and the Cobb angle was corrected from an average of 18.9° preoperatively to an average of 6.2° postoperatively.[85] Pimenta et al[80] reported on 39 patients treated with direct lateral interbody fusion at an average of two levels. Scoliosis improved from an average of 18° preoperatively to an average of 8° postoperatively, and lumbar lordosis increased from an average of 34° preoperatively to an average of 41° postoperatively. All patients were walking and tolerating a regular diet on the day of the surgery. The average blood loss was less than 100 mL, and the average operative time was 200 minutes. The average duration of hospitalization was 2.2 days. Pain scores and functional scores improved. In a larger study, the results of extreme lateral interbody fusion in 145 patients treated for degenerative disk disease at multiple institutions were reported (N Wright, MD, Banff, Canada, unpublished data presented at the International Meeting on Advanced Spinal Techniques, 2005). The number of levels treated ranged from one to four (72% of the procedures were at a single level; 22% at two levels; 5% at three levels; and 1% at four levels). Interbody spacers (polyetheretherketone in 86%, allograft in 8%, and a cage in 6%) were used in conjunction with bone morphogenetic protein (52%), demineralized bone matrix (39%), or autograft (9%). Twenty percent of the operations were stand-alone interbody fusions, 23% used a lateral rod-screw construct, and 58% used posterior pedicle screws. The average time for surgery was 74 minutes, and the average blood loss was 88 mL. There were two transient genitofemoral injuries, and five patients experienced transient

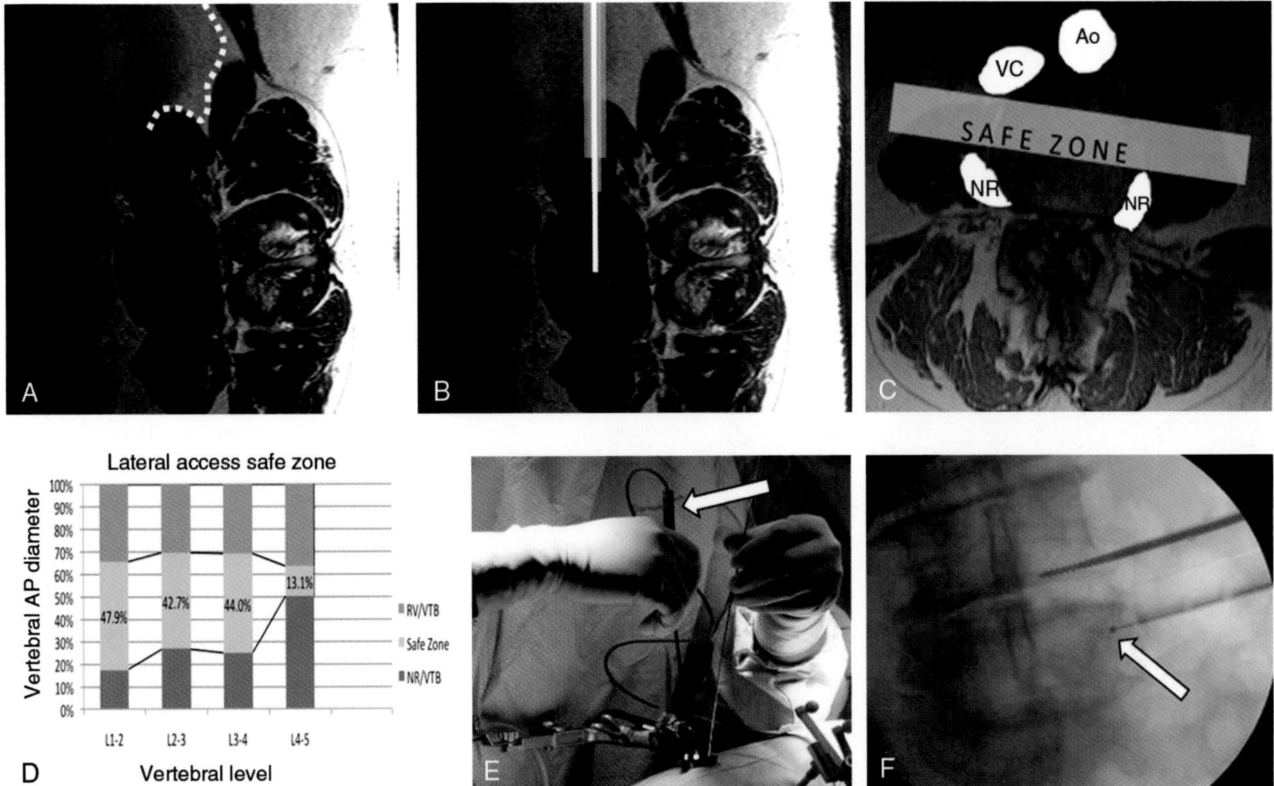

Figure 7 Direct lateral transpsoas approach and the safe zone. **A,** Axial T2-weighted MRI scan at the L4-L5 level showing the plane of dissection (dashed white line). **B,** Axial T2-weighted MRI scan at the L4-L5 level showing the sequence of psoas dilation beginning with insertion of the guidewire (white line) followed by sequential insertion of dilators (yellow tubes). **C,** Axial T1-weighted MRI scan showing the safe zone bounded posteriorly by the nerve roots (NR) and anteriorly by the vena cava (VC). The aorta (Ao) is anterior. **D,** Graph showing the limits of the safe zone from L4-L5 to L1-L2. The safe zone at L4-L5 is substantially narrower than that at the other levels, making the L4-L5 level the most challenging for direct lateral approaches. AP = anteroposterior, NR/VTB = nerve root/vertebral body, and RV/VTB = vena cava/vertebral body. **E,** Intraoperative photograph showing a ball-tipped probe being used for neurophysiologic monitoring (arrow). **F,** Intraoperative AP radiograph showing the position of the ball-tipped probe through the retractor slot (arrow).

hip flexor weakness. Most patients walked on the day of surgery and were discharged on the first postoperative day.

The outcomes of 13 patients treated with multilevel extreme lateral interbody fusion for adult lumbar scoliosis of greater than 30° were described (BA Akbarnia, MD, et al, Hong Kong, China, unpublished data presented at the 15th International Meeting on Advanced Spine Techniques, 2008). A mean of three levels were treated, and all procedures were combined with posterior spinal fusion and instrumentation. Substantial improvements in lumbar scoliosis and lordosis were reported at a mean of 9 months. One graft required revision because of migration, and one hernia occurred at the level of the incision for the extreme lateral interbody fusion. All cases of psoas muscle weakness or thigh numbness or pain resolved within 6 months. Short-term postoperative visual analog scale, Scoliosis Research Society-22, and Oswestry Disability Index scores were improved compared with preoperative scores. Similar results were shown by Anand et al[85] in a series of 12 patients. The number of levels treated ranged from 2 to 8 (mean, 3.64). The mean blood loss was 163.89 mL (SD, 105.41 mL) for anterior procedures and 93.33 mL (SD, 101.43 mL) for posterior percutaneous pedicle screw fixation. The mean surgical time was 4.01 hours (SD, 1.88 hours) for anterior procedures and 3.99 hours (SD, 1.19 hours) for posterior procedures. The mean Cobb angle improved significantly from 18.93° (SD, 10.48°) preoperatively to 6.19° (SD, 7.20°) at a mean of 75 days postoperatively.

Minimally Invasive Posterior Instrumentation

The rationale for minimally invasive pedicle screw insertion into the spine, which can be performed percutane-

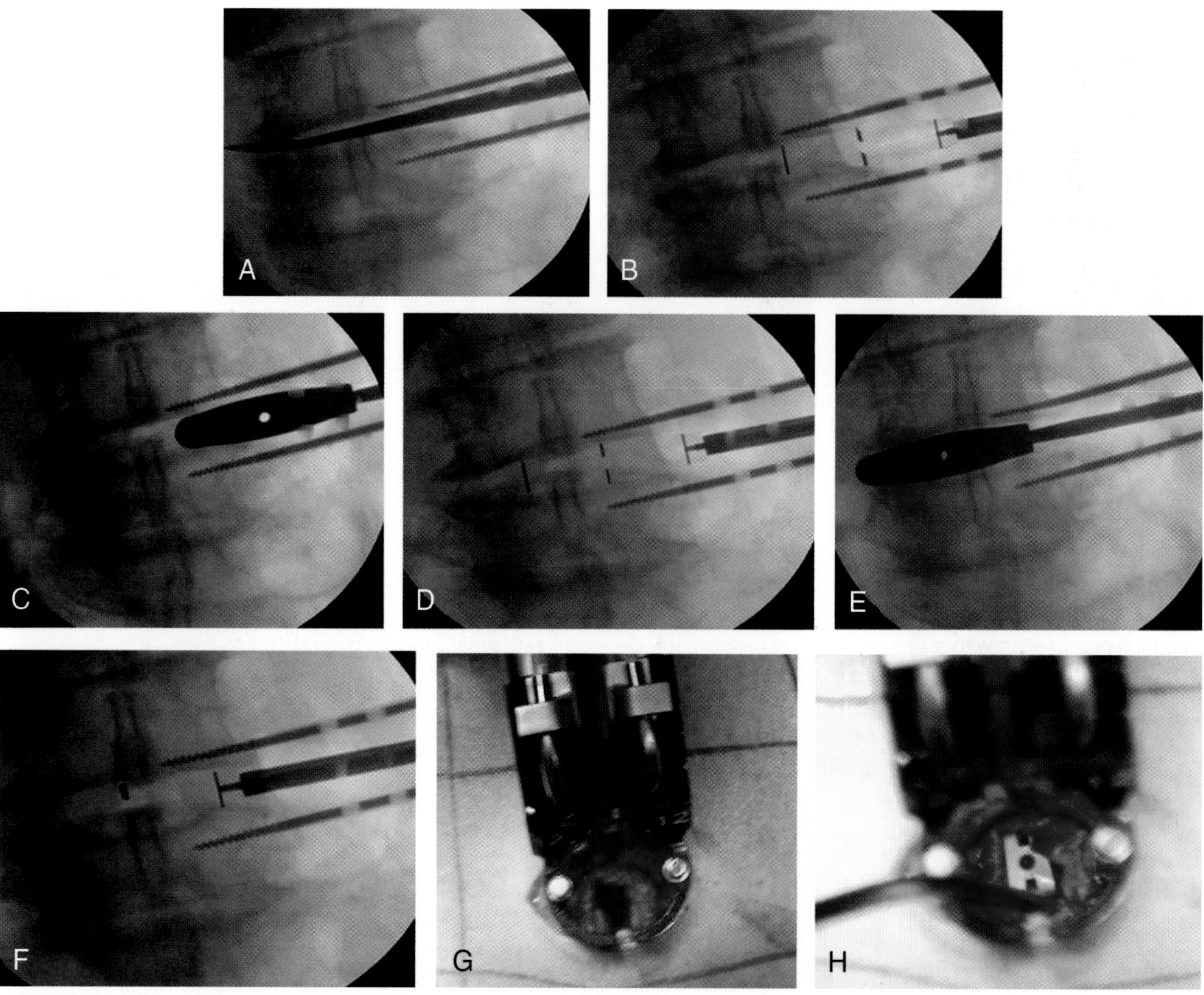

Figure 8 Direct lateral diskectomy and insertion of an interbody cage. Intraoperative AP radiographs showing release of the contralateral anulus with use of a periosteal elevator (**A**); insertion of a blunt dilator/sizer (**B** and **C**); and insertion of a synthetic interbody cage, which spans the entire disk space from cortical rim to cortical rim (**D, E,** and **F**). Intraoperative photographs showing the surgical corridor and surgical target site after diskectomy (**G**) and after cage insertion (**H**).

ously or via a paramedian mini-open technique, is to preserve multifidus muscle function. With the percutaneous technique, the pedicle is entered with the use of a Jamshidi-type trocar needle under fluoroscopic control (**Figure 10**). Once the needles are within the pedicles, the stylets are removed, and guidewires are inserted. Sequential soft-tissue dilators are used to create a path for the tap and screw. The outermost dilator can be used as a protective sleeve during pedicle tapping. The guidewire is then used to direct cannulated taps and screws into the pedicle. A cannulated pedicle screw is placed over the guidewire. Rods are inserted percutaneously to minimize soft-tissue trauma (**Figure 11**).

With the mini-open technique, a longitudinal, paramedian incision is placed slightly lateral to the lateral edge of the pedicles. Dissection is performed through the intermuscular plane between the multifidus and longissimus muscles. A tubular retractor system is subsequently deployed after tissue dilation is performed. The pars interarticularis and the mammillary processes of the cephalad and caudad levels are exposed. A high-speed burr is used to create a starting point, and pedicle probes are used to enter the pedicle. Cannulated or noncannulated pedicle screws can be used with this technique. The exposure allows for decortication of the pars, facet joint, and transverse processes for bone grafting and fusion.

The mini-open technique offers several advantages over the percutaneous method. It allows direct visualization of the anatomy and the choice of using either cannulated or noncannu-

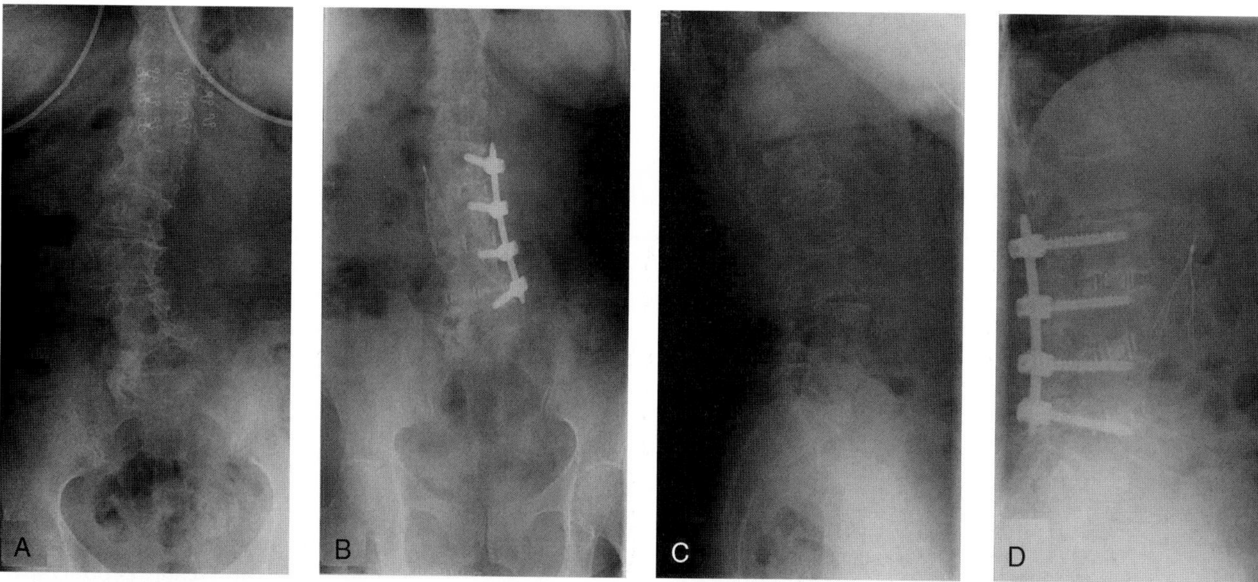

Figure 9 Preoperative (**A** and **C**) and postoperative (**B** and **D**) radiographs showing the magnitude of curve correction in a 68-year-old woman who presented with a long-standing history of low back pain and left anterior thigh pain. The patient was treated with a direct lateral approach with L2-L3, L3-L4, and L4-L5 diskectomies and interbody fusion resulting in indirect foraminal decompression. This was followed by unilateral pedicle screw instrumentation, which was performed with the patient in the lateral decubitus position, obviating the need for changing the patient's position.

lated pedicle-screw systems. The mini-open technique also allows greater access for bone grafting posteriorly. However, the mini-open technique threatens the medial branch of the dorsal rami, which extends downward to the transverse process of the caudad level. The nerve then curves posteriorly, where it branches to supply the multifidus muscle, the intertransverse muscles and ligaments, and the facet joint of the cephalad level. As a result, insertion of a pedicle screw through the mammillary process at one level can cause injury to the medial branch of the dorsal rami that supplies the adjacent cephalad level. In a cadaver study comparing these minimally invasive spine techniques, Regev et al[86] found that the mini-open technique causes injury to the medial branch of the dorsal rami more frequently than does the percutaneous technique. The authors recommended that pedicle screw insertion at the cephalad level be performed percutaneously if minimization of denervation of the multifidus complex at the cephalad adjacent level is desired.

Overall safety and accuracy have been reported for minimally invasive pedicle screw insertion. Ringel et al[87] assessed 488 pedicle screws implanted in a total of 103 patients via a percutaneous technique and found that only 3% of the screws were rated as unacceptable, leading to 9 screw-revision surgical procedures. These results mirror a growing body of evidence that reflect the safety and efficacy of minimally invasive posterior spinal instrumentation.[88-90] In a meta-analysis of 130 studies and 37,337 pedicle screws placed, the overall screw placement accuracy was 91.3%.[91]

Limitations and Drawbacks

Radiation Exposure

There are several techniques for minimally invasive posterior screw insertion, but the percutaneous pedicle screw technique is the least disruptive to tissue and has been adapted by some for single or multilevel fusions. Its use, however, depends on intraoperative multiplanar fluoroscopy. The surgical time for inserting two screws at the same vertebral level is 10 minutes or longer with the use of advanced fluoroscopic techniques, whereas lateral-only fluoroscopic methods require fewer than 5 minutes per level.[92-94] With increased insertion times associated with advanced fluoroscopic guidance, the cumulative radiation exposure increases concomitantly.

Studies have shown that fluoroscopically guided pedicle screw placement exposes surgeons to a dose of radiation that is 10 to 12 times the dose associated with nonspinal musculoskeletal procedures.[95] Despite these concerns, the convenience of the C-arm, combined with a high degree of accuracy, has made intraoperative fluoroscopy an increasingly necessary part of advanced minimally invasive spine surgery. Exposure of both the surgeon and the patient to radiation was analyzed in a prospective study of 24 consecutive patients treated with

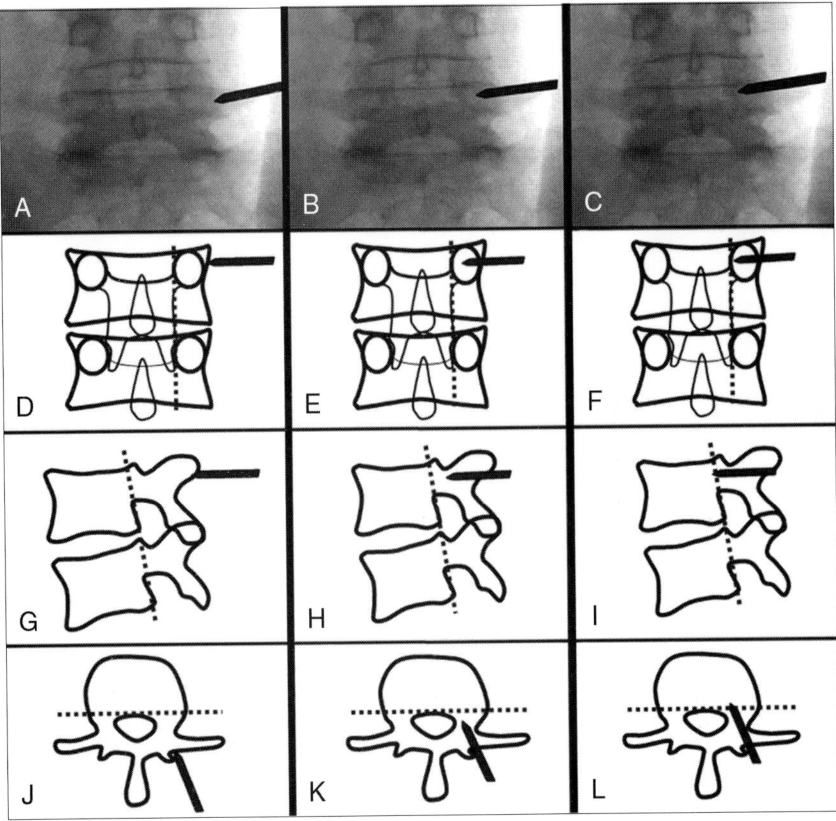

Figure 10 Percutaneous pedicle screw insertion requires scrupulous intraoperative imaging. **A** through **C,** The trocar needle is inserted with the use of a perfect en face AP image of the pedicle. **D** through **F,** The needle is inserted from a lateral to medial direction until the tip reaches the medial border of the pedicle. **G** through **I,** The C-arm is used for a lateral view. **J** through **L,** If the needle is correctly inserted into the pedicle, the tip should be past the posterior vertebral body line. Panels **D, G,** and **J** show the initial position of the needle in the AP, lateral, and axial planes, respectively. Panels **E, H,** and **K** show the needle halfway across the pedicle. Panels **F, I,** and **L** show the needle at the medial border of the pedicle. Once past the posterior vertebral body line, the needle can be inserted another 5 mm, in preparation for insertion of the guidewire.

minimally invasive transforaminal lumbar interbody fusion.[96] The mean fluoroscopy time was 1.69 minutes (range, 0.82 to 3.73 minutes) per case. The authors concluded that patient exposures were low and compared favorably with those associated with other common interventional fluoroscopically guided procedures. Kim et al[97] showed that the use of navigation-assisted fluoroscopy for minimally invasive transforaminal lumbar interbody fusion markedly decreases direct exposure to radiation by allowing the surgeon to step away from the surgical field during image acquisition. In addition to reducing radiation exposure, navigation eliminates the need for cumbersome protective lead gear and eliminates the need for fluoroscopy during surgery.

Learning Curve for Minimally Invasive Spine Surgery

The barriers to widespread adoption of minimally invasive techniques appear to be related to the technical difficulties of the procedures and a lack of adequate training opportunities. Webb et al[98] showed that most spinal surgeons perceive minimally invasive spine surgery to be efficacious, and most wish to perform more procedures. However, most surgeons have not pursued minimally invasive spine surgery because of concerns about the technical difficulties of the procedure and a lack of adequate training opportunities. Nowitzke[99] evaluated the learning curve for tubular decompression and noted that 3 of the first 7 cases performed in the series, but none of the subsequent 28 cases, required conversion to open surgery. Villavicencio et al[100] noted a higher rate of overall perioperative complications, Dhall et al[72] found a higher rate of instrumentation-related complications, and Peng et al[71] reported longer surgical times when comparing minimally invasive transforaminal lumbar interbody fusion with open transforaminal lumbar interbody fusion. Improving the learning curve for minimally invasive spine surgery requires studies to allow a better understanding of the specific portions of the procedure that are most challenging and to develop appropriate instrumentation and improved training techniques.

Summary

The posterior spine is dynamically stabilized by a diverse group of muscles that lie in close proximity to the vertebrae and possess multiple tendon insertion sites. In humans, stability and motion are controlled by active and passive means. The multifidus muscle is a powerful spine stabilizer because it has short and powerful fibers that enable it to produce large forces over short distances. Traditional posterior midline open approaches disrupt the function of this muscle through tendon detachment, devascularization, and crush injury. Minimally invasive spine surgery techniques were devel-

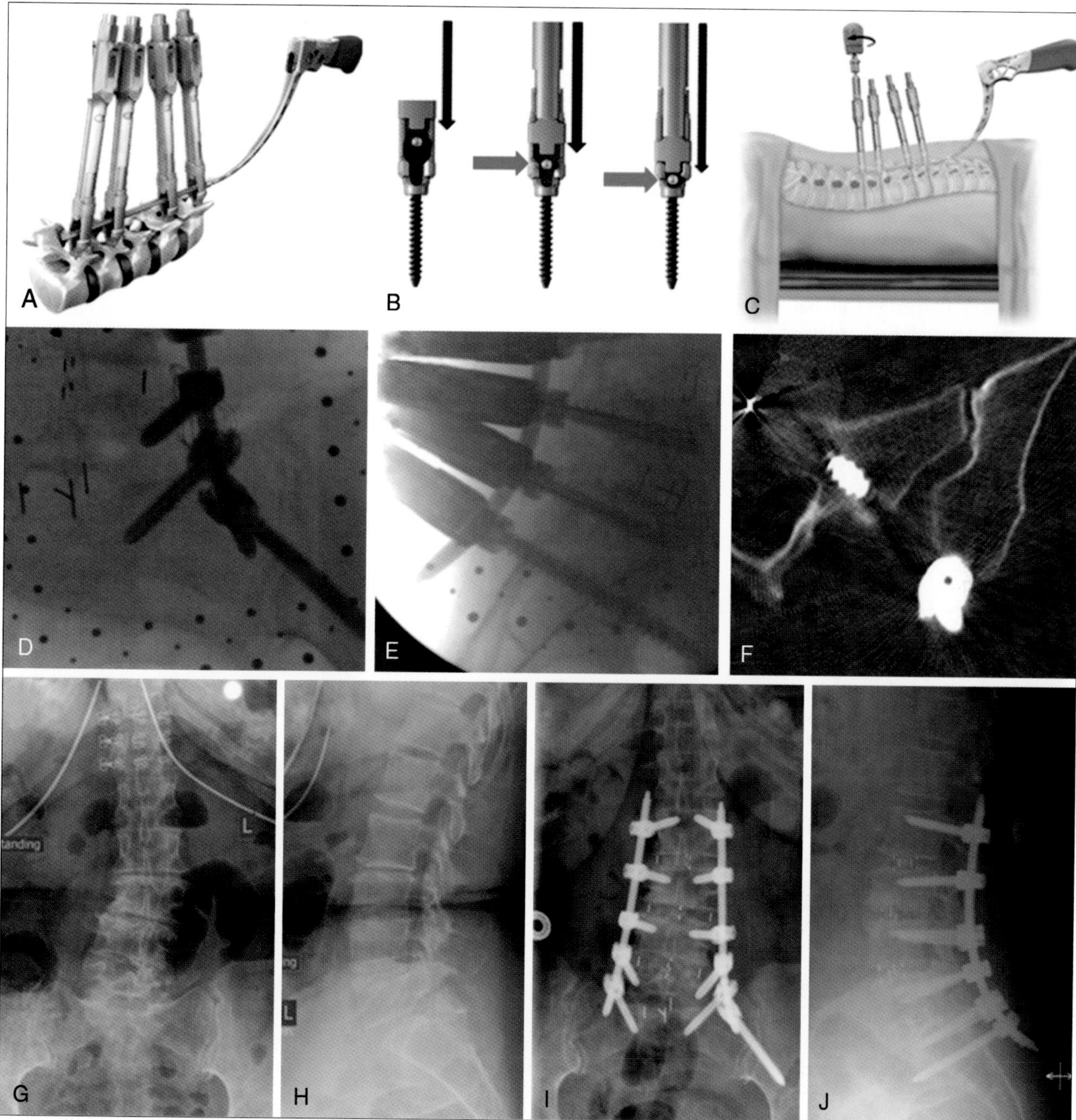

Figure 11 Minimally invasive rod insertion and deformity correction. Illustrations showing the technique of rod insertion through pedicle screw sleeves (**A**), which can then be used to reduce the rod to the tulip of the pedicle screw (**B**) with the use of a simple, threaded, sleeve reduction system that can be deployed outside the body (**C**). Intraoperative radiographs showing the construct in the AP (**D**) and lateral (**E**) planes. Pelvic fixation can be achieved by inserting the pelvic polyaxial screw in line with the S1 screw, as shown in the axial CT image (**F**). A comparison of preoperative radiographs (**G** and **H**) with postoperative standing radiographs (**I** and **J**) shows the final construct and the degree of deformity correction.

oped in an attempt to minimize surgical damage and preserve normal function. The rationale of this approach relies on limiting the surgical corridor to the minimum necessary to safely expose the surgical target site and minimize injury to the anatomic structures necessary for normal function. The traditional use of self-retaining retractors, which can induce crush injuries to muscle, has been supplanted by table-mounted, tubular-type retractors that minimize pressure on muscles, vessels, and nerves. As minimally invasive spine surgery continues to evolve, it is important to properly evaluate the risks and benefits of various minimally invasive techniques with prospective, long-term clinical studies.

References

1. Datta G, Gnanalingham KK, Peterson D, et al: Back pain and disability after lumbar laminectomy: Is there a relationship to muscle retraction? *Neurosurgery* 2004;54(6):1413-1420.
2. Gejo R, Kawaguchi Y, Kondoh T, et al: Magnetic resonance imaging and histologic evidence of postoperative back muscle injury in rats. *Spine (Phila Pa 1976)* 2000;25(8): 941-946.
3. Gejo R, Matsui H, Kawaguchi Y, Ishihara H, Tsuji H: Serial changes in trunk muscle performance after posterior lumbar surgery. *Spine (Phila Pa 1976)* 1999; 24(10):1023-1028.
4. Gille O, Jolivet E, Dousset V, et al: Erector spinae muscle changes on magnetic resonance imaging following lumbar surgery through a posterior approach. *Spine (Phila Pa 1976)* 2007; 32(11):1236-1241.
5. Hyun SJ, Kim YB, Kim YS, et al: Postoperative changes in paraspinal muscle volume: Comparison between paramedian interfascial and midline approaches for lumbar fusion. *J Korean Med Sci* 2007;22(4):646-651.
6. Kawaguchi Y, Matsui H, Gejo R, Tsuji H: Preventive measures of back muscle injury after posterior lumbar spine surgery in rats. *Spine (Phila Pa 1976)* 1998;23(21): 2282-2288.
7. Mayer TG, Vanharanta H, Gatchel RJ, et al: Comparison of CT scan muscle measurements and isokinetic trunk strength in postoperative patients. *Spine (Phila Pa 1976)* 1989;14(1): 33-36.
8. Motosuneya T, Asazuma T, Tsuji T, Watanabe H, Nakayama Y, Nemoto K: Postoperative change of the cross-sectional area of back musculature after 5 surgical procedures as assessed by magnetic resonance imaging. *J Spinal Disord Tech* 2006;19(5):318-322.
9. Rantanen J, Hurme M, Falck B, et al: The lumbar multifidus muscle five years after surgery for a lumbar intervertebral disc herniation. *Spine (Phila Pa 1976)* 1993; 18(5):568-574.
10. Granata KP, Marras WS: An EMG-assisted model of loads on the lumbar spine during asymmetric trunk extensions. *J Biomech* 1993;26(12):1429-1438.
11. Marras WS, Davis KG, Granata KP: Trunk muscle activities during asymmetric twisting motions. *J Electromyogr Kinesiol* 1998;8(4):247-256.
12. Kim DY, Lee SH, Chung SK, Lee HY: Comparison of multifidus muscle atrophy and trunk extension muscle strength: Percutaneous versus open pedicle screw fixation. *Spine (Phila Pa 1976)* 2005;30(1):123-129.
13. Mattila M, Hurme M, Alaranta H, et al: The multifidus muscle in patients with lumbar disc herniation: A histochemical and morphometric analysis of intraoperative biopsies. *Spine (Phila Pa 1976)* 1986;11(7): 732-738.
14. Kawaguchi Y, Matsui H, Tsuji H: Back muscle injury after posterior lumbar spine surgery: Part 2. Histologic and histochemical analyses in humans. *Spine (Phila Pa 1976)* 1994;19(22):2598-2602.
15. Kawaguchi Y, Matsui H, Tsuji H: Back muscle injury after posterior lumbar spine surgery: Part 1. Histologic and histochemical analyses in rats. *Spine (Phila Pa 1976)* 1994;19(22):2590-2597.
16. Kawaguchi Y, Matsui H, Tsuji H: Back muscle injury after posterior lumbar spine surgery: A histologic and enzymatic analysis. *Spine (Phila Pa 1976)* 1996;21(8): 941-944.
17. Kawaguchi Y, Yabuki S, Styf J, et al: Back muscle injury after posterior lumbar spine surgery: Topographic evaluation of intramuscular pressure and blood flow in the porcine back muscle during surgery. *Spine (Phila Pa 1976)* 1996;21(22):2683-2688.
18. Taylor H, McGregor AH, Medhi-Zadeh S, et al: The impact of self-retaining retractors on the paraspinal muscles during posterior spinal surgery. *Spine (Phila Pa 1976)* 2002;27(24):2758-2762.
19. Styf JR, Willén J: The effects of external compression by three different retractors on pressure in the erector spine muscles during and after posterior lumbar spine surgery in humans. *Spine (Phila Pa 1976)* 1998;23(3):354-358.
20. Stevens KJ, Spenciner DB, Griffiths KL, et al: Comparison of minimally invasive and conventional open posterolateral lumbar fusion using magnetic resonance imaging and retraction pressure studies. *J Spinal Disord Tech* 2006;19(2):77-86.
21. Tsutsumimoto T, Shimogata M, Ohta H, Misawa H: Mini-open versus conventional open posterior lumbar interbody fusion for the treatment of lumbar degenerative spondylolisthesis: Comparison of paraspinal muscle damage and slip reduction. *Spine (Phila Pa 1976)* 2009;34(18):1923-1928.
22. Macintosh JE, Bogduk N: 1987 Volvo award in basic science: The morphology of the lumbar erector spinae. *Spine (Phila Pa 1976)* 1987;12(7):658-668.
23. Macintosh JE, Bogduk N: The attachments of the lumbar erector spinae. *Spine (Phila Pa 1976)* 1991;16(7):783-792.

24. Sihvonen T, Herno A, Paljärvi L, Airaksinen O, Partanen J, Tapaninaho A: Local denervation atrophy of paraspinal muscles in postoperative failed back syndrome. *Spine (Phila Pa 1976)* 1993;18(5):575-581.
25. Kim KT, Lee SH, Suk KS, Bae SC: The quantitative analysis of tissue injury markers after mini-open lumbar fusion. *Spine (Phila Pa 1976)* 2006;31(6):712-716.
26. Ren G, Eiskjaer S, Kaspersen J, Christensen FB, Rasmussen S: Microdialysis of paraspinal muscle in healthy volunteers and patients underwent posterior lumbar fusion surgery. *Eur Spine J* 2009; 18(11):1604-1609.
27. Zander T, Rohlmann A, Klöckner C, Bergmann G: Influence of graded facetectomy and laminectomy on spinal biomechanics. *Eur Spine J* 2003;12(4):427-434.
28. Abumi K, Panjabi MM, Kramer KM, Duranceau J, Oxland T, Crisco JJ: Biomechanical evaluation of lumbar spinal stability after graded facetectomies. *Spine (Phila Pa 1976)* 1990;15(11): 1142-1147.
29. Tuite GF, Doran SE, Stern JD, et al: Outcome after laminectomy for lumbar spinal stenosis: Part II. Radiographic changes and clinical correlations. *J Neurosurg* 1994; 81(5):707-715.
30. Tuite GF, Stern JD, Doran SE, et al: Outcome after laminectomy for lumbar spinal stenosis: Part I. Clinical correlations. *J Neurosurg* 1994;81(5):699-706.
31. Johnsson KE, Willner S, Johnsson K: Postoperative instability after decompression for lumbar spinal stenosis. *Spine (Phila Pa 1976)* 1986;11(2):107-110.
32. Bresnahan L, Ogden AT, Natarajan RN, Fessler RG: A biomechanical evaluation of graded posterior element removal for treatment of lumbar stenosis: Comparison of a minimally invasive approach with two standard laminectomy techniques. *Spine (Phila Pa 1976)* 2009;34(1): 17-23.
33. Foley KT, Smith MM: Microendoscopic discectomy. *Tech Neurosurg* 1997;3:301-307.
34. Foley KT, Smith MM, Rampersaud YR: Microendoscopic approach to far-lateral lumbar disc herniation. *Neurosurg Focus* 1999; 7(5):e5.
35. Perez-Cruet MJ, Foley KT, Isaacs RE, et al: Microendoscopic lumbar discectomy: Technical note. *Neurosurgery* 2002;51(5, Suppl):S129-S136.
36. Schick U, Döhnert J, Richter A, König A, Vitzthum HE: Microendoscopic lumbar discectomy versus open surgery: An intraoperative EMG study. *Eur Spine J* 2002;11(1):20-26.
37. Muramatsu K, Hachiya Y, Morita C: Postoperative magnetic resonance imaging of lumbar disc herniation: Comparison of microendoscopic discectomy and Love's method. *Spine (Phila Pa 1976)* 2001;26(14):1599-1605.
38. Wu X, Zhuang S, Mao Z, Chen H: Microendoscopic discectomy for lumbar disc herniation: Surgical technique and outcome in 873 consecutive cases. *Spine (Phila Pa 1976)* 2006;31(23): 2689-2694.
39. Katayama Y, Matsuyama Y, Yoshihara H, et al: Comparison of surgical outcomes between macro discectomy and micro discectomy for lumbar disc herniation: A prospective randomized study with surgery performed by the same spine surgeon. *J Spinal Disord Tech* 2006;19(5):344-347.
40. Cole JS IV, Jackson TR: Minimally invasive lumbar discectomy in obese patients. *Neurosurgery* 2007;61(3):539-544.
41. Arts MP, Brand R, van den Akker ME, et al: Tubular diskectomy vs conventional microdiskectomy for sciatica: A randomized controlled trial. *JAMA* 2009;302(2): 149-158.
42. Ryang YM, Oertel MF, Mayfrank L, Gilsbach JM, Rohde V: Standard open microdiscectomy versus minimal access trocar microdiscectomy: Results of a prospective randomized study. *Neurosurgery* 2008;62(1):174-182.
43. Righesso O, Falavigna A, Avanzi O: Comparison of open discectomy with microendoscopic discectomy in lumbar disc herniations: Results of a randomized controlled trial. *Neurosurgery* 2007;61(3):545-549.
44. Weiner BK, Walker M, Brower RS, McCulloch JA: Microdecompression for lumbar spinal canal stenosis. *Spine (Phila Pa 1976)* 1999;24(21):2268-2272.
45. Palmer S, Turner R, Palmer R: Bilateral decompressive surgery in lumbar spinal stenosis associated with spondylolisthesis: Unilateral approach and use of a microscope and tubular retractor system. *Neurosurg Focus* 2002;13(1):E4.
46. Palmer S, Turner R, Palmer R: Bilateral decompression of lumbar spinal stenosis involving a unilateral approach with microscope and tubular retractor system. *J Neurosurg* 2002;97(2, Suppl): 213-217.
47. Costa F, Sassi M, Cardia A, et al: Degenerative lumbar spinal stenosis: Analysis of results in a series of 374 patients treated with unilateral laminotomy for bilateral microdecompression. *J Neurosurg Spine* 2007;7(6):579-586.
48. Iwatsuki K, Yoshimine T, Aoki M: Bilateral interlaminar fenestration and unroofing for the decompression of nerve roots by using a unilateral approach in lumbar canal stenosis. *Surg Neurol* 2007;68(5):487-492.
49. Khoo LT, Fessler RG: Microendoscopic decompressive laminotomy for the treatment of lumbar steno-

sis. *Neurosurgery* 2002;51(5, Suppl):S146-S154.

50. Rahman M, Summers LE, Richter B, Mimran RI, Jacob RP: Comparison of techniques for decompressive lumbar laminectomy: The minimally invasive versus the "classic" open approach. *Minim Invasive Neurosurg* 2008; 51(2):100-105.
51. Thomé C, Zevgaridis D, Leheta O, et al: Outcome after less-invasive decompression of lumbar spinal stenosis: A randomized comparison of unilateral laminotomy, bilateral laminotomy, and laminectomy. *J Neurosurg Spine* 2005;3(2):129-141.
52. Ikuta K, Arima J, Tanaka T, et al: Short-term results of microendoscopic posterior decompression for lumbar spinal stenosis: Technical note. *J Neurosurg Spine* 2005; 2(5):624-633.
53. Oertel MF, Ryang YM, Korinth MC, Gilsbach JM, Rohde V: Long-term results of microsurgical treatment of lumbar spinal stenosis by unilateral laminotomy for bilateral decompression. *Neurosurgery* 2006;59(6):1264-1270.
54. Ikuta K, Tono O, Tanaka T, et al: Surgical complications of microendoscopic procedures for lumbar spinal stenosis. *Minim Invasive Neurosurg* 2007;50(3): 145-149.
55. Yagi M, Okada E, Ninomiya K, Kihara M: Postoperative outcome after modified unilateral-approach microendoscopic midline decompression for degenerative spinal stenosis. *J Neurosurg Spine* 2009; 10(4):293-299.
56. Castro-Menéndez M, Bravo-Ricoy JA, Casal-Moro R, Hernández-Blanco M, Jorge-Barreiro FJ: Midterm outcome after microendoscopic decompressive laminotomy for lumbar spinal stenosis: 4-year prospective study. *Neurosurgery* 2009;65(1):100-110.
57. Asgarzadie F, Khoo LT: Minimally invasive operative management for lumbar spinal stenosis: Overview of early and long-term outcomes. *Orthop Clin North Am* 2007;38(3):387-399.
58. Podichetty VK, Spears J, Isaacs RE, Booher J, Biscup RS: Complications associated with minimally invasive decompression for lumbar spinal stenosis. *J Spinal Disord Tech* 2006;19(3):161-166.
59. Rosen DS, O'Toole JE, Eichholz KM, et al: Minimally invasive lumbar spinal decompression in the elderly: Outcomes of 50 patients aged 75 years and older. *Neurosurgery* 2007;60(3):503-510.
60. Sasaki M, Abekura M, Morris S, et al: Microscopic bilateral decompression through unilateral laminotomy for lumbar canal stenosis in patients undergoing hemodialysis. *J Neurosurg Spine* 2006;5(6):494-499.
61. Tomasino A, Parikh K, Steinberger J, Knopman J, Boockvar J, Härtl R: Tubular microsurgery for lumbar discectomies and laminectomies in obese patients: Operative results and outcome. *Spine (Phila Pa 1976)* 2009;34(18): E664-E672.
62. Pao JL, Chen WC, Chen PQ: Clinical outcomes of microendoscopic decompressive laminotomy for degenerative lumbar spinal stenosis. *Eur Spine J* 2009;18(5): 672-678.
63. Sasai K, Umeda M, Maruyama T, Wakabayashi E, Iida H: Microsurgical bilateral decompression via a unilateral approach for lumbar spinal canal stenosis including degenerative spondylolisthesis. *J Neurosurg Spine* 2008;9(6): 554-559.
64. Kleeman TJ, Hiscoe AC, Berg EE: Patient outcomes after minimally destabilizing lumbar stenosis decompression: The "Port-Hole" technique. *Spine (Phila Pa 1976)* 2000;25(7):865-870.
65. Blume H, Rojas C: Unilateral lumbar interbody fusion (posterior approach) utilizing dowel grafts: Experience in over 200 patients. *J Neurol Orthop Surg* 1981;2:171.
66. Harms JG, Jeszensky D: The unilateral, transforaminal approach for posterior lumbar interbody fusion. *Orthop Traumatol* 1998;6: 88-99.
67. Cloward RB: The treatment of ruptured lumbar intervertebral discs by vertebral body fusion: I. Indications, operative technique, after care. *J Neurosurg* 1953;10(2): 154-168.
68. Foley KT, Holly LT, Schwender JD: Minimally invasive lumbar fusion. *Spine (Phila Pa 1976)* 2003;28(15, Suppl):S26-S35.
69. Hee HT, Castro FP Jr, Majd ME, Holt RT, Myers L: Anterior/posterior lumbar fusion versus transforaminal lumbar interbody fusion: Analysis of complications and predictive factors. *J Spinal Disord* 2001;14(6):533-540.
70. Whitecloud TS III, Roesch WW, Ricciardi JE: Transforaminal interbody fusion versus anterior-posterior interbody fusion of the lumbar spine: A financial analysis. *J Spinal Disord* 2001;14(2): 100-103.
71. Peng CW, Yue WM, Poh SY, Yeo W, Tan SB: Clinical and radiological outcomes of minimally invasive versus open transforaminal lumbar interbody fusion. *Spine (Phila Pa 1976)* 2009;34(13): 1385-1389.
72. Dhall SS, Wang MY, Mummaneni PV: Clinical and radiographic comparison of mini-open transforaminal lumbar interbody fusion with open transforaminal lumbar interbody fusion in 42 patients with long-term follow-up. *J Neurosurg Spine* 2008;9(6):560-565.
73. Selznick LA, Shamji MF, Isaacs RE: Minimally invasive

interbody fusion for revision lumbar surgery: Technical feasibility and safety. *J Spinal Disord Tech* 2009;22(3):207-213.

74. Kasis AG, Marshman LA, Krishna M, Bhatia CK: Significantly improved outcomes with a less invasive posterior lumbar interbody fusion incorporating total facetectomy. *Spine (Phila Pa 1976)* 2009;34(6):572-577.
75. Molinari RW, Gerlinger T: Functional outcomes of instrumented posterior lumbar interbody fusion in active-duty US servicemen: A comparison with nonoperative management. *Spine J* 2001;1(3): 215-224.
76. Fritzell P, Hägg O, Wessberg P, Nordwall A: 2001 Volvo Award Winner in Clinical Studies: Lumbar fusion versus nonsurgical treatment for chronic low back pain. A multicenter randomized controlled trial from the Swedish Lumbar Spine Study Group. *Spine (Phila Pa 1976)* 2001;26(23): 2521-2534.
77. Christensen FB, Hansen ES, Eiskjaer SP, et al: Circumferential lumbar spinal fusion with Brantigan cage versus posterolateral fusion with titanium Cotrel-Dubousset instrumentation: A prospective, randomized clinical study of 146 patients. *Spine (Phila Pa 1976)* 2002;27(23):2674-2683.
78. McAfee PC, Regan JJ, Geis WP, Fedder IL: Minimally invasive anterior retroperitoneal approach to the lumbar spine: Emphasis on the lateral BAK. *Spine (Phila Pa 1976)* 1998;23(13):1476-1484.
79. Ozgur BM, Hughes SA, Baird LC, Taylor WR: Minimally disruptive decompression and transforaminal lumbar interbody fusion. *Spine J* 2006;6(1):27-33.
80. Pimenta L, Lhamby J, Gharzedine I, Coutinho E: XLIF approach for the treatment of adult scoliosis: 2 year follow-up. *Spine J* 2004;7(Suppl):52S-53S.
81. Saraph V, Lerch C, Walochnik N, Bach CM, Krismer M, Wimmer C: Comparison of conventional versus minimally invasive extraperitoneal approach for anterior lumbar interbody fusion. *Eur Spine J* 2004;13(5):425-431.
82. Regev GJ, Chen L, Dhawan M, Lee YP, Garfin SR, Kim CW: Morphometric analysis of the ventral nerve roots and retroperitoneal vessels with respect to the minimally invasive lateral approach in normal and deformed spines. *Spine (Phila Pa 1976)* 2009;34(12):1330-1335.
83. Bose B, Wierzbowski LR, Sestokas AK: Neurophysiologic monitoring of spinal nerve root function during instrumented posterior lumbar spine surgery. *Spine (Phila Pa 1976)* 2002; 27(13):1444-1450.
84. Knight RQ, Schwaegler P, Hanscom D, Roh J: Direct lateral lumbar interbody fusion for degenerative conditions: Early complication profile. *J Spinal Disord Tech* 2009;22(1):34-37.
85. Anand N, Baron EM, Thaiyananthan G, Khalsa K, Goldstein TB: Minimally invasive multilevel percutaneous correction and fusion for adult lumbar degenerative scoliosis: A technique and feasibility study. *J Spinal Disord Tech* 2008;21(7):459-467.
86. Regev GJ, Lee YP, Taylor WR, Garfin SR, Kim CW: Nerve injury to the posterior rami medial branch during the insertion of pedicle screws: Comparison of mini-open versus percutaneous pedicle screw insertion techniques. *Spine (Phila Pa 1976)* 2009;34(11):1239-1242.
87. Ringel F, Stoffel M, Stüer C, Meyer B: Minimally invasive transmuscular pedicle screw fixation of the thoracic and lumbar spine. *Neurosurgery* 2006;59(4, Suppl 2):ONS361-ONS3667.
88. Foley KT, Gupta SK: Percutaneous pedicle screw fixation of the lumbar spine: Preliminary clinical results. *J Neurosurg* 2002;97(1, Suppl):7-12.
89. Schwender JD, Holly LT, Rouben DP, Foley KT: Minimally invasive transforaminal lumbar interbody fusion (TLIF): Technical feasibility and initial results. *J Spinal Disord Tech* 2005; 18(Suppl):S1-S6.
90. Eck JC, Hodges S, Humphreys SC: Minimally invasive lumbar spinal fusion. *J Am Acad Orthop Surg* 2007;15(6):321-329.
91. Kosmopoulos V, Schizas C: Pedicle screw placement accuracy: A meta-analysis. *Spine (Phila Pa 1976)* 2007;32(3):E111-E120.
92. Merloz P, Troccaz J, Vouaillat H, et al: Fluoroscopy-based navigation system in spine surgery. *Proc Inst Mech Eng H* 2007;221(7): 813-820.
93. Assaker R, Cinquin P, Cotten A, Lejeune JP: Image-guided endoscopic spine surgery: Part I. A feasibility study. *Spine (Phila Pa 1976)* 2001;26(15):1705-1710.
94. Assaker R, Reyns N, Pertruzon B, Lejeune JP: Image-guided endoscopic spine surgery: Part II. Clinical applications. *Spine (Phila Pa 1976)* 2001;26(15):1711-1718.
95. Rampersaud YR, Foley KT, Shen AC, Williams S, Solomito M: Radiation exposure to the spine surgeon during fluoroscopically assisted pedicle screw insertion. *Spine (Phila Pa 1976)* 2000;25(20):2637-2645.
96. Bindal RK, Glaze S, Ognoskie M, Tunner V, Malone R, Ghosh S: Surgeon and patient radiation exposure in minimally invasive transforaminal lumbar interbody fusion. *J Neurosurg Spine* 2008; 9(6):570-573.
97. Kim CW, Lee YP, Taylor W, Oygar A, Kim WK: Use of navigation-assisted fluoroscopy to decrease radiation exposure during minimally invasive spine surgery. *Spine J* 2008;8(4):584-590.

98. Webb J, Gottschalk L, Lee YP, Garfin S, Kim C: Surgeon perceptions of minimally invasive spine surgery. *SAS J* 2008;2(3):145.

99. Nowitzke AM: Assessment of the learning curve for lumbar microendoscopic discectomy. *Neurosurgery* 2005;56(4):755-762.

100. Villavicencio AT, Burneikiene S, Bulsara KR, Thramann JJ: Perioperative complications in transforaminal lumbar interbody fusion versus anterior-posterior reconstruction for lumbar disc degeneration and instability. *J Spinal Disord Tech* 2006;19(2):92-97.

Video Reference

30.1: Kim CW: Video. Excerpt. *MIS Transforaminal Lumbar Interbody Fusion Technique.* San Diego, CA, 2010.

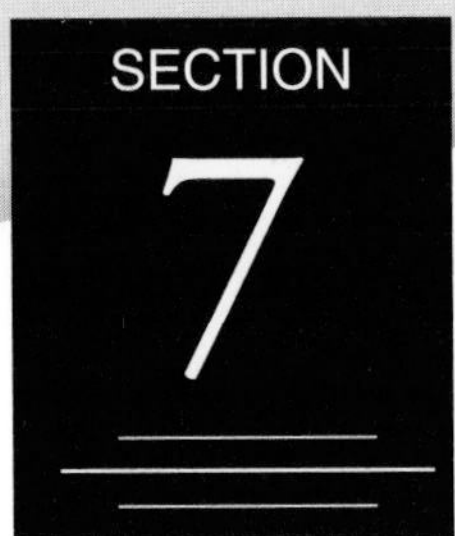

Section 7

Pediatrics

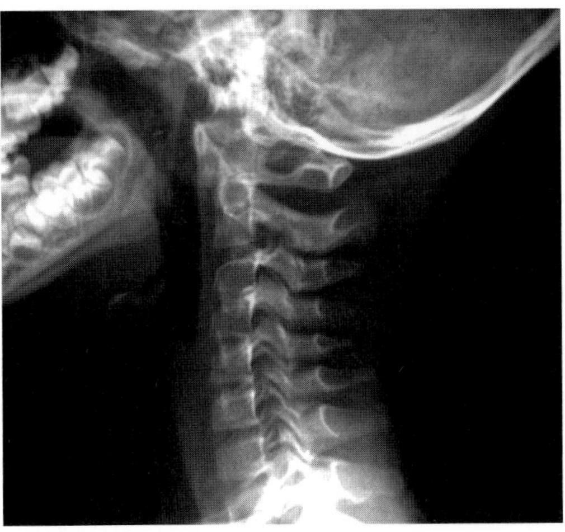

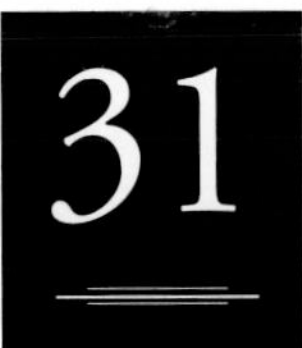

Top 10 Pediatric Orthopaedic Surgical Emergencies: A Case-Based Approach for the Surgeon On Call

Martin J. Herman, MD
James McCarthy, MD
R. Baxter Willis, MD, FRCSC
Peter D. Pizzutillo, MD

Abstract

Pediatric patients who require orthopaedic surgical emergency care are often treated by orthopaedic surgeons who primarily treat adult patients. Essential information is needed to safely evaluate and treat the most common surgical emergencies in pediatric patients, including hip fractures; supracondylar humeral, femoral, and tibial conditions of the hip (such as slipped capital femoral epiphysis and septic arthritis); and limb- and life-threatening pathologies, including compartment syndrome, the dysvascular limb, cervical spine trauma, and the polytraumatized child. To provide optimal care to pediatric patients, it is important to be aware of the key points in patient evaluation and surgical care as well as expected complications.

Instr Course Lect 2011;60:373-395.

As the number of pediatric orthopaedic surgeons practicing in the United States continues to decline, the management of pediatric surgical emergency patients is becoming the responsibility of orthopaedic surgeons who primarily treat adults. Although all orthopaedic surgeons are trained in emergency care, most do not routinely treat pediatric patients in their practices. In many regions, reliable or convenient transfer to the care of a pediatric orthopaedic surgeon is not an available option. This chapter will discuss essential information that is needed "in the middle of the night" to adequately assess and safely treat the most common pediatric orthopaedic surgical emergencies. Each emergency scenario (not listed in the order of severity) includes a discussion of the patient evaluation; surgical considerations, including equipment needs and surgical techniques; and expected complications, with tips on how to avoid them.

Unstable Slipped Capital Femoral Epiphysis

Slipped capital femoral epiphysis (SCFE) is a condition in which the femoral neck displaces anteriorly and proximally through the proximal femoral capital physis, tipping the femoral head posteriorly and into varus (**Figure 1**). It is an uncommon but potentially devastating disorder that requires accurate assessment and urgent treatment. Although there is controversy regarding the optimal treatment method, there is a general consensus regarding basic treatment principles. The potential loss of blood flow to the femoral head is of great concern and urgency in treating patients with unstable SCFE.

The anatomy of the vascular supply to the femoral head is well described.[1] Unlike the more common stable

Dr. McCarthy or an immediate family member has received research or institutional support from EBI/Biomet and Aesculap/B. Braun and has received nonincome support (such as equipment or services), commercially derived honoraria, or other non–research-related funding (such as paid travel) from Wolters Kluwer Health–Lippincott Williams & Wilkins. Dr. Willis or an immediate family member serves as a board member, owner, officer, or committee member of the Pediatric Orthopaedic Society of North America and serves as an unpaid consultant to Orthopediatrics. Neither of the following authors or any immediate family member has received anything of value from or owns stock in a commercial company or institution related directly or indirectly to the subject of this chapter: Dr. Herman and Dr. Pizzutillo.

Table 1
Methods of Classifying Stable Versus Unstable SCFEs

Stable	Unstable
(-) effusion, (+) metaphyseal remodeling	(+) effusion, (-) metaphyseal remodeling
No movement with fluoroscopy	Movement with fluoroscopy
Patient presents in clinic	Patient presents in emergency room

SCFE = slipped capital femoral epiphysis

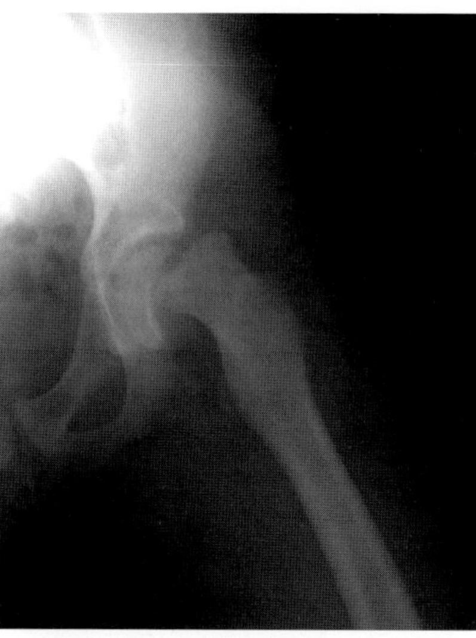

Figure 1 AP radiograph of an unstable grade II SCFE in an 11-year-old boy who tripped on a curb and was unable to walk.

Table 2
Underlying Conditions That May Be Associated With SCFE

Systemic Disorders
Hypothyroidism
Panhypopituitarism
Growth hormone abnormalities
Hypogonadism
Anatomic Variations
Femoral retroversion
Coxa vara
Increased physeal slope
Deep acetabuli
Other
Radiation therapy
Renal osteodystrophy (caused by secondary hyperparathyroidism)
Down syndrome (resulting from hypothyroidism)
Genetic causes: increased incidence in family members

SCFE = slipped capital femoral epiphysis

SCFE, disruption of the blood supply appears to be common in unstable SCFE and may be reconstituted with reduction.[2] Increased intracapsular pressure, which also occurs in SCFE, is further increased with reduction, indicating that a tamponade effect may lead to decreased blood flow in a manner similar to that which occurs in compartment syndrome.[3] Urgent capsulotomy should be performed at the time of stabilization.

Patient Assessment

SCFEs have been classified based on the degree of displacement, the acuity of the slip, and, more recently, the stability of the slip. A SCFE is defined as unstable if the patient is unable to ambulate, even with crutches.[4] **Table 1** shows several other methods used to classify stable versus unstable SCFEs. Patients with unstable SCFE need urgent treatment and have a high rate of poor outcomes. Up to 50% of unstable SCFEs have poor outcomes that primarily result from osteonecrosis of the femoral head.

A patient with unstable SCFE often presents with a sudden onset of groin or knee pain, obligatory external rotation, and the inability to ambulate. Many patients have a history of prodromal symptoms. Typically, unstable SCFE is obvious on radiographic studies. Cross-table lateral views should be obtained; frog-lateral views may cause the patient discomfort and may potentially further displace the SCFE. Other underlying conditions, such as endocrine dysfunction, may be associated with SCFE in 5% to 8% of patients[5] (**Table 2**). An endocrine workup should be considered for children who appear slimmer or shorter than would be expected based on their age. The 10-10-15-50 rule (children in less than the 10th percentile for height and those younger than 10 years or older than 15 years who are in less than the 50th percentile for weight) can be used as a guide when considering the need for an endocrine workup. The opposite hip should be carefully assessed for signs of early SCFE, which is usually a nontraumatic disorder. If a slip is found, pinning of the contralateral side is warranted. However, even if there is no slip, some patients, such as those with endocrine abnormalities, girls younger than 10 years or boys younger than 12 years, or patients in whom follow-up care is unlikely, may warrant pinning of the contralateral hip.[6]

Surgical Considerations

The initial surgical setup is critical. Children with SCFE are often obese, and fluoroscopic images, especially the lateral view, can be difficult to clearly assess. A fracture table is used, and little traction is typically needed. Before prepping the patient, the C-arm should be manipulated to ensure that the appropriate views can be obtained. If two C-arms are used, the lateral C-arm should be positioned first and should not be moved for the remainder of the surgical procedure. Because an AP view can usually be easily obtained, the C-arm is positioned after the patient is prepped and draped.[7]

Cannulated stainless steel 7.3-mm screws are preferred. Smaller 6.5-mm screws can be used, but the smaller and more flexible guide pin makes redirecting the pin more difficult.

In situ pinning of an unstable SCFE should be performed urgently. Osteonecrosis is less likely to occur if surgery is done within the first 24 hours; most surgeons believe that it should be performed as soon as possible. The procedure involves positioning the patient without a forceful reduction maneuver, decompressing the capsule, and placing one or two screws.[8] With unstable SCFE, there may be an "incidental" reduction when positioning the patient on the fracture table. This incidental reduction will rarely result in reducing the original anatomic shape because the proximal femur often has undergone some chronic changes, even in a patient without prodromal symptoms; this deformity will block full reduction. The chronic deformity may also explain why forced closed reduction leads to a higher risk of osteonecrosis.

For surgeons more familiar with pinning in adult hips, the hip anatomy of a pediatric patient may present a challenge. The goal is to get at least one pin in the center-center position of the femoral head, crossing perpendicular to the physis in all planes, with three to five threads across the neck in a center-center position and the tip of the pin staying 8 to 10 mm from the subchondral bone. To accomplish this goal, it is necessary to start more anteriorly and proximally on the femur. The starting point is estimated by laying the guide pin on the thigh in both the AP and lateral C-arm views and then marking the starting point just proximal to where the two pins cross. A small Kirschner wire (0.065-inch) can be used as a sound, placed through the skin (before the incision), to ensure that the correct location has been found. A 1-cm incision is made, and the larger guide pin for the 7.3-mm cannulated screw is inserted. This pin is stout enough so that it can be tapped into place to obtain the bony starting point and subsequently drilled when the starting position and trajectory are believed to be adequate.

Occasionally the deformity is so large that if the pin is placed just proximal to where the two pins cross (as previously described), it will be in the femoral neck, which provides little fixation and can result in impingement of the screw head with the hip in flexion.[9] In this instance, the starting point should be lateral to the intertrochanteric line. If prophylactic pinning is performed, the tendency is to place the pin more laterally and distally, which is appropriate; however, the starting point should never be placed below the lesser trochanter because such placement may result in a subtrochanteric fracture.

With the pin across the physis, positioning can be confirmed by several methods to ensure that the hip joint was not violated. The approach-withdrawal technique, in which the hip is rotated in varying degrees of flexion, is commonly used. As the hip is rotated, the screw tip should appear to approach the subchondral bone, then begin to withdraw as hip rotation is continued. The bulls-eye view also can be used as a supplemental orthogonal view.[10] If there is any concern about appropriate screw placement, a postoperative CT can be obtained. Two screws provide marginally stronger fixation and may prevent rotation but can be difficult to place in a patient with significant displacement. Capsular decompression is always indicated and can be done by either sliding a periosteal elevator along the anterior neck of the femur, opening the capsule, or by inserting a large-bore catheter into the hip joint. These methods have been found to be effective.

Postoperatively, the patient is instructed to use crutches for up to 3 months (compared with up to 6 weeks for a stable SCFE). Follow-up radiographs should always include complete views of both hips; attention also should be focused on the contralateral hip to identify early SCFE.

Complications

There are many possible long-term complications of SCFE, many of which are the result of the initial injury. Prior to surgery, the patient and parents should be counseled regarding possible complications. Technical problems, such as improper placement of intra-articular screws, screw head impingement, and subtrochanteric fractures, can be diminished by following appropriate surgical guidelines. Osteonecrosis, which occurs at a rate as high as 47%, is the most serious and significant complication. Care should be taken to avoid screw placement in the superior-posterior femoral head because the lateral epiphyseal vessels enter this region. Greater trochanteric overgrowth, leg-length inequality, and chondrolysis are much less likely. Long-term osteoarthrosis can occur, especially if there is significant residual deformity. The incidence of osteoarthritis after SCFE and the clinical significance of SCFE is more controversial.[11,12] Because of the risk of osteoarthritis, some surgeons recommend more aggressive initial treatment of children with an unstable SCFE, including performing a surgical dislocation with urgent reduction, resection of the femoral neck, and fixation. Preliminary reports have shown very low osteonecrosis rates (DJ Sucato, MD, and DA Podeszwa, MD, Hollywood FL, unpublished data presented at the Pediatric Orthopaedic Society of North America meeting, 2007). Some surgeons have used gradual distraction in an attempt to provide reduction,

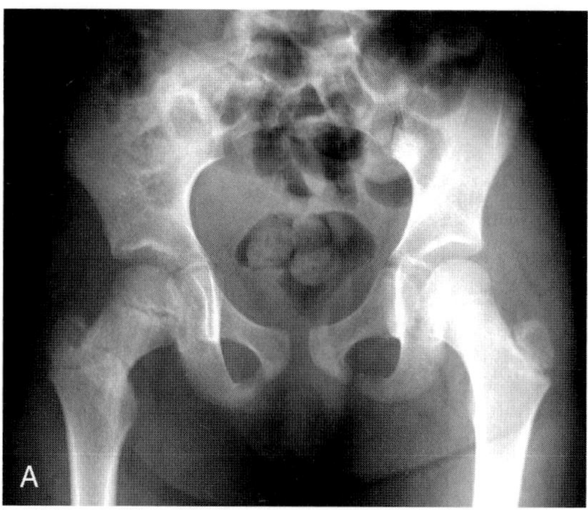

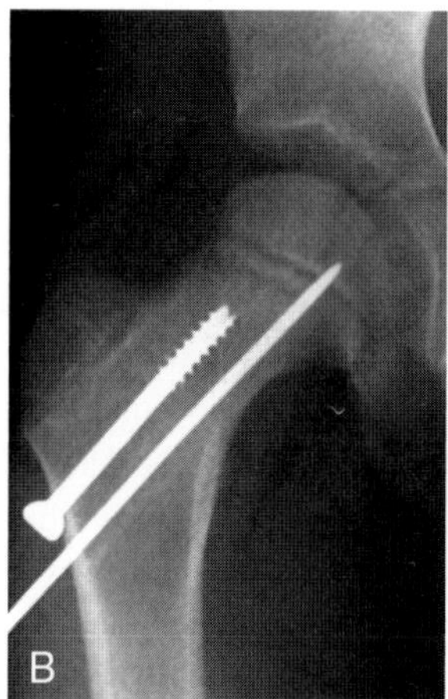

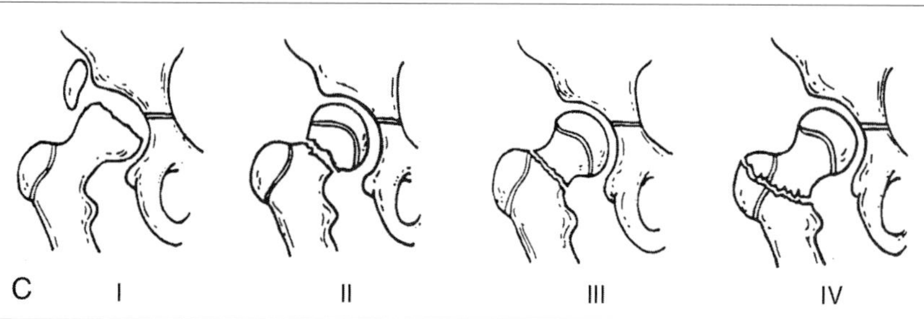

Figure 2 **A,** AP radiograph shows a minimally displaced femoral neck fracture in a 7-year-old girl. The injury occurred when the girl fell from a window, and she was unable to stand because of pain.. **B,** Radiograph after closed reduction and fixation. The hip was aspirated of blood after reduction, and the girl was placed in a spica cast. **C,** The injury is a type II hip fracture based on the Delbert and Colonna classification system. The characteristics of the four fracture types are described in the text.

whereas others use early detection of osteonecrosis and subsequent treatment with bisphosphonates to decrease the rate and degree of femoral head collapse.[13,14]

Hip Fractures and Dislocations

Pediatric femoral neck fractures, unlike adult hip fractures, are uncommon, accounting for less than 1% of all pediatric fractures[15-17] (**Figure 2**). Identifying these fractures is important because of their high complication rate (up to 60%). Pediatric femoral neck fractures can be difficult to manage, require urgent treatment, and have the potential for causing long-term disability. These fractures involve some of the same concerns as SCFE, including a precarious blood supply and issues of capsular distention, both leading to the potential interruption of blood flow and osteonecrosis. Pediatric femoral neck fractures differ from SCFE in that they are predominately extraphyseal, are acute with no chronic bony changes, and result from high-energy injuries.

Patient Assessment

The classification of pediatric hip fractures, described by Delbert and Colonna in 1929, is simple, is anatomically based, and has prognostic and treatment implications (**Figure 2, C**). Type I fractures are transepiphyseal (as are SCFEs), but unlike SCFEs, these fractures are associated with a high-energy traumatic event. Type I fractures are rare, accounting for less than 10% of all pediatric hip fractures, but carry the highest risk of osteonecrosis. In approximately 50% of type I fractures, the femoral head is dislocated and rests outside the acetabulum. In such instances, the risk of osteonecrosis approaches 100%.

In type II (transcervical) and type III (basicervical) hip fractures, the fracture occurs through the femoral neck. These fractures make up approximately 80% of all pediatric hip fractures. The risk of osteonecrosis is 30% to 50% and probably increases in more proximal fractures. Varus hip fractures are one of the few fractures in children that have a relatively high risk of nonunion (15% to 30%).

Type IV fractures occur through the intertrochanteric region and make up the remaining 10% to 15% of pediatric hip fractures. Osteonecrosis is uncommon; however, the possibility of a pathologic fracture must always be considered, especially with lower-energy injuries.

Surgical Considerations

Treatment guidelines for all pediatric hip fractures include urgent reduction, joint decompression, and stable fixation; treatment should be performed as soon as possible (< 24 hours after injury) for type I to III fractures. Prompt treatment may decrease the rate of osteonecrosis.[17]

Most orthopaedic surgeons are comfortable treating pediatric hip fractures; aside from type I fractures, the techniques are similar to those used in adults. A fracture table is used for older children, with gentle traction, abduction, and internal rotation. Younger children may be treated with manual traction on a fluoroscopy table. The goal is to prevent residual varus and achieve less than 10% to 20% displacement. The anterolateral approach should be used for an open reduction (if needed), and the physis should be avoided if possible; however, stability is more important than avoiding the physis, which provides excellent fixation. If the patient is younger than 3 years and it is necessary to cross the physis, smooth pins should be considered along with a spica cast. Trochanteric overgrowth should be carefully assessed. If there are indications of early growth arrest, a greater trochanteric epiphysiodesis should be considered. If the head fragment is unstable, a large screw may rotate the proximal fragment when being advanced and can potentially tear or kink the retinacular vessels. Head fragment rotation can be avoided by placing two guide pins before inserting the screws.

Fracture-Specific Care

Because type I fractures have a high risk of osteonecrosis and can occur in very young children, it is important that the family be informed of this complication before treatment. If the femoral head can be reduced closed, then smooth pinning and spica cast treatment should be used. If the proximal femur is large enough, the use of cannulated screws is an option. As with all type I to III pediatric hip fractures, the capsule should be decompressed by a large bore needle or by opening the capsule. Unlike in a patient with SCFE, the anatomy is not distorted, and the direction of the screws or pins is similar to pinning in an adult hip. Varus malunion and fracture nonunion is uncommon.

Type II and III fractures are treated much like adult femoral neck fractures. Type II fracture fixation often requires crossing the physis. Multiple threaded screws are used to stabilize the fracture, and a capsulotomy is performed.[2,3] Accurate reduction is important because these fractures have the potential for nonunion, especially if reduced and fixed in varus. In younger children, the hip can be placed in a spica cast for additional immobilization.

If the fracture is nondisplaced, traction or a cast may be used to treat type IV fractures; however, close follow-up is needed to ensure that varus positioning does not occur. If the fracture is displaced, it should be reduced and stabilized with a hip screw and a side-plate construct. Rotational stability should be achieved with two guide pins before placing the large hip screw if there is concern regarding proximal fragment stability. All fractures should be assessed for underlying pathology by carefully examining the preoperative radiographs.

Complications

Osteonecrosis is the most devastating of several complications that can occur after a hip fracture. After a fracture, osteonecrosis is usually noted radiographically by 9 to 12 months or 2 to 4 weeks with MRI. The prevalence of osteonecrosis increases with increased displacement, is more common in children older than 10 years, and is more prevalent in certain fracture types (for example, more prevalent in type I than type II fractures).[18] If osteonecrosis occurs, most patients require further treatment. In patients younger than 12 years, the treatment protocol is similar to that of Legg-Calvé-Perthes disease; whereas in children older than 12 years, the treatment is similar to that of osteonecrosis in adults. If osteonecrosis is diagnosed early, medical treatment with bisphosphonates can be considered.

A growth arrest of the proximal femoral epiphysis may occur in 10% to 60% of patients, secondary to injury to the proximal femoral physeal fracture, osteonecrosis, or fixation across the physis. Trochanteric overgrowth can be treated with a greater trochanteric epiphysiodesis. Limb-length discrepancy can be treated with a contralateral distal femoral epiphysiodesis if the projected limb-length discrepancy warrants intervention (usually a projected limb-length inequality exceeding 2 cm).

Varus malunion, which may occur in up to 20% of fractures, is primarily caused by inadequate reduction or fixation. A valgus osteotomy should be considered, especially in older children with varus of 110° or less. Nonunions occur in 5% to 8% of pediatric hip fractures, typically in type II or III fractures. Nonunion is primarily caused by failure to obtain and maintain reduction. Treatment options include bone grafting and valgus osteotomy if associated with a varus malunion.

Pediatric hip dislocations are more common than hip fractures; most are posterior (85% to 90%). High-energy dislocations, with a mechanism similar to that seen in adult hip dislocations, are more common and account for 75% of pediatric hip dislocations.[19] Unlike adult hip dislocations, a low-energy injury, such as a fall while walking, can lead to a hip dislocation, especially in very young children.

Hip dislocations should be treated with reduction within 6 hours. A closed reduction using a muscle relaxant, gentle traction, and flexion and adduction of the leg is performed. In adolescents, fluoroscopy should be considered to ensure that physeal separation does not occur during the attempted reduction.[20] CT or MRI of the hip should always be done after the reduction to evaluate for intra-articular fragments. Open reduction of the hip joint is considered if the initial reduction appears nonconcentric, there is a fracture of the proximal femur, or closed reduction is unsuccessful.

Complications following hip dislocation include osteonecrosis in 3% to

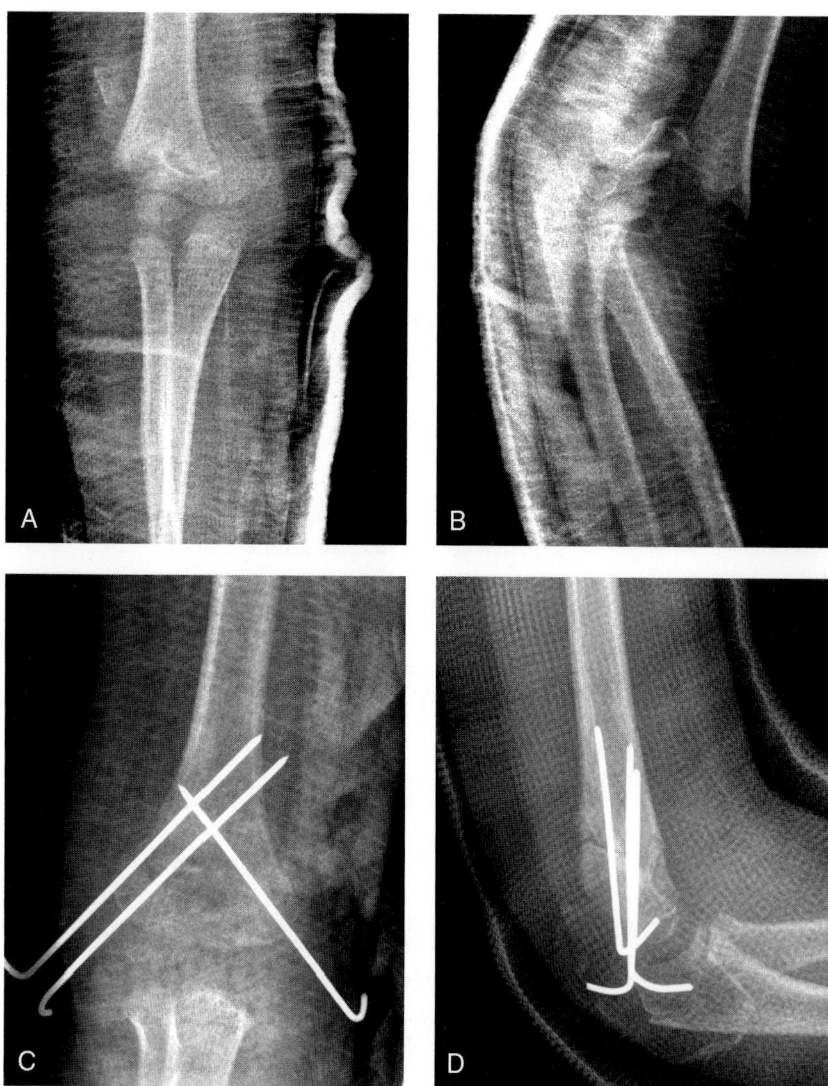

Figure 3 **A** through **D,** Radiographic studies of a 5-year-old boy who was taken to the emergency department 3 hours after falling from monkey bars directly onto his outstretched left hand. Examination showed significant swelling in the antecubital fossa; the patient was unwilling to move his elbow. The neurovascular status was intact. AP **(A)** and lateral radiographs **(B)** of the elbow. AP **(C)** and lateral **(D)** radiographs after the patient was treated with closed reduction and percutaneous pinning the following morning. The patient had an excellent outcome.

10% of patients (less common than in adult hip dislocations), myositis ossificans, redislocation, neurovascular injury (in 5%), and premature degenerative joint disease.[21]

Displaced Supracondylar Humeral Fractures

Supracondylar fractures of the humerus are one of the most common fractures in children, making up 85% of elbow fractures and 15% of all pediatric fractures[22] (**Figure 3**). For many orthopaedic surgeons, this fracture provokes anxiety because of the associated complications, including neurovascular injury, compartment syndrome, and malunion. Historically, displaced supracondylar fractures have been treated as a surgical emergency because of the concern for increased complications if treatment is delayed. Several recent studies, however, have indicated that there is no increase in the need for open reduction and no increase in complications for those fractures treated in a delayed fashion compared with those treated emergently.[23-25] Delaying treatment 8 to 12 hours is safe if the skin is not compromised and the neurovascular status of the limb is normal.

Patient Assessment

Most children sustain isolated supracondylar fractures from falls onto an outstretched hand. If the patient history suggests a high-energy mechanism, the child should be fully assessed for associated injuries. The elbow should be examined for deformity, skin lacerations with exposed bone, and tenting or puckering seen just proximal to the antecubital fossa from impalement of the distal end of the shaft fragment in the dermis. In a child who can cooperate with the examiner, careful motor and sensory testing is critical. In an uncooperative child, observational examination of motor function may be the only means of assessing neurologic injury. For example, a child with a palsy of the anterior interosseous nerve, a branch of the median nerve that is most commonly injured, will keep the index finger extended when grasping or making a fist. The vascular status of the limb also must be carefully assessed. Documenting the radial pulses and overall perfusion by assessing capillary refill in the fingers is crucial to decision making regarding the timing of treatment; emergency surgery should be considered when the child has an absent pulse, even if perfusion of the hand is normal. Prior to splinting the elbow in moderate flexion, the compartments of the arm and forearm are palpated for tenderness or swelling.

High-quality AP and lateral radiographs of the elbow are obtained after splinting to prevent further injury of the fractured limb while imaging is completed. Extension-type fractures are most common, but 3% to 5% of injuries are flexion-type (the distal fragment is flexed or displaced anteriorly with apex posterior angulation).

The Gartland classification system describes extension-type supracondylar fractures (**Table 3**). Most type II fractures and all type III fractures are best treated surgically.

Table 3
Gartland Classification for Supracondylar Fractures

Type	Description
I	Nondisplaced fracture
II	Displaced, with bony contact
III	Displaced, no bony contact

Surgical Considerations

Although closed treatment methods (closed reduction and casting) and traction methods have been used with success in the past, the standard of treatment is closed reduction and percutaneous pinning in the operating room for Gartland type III fractures. In most patients, closed reduction is successful. Open reduction is reserved for patients with open fractures or if satisfactory closed reduction cannot be achieved (approximately 5% of patients). Open reduction is best done through an anterior approach.

Closed reduction is best accomplished with the patient under general anesthesia, in the operating room, and under sterile conditions. Closed reduction is performed with fluoroscopic control after the involved arm is prepped and draped. The reduction is accomplished by applying longitudinal traction first, correcting the medial or lateral translation next, followed by acute flexion of the elbow. The reduction is confirmed fluoroscopically. In the coronal plane, an acceptable reduction is one in which the elbow carrying angle is zero or ideally in mild valgus; varus is unacceptable. In the sagittal plane, the anterior humeral line should pass through the anterior or middle third of the capitellum. As much as 50% translation of the distal fragment in either plane is acceptable.

Stabilization is then performed using 0.062-mm diameter Kirschner wires (pins), except in very young children in whom smaller diameter wires may be necessary. A lateral pin is placed first, starting in the center of the capitellum or at the junction of the capitellum and metaphysis. A second pin is inserted either laterally or medially. A second lateral pin may be placed parallel to the first pin or slightly divergent from it.[26] Placement of a medial pin is an option used predominantly for unstable fracture patterns. To avoid iatrogenic injury to the ulnar nerve, the medial pin is best placed with the elbow held in extension through a small incision over the medial epicondyle anterior to the ulnar groove.[27] It is critical that the pins do not intersect at the fracture site and are bicortical to ensure maximum stability and prevent rotation of the distal fragment.[28] Placement of a third pin, usually laterally, is indicated if fracture stability is in question after clinical and fluoroscopic assessment with two pins in place. After pinning, the arm is splinted with the elbow held in 60° to 80° of flexion.

Complications

Cubitus varus is the most common complication. Cubitus varus is a rotational and varus malunion that does not remodel, sometimes requiring late osteotomy. It results from unstable fractures treated without fixation, inadequate fracture reduction, or loss of reduction secondary to poor fixation. Nerve palsies also occur (anterior interosseous more often than median nerve, median nerve more often than radial nerve, radial nerve more often than ulnar nerve) but usually resolve within 6 to 12 weeks. Compartment syndrome of the forearm is an uncommon but devastating complication. Brachial artery entrapment and laceration are rarely associated with supracondylar humeral fractures.

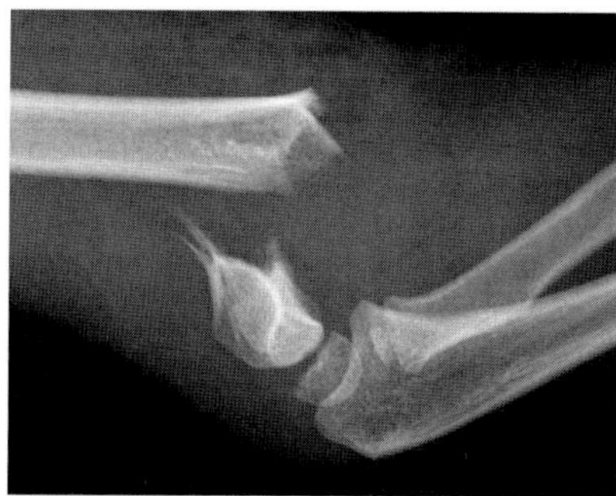

Figure 4 A lateral radiograph of the elbow of a 6-year-old girl who fell off a balance beam and had extreme swelling, absent radial pulse, and inability to flex the distal interphalangeal joint of the index finger. A severely displaced type III supracondylar fracture is shown. The patient was treated with emergency closed reduction and pinning. The radial pulse returned after reduction in the operating room. The anterior interosseous nerve palsy resolved in 4 weeks.

The Pulseless Supracondylar Fracture

The pulseless supracondylar fracture is rare because vascular compromise after fracture is uncommon in children (**Figure 4**). Although vessel laceration sometimes occurs, most instances of vascular compromise are the result of vessel impingement, kinking, or spasm from fracture displacement or traction. Physeal fractures of the distal femur and proximal tibia that displace anteriorly (apex posterior angulation) and

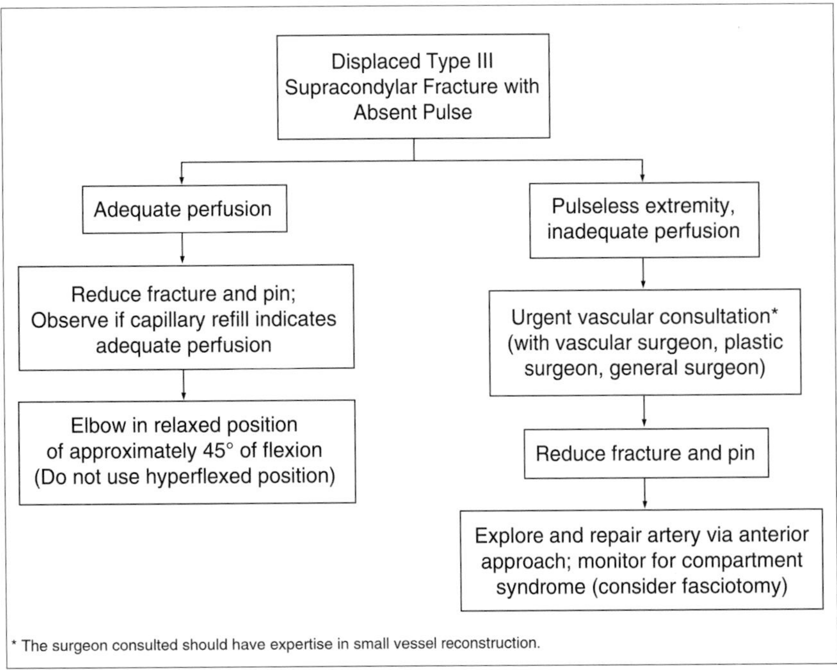

Figure 5 Algorithm for managing a pulseless supracondylar fracture.

extension-type displaced supracondylar humeral fractures are the injuries most frequently associated with vascular compromise. These injuries demand emergency management to avoid disastrous complications, such as muscle ischemia and necrosis, compartment syndrome, and the loss of a limb.

Patient Assessment

It is important to determine the mechanism of injury. A high-energy mechanism is the likely cause of a pulseless limb from a fracture (especially a knee fracture) or a mangled limb in a child. The surgeon should rule out associated injuries while maintaining focus on the dysvascular limb. Lacerations and open wounds should be inspected for evidence of bleeding, a sign of a potential vessel laceration, and a compressive dressing or tourniquet should be applied to prevent exsanguination of the patient. The grossly malaligned limb is gently realigned by applying longitudinal traction; then a splint is placed.

The vascular status of the limb is then determined. Distal pulses are assessed by palpation and Doppler ultrasound if necessary. Perfusion may be preserved despite a loss of pulses. Pale skin tone, coolness to touch, and a sluggish or absent capillary refill are signs that distal perfusion is not preserved and the condition is limb threatening. For a patient with a perfused limb, radiographs and other imaging studies may be done in the emergency department; critical studies should be done for the patient with a dysvascular extremity.

Surgical Considerations

For a pulseless supracondylar fracture, reduction and stabilization should be done first. After reduction, the radial pulse is careful reassessed. If a radial pulse is not detected, Doppler ultrasound is used to assess vascularity, noting flow that is synchronous with pulse oximetry measured on one of the unaffected limbs. With warming of the limb and within approximately 20 minutes of reduction, flow will return if the dysvascularity was secondary to vessel kinking or spasm, the most common scenarios.

If the pulse does not return, it is imperative to differentiate between a pulseless extremity that is pink and viable and an extremity that is pulseless, cold, and with definite vascular insufficiency. For most patients with displaced supracondylar fractures, reduction will restore the arterial circulation and limb perfusion.[29-31] Supracondylar fractures occur below the site of origin of abundant collateral circulation to the forearm and hand, allowing adequate inflow of blood despite the absence of a radial pulse. If the fracture has been adequately reduced and the hand is warm, is normal in color, and has brisk capillary refill, the fracture is placed in a splint and the child is admitted for 48 hours of careful monitoring of the vascular status of the limb. Arteriography or exploration of the brachial artery is not indicated.[29-31]

After fracture reduction, the extremity that remains pulseless, pale, and cool to touch must be explored. In most instances, the vessel is compromised at the apex of the fracture deformity, making a preoperative arteriogram unnecessary except when the limb has multiple fractures or lacerations. For the patient with a displaced extension-type supracondylar fracture, the brachial artery is explored through an anterior approach to the elbow. Surgical repair or bypass of the injured segment is best performed by a surgeon competent in repairing and reconstructing small caliber peripheral vessels[29,32,33] (generally a plastic, hand, or vascular surgeon). Fasciotomies of the distal limb are indicated in conjunction with the vascular repair if flow has been absent for 6 hours or more. As an example, an algorithm for managing a pulseless displaced type III supracondylar fracture is shown in **Figure 5**.

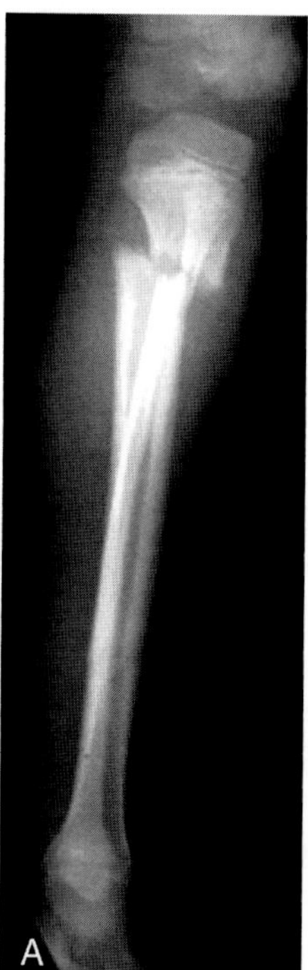

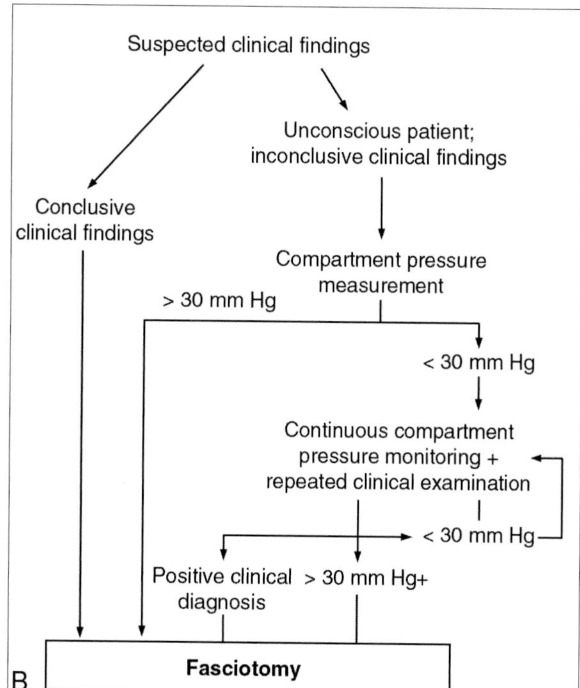

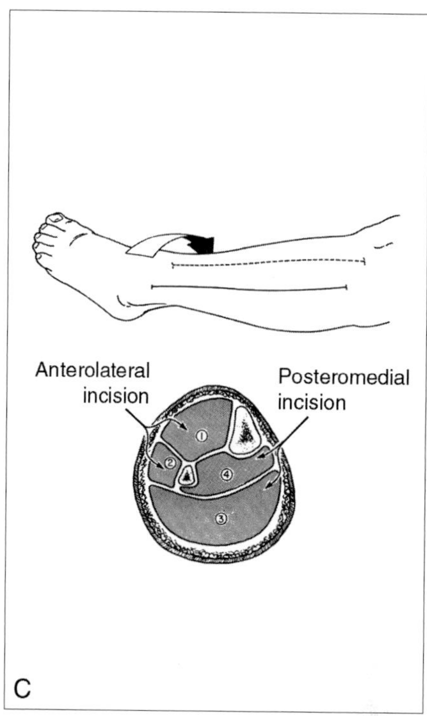

Figure 6 **A,** A lateral radiograph showing a closed fracture of the proximal third of the tibia and fibula, the only injury in a 7-year-old boy who was struck by an automobile while riding his bicycle. The child was in severe pain and unable to cooperate with sensorimotor testing. His calf was tense and painful to touch. The pain was aggravated by passive dorsiflexion and plantar flexion of his toes and foot. Because of the clinical findings, the patient was taken to the operating room where compartment pressures were measured at 65 mm Hg in the deep posterior compartment, an indicator of compartment syndrome based on an algorithm for diagnosing and treating this condition (**B**). Emergency fasciotomies of the leg were performed through medial and lateral incisions (**C**).

Complications

Cold claudication, which manifests in some children as skin mottling or pain when exposed to low temperatures, is a potential complication of a brachial artery injury with little clinical disability. Compartment syndrome, Volkmann contracture of the forearm, and limb loss are other complications of missed or untreated vascular injury associated with a displaced supracondylar fracture.

Compartment Syndrome

Compartment syndrome is a symptom complex caused by elevated pressure of tissue fluid in an enclosed osseofascial compartment of the limb that interferes with circulation to the muscles and nerves of that compartment.[34] This condition is uncommon in children but can result from several etiologies, including fractures (**Figure 6, A**) and crush injuries of the extremities, postoperative swelling from osteotomies and other procedures, constrictive casts or splints, burns, extravasation of fluid from intravenous line infiltration, infections, and insect or snake bites. The most common sites are the leg and forearm, in association with tibial shaft and supracondylar humeral fractures, respectively.[35] Because the examination of children, especially, younger nonverbal or uncooperative children, is difficult, the classic findings of compartment syndrome in adults are not readily detectable. Escalating pain is perhaps the most reliable sign of an evolving compartment syndrome in children.[36]

Patient Assessment

The classic findings of compartment syndrome should be carefully determined. Severe pain despite adequate splinting and analgesia is the most important early clinical sign. The calf or forearm and the distal extremity appear swollen, with the soft-tissue compartments tense and tender when palpated. Passive stretching of muscles within the swollen compartment(s) elicits pain. Decreased sensation and weak or absent motor function in the limb are other important signs. In children, anxiety, pain, and difficulty understanding directions or commands makes sensorimotor assessment challenging and unreliable. Neurapraxia associated with the injury also makes the function of a particular nerve impossible to use as a guide to the development of compartment syndrome. It should also be remembered that distal perfusion is often preserved in patients with compartment syndrome; pulselessness is a late manifestation of the condition. The measurement of compartment pressures is useful for diagnosing compartment syndrome but is painful and technically difficult in a small limb. Intracompartmental pressures greater than 30 mm Hg or within 30 mm Hg of the child's diastolic pressure (delta $P < 30$) is indicative of the diagnosis (**Figure 6, B**). A review of the nursing record of narcotic administration that shows an increasing need for analgesia is the most valuable evidence of compartment syndrome.

Surgical Considerations

If compartment syndrome is suspected, confirmation of intracompartmental pressures in the operating room is sometimes helpful. Emergency release of the compartments should be done in all patients with suspected compartment syndrome regardless of the measurements. For the traumatically injured leg, decompression of all four compartments through a two-incision approach is recommended, even if all compartments do not show evidence of elevated pressures (**Figure 6, C**). In the forearm, volar decompression alone may be adequate based on the examination and pressure measurements.

The lower leg is the most common site for fasciotomies. A longitudinal lateral incision is made over the posterior third of the anterior compartment and is extended proximally and distally to allow decompression of the entire compartment. In the distal third of the incision, the superficial peroneal nerve under the fascia must be identified to avoid cutting it. Through the same incision, the lateral compartment is identified posterior to the intermuscular septum and decompressed in a similar fashion. A medial incision is then made behind the palpable posterior edge of the tibia, and a fasciotomy of the superficial posterior compartment is performed. The soleus muscle is then taken down from the posterior tibial shaft in its distal third, allowing exposure of the fascia of the deep posterior compartment. This compartment is incised and decompressed along its length.

After decompression, any associated fracture is reduced and stabilized, either with a splint or, more commonly, with fixation. Tibial fractures may be treated either with flexible nails or external fixation. The compartments are left open and dressed, or a vacuum-assisted closure system is applied. The wounds are closed on a delayed primary basis at 36 to 48 hours if possible. Skin grafting is usually unnecessary.

Complications

Splinting of the extremity after surgery and early initiation of physical therapy may prevent soft-tissue contractures and stiffness. The worst complication is a failure to recognize the diagnosis. Compartment release within 12 to 24 hours of injury, and sometimes even later if the evolution of symptoms was gradual, often results in satisfactory outcomes. Compartment release more than 72 hours after onset is not recommended because of the risk of infection.

The Polytraumatized Child

Blunt trauma is the result of high-energy injuries, such as a motor vehicle crash or fall from a height, and is the leading cause of death in children.[36] Although head injuries account for more than 80% of these deaths, injuries to the abdominal viscera, the thorax, and fractures (particularly of the pelvis and the femur) contribute to the morbidity associated with blunt trauma.[37-40] Unlike adults, children rarely have associated comorbidities, such as cardiopulmonary disease, and are better able to tolerate hypovolemia.[41] Careful surveillance for associated injuries, which are sometimes occult, and a systematic plan of resuscitation are critical in managing a child with long-bone fractures from high-energy trauma.

Early definitive orthopaedic management of polytraumatized patients had been advocated throughout the 1980s.[42] A paradigm shift occurred in the early 1990s when some centers used the principles of damage control orthopaedics (DCO) for the most severely injured patients.[43,44] With this approach, external fixation and splinting are emergently applied to provisionally stabilize fractures, allowing the patient's cardiopulmonary resuscitation to be completed and the patient's overall condition to stabilize.[45,46] Definitive orthopaedic surgery, such as intramedullary fixation and open reduction and fixation, proceeds after a recovery period, usually within 5 to 10 days of the initial injury. Advocates of DCO hypothesize that this delay reduces the physiologic stress of prolonged orthopaedic surgery immediately after the initial injury (the second hit), resulting in fewer complications related to inflammatory mediators, such as acute respiratory stress syndrome and multiorgan system failure.

Although not studied in children, the principles of DCO are applicable in many pediatric orthopaedic polytrauma patients (**Figure 7**). At Saint Christopher's Hospital for Children in Philadelphia, a child with a severe head injury whose intracranial pressures are more than 30 mm Hg or uncontrolled medically is best managed in a delayed fashion, with splint immobilization or skin traction for fractures that are not life- or limb-threatening; other indications for following DCO principles in children include hypothermia (core

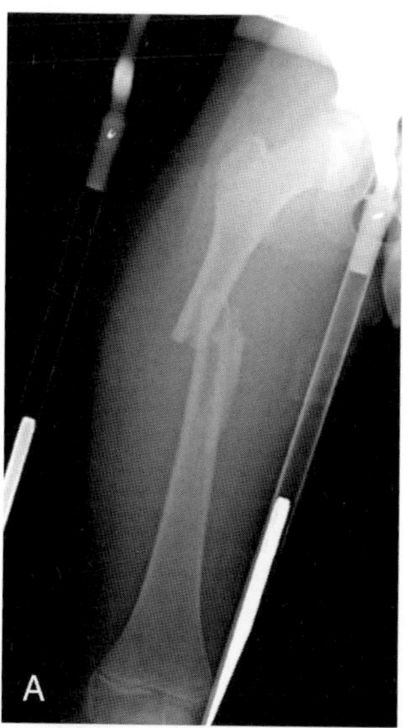

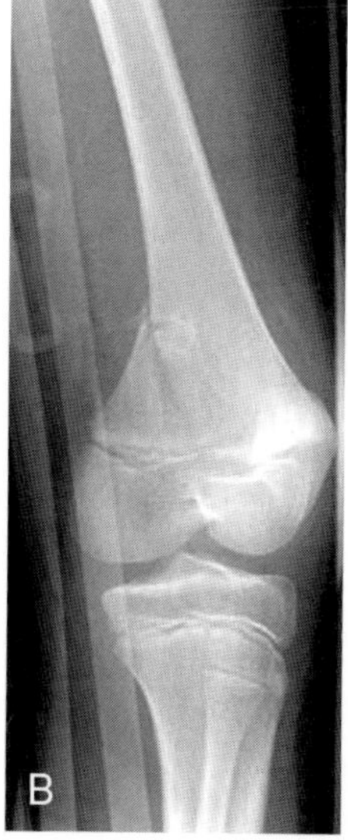

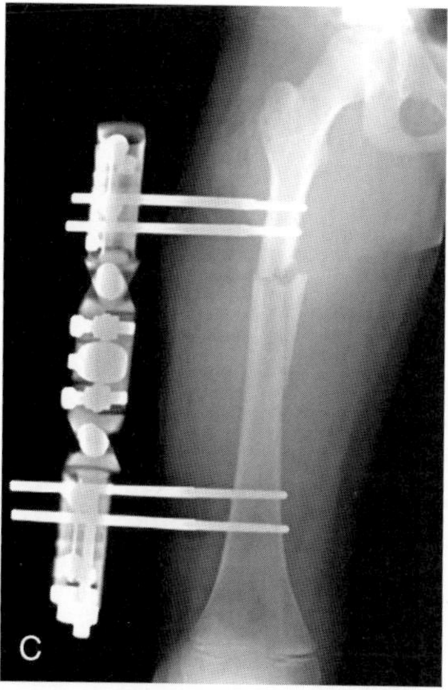

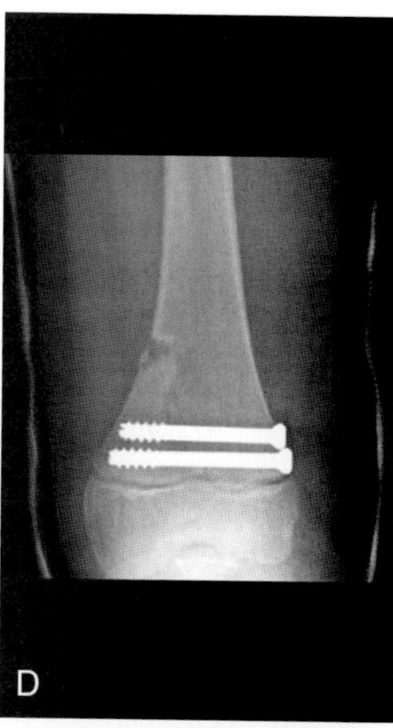

Figure 7 **A** through **D**, Imaging studies of a 12-year-old boy who was struck by a truck while riding his bicycle. He sustained a closed head injury, a type III supracondylar humeral fracture, a right comminuted femoral shaft fracture (**A**), and a displaced distal left femoral physeal fracture (**B**). On the night of admission, an intracranial pressure monitor was placed, and the elbow fracture was treated with closed reduction and percutaneous pinning. His intracranial pressure was 40 mm Hg. Two days later, when his intracranial pressure returned to normal, the patient was cleared for return to the operating room for external fixation of his right femoral shaft fracture (**C**) and closed reduction and percutaneous screw fixation of his left distal femoral fracture (**D**).

temperature less than 35.5°), coagulopathy (elevations of prothrombin time or partial thromboplastin time or diminished platelets) or metabolic acidosis (pH < 7.2) after initial resuscitation. Although early fracture fixation may reduce the length of the hospital stay for some children, delayed treatment, usually within 2 to 6 days of injury, rarely has a detrimental effect on the long-term outcome.[47]

Patient Assessment

Obtaining the patient's history, particularly the details about the mechanism of injury and preexisting medical conditions, is the necessary starting point that often sets in motion the appropriate trauma team response. Initial treatment in the trauma room focuses on airway management and cardiopulmonary resuscitation, followed by the primary clinical survey for head, thoracoabdominal, and obvious musculoskeletal injuries. The orthopaedic surgeon should identify the most severe injuries, such as a spinal injury, a dysvascular or mangled limb, or an unstable pelvic fracture,[48] which require early treatment. Applying a cervical collar, taking log-roll precautions, dressing severe open wounds, grossly realigning and splinting fractures, and placing a pelvic binder should be done in the trauma room when indicated.

During initial cardiopulmonary stabilization, plain radiographs of the chest, spine, pelvis, and obvious fractures are obtained as indicated. After initially stabilizing the patient, CT with rapid-sequencing techniques is often the best method for evaluating head and thoracoabdominal injuries as well as spinal and pelvic pathology. A complete secondary orthopaedic survey is done after secondary imaging and ideally before emergency surgical treatment.

Surgical Considerations

After a careful and thorough review of the physical findings and imaging studies, emergency management demands a team approach. The trauma/general surgeon, the orthopaedic surgeon, the neurosurgeon, and the anesthesiologist must identify the injuries that require immediate treatment and should frankly discuss the surgical time needed and the potential blood loss for any proposed procedures. Injuries that may require immediate orthopaedic treatment include compartment syndromes, mangled or dysvascular limbs, severe soft-tissue injuries, incomplete spinal cord injuries associated with a spinal column fracture, and unstable pelvic ring injuries that are unresponsive to pelvic binding or embolization.

Emergency surgery planning begins with careful equipment selection. The patient is best positioned on a radiolucent table or a fracture table that allows fluoroscopic access to all involved limbs. For fracture fixation, either titanium elastic nails or external fixation may be applied rapidly with limited

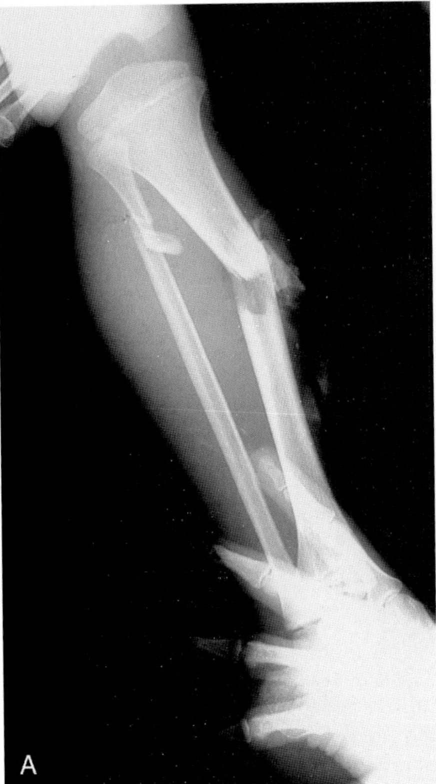

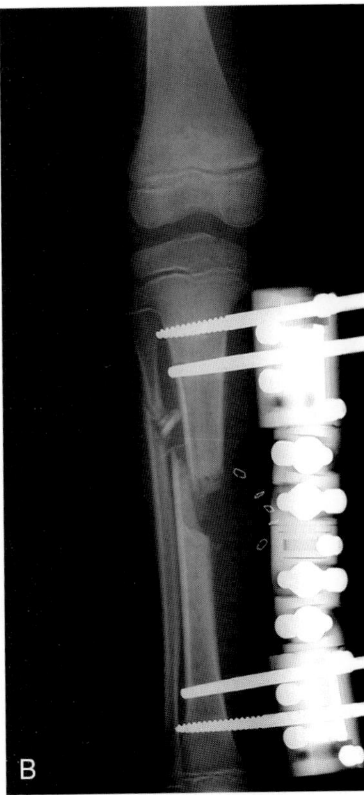

Figure 8 **A,** AP radiograph of the tibia of a 6-year-old boy who was struck by a motor vehicle while walking. An isolated grade IIIB open tibial-fibular fracture is seen. The neurovascular status of the limb was normal. The patient was treated with emergency irrigation and débridement and external fixation (**B**) of the comminuted diaphyseal tibial fracture.

exposure in many cases. Smooth wires placed percutaneously are best for stabilizing periarticular or physeal fractures and may also be used to stabilize some diaphyseal and metaphyseal fractures in younger children. High-volume, low-flow irrigation is recommended for cleaning contaminated wounds. Screw and/or plate fixation and reamed intramedullary nailing systems are sometimes used in the emergency operating room; however, because of the prolonged surgical time and exposure needed for these techniques, it is preferable to provide such definitive treatment after the patient's condition has improved. Emergency surgical care of the polytraumatized child must ultimately be individualized and practical. With the early and carefully use of DCO, late definitive management can be achieved without increasing complications.

Complications

Emergency care of the polytraumatized child is critical to survival, but ensuring good long-term outcomes and return of normal function requires vigilance in the immediate postinjury period. In the days following the trauma, the child must be reassessed for missed musculoskeletal and other injuries. Because of the capacity of children to heal, the orthopaedic surgeon must make the best effort to diagnose and appropriately manage all injuries regardless of the graveness of the child's injuries. Delayed or missed diagnoses of injuries or suboptimal management of fractures contribute to the likelihood of long-term disabilities in the polytraumatized child. If DCO was used, the surgeon must make plans with the care team for return to the operating room for definitive treatment of injuries.

The polytraumatized child is frequently treated within days of injury by an orthopaedic surgical team. Serious complications related to orthopaedic injuries include the development of compartment syndrome and skin breakdown under casts or splints, conditions that are particularly difficult to identify in the child with a severe head injury.[49] The orthopaedic team must also be mindful of potential medical complications, including fat emboli syndrome, pneumonia, urinary tract infection, and, uncommonly, deep venous thrombosis in older children. Because deep venous thrombosis is exceedingly uncommon in children, prophylaxis is rarely indicated. Early mobilization with physical therapy in the hospital and placement in specialized rehabilitation facilities on discharge may also speed recovery. Careful follow-up for months to years after injury is necessary to identify late complications, such as late infections, joint stiffness, heterotopic ossification, growth disturbance, and spasticity after head injury.

Open Tibial Fractures

Tibial shaft fractures in children are mostly closed injuries that result from low-energy mechanisms, such as sports injuries or falls, and are best managed by fracture reduction and cast immobilization.[50] Open tibial fractures are rare, comprising only 2% to 3% of all tibial fractures in children.[51] Because these injuries result from high-energy mechanisms, such as motor vehicle crashes, the child with a severe, open tibial fracture must be thoroughly assessed for associated injuries (**Figure 8**). The principles of treating open tibial fractures in children do not significantly differ from those used in adults. Although the outcomes of severe open tibial fractures in children are generally better than those in adults, serious complications can occur and must be treated appropriately to ensure healing and recovery of function.

Table 4
Recommended Antibiotic and Tetanus Prophylaxis for Open Fractures

Cefazolin (100 mg/kg/day divided into doses given every 8 hours) for all grades of open fractures
Gentamicin (5 to 7.5 mg/kg/day divided into doses given every 8 hours) for all grade 2 and 3 open fractures
Penicillin (150,000 units/kg/day divided into doses given every 6 hours) for farm injuries and patients at risk for clostridium and anaerobes
Tetanus toxoid given if immunization record is unknown or the last booster immunization was given more than 5 years prior; also consider tetanus immune globulin for injuries of unknown status and high-risk injuries

Patient Assessment

The evaluation begins with a thorough head-to-toe examination for other injuries. Once cardiopulmonary assessment and stabilization are achieved, the vascular status of the fractured limb is determined by assessing distal pulses and the capillary refill of the toes. The open wound is inspected for bleeding, skin and muscle laceration or defects, bone exposure, and gross contamination. The Gustilo and Anderson open fracture system is useful in evaluating open fractures in children. Particularly in a small limb, absolute wound size is not as important a factor in type assignment as the condition of the soft tissues and the degree of periosteal stripping. In the awake patient, distal motor and sensory function is determined, and the compartments are evaluated for swelling and tenderness. After the examination is completed, the wound is covered with a sterile dressing, and the limb is grossly realigned and splinted. A complete radiographic evaluation of the tibia should be done. Radiographs of the ipsilateral femur, ankle, and foot are obtained as clinically indicated to complete the evaluation.

The administration of antibiotics in the emergency department combined with a thorough irrigation and débridement in the operating room within 24 hours of injury is the best way to minimize the risk of infection in open fractures in children.[52] Immediately after the assessment, the child with an open tibial fracture is treated with intravenous antibiotics and the appropriate tetanus prophylaxis (**Table 4**). Definitive plans for patient management, based on the child's overall condition and the severity of the limb injury, are made in consultation with the trauma team. The decision to perform emergent care or to delay surgical treatment to the next day (but within 24 hours of injury) is based on the vascular status of the limb and the severity of the wound.

Surgical Considerations

The patient is positioned on a radiolucent operating table that allows access to the limb for fluoroscopic imaging, and a tourniquet is placed on the proximal thigh. Equipment is needed to perform both a thorough irrigation and débridement of the wound and fracture stabilization. Bulb irrigation is safest for cleansing small wounds, eliminating the risk of high-pressure extravasation of saline into fixed tissue compartments. Pulse-lavage systems, however, are best for treating large or grossly contaminated wounds. Although cast immobilization may be used for some open fractures with small wounds, this chapter's authors believe that surgical stabilization is indicated for most open tibial fractures in children that remain unstable after reduction. Flexible titanium nails and external fixation are most commonly used to stabilize these injuries. A vascular surgeon should be available if vascular injury is suspected.

Irrigation and débridement is performed to remove all debris introduced into the wound as well as devitalized soft tissue and bone. To accomplish this, extension of the open wound is always necessary to allow adequate exposure of both ends of the fracture site and the zone of soft-tissue injury. Devitalized tissue and circumferentially stripped fragments of cortical bone are débrided. Tissue of questionable viability, particularly large soft-tissue flaps, should be preserved when possible, especially during the initial washout. If the lower leg compartments are severely swollen or tense, intracompartmental pressure measurements can be obtained to assist the surgeon in assessing the need for four-compartment fasciotomies.

Flexible titanium nail stabilization has become a frequently used technique for children with noncomminuted (length-stable) diaphyseal tibial fractures with an open tibial tubercle.[53] Introduced through medial and lateral proximal metaphyseal drill holes placed just posterior to the tibial tubercle and approximately 2 cm distal to the physis, two intramedullary nails of the same diameter are passed anterograde across the fracture site into the distal metaphysis. For most fractures in children, nails measuring 3.0 to 4.0 mm in diameter, ideally filling together 80% of the canal at the isthmus, are adequate. The nails may be prebent to promote maximal separation at the fracture site and three-point contact within the bone, which are the keys to stable fixation with flexible nails. Supplemental splint or cast immobilization is frequently used, particularly immediately after surgery, to control rotation and for comfort. Fixation with flexible nails is indicated for children and adolescents with open physes. Locked nails are best used for tibial fractures in skeletally mature patients.

External fixation remains the most versatile option and, for many orthopaedic surgeons, the most familiar one. A simple monolateral frame secured with four to six cortical screws is effective for stabilizing most diaphyseal fracture patterns in children of all ages. The bone screw size varies from 3.5 to 4.5 mm, depending on the diameter of the bone. The best indications for external fixation are fractures with severe comminution (length-unstable patterns), those with segmental bone loss, and those with extensive soft-tissue damage or loss.[54] External fixation, however, is more painful for children compared with fixation with flexible titanium nails and may compromise soft-tissue reconstructive options, such as flaps.[55] It is also associated with other complications, including infection at the pin sites and refractures after removal, a risk that may be diminished by frame dynamization and early protection during weight bearing. Other options for tibial stabilization include smooth wire fixation for younger children and reamed, locked intramedullary nail fixation in skeletally mature older children and adolescents.[56]

Complications

In the immediate postoperative period, the child must be carefully monitored for the development of compartment syndrome. A 48-hour course of intravenous antibiotics is routinely prescribed after injury. For children with severe soft-tissue damage, repeat irrigation and débridement at 2- to 3-day intervals may be necessary to ensure that all devitalized tissue is removed and to diminish the risk of infection. The initial application of vacuum-assisted closure systems (often coupled with delayed primary wound closure) and flap coverage are options for soft-tissue management in children.[57] Because loss of reduction can occur after stabilization with both flexible titanium nails and external fixation, radiographs are routinely done at weekly intervals for several weeks after injury. Late complications of open tibial fractures include osteomyelitis, delayed union, and nonunion.

Septic Arthritis of the Hip

In the age of antibiotics, the focus in treating septic arthritis of the hip shifted from the preservation of life to the preservation of normal growth and function of the hip joint. Septic arthritis of the hip occurs most commonly in the first decade of life and is more common in males. Although a primary source of infection is infrequently identified, it is believed that hematogenous spread of intra-articular bacteremia to the joint synovium is the primary method of infection in patients in this age group. Educational efforts by primary care providers have led to increased awareness of the serious clinical consequences of late diagnosis of this condition and have resulted in earlier diagnosis and intervention.

Patient Assessment

The child with septic arthritis of the hip typically presents with fever; an insidious history of limping or inability to bear weight; and limited, painful range of motion of the hip joint (**Figure 9**). In nonambulatory infants, the diagnosis may be delayed because of less acute expression of clinical symptoms and signs as well as equivocal laboratory studies. This is especially true in the neonate who may show no signs of sepsis besides anorexia. The classic signs of septic arthritis of the hip that involve flexion, abduction, and external rotation of the hip with marked swelling of the thigh are late findings and are often associated with significant sequelae. The physical examination includes evaluation of the abdomen and pelvis; assessment of range of motion of the hip, knee, and ankle; and palpation of the entire limb for tenderness of the long bones and the presence of joint effusions in the knee or ankle.

Early in the clinical presentation of septic arthritis, the differential diagnosis is broad and includes toxic synovitis, rheumatologic synovitis of the hip, Lyme disease, osteomyelitis of the proximal femur or pelvis, septic arthritis of the sacroiliac joint, vertebral osteomyelitis, psoas muscle or retroperitoneal abscesses, and abdominal or pelvic lymphadenitis and neoplasm (such as leukemia). Narrowing of the differential diagnoses is challenging but must be done expeditiously to avoid delaying urgent treatment of septic arthritis of the hip.

Diagnostic testing includes radiographs of the pelvis and femur to identify fractures, bone lesions or periosteal reaction indicative of osteomyelitis or tumor, and widening of the hip joint space suggestive of septic arthritis or other conditions associated with a joint effusion.[58] When initial laboratory tests, such as white blood cell (WBC) count, erythrocyte sedimentation rate (ESR), and C-reactive protein (CRP), are obtained, blood cultures are also drawn to identify an organism before antibiotic treatment is started. When ultrasonography confirms the presence of fluid within the joint, aspiration of the hip joint is indicated to expedite the diagnosis of septic arthri-

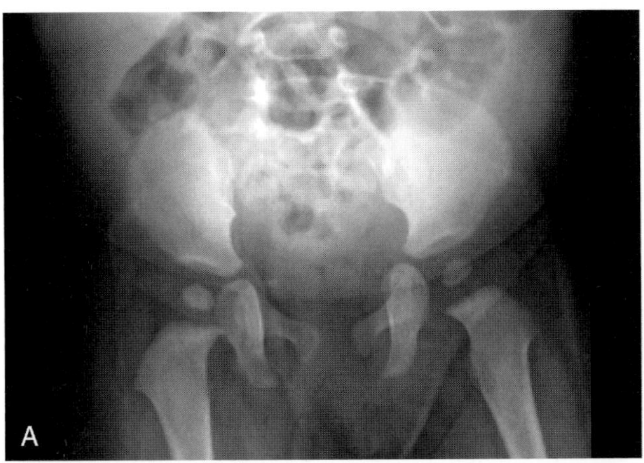

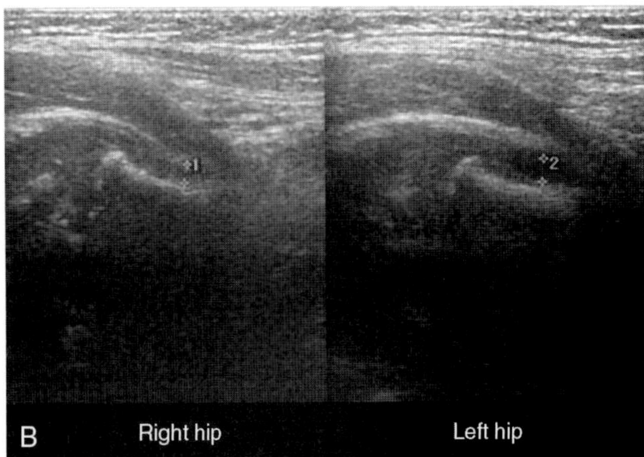

Figure 9 **A** and **B,** Radiograph and ultrasound from an 18-month-old girl who stopped walking. At presentation her temperature measured 102°, and she held her hip flexed and externally rotated. WBC count was normal, ESR was 50 mm/hour, and C–reactive protein (CRP) was 4 mg/L. **A,** AP radiograph of the hips and pelvis was unremarkable. **B,** Ultrasound evaluation of the hips showed a significant increase in intracapsular distance in the involved hip. The hip was aspirated, and the 3 mL of cloudy fluid was analyzed; the Gram stain was negative but 80,000/µL WBCs were identified. The child was diagnosed with septic arthritis of the hip and urgently treated in the operating room with incision and drainage of the hip through an anterior hip approach.

tis.[59,60] In addition to providing an important source for bacterial culture and sensitivity, the gross appearance and analysis of the fluid, including cell count and Gram stain, provide important clues to the diagnosis. When a definite diagnosis of septic arthritis of the hip cannot be made with initial studies, Lyme titers, rheumatologic studies, and MRI of the pelvis and femur to rule out inflammatory disease, osteomyelitis, myositis, or abscess formation are helpful in clarifying the diagnosis.

Toxic synovitis of the hip is the most common condition in the differential diagnosis of hip inflammation. The child with toxic synovitis typically presents with a limp for several days, is less ill appearing than the child with septic arthritis, and exhibits only minimal limitation of hip motion. Medical history will often reveal a recent viral infection. Radiographs of the hip and pelvis and laboratory studies are usually normal or show mild elevations of WBC, ESR, and CRP. Ultrasound evaluation of the hip will show a small amount of intracapsular fluid.

Differentiating early septic arthritis of the hip from toxic synovitis is sometimes difficult. The child who is unable to bear weight on the affected limb, has a temperature higher than 38.5°C, a WBC greater than 12,000/µL, an ESR greater than 40 mm/hour, and a CRP greater than 2.0 mg/L has a high likelihood of septic arthritis.[61,62] Aspiration of the hip joint is indicated to confirm the diagnosis. Cloudy or purulent fluid with more than 50,000/µL WBCs composed of greater than 75% polymorphonuclear cells or a positive Gram stain of the aspirate are diagnostic findings for septic arthritis.

Surgical Considerations

Once the diagnosis of septic arthritis of the hip is made, urgent surgical drainage of the hip is indicated. Although there are multiple approaches to the hip joint, the anterior (Smith-Peterson) approach is most commonly used. The child is positioned supine with a small bolster placed under the involved hip, and the entire limb is prepped and draped free. A 4-cm obliquely oriented skin incision is made in line with the inguinal ligament and 2 cm below the anterosuperior iliac spine. The superficial fascia is incised, and the interval between the tensor fascia lata and the sartorius muscles is identified. The lateral femoral cutaneous nerve is often seen in the field and can be retracted. The lateral border of the rectus femoris is then identified and retracted medially, revealing the anterior capsule of the hip joint. Excision of a 1-cm square area of capsule, as opposed to incision alone, is recommended to ensure continued drainage from the joint. After obtaining cultures from the hip joint, it is irrigated with saline infused through a large intravenous or small rubber catheter until the joint is clear of debris. A drain, usually a 0.25-inch diameter Penrose drain, is placed in the joint and secured to the capsular edge or deep fascia with absorbable sutures. The skin incision is loosely closed around the drain, and a dressing is applied. The drain is later pulled approximately 48 hours postoperatively. Postoperative immobilization or traction is

Table 5
Most Common Causative Organisms for Septic Arthritis in Children by Age

Age of Child	Organisms
Age < 3 months	*Staphylococcus aureus* Group B streptococcus Gram-negative bacilli
Age 3 months to 5 years	*S aureus* Group A streptococcus *Streptococcus pneumoniae* *Haemophilus influenzae* *Kingella kingae*
Age ≥ 5 years	*S aureus* Group A streptococcus *S pneumoniae*

Table 6
Empiric Antibiotic Choices for Septic Arthritis by Age at Saint Christopher's Hospital for Children

Age < 3 months	Nafcillin + gentamicin[a]
Age 3 months to 5 years	Ampicillin-sulbactam + clindamycin[b]
Age ≥ 5 years	Nafcillin + clindamycin[a]

[a]Substitute vancomycin for nafcillin (Note: Clindamycin is contraindicated in infants younger than 3 months.)
[b]Add vancomycin if concomitant staph-like skin or soft-tissue infection, history of methicillin-resistant *S aureus*, toxic or septic clinical appearance

unnecessary, and active motion of the hip joint is encouraged. Following surgical drainage of the hip, osteomyelitis of the proximal femur is ruled out by MRI evaluation.

Arthroscopic drainage and irrigation is effective but is best reserved for older children and adolescents. Drainage of the hip joint by serial aspiration is not an acceptable method of treatment. This technique involves repeated daily aspiration of the hip joint, which results in increased pain and anxiety for the patient; additionally, the surgeon is not able to fully examine, decompress, and irrigate the joint.

Immediately after surgery, intravenous antibiotics are administered. Empiric drug choices are based on the age of the child, the most likely causative organisms (**Table 5**), and the known resistance patterns of organisms in the treating institution or local community. The antibiotic recommendations shown in **Table 6** are based on the 2008 practices at Saint Christopher's Hospital for Children in Philadelphia. For septic arthritis without osteomyelitis, a 3-week course of antibiotics (initially given intravenously and then orally if possible based on the organism's susceptibility and patient compliance) is adequate therapy.[63] When coexistent osteomyelitis of the proximal femur is documented, intravenous antibiotics for a 4- to 6-week duration is indicated. This regimen necessitates placing a peripherally inserted central catheter.

Complications

Rapid improvements in the clinical state and laboratory studies, especially the CRP, are usually noted within 36 hours of drainage. If symptoms and laboratory studies do not progressively improve, other sources of infection, the possibility of inadequate surgical drainage of the hip joint, or the choice of an ineffective antibiotic regimen must be considered.

Although most children with septic arthritis of the hip who are diagnosed early and treated appropriately have no complications, poor outcomes may occur and have been correlated with patient age younger than 6 months at the time of diagnosis, a delay in treatment longer than 72 hours, inadequate irrigation and drainage, inappropriate antibiotic therapy, concomitant osteomyelitis of the proximal femur, and septic dislocation of the hip.[64] These poor outcomes most commonly result from articular and physeal cartilage injuries. The growing hip joint will sustain direct cartilage injury from bacterial enzymes and the patient's own inflammatory cascade as well as vascular insult caused by prolonged increased intracapsular pressure and vessel thrombosis from septic emboli. Joint stiffness and chondrolysis, osteonecrosis of the femoral head, partial or complete early closure of the physis of the proximal femur and of the triradiate cartilage, limb-length discrepancy, acetabular insufficiency, dissolution of the femoral neck with pseudarthrosis formation, and complete destruction of the femoral head and neck are potential complications.[65-67]

Necrotizing Fasciitis

Necrotizing fasciitis is an insidious and life-threatening condition that occurs in both children and adults. The hallmark of the clinical disease is necrosis of muscle fascia, often with concomitant cellulitis, myositis, or osteomyelitis, caused by a bacterial infection, most commonly *Streptococcus* or *Staphylococcus* species, which spreads along fascial planes.[68] Although uncommon, approximately 1,500 cases per year are reported in the United States; the mortality rate for the pediatric population is 5% and 20% in the adult population.[69] Necrotizing fasciitis results from the release of superantigens, which have now been associated with more than 40 different bacteria that infect humans.[70] Superantigens are powerful T cell mitogens that initiate the release of massive amounts of cytokines, such as tumor necrosis factor-α, interleukin-β, and T cell mediators. The toxic release results in a rapidly progressing inflammatory state in skin, muscle, fascia, and/or bone that is reflected clinically by the rapid onset of pain in the involved extremity as well as systemic signs and symptoms of sepsis. Aggressive treatment is necessary to limit disability and, in some cases, save the life of the child.

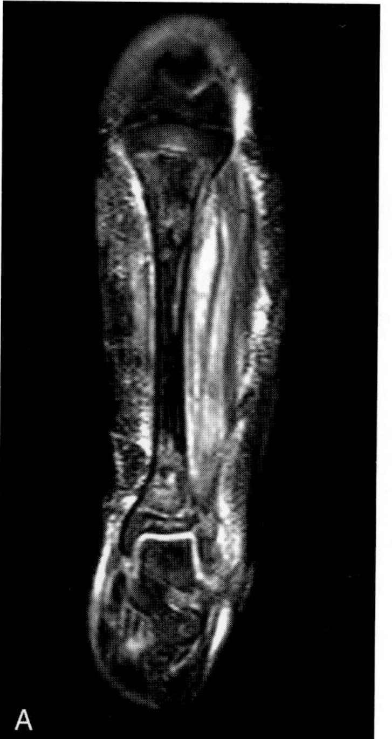

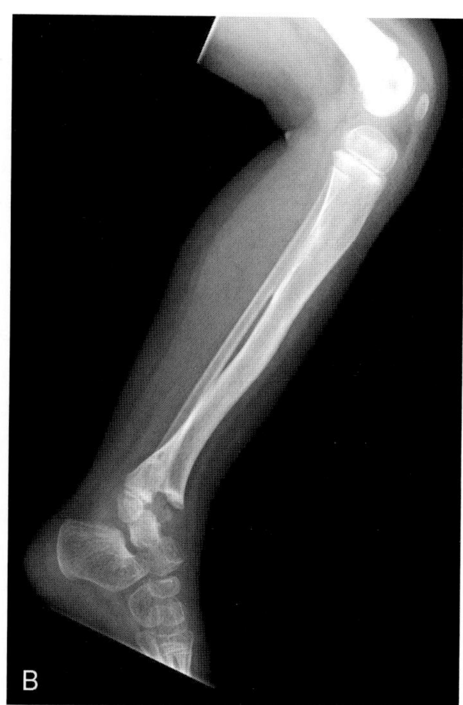

Figure 10 **A** and **B**, Imaging studies of a 4-year-old girl who presented for treatment with limping and a 2-day fever. The patient was lethargic with a temperature of 102.3° and labile blood pressure. Her lower leg was severely swollen and circumferentially tender. Her ESR was 60 mm/hour, CRP was 6.5 mg/L, and WBC was 15,000/µL. Initial radiographs were normal. **A,** MRI was consistent with cellulitis circumferentially. Myositis is evident within the muscles of the calf. The fascia was bright on T2 imaging, a finding suspicious for fasciitis. The patient was treated with emergency fasciotomies with subtotal fasciectomies of the leg. The patient remained in the intensive care unit for 1 week, had three subsequent irrigations and débridements before wound closure, and received a prolonged course of antibiotic therapy. **B,** A radiograph of the lower leg at 9-month follow-up showed sequelae of osteomyelitis of the tibia with injury to the distal tibial physis and the talus.

Patient Assessment

The diagnosis of necrotizing fasciitis requires a high index of suspicion. There is usually no history of antecedent trauma or infections in children with necrotizing fasciitis, but immunologic incompetence and generalized metabolic disorders have been associated with the diagnosis in adult patients. The child typically presents with mild swelling of a portion of the upper or lower extremity or an insidious onset of limp (**Figure 10**). Early in the course of the disease, few systemic findings are apparent. Necrotizing fasciitis often is diagnosed initially as cellulitis by the primary care clinician. Within a short period of time, usually less than 48 hours, fever develops and pain and swelling are markedly increased. The physical examination is notable for local tenderness to palpation and tense edema beyond the initial area of swelling and pain. As the process evolves, the apparent cellulitis worsens with the development of more extensive erythema, skin blisters, and bullae. Circumferential limb swelling develops, and distal limb perfusion may be compromised as evidenced by diminished capillary refill and pulses. The patient may appear diaphoretic, pale, and anxious. A critical part of evaluating a child with suspected necrotizing fasciitis is assessing vital signs. Tachycardia and hypotension are indicators of evolving sepsis and support the diagnosis of necrotizing fasciitis.[71]

When necrotizing fasciitis is considered in a differential diagnosis, the patient should be immediately admitted to an intensive care unit. After laboratory studies and blood cultures are urgently obtained, the patient is prepared for anesthesia with physiologic support and broad spectrum intravenous antibiotics. In advanced cases, pressors may be necessary to ensure adequate limb perfusion. Radiographic imaging of the involved limb may be helpful. In an effort to treat patients expeditiously, limited MRI evaluation of the involved limb is extremely helpful and is obtained on an emergent basis.

The differential diagnoses include cellulitis, myositis, muscle abscess, and osteomyelitis. Evaluating MRI studies is most helpful in differentiating these entities and will result in meaningful treatment recommendations. Cellulitis typically is diagnosed by identifying edema of subcutaneous fat only. When subcutaneous fat and fascial planes show significant involvement on T2-weighted MRIs, necrotizing fasciitis must be ruled out. The presence of subcutaneous gas is pathognomonic of fasciitis but is seen in only 34% to 67% of cases at later stages of the disease. MRI will identify myositis, abscess, and osteomyelitis more specifically. Although each condition may coexist with the others, MRI is helpful in guiding nonsurgical medical treatment of cellulitis, myositis, and osteomyelitis in the early stages. MRI also aids in localizing abscesses to plan for surgical drainage.

Surgical Considerations

Once the diagnosis of necrotizing fasciitis is suspected or confirmed, emergent surgical intervention is indicated. When treatment has been delayed more than 24 hours after the onset of symptoms, the mortality rate will increase with increasing time to treatment. The goals of surgery are to débride necrotic tissue and decompress the soft tissues. Aggressive surgical débridement and extensile exposures are necessary to effectively treat this condition.[72]

In the lower limb, for example, midline medial and lateral longitudinal incisions are made in the skin, similar to those used to perform fasciotomies for compartment syndrome. The fascia is incised, and the underlying muscle and bone are inspected for evidence of necrotic muscle, abscesses, and osteomyelitis, with débridement performed as necessary. Dull, gray, or obviously necrotic fascia must be removed. In many instances, subtotal or total fasciectomy of the involved limb is necessary to control the infection. The exposure must be extended proximally or distally as necessary until normal tissue is identified. After débridement, the wound is cultured and the débrided tissue is sent for pathologic analysis. The wound is then irrigated copiously with saline, often with pulsatile lavage. Vacuum-assisted wound closure reduces swelling, promotes continuous drainage, and facilitates closure of these extensive wounds. Vacuum-assisted closure dressing change, repeat débridement, and wound irrigation are scheduled in the operating room every 48 to 72 hours until all necrotic tissue is removed and the infection is controlled. Secondary skin closure may then be performed.

Complications

Once the acute disease process has been successfully managed with a combination of intravenous antibiotics and surgery, the skeletally immature patient will require serial clinical and imaging follow-up until skeletal maturity to monitor alterations in growth. Even when early evaluations suggest that growth of the involved limb is proceeding at a normal rate, serial examinations throughout growth may detect a more insidious growth inhibition, a so-called sick physis, in which involved physes slowly halt normal growth when compared with the opposite, uninvolved limb. Complications that may result from necrotizing fasciitis include permanent loss of muscle tissue, physeal injury or destruction resulting in progressive limb deformity or length discrepancy, joint destruction, gangrene requiring amputation, and death.[73,74] Increased mortality is associated with inadequate surgical débridement, inappropriate antibiotics, chickenpox, and the extension of necrotizing fasciitis of the lower extremity to the abdomen or back.

Cervical Spine Injury

Acute cervical spine injuries in children younger than 15 years account for only 1.9% of all children and adolescents with cervical spine injuries.[75,76] In children younger than 8 years, most cervical spine injuries are the result of high-energy mechanisms, such as a motor vehicle crash, a fall, or child abuse; however, in the toddler such injuries can result from minor trauma.[77,78] Older children and adolescents are more likely to be injured during sports or recreational activities, such as diving. The injury severity is greater in younger patients than in adults, with an increased risk of permanent neurologic deficits and a higher mortality rate. Because the occurrence of cervical spine injury in children is uncommon, a higher index of suspicion for injury is required for early diagnosis and treatment. Children younger than 8 years most commonly sustain injuries to the upper cervical spine, whereas older children and adolescents are more likely to have injuries of the subaxial cervical spine.[79-81]

Patient Assessment

Evaluating a child with a sudden onset of neck pain requires a detailed history to determine the mechanism of injury as well as loss of consciousness, pain, paresthesias, weakness of the extremities, or sphincter dysfunction. For those who sustained injury as a result of a high-energy mechanism, cardiopulmonary stabilization and a primary assessment for associated head, thoracoabdominal, and pelvic injuries is performed emergently. The orthopaedic examination begins with a careful evaluation of the head and neck, noting skull or facial injuries and the position of the head, such as lateral tilting or rotation (**Figure 11**). The neck is palpated for local tenderness at the posterior midline of the cervical spine and spasm of the neck muscles. A thorough neurologic examination is mandatory for all patients with a suspected cervical spine injury. Sensory and motor testing and assessing reflexes is performed and carefully documented. A complete evaluation of the thoracolumbar spine, pelvis, and extremities to rule out other musculoskeletal injuries completes the examination.

After the evaluation, a cervical collar is applied. The child is also transported on a spine board with an occipital recess to accommodate the head or a board modified with pads or sheets that elevate the thorax while diagnostic testing is performed.[82] Radiographs and CT of the cervical spine, including coronal axial and reconstructed images, are routinely obtained in the emergency department. MRI may be performed to directly evaluate the neural axis if clinically indicated but is not typically a part of the initial workup.[83]

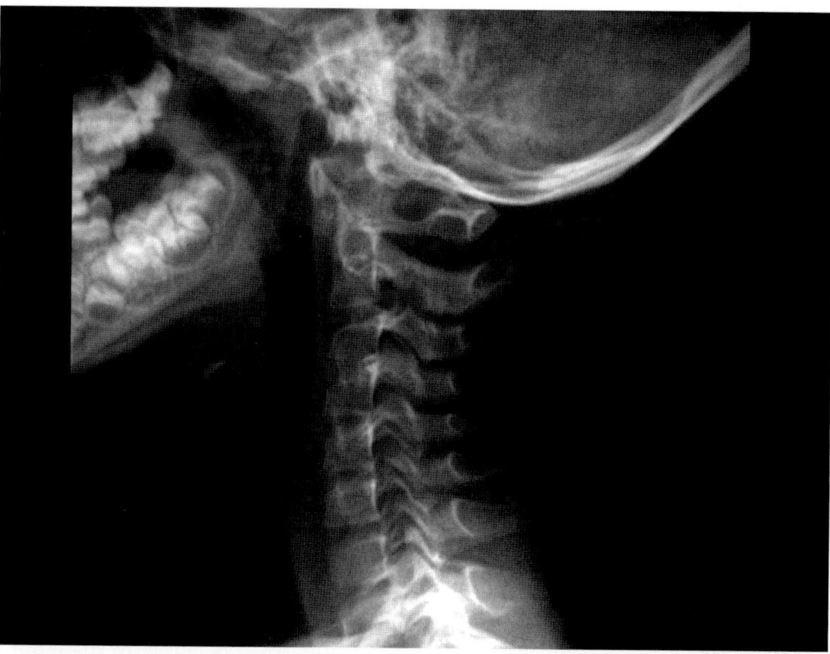

Figure 11 A lateral radiograph of the cervical spine of an 11-year-old boy who was injured while wrestling confirmed the suspected diagnosis of traumatic atlantoaxial rotatory instability. The patient was treated with head-halter traction for 3 days followed by immobilization in a Minerva cast for 8 weeks. At 3-month follow-up the flexion-extension radiographs were normal.

Treatment Considerations

The type of cervical spine injury and the neurologic status of the patient determine the type of treatment. Definitive treatment of cervical spine injuries can often be delayed unless incomplete neurologic injury has occurred that warrants emergent decompression and stabilization. This is an uncommon scenario in children. For patients with normal neurologic function, the emergency management goal for the surgeon is to stabilize the spinal column until delayed definitive treatment can be executed. For stable injuries, a well-fitted cervical collar is adequate for protection. For patients with instability or potential instability, such as traumatic atlantoaxial rotatory instability or fracture of the odontoid, more control of the cervical spine is necessary to prevent progressive injury.

Head-halter traction is a safe, noninvasive method of immobilizing the child's head and neck and is easily applied.[77] With the patient lying supine, traction is applied through a commercially available head-chin strap halter system that applies force to the head and neck in neutral alignment. Attention to detail is necessary to assure safe application. A small rolled towel is placed under the shoulders of children 8 years and younger to avoid forced flexion of the cervical spine imposed by their relatively large skulls.[82] The posterior pad of the halter cups the occiput while the anterior pad secures the mandible. The halter cords, which allow attachment to traction weights at the head of the bed, must not contact the ears because this is irritating to the patient. Placing marking tapes on the side rails of the hospital bed that indicate the patient's shoulder levels will alert all health providers to the proper alignment of the traction and the ideal position for the patient in bed. Elevation of the head of the bed by 20° will provide body weight countertraction and aid in maintaining the patient at the appropriate position in bed. In younger children, a Posey chest-abdominal restraint is necessary to maintain proper positioning in bed and to prevent sudden movements that could result in cervical spine or cord damage. When the upper cervical spine is involved, only 2 to 4 lb of traction are required. The child's neurologic status, including the cranial nerve motor and sensory examination, is monitored at 1-hour intervals while in traction. A clearly marked sign over the patient's bed stipulates that the traction must remain in place at all times, and any adjustments to the halter traction should be performed by the treating surgeon and staff.

Halo traction also can be used but is not usually required in younger patients. Tong traction is more appropriate for the adolescent patient. When halo traction is used in younger patients, the number of halo pins used and the torque applied will differ for varying age groups. In the toddler, 8 to 10 pins may be necessary. Loosening, skull penetration of thin bone, and local infection at the pin sites are possible complications.[84,85] In the child younger than 8 years, the benefits of halo traction are outweighed by the risks, especially when halter traction and Posey restraint have proved successful.

The patient with traumatic atlantoaxial rotatory instability is assessed on a frequent basis to determine improvement in head position, decreasing discomfort, and improved range of voluntary motion of the neck in lateral rotation. If atlantoaxial rotatory subluxation is not resolved within 24 hours, lateral cervical spine radiographs in traction are repeated to confirm the diagnosis and to more critically evaluate the position of the cervical spine. Once normal active lateral rotation of the neck is achieved, lateral radiographs of the cervical spine are repeated in traction. This will show normal rotational alignment of the atlas and the axis. If the atlanto-dens interval is normal, the patient can be treated in a halo vest or Minerva cast. CT is used to confirm cervical alignment after application of the halo vest or cast. After 6 to 8 weeks of immobilization, lateral radiographs of the cervical spine are repeated. If normal alignment has been maintained, the patient is weaned from immobilization to a cervical collar, and physical therapy is initiated for strengthening and range of motion. Subsequent active flexion-extension lateral radiographs of the cervical spine are performed to document stability. Recurrent subluxation or persistent atlantoaxial instability are treated with spinal fusion.[86-88]

Complications

Progression of neurologic injury is the most feared complication. A high index of suspicion for a potentially missed injury based on the patient's history and examination must be maintained. This is particularly important if the patient with a head injury is unable to cooperate with the neurologic examination. Repeat clinical assessment as the patient becomes more lucid and thorough imaging of the spinal column will reduce the incidence of missed injuries. Progression of neurologic injury in the child with an unstable cervical spine injury is a complication that is potentially preventable. Careful emergency spinal immobilization and close consultation with the surgeon or team that is to provide definitive care of the injury offers the best chance for a successful outcome.

Summary

The orthopaedic surgeon responsible for the care of pediatric orthopaedic conditions must be aware of the essential information needed to manage the most common emergencies. Combining the skill sets for evaluating and managing general orthopaedic patients with the basic knowledge presented in this chapter for evaluating and treating 10 common pediatric orthopaedic emergencies will assist orthopaedic surgeons who primarily treats adults to safely and effectively care for pediatric patients.

References

1. Gautier E, Ganz K, Krügel N, Gill T, Ganz R: Anatomy of the medial femoral circumflex artery and its surgical implications. *J Bone Joint Surg Br* 2000;82(5): 679-683.
2. Maeda S, Kita A, Funayama K, Kokubun S: Vascular supply to slipped capital femoral epiphysis. *J Pediatr Orthop* 2001;21(5): 664-667.
3. Herrera-Soto JA, Duffy MF, Birnbaum MA, Vander Have KL: Increased intracapsular pressures after unstable slipped capital femoral epiphysis. *J Pediatr Orthop* 2008;28(7):723-728.
4. Loder RT, Richards BS, Shapiro PS, Reznick LR, Aronson DD: Acute slipped capital femoral epiphysis: The importance of physeal stability. *J Bone Joint Surg Am* 1993;75(8): 1134-1140.
5. Loder RT, Wittenberg B, DeSilva G: Slipped capital femoral epiphysis associated with endocrine disorders. *J Pediatr Orthop* 1995;15(3):349-356.
6. Riad J, Bajelidze G, Gabos PG: Bilateral slipped capital femoral epiphysis: Predictive factors for contralateral slip. *J Pediatr Orthop* 2007;27(4):411-414.
7. Klug R, McCarthy JJ, Eilert RE: The use of a two C-arm technique in the treatment of slipped capital femoral epiphysis. *Orthopedics* 2004;27(10):1041-1042.
8. Aronson DD, Carlson WE: Slipped capital femoral epiphysis: A prospective study of fixation with a single screw. *J Bone Joint Surg Am* 1992;74(6):810-819.
9. Goodwin RC, Mahar AT, Oswald TS, Wenger DR: Screw head impingement after in situ fixation in moderate and severe slipped capital femoral epiphysis. *J Pediatr Orthop* 2007;27(3):319-325.
10. McCarthy JJ: The bull's eye view in slipped capital femoral epiphysis. *Orthopedics* 2008;31(2): 137-139.
11. Boyer DW, Mickelson MR, Ponseti IV: Slipped capital femoral epiphysis: Long-term follow-up study of one hundred and twenty-one patients. *J Bone Joint Surg Am* 1981;63(1):85-95.
12. Leunig M, Casillas MM, Hamlet M, et al: Slipped capital femoral epiphysis: Early mechanical damage to the acetabular cartilage by a prominent femoral metaphysis. *Acta Orthop Scand* 2000; 71(4):370-375.
13. Song HR, Myrboh V, Lee SH: Unstable slipped capital femoral epiphysis: Reduction by gradual distraction with external fixator. A case report. *J Pediatr Orthop B* 2005;14(6):426-428.

14. Ramachandran M, Ward K, Brown RR, Munns CF, Cowell CT, Little DG: Intravenous bisphosphonate therapy for traumatic osteonecrosis of the femoral head in adolescents. *J Bone Joint Surg Am* 2007;89(8):1727-1734.

15. Beaty JH: Fractures of the hip in children. *Orthop Clin North Am* 2006;37(2):223-232, vii.

16. Quick TJ, Eastwood DM: Pediatric fractures and dislocations of the hip and pelvis. *Clin Orthop Relat Res* 2005;432:87-96.

17. Shrader MW, Jacofsky DJ, Stans AA, Shaughnessy WJ, Haidukewych GJ: Femoral neck fractures in pediatric patients: 30 years experience at a level 1 trauma center. *Clin Orthop Relat Res* 2007;454:169-173.

18. Moon ES, Mehlman CT: Risk factors for avascular necrosis after femoral neck fractures in children: 25 Cincinnati cases and meta-analysis of 360 cases. *J Orthop Trauma* 2006;20(5):323-329.

19. Vialle R, Odent T, Pannier S, Pauthier F, Laumonier F, Glorion C: Traumatic hip dislocation in childhood. *J Pediatr Orthop* 2005;25(2):138-144.

20. Odent T, Glorion C, Pannier S, Bronfen C, Langlais J, Pouliquen JC: Traumatic dislocation of the hip with separation of the capital epiphysis: 5 adolescent patients with 3-9 years of follow-up. *Acta Orthop Scand* 2003; 74(1):49-52.

21. Mehlman CT, Hubbard GW, Crawford AH, Roy DR, Wall EJ: Traumatic hip dislocation in children. Long-term followup of 42 patients. *Clin Orthop Relat Res* 2000;376:68-79.

22. Shrader MW: Pediatric supracondylar fractures and pediatric physeal elbow fractures. *Orthop Clin North Am* 2008;39(2):163-171, v.

23. Mehlman CT, Strub WM, Roy DR, Wall EJ, Crawford AH: The effect of surgical timing on the perioperative complications of treatment of supracondylar humeral fractures in children. *J Bone Joint Surg Am* 2001;83-A(3): 323-327.

24. Alburger PD, Weidner PL, Betz RR: Supracondylar fractures of the humerus in children. *J Pediatr Orthop* 1992;12(1):16-19.

25. Green NE: Overnight delay in the reduction of supracondylar fractures of the humerus in children. *J Bone Joint Surg Am* 2001; 83-A(3):321-322.

26. Skaggs DL, Cluck MW, Mostofi A, Flynn JM, Kay RM: Lateral-entry pin fixation in the management of supracondylar fractures in children. *J Bone Joint Surg Am* 2004;86-A(4):702-707.

27. Green DW, Widmann RF, Frank JS, Gardner MJ: Low incidence of ulnar nerve injury with crossed pin placement for pediatric supracondylar humerus fractures using a mini-open technique. *J Orthop Trauma* 2005; 19(3):158-163.

28. Sankar WN, Hebela NM, Skaggs DL, Flynn JM: Loss of pin fixation in displaced supracondylar humeral fractures in children: Causes and prevention. *J Bone Joint Surg Am* 2007;89(4): 713-717.

29. Shaw BA, Kasser JR, Emans JB, Rand FF: Management of vascular injuries in displaced supracondylar humerus fractures without arteriography. *J Orthop Trauma* 1990;4(1):25-29.

30. Garbuz DS, Leitch K, Wright JG: The treatment of supracondylar fractures in children with an absent radial pulse. *J Pediatr Orthop* 1996;16(5):594-596.

31. Sabharwal S, Tredwell SJ, Beauchamp RD, et al: Management of pulseless pink hand in pediatric supracondylar fractures of humerus. *J Pediatr Orthop* 1997; 17(3):303-310.

32. Lipscomb PR, Burleson RJ: Vascular and neural complications in supracondylar fractures of the humerus in children. *J Bone Joint Surg Am* 1955;37-A(3):487-492.

33. Schoenecker PL, Delgado E, Rotman M, Sicard GA, Capelli AM: Pulseless arm in association with totally displaced supracondylar fracture. *J Orthop Trauma* 1996; 10(6):410-415.

34. Willis RB, Rorabeck CH: Treatment of compartment syndrome in children. *Orthop Clin North Am* 1990;21(2):401-412.

35. Bae DS, Kadiyala RK, Waters PM: Acute compartment syndrome in children: Contemporary diagnosis, treatment, and outcome. *J Pediatr Orthop* 2001; 21(5):680-688.

36. Buckley SL, Gotschall C, Robertson W Jr, et al: The relationships of skeletal injuries with trauma score, injury severity score, length of hospital stay, hospital charges, and mortality in children admitted to a regional pediatric trauma center. *J Pediatr Orthop* 1994; 14(4):449-453.

37. Jawadi AH, Letts M: Injuries associated with fracture of the femur secondary to motor vehicle accidents in children. *Am J Orthop (Belle Mead NJ)* 2003;32(9):459-462, discussion 462.

38. Letts M, Davidson D, Lapner P: Multiple trauma in children: Predicting outcome and long-term results. *Can J Surg* 2002;45(2): 126-131.

39. Sullivan T, Haider A, DiRusso SM, Nealon P, Shaukat A, Slim M: Prediction of mortality in pediatric trauma patients: New injury severity score outperforms injury severity score in the severely injured. *J Trauma* 2003;55(6): 1083-1087, discussion 1087-1088.

40. Yian EH, Gullahorn LJ, Loder RT: Scoring of pediatric orthopaedic polytrauma: Correlations of

different injury scoring systems and prognosis for hospital course. *J Pediatr Orthop* 2000;20(2): 203-209.

41. Armstrong PF: Initial management of the multiply injured child: The ABCs. *Instr Course Lect* 1992;41:347-350.
42. Bone LB, Johnson KD, Weigelt J, Scheinberg R: Early versus delayed stabilization of femoral fractures: A prospective randomized study. *J Bone Joint Surg Am* 1989; 71(3):336-340.
43. Pape HC, Giannoudis P, Krettek C: The timing of fracture treatment in polytrauma patients: Relevance of damage control orthopedic surgery. *Am J Surg* 2002; 183(6):622-629.
44. Pape HC, Hildebrand F, Pertschy S, et al: Changes in the management of femoral shaft fractures in polytrauma patients: From early total care to damage control orthopedic surgery. *J Trauma* 2002;53(3):452-461, discussion 461-462.
45. Nowotarski PJ, Turen CH, Brumback RJ, Scarboro JM: Conversion of external fixation to intramedullary nailing for fractures of the shaft of the femur in multiply injured patients. *J Bone Joint Surg Am* 2000;82(6):781-788.
46. Scalea TM, Boswell SA, Scott JD, Mitchell KA, Kramer ME, Pollak AN: External fixation as a bridge to intramedullary nailing for patients with multiple injuries and with femur fractures: Damage control orthopedics. *J Trauma* 2000;48(4):613-621, discussion 621-623.
47. Loder RT: Pediatric polytrauma: Orthopaedic care and hospital course. *J Orthop Trauma* 1987; 1(1):48-54.
48. Blasier RD, McAtee J, White R, Mitchell DT: Disruption of the pelvic ring in pediatric patients. *Clin Orthop Relat Res* 2000; 376:87-95.
49. Loder RT, Gullahorn LJ, Yian EH, Ferrick MR, Raskas DS, Greenfield ML: Factors predictive of immobilization complications in pediatric polytrauma. *J Orthop Trauma* 2001;15(5):338-341.
50. Kreder HJ, Armstrong P: A review of open tibia fractures in children. *J Pediatr Orthop* 1995;15(4): 482-488.
51. Robertson P, Karol LA, Rab GT: Open fractures of the tibia and femur in children. *J Pediatr Orthop* 1996;16(5):621-626.
52. Skaggs DL, Friend L, Alman B, et al: The effect of surgical delay on acute infection following 554 open fractures in children. *J Bone Joint Surg Am* 2005;87 (1):8-12.
53. Srivastava AK, Mehlman CT, Wall EJ, Do TT: Elastic stable intramedullary nailing of tibial shaft fractures in children. *J Pediatr Orthop* 2008;28(2):152-158.
54. Myers SH, Spiegel D, Flynn JM: External fixation of high-energy tibia fractures. *J Pediatr Orthop* 2007;27(5):537-539.
55. Kubiak EN, Egol KA, Scher D, Wasserman B, Feldman D, Koval KJ: Operative treatment of tibial fractures in children: Are elastic stable intramedullary nails an improvement over external fixation? *J Bone Joint Surg Am* 2005;87(8):1761-1768.
56. Cullen MC, Roy DR, Crawford AH, Assenmacher J, Levy MS, Wen D: Open fracture of the tibia in children. *J Bone Joint Surg Am* 1996;78(7):1039-1047.
57. Mooney JF III, Argenta LC, Marks MW, et al: Treatment of soft tissue defects in pediatric patients using the V.A.C. system. *Clin Orthop Relat Res* 2003;376:26-31.
58. Jaramillo D, Treves ST, Kasser JR, Harper M, Sundel R, Laor T: Osteomyelitis and septic arthritis in children: Appropriate use of imaging to guide treatment. *ARJ Am J Roentgenol* 1995;165(2): 399-403.
59. Zamzam MM: The role of ultrasound in differentiating septic arthritis from transient synovitis of the hip in children. *J Pediatr Orthop B* 2006;15(6):418-422.
60. Cavalier R, Herman MJ, Pizzutillo PD, Geller E: Ultrasound-guided aspiration of the hip in children: A new technique. *Clin Orthop Relat Res* 2003;415: 244-247.
61. Kocher MS, Zurakowski D, Kasser JR: Differentiating between septic arthritis and transient synovitis of the hip in children: An evidence-based clinical prediction algorithm. *J Bone Joint Surg Am* 1999;81(12):1662-1670.
62. Caird MS, Flynn JM, Leung YL, Millman JE, D'Italia JG, Dormans JP: Factors distinguishing septic arthritis from transient synovitis of the hip in children: A prospective study. *J Bone Joint Surg Am* 2006;88(6):1251-1257.
63. Kim HK, Alman B, Cole WG: A shortened course of parenteral antibiotic therapy in the management of acute septic arthritis of the hip. *J Pediatr Orthop* 2000; 20(1):44-47.
64. Griffin PP, Green WT Sr: Hip joint infections in infants and children. *Orthop Clin North Am* 1978;9(1):123-134.
65. Choi IH, Pizzutillo PD, Bowen JR, Dragann R, Malhis T: Sequelae and reconstruction after septic arthritis of the hip in infants. *J Bone Joint Surg Am* 1990; 72(8):1150-1165.
66. Peters W, Irving J, Letts M: Long-term effects of neonatal bone and joint infection on adjacent growth plates. *J Pediatr Orthop* 1992; 12(6):806-810.
67. Choi IH, Yoo WJ, Cho TJ, Chung CY: Operative reconstruction for septic arthritis of the hip. *Orthop Clin North Am* 2006; 37(2):173-183, vi.

68. Liu YM, Chi CY, Ho MW, et al: Microbiology and factors affecting mortality in necrotizing fasciitis. *J Microbiol Immunol Infect* 2005; 38(6):430-435.

69. Eneli I, Davies HD: Epidemiology and outcome of necrotizing fasciitis in children: An active surveillance study of the Canadian Paediatric Surveillance Program. *J Pediatr* 2007;151(1):79-84 .

70. Wong CH, Chang HC, Pasupathy S, Khin LW, Tan JL, Low CO: Necrotizing fasciitis: Clinical presentation, microbiology, and determinants of mortality. *J Bone Joint Surg Am* 2003; 85-A(8):1454-1460.

71. Ozalay M, Ozkoc G, Akpinar S, Hersekli MA, Tandogan RN: Necrotizing soft-tissue infection of a limb: Clinical presentation and factors related to mortality. *Foot Ankle Int* 2006;27(8):598-605.

72. Muqim R: Necrotizing fasciitis: Management and outcome. *J Coll Physicians Surg Pak* 2003;13(12): 711-714.

73. Golger A, Ching S, Goldsmith CH, Pennie RA, Bain JR: Mortality in patients with necrotizing fasciitis. *Plast Reconstr Surg* 2007; 119(6):1803-1807.

74. Mulla ZD: Clinical and epidemiologic features of invasive group A streptococcal infections in children. *Pediatr Int* 2007;49(3): 355-358.

75. Henrys P, Lyne ED, Lifton C, Salciccioli G: Clinical review of cervical spine injuries in children. *Clin Orthop Relat Res* 1977;129: 172-176.

76. Brown RL, Brunn MA, Garcia VF: Cervical spine injuries in children: A review of 103 patients treated consecutively at a level 1 pediatric trauma center. *J Pediatr Surg* 2001;36(8):1107-1114.

77. Pizzutillo PD, Rocha EF, D'Astous J, Kling TF Jr , McCarthy RE: Bilateral fracture of the pedicle of the second cervical vertebra in the young child. *J Bone Joint Surg Am* 1986;68(6): 892-896.

78. Herman MJ, Pizzutillo PD: Cervical spine disorders in children. *Orthop Clin North Am* 1999; 30(3):457-466, ix.

79. Bucholz RW, Burkhead WZ: The pathological anatomy of fatal atlanto-occipital dislocations. *J Bone Joint Surg Am* 1979;61(2): 248-250.

80. McGrory BJ, Klassen RA, Chao EY, Staeheli JW, Weaver AL: Acute fractures and dislocations of the cervical spine in children and adolescents. *J Bone Joint Surg Am* 1993;75(7): 988-995.

81. Georgopoulos G, Pizzutillo PD, Lee MS: Occipito-atlantal instability in children. A report of five cases and review of the literature. *J Bone Joint Surg Am* 1987;69(3): 429-436.

82. Herzenberg JE, Hensinger RN, Dedrick DK, Phillips WA: Emergency transport and positioning of young children who have an injury of the cervical spine: The standard backboard may be hazardous. *J Bone Joint Surg Am* 1989;71(1):15-22.

83. Pang D, Pollack IF: Spinal cord injury without radiographic abnormality in children: The SCIWORA syndrome. *J Trauma* 1989;29(5):654-664.

84. Dormans JP, Criscitiello AA, Drummond DS, Davidson RS: Complications in children managed with immobilization in a halo vest. *J Bone Joint Surg Am* 1995;77(9):1370-1373.

85. Caird MS, Hensinger RN, Weiss N, Farley FA: Complications and problems in halo treatment of toddlers: Limited ambulation is recommended. *J Pediatr Orthop* 2006;26(6):750-752.

86. Koop SE, Winter RB, Lonstein JE: The surgical treatment of instability of the upper part of the cervical spine in children and adolescents. *J Bone Joint Surg Am* 1984;66(3):403-411.

87. Pizzutillo PD, Herman MJ: Injuries of the pediatric cervical spine, in Cotler J, ed: *Surgery of Spine Trauma*. Philadelphia, PA, Williams & Wilkins, 2000, pp 333-354.

88. Dormans JP, Drummond DS, Sutton LN, Ecker ML, Kopacz KJ: Occipitocervical arthrodesis in children: A new technique and analysis of results. *J Bone Joint Surg Am* 1995;77(8):1234-1240.

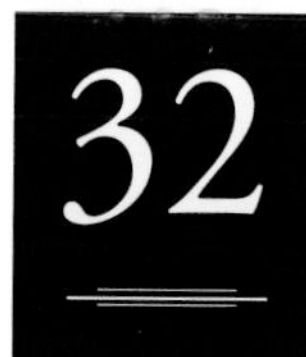

Management of Fractures in Adolescents

Shital N. Parikh, MD
Lawrence Wells, MD
Charles T. Mehlman, DO, MPH
Susan A. Scherl, MD

Abstract

There are well-established treatment standards for adults who sustain fractures; however, these treatment standards are not always applicable when treating adolescents with similar fractures because of the presence of physes. Fractures in adolescents are treated by pediatric orthopaedic surgeons, adult orthopaedic traumatologists, or general orthopaedic surgeons. It is imperative that the principles of fracture management are well defined and discussed in both the pediatric and adult orthopaedic community.

Controversial topics include the youngest age at which an adolescent can be treated as an adult and acceptable fracture reduction criteria. The general principles of managing fractures in adolescents regarding classification, treatment options, complications, and estimating skeletal age should be understood by the treating physician.

Instr Course Lect 2011;60:397-411.

Adolescence is defined as a transition phase between childhood and adulthood. It encompasses puberty (a period of rapid growth and hormonal changes), which includes an acceleration phase of growth (for approximately 2 years), a peak (peak height velocity), and a deceleration phase (for 1 to 2 years). The mean age at the time of the peak height velocity is 12 years (typical range, 10 to 14 years) for girls and 14 years (typical range, 12 to 16 years) for boys. Typically, girls who are older than 14 years and boys who are older than 16 years are considered skeletally mature and can undergo treatment similar to that for their adult counterparts. In this chapter, girls from 8 to 14 years old and boys from 10 to 16 years old will be considered adolescents.[1,2]

The gold standard for fracture treatment in adults is often not applicable to an adolescent. Similarly, what is considered appropriate for a child is not considered acceptable for an adolescent; for example, the use of a hip spica cast is considered appropriate for a femoral shaft fracture in a child but not for such a fracture in an adolescent.

A primary difference between adults and skeletally immature patients is the quality of the bone. Because the bones of an adolescent are less mineralized, more vascular, more porous, and more elastic than the bones of an adult, the bones of an adolescent absorb more energy before they fracture, heal more quickly, and produce greater callus. The immature skeleton dissipates energy better than does the adult skeleton, and this decreases the severity of the comminution of fractures.[3] Physes are present in adolescents, and they are the weakest link in the bone. Physeal fractures occur in adolescents,

Dr. Mehlman or an immediate family member serves as a board member, owner, officer, or committee member of the Pediatric Orthopaedic Society of North America, the Scoliosis Research Society, the Ohio University COM Alumni Association, and the American Osteopathic Academy of Orthopedics and has received research or institutional support from Abbott, DePuy, Globus Medical, Medtronic Sofamor Danek, the National Institutes of Health (NIAMS & NICHD), Synthes, the University of Cincinnati, and the Scoliosis Research Society. Dr. Scherl or an immediate family member serves as a board member, owner, officer, or committee member of the Orthopaedic Trauma Association and the Pediatric Orthopaedic Society of North America and has received research or institutional support from Arthrex, the National Institutes of Health (NIAMS & NICHD), Tornier, and ESKA. Neither of the following authors nor any immediate family member has received anything of value from or owns stock in a commercial company or institution related directly or indirectly to the subject of this chapter: Dr. Parikh and Dr. Wells.

whereas dislocations and ligamentous injuries would occur in adults. The pattern of physeal closure in adolescents determines the physeal fracture pattern, which explains the Tillaux fracture of the distal part of the tibia and tibial tuberosity avulsion in the proximal part of the tibia. It is essential to consider the presence of an open physis during the treatment of nonphyseal fractures in adolescents to avoid iatrogenic physeal injury and possible growth disturbances. Other issues, including compliance, emotional outbursts, peer pressure, aesthetics, and other psychosocial and behavioral elements, should be considered when treating an adolescent.[4,5]

Specific implants and instruments are now available to treat certain fractures in adolescents. However, this is not true for all fractures in adolescents, and it is not uncommon for fractures in adolescents to be fixed with implants and instruments from an orthopaedic set meant for adults. Tibial nails have been used to treat femoral shaft fractures in adolescents, and the feasibility of using humeral nails for femoral and tibial shaft fractures has been explored.[6,7]

Estimating Skeletal Maturity

Chronologic age does not necessarily correlate with skeletal maturity or allow sufficient prediction of remaining growth. Determining skeletal age is the preferred method for estimating the years of growth remaining. The Greulich and Pyle[8] atlas (hand and wrist radiographs), the Pyle and Hoerr[9] atlas (knee radiographs), the Sauvegrain method[10] (elbow radiographs), the Risser sign[11] (iliac apophyseal ossification), the Oxford score[12] (hip and pelvic radiographs), and the Tanner-Whitehouse-III score[13] (radiographs of the radius, ulna, and small bones of the hand or RUS score) are all used to estimate skeletal age. This chapter's authors find it simple to use the method described by Sanders et al,[14] which is based on a simplified Tanner-Whitehouse-III maturity assessment. According to this method, if the physes of the distal phalanges of the hand are wide open, the patient is skeletally immature; if these physes are partially closed, the patient is approaching peak height velocity; and once these physes are closed, the patient has reached peak height velocity. Biologic age estimation using the traditional Tanner staging method or based on secondary sexual characteristics or menarche is important but less commonly used.[2,15]

Classification of Physeal Fractures

Although each anatomic region has a separate fracture classification, all injuries around the physis can be classified with the commonly used Salter-Harris system[16] (**Figure 1**). Salter-Harris types I and II are extra-articular fractures, Salter-Harris types III and IV are intra-articular fractures, and Salter-Harris type V is a retrospective diagnosis. Rang et al[17] described a type VI fracture, which involves injury to the perichondral ring of LaCroix. The other two commonly seen physeal fracture patterns not described by the Salter-Harris classification are the Peterson type I fracture (a fracture of the metaphysis extending into the physis) and the Peterson type VI fracture (a fracture with a portion of the physis missing).[18] A Peterson type VI fracture is similar to a Rang type VI fracture. These classification systems help to predict the extent and prognosis of physeal injury, aid in decision making for its management, and allow better communication for clinical and research purposes.

Imaging

General principles of fracture imaging and the inclusion of joints above and below the fractures should be followed. Comparison views of the contralateral extremity may be useful for the evaluation of physeal fractures or minimally displaced or nondisplaced fractures, or to delineate ossification patterns. Stress radiographs are not recommended because of the pain involved and the risk of iatrogenic physeal injury. A CT scan is recommended for evaluating certain intra-articular fractures in the knee or ankle region to better define the fracture pattern and aid in management. MRI is used for the evaluation of suspected ligamentous injuries, chondral injuries, and osteochondral injuries or to determine the "health" of physes.[3,19-21]

Principles of Treating Physeal Fractures in Adolescents

The following principles should be followed in treating physeal fractures in adolescent patients. (1) Displaced physeal fractures should be reduced with traction and very gentle manipulation. Open reduction is better than multiple attempts at closed reduction to avoid iatrogenic physeal injury. (2) Physeal fracture reduction should not be attempted later than 7 to 10 days after injury, unless there is an intra-articular step-off of more than 2 mm. (3) Pins or screws used for internal fixation should be placed parallel to the physis. Smooth pins should be used if they must cross the physis. The pins crossing the physis are removed as soon as early signs of fracture healing appear. (4) Arthroscopic examination during internal fixation of intra-articular fractures can improve the accuracy of a reduction. (5) Resecting a small portion of periosteum on either side of the physis during an open fracture reduction requiring elevation of the periosteum near the physis reduces the risk of osseous bar formation across the physis. (6) For an

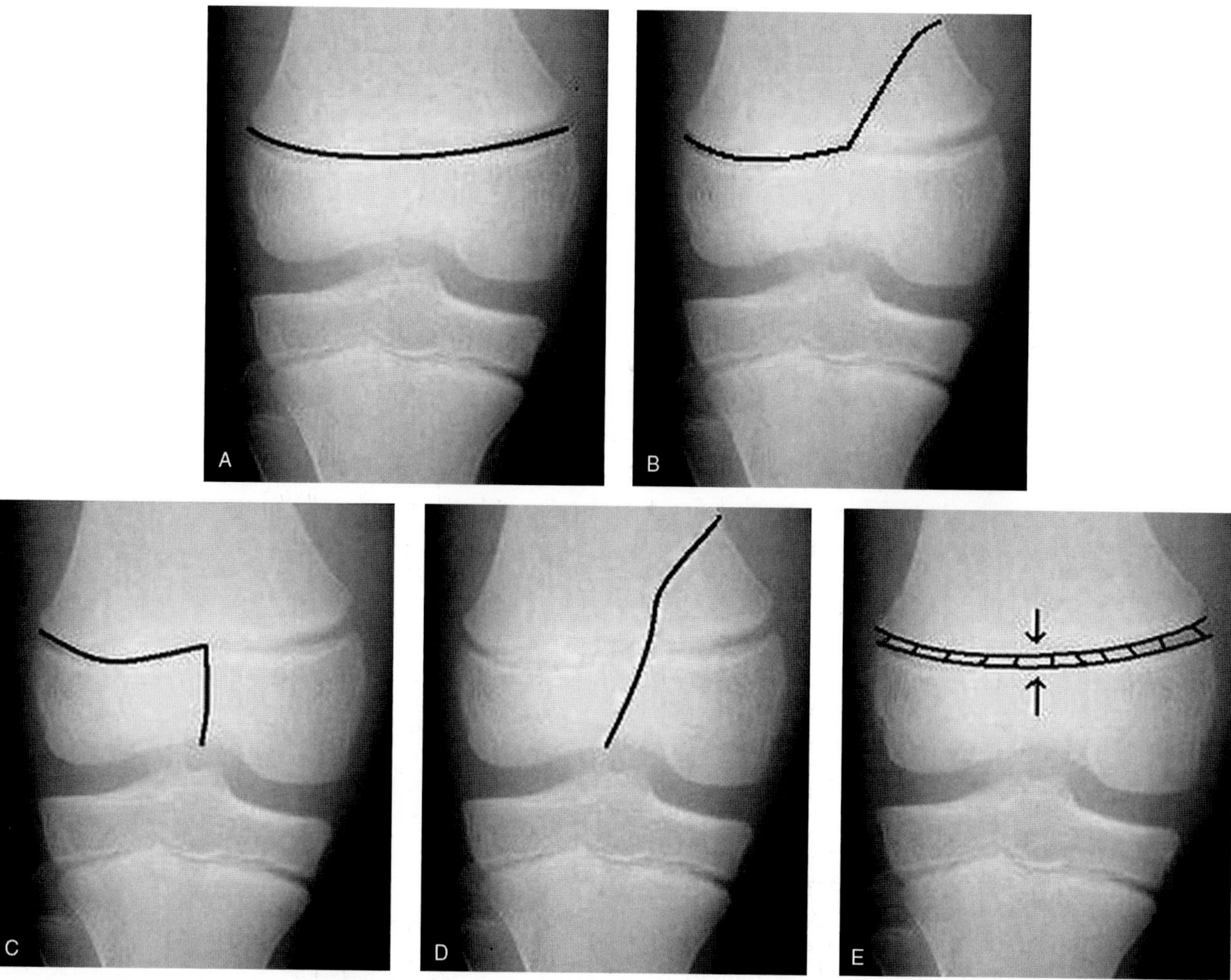

Figure 1 Salter-Harris classification system for physeal fractures. **A**, Type I is a fracture through the hypertrophic zone of the physis with no involvement of the surrounding bone. **B**, Type II is similar to type I but has a metaphyseal fragment on the compression side of the fracture (the Thurston-Holland sign). **C**, Type III involves physeal separation with fracture through the epiphysis into the joint. **D**, Type IV is a fracture through the metaphysis, physis, and epiphysis. **E**, Type V is a compression or crushing injury to the physis.

exposed or crushed physeal injury, an acute Langenskiöld procedure (using free fat interpositional graft) can be performed to help prevent growth arrest.[22,23] (7) Most physeal fractures heal in 3 weeks. (8) Once a physeal fracture has healed, the patient should be monitored for growth disturbances for at least 6 months or until the patient is skeletally mature. (9) Growth arrest lines (Park-Harris lines) are transverse lines seen in the metaphysis. Their orientation and relationship to the physis are used to assess growth.[24,25]

The sequelae and complications of physeal fractures and their management are described in **Figure 2**. This algorithm is applicable when a patient has at least 2 years of growth remaining.[23,26-31]

Principles of Treating Nonphyseal Fractures in Adolescents

The following principles should be followed in treating nonphyseal fractures in adolescent patients. (1) Following a fracture, the bone in adolescent patients does not remodel as it does in young children. The acceptable fracture reduction parameters in adolescents are similar to those used for adults. (2) Besides age, the weight of the patient and the fracture characteristics help to determine the optimal fracture fixation method and postoperative management. (3) For most displaced diaphyseal fractures of long bones, elastic stable intramedullary nails are the implants of choice, and (4) locking plates are usually not needed. (5) For most displaced metaphyseal fractures, percutaneous pin fixation is adequate. These pins can be cut and

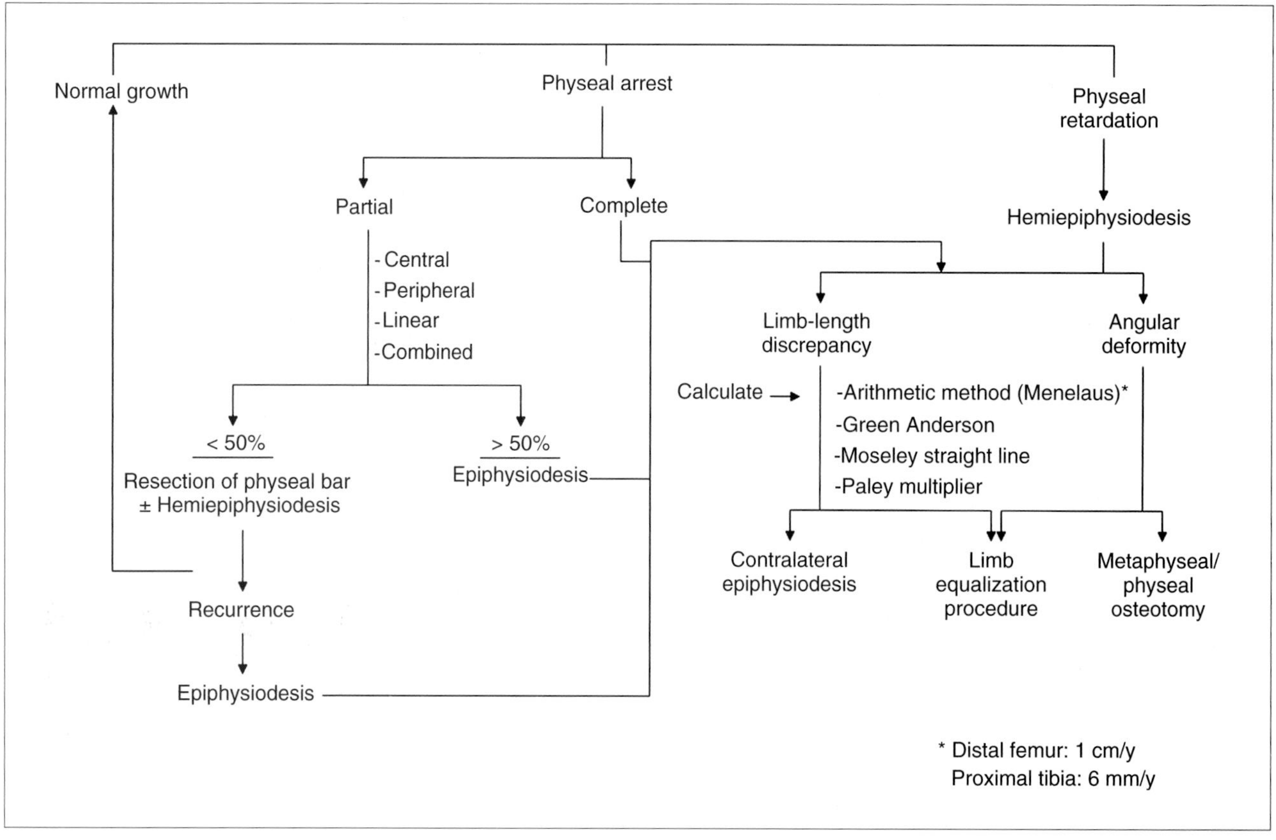

Figure 2 Algorithm for managing physeal injuries and their complications.

left outside the skin for later removal in the physician's office. (6) Fracture fixation is usually supplemented with a splint, cast, or brace. (7) Implant removal is optional, although it is recommended that elastic stable intramedullary nails be removed after the fracture heals.

Clavicle Shaft

The clavicle is the first bone to start the ossification process and the last to finish it.[32] Incomplete and minimally displaced fractures of the clavicle shaft are treated nonsurgically. The healing and remodeling capacities of the clavicle are excellent, and this is a major reason for nonsurgical care of nearly all clavicle fractures. However, it has been shown that most clavicle growth has been completed by adolescence, with 80% of longitudinal growth completed by 9 years of age in girls and by 12 years of age in boys; thus, the remodeling potential beyond these ages may be limited.[33] The discussion between the family and the pediatric orthopaedic surgeon regarding an adolescent with a completely displaced clavicle shaft fracture has changed substantially in the last several years. Recent published evidence regarding the treatment of adults with clavicle fractures has expanded the discussion of the treatment of completely displaced clavicle shaft fractures to include the possibility of open reduction and internal fixation.[34-36] Two centimeters or more of fracture fragment displacement has been suggested as an important threshold in adults. However, in the level I comparative study performed by the Canadian Orthopaedic Trauma Society that showed superiority of treatment with open reduction and internal fixation with a plate and screws, the authors simply used "completely displaced" as a criterion for entry into the study.[34]

Currently, the most common procedure for surgical treatment of a displaced clavicle shaft fracture in an adolescent is open reduction and internal fixation with a plate and screws. A transverse incision is placed near or slightly below the anticipated lower border of the reconstructed clavicle shaft. The surgical approach involves progressive exposure of the fracture fragments through subcutaneous tissue, platysma, and the clavipectoral fascia and periosteal layers, with protection of crossing branches of the supraclavicular nerve.[35,37] Standard fixation principles, including selective use of interfragmentary lag screws as indicated, are applied. Careful drilling and a depth gauge technique are advised for all portions of the procedure, but, more medially, the subclavian neurovascular bundle is only about 10 mm away from the clavicle.[38] Open reduction and plate fixation allows adolescents to return to full activities about 4 weeks sooner than would be possible with nonsurgical treatment (at 12 weeks rather than 16 weeks).[36]

Radial and Ulnar Shafts

Forearm shaft fractures are the third most common fracture in children. The literature reflects a strong and positive precedent for nonsurgical care, but the outcomes of many of the studies may be biased by the inclusion of very young patients and distal metaphyseal radial fractures under the heading of "forearm fracture." Analysis of the outcomes of forearm shaft fractures in adolescents has shown that these fractures are more difficult to manage with nonsurgical methods than has been generally believed.[39,40]

The shaft of the radius is that portion extending from the proximal base of the tubercle of Lister to the proximal base of the bicipital tuberosity, with the ulnar shaft defined in a similar manner. A practical classification of shaft fractures of the forearm in the pediatric population recognizes the existence of two bones, three levels (the proximal, middle, and distal thirds), and four fracture patterns (plastic deformation, greenstick, complete, and comminuted).[41] Good-quality radiographs should be obtained in two orthogonal planes. If there is angulation in both planes, the true angulation will be greater than either single view reveals. The proximal and distal radioulnar joints should be carefully inspected in a patient who has what appears to be a single-bone shaft fracture.

Greenstick fractures have continuity of at least one cortex and may be reduced by derotating the forearm. A complete shaft fracture of both forearm bones in a child who is younger than 10 years can usually be successfully managed with closed methods. Angulation of more than 20° in the distal third, 15° in the middle third, or 10° in the proximal third is not acceptable even in patients younger than 10 years.[42,43] Bayonet apposition is acceptable in these young patients provided that satisfactory angular, rotational, and interosseous space alignment is maintained. In children older than 10 years, angulation of more than 10° is usually unacceptable. The most common indications for surgical fixation are an open fracture and an inadequately reduced fracture involving both the radial and the ulnar shaft in an adolescent. Intramedullary flexible nails (elastic stable intramedullary nails) are the fixation implants of choice. A closed reduction and elastic nail fixation should be tried initially, but if this cannot be achieved within the first 10 minutes, it should be converted to a minimally open reduction and elastic nail fixation. Elastic stable intramedullary nails (1.5 to 2.0 mm) are adequate, and, if needed, smaller smooth Steinmann pins are used. The radial nail is contoured to reestablish the radial bow, while the ulnar nail is minimally contoured. The narrowest portion of the intramedullary canal of the radius is central, near the isthmus, whereas the narrowest portion of the ulna is near its distal third. Internal fixation of the radius should be performed first. The radial entry point is the floor of the first dorsal compartment or the bare area just proximal to the Lister tubercle between the second and third dorsal compartments. Appropriate rotation of the contoured radial implant is necessary to properly restore the radial bow. The ulnar entry point is the anconeus starting point along the lateral edge of the proximal part of the ulna, just distal to the growth plate. The intramedullary fixation devices should not violate either of the physes, and the extensor tendons should be protected from the sharp edges of the distal aspect of the radial elastic nails. The intramedullary nails are removed after 6 or more months. The potential complications of elastic stable intramedullary nailing include nail migration, delayed union or nonunion, loss of reduction, loss of motion, infection, nerve injury, muscle entrapment, extensor tendon injury, a reoperation, physeal injury, and compartment syndrome (**Figure 3**).

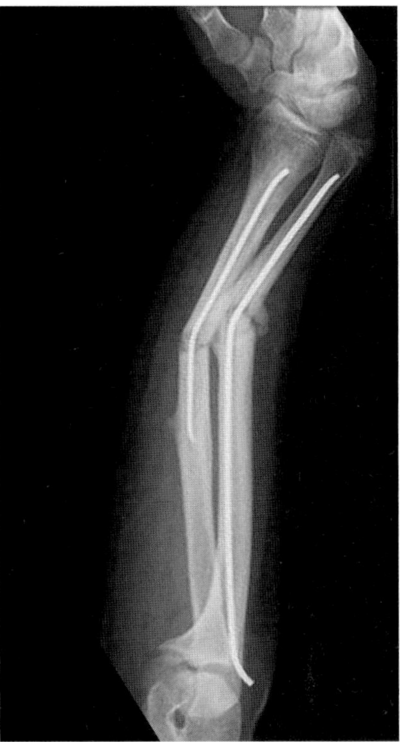

Figure 3 Radiograph showing complications of nailing of radial and ulnar shaft fractures, including nonunion, a short radial nail, and the need for a reoperation. The patient underwent removal of the nails, bone grafting, and plate fixation of both fractures.

Femoral Shaft

The goals for treating femoral shaft fractures are timely union, no rotational deformity, less than 2 cm of shortening, and angular alignment within the acceptable parameters of

10° to 20° in the sagittal plane and 5° to 10° in the frontal plane. Valgus and procurvatum are tolerated better than varus and recurvatum deformity. Numerous treatment options are available, and the surgeon must base his or her decision on a combination of patient factors, such as age and size, fracture morphology, and type and extent of other injuries and morbidities; surgeon factors, such as familiarity with and preference for a particular technique and availability of equipment; and social factors, such as the psychologic impact on the patient, disruption to the family, loss of time from school, and cost.

For adolescents, surgical treatment of femoral shaft fractures is favored over nonsurgical treatment. The benefits of surgery are lower rates of malunion, shorter hospitalization, earlier mobilization, and better social acceptance and cost-effectiveness. The potential disadvantages are the risks of surgery, scars, infection, bleeding, the need for implant removal, and the risk of damage to the physis. The various surgical treatment options include external fixation, plating, the use of elastic stable intramedullary nails, and the use of rigid intramedullary nails. This chapter's authors are not aware of any prospective randomized trials comparing operative treatments, but the many retrospective studies of the various options all have demonstrated acceptable results.[44-60] Recently, the American Academy of Orthopaedic Surgeons (AAOS) published clinical practice guidelines for pediatric femoral fractures.[61] The use of elastic stable intramedullary nails is a treatment option for patients 11 years or younger, whereas surgical treatment with elastic stable intramedullary nails, trochanteric antegrade nails, or plating are options for those 11 years or older.

External fixation is simple and quick to apply, it can be applied at the bedside if necessary, and the technique is familiar to most orthopaedic surgeons.[45,46,48,62,63] It is used primarily in patients with soft-tissue injury, multiple traumatic injuries, or severe shortening. Compared with some other treatment options, it is not as well accepted by patients and families, and the cosmetic appearance of the pin site scars can be an issue. Pin site irritation and infection are common, and a relatively high refracture rate and loss of knee range of motion and quadriceps strength have been reported.[64,65]

Plate and screw fixation is useful for very proximal or distal fractures and when the medullary canal is too small for a nail.[44,49,54,59,66] The plate is inserted through a straight lateral approach. Alternatively, a minimally invasive technique with submuscular plating through small, transverse incisions may be used. Locking screws may be used for very proximal or distal fractures, to convert the construct to a fixed-angle construct. In a growing child, the plate generally must be removed before it is overgrown with bone. It is unclear whether or not the plate or screw holes act as a stress riser leading to an increased refracture rate in these patients.

Elastic stable intramedullary nails have become the treatment of choice for adolescent femoral fractures because they are simple and quick to insert, the incisions are small, and family acceptance is high.[52,55,56,60] The original indications for elastic stable intramedullary nails were type 0 or 1 Winquist middiaphyseal fractures, but good results can be achieved when the devices are used for proximal, distal, and comminuted fractures. However, complications and loss of reduction are more likely in children who are 11 years or older, who are heavier than 108 lb (49 kg), who have a distal or (especially) proximal fracture, and who have a comminuted or "length unstable" fracture.[67-71] Adjunctive immobilization or alternate treatment options should be considered in those cases. When flexible nails are chosen, the surgeon should always use two nails of the same diameter. Failure to do so will lead to angulation. The width of each nail should be 40% of the diameter of the diaphysis at its narrowest point. The canal should never be more than 80% filled. The nails are bent before insertion, such that the apex of the bend is at the fracture site. For middiaphyseal fractures being treated with retrograde insertion, the nails should be contoured into two C shapes. For proximal fractures being treated with antegrade insertion, the medial nail should be contoured into a C and the lateral nail, into an S. The nails should be removed 6 months to 1 year after insertion. Overgrowth at the fracture site has not been a substantial problem with the use of elastic stable intramedullary nails. Complications include irritation at the insertion sites, the tendency for the fracture to fall into varus, and the potential for intra-articular nail penetration.

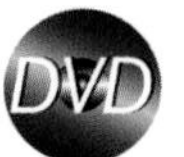

Video 32.1: Elastic Stable Intramedullary Nailing (ESIN) for Femoral Shaft Fracture. Shital N. Parikh, MD (16 min)

Trochanteric antegrade nails can be used in older, heavier children and for unstable fracture patterns.[47,53,58,72-75] The technique is generally familiar to orthopaedic surgeons who treat adults, although there are some variations among available systems. These variations include cannulated versus noncannulated nails, universal versus right and left nails, and nails that are prebent versus those requiring custom bending. The differences are not critical, but the surgeon should know the details of the system being used. Trochanteric antegrade nails generally do not require reaming; however, the nails are typically wider proximally than distally, and the proximal part of the canal may need to be reamed to accommodate this. Complications include potential harm to the hip abductors, potential osteonecrosis of the greater trochanter, and "explosion" of the proximal part of the femur during insertion.[76-81] The piriformis entry point is reserved for patients with closed physes because cases of osteonecrosis of the femoral head have been reported in children with open physes.[76,80,81]

Distal Part of Femur

Distal femoral fractures in adolescents are caused by either high-energy trauma or a sports-related injury.[82-86] A careful neurovascular examination of the injured extremity is necessary. Fractures of the distal part of the femur are either metaphyseal or physeal.

Metaphyseal fractures are classified by the direction of the apex of angulation. The gastrocnemius muscles pull the distal fragment posteriorly, producing an apex-posterior angulation. In patients who are younger than 10 years, closed reduction, percutaneous cross-pin fixation, and a long leg cast are satisfactory treatments. Loss of reduction is a risk, and the patient should be evaluated every week for at least the first 3 weeks. In patients 10 years or older or those with a comminuted and/or unstable fracture, submuscular plating or external fixation is recommended. For distal fractures, locking screws may be used with the submuscular plate to achieve a fixed-angle device. For open fractures, patients with multiple injuries, or a floating knee, external fixation should be used.

Physeal fractures of the distal part of the femur are classified with the Salter-Harris system.[83,84,86] For intra-articular fractures, a CT scan may help to identify fracture lines and aid in preoperative planning. Vascular and nerve injuries are not infrequent. CT angiography is recommended if a vascular injury is suspected. Reduction of the fracture into anatomic alignment and maintenance of reduction are the goals of treatment for displaced fractures. For nondisplaced Salter-Harris type I and II physeal fractures, a long leg cast is usually adequate. If a cast alone is inadequate, stabilization with percutaneously placed, crossed, transphyseal, smooth pins is recommended; this is similar to the treatment of displaced Salter-Harris type I or II fractures with a small metaphyseal fragment after closed reduction. A long leg cast and close follow-up are recommended. The pins are removed at approximately 4 weeks. A Salter-Harris type II fracture with a large metaphyseal fragment can be stabilized with cannulated screws through the metaphyseal fragment into the metaphyseal bone and application of a long leg cast, avoiding transphyseal fixation. Displaced Salter-Harris type III and IV fractures should be anatomically reduced and internally fixed with cannulated compression screws placed across the fracture and parallel to the physis. All patients with a fracture of the distal femoral physis should not bear weight until the fracture has healed. About 50% of all distal femoral physeal fractures lead to a growth disturbance, and patients with a Salter-Harris type II injury have the greatest risk of limb-length inequality or angular deformity[87,88] (**Figure 4**). Other potential complications include nonunion, which is treated with bone graft and rigid fixation, and arthrofibrosis, which is treated with knee manipulation and aggressive physical therapy after the fracture heals.[89,90]

Proximal Part of Tibia

In adolescents, tibial spine fractures occur with hyperextension of the knee, typically during bicycling. The pull of the anterior cruciate ligament (ACL) leads to an avulsion fracture of the tibial spine, which may extend into the medial or lateral tibial plateau. Pain, swelling caused by hemarthrosis, and a positive Lachman test are present. The avulsed tibial spine fracture is best seen on the lateral radiograph. An MRI may be necessary for a patient younger than 10 years, as much of the eminence is still cartilaginous. Tibial eminence fractures were classified by Meyers and McKeever into three types.[91] Type I is minimally displaced, type II is displacement of the anterior part of the tibial spine with an intact posterior hinge, and type III is complete separation of the avulsed fragment from the proximal tibial epiphysis. Zaricznyj[92] described a type IV fracture, which is a comminuted tibial spine fracture fragment (**Figure 5**). Type I is managed with a long leg cast with the limb flexed approximately 10° to 15° to avoid excessive tension on the ACL and further displacement of the tibial spine. If anatomic reduction of a type II fracture can be achieved by aspiration of the hemarthrosis and extension of the leg, then, like type I fractures, the type II fracture can be treated with a long leg cast, with weekly radiographs to ensure maintenance of reduction. For irreducible type II and type III fractures, arthroscopic or open reduction is recommended. An entrapped meniscus may be seen during arthroscopic surgery.[93] This chapter's authors prefer arthroscopic epiphyseal or transphyseal screw fixation for type II and type III fractures with a large fracture fragment and recommend suture fixation woven through the base of the ACL and tied over the metaphyseal bridge on the proximal part of the tibia for treatment of a type IV or small fracture fragment.[94] A transphyseal screw, if used, should be removed after 3 months to prevent

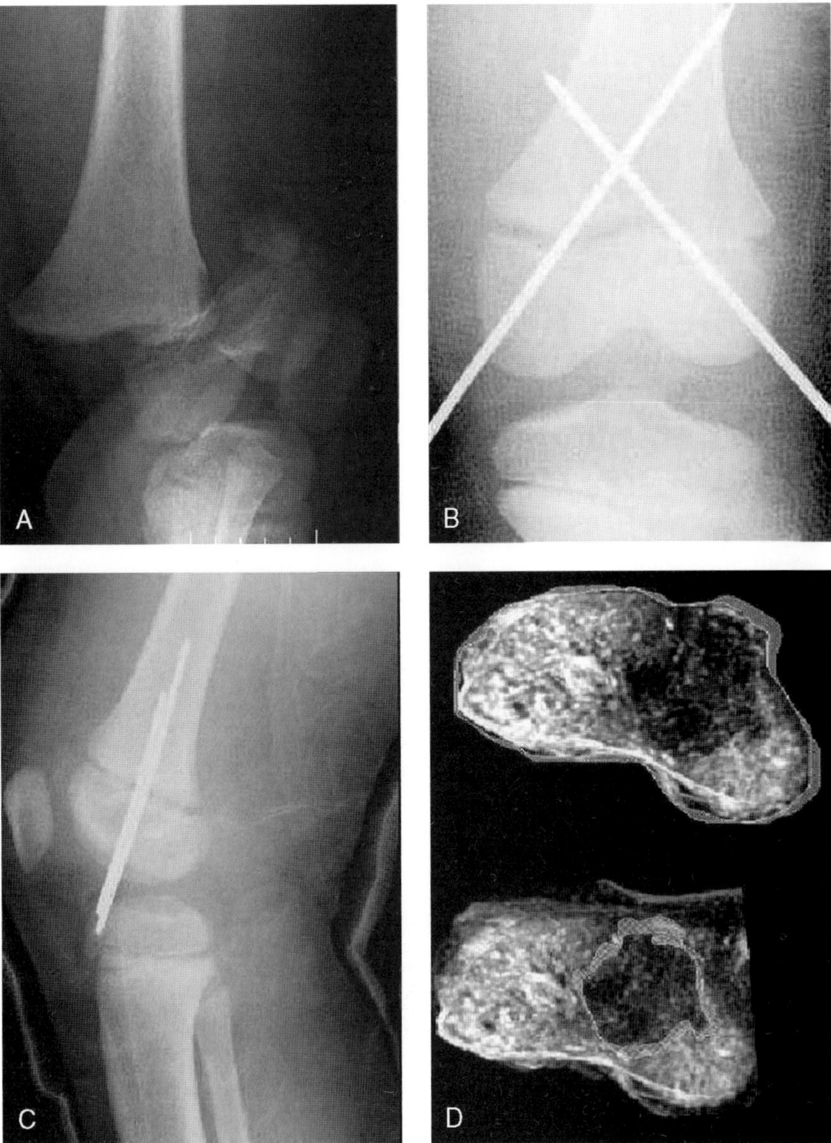

Figure 4 Salter-Harris type II fracture of the distal part of the femur (**A**), treated with open reduction and percutaneous pinning (**B** and **C**). An attempt at closed reduction showed a persistent gap over the medial part of the distal femoral physis cause by the interposed periosteum, which was removed during open reduction. Although the fracture healed, the patient had a physeal bar. The CT scan (**D**) shows the area of the physis and the area of physeal arrest. The physeal arrest is a central type.

growth disturbances.[95] The ACL may be stretched during this injury, but symptomatic instability is uncommon. Other potential complications include nonunion, malunion with resultant notch impingement, and arthrofibrosis.

Proximal tibial physeal fractures are categorized with the Salter-Harris classification. In adolescents, these fractures occur during sports activities or motor vehicle crashes, with a valgus or a hyperextension force on a fixed knee.[83,86,96] A CT scan is recommended for complex, high-energy injuries such as Salter-Harris type III and IV fractures involving the tibial plateau. Neurovascular injuries and compartment syndromes are not uncommon, and the possibility that they are present should be considered for every patient. The principles of treatment for proximal tibial physeal fractures are similar to those for distal femoral physeal fractures. Potential complications include neurovascular injuries, compartment syndrome, and growth disturbances.

Metaphyseal fractures of the proximal part of the tibia are usually treated with closed reduction and a long leg cast. With low-energy fractures in patients younger than 10 years, so-called Cozen fractures,[97] the most common complication is genu valgum in the first 6 to 12 months after the fracture caused by medial proximal tibial overgrowth. No treatment is needed for this deformity, as it usually corrects spontaneously. For high-energy fractures in patients 10 years or older, closed or open reduction and internal fixation with buttress plates and/or interfragmentary compression screws is used if the reduction cannot be held with a cast or if the patient cannot be treated with a long leg cast. Neurovascular injuries, compartment syndrome, and malunion are potential complications.

Tibial tubercle fractures occur most commonly in teenaged males who participate in repetitive jumping sports, and these injuries usually cause pain, swelling, and an inability to extend the knee against gravity. The fractures are classified according to the Watson-Jones classification, as modified by Ogden et al[98] (**Figure 6**). Nondisplaced type I fractures without an extensor lag can be treated in a cylinder cast with the knee in extension for 4 to 6 weeks, followed by rehabilitation. All displaced fractures (types II, III, and IV) require open anatomic reduction and internal fixation with 4.5- or 6-mm screws. For type III fractures, arthroscopic or open joint visualiza-

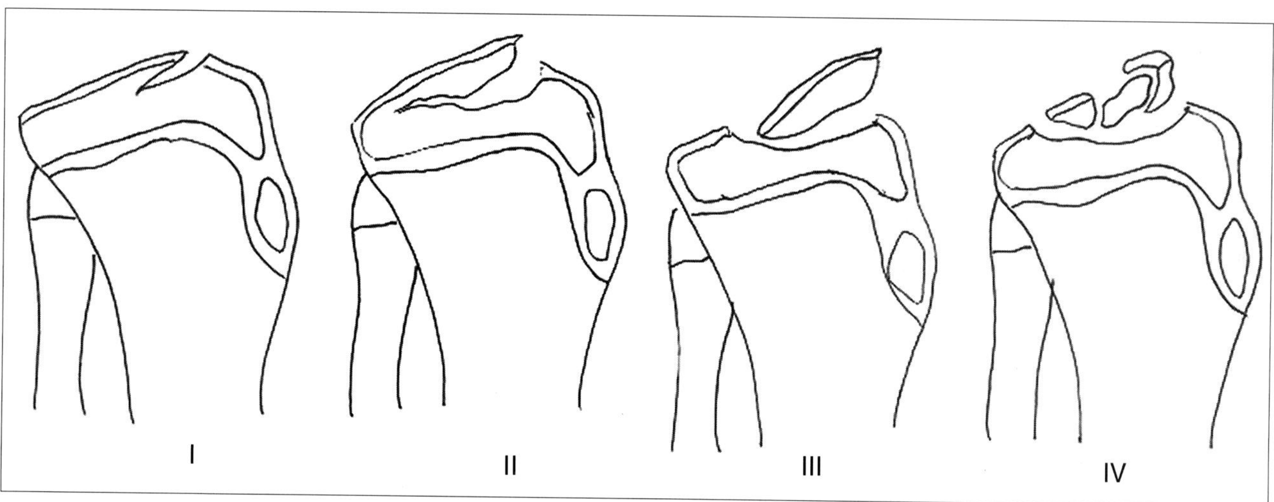

Figure 5 Classification of tibial spine fractures.

I
II
III
IV
V

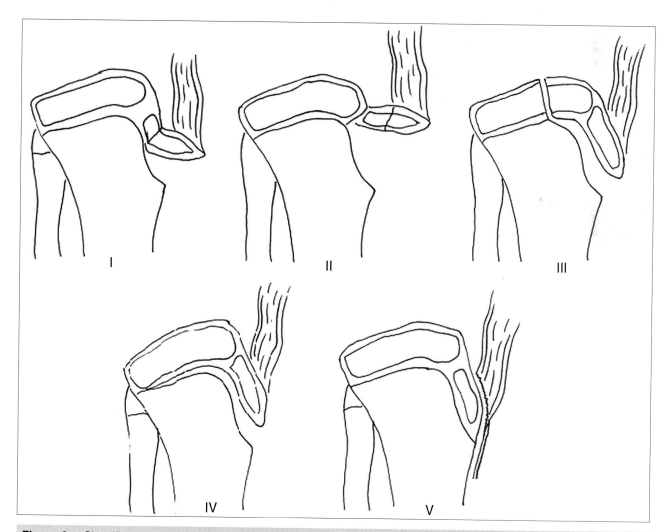

Figure 6 Classification of tibial tuberosity fractures.

tion should be performed to ensure adequate joint-surface reduction. Type IV fractures are similar to Salter-Harris type I or II fractures of the proximal part of the tibia, with a potential for neurovascular injuries. For type V fractures, the periosteal sleeve should be reattached with sutures or suture anchors. Prophylactic anterior compartment fasciotomy should be performed. Postoperatively, the knee should be immobilized until the bone heals. Potential complications include prominent implants requiring removal, compartment syndrome, and genu recurvatum caused by premature closure of the tibial apophysis.

Ankle

Physeal injuries to the ankle account for 15% to 38% of all physeal injuries.[99-102] The distal tibial physis appears by age 1 year and closes by age 12 to 14 years in girls and by age 15 to 18 years in boys. The distal fibular physis appears by age 2 years and closes somewhat later than the distal tibial physis (by age 19 to 20 years). The medial malleolus projection appears by age 7 years and is fully formed by age 10 years. Ankle physeal injury patterns are partly caused by the physeal anatomy as it relates to the patient's age. The distal tibial physis closes in a circular pattern that proceeds from the center to medial to lateral, and the fracture patterns reflect the areas of the physis that are still open. A CT scan is recommended for intra-articular fractures to evaluate for articular displacement, physeal congruity, and surgical planning.[103,104] A CT scan is also recommended after initial reduction if there are concerns about persistent or recurrent displacement. The ankle fracture classifications commonly used for adults, such as the Weber and Lauge-Hansen systems, are not useful for adolescents.[105-110] The Dias and Tachdjian[111] classification incorporates the Salter-Harris classification; the first word in each descriptor indicates the position of the foot, and the second indicates the direction of the force. The Vahvanen and Aalto[112] classification stratifies physeal ankle fractures into two groups: group I is low-risk avulsion fractures and epiphyseal separations, and group II is high-risk transphyseal fractures.

Patients with a nondisplaced Salter-Harris type I or II fracture should be treated with a below-knee walking cast for 3 to 4 weeks. Patients with a displaced Salter-Harris type I or II fracture should have a closed reduction under appropriate sedation followed by application of a well-molded above-knee cast, which can be switched to a below-knee cast after 3 weeks. If there is a physeal gap or translation of more than 2 mm after a closed reduction, an open reduction and fixation is indicated. A periosteal flap often prevents an anatomic reduction and, if it is not removed, there is a 60% incidence of premature physeal closure.[113] In children younger than 10 years, the acceptable reduction parameters are less than 10° of flexion or extension and less than 20° of varus or valgus angulation. In children 10 years or older, no more than 5° of angulation in any direction should be accepted. Most Salter-Harris type III and IV fractures require open reduction and internal fixation to obtain and maintain an anatomic reduction and joint congruity. An accurate reduction helps prevent premature growth arrest.[99,112,114,115] Pins or screws can be used for fixation. Transphyseal fixation should be avoided if possible, but, if transphyseal fixation is necessary, smooth pins should be used and then removed at 3 to 4 weeks. Use of a short leg cast or splint for 4 to 6 weeks is recommended. Once the cast is removed, motion and proprioception exercises should be performed before the patient returns to full activity. Radiographs should be obtained at 3-month intervals for at least 1 year to check for growth arrest.[116-118]

The Tillaux fracture is a Salter-Harris type III fracture of the anterolateral portion of the distal tibial epiphysis, which is the final tibial physeal area to close.[119] It appears on the AP radiograph as a vertical line through the epiphysis. The appropriate closed reduction maneuver is internal rotation of the foot; however, these fractures may require open reduction to restore the joint surface and prevent articular degeneration. One or two pins or screws placed through the epiphysis are usually sufficient. Tillaux fractures occur toward the conclusion of physeal closure, and symptomatic growth arrest is rare.

A triplane fracture is a multiplanar Salter-Harris type IV fracture,[120] which appears as a Salter-Harris type II fracture on the lateral radiograph and a Salter-Harris type III fracture on the AP radiograph. Patients with such a fracture are usually younger than those who have a Tillaux fracture and more of the physis is open, but a growth arrest is clinically unimportant. These fractures are usually described as being in two or three parts, but they may also be in four parts. Because these patterns are so complicated, a CT scan helps assess the fracture pattern, and it is suggested that CT be performed before surgery.

The closed reduction maneuver for a typical triplane fracture is flexion of the knee to 90°, and plantar flexion and internal rotation of the foot, with the patient under adequate sedation or general anesthesia. Multiple or forceful reduction attempts should be avoided. If the reduction is acceptable, the limb is immobilized in a long leg cast for 3 weeks, after which a short leg cast is worn for 3 weeks. If there is a concern about redisplacement, percutaneous screw fixation in a medial-lateral plane in the epiphysis and in the anterior-posterior plane in the metaphysis should be performed at the time of the initial reduction. If closed reduction is unacceptable, open reduction should be performed with use of an anterolateral or anteromedial incision and a posterolateral or posteromedial incision. The goal of open reduction is to obtain a congruous joint surface.

Summary

The challenges in the management of fractures in adolescents are unique and should be recognized. These fractures should not be grouped with pediatric fractures, for which nonsurgical treatment often suffices. The presence of physes and unique bone characteristics should differentiate the fracture management in adolescents from that of their adult counterparts.

References

1. Dimeglio A: Growth in pediatric orthopaedics. *J Pediatr Orthop* 2001;21(4):549-555.
2. Tanner JM, Whitehouse RH: Clinical longitudinal standards for height, weight, height velocity, weight velocity, and stages of puberty. *Arch Dis Child* 1976;51(3):170-179.
3. Rathjen KE, Birch JG: Physeal injuries and growth disturbances, in Beaty JH, Kasser JR, eds: *Rockwood and Wilkins' Fractures in Children*, ed 6. Philadelphia, PA, Lippincott Williams & Wilkins, 2006, pp 99-131.
4. Pattussi MP, Lalloo R, Bassani DG, Olinto MT: The role of psychosocial, behavioural and emotional factors on self-reported major injuries in Brazilian adolescents: A case-control study. *Injury* 2008;39(5):561-569.
5. Valovich McLeod TC, Bay RC, Parsons JT, Sauers EL, Snyder AR: Recent injury and health-related quality of life in adolescent athletes. *J Athl Train* 2009;44(6):603-610.
6. Bienkowski P, Harvey EJ, Reindl R, Berry GK, Benaroch TE, Ouellet JA: The locked flexible intramedullary humerus nail in pediatric femur and tibia shaft fractures: A feasibility study. *J Pediatr Orthop* 2004;24(6):634-637.
7. Mehlman CT, Bishai SK: Tibial nails for femoral shaft fractures in large adolescents with open femoral physes. *J Trauma* 2007;63(2):424-428.
8. Greulich WW, Pyle SI: *Radiographic Atlas of Skeletal Development of the Hand and Wrist*, ed 2. Stanford, CA, Stanford University Press, 1959.
9. Pyle SI, Hoerr NL: *Radiographic Atlas of Skeletal Development of the Knee: A Standard of Reference.* Springfield, IL, Charles C. Thomas, 1955.
10. Diméglio A, Charles YP, Daures JP, de Rosa V, Kaboré B: Accuracy of the Sauvegrain method in determining skeletal age during puberty. *J Bone Joint Surg Am* 2005;87(8):1689-1696.
11. Risser JC: The iliac apophysis: An invaluable sign in the management of scoliosis. *Clin Orthop* 1958;11:111-119.
12. Acheson RM: The Oxford method of assessing skeletal maturity. *Clin Orthop* 1957;10:19-39.
13. Tanner JM, Healy MJ, Goldstein H, Cameron N: *Assessment of Skeletal Maturity and Prediction of Adult Height (TW3 method)*, ed 3. London, England, WB Saunders, 2001.
14. Sanders JO, Khoury JG, Kishan S, et al: Predicting scoliosis progression from skeletal maturity: A simplified classification during adolescence. *J Bone Joint Surg Am* 2008;90(3):540-553.
15. Sanders JO: Maturity indicators in spinal deformity. *J Bone Joint Surg Am* 2007;89(Suppl 1):14-20.
16. Salter RB, Harris WR: Injuries involving the epiphyseal plate. *J Bone Joint Surg Am* 1963;45:587-622.
17. Rang M, Pring ME, Wenger DR: *Rang's Children's Fractures*, ed 3. Philadelphia, PA, Lippincott Williams & Wilkins, 2005.
18. Peterson HA: Physeal fractures: Part 2. Two previously unclassified types. *J Pediatr Orthop* 1994;14(4):431-438.
19. Boutis K, Narayanan UG, Dong FF, et al: Magnetic resonance imaging of clinically suspected Salter-Harris I fracture of the distal fibula. *Injury* 2010;41(8):852-856.
20. Carey J, Spence L, Blickman H, Eustace S: MRI of pediatric growth plate injury: Correlation with plain film radiographs and clinical outcome. *Skeletal Radiol* 1998;27(5):250-255.
21. Havránek P, Lízler J: Magnetic resonance imaging in the evaluation of partial growth arrest after physeal injuries in children. *J Bone Joint Surg Am* 1991;73(8):1234-1241.
22. Foster BK, John B, Hasler C: Free fat interpositional graft in acute physeal injuries: The anticipatory Langenskiöld procedure. *J Pediatr Orthop* 2000;20(3):282-285.
23. Langenskiöld A: The possibilities of eliminating premature partial closure of an epiphyseal plate caused by trauma or disease. *Acta Orthop Scand* 1967;38:267-279.
24. Lee TM, Mehlman CT: Hyphenated history: Park-Harris growth arrest lines. *Am J Orthop (Belle Mead NJ)* 2003;32(8):408-411.
25. Ogden JA: Growth slowdown and arrest lines. *J Pediatr Orthop* 1984;4(4):409-415.
26. Anderson M, Messner MB, Green WT: Distribution of

lengths of the normal femur and tibia in children from one to eighteen years of age. *J Bone Joint Surg Am* 1964;46:1197-1202.

27. Menelaus MB: Correction of leg length discrepancy by epiphysial arrest. *J Bone Joint Surg Br* 1966; 48(2):336-339.

28. Moseley CF: A straight-line graph for leg-length discrepancies. *J Bone Joint Surg Am* 1977;59(2): 174-179.

29. Ogden JA: The evaluation and treatment of partial physeal arrest. *J Bone Joint Surg Am* 1987;69(8): 1297-1302.

30. Paley D, Bhave A, Herzenberg JE, Bowen JR: Multiplier method for predicting limb-length discrepancy. *J Bone Joint Surg Am* 2000; 82-A(10):1432-1446.

31. Peterson HA: Partial growth plate arrest and its treatment. *J Pediatr Orthop* 1984;4(2):246-258.

32. Mehlman CT: Injuries to the lateral end of the clavicle and AC joint: A pediatric perspective. *J Am Osteo Acad Orthop* 1996; 33(3):82-90.

33. McGraw MA, Mehlman CT, Lindsell CJ, Kirby CL: Postnatal growth of the clavicle: Birth to 18 years of age. *J Pediatr Orthop* 2009;29(8):937-943.

34. Canadian Orthopaedic Trauma Society: Nonoperative treatment compared with plate fixation of displaced midshaft clavicular fractures: A multicenter, randomized clinical trial. *J Bone Joint Surg Am* 2007;89(1):1-10.

35. Mehlman CT, Yihua G, Bochang C, Zhigang W: Operative treatment of completely displaced clavicle shaft fractures in children. *J Pediatr Orthop* 2009;29(8): 851-855.

36. Vander Have KL, Perdue AM, Caird MS, Farley FA: Operative versus nonoperative treatment of midshaft clavicle fractures in adolescents. *J Pediatr Orthop* 2010; 30(4):307-312.

37. Altamimi SA, McKee MD; Canadian Orthopaedic Trauma Society: Nonoperative treatment compared with plate fixation of displaced midshaft clavicular fractures: Surgical technique. *J Bone Joint Surg Am* 2008;90(Suppl 2 Pt 1):1-8.

38. Qin D, Zhang Q, Zhang YZ, Pan JS, Chen W: Safe drilling angles and depths for plate-screw fixation of the clavicle: Avoidance of inadvertent iatrogenic subclavian neurovascular bundle injury. *J Trauma* 2010;69(1):162-168.

39. Mehlman CT, Wall EJ: Injuries to the shafts of the radius and ulna, in Beaty JH, Kasser JR, eds: *Rockwood and Wilkins' Fractures in Children*, ed 6. Philadelphia, PA, Lippincott Williams & Wilkins, 2006, pp 399-441.

40. Price CT, Scott DS, Kurzner ME, Flynn JC: Malunited forearm fractures in children. *J Pediatr Orthop* 1990;10(6):705-712.

41. Mehlman CT, Wall EJ: Injuries to the shafts of the radius and ulna, in Beaty JH, Kasser JR, eds: *Rockwood and Wilkins' Fractures in Children*, ed 7. Philadelphia, PA, Lippincott Williams & Wilkins, 2010, pp 347-402.

42. Younger AS, Tredwell SJ, Mackenzie WG, Orr JD, King PM, Tennant W: Accurate prediction of outcome after pediatric forearm fracture. *J Pediatr Orthop* 1994; 14(2):200-206.

43. Zionts LE, Zalavras CG, Gerhardt MB: Closed treatment of displaced diaphyseal both-bone forearm fractures in older children and adolescents. *J Pediatr Orthop* 2005;25(4):507-512.

44. Ağuş H, Kalenderer O, Eryanilmaz G, Omeroğlu H: Biological internal fixation of comminuted femur shaft fractures by bridge plating in children. *J Pediatr Orthop* 2003;23(2):184-189.

45. Aronson J, Tursky EA: External fixation of femur fractures in children. *J Pediatr Orthop* 1992; 12(2):157-163.

46. Bar-On E, Sagiv S, Porat S: External fixation or flexible intramedullary nailing for femoral shaft fractures in children: A prospective, randomised study. *J Bone Joint Surg Br* 1997;79(6):975-978.

47. Beaty JH, Austin SM, Warner WC, Canale ST, Nichols L: Interlocking intramedullary nailing of femoral-shaft fractures in adolescents: Preliminary results and complications. *J Pediatr Orthop* 1994;14(2):178-183.

48. Blasier RD, Aronson J, Tursky EA: External fixation of pediatric femur fractures. *J Pediatr Orthop* 1997;17(3):342-346.

49. Caird MS, Mueller KA, Puryear A, Farley FA: Compression plating of pediatric femoral shaft fractures. *J Pediatr Orthop* 2003; 23(4):448-452.

50. Czertak DJ, Hennrikus WL: The treatment of pediatric femur fractures with early 90-90 spica casting. *J Pediatr Orthop* 1999;19(2): 229-232.

51. Ferguson J, Nicol RO: Early spica treatment of pediatric femoral shaft fractures. *J Pediatr Orthop* 2000;20(2):189-192.

52. Flynn JM, Hresko T, Reynolds RA, Blasier RD, Davidson R, Kasser J: Titanium elastic nails for pediatric femur fractures: A multicenter study of early results with analysis of complications. *J Pediatr Orthop* 2001;21(1):4-8.

53. Kanellopoulos AD, Yiannakopoulos CK, Soucacos PN: Closed, locked intramedullary nailing of pediatric femoral shaft fractures through the tip of the greater trochanter. *J Trauma* 2006;60(1): 217-223.

54. Kregor PJ, Song KM, Routt ML Jr , Sangeorzan BJ, Liddell RM, Hansen ST Jr: Plate fixation of femoral shaft fractures

in multiply injured children. *J Bone Joint Surg Am* 1993; 75(12):1774-1780.

55. Ligier JN, Metaizeau JP, Prévot J, Lascombes P: Elastic stable intramedullary pinning of long bone shaft fractures in children. *Z Kinderchir* 1985;40(4):209-212.

56. Ligier JN, Metaizeau JP, Prévot J, Lascombes P: Elastic stable intramedullary nailing of femoral shaft fractures in children. *J Bone Joint Surg Br* 1988;70(1):74-77.

57. Stans AA, Morrissy RT, Renwick SE: Femoral shaft fracture treatment in patients age 6 to 16 years. *J Pediatr Orthop* 1999; 19(2):222-228.

58. Townsend DR, Hoffinger S: Intramedullary nailing of femoral shaft fractures in children via the trochanter tip. *Clin Orthop Relat Res* 2000;376:113-118.

59. Ward WT, Levy J, Kaye A: Compression plating for child and adolescent femur fractures. *J Pediatr Orthop* 1992;12(5):626-632.

60. Ziv I, Blackburn N, Rang M: Femoral intramedullary nailing in the growing child. *J Trauma* 1984;24(5):432-434.

61. Kocher MS, Sink EL, Blasier RD, et al: *Treatment of Pediatric Diaphyseal Femur Fractures: Guideline and Evidence Report.* Rosemont, IL, American Academy of Orthopaedic Surgeons, 2009.

62. Domb BG, Sponseller PD, Ain M, Miller NH: Comparison of dynamic versus static external fixation for pediatric femur fractures. *J Pediatr Orthop* 2002; 22(4):428-430.

63. Nork SE, Hoffinger SA: Skeletal traction versus external fixation for pediatric femoral shaft fractures: A comparison of hospital costs and charges. *J Orthop Trauma* 1998;12(8):563-568.

64. Miner T, Carroll KL: Outcomes of external fixation of pediatric femoral shaft fractures. *J Pediatr Orthop* 2000;20(3):405-410.

65. Skaggs DL, Leet AI, Money MD, Shaw BA, Hale JM, Tolo VT: Secondary fractures associated with external fixation in pediatric femur fractures. *J Pediatr Orthop* 1999;19(5):582-586.

66. Eren OT, Kucukkaya M, Kockesen C, Kabukcuoglu Y, Kuzgun U: Open reduction and plate fixation of femoral shaft fractures in children aged 4 to 10. *J Pediatr Orthop* 2003;23(2):190-193.

67. Flynn JM, Luedtke L, Ganley TJ, Pill SG: Titanium elastic nails for pediatric femur fractures: Lessons from the learning curve. *Am J Orthop (Belle Mead NJ)* 2002; 31(2):71-74.

68. Luhmann SJ, Schootman M, Schoenecker PL, Dobbs MB, Gordon JE: Complications of titanium elastic nails for pediatric femoral shaft fractures. *J Pediatr Orthop* 2003;23(4):443-447.

69. Moroz LA, Launay F, Kocher MS, et al: Titanium elastic nailing of fractures of the femur in children: Predictors of complications and poor outcome. *J Bone Joint Surg Br* 2006;88(10):1361-1366.

70. Rohde RS, Mendelson SA, Grudziak JS: Acute synovitis of the knee resulting from intra-articular knee penetration as a complication of flexible intramedullary nailing of pediatric femur fractures: Report of two cases. *J Pediatr Orthop* 2003;23(5):635-638.

71. Wall EJ, Jain V, Vora V, Mehlman CT, Crawford AH: Complications of titanium and stainless steel elastic nail fixation of pediatric femoral fractures. *J Bone Joint Surg Am* 2008;90(6):1305-1313.

72. Jencikova-Celerin L, Phillips JH, Werk LN, Wiltrout SA, Nathanson I: Flexible interlocked nailing of pediatric femoral fractures: Experience with a new flexible interlocking intramedullary nail compared with other fixation procedures. *J Pediatr Orthop* 2008; 28(8):864-873.

73. Keeler KA, Dart B, Luhmann SJ, et al: Antegrade intramedullary nailing of pediatric femoral fractures using an interlocking pediatric femoral nail and a lateral trochanteric entry point. *J Pediatr Orthop* 2009;29(4):345-351.

74. Momberger N, Stevens P, Smith J, Santora S, Scott S, Anderson J: Intramedullary nailing of femoral fractures in adolescents. *J Pediatr Orthop* 2000; 20(4):482-484.

75. Timmerman LA, Rab GT: Intramedullary nailing of femoral shaft fractures in adolescents. *J Orthop Trauma* 1993;7(4): 331-337.

76. Buckaloo JM, Iwinski HJ, Bertrand SL: Avascular necrosis of the femoral head after intramedullary nailing of a femoral shaft fracture in a male adolescent. *J South Orthop Assoc* 1997;6(2):97-100.

77. González-Herranz P, Burgos-Flores J, Rapariz JM, Lopez-Mondejar JA, Ocete JG, Amaya S: Intramedullary nailing of the femur in children: Effects on its proximal end. *J Bone Joint Surg Br* 1995;77(2):262-266.

78. Gordon JE, Swenning TA, Burd TA, Szymanski DA, Schoenecker PL: Proximal femoral radiographic changes after lateral transtrochanteric intramedullary nail placement in children. *J Bone Joint Surg Am* 2003;85-A(7): 1295-1301.

79. Letts M, Jarvis J, Lawton L, Davidson D: Complications of rigid intramedullary rodding of femoral shaft fractures in children. *J Trauma* 2002;52(3):504-516.

80. Mileski RA, Garvin KL, Huurman WW: Avascular necrosis of the femoral head after closed intramedullary shortening in an adolescent. *J Pediatr Orthop* 1995; 15(1):24-26.

81. Raney EM, Ogden JA, Grogan DP: Premature greater trochanteric epiphysiodesis secondary to intramedullary femoral rodding. *J Pediatr Orthop* 1993; 13(4):516-520.

82. Riseborough EJ, Barrett IR, Shapiro F: Growth disturbances following distal femoral physeal fracture-separations. *J Bone Joint Surg Am* 1983;65(7):885-893.

83. Edwards PH Jr , Grana WA: Physeal fractures about the knee. *J Am Acad Orthop Surg* 1995;3(2): 63-69.

84. Eid AM, Hafez MA: Traumatic injuries of the distal femoral physis: Retrospective study on 151 cases. *Injury* 2002;33(3):251-255.

85. Sferopoulos NK: Concomitant physeal fractures of the distal femur and proximal tibia. *Skeletal Radiol* 2005;34(7):427-430.

86. Zionts LE: Fractures around the knee in children. *J Am Acad Orthop Surg* 2002;10(5):345-355.

87. Basener CJ, Mehlman CT, DiPasquale TG: Growth disturbance after distal femoral growth plate fractures in children: A meta-analysis. *J Orthop Trauma* 2009; 23(9):663-667.

88. Ilharreborde B, Raquillet C, Morel E, et al: Long-term prognosis of Salter-Harris type 2 injuries of the distal femoral physis. *J Pediatr Orthop B* 2006;15(6):433-438.

89. Goldberg BA, Mansfield DS, Davino NA: Nonunion of a distal femoral epiphyseal fracture-separation. *Am J Orthop (Belle Mead NJ)* 1996;25(11):773-777.

90. Hart AJ, Eastwood DM, Dowd GS: Fixed flexion deformity of the knee following femoral physeal fracture: The Inverted Cyclops lesion. *Injury* 2004; 35(12):1330-1333.

91. Meyers MH, McKeever FM: Fracture of the intercondylar eminence of the tibia. *J Bone Joint Surg Am* 1959;41-A(2):209-222.

92. Zaricznyj B: Avulsion fracture of the tibial eminence: Treatment by open reduction and pinning. *J Bone Joint Surg Am* 1977;59(8): 1111-1114.

93. Kocher MS, Micheli LJ, Gerbino P, Hresko MT: Tibial eminence fractures in children: Prevalence of meniscal entrapment. *Am J Sports Med* 2003; 31(3):404-407.

94. Hirschmann MT, Mayer RR, Kentsch A, Friederich NF: Physeal sparing arthroscopic fixation of displaced tibial eminence fractures: A new surgical technique. *Knee Surg Sports Traumatol Arthrosc* 2009;17(7):741-747.

95. Kocher MS, Saxon HS, Hovis WD, Hawkins RJ: Management and complications of anterior cruciate ligament injuries in skeletally immature patients: Survey of the Herodicus Society and the ACL Study Group. *J Pediatr Orthop* 2002;22(4):452-457.

96. Mubarak SJ, Kim JR, Edmonds EW, Pring ME, Bastrom TP: Classification of proximal tibial fractures in children. *J Child Orthop* 2009;3(3): 191-197.

97. Cozen L: Fracture of the proximal portion of the tibia in children followed by valgus deformity. *Surg Gynecol Obstet* 1953;97(2):183-188.

98. Ogden JA, Tross RB, Murphy MJ: Fractures of the tibial tuberosity in adolescents. *J Bone Joint Surg Am* 1980;62(2):205-215.

99. Kay RM, Matthys GA: Pediatric ankle fractures: Evaluation and treatment. *J Am Acad Orthop Surg* 2001;9(4):268-278.

100. Mann DC, Rajmaira S: Distribution of physeal and nonphyseal fractures in 2,650 long-bone fractures in children aged 0-16 years. *J Pediatr Orthop* 1990;10(6): 713-716.

101. Rogers LF: The radiography of epiphyseal injuries. *Radiology* 1970;96(2):289-299.

102. Crawford AH, Al-Sayyad MJ, Mehlman CT: Fractures and dislocations of the foot and ankle, in Green NE, Swiontkowski MF, eds: *Skeletal Trauma in Children*, ed 4. Philadelphia, PA, Saunders, 2008, pp 507-584.

103. Cutler L, Molloy A, Dhukuram V, Bass A: Do CT scans aid assessment of distal tibial physeal fractures? *J Bone Joint Surg Br* 2004;86(2):239-243.

104. Horn BD, Crisci K, Krug M, Pizzutillo PD, MacEwen GD: Radiologic evaluation of juvenile tillaux fractures of the distal tibia. *J Pediatr Orthop* 2001;21(2):162-164.

105. Weber BG: *Die Verletzungen des oberen Sprunggelenkes.* Bern, Germany, Huber, 1966.

106. Danis R: Les fractures malleolaires, in Danis R, ed: *Théorie et Pratique de l'Osteosynthese.* Paris, France, Masson, 1949.

107. Lauge-Hansen N: Fractures of the ankle: II. Combined experimental-surgical and experimental-roentgenologic investigations. *Arch Surg* 1950; 60(5):957-985.

108. Lauge-Hansen N: Fractures of the ankle: IV. Clinical use of genetic roentgen diagnosis and genetic reduction. *AMA Arch Surg* 1952; 64(4):488-500.

109. Lauge-Hansen N: Fractures of the ankle: V. Pronation-dorsiflexion fracture. *AMA Arch Surg* 1953; 67(6):813-820.

110. Lauge-Hansen N: Fractures of the ankle: III. Genetic roentgenologic diagnosis of fractures of the ankle. *Am J Roentgenol Radium Ther Nucl Med* 1954;71(3):456-471.

111. Dias LS, Tachdjian MO: Physeal injuries of the ankle in children: Classification. *Clin Orthop Relat Res* 1978;136:230-233.

112. Vahvanen V, Aalto K: Classification of ankle fractures in children. *Arch Orthop Trauma Surg* 1980; 97(1):1-5.

113. Barmada A, Gaynor T, Mubarak SJ: Premature physeal closure following distal tibia physeal fractures: A new radiographic predictor. *J Pediatr Orthop* 2003;23(6): 733-739.

114. Kling TF Jr, Bright RW, Hensinger RN: Distal tibial physeal fractures in children that may require open reduction. *J Bone Joint Surg Am* 1984;66(5): 647-657.

115. Spiegel PG, Cooperman DR, Laros GS: Epiphyseal fractures of the distal ends of the tibia and fibula: A retrospective study of two hundred and thirty-seven cases in children. *J Bone Joint Surg Am* 1978; 60(8):1046-1050.

116. Berson L, Davidson RS, Dormans JP, Drummond DS, Gregg JR: Growth disturbances after distal tibial physeal fractures. *Foot Ankle Int* 2000;21(1):54-58.

117. Kärrholm J, Hansson LI, Laurin S, Selvik G: Post-traumatic growth disturbance of the ankle treated by the Langenskiöld procedure: Evaluation by radiography, roentgen stereophotogrammetry, scintimetry and histology. Case report. *Acta Orthop Scand* 1983;54(5):721-729.

118. Leary JT, Handling M, Talerico M, Yong L, Bowe JA: Physeal fractures of the distal tibia: Predictive factors of premature physeal closure and growth arrest. *J Pediatr Orthop* 2009;29(4):356-361.

119. Kleiger B, Mankin HJ: Fracture of the lateral portion of the distal tibial epiphysis. *J Bone Joint Surg Am* 1964;46:25-32.

120. Cooperman DR, Spiegel PG, Laros GS: Tibial fractures involving the ankle in children: The so-called triplane epiphyseal fracture. *J Bone Joint Surg Am* 1978;60(8): 1040-1046.

Video Reference

32.1: Parikh SN: Video. *Elastic Stable Intramedullary Nailing (ESIN) for Femoral Shaft Fracture.* Cincinnati, OH, 2010.

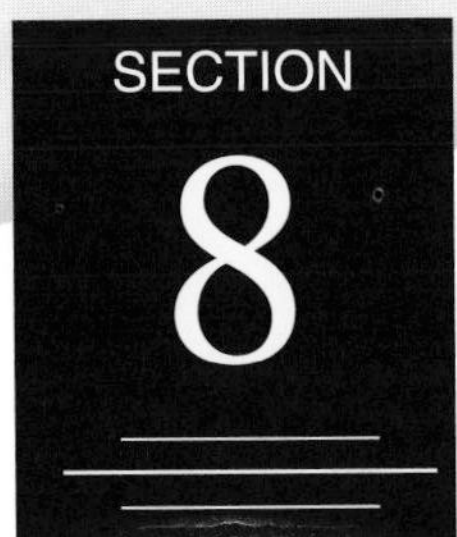

Sports Medicine

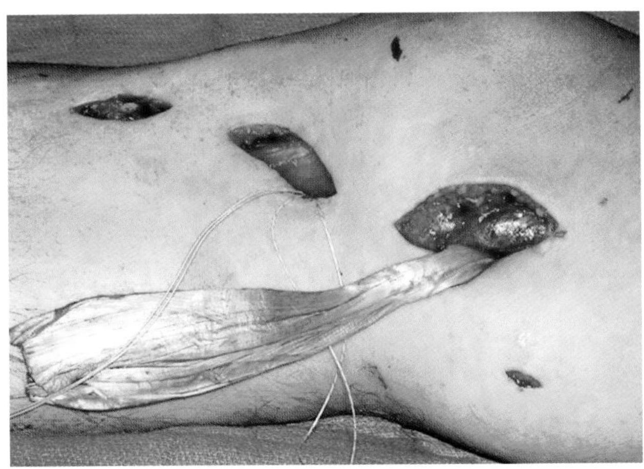

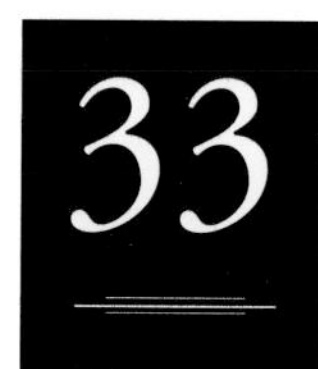

Repair of Complex and Avascular Meniscal Tears and Meniscal Transplantation

Frank R. Noyes, MD
Sue D. Barber-Westin, BS
Ryan C. Chen, MD

Abstract

A functional meniscus is critical to the long-term health of the knee joint. The repair of meniscal tears that extend into the central avascular region requires understanding the appropriate indications, contraindications, surgical techniques, and postoperative rehabilitation protocols. An inside-out repair technique using multiple vertical divergent sutures with an accessory posteromedial or posterolateral incision is recommended for optimal stability. In young, active patients, the risk of repair failure and the need for revision are outweighed by the benefit of meniscal preservation.

Although many meniscal tears are repairable, not all are salvageable, especially if considerable tissue damage has occurred. The goals of transplantation of human menisci are to restore partial load-bearing meniscal function, decrease patient symptoms, and provide chondroprotective effects. Clinical studies have shown that meniscal transplantation decreases tibiofemoral joint pain in the short term. The procedure remains in an evolving state with an unpredictable long-term outcome; however, most meniscal transplants gradually deteriorate, tear, or shrink in size over time, thereby losing the ability to provide function. The current goal is to provide short-term benefits to the patient until a superior meniscal transplant is clinically available.

Instr Course Lect 2011;60:415-437.

The importance of the menisci in the human knee is well understood. The menisci occupy 60% of the contact area between the tibial and femoral cartilage surfaces and transmit more than 50% of joint compression forces. Following meniscectomy, the tibiofemoral contact area decreases by approximately 50%, whereas the contact forces increase twofold to threefold.[1-6] The removal of as little as 15% to 34% of a meniscus increases contact pressures by more than 350%.[7] Total lateral meniscectomy results in a 45% to 50% decrease in the total contact area and a 235% to 335% increase in the peak local contact pressure.[8]

Meniscectomy frequently leads to irreparable joint damage, including degeneration of the articular cartilage, flattening of the articular surfaces, and subchondral bone sclerosis. Poor long-term clinical results following partial and total meniscectomy have been reported by many authors.[9-12] Trauma is one of the most common etiologies of meniscal tears. For example, 40% to 60% of patients who sustain a rupture of the anterior cruciate ligament also sustain a meniscal tear.[13,14] Many of these tears extend into the middle-third avascular region and are amenable to inside-out suture repair.

Meniscal tears are classified according to their location and type and the integrity of the tissue.[15] The meniscus is divided into anterior, middle, and posterior thirds as well as inner, middle, and outer thirds. Tears located at the peripheral attachment sites (meniscofemoral and meniscotibial) are referred to as outer-third, or red-red, tears. Tears located in the middle third are classified as either red-white or white-white tears. Red-white tears occur at the junction of the outer and middle thirds, approximately 4 mm from the meniscal attachment, with a vascular supply only in the outer third of the tear. White-white tears are located in the inner third, where there is no blood supply.

Single meniscal tears that occur in one plane are classified on the basis of

Dr. Noyes or an immediate family member serves as a board member, owner, officer, or committee member of the Cincinnati Sports Medicine Research and Education Foundation; has received royalties from Smith & Nephew; and has received research or institutional support from Arthrex, DePuy, DJ Orthopaedics, Genzyme, Mitek, Regeneration Technologies, Stryker, and AlloSource. Neither of the following authors nor any immediate family member has received anything of value from or owns stock in a commercial company or institution related directly or indirectly to the subject of this chapter: Ms. Barber-Westin and Dr. Chen.

Table 1
Indications and Contraindications for Meniscal Repair

Indications	Contraindications
Meniscal tear with tibiofemoral joint line pain	Tear in inner-third region (white-white)
Active patient younger than 60 years	Patient older than 60 years or sedentary (except those with a traumatic red-red tear that must be repaired to save the meniscus)
Concurrent knee ligament reconstruction or osteotomy	Patient unwilling to follow postoperative rehabilitation program
Meniscal tear reducible, good tissue integrity, normal position in joint once repaired	Chronic degenerative tear with tissue of poor quality not amenable to suture repair
Peripheral single longitudinal tear (red-red) in one plane; repairable in all cases, with high success rates	Longitudinal tear of < 10 mm in length
Red-white tear in middle-third region with vascular supply present	Incomplete radial tear that does not extend into outer-third region
Tear in outer- and middle-third regions (red-white) in one plane (longitudinal, radial, or horizontal); often repairable	
Complex tear in multiple planes (double or triple longitudinal or flap tear) in outer-third and middle-third regions (red-white); repair rather than excision	

their configuration, such as horizontal, radial, or longitudinal. Complex meniscal tears have components in multiple planes, including the vertical plane (double or triple longitudinal), vertical and horizontal planes, and vertical and radial planes (flap tears). MRI provides important information regarding the type of meniscal tear and the potential for repair to preserve function.[16]

Meniscal Repair

Indications and Contraindications

A comprehensive examination is conducted to assess gait, range of motion, tibiofemoral pain and crepitus, muscle strength, and ligament stability. Tibiofemoral joint-line tenderness is the primary indicator of a meniscal tear. Other clinical signs include pain on forced flexion, obvious meniscal displacement during joint compression, a lack of full extension, and a positive McMurray test.

Radiography should include a lateral view at 30° of flexion, a patellofemoral axial view, and a weight-bearing PA view at 45° of flexion. Full-length standing hip-knee-ankle weight-bearing radiographs are used as indicated to quantify varus or valgus malalignment. MRI may be done with a proton-density-weighted, high-resolution, fast spin-echo sequence to determine the status of the articular cartilage and the menisci.

The indications and contraindications for meniscal repair are shown in **Table 1**. Active patients in their second, third, or fourth decade of life are excellent candidates. Unstable red-white tears longer than 10 to 12 mm in the middle third of the meniscus should be considered for repair. The meniscal tissue should appear nearly normal, without secondary tears or fragmentation. The tear must be reducible at the time of arthroscopy, with adequate tear-site apposition. Patients must agree to comply with the postoperative rehabilitation program and avoid strenuous activities and deep knee flexion for 4 to 6 months.

Older, sedentary patients or those unwilling to comply with the postoperative rehabilitation protocol are treated with partial meniscectomy. Repair of inner-third white-white tears is not recommended. Middle-third white-white tears are repaired only when there is extension into this region from a red-red or red-white tear (a large flap tear). Repair is not appropriate for chronic degenerative tears, partial tears, or stable longitudinal tears less than 10 mm in length.

Surgical Techniques

Complications and deteriorating results have been reported following the use of all-inside meniscal fixation devices,[17-22] which have inferior failure, stiffness, and displacement properties compared with vertical sutures.[23,24] The lack of prospective, randomized level I clinical studies precludes definitive recommendations regarding the various devices that are currently available.[22,25] Therefore, this chapter focuses on suture repair techniques and outcomes. The surgical procedure has been described in the literature.[15]

A 30° arthroscope is used for standard intra-articular evaluation. A 70° arthroscope inserted through the notch allows visualization of the posterior peripheral meniscal attachment. The inside-out repair technique requires an accessory 3-cm posteromedial (**Figure 1**) or posterolateral (**Figure 2**) incision for safe suture retrieval. This exposure protects the neurovascular structures during suture retrieval and knot tying. The approach is per-

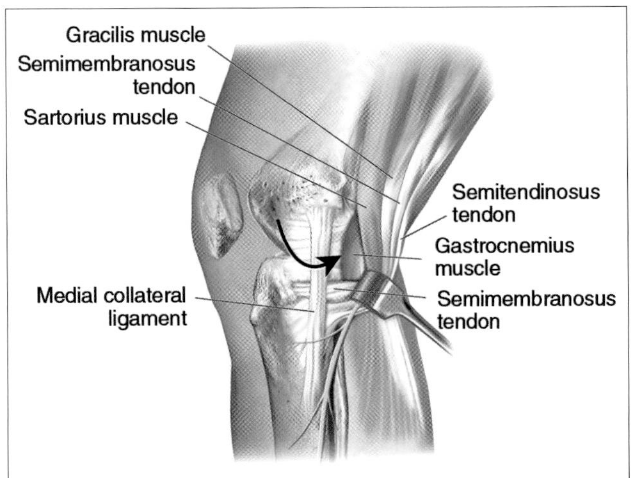

Figure 1 The accessory posteromedial approach for a repair of the medial meniscus. The interval is opened between the posteromedial aspect of the capsule and the gastrocnemius tendon, just proximal to the semimembranosus tendon (arrow). The fascia over the semimembranosus tendon is excised to its tibial attachment to facilitate retrieval of the posterior meniscal sutures. (Reproduced with permission from Noyes FR, Barber-Westin SD: Meniscus tears: Diagnosis, repair techniques, clinical outcomes, in Noyes FR, Barber-Westin SD, eds: *Noyes' Knee Disorders: Surgery, Rehabilitation, Clinical Outcomes*. Philadelphia, PA, WB Saunders, 2009, pp 733-771.)

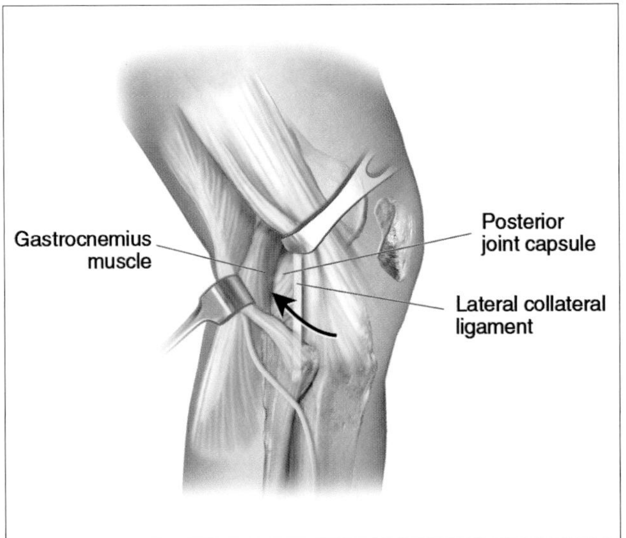

Figure 2 The accessory posterolateral approach for a repair of the lateral meniscus. The interval between the lateral aspect of the gastrocnemius and the posterolateral aspect of the capsule is opened bluntly, just proximal to the fibular head (arrow), avoiding penetration of the joint capsule. (Reproduced with permission from Noyes FR, Barber-Westin SD: Meniscus tears: Diagnosis, repair techniques, clinical outcomes, in Noyes FR, Barber-Westin SD, eds: *Noyes' Knee Disorders: Surgery, Rehabilitation, Clinical Outcomes*. Philadelphia, PA, WB Saunders, 2009, pp 733-771.)

formed under tourniquet control with the surgeon seated and using a headlight and the sterile prepared foot placed in the surgeon's lap. A popliteal retractor (Stryker, Kalamazoo, MI) is used to protect the popliteal neurovascular structures (**Figure 3**).

The 30° arthroscope is placed through the anteromedial portal for repairs of the medial meniscus and through the anterolateral portal for repairs of tears of the posterior third of the lateral meniscus. The meniscal tear is first carefully inspected to determine that good-quality meniscal tissue remains. The superior and inferior synovial attachments of the meniscus are rasped, and the tear edges are débrided to remove loose fragments. Often, there are remaining meniscal fragments at the outer meniscal tear region that require débridement to obtain a good perpendicular meniscal bed for suture fixation.

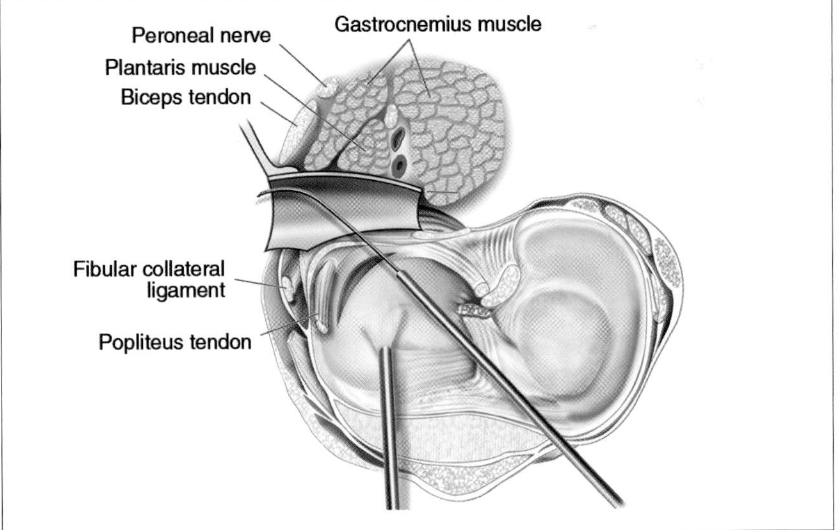

Figure 3 Cross section showing a popliteal retractor between the lateral aspect of the gastrocnemius and the posterior aspect of the capsule. A curved suture cannula is also used to angle the needles away from the neurovascular structures. (Reproduced with permission from Noyes FR, Barber-Westin SD: Meniscus tears: Diagnosis, repair techniques, clinical outcomes, in Noyes FR, Barber-Westin SD, eds: *Noyes' Knee Disorders: Surgery, Rehabilitation, Clinical Outcomes*. Philadelphia, PA, WB Saunders, 2009, pp 733-771.)

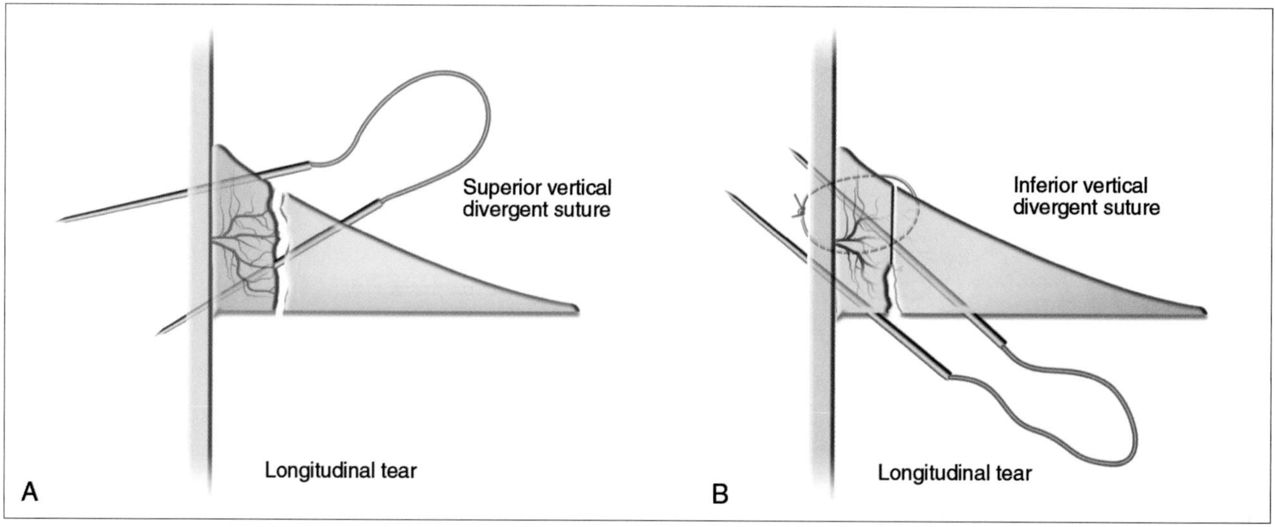

Figure 4 Double-stacked vertical suture pattern used for the repair of longitudinal meniscal tears. **A,** The superior sutures are placed first to close the superior gap and reduce the meniscus to its bed. **B,** The inferior sutures are then placed through the tear to close the inferior gap. (Reproduced with permission from Noyes FR, Barber-Westin SD: Meniscus tears: Diagnosis, repair techniques, clinical outcomes, in Noyes FR, Barber-Westin SD, eds: *Noyes' Knee Disorders: Surgery, Rehabilitation, Clinical Outcomes.* Philadelphia, PA, WB Saunders, 2009, pp 733-771.)

A single-barrel curved or straight cannula (Richard Wolf Medical Instruments, Vernon Hills, IL) is placed in the opposite portal for suture advancement. Curved cannulae are used to direct suture needles away from the midline neurovascular structures. After anatomic reduction of the tear edges, multiple vertical divergent sutures are advanced, retrieved through the accessory posterior incision, and tied directly to the posterior aspect of the capsule. The first vertical sutures are placed at the superior border of the meniscal tear to reduce the meniscus and prevent superior migration when inferior sutures are placed. Sutures are placed every 3 to 5 mm along the tear edges in both a superior and an inferior plane. The close interval between the sutures is required to maintain tear-site reduction during the prolonged time needed for healing of these avascular repairs. The repair is performed with multiple No. 2-0 braided polyester nonabsorbable sutures (Ticron; Davis and Geck, Danbury, CT) or Ethibond (Ethicon, Somerville, NJ) on double-loaded 10-inch (25.4-cm) needles.

For tears in the middle third of the meniscus, sutures are passed through the opposite portal with use of a 60° curved suture passer. The skin is undermined for suture retrieval. Tears in the anterior third are managed with a small skin incision, dissection down to the anterior meniscal attachment, and an outside-in repair.

A double-stacked technique is used for single longitudinal tears (**Figure 4**). Superior (femoral surface) sutures are placed first to reduce the meniscus to its bed, and inferior (tibial surface) sutures are then placed to approximate the inferior portion of the tear. The same technique is used for double longitudinal tears in which the outer tear is near the meniscocapsular junction and the inner tear is near the red-white junction (**Figure 5**). The peripheral tear is repaired first, followed by the central tear, which is repaired with vertical divergent sutures that span both tear sites (**Figure 6**).

Radial tears that extend to the outer third of the meniscus and the periphery of the meniscal attachment may be repaired. Horizontal sutures are used to reduce these tears anatomically and are placed at 2- to 4-mm intervals. Three or four sutures are placed superiorly, and one or two sutures are placed inferiorly. The inner tear is repaired first, after which the peripheral tear is repaired (**Figure 7**). Repair of a flap tear is indicated when the tear extends to the red-white junction or the periphery. Flap tears are managed by first repairing the radial component with horizontal sutures and then repairing the longitudinal component (**Figure 8**).

Strategies to Augment Healing

Experimental studies have demonstrated that avascular meniscal tears do not heal spontaneously.[26-29] Therefore, techniques to promote a healing response are considered essential in the management of these injuries. A fibrin clot has been used, with varying success, by some authors[29-31] to provide a reparative scaffold that supplies growth factors to promote chemotaxis, cell proliferation, and matrix synthesis to the tear site. Another technique is

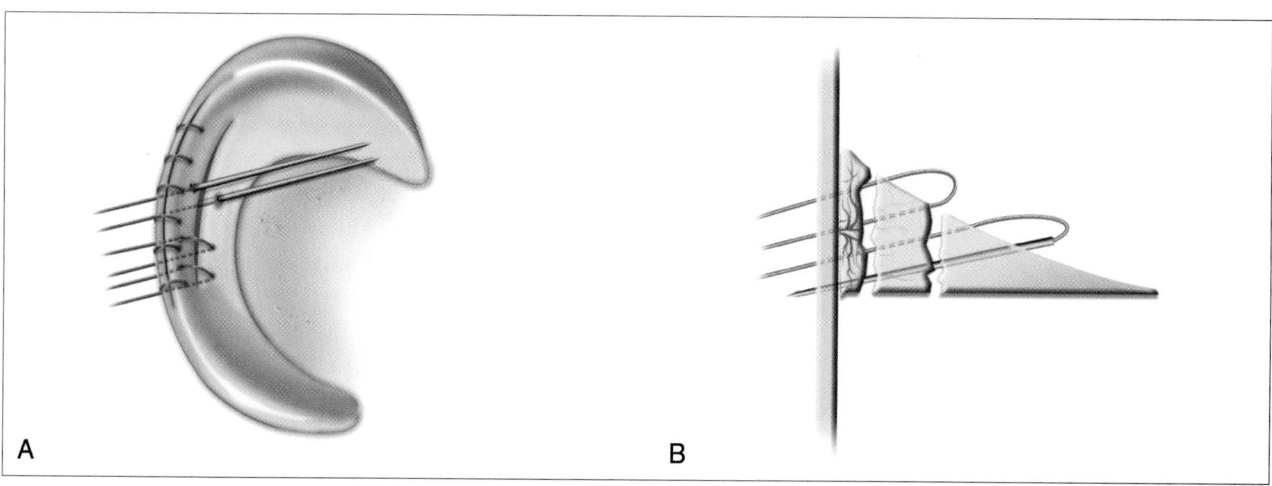

Figure 5 Double-stacked repair technique for double longitudinal tears. **A,** The peripheral tear is stabilized first with superior vertical divergent sutures. **B,** This is followed by repair of the inner tear in the same fashion. (Reproduced with permission from Noyes FR, Barber-Westin SD: Meniscus tears: Diagnosis, repair techniques, clinical outcomes, in Noyes FR, Barber-Westin SD, eds: *Noyes' Knee Disorders: Surgery, Rehabilitation, Clinical Outcomes*. Philadelphia, PA, WB Saunders, 2009, pp 733-771.)

trephination, in which radially oriented channels to the peripheral vascular supply are created to encourage vascular and cell migration to the tear site. Again, reports on healing after this technique have demonstrated variable outcomes. For example, Scott et al[32] reported an increase in the overall rate of healing of both medial and lateral menisci from 54.8% to 64% after the introduction of a technique involving dissection of the parameniscal synovial membrane. Zhang et al[33] reported a rerupture rate of only 5% in a group of 36 patients treated with suture repair as well as trephination.

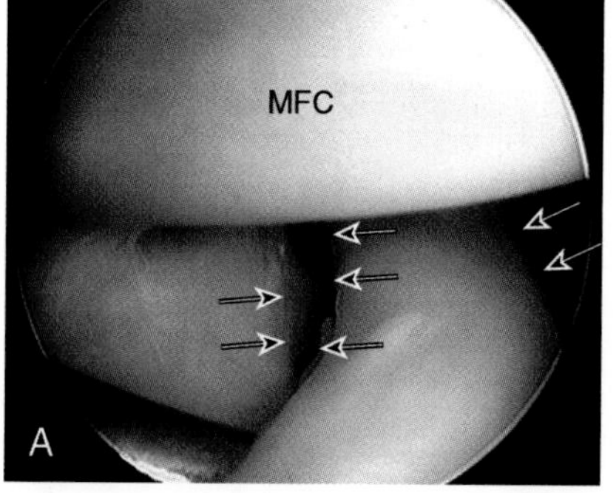

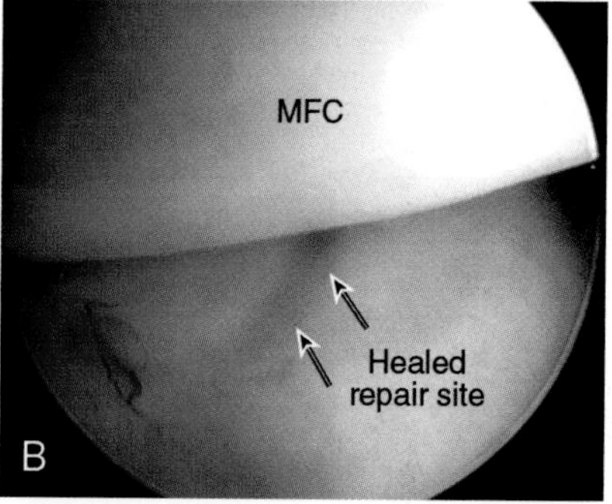

Figure 6 **A,** A double longitudinal medial meniscal tear consisting of a peripheral tear and another tear at the red-white junction (arrows). Because removal of the red-white tear and repair of the peripheral tear would have resulted in substantial loss of meniscal function, both tears were repaired. **B,** Healing of the tears was seen on arthroscopy performed 1 year later. MFC = medial femoral condyle. (Reproduced with permission from Noyes FR, Barber-Westin SD: Meniscus tears: Diagnosis, repair techniques, clinical outcomes, in Noyes FR, Barber-Westin SD, eds: *Noyes' Knee Disorders: Surgery, Rehabilitation, Clinical Outcomes*. Philadelphia, PA, WB Saunders, 2009, pp 733-771.)

Rasping of the vascularized parameniscal synovium promotes an injury response to assist healing. A few studies have shown that, following the use of this technique, synovial cells migrate to the site of an avascular meniscal tear[26,34] and result in superior healing compared with that following the use of a fibrin clot.[31] In a clinical study of the results of 81 inside-out repairs with parameniscal synovial rasping for tears with a 3- to 5-mm rim, Henning et al[35] reported a failure rate of only 9%. Rasping of the meniscal surface has been shown to induce the expression of cytokines, such as interleukin-1α, platelet-derived growth factor, and transforming growth factor-β1.[36] The expression of these chemotactic and mitogenic factors may facilitate meniscal healing.

Cell-based therapy involves transfer of tissue-engineered cells seeded onto scaffolds to augment healing. One study showed that implantation of an allogenic meniscal scaffold seeded with autologous articular chondrocytes along with a repair in a porcine model resulted in gross and histologic evidence of healing in all specimens.[37] In contrast, no healing was seen in three control groups: one treated with a scaf-

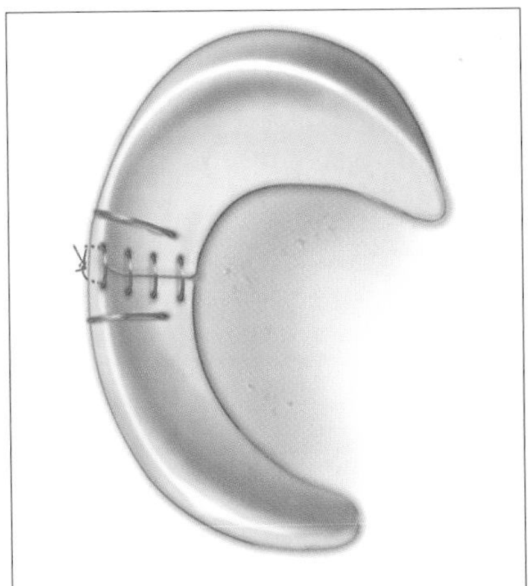

Figure 7 Repair technique for radial meniscal tears. The inner sutures are placed first, followed by the peripheral sutures. The first suture needle is placed midway through the meniscal body and then used to apply circumferential tension to reduce the tear gap; it is then advanced through the posterior aspect of the meniscal bed. The second suture needle is placed in a similar manner. This reduces the radial gap, allowing subsequent sutures to be placed. Usually, three or four sutures are placed superiorly and two sutures are placed inferiorly. Occasionally, superior vertical divergent sutures are placed along the tear site to help stabilize the repair. (Reproduced with permission from Noyes FR, Barber-Westin SD: Meniscus tears: Diagnosis, repair techniques, clinical outcomes, in Noyes FR, Barber-Westin SD, eds: *Noyes' Knee Disorders: Surgery, Rehabilitation, Clinical Outcomes.* Philadelphia, PA, WB Saunders, 2009, pp 733-771.)

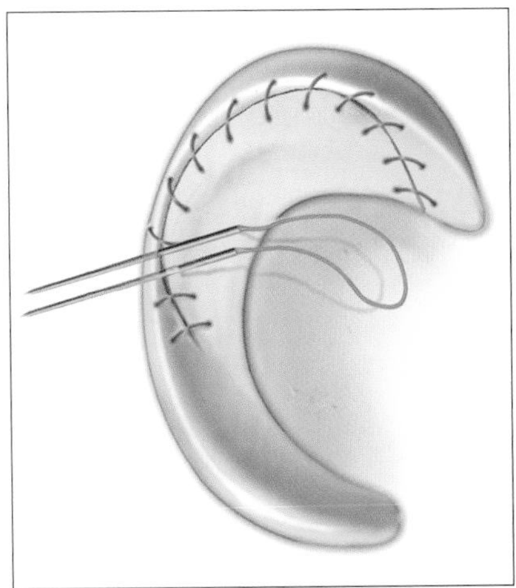

Figure 8 Repair technique for flap tears. The tear is identified and reduced. Horizontal tension sutures are placed first to anchor the radial component of the tear. The longitudinal component is then sutured with use of the double-stacked suture technique. (Reproduced with permission from Noyes FR, Barber-Westin SD: Meniscus tears: Diagnosis, repair techniques, clinical outcomes, in Noyes FR, Barber-Westin SD, eds: *Noyes' Knee Disorders: Surgery, Rehabilitation, Clinical Outcomes.* Philadelphia, PA, WB Saunders, 2009, pp 733-771.)

fold with repair, one treated with a repair alone, and one treated with no repair. In another study,[38] autologous and allogenic chondrocytes were seeded onto a bioabsorbable mesh to treat avascular porcine meniscal lesions; there was complete or partial healing in all animals, whereas there was no healing with repair alone or no treatment. Mesenchymal stem cells are appealing because of their potentially unlimited supply and ability to differentiate into specific therapeutic cell types.[39,40] Steinert et al[40] genetically modified bovine meniscal and mesenchymal stem cells to produce transforming growth factor-β1. The cells were inserted by means of a scaffold into explanted avascular meniscal repair sites. Both cell types resulted in cell proliferation, increased synthesis of proteoglycan and collagen, and histologic evidence of healing.

Growth factors promote cell maturation, differentiation, and proliferation and hold promise for healing of avascular tears. In a sheep model, meniscal fibrochondrocytes from the avascular region responded to basic fibroblast growth factor by proliferating and creating a new extracellular matrix.[41] DNA formation increased sevenfold, and protein synthesis increased 15-fold. Other authors have identified transforming growth factor-β1 as being effective at stimulating extracellular matrix production by rabbit meniscal fibrochondrocytes.[42]

The use of platelet-rich plasma as a healing adjunct has recently generated interest. Platelet-rich plasma contains a multitude of growth factors in physiologic proportions, which may be better than using isolated growth factors. Platelet-rich plasma may stimulate chemotaxis, cell proliferation, and angiogenesis. Ishida et al[43] reported that platelet-rich plasma improved healing of avascular meniscal defects, as determined on the basis of histologic criteria, in a rabbit model. Furthermore, in vitro analysis revealed enhanced extracellular matrix synthesis and proliferative behavior with platelet-rich plasma. Not all growth factors have been successful at promoting meniscal healing.[44,45] The ideal growth factor or combination of factors, dosage, and delivery mechanism as well as the potential side effects require further study. More information on techniques to enhance healing potential in avascular meniscal tears is available in chapter 35.

Postoperative Rehabilitation

The rehabilitation program following the repair of complex and avascular meniscal tears is summarized in **Table 2.**[46] Immediate knee motion from 0° to 90° is permitted. The goal is a range of motion of 0° to 90° by 7 to 10 days, 120° by 3 to 4 weeks, and 135° by 5 to 6 weeks. Protected, partial weight bearing for 4 weeks is recommended, with up to 6 weeks of toe-touch weight bearing when the patient had a radial tear. No squatting or deep flexion activities are permitted for 4 to 6 months, and running, jumping, and cutting are restricted for 6 months.

Table 2
Summary of Rehabilitation Protocol Following Repair of Meniscus Tears Extending Into the Avascular Region

	Postoperative Weeks					Postoperative Months			
	1-2	3-4	5-6	7-8	9-12	4	5	6	7-12
Brace: long-leg postoperative	X	X	X						
Range of motion minimum goals:									
0°-90°	X								
0°-120°		X							
0°-135°			X						
Weight bearing:									
Toe touch to one fourth body weight	X								
One half to three fourths body weight		X							
Full			X						
Patella mobilization	X	X	X						
Stretching: hamstring, gastrocnemius-soleus, iliotibial band, quadriceps	X	X	X	X	X	X	X	X	X
Strengthening:									
Quadriceps isometrics, straight leg raises, active knee extension	X	X	X	X	X	X	X	X	X
Closed-chain: gait retraining, toe raises, wall sits, minisquats			X	X	X	X	X	X	
Knee flexion hamstring curls (90°)				X	X	X	X	X	X
Knee extension quadriceps exercises (90°-30°)			X	X	X	X	X	X	X
Hip abduction-adduction			X	X	X	X	X	X	X
Leg press (70°-10°)					X	X	X	X	X
Balance-proprioceptive training: weight-shifting, minitrampoline, BAPS, BBS, plyometrics			X	X	X	X	X	X	X
Conditioning:									
Upper body ergometer		X	X	X					
Stationary bicycle				X	X	X	X	X	X
Aquatic program					X	X	X	X	X
Swimming (kicking)					X	X	X	X	X
Walking					X	X	X	X	X
Stair-climbing machine					X	X	X	X	X
Ski machine								X	X
Running: straight[a]								X	X
Cutting: lateral carioca, figure-of-8[a]									X
Full sports activity[a]									X

BAPS = Biomechanical Ankle Platform System (Camp, Jackson, MI), BBS = Biodex Balance System (Biodex, Shirley, NY).

[a]The return to running, cutting, and full sports activity is based on multiple criteria. Patients with noteworthy damage to the articular cartilage are advised to return to only light recreational activities.

(Reproduced with permission from Heckmann T, Noyes FR, Barber-Westin SD: Rehabilitation of meniscus repair and transplantation procedures, in Noyes FR, Barber-Westin SD, eds: *Noyes' Knee Disorders: Surgery, Rehabilitation, Clinical Outcomes.* Philadelphia, PA, WB Saunders, 2009, pp 806-817.)

Table 3
Rates of Reoperation Caused by Tibiofemoral Joint Symptoms Following Meniscal Repairs

Type of Meniscal Tear	Total No. of Meniscal Tears	No. Requiring Reoperation
Single longitudinal	92	11 (12%)
Double longitudinal	40	11 (28%)
Complex multiplanar	26	7 (27%)
Radial	15	4 (27%)
Horizontal	14	4 (29%)
Flap	9	2 (22%)
Triple longitudinal	2	0
Total	198	39 (20%)

(Adapted with permission from Rubman MH, Noyes FR, Barber-Westin SD: Arthroscopic repair of the meniscal tears that extend into the avascular zone: A review of 198 single and complex tears. Am J Sports Med 1998;26(1):87-95.)

Clinical Outcomes

Several prospective studies have documented the experiences of two of this chapter's authors (FRN and SDB-W) and other researchers with inside-out avascular meniscal repair, beginning in 1983. The first investigation included 66 patients who underwent a concomitant meniscal repair and anterior cruciate ligament reconstruction, followed by arthroscopy 6 to 25 months postoperatively.[47] There were a total of 79 meniscal repairs; 51 were done for tears located in the outer third of the meniscus, and 28 were done for complex tears that extended into the middle third. Follow-up arthroscopy was indicated for symptoms related to either tibial hardware or tibiofemoral joint pain. A surgeon who had not been involved in the care of the patients reviewed the arthroscopic videotapes and surgical records.

Of the repaired tears located in the outer third of the meniscus, 94% were classified as completely healed; 4% as partially healed; and 2% as failed. Of the repaired tears in the middle third, 54% were classified as completely healed; 32% as partially healed; and 14% as failed. The use of immediate knee motion and early weight bearing was not deleterious to the healing of the meniscal repairs. This was one of the first investigations to demonstrate that the repair of meniscal tears that are located either in the outer third or extend into the middle third have a satisfactory rate of healing when the procedure is warranted on clinical grounds.

Another prospective study determined the clinical outcomes of treatment of 198 meniscal tears (in 177 patients) that extended into the middle third of the meniscus or that had a rim width of 4 mm or more.[48] Either a clinical examination at a minimum of 2 years postoperatively or follow-up arthroscopy was necessary for inclusion in the study. One hundred twenty-six of the patients (71%) were treated with anterior cruciate ligament reconstruction at the time of the meniscal repair (96 patients) or at a mean of 22 weeks after the repair (30 patients).

The overall rate of reoperations because of tibiofemoral symptoms was 20% (39 meniscal repairs). All patients who had tibiofemoral pain had follow-up arthroscopy. The reoperation rates according to the type of tear are shown in **Table 3**.[48] The limited number of meniscal tears in the individual classification categories prevented the formulation of specific conclusions regarding the outcome for each tear pattern.

The effect of six factors on healing rates of meniscal repairs was evaluated in the study[48] (**Table 4**). The rates of healing were significantly affected by three factors: the tibiofemoral compartment of the meniscal repair (with the healing rate being higher after the lateral meniscal repairs than after the medial meniscal repairs), the time from the repair to the follow-up arthroscopy (with the patients evaluated 12 months or less postoperatively having a higher healing rate than those evaluated more than 12 months postoperatively), and the presence of tibiofemoral symptoms at the time of follow-up (with asymptomatic patients having a higher healing rate than symptomatic patients). The results of this investigation support a recommendation of repairing meniscal tears that extend into the middle third of the meniscus, especially in patients in their third or fourth decade of life and in competitive athletes. The reoperation rate in the study should not be interpreted as the rate of meniscal healing.

A third prospective study was performed to determine the outcome of meniscal tears that extended into the avascular region in patients age 40 years or older.[49] Thirty of 31 consecutive meniscal repairs in 29 patients were followed with either a clinical examination or arthroscopy. Anterior cruciate ligament reconstruction was performed at the time of the meniscal repair in 21 patients (72%).

There were no tibiofemoral joint symptoms and no need for additional surgery at the time of follow-up after 26 meniscal repairs (87%). The tibiofemoral compartment of the meniscal repair, the chronicity of the injury, concomitant anterior cruciate ligament reconstruction, or the condition

Table 4
Effect of Various Factors on Healing Rates of Meniscal Repairs That Had Follow-up Arthroscopy

Factor	Number of Tears		
	Healed	Partially Healed	Failed
Tibiofemoral compartment of meniscal repair[a]			
Medial (n = 47)	8	15	24
Lateral (n = 44)	15	20	9
Time from meniscal repair to follow-up arthroscopy[b]			
≤ 12 months (n = 61)	18	27	16
> 12 months (n = 30)	5	8	17
Timing of anterior cruciate ligament reconstruction			
With meniscal repair (n = 39)	12	18	9
After meniscal repair (n = 27)	9	11	7
Presence of tibiofemoral compartment symptoms at time of follow-up[c]			
Symptomatic (n = 39)	2	13	24
Asymptomatic (n = 52)	21	22	9
Time from original knee injury to meniscal repair[d]			
≤ 10 weeks (n = 33)	13	10	10
> 10 weeks (n = 58)	10	25	23
Patient age			
< 25 years (n = 44)	13	17	14
≥ 25 years (n = 47)	10	18	19

[a]The success rate for lateral compartment tears was significantly higher than that for medial compartment tears ($P = 0.008$).
[b]The success rate was significantly higher when the follow-up arthroscopy was done at 12 months or earlier than when it was done at more than 12 months ($P = 0.02$).
[c]The success rate was significantly higher when there were no tibiofemoral symptoms than when there were symptoms ($P = 0.0001$).
[d]The success rate was higher when the time from the original knee injury had been less than or equal to 10 weeks than when it had been more than 10 weeks ($P = 0.06$).

of the articular cartilage was not found to have a significant association with the presence of tibiofemoral pain at the time of follow-up or the need for a meniscal resection. There were no infections, knee motion problems, cases of saphenous neuritis, or other major complications. This study showed that repair of complex tears in older adults is feasible, and that most patients do not have tibiofemoral joint symptoms at an average of 3 years postoperatively.

In a fourth prospective study, the results of 71 of 74 consecutive meniscal repairs (a 96% follow-up rate) that had been done in 58 patients (64 knees) younger than 20 years were evaluated.[50] Fifty-four knees (84%) were in patients who had reached skeletal maturity. Forty-three meniscal repairs (61%) in 36 knees were performed concurrently with an anterior cruciate ligament reconstruction, and 14 meniscal repairs (20%) in 11 knees were done at a mean of 34 weeks before an anterior cruciate ligament reconstruction. All patients who had an anterior cruciate ligament reconstruction were skeletally mature. The initial follow-up evaluation, at a mean of 51 months postoperatively, showed no tibiofemoral symptoms or failure requiring resection after 53 (75%) of the 71 meniscal repairs.

From this study, a subgroup of 29 meniscal repairs of single longitudinal tears that extended into the avascular zone were further evaluated.[50] Clinical evaluation was conducted in 19 cases (at a mean of 16.8 ± 3.3 years postoperatively), MRI was done in 17 (at a mean of 17.2 years), and weight-bearing PA radiographs were made in 22 (at a mean of 16.8 ± 3.2 years). The results were determined with two validated knee rating systems and the assessment of radiographs and medical records by independent physicians and researchers. A 3-tesla MRI scanner with cartilage-sensitive pulse sequences, including T2 mapping, was used to study cartilage degeneration and repair site characteristics. Eighteen of the 29 meniscal repairs (62%) were successful, with retention of a meniscus that appeared to be functional. Six repairs required meniscal resection, two knees showed loss of joint space on radiographs, and three repairs failed according to MRI criteria. There were no significant differences between the short- and long-term results in terms of the mean scores for pain, swelling, and jumping; the patient's grade of the overall knee condition; or the overall Cincinnati knee rating score.

The results of this long-term evaluation support the recommendation of repair of simple or complex meniscal tears that extend into the avascular zone when the appropriate indications are present.[50] This recommendation is particularly appropriate for young, active individuals in whom removal of a meniscal tear that extends into the middle avascular region would result in major loss of meniscal function and an increased risk of future joint arthritis. Advanced MRI and weight-bearing PA radiographs are essential in determining the actual failure rate and chondroprotective effects of meniscal repairs.

The clinical outcomes of meniscal repairs from other recently published investigations[20,21,51-66] are summarized in **Table 5**. Most of these studies focused on vertical meniscal suture repair techniques; few authors reported on the outcome of horizontal suture repair or all-inside fixators. The rates of failure of vertical and horizontal suture repairs vary greatly, as do correlations with the side of the meniscal tear, concurrent anterior cruciate ligament reconstruction, the location of the meniscal tear, and patient age and sex.

Investigations of newer all-inside suture systems such as the RapidLoc (DePuy Mitek, Raynham, MA), the MaxFire Meniscal Repair Device (Biomet, Warsaw, IN), and FasT-Fix (Smith & Nephew Endoscopy, Andover, MA) have shown acceptable failure rates between 9% and 13%.[51,52,58,60,66-68] However, longer-term follow-up of the results associated with these systems is required to ensure that the rate of failure does not increase with time. In addition, this chapter's authors believe that the use of only two or three sutures, as practiced with all-inside suture systems, provides inadequate stabilization and is inferior to the use of multiple vertical divergent sutures.

Complications and deteriorating results were reported following the early use of all-inside fixation devices.[17-21,67] Lee and Diduch[17] reported an increasing rate of failure with time in 28 patients who had undergone meniscal repair with the Meniscus Arrow (Bionx Implants, Blue Bell, PA) and a concomitant anterior cruciate ligament reconstruction. The initial success rate of 90.6% reported at a mean of 2.3 years postoperatively decreased to 71.4% at 6.6 years. Complications with this device, such as chondral damage, cyst formation, chronic effusions, joint irritation, synovitis, and device breakage and migration into the extra-articular soft tissues, have been reported by several authors.[18-20,69-74]

The question of whether meniscal repair is effective in preventing joint deterioration remains unanswered. However, the well-documented irreparable joint damage and the poor results of long-term clinical studies following partial and total meniscectomy indicate that preservation of meniscal tissue is paramount for long-term joint function. It is our opinion that the gold standard technique is a meticulous inside-out repair with multiple vertical divergent sutures and an accessory posteromedial or posterolateral approach to tie the sutures directly posterior to the meniscus attachment. Meniscal repair is as important as, if not more important than, an anterior cruciate ligament reconstruction with regard to the long-term knee function of patients who sustain these concomitant injuries. Often, a complex meniscal repair will take as long as an anterior cruciate ligament reconstruction, and the surgeon should allow for sufficient time when planning the surgical procedure.

The approach of leaving a meniscal tear that is longer than 10 to 12 mm untreated at the time of anterior cruciate ligament reconstruction is not recommended. To use a conservative approach and hope for healing may risk further tearing and subsequent loss of meniscal function. Once a meniscectomy has been performed in a young patient, there are few additional options. It is unfortunate that many patients requiring meniscal transplantation had ineffective original treatment of the meniscal tear; either a large tear was not treated or was repaired with too few sutures or with fixators that provided only limited stability, or a major tear that extended into the middle avascular region was removed when it could have been repaired.

A fibrin clot technique was not used in studies conducted by two of this chapter's authors (FRN and SDB-W) because the clot would have interfered with the exact millimeter-to-millimeter reduction and fixation at the meniscal tear site with the suture technique that was performed.[47-50] In the future, tissue engineering may increase the success rates of meniscal repairs of tears that extend into the avascular region.[75-79] Cell-based therapy involving meniscal fibrochondrocytes, articular chondrocytes, or mesenchymal stem cells seeded onto scaffolds offer promise, as does the introduction of growth factors into the repair site.[80,81]

Meniscal Transplantation

Concepts

Although many meniscal tears are repairable, as previously discussed, not all torn menisci are salvageable, especially if considerable tissue damage has occurred. The goals of transplantation of human menisci are to restore the load-bearing function of the meniscus, decrease symptoms, and provide chondroprotective effects.[82-86] Even though the procedure was first described more than 25 years ago,[87] it remains in an evolving state with unpredictable and often undesirable long-term outcomes. Clinical studies have shown that meniscal transplantation decreases tibiofemoral joint pain in the short term. However, most meniscal transplants gradually deteriorate, tear, or shrink, thereby losing the ability to provide function. Therefore, the current goal is to provide short-term benefits to the patient until a superior meniscal transplant is clinically available.

Indications and Contraindications

The clinical evaluation of a candidate for meniscal transplantation is the same as that described for a candidate for meniscal repair. The indications and contraindications for this procedure are shown in **Table 6**. The optimal candidate is a patient 50 years or younger who had a total meniscectomy, has pain with daily activities, and demonstrates early deterioration of the articular cartilage in the involved tibiofemoral compartment. There should be no radiographic evidence of advanced arthritis in the tibiofemoral joint. At least 2 mm of tibiofemoral joint space should be visible on the 45° weight-bearing PA radiograph.[88] Arthroscopic examination confirms that a patient is a suitable candidate for meniscal transplantation. Normal axial alignment and a stable joint are required. The body mass index must be within the normal range.

Advanced knee joint arthritis with flattening of the femoral condyle, concavity of the tibial plateau, and osteophytes that prevent anatomic seating of the meniscal transplant are contraindications. Untreated lower limb malalignment and knee joint instability are associated with poor outcomes of meniscal transplantation. Preexisting knee arthrofibrosis, severe lower limb muscular atrophy, and a history of joint infection with subsequent arthritis are all contraindications. Symptomatic noteworthy deterioration of the patellofemoral articular cartilage (exposure of subchondral bone) and obesity (a body mass index of > 30 kg/m^2) are also contraindications.

Transplant Sizing

Radiographic criteria for the sizing of meniscal transplants established by Pollard et al[89] is used, and secondary sterilization with irradiation is avoided. The medial meniscal transplant cannot be oversized in its medial-to-lateral dimension because this would prevent use of the slot technique and the preferable bone-bridge transplant technique, which maintains the native geometry of the implant. The medial meniscus may have a thin or narrow anterior-third attachment distal to the tibial joint surface, which is not acceptable. The lateral meniscus may have a diminutive (8- to 10-mm) middle-third anatomic configuration, which also is not suitable for transplantation. The transplant is inspected before the patient is anesthetized, and preoperative planning involves advising the patient that, in rare instances, the transplant may not be suitable and thus may prevent the surgical procedure from commencing.

Surgical Management

Transplantation of the Lateral Meniscus

The surgical technique has been described in detail elsewhere.[90,91] The patient is placed in a supine position on the operating room table with a tourniquet applied with a leg holder, and the table is adjusted to allow 90° of knee flexion. A meniscal bed of 3 mm is retained when possible. The meniscal bed and the adjacent synovium are rasped in an attempt to aid in revascularization.

A limited 3-cm lateral arthrotomy is performed just adjacent to the patellar tendon and is preferred over an all-arthroscopic technique. A second 3-cm incision is made posterolaterally, and the approach is the same as that used for a repair of the lateral meniscus, as already described. An appropriately sized popliteal retractor is placed directly behind the lateral meniscus bed and anterior to the lateral head of the gastrocnemius.

The width of the transplant is determined. A template, made out of aluminum foil, of the transplant's width and length is cut and is inserted into the lateral compartment to determine the proper placement of the bone slot. This sizing step is important to ensure that no lateral overhang (extrusion) of the meniscal body is produced by placing the bone slot too far laterally. A rectangular bone slot is prepared at the anterior and posterior meniscal tibial attachment sites to match the dimensions of the prepared transplant.

The tibial bone slot is 1 to 2 mm wider than the transplant to facilitate implantation. A tibial slot sizing guide is used to check the length and depth. A sizing block confirms that the transplant bone bridge has the correct width and depth.

Use of a dovetail technique, which has the advantage of providing additional stability to the fixation at the tibial bone portion of the transplant, may also be considered. This procedure entails cutting a trapezoidal bone block that includes a narrower 7-mm bone bridge. This procedure requires additional time to prepare the transplant.

Table 5
Clinical Outcomes of Meniscal Repair

Study (Year)	No. and Type of Meniscal Tears; Anterior Cruciate Ligament Reconstruction	Surgical Details
Billante et al[51] (2008)	38 tears (9 red-red, 28 red-white, 1 white-white); all with anterior cruciate ligament reconstruction	All-inside, RapidLoc: mean, 1.97 devices (range, 1-4)
Krych et al[53] (2008)	47 patients younger than 18 years; simple, displaced bucket-handle, complex tears, all isolated	Variety of techniques: arrows, inside-out sutures
Bryant et al[54] (2007)	49 tears treated with inside-out suture, 51 treated with arrows; all vertical tears at meniscal synovial junction (red-red or red-white); prospective, randomized; anterior cruciate ligament reconstruction (31 in suture group, 34 arrow group)	Sutures and arrows placed every 5 mm; 10-mm or 13-mm arrows
Siebold et al[21] (2007)	113 longitudinal 10- to 25-mm tears (red-red or red-white); 75 with anterior cruciate ligament reconstruction	13-mm or 16-mm arrows; mean, 2 (range, 1-4) per repair
Barber et al[55] (2006)	32 longitudinal posterior horn tears (11 red-red, 21 red-white); 23 with anterior cruciate ligament reconstruction	All-inside, RapidLoc: mean, 2.2 devices (range, 1-4)
Majewski et al[57] (2006)	88 single longitudinal isolated tears	Outside-in; 3 to 6 sutures
Kotsovolos et al[58] (2006)	61 longitudinal > 10 mm tears (22 red-red, 39 red-white); 39 with anterior cruciate ligament reconstruction	All-inside, FasT-Fix: mean, 4.4 anchors
Barber and Coons[56] (2006)	41 longitudinal tears (31 red-red, 10 red-white); 35 with anterior cruciate ligament reconstruction	All-inside, BioStinger[a]: mean, 2.1 devices (range, 1-4)
Quinby et al[52] (2006)	54 tears (5 red-red, 49 red-white); all with anterior cruciate ligament reconstruction	All-inside, RapidLoc: mean, 1.8 devices (range, 1-4)
Kurzweil et al[20] (2005)	60 vertical longitudinal tears (red-red or red-white); 45 with anterior cruciate ligament reconstruction	Arrows
Haas et al[66] (2005)	42 peripheral longitudinal > 10-mm tears (red-red or red-white); 22 with anterior cruciate ligament reconstruction	All-inside, FasT-Fix: mean, 2.8 anchors—vertical, horizontal, or oblique positions used depending on tear
Barber et al[59] (2005)	89 longitudinal tears (60 red-red, 26 red-white, 3 white-white); mean, 20 mm; 73 with anterior cruciate ligament reconstruction	BioStinger in 47, vertical sutures in 29, BioStinger + sutures in 13
Kocabey et al[60] (2004)	55 longitudinal tears (29 red-red, 26 red-white); most 1-2 cm; 32 with anterior cruciate ligament reconstruction	All-inside, T-Fix: 2-6 devices used, horizontal mattress suture configuration
Steenbrugge et al[61] (2004)	45 tears (15 red-red, 28 red-white, 2 white-white); anterior cruciate ligament torn in 7 in inside-out group, not reconstructed; anterior cruciate ligament torn in 9 in arrow group, 6 reconstructed	Inside-out vertical sutures placed 3-4 mm intervals in 20; all-inside arrows inserted every 5-10 mm in 25
Spindler et al[62] (2003)	125 medial meniscus tears; most in periphery; all with anterior cruciate ligament reconstruction	Inside-out horizontal sutures in 40; all-inside arrows in 85
O'Shea and Shelbourne[63] (2003)	55 locked bucket-handle tears (1 red-red, 11 red-white, 43 white-white); staged anterior cruciate ligament reconstruction at mean of 77 days after meniscal repair	Inside-out, 3 to 6 vertical mattress sutures
Kurosaka et al[64] (2002)	114 chronic vertical or vertical-oblique tears in periphery; > 1 cm in length; anterior cruciate ligament reconstruction in 102 of 111 patients (92%)	Inside-out, vertical sutures
Rodeo[65] (2000)	90 tears (78 red-red, 10 red/white, 2 white/white); 38 with anterior cruciate ligament reconstruction	Outside-in, vertical sutures placed every 3-4 mm

[a]BioStinger (ConMed Linvatec, Largo, FL)

(Adapted with permission from Noyes FR, Barber-Westin SD: Meniscus tears: Diagnosis, repair techniques, clinical outcomes, in Noyes FR, Barber-Westin SD, eds: *Noyes' Knee Disorders: Surgery, Rehabilitation, Clinical Outcomes*. Philadelphia, PA, WB Saunders, 2009, pp 733-771.)

Table 5
Clinical Outcomes of Meniscal Repair (cont)

Evaluation Methods	Failure Rate	Other Results
Physical examination: mean, 30.4 months (range, 21-56)	13%	Failures associated only with sex (male)
Physical examination: mean, 5.8 years; retrospective chart review	38%	Failures associated with complex tears, rim width of > 3 mm
Physical examination: 2 years	Suture: 22% Arrow: 21.5%	3 arrows protruded into subcutaneous tissue, 1 removed; 1 suture required revision; 34 patients could not be randomized because of surgeons' opinions on indications for procedures
Physical examination: mean, 6 years (minimum, 5 years)	28.4%	81.5% with failure within 3 years postoperatively
Physical examination: mean, 31 months (range, 18-48)	12.5%	Chondral grooving observed in 1 knee; surgeon learning curve to avoid cutting suture during device insertion
Physical examination: 5-17 years	24%	8% with radiographic grade 2 or 3 arthrosis on involved side compared with grade 0 or 1 on uninvolved side
Physical examination: 14-28 months	9.8%	
Physical examination: 24-69 months	5%	Device migration in 4 knees, 3 with repeat surgery; chondral grooving in 1 knee
Physical examination: mean, 34.8 months (range, 24-50)	9%	
Physical examination 36-70 months	28%	20% rate of failure in knees with anterior cruciate ligament reconstruction, normal stability restored; 11% with damage to femoral articular cartilage; 13% of arrows broke during insertion
Physical examination: 22-27 months	12%	Failures associated with bucket-handle tears, multiplanar tears, tears longer than 2 cm, tears of > 3-month duration
Physical examination: 12-56 months	Vertical sutures: 0% BioStinger: 8% BioStinger + sutures: 15%	BioStinger unable to repair larger and anteriorly located tears
Physical examination: 4-24 months	13%	Rehabilitation program altered depending on type and size of tear
Physical examination: 6-15 years	Sutures: 0% arrows: 12%	
Physical examination: median, 68 months in suture group and 27 months in arrow group	Sutures: 12.5% arrow: 11%	
Follow-up arthroscopy: mean, 77 days postoperatively; physical examination: mean, 4.3 years postoperatively	Red-red: 0% red-white: 9% white-white: 19%	
Follow-up arthroscopy: mean, 13 months (range, 2 to 32); physical examination: mean, 54 months (range, 17-84) after follow-up arthroscopy	32%	Follow-up arthroscopy showed 79% healed; 13 repairs that initially healed failed later postoperatively
Physical examination: mean, 46 months (range, 36-89); MRI, CT, or arthroscopy in 86	13% (red/white: 40%)	Failures correlated with uncorrected anterior cruciate ligament deficiency, tears in middle-third region, tears in posterior horn of medial meniscus

Table 6
Indications and Contraindications for Meniscal Transplantation

Indications	Contraindications
Prior meniscectomy	Advanced knee joint arthrosis with flattening of femoral condyle, concavity of the tibial plateau, and osteophytes that prevent anatomic seating of meniscal transplant
Patient 50 years or younger	Uncorrected varus or valgus axial malalignment
Pain in tibiofemoral compartment in which meniscectomy performed	Uncorrected knee joint instability, anterior cruciate ligament deficiency
No radiographic evidence of advanced joint deterioration, ≥ 2 mm of tibiofemoral joint space on 45° weight-bearing PA radiographs	Knee arthrofibrosis
No or only minimal bone exposed on tibiofemoral surfaces	Substantial muscular atrophy
Normal axial alignment	Prior joint infection with subsequent arthritis
	Symptomatic noteworthy deterioration of patellofemoral articular cartilage
	Obesity (body mass index > 30 kg/m^2)
	Prophylactic procedure (asymptomatic patient with no articular cartilage damage)

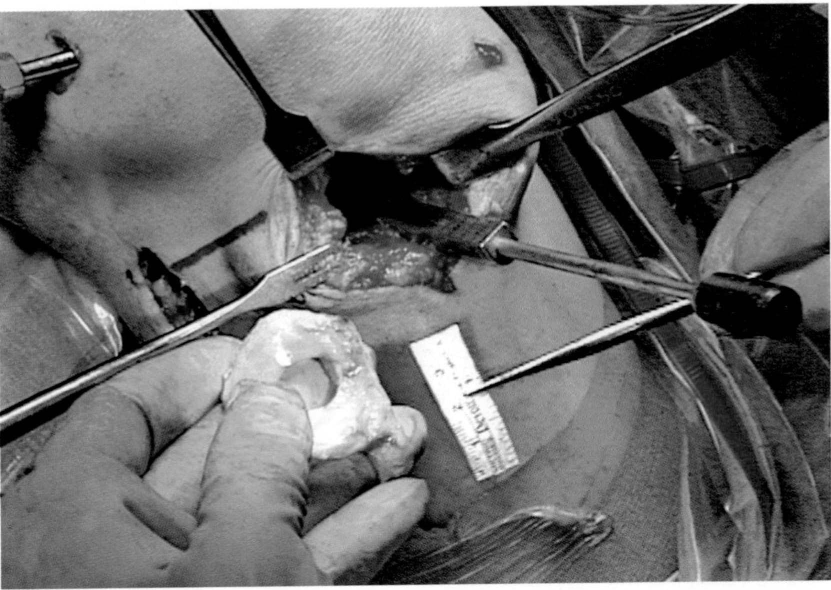

Figure 9 A lateral meniscal transplant with a central bone bridge ready to be placed into the tibial slot. (Reproduced with permission from Noyes FR, Barber-Westin SD, Rankin M: Meniscal transplantation in symptomatic patients less than fifty years old: Surgical technique. *J Bone Joint Surg Am* 2005;87 [Suppl 1 Pt 2]:149-165.)

The transplant is inserted into the slot (**Figure 9**), and the bone portion of the graft is seated against a retained posterior bone buttress at the tibia to achieve correct anterior-to-posterior placement of the attachment sites. A vertical suture in the posterior aspect of the meniscal body is passed posteriorly to provide tension and facilitate placement of the transplant. The knee is flexed, extended, and rotated to confirm that the placement of the transplant is correct. Sutures are placed into the anterior third of the meniscus, attaching it to the prepared meniscal rim under direct visualization.

Two No. 2-0 nonabsorbable sutures passed retrograde into the tibial slot over the central bone bridge (before passage of the transplant) hold the transplant securely in the tibial slot and are tied over a tibial post. The arthrotomy site is closed, and the inside-out meniscal repair is completed with multiple vertical divergent sutures, which are placed first superiorly to reduce the meniscus and then inferiorly in the outer third of the transplant. Sutures are not placed in the middle and inner thirds to avoid weakening the transplant, which has limited healing capability in those regions (**Figure 10**).

Transplantation of the Medial Meniscus

A 4-cm anteromedial skin incision is made adjacent to the patellar tendon for the anterior arthrotomy and a second 3-cm vertical incision is made posteromedially, in a manner similar to that described for inside-out meniscal repairs. A meniscal retractor is placed in the interval anterior to the gastrocnemius tendon and directly posterior to the meniscal bed and the posterior aspect of the capsule. The two approaches are performed with the tourniquet inflated to

275 mm Hg. The approaches usually require less than 15 minutes; otherwise, the tourniquet is not used.

The goal of the surgical procedure is to transplant the medial meniscus and bone attachments into the normal anterior and posterior attachments and suture the transplant to maintain the desired position in the knee joint. An aluminum foil template of the medial meniscus transplant is measured according to its anterior-posterior and medial-lateral dimensions and is inserted through the anterior arthrotomy site to measure the medial tibial plateau.

It is verified that the anterior and posterior meniscal attachment locations are at the anatomically correct sites. The central bone-bridge technique removes 4 to 6 mm of the medial intercondylar tubercle. If the transplant is suitable and no medial tibial overhang is present, then the central bone-bridge technique is preferred. If the transplant needs to be adjusted and tensioned to fit to the medial tibial plateau, then the two-tunnel technique is selected. This sizing step is critical to obtain proper placement of the medial meniscal transplant into the host tibia. In some knees, the central slot technique is not possible because of a sizing problem that results in excessive medial displacement of the meniscal body or that compromises the tibial attachment of the anterior cruciate ligament.

Central Bone-Bridge Technique for Transplantation of the Medial Meniscus

The meniscal transplant is prepared using either a rectangular or a dovetail technique. A reference slot is first made on the tibial plateau in the anteroposterior direction. A guide pin is positioned in the slot, inferiorly on the tibia, and a cannulated drill bit is placed over the pin to drill a tunnel.

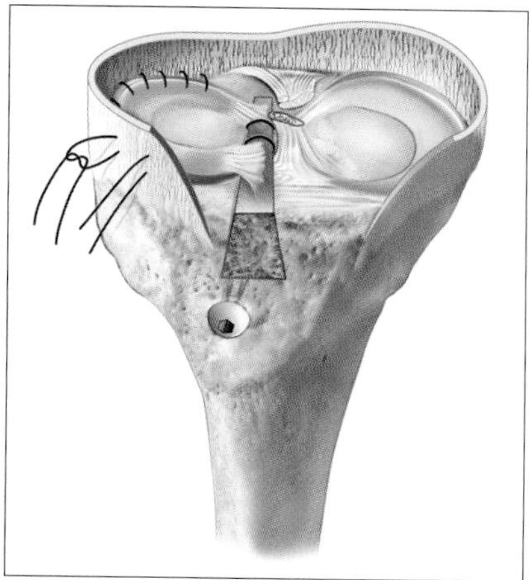

Figure 10 Lateral meniscus graft in place and sutured. (Reproduced with permission from Noyes FR, Barber-Westin SD: Meniscus transplantation: Diagnosis, operative techniques, and clinical outcomes, in Noyes FR, Barber-Westin SD, eds: *Noyes' Knee Disorders: Surgery, Rehabilitation, Clinical Outcomes.* Philadelphia, PA, WB Saunders, 2009, pp 772-805.)

Osteotomes and chisels are then used to prepare the tibial slot. The anterior cruciate ligament attachment is located directly lateral to the tibial slot, and no more than 2 mm of its attachment should be compromised. The final tibial slot is 8 to 9 mm in width and 10 mm in depth. A rasp is used to smooth the slot to allow insertion of the transplant's central bone bridge.

A vertical suture is placed through the posterior meniscal horn and advanced through the capsule to exit through the posteromedial incision. The meniscus is passed through the arthrotomy site into the knee, with tension placed on the posterior suture to facilitate the proper positioning of the meniscus in the knee joint. The position of the central bone bridge is adjusted in the anteroposterior direction to be anatomically correct relative to the femoral condyle. The knee is moved through flexion and extension and tibial rotation to align the transplant. Occasionally, there is an osteophyte on the anterior portion of the medial tibial plateau that must be resected to avoid compression of the meniscal transplant.

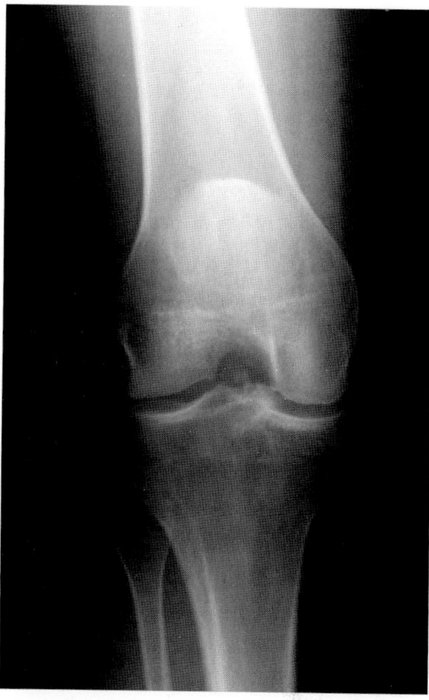

Figure 11 Weight-bearing PA radiograph of the knee of a 36-year-old woman, made 6 years after medial meniscus transplantation with a central bone bridge, showing incorporation of the bone bridge into the host with preservation of the medial joint space. (Reproduced with permission from Noyes FR, Barber-Westin SD, Rankin M: Meniscal transplantation in symptomatic patients less than fifty years old: Surgical technique. *J Bone Joint Surg Am* 2005;87[Suppl 1 Pt 2]:149-165.)

The suture fixation of the meniscal transplant is the same as that described for the lateral meniscus transplant (**Figure 11**).

Two-Tunnel Technique for Transplantation of the Medial Meniscus

If it is determined that the central bone-bridge technique cannot be used, the surgeon must prepare separate anterior and posterior bone attachments for the meniscal transplant that will be secured to the normal anatomic attachment sites. Using a meniscal implant from which one or both bone plugs have been removed, leaving only a soft-tissue graft without bone fixation, is not recommended because this compromises fixation at the anatomic attachment sites and meniscal extrusion is usually the end result. The transplant is prepared with a posterior bone plug 8 mm in diameter and 12 mm in length. The anterior bone attachment is 12 mm in width, length, and depth. Two No. 2-0 nonabsorbable sutures are passed retrograde through each bone attachment, with two additional locking sutures placed in the meniscus adjacent to the bone attachment for secure fixation.

The anteromedial and posteromedial approaches are performed as described. A guidewire is placed adjacent to the tibial tubercle and is directed to the anatomic posterior meniscal attachment. A tibial tunnel is drilled over the guidewire to a diameter of 9 mm. The bone tunnel edges are chamfered and slightly enlarged with a curet to allow easier passage of the graft into the tibial tunnel. A limited medial femoral condyle notchplasty is usually required. At least 8 mm of opening adjacent to the posterior cruciate ligament and medial femoral condyle is required to pass the posterior bone attachment of the graft. Rarely, a subperiosteal release of the long fibers of the tibial attachment of the distal part of the medial collateral ligament (with later suture anchor repair) is required to sufficiently open the medial aspect of the tibiofemoral joint.

The graft is passed through the anteromedial arthrotomy site. The surgeon is seated with a headlight in place, and the patient's knee is flexed 90°. A guidewire is passed retrograde through the tibial tunnel, and the sutures attached to the posterior bone plug are retrieved. A second suture is placed in the posterior horn and is passed inside out through the posteromedial approach to guide the meniscus.

The knee is flexed 20° under a maximum valgus load to facilitate passage of the posterior bone plug with the meniscal body suture held by an assistant. A nerve hook or other blunt instrument is used to gently assist the passage of the graft. With direct visualization, it is possible to confirm appropriate passage of the meniscal graft and positioning into the medial tibiofemoral compartment. Care is taken to not advance the posterior part of the meniscal body too far into the tibial tunnel and to seat only the osseous portion of the graft to avoid shortening the overall circumference of the meniscal graft.

The posterior meniscal bone attachment sutures are tied over the tibial post to provide tension to the posterior bone attachment. One or two sutures are passed to secure the posterior horn. The knee is flexed and extended to assess meniscal fit and displacement. The optimal location for the anterior meniscal bone attachment is identified to restore proper meniscal position and prevent medial overhang of the transplant. The knee is placed in full extension, and the position of the transplant is verified as being correct.

A 12-mm rectangular bone attachment is fashioned in the tibia to correspond to the anterior bone plug of the meniscal graft. A 4-mm bone tunnel is placed at the base of this bone slot to exit at the anterior aspect of the tibia just proximal to the posterior bone tunnel. The sutures are passed through the bone tunnel, and the anterior horn is seated. Full knee flexion and extension are again performed to determine proper graft placement and fit. Tension is applied to the anterior bone sutures, which are not tied at this point but are used to maintain tension in the graft during the inside-out suture repair. This meticulous seating of the meniscal transplant under circumferential tension with bone attachments for both the anterior and the posterior horn is believed to be crucial for an effective weight-bearing position and function of the meniscus.

The anterior arthrotomy site is closed, and the suture cannula is inserted into the lateral portal for the meniscal repair. The meniscal repair is performed in an inside-out fashion, starting with the posterior horn, with use of multiple vertical divergent sutures of No. 2-0 nonabsorbable material both superiorly and inferiorly and constant tensioning of the meniscus from posterior to anterior to establish circumferential tension.

Alternative techniques, such as the use of meniscal fixators, are not recommended because these devices lessen the ability to precisely secure and restore tension to the meniscal transplant. Finally, the anterior arthrotomy site is opened, and final tensioning and fixation of the anterior horn bone attachment are performed. Additional sutures are required to secure, under direct vision, the most anterior third of the meniscus to the capsular attachments (**Figure 12**).

Clinical Outcomes

Two prospective clinical studies of 96 fresh-frozen irradiated and 40 consecutive cryopreserved medial and lateral meniscal transplants were conducted.[82,92] The follow-up rate was 100% in both prospective studies.

In the first investigation, the outcomes after implantation of a total of 96 consecutive irradiated meniscal transplants in 82 patients were analyzed.[92] Twenty-eight menisci in 27 patients required early arthroscopic resection because of a lack of healing at a mean of 10 months postoperatively. These 28 menisci were included in the overall failure rate. One patient died of causes unrelated to the knee condition before the 2-year follow-up point. This left 67 menisci (57 medial and 10 lateral) in 54 patients, who all returned for follow-up at a mean of 44 months (range, 22 to 111 months) postoperatively.

The meniscal transplant failed in 1 of 18 knees (6%) with normal or only mild arthritis as seen on MRI, in 14 of 31 knees (45%) with moderate arthritis, and in 12 of 15 knees (80%) with advanced arthritis ($P < 0.001$). (MRI was not performed on three knees.)

Independent examiners conducted histologic evaluations of the 28 meniscal allografts that had failed early. There was no evidence of a cellular reaction suggestive of a rejection phenomenon in any of the tissues examined. The specimens consistently showed minimal, if any, cellular repopulation of any portion of the meniscus. The predominant cell type was a fibrocyte. Remodeling with abnormal collagen orientation was found in six specimens. The remodeling phenomenon resulted in a loss of the normal surface radial collagen architecture and a loss of the normal circumferential fibers within the meniscal substance. In essence, the tissue represented a fibrous tissue interposition arthroplasty with little to no remaining true meniscus properties.

It is not known if low-dose irradiation (2.0 to 2.5 mrad [20,000 to 25,000 Gy]) affects the failure rate of meniscal transplantation. This study suggested that patients with advanced arthritis and alterations in joint geometry (a major tibial concavity and femoral condyle flattening) with exposed bone surfaces over most of the tibiofemoral compartment are not candidates for meniscal transplantation.[92]

In the second prospective study, designed to avoid graft irradiation, a total of 40 cryopreserved meniscal transplants were implanted in 38 patients, who were then followed for a mean of 40 months (range, 24 to 69 months) postoperatively.[82] There were 20 male and 18 female patients whose mean age at surgery was 30 years. At the time of the lateral meniscus transplant, a concurrent osteochondral autograft transfer of the lateral femoral condyle was done in 13 knees to treat a full-thickness articular cartilage defect. Knee ligament reconstruction was done before the meniscal transplant in four knees and at the same time as the transplant in four knees.

Twenty-nine of the 40 meniscal transplants (73%) were analyzed with MRI at an average of 35 months (range, 12 to 67 months) postoperatively. Independent orthopaedic surgeons who were blinded with regard to patient information reviewed these images, measuring the height, width, and displacement of the transplant during full or partial weight-bearing conditions.[93] A system for the classification of meniscal transplant characteristics was developed on the basis of the findings on MRI, clinical examination, follow-up arthroscopy (when performed), and tibiofemoral symptoms.

Before surgery, 30 of the 38 patients (79%) had moderate to severe pain with daily activities, but only 4 (11%) had pain with daily activities at the time of follow-up. All patients had preoperative pain in the tibiofemoral compartment in which the meniscectomy was performed, but at the time of follow-up, 27 of 40 knees (68%) had no tibiofemoral compartment pain and 13 of 40 (33%) were improved and had only mild pain. Thirty-four of the 38 patients (89%) stated that the condition of the knee had improved. Preoperatively, only one patient was able to participate in sports without problems. At the time of follow-up, 29 of 38 patients (76%) were participating in light, low-impact sports without problems, and 1 patient was participating with symptoms, against advice.

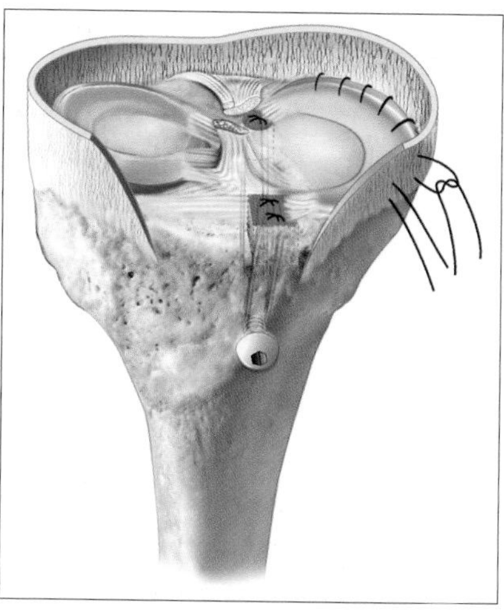

Figure 12 Appearance of the final anterior and posterior tunnel fixation of a medial meniscus transplant and vertical divergent sutures. An allograft bone trough technique is preferred; however, if there is a medial offset or overhang of the transplant, then a two-tunnel technique is required for adequate graft positioning. (Reproduced with permission from Noyes FR, Barber-Westin SD: Meniscus transplantation: Diagnosis, operative techniques, and clinical outcomes, in Noyes FR, Barber-Westin SD, eds: *Noyes' Knee Disorders: Surgery, Rehabilitation, Clinical Outcomes.* Philadelphia, PA, WB Saunders, 2009, pp 772-805.)

One patient had signs of a meniscal transplant tear at the time of follow-up. One patient had tibiofemoral joint line pain and increased palpable crepitus compared with the findings of the preoperative examination. All patients had a normal range of knee motion.

Five patients had follow-up arthroscopy because of symptoms related to the transplant. A tear in the periphery of the meniscal transplant, at the capsular junction, was successfully repaired in three patients, and small tears in the transplant were resected in two patients. None of these patients had additional symptoms. One other patient had a total knee replacement 35 months following the meniscal transplant because of unresolved knee pain.

The mean displacement of the 29 meniscal transplants examined with MRI was 2.2 ± 1.5 mm (range, 0 to 5 mm) in the coronal plane. In the sagittal plane, the mean displacement of the posterior horn of the transplants was 1.1 ± 2.0 mm (range, 0 to 9 mm), and the mean displacement of the anterior horn was 1.2 ± 1.7 mm (range, 0 to 6 mm). Intrameniscal signal intensity was normal in 1 case, grade 1 in 13 cases, grade 2 in 11 cases, grade 3 in 3 cases, and could not be evaluated in 1 case.

There was a correlation between the arthritis rating on MRI and the transplant characteristics. Of the 16 transplants in knees with mild arthritis, 10 had normal characteristics, and 6 had altered characteristics. Of the 12 transplants in knees with moderate arthritis, 3 had normal characteristics, 4 had altered characteristics, and 5 failed.

Studies of cryopreserved meniscal transplants conducted by others have reported a failure rate of approximately 30%. Stollsteimer et al[94] followed 23 patients for 13 to 69 months after implantation of a cryopreserved meniscal transplant. Eight of 23 patients (35%) required a second operation because of meniscal symptoms 5 to 28 months postoperatively. Although good pain relief was obtained in 18 knees, MRI in 12 knees showed some shrinkage of the transplants, which were an average of 63% of the size of the contralateral normal menisci.

Rath et al[95] reported the results 2 to 8 years following implantation of 22 cryopreserved meniscal transplants. A concomitant anterior cruciate ligament reconstruction was done in 11 of the 18 patients. Eight of the 22 menisci (36%) failed and were removed at an average of 31 months after implantation. Histologic analysis of the torn transplants demonstrated a more than 50% reduction in the number of meniscal fibrochondrocytes at the periphery compared with the number in the torn native menisci. Even so, all patients except one had significant improvements in outcome scores ($P < 0.0001$). Nine to 13 years following implantation of 20 cryopreserved meniscal transplants, Hommen et al[96] reported a 10-year survival rate of only 45%. The failures were identified on the basis of low Lysholm scores (< 65 points), no reduction in pain, findings on MRI, and second-look arthroscopy data.

Van Arkel et al[97] reported the results of 19 cryopreserved meniscal transplants followed for 14 to 55 months postoperatively with MRI, arthroscopy, and clinical examination. Sixteen transplants were successful, and 3 failed as indicated by clinical findings. However, MRI criteria showed eight failures, based on four transplants with severe shrinkage and four with moderate shrinkage. None of the transplants were in a normal position; 11 showed partial extrusion, 6 demonstrated extrusion, and 2 had a bucket-handle-like appearance. The authors did not provide details on the surgical technique, including whether attachment of the anterior and posterior horns was performed.

Two survival analyses of meniscal transplantation have been published based on the knowledge of this chapter's authors. Van Arkel and de Boer[98] conducted such an analysis of 63 consecutive cryopreserved meniscal transplants followed for 4 to 126 months postoperatively. Persistent pain or mechanical damage (a detached or torn transplant) was used to determine transplant failure. The cumulative 10-year survival rates of lateral transplants, medial transplants, and combined transplants in the same knee were 76%, 50%, and 67%, respectively. Lateral transplants failed at an average of 53 months after implantation, and medial transplants failed at an average of 25 months.

Verdonk et al[84] performed a follow-up study of 100 fresh meniscal transplants at a mean of 7.2 years postoperatively. The failure rate was 28% for medial meniscus transplants (mean time to failure, 6.0 ± 8.8 years) and 16% for lateral meniscus transplants (mean time to failure, 4.8 ± 2.8 years). The average cumulative survival time (11.6 years) was identical for the medial and lateral transplants. The cumulative survival rates at 10 years were 74.2% for the medial transplants and 69.8% for the lateral transplants. Medial meniscus transplants done concurrently with a high tibial osteotomy had a higher cumulative survival rate of 83.3% at 10 years.

Postoperative alterations in the signal intensity of meniscal transplants on MRI have been frequently reported.[94,97,99,100] Potter et al[99] evaluated 29 meniscal transplants with MRI and clinical examination 3 to 41 months postoperatively. Increased signal intensity was detected in the posterior horn in 15 knees, and peripheral displacement at the body was noted in 11; all of these knees had moderate or severe chondral degeneration. Histologic analysis showed peripheral cellular repopulation but a central core that was acellular or hypocellular with evidence of disorganized collagen fibers. Knees with mild chondral degeneration had no abnormalities noted in the meniscal transplant and showed clinical results that were superior to those with severe chondral degeneration.

Verdonk et al[101] followed 38 patients with a total of 39 fresh meniscal allografts for 10 to 14.8 years postoperatively. Standing PA radiographs of 32 knees made at the time of follow-up revealed no further decrease in the tibiofemoral joint space in 13 knees (41%), a grade 1 decrease in 11 (34%), a grade 2 decrease in 7 (22%), and a grade 3 decrease in 1 (3%). MRI was performed on 17 knees and showed partial extrusion of the transplant in 12 (71%). Grade 3 signal intensity was reported in 7 transplants at 1 year and in 10 transplants at the final follow-up evaluation. The authors concluded that the surgical procedure had a potentially chondroprotective effect on the basis of the absence of additional joint-space narrowing in 41% of the cases.

Meniscal transplantation is acceptable for younger patients, especially those who have symptoms with daily activities because there are few if any other available treatment options for such patients. Short-term results have shown that most patients have improved knee function and relief of pain. However, whether this surgical procedure provides a chondroprotective effect remains unknown. For this reason, meniscal transplantation is not recommended after meniscectomy in asymptomatic patients. Rather, patients should be followed yearly, and MRI of the articular cartilage to detect early deterioration should be performed before substantial symptoms occur to provide a relative indication for a meniscal transplant procedure. The long-term outcome appears to be eventual deterioration, degeneration, and loss of function. Patients should be advised that the procedure has only short-term benefits and, in the long term, additional surgery will likely be required. This chapter's authors believe it reasonable to consider a second meniscal transplant procedure after the first transplant has undergone the expected deterioration and symptoms have returned.

There are several areas in which advances may improve the success rates of meniscal transplantation. These include issues related to transplant remodeling; collagen fiber restoration to resist tensile, compressive, and shear forces; changes in the transplant collagen matrix with altered material and structural properties; cellular repopulation and function with regard to maintaining transplant homeostasis; and the use of fresh transplants with viable cells and meniscal scaffolds.

References

1. Ahmed AM, Burke DL: In-vitro measurement of static pressure distribution in synovial joints: Part I. Tibial surface of the knee. *J Biomech Eng* 1983;105(3): 216-225.
2. Fukubayashi T, Kurosawa H: The contact area and pressure distribution pattern of the knee: A study of normal and osteoarthrotic knee joints. *Acta Orthop Scand* 1980; 51(6):871-879.
3. Kettelkamp DB, Jacobs AW: Tibiofemoral contact area: Determination and implications. *J Bone Joint Surg Am* 1972;54(2): 349-356.
4. Kurosawa H, Fukubayashi T, Nakajima H: Load-bearing mode of the knee joint: Physical behavior of the knee joint with or without menisci. *Clin Orthop Relat Res* 1980;149:283-290.
5. Verma NN, Kolb E, Cole BJ, et al: The effects of medial meniscal transplantation techniques on intra-articular contact pressures. *J Knee Surg* 2008;21(1):20-26.
6. McDermott ID, Lie DT, Edwards A, Bull AM, Amis AA: The effects of lateral meniscal allograft transplantation techniques on tibio-femoral contact pressures. *Knee Surg Sports Traumatol Arthrosc* 2008;16(6):553-560.
7. Seedhom BB, Hargreaves DJ: Transmission of the load in the knee joint with special reference to the role of the menisci: Part II. Experimental results, discussion, and conclusions. *Eng Med* 1979;8: 220-228.
8. Paletta GA Jr, Manning T, Snell E, Parker R, Bergfeld J: The effect of allograft meniscal replacement on intraarticular contact area and pressures in the human knee: A biomechanical study. *Am J Sports Med* 1997;25(5):692-698.
9. Andersson-Molina H, Karlsson H, Rockborn P: Arthroscopic partial and total meniscectomy: A long-term follow-up study with matched controls. *Arthroscopy* 2002;18(2):183-189.
10. Roos EM, Ostenberg A, Roos H, Ekdahl C, Lohmander LS: Long-term outcome of meniscectomy: Symptoms, function, and performance tests in patients with or without radiographic osteoarthritis compared to matched controls. *Osteoarthritis Cartilage* 2001;9(4): 316-324.
11. Scheller G, Sobau C, Bülow JU: Arthroscopic partial lateral meniscectomy in an otherwise normal knee: Clinical, functional, and radiographic results of a long-term follow-up study. *Arthroscopy* 2001; 17(9):946-952.
12. McNicholas MJ, Rowley DI, McGurty D, et al: Total meniscectomy in adolescence: A thirty-year follow-up. *J Bone Joint Surg Br* 2000;82(2):217-221.
13. Levy AS, Meier SW: Approach to cartilage injury in the anterior cruciate ligament-deficient knee. *Orthop Clin North Am* 2003; 34(1):149-167.
14. Noyes FR, Bassett RW, Grood ES, Butler DL: Arthroscopy in acute traumatic hemarthrosis of the knee: Incidence of anterior cruciate tears and other injuries. *J Bone Joint Surg Am* 1980;62(5):687-695, 757.

15. Noyes FR, Barber-Westin SD: Meniscus tears: Diagnosis, repair techniques, clinical outcomes, in Noyes FR, Barber-Westin SD, eds: *Noyes' Knee Disorders: Surgery, Rehabilitation, Clinical Outcomes.* Philadelphia, PA, Saunders, 2009, pp 733-771.

16. Fox MG: MR imaging of the meniscus: Review, current trends, and clinical implications. *Radiol Clin North Am* 2007;45(6):1033-1053, vii.

17. Lee GP, Diduch DR: Deteriorating outcomes after meniscal repair using the Meniscus Arrow in knees undergoing concurrent anterior cruciate ligament reconstruction: Increased failure rate with long-term follow-up. *Am J Sports Med* 2005;33(8): 1138-1141.

18. Ménétrey J, Seil R, Rupp S, Fritschy D: Chondral damage after meniscal repair with the use of a bioabsorbable implant. *Am J Sports Med* 2002;30(6):896-899.

19. Tingstad EM, Teitz CC, Simonian PT: Complications associated with the use of meniscal arrows. *Am J Sports Med* 2001;29(1): 96-98.

20. Kurzweil PR, Tifford CD, Ignacio EM: Unsatisfactory clinical results of meniscal repair using the meniscus arrow. *Arthroscopy* 2005; 21(8):905.

21. Siebold R, Dehler C, Boes L, Ellermann A: Arthroscopic all-inside repair using the Meniscus Arrow: Long-term clinical follow-up of 113 patients. *Arthroscopy* 2007;23(4):394-399.

22. Lozano J, Ma CB, Cannon WD: All-inside meniscus repair: A systematic review. *Clin Orthop Relat Res* 2007;455:134-141.

23. Borden P, Nyland J, Caborn DN, Pienkowski D: Biomechanical comparison of the FasT-Fix meniscal repair suture system with vertical mattress sutures ande meniscus arrows. *Am J Sports Med* 2003;31(3):374-378.

24. Rankin CC, Lintner DM, Noble PC, Paravic V, Greer E: A biomechanical analysis of meniscal repair techniques. *Am J Sports Med* 2002;30(4):492-497.

25. Farng E, Sherman O: Meniscal repair devices: A clinical and biomechanical literature review. *Arthroscopy* 2004;20(3):273-286.

26. Arnoczky SP, Warren RF: The microvasculature of the meniscus and its response to injury: An experimental study in the dog. *Am J Sports Med* 1983;11(3):131-141.

27. Hashimoto J, Kurosaka M, Yoshiya S, Hirohata K: Meniscal repair using fibrin sealant and endothelial cell growth factor: An experimental study in dogs. *Am J Sports Med* 1992;20(5):537-541.

28. Zhang ZN, Tu KY, Xu YK, Zhang WM, Liu ZT, Ou SH: Treatment of longitudinal injuries in avascular area of meniscus in dogs by trephination. *Arthroscopy* 1988;4(3):151-159.

29. Port J, Jackson DW, Lee TQ, Simon TM: Meniscal repair supplemented with exogenous fibrin clot and autogenous cultured marrow cells in the goat model. *Am J Sports Med* 1996;24(4):547-555.

30. Arnoczky SP, Warren RF, Spivak JM: Meniscal repair using an exogenous fibrin clot: An experimental study in dogs. *J Bone Joint Surg Am* 1988;70(8):1209-1217.

31. Ritchie JR, Miller MD, Bents RT, Smith DK: Meniscal repair in the goat model: The use of healing adjuncts on central tears and the role of magnetic resonance arthrography in repair evaluation. *Am J Sports Med* 1998;26(2): 278-284.

32. Scott GA, Jolly BL, Henning CE: Combined posterior incision and arthroscopic intra-articular repair of the meniscus: An examination of factors affecting healing. *J Bone Joint Surg Am* 1986;68(6): 847-861.

33. Zhang Z, Arnold JA, Williams T, McCann B: Repairs by trephination and suturing of longitudinal injuries in the avascular area of the meniscus in goats. *Am J Sports Med* 1995;23(1):35-41.

34. Okuda K, Ochi M, Shu N, Uchio Y: Meniscal rasping for repair of meniscal tear in the avascular zone. *Arthroscopy* 1999;15 (3):281-286.

35. Henning CE, Lynch MA, Clark JR: Vascularity for healing of meniscus repairs. *Arthroscopy* 1987;3(1):13-18.

36. Ochi M, Uchio Y, Okuda K, Shu N, Yamaguchi H, Sakai Y: Expression of cytokines after meniscal rasping to promote meniscal healing. *Arthroscopy* 2001;17 (7):724-731.

37. Peretti GM, Gill TJ, Xu JW, Randolph MA, Morse KR, Zaleske DJ: Cell-based therapy for meniscal repair: A large animal study. *Am J Sports Med* 2004; 32(1):146-158.

38. Weinand C, Peretti GM, Adams SB Jr, Bonassar LJ, Randolph MA, Gill TJ: An allogenic cell-based implant for meniscal lesions. *Am J Sports Med* 2006; 34(11):1779-1789.

39. Izuta Y, Ochi M, Adachi N, Deie M, Yamasaki T, Shinomiya R: Meniscal repair using bone marrow-derived mesenchymal stem cells: Experimental study using green fluorescent protein transgenic rats. *Knee* 2005; 12(3):217-223.

40. Steinert AF, Palmer GD, Capito R, et al: Genetically enhanced engineering of meniscus tissue using ex vivo delivery of transforming growth factor-beta 1 complementary deoxyribonucleic acid. *Tissue Eng* 2007;13(9): 2227-2237.

41. Tumia NS, Johnstone AJ: Promoting the proliferative and synthetic activity of knee meniscal fibrochondrocytes using basic fibro-

blast growth factor in vitro. *Am J Sports Med* 2004;32(4):915-920.

42. Pangborn CA, Athanasiou KA: Growth factors and fibrochondrocytes in scaffolds. *J Orthop Res* 2005;23(5):1184-1190.
43. Ishida K, Kuroda R, Miwa M, et al: The regenerative effects of platelet-rich plasma on meniscal cells in vitro and its in vivo application with biodegradable gelatin hydrogel. *Tissue Eng* 2007;13(5): 1103-1112.
44. Petersen W, Pufe T, Stärke C, et al: The effect of locally applied vascular endothelial growth factor on meniscus healing: Gross and histological findings. *Arch Orthop Trauma Surg* 2007;127(4): 235-240.
45. Spindler KP, Mayes CE, Miller RR, Imro AK, Davidson JM: Regional mitogenic response of the meniscus to platelet-derived growth factor (PDGF-AB). *J Orthop Res* 1995;13(2):201-207.
46. Heckmann TP, Noyes FR, Barber-Westin SD: Rehabilitation of meniscus repair and transplantation procedures, in Noyes FR, Barber-Westin SD, eds: *Noyes' Knee Disorders: Surgery, Rehabilitation, Clinical Outcomes.* Philadelphia, PA, Saunders, 2009, pp 806-817.
47. Buseck MS, Noyes FR: Arthroscopic evaluation of meniscal repairs after anterior cruciate ligament reconstruction and immediate motion. *Am J Sports Med* 1991;19(5):489-494.
48. Rubman MH, Noyes FR, Barber-Westin SD: Arthroscopic repair of meniscal tears that extend into the avascular zone: A review of 198 single and complex tears. *Am J Sports Med* 1998;26(1):87-95.
49. Noyes FR, Barber-Westin SD: Arthroscopic repair of meniscus tears extending into the avascular zone with or without anterior cruciate ligament reconstruction in patients 40 years of age and older. *Arthroscopy* 2000;16(8): 822-829.
50. Noyes FR, Barber-Westin SD: Arthroscopic repair of meniscal tears extending into the avascular zone in patients younger than twenty years of age. *Am J Sports Med* 2002;30(4):589-600.
51. Billante MJ, Diduch DR, Lunardini DJ, Treme GP, Miller MD, Hart JM: Meniscal repair using an all-inside, rapidly absorbing, tensionable device. *Arthroscopy* 2008; 24(7):779-785.
52. Quinby JS, Golish SR, Hart JA, Diduch DR: All-inside meniscal repair using a new flexible, tensionable device. *Am J Sports Med* 2006;34(8):1281-1286.
53. Krych AJ, McIntosh AL, Voll AE, Stuart MJ, Dahm DL: Arthroscopic repair of isolated meniscal tears in patients 18 years and younger. *Am J Sports Med* 2008; 36(7):1283-1289.
54. Bryant D, Dill J, Litchfield R, et al: Effectiveness of bioabsorbable arrows compared with inside-out suturing for vertical, reparable meniscal lesions: A randomized clinical trial. *Am J Sports Med* 2007;35(6):889-896.
55. Barber FA, Coons DA, Ruiz-Suarez M: Meniscal repair with the RapidLoc meniscal repair device. *Arthroscopy* 2006;22(9): 962-966.
56. Barber FA, Coons DA: Midterm results of meniscal repair using the BioStinger meniscal repair device. *Arthroscopy* 2006;22(4):400-405.
57. Majewski M, Stoll R, Widmer H, Müller W, Friederich NF: Midterm and long-term results after arthroscopic suture repair of isolated, longitudinal, vertical meniscal tears in stable knees. *Am J Sports Med* 2006;34(7):1072-1076.
58. Kotsovolos ES, Hantes ME, Mastrokalos DS, Lorbach O, Paessler HH: Results of all-inside meniscal repair with the FasT-Fix meniscal repair system. *Arthroscopy* 2006;22(1):3-9.
59. Barber FA, Johnson DH, Halbrecht JL: Arthroscopic meniscal repair using the BioStinger. *Arthroscopy* 2005;21(6):744-750.
60. Kocabey Y, Nyland J, Isbell WM, Caborn DN: Patient outcomes following T-Fix meniscal repair and a modifiable, progressive rehabilitation program, a retrospective study. *Arch Orthop Trauma Surg* 2004;124(9):592-596.
61. Steenbrugge F, Verdonk R, Hürel C, Verstraete K: Arthroscopic meniscus repair: Inside-out technique vs. Biofix meniscus arrow. *Knee Surg Sports Traumatol Arthrosc* 2004;12(1): 43-49.
62. Spindler KP, McCarty EC, Warren TA, Devin C, Connor JT: Prospective comparison of arthroscopic medial meniscal repair technique: Inside-out suture versus entirely arthroscopic arrows. *Am J Sports Med* 2003;31(6): 929-934.
63. O'Shea JJ, Shelbourne KD: Repair of locked bucket-handle meniscal tears in knees with chronic anterior cruciate ligament deficiency. *Am J Sports Med* 2003; 31(2):216-220.
64. Kurosaka M, Yoshiya S, Kuroda R, Matsui N, Yamamoto T, Tanaka J: Repeat tears of repaired menisci after arthroscopic confirmation of healing. *J Bone Joint Surg Br* 2002;84(1):34-37.
65. Rodeo SA: Arthroscopic meniscal repair with use of the outside-in technique. *Instr Course Lect* 2000; 49:195-206.
66. Haas AL, Schepsis AA, Hornstein J, Edgar CM: Meniscal repair using the FasT-Fix all-inside meniscal repair device. *Arthroscopy* 2005;21(2):167-175.
67. Kalliakmanis A, Zourntos S, Bousgas D, Nikolaou P: Comparison of arthroscopic meniscal repair results using 3 different me-

niscal repair devices in anterior cruciate ligament reconstruction patients. *Arthroscopy* 2008;24(7): 810-816.

68. Asik M, Sen C, Erginsu M: Arthroscopic meniscal repair using T-fix. *Knee Surg Sports Traumatol Arthrosc* 2002;10(5):284-288.

69. Hürel C, Mertens F, Verdonk R: Biofix resorbable meniscus arrow for meniscal ruptures: Results of a 1-year follow-up. *Knee Surg Sports Traumatol Arthrosc* 2000;8(1): 46-52.

70. Albrecht-Olsen PM, Bak K: Arthroscopic repair of the bucket-handle meniscus: 10 failures in 27 stable knees followed for 3 years. *Acta Orthop Scand* 1993;64(4): 446-448.

71. Menche DS, Phillips GI, Pitman MI, Steiner GC: Inflammatory foreign-body reaction to an arthroscopic bioabsorbable meniscal arrow repair. *Arthroscopy* 1999; 15(7):770-772.

72. Hutchinson MR, Ash SA: Failure of a biodegradable meniscal arrow: A case report. *Am J Sports Med* 1999;27(1):101-103.

73. Oliverson TJ, Lintner DM: Biofix arrow appearing as a subcutaneous foreign body. *Arthroscopy* 2000; 16(6):652-655.

74. Calder SJ, Myers PT: Broken arrow: A complication of meniscal repair. *Arthroscopy* 1999;15(6): 651-652.

75. Sweigart MA, Athanasiou KA: Toward tissue engineering of the knee meniscus. *Tissue Eng* 2001; 7(2):111-129.

76. Evans CH, Ghivizzani SC, Robbins PD: Orthopaedic gene therapy. *Clin Orthop Relat Res* 2004; 429:316-329.

77. Adams SB Jr, Randolph MA, Gill TJ: Tissue engineering for meniscus repair. *J Knee Surg* 2005; 18(1):25-30.

78. Buma P, Ramrattan NN, van Tienen TG, Veth RP: Tissue engineering of the meniscus. *Biomaterials* 2004;25(9):1523-1532.

79. Caplan AI: Adult mesenchymal stem cells for tissue engineering versus regenerative medicine. *J Cell Physiol* 2007;213(2): 341-347.

80. Stone KR, Rodkey WG, Webber R, McKinney L, Steadman JR: Meniscal regeneration with copolymeric collagen scaffolds: In vitro and in vivo studies evaluated clinically, histologically, and biochemically. *Am J Sports Med* 1992; 20(2):104-111.

81. Rodkey WG, Steadman JR, Li ST: A clinical study of collagen meniscus implants to restore the injured meniscus. *Clin Orthop Relat Res* 1999;367(Suppl): S281-S292.

82. Noyes FR, Barber-Westin SD, Rankin M: Meniscal transplantation in symptomatic patients less than fifty years old. *J Bone Joint Surg Am* 2004;86-A(7):1392-1404.

83. Cole BJ, Carter TR, Rodeo SA: Allograft meniscal transplantation: Background, techniques, and results. *Instr Course Lect* 2003;52: 383-396.

84. Verdonk PC, Demurie A, Almqvist KF, Veys EM, Verbruggen G, Verdonk R: Transplantation of viable meniscal allograft: Survivorship analysis and clinical outcome of one hundred cases. *J Bone Joint Surg Am* 2005;87(4):715-724.

85. Kelly BT, Potter HG, Deng XH, et al: Meniscal allograft transplantation in the sheep knee: Evaluation of chondroprotective effects. *Am J Sports Med* 2006;34(9): 1464-1477.

86. Szomor ZL, Martin TE, Bonar F, Murrell GA: The protective effects of meniscal transplantation on cartilage: An experimental study in sheep. *J Bone Joint Surg Am* 2000;82(1):80-88.

87. Locht RC, Gross AE, Langer F: Late osteochondral allograft resurfacing for tibial plateau fractures. *J Bone Joint Surg Am* 1984;66(3): 328-335.

88. Rosenberg TD, Paulos LE, Parker RD, Coward DB, Scott SM: The forty-five-degree posteroanterior flexion weight-bearing radiograph of the knee. *J Bone Joint Surg Am* 1988;70(10):1479-1483.

89. Pollard ME, Kang Q, Berg EE: Radiographic sizing for meniscal transplantation. *Arthroscopy* 1995; 11(6):684-687.

90. Noyes FR, Barber-Westin SD, Rankin M: Meniscal transplantation in symptomatic patients less than fifty years old. *J Bone Joint Surg Am* 2005;87(Suppl 1, Pt 2): 149-165.

91. Noyes FR, Barber-Westin SD: Meniscus transplantation: Diagnosis, operative techniques, and clinical outcomes, in Noyes FR, Barber-Westin SD, eds: *Noyes' Knee Disorders: Surgery, Rehabilitation, Clinical Outcomes*. Philadelphia, PA, Saunders, 2009, pp 772-805.

92. Noyes FR, Barber-Westin SD, Butler DL, Wilkins RM: The role of allografts in repair and reconstruction of knee joint ligaments and menisci. *Instr Course Lect* 1998;47:379-396.

93. Rankin M, Noyes FR, Barber-Westin SD, Hushek SG, Seow A: Human meniscus allografts' in vivo size and motion characteristics: Magnetic resonance imaging assessment under weightbearing conditions. *Am J Sports Med* 2006;34(1):98-107.

94. Stollsteimer GT, Shelton WR, Dukes A, Bomboy AL: Meniscal allograft transplantation: A 1- to 5-year follow-up of 22 patients. *Arthroscopy* 2000;16(4):343-347.

95. Rath E, Richmond JC, Yassir W, Albright JD, Gundogan F: Meniscal allograft transplantation: Two- to eight-year results. *Am J Sports Med* 2001;29(4):410-414.

96. Hommen JP, Applegate GR, Del Pizzo W: Meniscus allograft transplantation: Ten-year results of cryopreserved allografts. *Arthroscopy* 2007;23(4):388-393.

97. van Arkel ER, Goei R, de Ploeg I, de Boer HH: Meniscal allografts: Evaluation with magnetic resonance imaging and correlation with arthroscopy. *Arthroscopy* 2000;16(5):517-521.

98. van Arkel ER, de Boer HH: Survival analysis of human meniscal transplantations. *J Bone Joint Surg Br* 2002;84(2):227-231.

99. Potter HG, Rodeo SA, Wickiewicz TL, Warren RF: MR imaging of meniscal allografts: Correlation with clinical and arthroscopic outcomes. *Radiology* 1996;198(2):509-514.

100. Wirth CJ, Peters G, Milachowski KA, Weismeier KG, Kohn D: Long-term results of meniscal allograft transplantation. *Am J Sports Med* 2002;30(2):174-181.

101. Verdonk PC, Verstraete KL, Almqvist KF, et al: Meniscal allograft transplantation: Long-term clinical results with radiological and magnetic resonance imaging correlations. *Knee Surg Sports Traumatol Arthrosc* 2006;14(8):694-706.

All-Arthroscopic Meniscus Repair of Avascular and Biologically At-Risk Meniscal Tears

Michael W. Kessler, MD, MPH
Nicholas A. Sgaglione, MD

Abstract

Meniscal repair strategies have evolved over time from a more invasive open method to less invasive, all-arthroscopic approaches. Novel devices and surgical techniques currently enable the successful arthroscopic placement of biomechanically optimal sutures that provide compression across the tear site with less potential surgical morbidity. Current techniques do not require accessory posteromedial or posterolateral incisions and significantly reduce the incidence of complications and pain associated with more invasive surgery. Along with these improved methods, the indications for meniscal repair are expanding to include tear patterns previously considered biologically at risk for poor healing. More recently, with the addition of biologic augmentation methods, such as the introduction of platelet-rich plasma as well as reported tissue engineering advances, it may be possible to continue to broaden the indications and success of meniscal preservation through repair and replacement.

Instr Course Lect 2011;60:439-452.

Meniscal repair techniques have been evolving and now include open, outside-in, inside-out, all-inside, and all-arthroscopic implant fixators and all-arthroscopic suture-based devices. Improved surgical techniques and longer-term outcomes have expanded the emphasis on meniscal preservation and native meniscal tissue.

Total and select partial meniscectomies have deleterious effects on knee joint biomechanics, leading to the earlier onset of cartilage degeneration. To reduce the risks of articular cartilage breakdown and postmeniscectomy joint pain, meniscal repair is important in younger, active patients. All-arthroscopic suture-based meniscal repair devices allow the surgeon to achieve compression across the meniscal tear site while avoiding accessory incisions that may place neurovascular structures at risk for injury. These devices have yielded biomechanical and clinical outcomes that approach those of vertical mattress sutures placed using inside-out techniques. Future directions include using advanced biologic solutions, such as fibrin clots, adjunctive autogenous platelet-rich fibrin matrices, marrow stimulation techniques, exogenous growth factors, and novel tissue engineering.[1-3] More information on advanced biologic solutions in meniscal repair is available in chapter 35.

Clinical Evaluation

Clinical assessment of meniscal pathology begins with a thorough patient history and physical examination. Common presentations include focal joint line pain, swelling, and mechanical symptoms such as catching and locking. The physical examination should assess alignment and the level of inflammation and should include specific tests for ligament patholaxity, patellofemoral pathology, and articular cartilage lesions. Meniscal evaluation includes palpating for joint line tenderness, assessing range of motion, and

Neither Dr. Kessler nor an immediate family member has received anything of value from or owns stock in a commercial company or institution related directly or indirectly to the subject of this chapter. Dr. Sgaglione or an immediate family member serves as a board member, owner, officer, or committee member of the Arthroscopy Association of North America and serves as a paid consultant to or is an employee of Biomet, CONMED Linvatec, and Smith & Nephew.

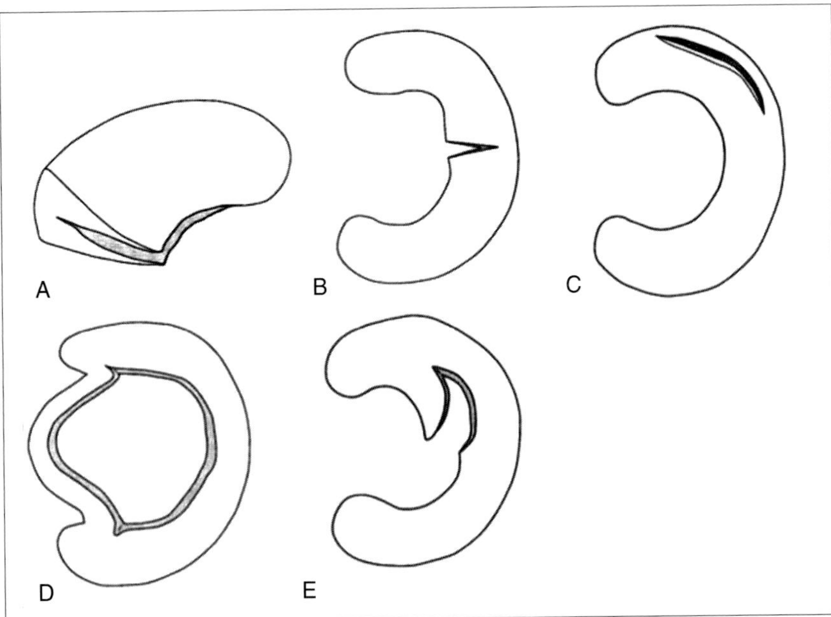

Figure 1 Types of meniscal tear configurations. **A,** Horizontal tear. **B,** Vertical radial tear. **C,** Vertical longitudinal tear. **D,** Bucket-handle tear. **E,** Flap tear. (Adapted with permission from Newman AP, Daniels AV, Burkes AT: Principles and decision making in meniscal surgery. *Arthroscopy* 1993;9:33-51.)

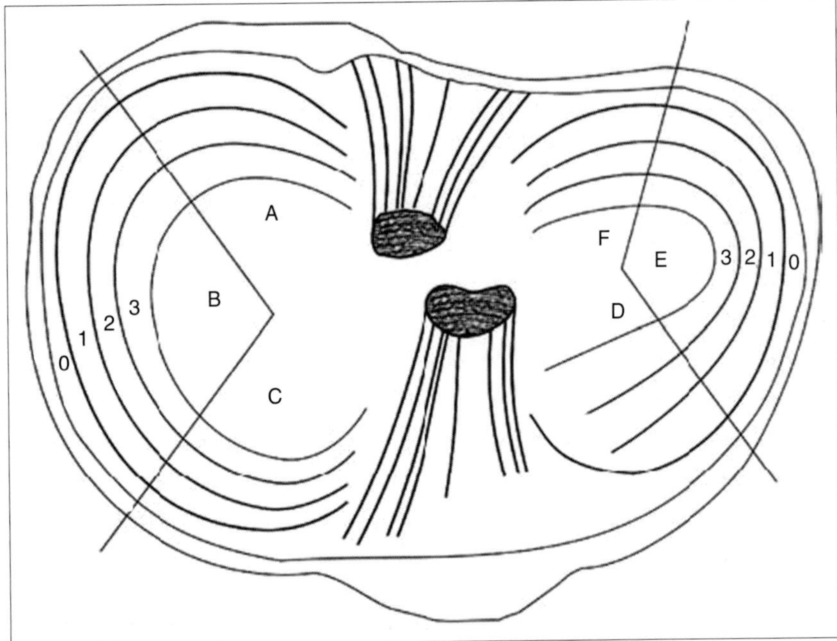

Figure 2 The Cooper tear classification system divides each meniscus into three radial zones and four circumferential zones. The medial meniscal radial zones are A, B, C, with A indicating the posterior horn. The lateral meniscal radial zones are D, E, and F, with F indicating the posterior horn of the lateral meniscus. The circumferential zones are 0, meniscocapsular; 1, outer third; 2, middle third; and 3, inner third. (Adapted with permission from Terzides IP, Christodoula A, Plournis A, et al: Meniscal tear characteristics in young athletes with a stable knee. *Am J Sports Med* 2006;34:1170-1175.)

performing specific axial compression rotation tests.[4,5]

Routine examination of the knee should include plain radiographs to identify associated osteoarthritis, chondrocalcinosis, osteochondral defects, or osteonecrosis. A standard knee series should include weight-bearing AP, lateral, notch, and sunrise radiographic views, as well as a standing flexed PA view to better define joint-space narrowing. MRI may not be routinely required; however, it has an accuracy rate of 98% in diagnosing meniscal injury and plays a role in the comprehensive evaluation of the entire joint.[6,7]

Meniscal Pathoanatomy

Meniscal tear configurations and patterns can be categorized into vertical longitudinal, bucket-handle, oblique, radial, and horizontal tears[1,8] (**Figure 1**). A zonal classification has been described by Cooper et al,[9] with each meniscus divided into three radial zones and four circumferential zones (**Figure 2**).

The vascular anatomy of the meniscus has been well described, with the meniscus split into three distinct vascular zones.[10] The vascular supply originates from the superior and inferior branches of the medial and lateral geniculate arteries.[11] The peripheral zone has the most significant and predictable vascular supply and is known as the red-red zone; the middle third of the meniscus is a combination of both vascularized and nonvascularized areas and is known as the red-white zone. The inner third, with the least viable vascular penetration, is known as the white-white zone.[10] This zone is believed to have the least likelihood of healing after an attempted meniscal repair; tears in this avascular zone have been termed biologically at risk for healing.

Table 1
Indications for Meniscal Resection, Rasping, and Repair

Indication	Resection	Rasping	Repair
Chronicity	Degenerative, nonclinically correlative tears in older patients	NA	Acute, symptomatic tears
Pattern	Oblique flaps, radial, degenerative complex, horizontal	Incomplete longitudinal	Longitudinal/vertical bucket-handle tears
Site	Inner (white-white)	Red-red posterior horn, lateral meniscus	Peripheral (red-red), middle (red-white), inner (white-white)
Size	NA	< 7 to 10 mm	> 7 to 10 mm
Excursion	NA	Stable, incomplete tears, < 3 to 5 mm displaced into notch	Unstable, > 5 mm displaced into notch
Tissue Viability	Deformed, frayed, nonviable	Viable	Minimal deformation, holds repair device, viable
Prognosticators	ACL intact, no malalignment or chondral lesions; associated infectious, rheumatoid, or collagen vascular diseases	ACL intact, well-aligned, no chondral lesions	Associated ACL repair or chondral procedure, axially malaligned
Patient Compliance and/or Preference	Recovery or rehabilitation is an issue	NA	Patient preferred

ACL = anterior cruciate ligament, NA = not applicable
(Adapted with permission from Sgaglione NA, Steadman JR, Shaffer B, Miller MD, Fu FH: Current concepts in meniscus surgery: Resection to replacement. *Arthroscopy* 2003;19(Suppl 1):161-188.)

Repair Versus Resection

The decision to repair a torn meniscus or perform a partial meniscectomy is dependent on several variables, including the pattern, geometry, site, vascularity, size, and stability of the tear. Tissue viability or quality, associated pathology, concomitant injuries, and the patient's preferences and goals also play an important role in this decision[12] (**Table 1**). In a study investigating the effects of arthroscopic partial medial meniscectomy, Faunø[13] reported that patients had a significantly greater chance of postoperative osteoarthritic changes in the operated knee when compared with the control knee. In addition, a significantly higher number of patients with varus knee alignment had signs of arthrosis after the procedure when compared with patients with normal or valgus knee alignment. The authors concluded that a medial meniscal repair may be more strongly indicated in patients with varus knee malalignment.

Other studies reported that, as early as 4.5 years after meniscectomy, degenerative changes can be seen on plain radiographs.[14,15] At 12 years postoperatively, patients with less than 50% of a meniscal rim remaining have worse radiographic progression of osteoarthritis than do patients with a greater amount of remaining meniscus. Female sex and chondral pathology are associated with worse short-term outcomes, including knee pain, knee function, and overall physical knee status.[16] A better prognosis is associated with certain tear characteristics, such as an isolated medial meniscal tear, vertical tear patterns, and an intact meniscal rim, and with other factors, such as patient age younger than 35 years and the absence of articular cartilage pathology.[17]

Meniscal resection may have a significant impact on other aspects of knee function, as shown in various biomechanical models. Levy et al[18] reported that medial meniscectomy in association with anterior cruciate ligament (ACL) deficiency resulted in significantly increased anterior displacement when compared with meniscectomy in a knee with an intact ACL. Sturnieks et al[19] reported that after an arthroscopic partial medial meniscectomy, patients exhibited increased knee medial adduction moments during stance when compared with control groups. These adduction moments concentrate load on the medial tibiofemoral compartment, which can lead to hyaline tissue breakdown.

Allaire et al[20] reported on the biomechanical consequences of a tear of the posterior root of the medial meniscus and found that there was a 25% increase in peak contact pressure at 30°, 60°, and 90° of flexion. They also found that the affected knees exhibited significant increases in external rotation and lateral tibial translation compared with intact knees; these changes were reversed with repair of the posterior root. The authors concluded that a posterior root tear of the medial meniscus resulted in a "functional meniscectomy" via a complete disruption of the circumferential fibers, thereby negating the resistance to extrusion and functional hoop stresses and increasing the pathologic loads. Conversely, incomplete horizontal or vertical circumferential tears may cause mechanical symptoms and pain but tend to not violate the circumferential fibers.[21]

Cadaver studies have shown that the loss of the medial meniscus will decrease contact areas by 75% and subsequently increase peak contact pressures by 235%.[22,23] A linear correlation between the amount of meniscus removed and the increased peak stresses on the tibial surfaces has been observed. Although this is true in medial compartment disease, both the lateral tibial plateau and the lateral femoral condyle are convex, resulting in increased point loading and peak contact pressures in the lateral compartment after meniscectomy compared with the medial compartment.[24]

Not all meniscal tears require repair or resection. Certain tears may be left untreated or may be treated with trephination or rasping to promote a healing response. This is especially true if these procedures are performed concurrently with ACL reconstruction. Shelbourne and Heinrich[25] reported that lateral meniscal tears in the posterior horn, stable and incomplete radial tears, and posterior third tears that do not extend more than 1 cm may be treated with abrasion and trephination alone. The authors reported normal postoperative International Knee Documentation Committee (IKDC) scores and a normal radiographic appearance at follow-up in 95% of patients treated with abrasion and trephination.

In studying the timing of surgery, some authors have found that earlier repairs yield improved results. Tenuta and Arciero[26] reported that repairs performed at 19 weeks after injury had enhanced healing results compared with repairs done after 60 weeks. Henning et al[1] and Cannon and Vittori[27] found a difference in repairs performed earlier or later than 8 weeks after injury. Conversely, Scott et al[28] reported no difference in healing rates for patients with repairs earlier or later than 3 weeks after injury. Noyes and Barber-Westin,[29,30] in two separate studies, found that the length of time from injury to repair had no effect on healing and clinical outcomes for older patients (40 years or older) or for young patients (19 years or younger).

Krych et al[31] reported on the outcomes of isolated meniscal repairs in patients 18 years or younger treated with a suture technique. At a mean follow-up of 5.8 years, the overall clinical success rate was 62%, with an 80% success rate for simple tears, 68% for displaced bucket-handle tears, and 13% for complex tears. Significant variables associated with failed outcomes were tears with a rim width greater than 3 to 6 mm (red-white boundary) and more complex tear patterns.

Surgical Techniques

Meniscal repair can be arthroscopically assisted (inside-out, outside-in) and all-arthroscopic. The all-arthroscopic technique includes repairs performed either with meniscal fixator devices or suture-based devices. The use of implant fixators is no longer favored because of concerns about longer-term failures and complications associated with chondral abrasion. Each technique has advantages and disadvantages.

Outside-in repair techniques have been particularly useful for anterior horn and middle third meniscal repairs. The advantages of this technique include no large posterior incision and the ability to access anterior areas that may have limited access. The disadvantages include the use and seating of an intra-articular Mulberry knot (although more recent techniques have been described for placing vertical and horizontal mattress sutures with wire loop retrievers) and the placement of outside-in knots seated extrinsic to the capsule.[12,32]

Arthroscopically assisted inside-out repair techniques have been termed the gold standard of meniscal repair. The advantages of this technique include the ability to predictably place vertical, horizontal, and oblique suture patterns, with access to the middle third and posterior horns of the menisci. The knots are tied over the capsule, with direct visualization via a posteromedial or posterolateral incision used to capture exiting repair needles and protect the neurovascular bundle.[1,11,12,28] Biomechanical benefits from vertical mattress suturing result from the greater number of meniscal circumferential fibers vertically stabilized by the suture repair construct.[33,34]

The early generation all-arthroscopic meniscal repair techniques were initially developed to achieve simpler surgical techniques and eliminate accessory incisions using rigid implant fixators that achieved purchase on both sides of the meniscal fragments.[35,36] The disadvantages of these devices were that they performed inferiorly to the inside-out or outside-in suture methods on biomechanical testing and resulted in foreign body reactions and abrasive chondral injury.[37] The rigid implant fixators also have increased failure rates as the length of follow-up increases.[38]

All-arthroscopic suture-based repair devices combine traditional suture methods with the advancing technology of using suture and anchors to suture meniscal fragments. These devices can be placed using an all-inside truly arthroscopic technique to provide two-point fixation with a suture-based implant, which is placed through the meniscus and seated outside the capsule. This placement provides resistance to allow the suture to be cinched, thereby compressing the meniscal tear fragments. All-arthroscopic suture-based meniscal repair devices have been tested and have shown biomechanical stability characteristics similar to those of inside-out suturing techniques. The disadvantages of the suture-based meniscal fixators include the learning curve associated with use, soft-tissue irritation from extracapsular placement, and the absence of long-term outcome studies.[39] Assessment and technical treatments using tear preparation, fixation compression, biologic augmentation, and selective rehabilitation are essential.

Rehabilitation

The key considerations for selecting rehabilitation protocols include the type of meniscal tear, the type of repair, and concomitant surgical procedures. Some authors have recommended accelerated rehabilitation programs with good clinical results, whereas other authors have cited a more measured approach.[26,40,41] In patients with a biologically or biomechanically at-risk repair, or if the tear has a complex configuration, a more conservative rehabilitation program may be favored. In general, an immobilizer is placed postoperatively, but protected range of motion from 0° to 90° is initiated immediately. Initially, patients bear partial weight with crutches, advancing to full weight bearing as tolerated as early as 4 weeks postoperatively. After achieving clinical success, defined as no pain, no joint line tenderness, the ability to perform full range of motion, and no symptoms with sport-specific functional testing, the patient may return to sports participation, usually at 4 to 6 months postoperatively.

Current Generation Repair Devices

The current generation of all-arthroscopic meniscal repair devices is generally suture based, using integrated needle delivery insertion systems. The soft-tissue anchor is placed in an extracapsular position, and the suture is packaged with a pretied, self-sliding knot or tensioning construct. This construct allows the application of compression across the tear site between the knot and the extracapsular implant anchor.

Commonly used repair systems include integrated locking suture and anchor devices such as the RapidLoc Meniscal Repair System (DePuy Mitek, Raynham, MA), the Ultra FasT-Fix Meniscal Repair System (Smith & Nephew Endoscopy, Andover, MA), the Arthrex Meniscal Cinch (Arthrex, Naples, FL), and the MaxFire Meniscal Repair Device (Biomet, Warsaw, IN) and integrated locking suture-only devices such as the CrossFix Meniscal Repair System (Cayenne Medical, Scottsdale, AZ).

RapidLoc System

The RapidLoc Meniscal Repair System is an integrated delivery system consisting of a soft-tissue anchor called a backstop (5 × 1.5 mm poly-L-lactic acid), a connecting suture, and a "top hat" (polydioxanone), which compresses the meniscal tear against the backstop (**Figure 3**). The backstop is seated in an extracapsular position, and the top hat is compressed against the articular femoral side of the meniscus with a knot pusher and ultimately secured by a pretied knot. The three delivery needle options for the RapidLoc device include straight and 12° and 27° curved tips. Suture options have included 2-0 Ethibond (Ethicon, Sommerville, NJ), extended resorption 2-0 Panacryl (Ethicon), or, more recently, the RapidLoc A2 loaded with two polyether-ether-ketone implants and a 2-0 Orthocord (DePuy Mitek) high-strength suture.[35]

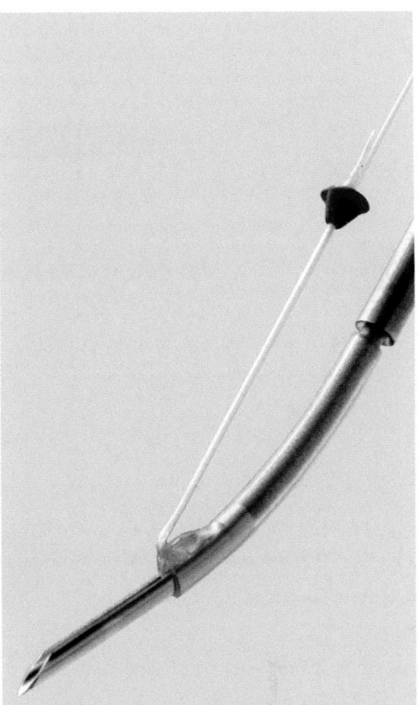

Figure 3 The RapidLoc Meniscal Repair device.

Ultra FasT-Fix System

The Ultra FasT-Fix Meniscal Repair System uses two 5-mm bioinert polyether-ether-ketone anchors attached to a nonabsorbable No. 0 Ultrabraid (Smith & Nephew) high-strength suture, pretied with a self-sliding knot (**Figure 4**). The delivery needle tip configuration options are either straight, 27° curved, or 15° reverse curved. More recently, a newer generation FasT-Fix 360 has been introduced with lower profile needles and anchors and a stiffer delivery calibrated-depth stop shaft, which allows more predictable and easier anchor deployment and the use of 2-0 Ultrabraid suture.[35]

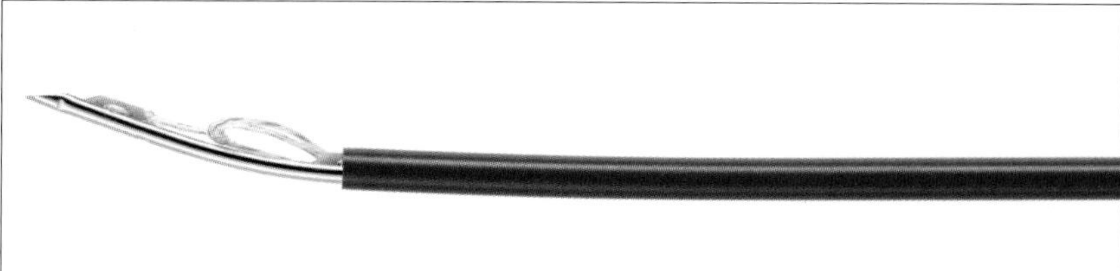

Figure 4 The Ultra FasT-Fix device.

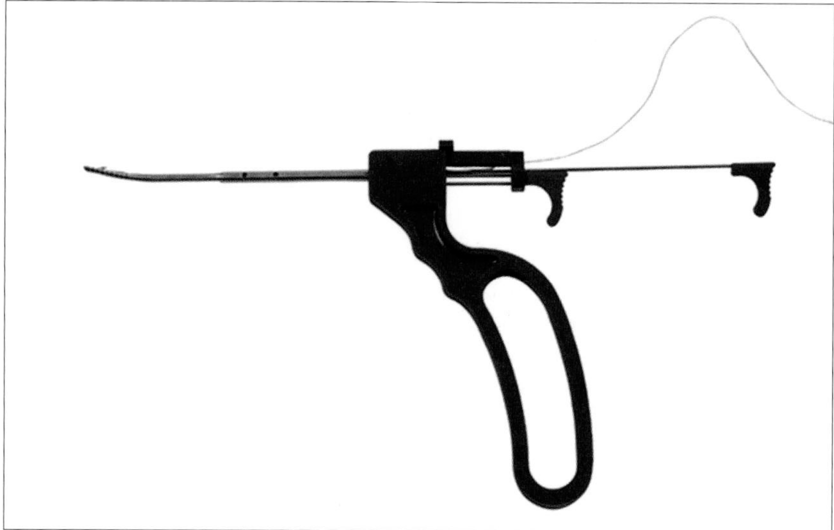

Figure 5 The Meniscal Cinch device.

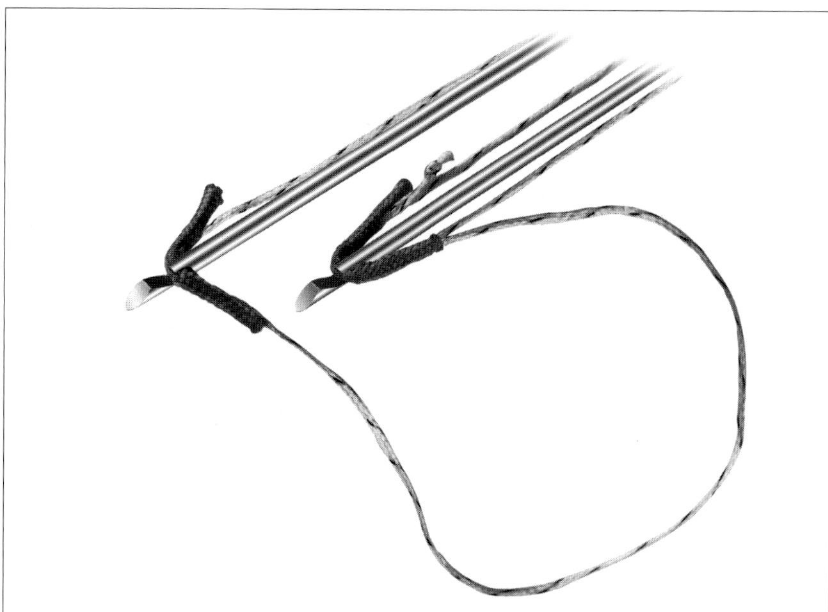

Figure 6 The MaxFire Meniscal Repair device.

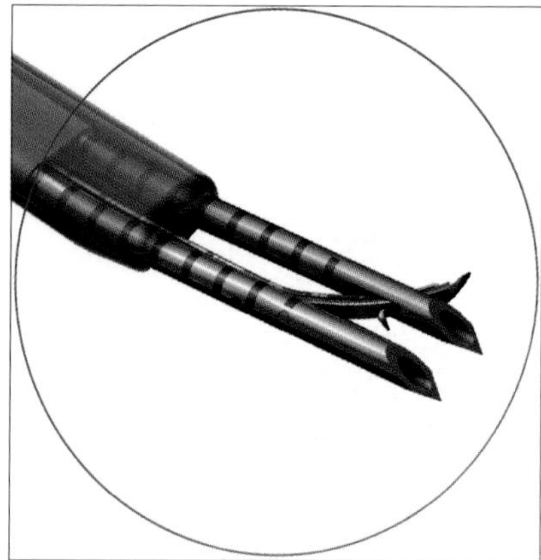

Figure 7 The CrossFix Meniscal Repair System.

Meniscal Cinch

The Arthrex Meniscal Cinch is a dual trocar, pistol grip system that contains two polyether-ether-ketone implants connected via a 2-0 FiberWire (Arthrex) suture (**Figure 5**). There is an incorporated adjustable depth limiter and a pretied self-sliding knot that can be countersunk into the meniscus.

MaxFire

The MaxFire Meniscal Repair Device contains two No. 5 braided polyester all-suture pledget anchors connected via a ZipLoop (Biomet) suture, which incorporates a weave in which a single strand of braided polyethylene suture is woven through itself twice in opposite directions (**Figure 6**). The loop is tensioned along the articular side of the meniscus, and no knots are necessary to maintain compression across the tear site. The integrated delivery device is ergonomic with sliding anchor deployment triggers.

CrossFix

The CrossFix Meniscal Repair System is a suture-only device with an incorporated adjustable depth limiter (**Figure 7**). The delivery system uses two needles (available in straight or up-curved) to deploy the suture across the meniscus tear site; it is then passed

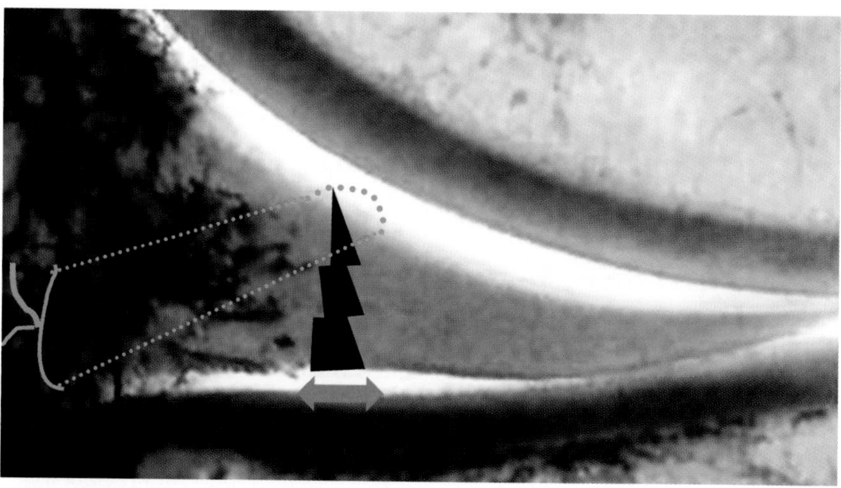

Figure 8 Image showing the microvasculature of a human meniscus. The dotted line shows the vertical mattress suture with circumferential band. The black area is the meniscal tear. The two-headed arrow shows the distance needed to be reduced by the suture.

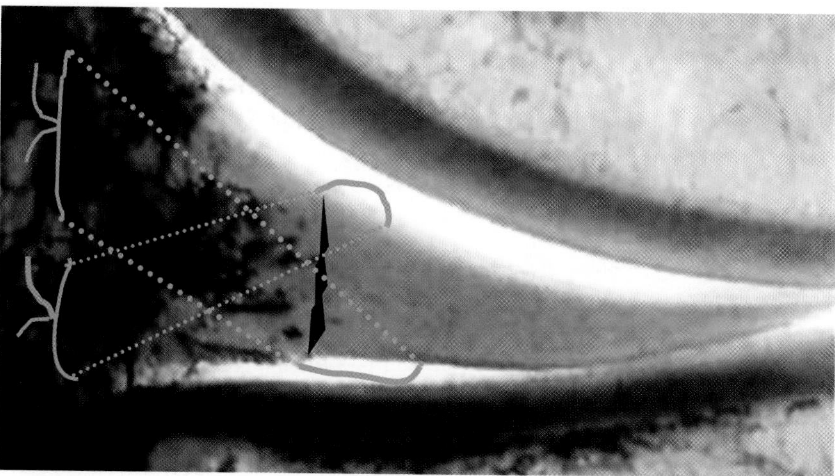

Figure 9 Image showing the microvasculature of a human meniscus. Dotted lines show a double vertical mattress suture. The black area shows a reduced meniscal tear.

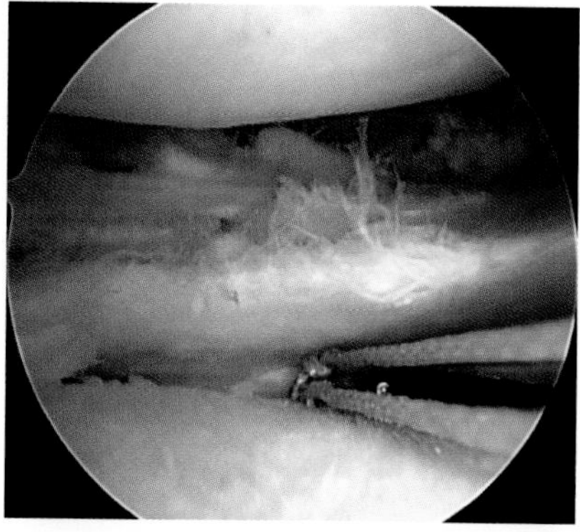

Figure 10 Arthroscopic view of tibial-side suturing of a longitudinal meniscal tear with an integrated locking suture and anchor device (FasT-Fix).

from one needle to the other via an integrated crossing needle. This creates a 3-mm, 10° oblique stitch that is then tensioned down onto the articular side of the meniscus with a pretied self-sliding knot.

Biomechanics

The goal of the suture-based meniscal repair devices is to provide a repair construct that is biomechanically optimal, approximating a vertical mattress suture construct. These devices offer the ability to impart compression across the tear site and create a much more stable repair when compared with early generation rigid barbed implant meniscal fixators.

Borden et al[39] investigated the biomechanical differences between an integrated locking suture and anchor device (FasT-Fix) in a horizontal mattress configuration, vertical mattress sutures (No. 0 Ti-Cron; Ethicon), and a polymer implant fixator device (Meniscus Arrow implants; ConMed Linvatec, Largo, FL). The human cadaver knees had a 2-cm anteroposterior vertical longitudinal incision placed 3 mm from the peripheral meniscal edge (**Figures 8** and **9**). The integrated locking suture and anchor device and the vertical mattress sutures performed equally well and showed significantly better performance than the polymer implant fixator in all aspects of biomechanical testing, including load at failure (100 N versus 50 N), stiffness (8 N/mm versus 6 N/mm), and displacement (17 mm versus 11 mm). During cyclic testing, all polymer implant fixator samples failed before the test was completed, whereas the integrated locking suture and anchor device and the vertical mattress sutures performed well, with no significant differences.

Barber et al[42] created a vertical longitudinal tear 3 mm from the periphery in porcine menisci and then biomechanically tested an integrated locking suture and anchor device (FasT-Fix; both vertical [**Figure 10**] and horizontal [**Figure 11**] configurations), two Meniscal Darts (Arthrex), a second integrated locking suture and anchor device (RapidLoc), an Arthrotek meniscal screw (Biomet), a single vertical suture, and a single hori-

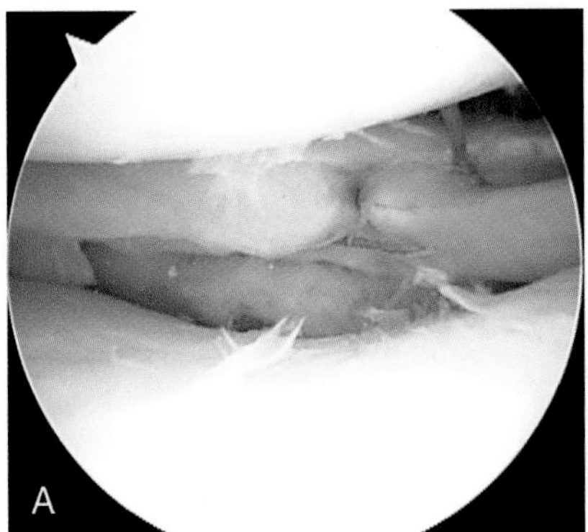

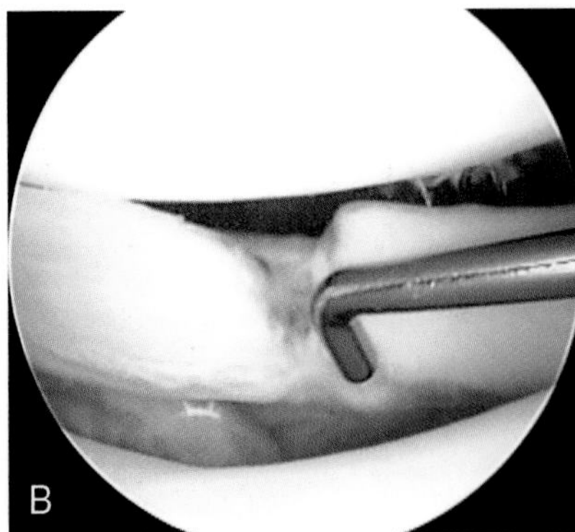

Figure 11 **A,** Arthroscopic image of a repaired radial meniscal tear. **B,** Second-look arthroscopy of a healed radial meniscal tear.

zontal suture (both 2-0 Mersilene [Ethicon] placed inside-out). The single vertical suture required the greatest load to failure; however, the integrated locking suture and anchor device tested in both the vertical and horizontal configurations performed better than the single horizontal suture and all other meniscal repair devices.

In a more recent study, the same investigators analyzed the biomechanical strength in load-to-failure and in cyclic loading of ultra-high-molecular-weight polyethylene suture compared to nonabsorbable braided polyester suture (Mersilene), ultra-high-molecular-weight polyethylene suture (Orthocord), multistranded long chain ultra-high-molecular-weight polyethylene core with a braided jacket of polyester suture (FiberWire), and ultra-high-molecular-weight polyethylene suture (Ultrabraid).[43] The meniscal repair devices (Ultra FasT-Fix, RapidLoc A2, and MaxFire) containing the ultra-high-molecular-weight polyethylene suture showed significantly greater pullout strength and less elongation over 500 cycles than the ultra-high-molecular-weight polyethylene suture (Ultrabraid) construct, which was placed and tied by hand. The ultra-high-molecular-weight polyethylene suture (Orthocord) placed in a vertical mattress orientation provided the strongest resistance to cyclic loading when compared to all the other suture configurations and suture devices.

Zantop et al[44] biomechanically tested and evaluated two integrated locking suture and anchor devices (FasT-Fix and RapidLoc), a polymer implant fixator (Meniscus Arrow), and both horizontal and vertical 2-0 Ethibond sutures (outside-in) in bovine meniscal tears. Repair constructs were studied, and the horizontal (87 N) and vertical (106 N) FasT-Fix repairs were not significantly different than the vertical mattress (85 N) repairs; however, all three had significantly stronger pullout strength than the horizontal mattress suture (63 N), the RapidLoc (45 N), and the Meniscus Arrow (49 N). With respect to stiffness, the horizontal (27 N/mm) and vertical (33 N/mm) FasT-Fix constructs were significantly different than the vertical sutures (16 N/mm), the horizontal (12 N/mm) sutures, the RapidLoc (13 N/mm), and the Meniscus Arrow (10 N/mm). The failure method for the vertical and horizontal sutures and the FasT-Fix constructs was at the knot, whereas the RapidLoc failed at the anchor site, and the Meniscus Arrow failed with pullout of the barbs from the peripheral meniscal tissue. In another study, the constructs were tested with cyclic loading to better represent in vivo loads.[45] After 1,000 cycles, there was no significant difference in displacement for any of the devices. The vertical and horizontal FasT-Fix devices were significantly stiffer than all other constructs, and the load to failure was significantly lower for the RapidLoc and the horizontal mattress suture than all other constructs.

In a study examining the biomechanical differences between the Meniscal Viper Repair System (Arthrex), the FasT-Fix (vertical orientation), and vertical mattress sutures, it was shown that the vertical mattress sutures had significantly greater stiffness and less mean displacement than the other devices during cyclic testing.[46] Both the vertical mattress suture and the FasT-Fix required a significantly higher load to failure than did the Meniscal Viper. The Meniscal Viper and FasT-Fix had significantly greater stiffness than the vertical mattress sutures on load-to-failure testing.

Biologic Augmentation

Successful healing and clinical meniscal stabilization remains a major concern for patients with biologically at-risk meniscal repairs, especially those not associated with a concomitant ACL reconstruction. Cannon and Vittori[27] reported that meniscal repairs in patients treated with ACL reconstruction had a 93% healing rate, whereas those performed in stable knees had a healing rate of 50%. The hematoma formation after an ACL reconstruction may trap platelets, which subsequently release growth factors and cytokines that attract pluripotent hematopoietic stem cells and direct their differentiation.[3] The acutely reconstructed ACL may protect the repair site from excessive forces that can affect the tear.[27]

Biologic augmentation of healing may be achieved by the addition of a fibrin clot, which has resulted in significantly increased healing rates of isolated meniscal repairs in stable knees.[1,47] The platelet-rich fibrin matrix differs from a fibrin clot in that it is a more concentrated and volume-stable material (**Figure 12**). The platelet-rich fibrin matrix is denser than the fibrin clot and is typically sewn into the meniscal tear between the meniscal fragments.[3]

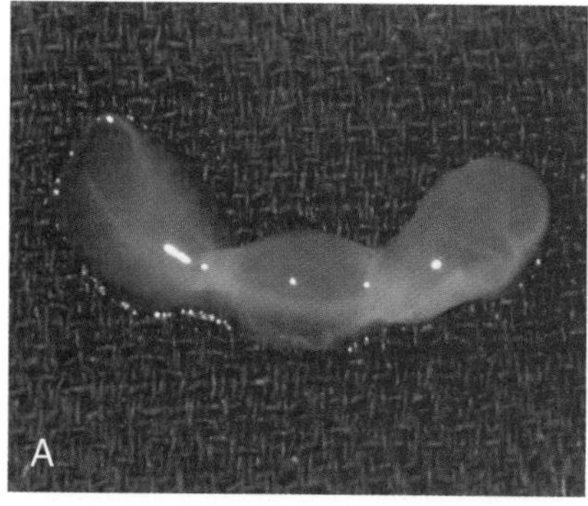

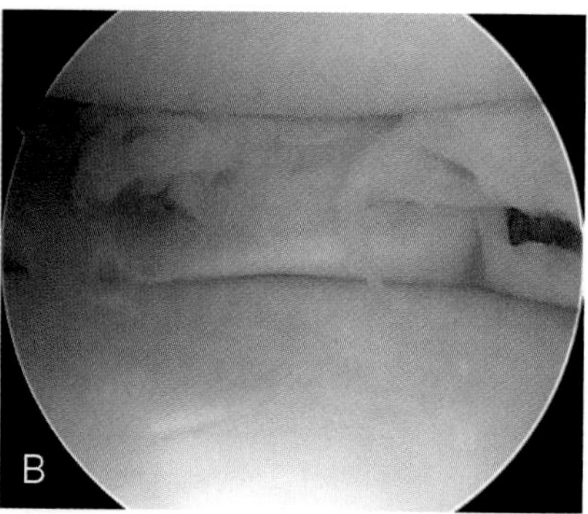

Figure 12 **A,** A platelet-rich fibrin matrix. **B,** Arthroscopic in situ view of a platelet-rich fibrin matrix.

Outcomes

In a prospective study, Kotsovolos et al[48] reported on 61 consecutive meniscal repairs with an integrated locking suture and anchor device, with an average 18-month follow-up. Results showed a 90.2% clinical success rate, with success defined as no joint line tenderness, locking, or swelling, and a negative McMurray test. The mean postoperative Lysholm scores significantly improved compared with preoperative scores, with 88% of the patients having good or excellent results. The patients also had significantly improved Tegner scores postoperatively. Clinical success was consistent for both isolated meniscal repairs and those associated with an ACL reconstruction. In a similar study, Barber et al[49] reported that patients had an 83% success rate for repairs with an integrated locking suture and anchor device.

Using CT arthrographic assessment to determine whether there are different rates of healing depending on the zone (anterior, middle, posterior) of the meniscus, Pujol et al[7] studied 53 consecutive meniscal repairs performed with an integrated locking suture and anchor device, outside-in sutures, or both devices, which were prospectively followed for 1 year. Tears extending from the posterior to middle segments had a significantly higher healing rate than that of an isolated posterior repair. Overall, patients had significantly increased IKDC scores postoperatively; those scores correlated well with the longitudinal healing rate.

In a study evaluating a first generation integrated locking suture and anchor device (RapidLoc with a poly-L-lactic acid top hat), Quinby et al[50] reported a 90.7% success rate in patients treated with a concomitant ACL reconstruction at a mean follow-up of 34.8 months. The authors also found a significant negative correlation with chronic tears of more than 3 months duration and lower IKDC scores. Billante et al[51] subsequently studied a newer integrated locking suture and anchor device (RapidLoc system with a polydioxanone top hat) and reported a clinical success rate of 86.8% at a mean follow-up of 30.4 months in patients who were treated with a concomitant ACL reconstruction. The only clinical factor that significantly differed between a successful outcome and a failed outcome was the Visual Analog Scale domain of self-reported perceived pain, with patients with clinical failures reporting higher pain levels. In addition, there were no chondral injuries noted during four second-look arthroscopies.

The repair of tears located in Cooper radial zones 1 and 2 with the RapidLoc, T-Fix (Acufex Microsurgical, Mansfield, MA), and FasT-Fix were studied and reported on by Kalliakmanis et al.[52] The clinical success rates were 92.4% for the FasT-Fix, 87% for the T-Fix, and 86.5% for the RapidLoc. All groups showed a significant increase in Lysholm and IKDC scores, with no significant differences in functional scores between the groups.

Complications

The complications associated with all-arthroscopic meniscal repairs include chondral injury, soft-tissue inflammation, painful implants, and failure to heal. For routine knee arthroscopy, the risk of infection has been shown to be 0.23% to 0.42%, with an increased risk for patients with extended tourniquet time, multiple procedures, and a history of prior surgery.[53,54] The risks of neurologic injury are greatest in the arthroscopically assisted methods of meniscal repair (0.059% to 4.9%), with medial meniscal repairs associated with saphenous neurapraxia (in up to 43% of patients) and lateral meniscal repairs associated with peroneal neuropathy.[55] Specifically, inside-out repairs of the medial meniscus with accessory incisions have been reported to carry an overall complication rate as high as 19%, with a rate of 13% for inside-out repairs of the lateral meniscus.[56]

The main complications associated with the use of all-arthroscopic rigid meniscal fixators were broken and prominent implants, retained polymer foreign bodies after failed resorption, inflammatory reactions, cyst formation, and chondral injuries.[55] These risks have been significantly decreased with the development of suture-based meniscal repair devices. Cohen et al[57] examined the proximity of implants to neurovascular structures about the knee and discovered that the needle of an integrated locking suture and anchor all-arthroscopic device without a depth limiter was as close as 0.5 mm from the popliteal artery on a lateral radiograph.

The complications most specific to the suture-based devices are soft-tissue irritation from the extracapsular placement of the anchors and the associated learning curve, which may lead to even greater increases in surgical and tourniquet time during a surgeon's initial experience with the devices.[39,55]

Future Directions

Okuda et al[58] studied the ability to expand the vascularity of the synovial tissue in tears of the avascular zone to improve healing rates. After creating a longitudinal tear in the avascular zone of rabbit menisci, meniscal rasping was performed from the parameniscal synovium to the inner portion of the tear. The same tear was created in the contralateral knee, but no rasping was performed to provide a controlled comparison. After 16 weeks, the rasped menisci showed significantly improved macroscopic and histologic healing results compared with the control menisci; at both 4 and 8 weeks, the rasped group showed statistically increased maximal tensile strength and stiffness.

O'Shea and Shelbourne[59] analyzed patients with displaced bucket-handle meniscal tears who were treated with a two-staged procedure of meniscal repair and subsequent ACL reconstruction. This method allowed the authors to investigate their meniscal repairs during the latter surgery. The meniscal repairs with vertical mattress sutures were performed after trephination of the tear site. The ACL reconstruction was performed only after the affected knee had the same range of motion as the uninvolved knee. At the time of the ACL reconstruction, only 6 of 55 meniscal repairs showed no signs of healing. After an average 4-year follow-up, 83.7% of white-white zone meniscal repairs remained asymptomatic, whereas all red-white and red-red zone repairs remained asymptomatic.

Rubman et al[60] evaluated 198 inside-out meniscal repairs of tears with a rim width of 4 mm or greater and a mean follow-up of 2 years. The sutures were placed in a vertical mattress or double vertical mattress configuration. Of the 91 patients who were treated with repeat arthroscopy, 64% had healed or partially healed menisci. There was a significant improvement in healing in patients who had the repair in the lateral tibiofemoral compartment compared with the medial compartment, in patients who had a shorter period of time from repair to follow-up arthroscopic examination and in those with no tibiofemoral compartment symptoms.

In an analysis of five patients with a tear of the posterolateral aspect of the lateral meniscus anterior to the popliteus fossa, van Trommel et al[61] reported excellent healing after meniscal repair with an outside-in technique with the addition of a fibrin clot. This area of the lateral meniscus is difficult to repair because of the extremely limited number of penetrating vessels. In this small study, MRI showed complete healing at the repair sites; all patients in the study regained their preoperative function.

Platelet-rich plasma and platelet-rich fibrin matrix have both shown promise in improving histologic outcomes of meniscal repair. Ishida et al[62] found that platelet-rich plasma improved healing rates in vivo and caused increased production of the extracellular matrix proteins biglycan and decorin. These proteins indicate the repopulation of appropriate meniscal extracellular matrix. The use of angiogenic suture material is being considered as a technique to improve the poor vascular supply to the central third of the meniscus. Angiogenic sutures directly supply biochemical agents or growth factors to an area that is known to be vascularly challenged. After trephination and débridement of the meniscocapsular junction, these growth factors may facilitate blood vessel proliferation in a previously avascular region.

Tissue engineering and gene therapy have directed pluripotent mesenchymal, adipose, and hematopoietic stem cells down a variety of pathways to facilitate regeneration of bone, cartilage, tendon, and ligaments.[63] These technologies may have the ability to improve meniscal repair outcomes and healing rates in biologically at-risk areas. Cell-based therapies may represent a promising source of future research to promote healing in the avascular portions of menisci. Weinand et al[64] harvested chondrocytes from porcine costal cartilage, seeded them onto scaffolds, and cultured the cells. After 1 week, the construct was implanted into a white-white tear of the porcine medial meniscus. After 12 weeks, the menisci were harvested and were found to have gross closure of the lesion, acceptable integration into the native meniscus, and were grossly mechanically stable. Histologically, no cellular rejection was noted. Peretti et al[65] reported similar results by using porcine menisci as a scaffold, which was then seeded with meniscal fibrochondrocytes. The meniscal scaffolds were then implanted into a longitudinal tear in the avascular portion of the medial meniscus that had been repaired with a vertical mattress suture. A similar tear was created and repaired in the contralateral knee to serve as a control. The repairs treated with the cell-based therapy showed improved healing characteristics, both grossly and histologically.

The Authors' Preferred Technique

Surgical meniscus repair is commonly performed with the patient under general anesthesia. The patient is placed supine on the operating table, and a lateral post is used to facilitate valgus stress of the knee when treating medial meniscal pathology. If additional procedures are planned, such as ACL reconstruction or cartilage resurfacing procedures, the meniscal pathology is treated primarily.

The characteristics of the meniscal tear, including tear size, length, geometry, stability, ease of reduction, and tissue viability must be assessed and are used by the surgeon to choose the most appropriate suturing technique. To achieve a safe delivery and approach, a contralateral portal is used for either all-arthroscopic or inside-out suturing.

If a concomitant ACL reconstruction is not performed, a fibrin clot or platelet-rich fibrin matrix technique is used, and autologous blood is procured sterilely and prepared by the surgical team.[35,36] The first essential step in the repair process is to débride the tear site, its edges, and the peripheral meniscocapsular junction. Additional vascular access channels can be created by performing trephination across the tear site directed to the periphery using an 18-gauge spinal needle. The tear is then reduced, and provisional fixation can be provided with an 18-gauge spinal needle or an outside-in No. 0 polydioxanone traction stitch. After appropriate reduction has been obtained, vertical mattress sutures are placed approximately 3 to 5 mm apart. Greater stability may be obtained with the introduction of a double vertical mattress suture using alternating femoral- and tibial-side divergent patterns. Anterior and middle third meniscal tears are generally treated with a hybridized technique using both all-arthroscopic meniscal suture devices and outside-in suturing using a vertical mattress suture configuration with 18-gauge needles and wire loop suture retrievers.

The platelet-rich fibrin matrix technique, which is used in cases of "isolated" meniscal repair, involves obtaining 9 mL of autologous blood that is then transferred to a collection kit (Cascade Autologous Platelet System; Musculoskeletal Transplant Foundation, Edison, NJ). The blood is centrifuged for 15 minutes to separate the red blood cells from the platelet-rich plasma, and then the plasma is centrifuged for 6 minutes to create a fibrin matrix that is stable enough for suture fixation. The volume stable platelet-rich fibrin matrix is then inserted during meniscal suturing and incorporated into the repair construct.[3]

Postoperative rehabilitation protocols are individualized for each patient and are based on the type of repaired tear. In the operating room, the knee is placed in an immobilizer or hinged brace that is locked in extension. It may be removed for range of motion therapy and when comfort allows at approximately 3 to 4 weeks postoperatively. Initially, weight bearing is limited to prevent excessive compressive or shear forces on the repair. After antalgic symptoms have subsided and quadriceps strength is adequate, full weight bearing is permitted. Range of motion of 0° to 90° is initiated on postoperative day 1, with progression to terminal flexion gradually increased over 8 weeks. Avascular and biologically at-risk tears may remain protected for a longer period of time with a more measured rehabilitation protocol.

Summary

The evolution of meniscal repair techniques has helped to place a greater emphasis on meniscus repair and preservation. Newer all-arthroscopic suture-based meniscal repair devices can provide biomechanical stability through compression across the tear site with associated equivalent mechanical properties compared with traditional arthroscopically assisted inside-out repairs. With newer implant development and less invasive arthroscopic techniques, learning curves for surgeons are decreasing and successful clinical outcomes are being maintained or improved. The potential addition and advances of biologic augmentation in the future may serve to broaden the indications and success of meniscal repair.

References

1. Henning CE, Lynch MA, Yearout KM, Vequist SW, Stallbaumer RJ, Decker KA: Arthroscopic meniscal repair using an exogenous fibrin clot. *Clin Orthop Relat Res* 1990;252:64-72.
2. Freedman KB, Nho SJ, Cole BJ: Marrow stimulating technique to augment meniscus repair. *Arthroscopy* 2003;19(7):794-798.
3. Angel MJ, Sgaglione NA, Grande DA: Clinical applications of bioactive factors in sports medicine: Current concepts and future trends. *Sports Med Arthrosc* 2006; 14(3):138-145.
4. Malanga GA, Andrus S, Nadler SF, McLean J: Physical examination of the knee: A review of the original test description and scientific validity of common orthopedic tests. *Arch Phys Med Rehabil* 2003;84(4):592-603.
5. Evans PJ, Bell GD, Frank C: Prospective evaluation of the McMurray test. *Am J Sports Med* 1993; 21(4):604-608.

6. Karachalios T, Hantes M, Zibis AH, Zachos V, Karantanas AH, Malizos KN: Diagnostic accuracy of a new clinical test (the Thessaly test) for early detection of meniscal tears. *J Bone Joint Surg Am* 2005;87(5):955-962.
7. Pujol N, Panarella L, Selmi TA, Neyret P, Fithian D, Beaufils P: Meniscal healing after meniscal repair: A CT arthrography assessment. *Am J Sports Med* 2008; 36(8):1489-1495.
8. Terzidis IP, Christodoulou A, Ploumis A, Givissis P, Natsis K, Koimtzis M: Meniscal tear characteristics in young athletes with a stable knee: Arthroscopic evaluation. *Am J Sports Med* 2006;34(7): 1170-1175.
9. Cooper DE, Arnoczky SP, Warren RF: Meniscal repair. *Clin Sports Med* 1991;10(3):529-548.
10. Arnoczky SP, Warren RF: Microvasculature of the human meniscus. *Am J Sports Med* 1982;10(2): 90-95.
11. Fazalare JJ, McCormick KR, Babins DB: Meniscal repair of the knee. *Orthopedics* 2009;32(3): 199-205.
12. Sgaglione NA, Steadman JR, Shaffer B, Miller MD, Fu FH: Current concepts in meniscus surgery: Resection to replacement. *Arthroscopy* 2003;19(10, Suppl 1): 161-188.
13. Faunø P, Nielsen AB: Arthroscopic partial meniscectomy: A long-term follow-up. *Arthroscopy* 1992;8(3):345-349.
14. Jørgensen U, Sonne-Holm S, Lauridsen F, Rosenklint A: Long-term follow-up of meniscectomy in athletes: A prospective longitudinal study. *J Bone Joint Surg Br* 1987;69(1):80-83.
15. Fabricant PD, Jokl P: Surgical outcomes after arthroscopic partial meniscectomy. *J Am Acad Orthop Surg* 2007;15(11): 647-653.
16. Fabricant PD, Rosenberger PH, Jokl P, Ickovics JR: Predictors of short-term recovery differ from those of long-term outcome after arthroscopic partial meniscectomy. *Arthroscopy* 2008;24(7): 769-778.
17. Chatain F, Adeleine P, Chambat P, Neyret P; Société Française d'Arthroscopie: A comparative study of medial versus lateral arthroscopic partial meniscectomy on stable knees: 10-year minimum follow-up. *Arthroscopy* 2003; 19(8):842-849.
18. Levy IM, Torzilli PA, Warren RF: The effect of medial meniscectomy on anterior-posterior motion of the knee. *J Bone Joint Surg Am* 1982;64(6):883-888.
19. Sturnieks DL, Besier TF, Mills PM, et al: Knee joint biomechanics following arthroscopic partial meniscectomy. *J Orthop Res* 2008;26(8):1075-1080.
20. Allaire R, Muriuki M, Gilbertson L, Harner CD: Biomechanical consequences of a tear of the posterior root of the medial meniscus: Similar to total meniscectomy. *J Bone Joint Surg Am* 2008;90(9): 1922-1931.
21. McDermott ID, Amis AA: The consequences of meniscectomy. *J Bone Joint Surg Br* 2006;88(12): 1549-1556.
22. Baratz ME, Fu FH, Mengato R: Meniscal tears: The effect of meniscectomy and of repair on intraarticular contact areas and stress in the human knee: A preliminary report. *Am J Sports Med* 1986;14(4):270-275.
23. Burke DL, Ahmed AM, Miller J: A biomechanical study of partial and total medial meniscectomy of the knee. *Trans Orthop Res Soc* 1978;3:91.
24. McNicholas MJ, Rowley DI, McGurty D, et al: Total meniscectomy in adolescence: A thirty-year follow-up. *J Bone Joint Surg Br* 2000;82(2):217-221.
25. Shelbourne KD, Heinrich J: The long-term evaluation of lateral meniscus tears left in situ at the time of anterior cruciate ligament reconstruction. *Arthroscopy* 2004; 20(4):346-351.
26. Tenuta JJ, Arciero RA: Arthroscopic evaluation of meniscal repairs: Factors that effect healing. *Am J Sports Med* 1994;22(6): 797-802.
27. Cannon WD Jr, Vittori JM: The incidence of healing in arthroscopic meniscal repairs in anterior cruciate ligament-reconstructed knees versus stable knees. *Am J Sports Med* 1992; 20(2):176-181.
28. Scott GA, Jolly BL, Henning CE: Combined posterior incision and arthroscopic intra-articular repair of the meniscus: An examination of factors affecting healing. *J Bone Joint Surg Am* 1986;68(6): 847-861.
29. Noyes FR, Barber-Westin SD: Arthroscopic repair of meniscus tears extending into the avascular zone with or without anterior cruciate ligament reconstruction in patients 40 years of age and older. *Arthroscopy* 2000;16(8): 822-829.
30. Noyes FR, Barber-Westin SD: Arthroscopic repair of meniscal tears extending into the avascular zone in patients younger than twenty years of age. *Am J Sports Med* 2002;30(4):589-600.
31. Krych AJ, McIntosh AL, Voll AE, Stuart MJ, Dahm DL: Arthroscopic repair of isolated meniscal tears in patients 18 years and younger. *Am J Sports Med* 2008;36(7):1283-1289.
32. Rodeo SA: Arthroscopic meniscal repair with use of the outside-in technique. *Instr Course Lect* 2000; 49:195-206.
33. Kohn D, Siebert W: Meniscus suture techniques: A comparative biomechanical cadaver study. *Arthroscopy* 1989;5(4):324-327.

34. Post WR, Akers SR, Kish V: Load to failure of common meniscal repair techniques: Effects of suture technique and suture material. *Arthroscopy* 1997;13(6):731-736.
35. Sgaglione NA: New generation meniscus fixator devices. *Sports Med Arthrosc* 2004;12(1):44-59.
36. Sgaglione NA: Meniscus repair update: Current concepts and new techniques. *Orthopedics* 2005;28(3):280-286.
37. Lozano J, Ma CB, Cannon WD: All-inside meniscus repair: A systematic review. *Clin Orthop Relat Res* 2007;455:134-141.
38. Lee GP, Diduch DR: Deteriorating outcomes after meniscal repair using the Meniscus Arrow in knees undergoing concurrent anterior cruciate ligament reconstruction: Increased failure rate with long-term follow-up. *Am J Sports Med* 2005;33(8):1138-1141.
39. Borden P, Nyland J, Caborn DN, Pienkowski D: Biomechanical comparison of the FasT-Fix meniscal repair suture system with vertical mattress sutures and meniscus arrows. *Am J Sports Med* 2003;31(3):374-378.
40. Barber FA: Accelerated rehabilitation for meniscus repairs. *Arthroscopy* 1994;10(2):206-210.
41. Mariani PP, Santori N, Adriani E, Mastantuono M: Accelerated rehabilitation after arthroscopic meniscal repair: A clinical and magnetic resonance imaging evaluation. *Arthroscopy* 1996;12(6):680-686.
42. Barber FA, Herbert MA, Richards DP: Load to failure testing of new meniscal repair devices. *Arthroscopy* 2004;20(1):45-50.
43. Barber FA, Herbert MA, Schroeder FA, Aziz-Jacobo J, Sutker MJ: Biomechanical testing of new meniscal repair techniques containing ultra high-molecular weight polyethylene suture. *Arthroscopy* 2009;25(9):959-967.
44. Zantop T, Eggers AK, Weimann A, Hassenpflug J, Petersen W: Initial fixation strength of flexible all-inside meniscus suture anchors in comparison to conventional suture technique and rigid anchors: Biomechanical evaluation of new meniscus refixation systems. *Am J Sports Med* 2004;32(4):863-869.
45. Zantop T, Eggers AK, Musahl V, Weimann A, Petersen W: Cyclic testing of flexible all-inside meniscus suture anchors: Biomechanical analysis. *Am J Sports Med* 2005;33(3):388-394.
46. Chang HC, Nyland J, Caborn DN, Burden R: Biomechanical evaluation of meniscal repair systems: A comparison of the Meniscal Viper Repair System, the vertical mattress FasT-Fix Device, and vertical mattress ethibond sutures. *Am J Sports Med* 2005;33(12):1846-1852.
47. Arnoczky SP, Warren RF, Spivak JM: Meniscal repair using an exogenous fibrin clot: An experimental study in dogs. *J Bone Joint Surg Am* 1988;70(8):1209-1217.
48. Kotsovolos ES, Hantes ME, Mastrokalos DS, Lorbach O, Paessler HH: Results of all-inside meniscal repair with the FasT-Fix meniscal repair system. *Arthroscopy* 2006;22(1):3-9.
49. Barber FA, Schroeder FA, Oro FB, Beavis RC: FasT-Fix meniscal repair: mid-term results. *Arthroscopy* 2008;24(12):1342-1348.
50. Quinby JS, Golish SR, Hart JA, Diduch DR: All-inside meniscal repair using a new flexible, tensionable device. *Am J Sports Med* 2006;34(8):1281-1286.
51. Billante MJ, Diduch DR, Lunardini DJ, Treme GP, Miller MD, Hart JM: Meniscal repair using an all-inside, rapidly absorbing, tensionable device. *Arthroscopy* 2008;24(7):779-785.
52. Kalliakmanis A, Zourntos S, Bousgas D, Nikolaou P: Comparison of arthroscopic meniscal repair results using 3 different meniscal repair devices in anterior cruciate ligament reconstruction patients. *Arthroscopy* 2008;24(7):810-816.
53. Armstrong RW, Bolding F, Joseph R: Septic arthritis following arthroscopy: Clinical syndromes and analysis of risk factors. *Arthroscopy* 1992;8(2):213-223.
54. Wind WM, McGrath BE, Mindell ER: Infection following knee arthroscopy. *Arthroscopy* 2001;17(8):878-883.
55. Sgaglione NA: Complications of meniscus surgery. *Sports Med Arthrosc* 2004;12(3):148-159.
56. Austin KS, Sherman OH: Complications of arthroscopic meniscal repair. *Am J Sports Med* 1993;21(6):864-868, discussion 868-869.
57. Cohen SB, Boyd L, Miller MD: Vascular risk associated with meniscal repair using Rapidloc versus FasT-Fix: Comparison of two all-inside meniscal devices. *J Knee Surg* 2007;20(3):235-240.
58. Okuda K, Ochi M, Shu N, Uchio Y: Meniscal rasping for repair of meniscal tear in the avascular zone. *Arthroscopy* 1999;15(3): 281-286.
59. O'Shea JJ, Shelbourne KD: Repair of locked bucket-handle meniscal tears in knees with chronic anterior cruciate ligament deficiency. *Am J Sports Med* 2003;31(2):216-220.
60. Rubman MH, Noyes FR, Barber-Westin SD: Arthroscopic repair of meniscal tears that extend into the avascular zone: A review of 198 single and complex tears. *Am J Sports Med* 1998;26(1):87-95.
61. van Trommel MF, Simonian PT, Potter HG, Wickiewicz TL: Arthroscopic meniscal repair with fibrin clot of complete radial tears of the lateral meniscus in the avascular zone. *Arthroscopy* 1998;14(4):360-365.

62. Ishida K, Kuroda R, Miwa M, et al: The regenerative effects of platelet-rich plasma on meniscal cells in vitro and its in vivo application with biodegradable gelatin hydrogel. *Tissue Eng* 2007;13(5): 1103-1112.

63. Kessler MW, Ackerman G, Dines JS, Grande DA: Emerging technologies and fourth generation issues in cartilage repair. *Sports Med Arthrosc* 2008;16(4): 246-254.

64. Weinand C, Peretti GM, Adams SB Jr, Randolph MA, Savvidis E, Gill TJ: Healing potential of transplanted allogeneic chondrocytes of three different sources in lesions of the avascular zone of the meniscus: A pilot study. *Arch Orthop Trauma Surg* 2006; 126(9):599-605.

65. Peretti GM, Gill TJ, Xu JW, Randolph MA, Morse KR, Zaleske DJ: Cell-based therapy for meniscal repair: A large animal study. *Am J Sports Med* 2004;32(1): 146-158.

Enhancing Meniscal Repair Through Biology: Platelet-Rich Plasma as an Alternative Strategy

Demetris Delos, MD
Scott A. Rodeo, MD

Abstract

Meniscal tears are common orthopaedic injuries that can manifest with significant pain and mechanical symptoms. The treatment of meniscal tears has evolved from total meniscectomy to partial meniscectomy and meniscal repair. Preserving the meniscus is ideal because the loss of any portion of the meniscus can lead to significantly increased articular cartilage contact stresses compared with the intact state. However, most of the meniscus has a limited ability to heal because of poor vascularity. This has prompted a search for a better understanding of the biology of meniscal healing and methods to enhance the process.

Growth factors have been shown to positively affect meniscal cell function, including platelet-derived growth factor, fibroblast growth factor, basic fibroblast growth factor, transforming growth factor-β, insulin-like growth factor, bone morphogenetic protein, hepatocyte growth factor, and vascular endothelial growth factor. In vitro studies have shown that other cytokines, including interleukin-1, tumor necrosis factor-α, and the matrix metalloproteinases, negatively affect meniscal healing.

Identification of these growth factors has led to strategies to deliver serum-derived factors to the meniscus to improve healing. Platelet-rich plasma is the latest technique to be evaluated for augmenting meniscal healing. Activation of the platelets leads to the local release of growth factors from the alpha and dense granules located in the platelet cytoplasm. These growth factors have been associated with the initiation of a healing cascade leading to cellular chemotaxis, angiogenesis, collagen matrix synthesis, and cell proliferation.

Instr Course Lect 2011;60:453-460.

Dr. Rodeo or an immediate family member has received research or institutional support from Wyeth and owns stock or stock options in Cayenne Medical. Neither Dr. Delos nor any immediate family member has received anything of value from or owns stock in a commercial company or institution related directly or indirectly to the subject of this chapter.

Meniscal tears are common orthopaedic injuries. Patients often present with significant pain and mechanical symptoms. Historically, a total meniscectomy was advocated for treatment; however, surgeons are now aware of the critical function of the meniscus and emphasize meniscal preservation strategies. Because the effectiveness of meniscal repairs is limited by the avascularity of the central meniscus, new treatment strategies that can enhance the repair process are being investigated. In the past, fibrin clot was advocated for augmenting repairs; now, platelet-rich plasma (PRP) is being investigated for its potential therapeutic properties. This chapter will present an overview of the biology of meniscal healing and will review techniques that aim to translate that knowledge into improved meniscal healing, with an emphasis on the use of PRP.

The Clinical Problem

Meniscal tears are common injuries, with an estimated mean annual incidence of 60 to 70 per 100,000 individuals.[1,2] These tears can cause knee swelling and pain, along with occasional mechanical symptoms of locking or catching, clicking, and blocked extension. The critical role of the meniscus in knee function has been recognized for some time, with contemporary data showing poor long-term outcomes with rapidly advancing secondary osteoarthritis following meniscectomy.[3-5] This information has resulted in efforts aimed at preserving the meniscus, including partial meniscectomy and meniscal repair.

Evidence shows that all forms of meniscectomy can lead to an increased risk of osteoarthritis over time, and that the extent of resection correlates with the extent of radiographic osteoarthritis.[6,7] Partial meniscectomy also has been reported to significantly decrease contact areas and increase mean and peak loads, with peak loads in the knee elevated 65% compared with the intact state.[8-10] Total meniscectomy has been shown to increase peak loads up to 235%.[8] However, meniscal repair has not been proven superior to partial meniscectomy.[11,12] Although the causes for this appear to be multifactorial (including the type of repair and the integrity of the meniscal and articular cartilage at the time of injury and prior to injury), the healing capacity of the meniscus may be an important factor. The current standard of care is to preserve native tissue, if possible, rather than resect it. There is a great need for novel methods to augment meniscal repair. To devise these methods, it is necessary to understand the biology of meniscal healing.

The Biology of Meniscal Healing

Blood Supply and Vascularity

Seminal studies on the vascularity of the meniscus show that only the peripheral 10% to 25% of the adult meniscus is vascularized (by the superior and inferior medial and lateral geniculate arteries).[13,14] Most of the meniscus receives nutrients through local diffusion. This observation is often used to explain why peripheral tears display a more robust healing response compared with more central lesions, a finding noted as early as 1936.[15-19] More recent work provides further evidence that regional differences in meniscal healing may be primarily related to vascularity rather than intrinsic disparities. An in vitro porcine model of meniscal repair comparing explants from the outer, vascular, peripheral zone and the inner avascular zone showed similar healing potential, with no difference in repair strength between the two groups.[20]

Effect of Cytokines and Growth Factors on Meniscal Healing

Since the elucidation of the blood supply to the human meniscus, investigators have sought to enhance the healing response through a better understanding of the inflammatory cascade and the factors involved in meniscal repair. In 1985, Webber et al[21] reported that meniscal cells were capable of replication and matrix synthesis when introduced to an anabolic environment. They showed that fibrochondrocytes could be stimulated by the addition of either fibroblast growth factor (FGF) or human platelet lysate in a dose-dependent manner. Since that time, extensive research has been conducted on the various cytokines and growth factors that may play a role in meniscal healing.

Proinflammatory Cytokines

In vitro studies have shown that the proinflammatory cytokines, tumor necrosis factor-α and interleukin-1 (IL-1), can inhibit meniscal repair despite the presence of viable cells.[22,23] Even a single day of exposure to IL-1 was shown to reduce cell accumulation and repair shear strength.[23] IL-1 also has been associated with an increase in matrix metalloproteinase (MMP) activity.[23,24] Attempts to inhibit either IL-1 or tumor necrosis factor-α can promote integrative repair in an inflammatory environment.[25] In vitro work also has shown that the inhibition of MMPs can enhance meniscal repair. The broad-spectrum MMP inhibitor GM 6001 was reported to decrease MMP activity, increase in vitro meniscal repair shear strength, and enhance tissue repair at the healing interface.[26]

Growth Factors

Growth factors that have previously been shown to be involved in the repair and healing of musculoskeletal tissues include platelet-derived growth factor (PDGF), FGF, transforming growth factor β (TGF-β), and insulin-like growth factor (IGF).[27-30] Consequently, these factors are appealing targets for investigation in the context of meniscal repair. A recent report has shown that IGF-1, TGF-β1, and basic fibroblast growth factor (bFGF) can promote in vitro human fetal meniscal cell proliferation, and combinations of these growth factors show greater effects than growth factors in isolation.[31]

Growth Factors Can Increase DNA and Extracellular Matrix Synthesis in All Meniscal Zones

IGF-1 has been shown to increase the synthesis of DNA and extracellular matrix in all meniscal zones, with a greater response from cells in the avascular zone.[32] TGF-β, bFGF, and PDGF-AB have also been shown to promote cell proliferation and extracellular matrix formation in all zones of the meniscus.[33-35] Human meniscal specimens sutured with gelatin hydrogel-coated thread incorporating FGF-2 showed more proliferating cells and fewer apoptotic cells compared with control specimens.[36] An additional effect of FGF-2 includes increased gene expression of matrix-associated proteoglycans (biglycan and fibromodulin) by human meniscal cells, which was further enhanced by culture in a hypoxic (5% oxygen tension) environment.[37] A dose-dependent increase in proteoglycan synthesis has been previously reported for PDGF-AB, TGF-β1, and bone morphogenetic protein-7.[38]

Combining Factors

Combining growth factors also has been shown to have a positive effect on healing. In a recent in vitro study, the combination of hepatocyte growth factor and PDGF resulted in the alignment and migration of meniscal cells toward the meniscal defect. By 4 weeks, the combination of factors resulted in the formation of tissue suggestive of organized collagen.[39]

Differences in Response Based on Region

Other investigators have reported a differential response to factors based on the cellular region of origin.[40-42] In one study, cells from the outer (vascular) zone exhibited higher rates of DNA synthesis (maximum twofold) with exposure to PDGF-AB, hepatocyte growth factor, and bone morphogenetic protein-2 when compared with cells from the inner (avascular) zone.[40] In another study, meniscal explants obtained from the inner avascular zone were reported to lack the ability to proliferate in the presence of PDGF-AB, whereas explants from the outer vascular region showed a 2.5-fold increase in DNA synthesis in the presence of PDGF-AB.[41] In an in vitro rabbit model, meniscal tissue taken from the peripheral zone and implanted into a defect in the avascular zone showed better healing than defects in the avascular zone.[42]

These data conflict with the results of a study by Hennerbichler et al[20] in which no differences in healing between explants from the avascular and vascular zones in a porcine in vitro model were reported. After 6 weeks of culture, the authors reported the migration of cells to the repair site with subsequent bridging tissue formation at the healing interface in both groups. Therefore, it is not yet clear whether the differences in healing in the different zones of the meniscus can be completely attributed to vascularity.

Vascular Endothelial Growth Factor and Angiogenesis

The role of vascular endothelial growth factor (VEGF) in meniscal healing has been investigated. In a rabbit model of meniscal injury, 90% of meniscal lacerations had healed in 5 to 10 weeks, without any healing observed in the avascular area. Although VEGF expression was found to be greatest in the avascular region, true angiogenesis (blood vessel formation) was lacking.[43] Local application of VEGF in the form of sutures coated with VEGF and poly-DL-lactic acid also failed to promote meniscal healing in the avascular zone in a sheep model.[44,45] Although VEGF was observed to promote endothelial cell formation, vasculogenesis was not apparent. Of note, MMP-13 expression was found in the treated group, which could weaken the tissue because of matrix degradation.

Bone Marrow Stem Cells and Growth Factors

In a recently published study, human IGF-1 transfected into bone marrow stem cells and mixed with calcium alginate gel was shown to improve healing of full-thickness meniscal defects in the avascular zone in a goat in vivo model.[46] The experimental group showed filling of the defect with tissue resembling normal meniscal fibrocartilage and a higher proteoglycan content than the control group. In a 2007 study, transplantation of TGF-β1-transduced bone marrow stem cells seeded into type I collagen-glycosaminoglycan matrices in bovine meniscal lesions of the avascular zone resulted in filling of the lesions with repair tissue after 3 weeks of in vitro culture.[47]

These studies are some of the first to use tissue engineering to try to enhance meniscal healing and repair. The studies provide exciting new alternative approaches, which may hold great promise in the future.

Surgical Techniques to Enhance the Biologic Response

With more data showing the positive effects of specific growth factors on meniscal healing and repair and the inhibitory effects of certain cytokines and proinflammatory mediators, clinicians have attempted to translate that knowledge into techniques to enhance healing through neovascularization (trephination and rasping) or augmentation via the local application of growth factors (such as fibrin clot and PRP).

Neovascularization Techniques: Trephination and Rasping

Trephination (creating holes in the meniscus) and rasping are procedures that attempt to increase vascularity by stimulating vascular channel development and blood flow to the area of injury. Animal studies have reported evidence of partial or complete healing by trephination in artificially created longitudinal injuries in the avascular area of dog menisci, along with enhanced healing in goats with unstable lesions that were sutured and trephined.[48,49]

In stable, peripheral, vertical, medial meniscal tears treated with abrasion and trephination at the time of anterior cruciate ligament reconstruction surgery, up to 94% of patients remained asymptomatic without further stabilization.[11] Similarly good results were reported for patients with lateral meniscal tears; only 8 of 332 patients (2.4%) required subsequent surgery after using this technique.[50] Good or excellent results were reported in 90% of cases in one study of patients with symptomatic incomplete meniscal tears.[51]

Meniscal rasping has been shown to elevate levels of cytokines, such as IL-1α, TGF-β1, PDGF, and proliferating cell nuclear antigen (also known as cyclin, which functions as a cofactor for DNA polymerase-δ in DNA) in a rabbit model of meniscal injury in the avascular zone.[52] However, trephination and rasping have limited applicability to larger tears, and clinical data are limited regarding their effectiveness in treating tears in the avascular zone.

Augmentation

Fibrin Clot

The use of fibrin clot for the purpose of meniscal healing was first described by Arnoczky et al[53] in 1988. The authors observed that defects filled with fibrin clot healed through a proliferation of fibrous connective tissue that eventually modulated into fibrocartilaginous tissue. The fibrin clot appeared to act as a chemotactic and mitogenic stimulus for reparative cells while substituting as a scaffold for the reparative process. Their study in dogs showed the absence of healing tissue in the control subjects. Henning et al[54] reported an 8% tear failure rate with exogenous fibrin clot treatment versus 41% in repairs not treated with clot. Fibrin clot also has been reported to enhance healing in peripheral, radial, and lateral meniscal tears that extended to the popliteal tendon; however, results in tears in the inner avascular region have been less favorable and less predictable.[55-57]

Platelet-Rich Plasma

PRP is a new, exciting, locally administered agent that may hold potential in meniscal healing. PRP is a concentrated solution of platelets derived from a patient's own whole blood. Activation of the platelets, whether ex vivo (by thrombin and calcium) or in vivo by exposure to collagen,[58] leads to the local release of growth factors from the alpha and dense granules located in the platelet cytoplasm. Growth factors found within alpha granules include PDGF, VEGF, TGF-β1, epidermal growth factor, bFGF, and IGF-1.[59] These growth factors are associated with the initiation of a healing cascade leading to cellular chemotaxis, angiogenesis, collagen matrix synthesis, and cell proliferation. Adenosine, serotonin, histamine, and calcium are found in the dense granules. Growth factors found in the plasma include hepatocyte growth factor and IGF-1. The vast array of growth factors within PRP makes it an appealing alternative treatment.

The number of clinical applications of PRP is increasing, although the literature regarding its effects on soft-tissue healing is limited. Nevertheless, small case series have shown promising results. In a recent case-controlled study, Sánchez et al[60] reported that six athletes treated with open Achilles tendon repair along with PRP injection recovered range of motion sooner and were able to return to running and training in less time than six athletes treated with open Achilles repair without PRP injection. Mishra et al[61] reported significant pain relief in patients who received a single PRP injection for chronic elbow epicondylar pain at final follow-up. Virchenko and Aspenberg[62] proposed that the increased functional gains observed in a rat Achilles transection model after a single PRP treatment were caused by accelerated healing capacity leading to earlier mechanical stimulation.

PRP and Meniscal Healing

The literature on the effects of PRP on meniscal tissue is limited, with only one published study currently available. In a combination in vivo/in vitro study, Ishida et al[63] reported that PRP enhanced healing of rabbit meniscal defects. In the in vitro study, meniscal cells cultured with PRP showed greater expression of fibrocartilage-related genes. In the in vivo study, 1.5-mm-diameter full-thickness defects were created in the avascular region of rabbit menisci and filled with gelatin hydrogel along with PRP, platelet-poor plasma, or gelatin hydrogel alone. Histologic scoring of the defect sites at 12 weeks revealed significantly better meniscal repair in the rabbits receiving PRP with gelatin hydrogel than in the other two groups.

PRP and Meniscal Repair: Surgical Technique and Clinical Considerations

An important factor to consider in meniscal repair is the kinetics of growth factor release from the PRP implant. Augmentation of healing is probably most effective with the gradual release of cytokines over time, and it is likely that specific factors work best at different times. However, there are currently few data available about the optimal timing for specific factors. This chapter's authors have used the Cascade Platelet-Rich Fibrin Matrix (PRFM) (MTF Sports Medicine, a division of the Musculoskeletal Transplant Foundation, Edison, NJ) preparation for meniscus repair (**Figure 1**). This material can be sutured at the repair site, thus assuring delivery and retention at the tear.

After the repair is completed using the surgeon's favored technique, an additional suture is placed at the tear site. If this suture is placed using either an inside-out or an outside-in technique, it will exit the skin at the joint line. Alternatively, an arthroscopic suture passing device can be used for an all-inside technique. This suture is

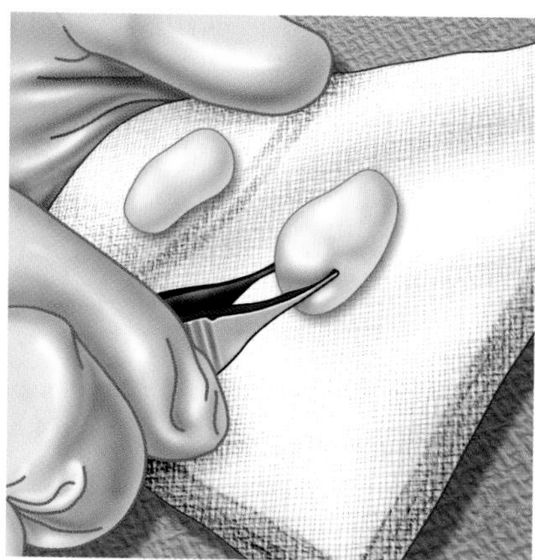

Figure 1 Illustration showing the preparation of the PRFM. (Reproduced with permission from the Musculoskeletal Transplant Foundation, Edison, NJ.)

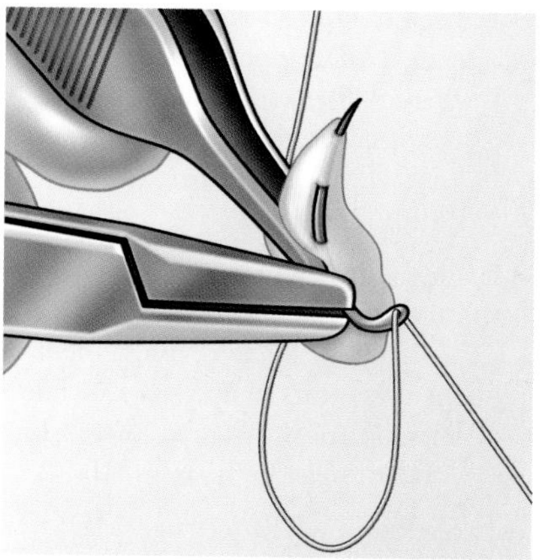

Figure 2 Illustration showing suture passing through the PRFM. (Reproduced with permission from the Musculoskeletal Transplant Foundation, Edison, NJ.)

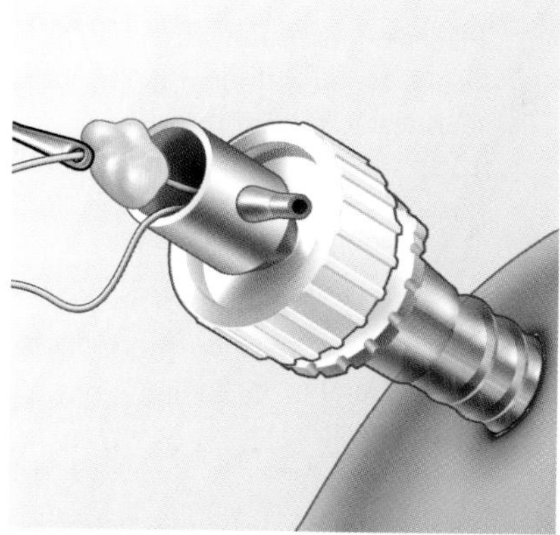

Figure 3 Illustration of the PRFM being shuttled through a cannula. (Reproduced with permission from the Musculoskeletal Transplant Foundation, Edison, NJ.)

brought out of an 8-mm cannula placed in an anterior portal. The PRFM material is attached to the suture (**Figure 2**). This suture is then used to shuttle the PRFM into the tear site (**Figure 3**). It is important to remove the diaphragm from the cannula before the PRFM is pulled through because the diaphragm may damage the PRFM as it is pulled into the joint.

After the PRFM has been shuttled into the joint, it is secured by tying the attached suture (**Figures 4** and **5**). If the suture exits the skin posteromedially or posterolaterally (passed using an inside-out or an outside-in technique), the extra-articular end of the suture is tied to an adjacent suture with the usual technique. If an all-inside technique is used, the suture end is tied to an adjacent suture using arthroscopic knot tying.

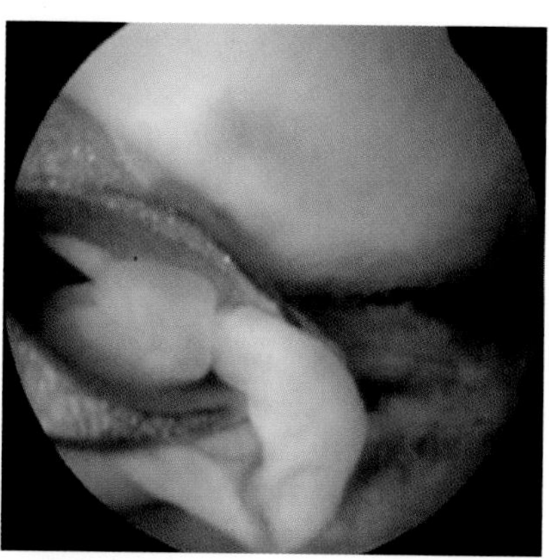

Figure 4 Arthroscopic view of the PRFM being shuttled to the tear site.

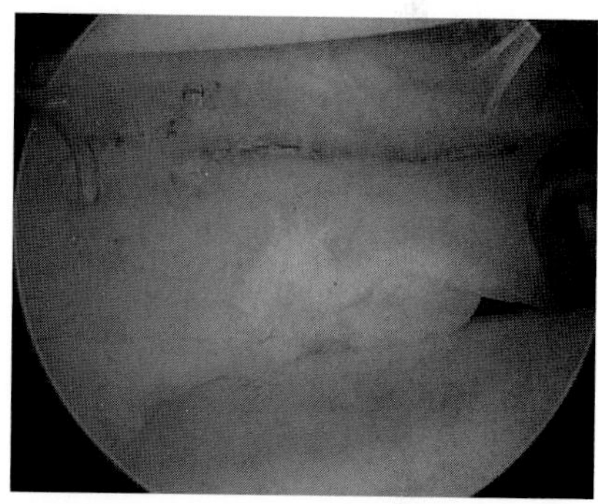

Figure 5 Arthroscopic view of the tear site repaired with PRFM augmentation.

Summary

Partial meniscectomy is usually required for treating a meniscal tear, but it involves the irreversible removal of native tissue with the consequent increase in peak contact stresses across the knee. Meniscal repair is an appealing alternative treatment, but its effectiveness is limited, especially with tears in the avascular zone. Attempts to improve outcomes in meniscal repairs have relied on an increasing working knowledge of the biology of meniscal healing. A variety of growth factors have been implicated for their anabolic effects on the healing process. Several proinflammatory cytokines have also been identified that appear to inhibit healing. Repair augmentation techniques that attempt to take advantage of these factors have evolved from using fibrin clot in the past to the current use of PRP.

PRP is an exciting, locally applied agent that uses a patient's own blood to derive the platelet-rich compound. Once platelets are activated, a host of growth factors, such as PDGF, IGF-1, VEGF, and others, are released into the local repair environment. In vitro studies have shown that these growth factors positively affect meniscal cell biology. The use of PRP to augment meniscal repairs is a technically simple procedure that holds great promise. Data are lacking regarding the clinical results of this treatment, but investigations of PRP to augment healing are currently being performed.

References

1. Hede A, Jensen DB, Blyme P, Sonne-Holm S: Epidemiology of meniscal lesions in the knee: 1,215 open operations in Copenhagen 1982-84. *Acta Orthop Scand* 1990;61(5):435-437.
2. Nielsen AB, Yde J: Epidemiology of acute knee injuries: A prospective hospital investigation. *J Trauma* 1991;31(12):1644-1648.
3. Fairbank TJ: Knee joint changes after meniscectomy. *J Bone Joint Surg Am* 1948;30(4):664-670.
4. Wroble RR, Henderson RC, Campion ER, el-Khoury GY, Albright JP: Meniscectomy in children and adolescents: A long-term follow-up study. *Clin Orthop Relat Res* 1992;279:180-189.
5. Jørgensen U, Sonne-Holm S, Lauridsen F, Rosenklint A: Long-term follow-up of meniscectomy in athletes: A prospective longitudinal study. *J Bone Joint Surg Br* 1987;69(1):80-83.
6. Roos H, Laurén M, Adalberth T, Roos EM, Jonsson K, Lohmander LS: Knee osteoarthritis after meniscectomy: Prevalence of radiographic changes after twenty-one years, compared with matched controls. *Arthritis Rheum* 1998;41(4):687-693.
7. Englund M, Lohmander LS: Risk factors for symptomatic knee osteoarthritis fifteen to twenty-two years after meniscectomy. *Arthritis Rheum* 2004;50(9):2811-2819.
8. Baratz ME, Fu FH, Mengato R: Meniscal tears: The effect of meniscectomy and of repair on intraarticular contact areas and stress in the human knee: A preliminary report. *Am J Sports Med* 1986;14(4):270-275.
9. Ihn JC, Kim SJ, Park IH: In vitro study of contact area and pressure distribution in the human knee after partial and total meniscectomy. *Int Orthop* 1993;17(4):214-218.
10. Lee SJ, Aadalen KJ, Malaviya P, et al: Tibiofemoral contact mechanics after serial medial meniscectomies in the human cadaveric knee. *Am J Sports Med* 2006;34(8):1334-1344.
11. Shelbourne KD, Carr DR: Meniscal repair compared with meniscectomy for bucket-handle medial meniscal tears in anterior cruciate ligament-reconstructed knees. *Am J Sports Med* 2003;31(5):718-723.
12. Shelbourne KD, Dersam MD: Comparison of partial meniscectomy versus meniscus repair for bucket-handle lateral meniscus tears in anterior cruciate ligament reconstructed knees. *Arthroscopy* 2004;20(6):581-585.
13. Arnoczky SP, Warren RF: Microvasculature of the human meniscus. *Am J Sports Med* 1982;10(2):90-95.
14. Arnoczky SP, Warren RF: The microvasculature of the meniscus and its response to injury: An experimental study in the dog. *Am J Sports Med* 1983;11(3):131-141.
15. King D: The healing of semilunar cartilages: 1936. *Clin Orthop Relat Res* 1990;252:4-7.
16. Heatley FW: The meniscus: Can it be repaired? An experimental investigation in rabbits. *J Bone Joint Surg Br* 1980;62(3):397-402.
17. Wirth CR: Meniscus repair. *Clin Orthop Relat Res* 1981;157:153-160.
18. Cassidy RE, Shaffer AJ: Repair of peripheral meniscus tears: A preliminary report. *Am J Sports Med* 1981;9(4):209-214.
19. Cabaud HE, Rodkey WG, Fitzwater JE: Medical meniscus repairs: An experimental and morphologic study. *Am J Sports Med* 1981;9(3):129-134.
20. Hennerbichler A, Moutos FT, Hennerbichler D, Weinberg JB, Guilak F: Repair response of the inner and outer regions of the porcine meniscus in vitro. *Am J Sports Med* 2007;35(5):754-762.
21. Webber RJ, Harris MG, Hough AJ Jr: Cell culture of rabbit meniscal fibrochondrocytes: Proliferative and synthetic response to growth factors and ascorbate. *J Orthop Res* 1985;3(1):36-42.
22. Hennerbichler A, Moutos FT, Hennerbichler D, Weinberg JB, Guilak F: Interleukin-1 and tumor necrosis factor alpha inhibit repair of the porcine meniscus in vitro. *Osteoarthritis Cartilage* 2007;15(9):1053-1060.
23. Wilusz RE, Weinberg JB, Guilak F, McNulty AL: Inhibition of integrative repair of the meniscus following acute exposure to interleukin-1 in vitro. *J Orthop Res* 2008;26(4):504-512.
24. Cao M, Stefanovic-Racic M, Georgescu HI, Miller LA, Evans CH: Generation of nitric oxide by lapine meniscal cells and its effect on matrix metabolism: Stimulation of collagen production by arginine. *J Orthop Res* 1998;16(1):104-111.
25. McNulty AL, Moutos FT, Weinberg JB, Guilak F: Enhanced integrative repair of the porcine meniscus in vitro by inhibition of interleukin-1 or tumor necrosis factor alpha. *Arthritis Rheum* 2007;56(9):3033-3042.
26. McNulty AL, Weinberg JB, Guilak F: Inhibition of matrix metalloproteinases enhances in vitro repair of the meniscus. *Clin Orthop Relat Res* 2009;467(6):1557-1567.
27. Hulth A, Johnell O, Miyazono K, Lindberg L, Heinegård D, Heldin CH: Effect of transforming growth factor-beta and platelet-derived growth factor-BB on articular cartilage in rats. *J Orthop Res* 1996;14(4):547-553.
28. Finesmith TH, Broadley KN, Davidson JM: Fibroblasts from wounds of different stages of re-

pair vary in their ability to contract a collagen gel in response to growth factors. *J Cell Physiol* 1990;144(1):99-107.

29. Letson AK, Dahners LE: The effect of combinations of growth factors on ligament healing. *Clin Orthop Relat Res* 1994;308: 207-212.
30. Schmidt CC, Georgescu HI, Kwoh CK, et al: Effect of growth factors on the proliferation of fibroblasts from the medial collateral and anterior cruciate ligaments. *J Orthop Res* 1995;13(2): 184-190.
31. Ye C, Deng Z, Li B: Effect of three growth factors on proliferation and cell phenotype of human fetal meniscal cells. *Zhongguo Xiu Fu Chong Jian Wai Ke Za Zhi* 2007;21(10):1137-1141.
32. Tumia NS, Johnstone AJ: Regional regenerative potential of meniscal cartilage exposed to recombinant insulin-like growth factor-I in vitro. *J Bone Joint Surg Br* 2004;86(7):1077-1081.
33. Tumia NS, Johnstone AJ: Promoting the proliferative and synthetic activity of knee meniscal fibrochondrocytes using basic fibroblast growth factor in vitro. *Am J Sports Med* 2004;32(4):915-920.
34. Collier S, Ghosh P: Effects of transforming growth factor beta on proteoglycan synthesis by cell and explant cultures derived from the knee joint meniscus. *Osteoarthritis Cartilage* 1995;3(2): 127-138.
35. Tumia NS, Johnstone AJ: Platelet derived growth factor-AB enhances knee meniscal cell activity in vitro. *Knee* 2009;16(1):73-76.
36. Narita A, Takahara M, Ogino T, Fukushima S, Kimura Y, Tabata Y: Effect of gelatin hydrogel incorporating fibroblast growth factor 2 on human meniscal cells in an organ culture model. *Knee* 2009;16(4):285-289.
37. Adesida AB, Grady LM, Khan WS, Hardingham TE: The matrix-forming phenotype of cultured human meniscus cells is enhanced after culture with fibroblast growth factor 2 and is further stimulated by hypoxia. *Arthritis Res Ther* 2006;8(3):R61.
38. Lietman SA, Hobbs W, Inoue N, Reddi AH: Effects of selected growth factors on porcine meniscus in chemically defined medium. *Orthopedics* 2003;26(8): 799-803.
39. Bhargava MM, Hidaka C, Hannafin JA, Doty S, Warren RF: Effects of hepatocyte growth factor and platelet-derived growth factor on the repair of meniscal defects in vitro. *In Vitro Cell Dev Biol Anim* 2005;41(8-9):305-310.
40. Bhargava MM, Attia ET, Murrell GA, Dolan MM, Warren RF, Hannafin JA: The effect of cytokines on the proliferation and migration of bovine meniscal cells. *Am J Sports Med* 1999;27(5): 636-643.
41. Spindler KP, Mayes CE, Miller RR, Imro AK, Davidson JM: Regional mitogenic response of the meniscus to platelet-derived growth factor (PDGF-AB). *J Orthop Res* 1995;13(2):201-207.
42. Kobayashi K, Fujimoto E, Deie M, Sumen Y, Ikuta Y, Ochi M: Regional differences in the healing potential of the meniscus: An organ culture model to eliminate the influence of microvasculature and the synovium. *Knee* 2004;11(4):271-278.
43. Becker R, Pufe T, Kulow S, et al: Expression of vascular endothelial growth factor during healing of the meniscus in a rabbit model. *J Bone Joint Surg Br* 2004;86(7): 1082-1087.
44. Petersen W, Pufe T, Stärke C, et al: Locally applied angiogenic factors: A new therapeutic tool for meniscal repair. *Ann Anat* 2005; 187(5-6):509-519.
45. Petersen W, Pufe T, Stärke C, et al: The effect of locally applied vascular endothelial growth factor on meniscus healing: Gross and histological findings. *Arch Orthop Trauma Surg* 2007;127(4): 235-240.
46. Zhang H, Leng P, Zhang J: Enhanced meniscal repair by overexpression of hIGF-1 in a full-thickness model. *Clin Orthop Relat Res* 2009;467(12):3165-3174.
47. Steinert AF, Palmer GD, Capito R, et al: Genetically enhanced engineering of meniscus tissue using ex vivo delivery of transforming growth factor-beta 1 complementary deoxyribonucleic acid. *Tissue Eng* 2007; 13(9):2227-2237.
48. Zhang ZN, Tu KY, Xu YK, Zhang WM, Liu ZT, Ou SH: Treatment of longitudinal injuries in avascular area of meniscus in dogs by trephination. *Arthroscopy* 1988;4(3):151-159.
49. Zhang Z, Arnold JA, Williams T, McCann B: Repairs by trephination and suturing of longitudinal injuries in the avascular area of the meniscus in goats. *Am J Sports Med* 1995;23(1):35-41.
50. Shelbourne KD, Heinrich J: The long-term evaluation of lateral meniscus tears left in situ at the time of anterior cruciate ligament reconstruction. *Arthroscopy* 2004; 20(4):346-351.
51. Fox JM, Rintz KG, Ferkel RD: Trephination of incomplete meniscal tears. *Arthroscopy* 1993;9(4): 451-455.
52. Ochi M, Uchio Y, Okuda K, Shu N, Yamaguchi H, Sakai Y: Expression of cytokines after meniscal rasping to promote meniscal healing. *Arthroscopy* 2001; 17(7):724-731.
53. Arnoczky SP, Warren RF, Spivak JM: Meniscal repair using an exogenous fibrin clot: An experimental study in dogs. *J Bone Joint Surg Am* 1988;70(8):1209-1217.

54. Henning CE, Lynch MA, Yearout KM, Vequist SW, Stallbaumer RJ, Decker KA: Arthroscopic meniscal repair using an exogenous fibrin clot. *Clin Orthop Relat Res* 1990;252:64-72.

55. van Trommel MF, Simonian PT, Potter HG, Wickiewicz TL: Arthroscopic meniscal repair with fibrin clot of complete radial tears of the lateral meniscus in the avascular zone. *Arthroscopy* 1998; 14(4):360-365.

56. McAndrews PT, Arnoczky SP: Meniscal repair enhancement techniques. *Clin Sports Med* 1996; 15(3):499-510.

57. Biedert RM: Treatment of intrasubstance meniscal lesions: A randomized prospective study of four different methods. *Knee Surg Sports Traumatol Arthrosc* 2000; 8(2):104-108.

58. Fufa D, Shealy B, Jacobson M, Kevy S, Murray MM: Activation of platelet-rich plasma using soluble type I collagen. *J Oral Maxillofac Surg* 2008;66(4):684-690.

59. Anitua E, Andia I, Ardanza B, Nurden P, Nurden AT: Autologous platelets as a source of proteins for healing and tissue regeneration. *Thromb Haemost* 2004; 91(1):4-15.

60. Sánchez M, Anitua E, Azofra J, Andía I, Padilla S, Mujika I: Comparison of surgically repaired Achilles tendon tears using platelet-rich fibrin matrices. *Am J Sports Med* 2007;35(2):245-251.

61. Mishra A, Pavelko T: Treatment of chronic elbow tendinosis with buffered platelet-rich plasma. *Am J Sports Med* 2006;34(11):1774-1778.

62. Virchenko O, Aspenberg P: How can one platelet injection after tendon injury lead to a stronger tendon after 4 weeks? Interplay between early regeneration and mechanical stimulation. *Acta Orthop* 2006;77(5):806-812.

63. Ishida K, Kuroda R, Miwa M, et al: The regenerative effects of platelet-rich plasma on meniscal cells in vitro and its in vivo application with biodegradable gelatin hydrogel. *Tissue Eng* 2007;13(5): 1103-1112.

Surgical Management of Articular Cartilage Defects of the Knee

Andreas H. Gomoll, MD
Jack Farr, MD
Scott D. Gillogly, MD
James S. Kercher, MD
Tom Minas, MD

Abstract

Articular cartilage defects of the knee present diagnostic and treatment challenges for orthopaedic surgeons. As new data and technologies become available, treatment algorithms are continually being refined. It is important to examine treatment recommendations from the current literature and understand surgical techniques for articular cartilage repair.

Instr Course Lect 2011;60:461-483.

Articular cartilage defects are often seen during knee arthroscopy. If they are symptomatic, they can cause disability comparable with that associated with advanced knee osteoarthritis.[1] The most difficult aspect of the assessment and treatment of articular cartilage injury is the surgical decision-making process, which involves the timing of cartilage repair surgery and choosing the most appropriate procedure for the individual patient.

Dr. Gomoll or an immediate family member is a member of a speakers' bureau or has made paid presentations on behalf of Arthrex and Genzyme; serves as a paid consultant to or is an employee of Genzyme, Tigenix, and Mentice; and has received research or institutional support from Genzyme and Conformis. Dr. Farr or an immediate family member has received royalties from DePuy, Mitek, and Stryker; is a member of a speakers' bureau or has made paid presentations on behalf of DePuy and Genzyme; serves as a paid consultant to or is an employee of DePuy, Genzyme, Mitek, Zimmer, VOT, Advanced Biosurfaces, Tigenix, and Arthrex; has received research or institutional support from DePuy, Eli Lilly, Genzyme, Mitek, Regeneration Technologies, Smith & Nephew, Zimmer, Advanced Biosurfaces, and Osiris; and owns stock or stock options in Advanced Biosurfaces and VOT. Dr. Gillogly or an immediate family member serves as a board member, owner, officer, or committee member of the Atlanta Sports Medicine Surgery Center; serves as a paid consultant to or is an employee of Genzyme, Carticept, MedShape Solutions, Exactech, Tornier, and the Musculoskeletal Transplant Foundation; has received research or institutional support from Genzyme, Smith & Nephew, MedShape Solutions, and Arthrex; and owns stock or stock options in Pfizer. Dr. Minas or an immediate family member is a member of a speakers' bureau or has made paid presentations on behalf of Genzyme and Conformis; serves as a paid consultant to or is an employee of Genzyme; has received research or institutional support from Genzyme and Conformis; and owns stock or stock options in Conformis. Neither Dr. Kercher nor any immediate family member has received anything of value from or owns stock in a commercial company or institution related directly or indirectly to the subject of this chapter.

Diagnosis of Articular Cartilage Defects

Patients with symptomatic cartilage defects typically have activity-related knee pain and swelling, although larger lesions can also cause symptoms of catching or locking. Defects on the femoral condyles cause pain at or close to the joint line with impact activities, such as running or descending stairs, unlike patellofemoral defects, which cause anterior knee pain during stair climbing, squatting, or rising from a chair. Unfortunately, there are no pathognomonic symptoms for cartilage defects, and frequently these defects coexist with meniscal tears, patellofemoral abnormalities, or early osteoarthritis.

If the patient had prior knee surgery, previous surgical reports can provide important clues pertaining to the condition of the articular cartilage at the time of that surgery.

Physical Findings

Patients with an articular cartilage defect do not have specific findings on examination. There may be a small or large knee effusion. Knee motion is usually preserved, although displaced osteochondral fragments can cause intermittent locking of the knee. Larger defects, particularly bipolar defects in the patellofemoral compartment, can cause reproducible catching or clicking on knee-motion examination and patellar manipulation. Tenderness on palpation of the femoral condyles and joint lines suggests the presence of synovial inflammation. Additional important findings are overall alignment of the knee, tracking of the patella with flexion and extension, and ligamentous laxity.

Diagnostic Imaging

Radiographs are important for evaluating malalignment and degenerative changes of the knee joint. The most commonly used radiographs include weight-bearing AP views in full extension and PA views in flexion,[2] lateral and patellofemoral views, and a full-length hip-to-ankle AP view. Sizing radiographs are required before meniscal or osteochondral allograft transplantation, if either treatment approach is selected; a marker of known size is included in the radiographic view to account for image magnification.

High-resolution MRI (1.5 tesla or greater) is a reliable means with which to evaluate articular cartilage defects. The recent introduction of cartilage-specific imaging protocols has dramatically improved the quality of MRI scans and allows noninvasive monitoring after cartilage repair procedures.[3]

CT arthrography is useful for evaluating conditions affecting the entire osteochondral unit, such as osteochondritis dissecans, or after failed prior cartilage repair to assess changes in the subchondral bone. Both MRI and CT allow evaluation of the patellofemoral compartment for trochlear dysplasia, patellar subluxation, and patellar tilt. The tibial tubercle-to-trochlear groove distance can be calculated from axial images to determine the need for (antero) medialization tibial tubercle osteotomy.

Cartilage Repair

Indications

Not all articular cartilage defects are symptomatic, so careful assessment of other potential causes of knee pain is crucial. Nonsurgical treatment with physical therapy, especially for patellofemoral defects, should be continued for at least 3 to 6 months in conjunction with activity modification and weight loss. Therapy should include patellofemoral strengthening as well as a four-way hip program. Older patients who are within a few years of age eligibility for knee replacement surgery should also undergo a trial of injection therapy with steroids and/or viscosupplementation. Extensive counseling about how the recovery period after cartilage repair is relatively longer than that after total knee arthroplasty is particularly important for patients in this age group to avoid unrealistic expectations and disappointment.

Surgery is considered after establishing that the patient's symptoms are consistent with a full-thickness (grade 3 or 4) cartilage defect and after adequate nonsurgical management has failed to provide acceptable pain relief. Patients must understand that rehabilitation is extensive, and they will not be able to return to activities for a prolonged period after cartilage repair.

Contraindications

Patients who smoke,[4] are obese (a body mass index of > 35 kg/m^2), have an inflammatory condition, or have an uncorrected articular comorbidity (such as knee malalignment, meniscal deficiency, or ligamentous laxity) are not good candidates for cartilage repair and usually are advised against having this surgery. Advanced degenerative change (> 50% joint-space narrowing) is considered a contraindication to cartilage repair in all but very young patients with intolerable knee pain and swelling and no other treatment options.

Treatment Algorithm Based on Published Results of Cartilage Repair Procedures

As indicated by multiple studies, including randomized controlled trials, treatment strategies for cartilage repair can be based primarily on the location and size of the defect, with age as a potential secondary consideration. The two most common locations for cartilage defects are the medial femoral condyle and the patellofemoral joint.[5] The tibiofemoral and patellofemoral compartments function quite differently; therefore, the treatment algorithms for these two locations differ as well[6,7] (**Table 1**).

Tibiofemoral Compartment

The choice of cartilage repair procedure for an articular cartilage defect in the tibiofemoral compartment is primarily determined by the defect size. In a randomized controlled trial, Knutsen et al[8] showed that the overall results of microfracture and autologous chondrocyte implantation were similar. However, cartilage defects larger than 4 cm^2 treated with microfracture had significantly worse results, while the size of the defect did not affect the results of autologous chondrocyte implantation. The authors therefore concluded that larger defects should be treated with autologous chondrocyte implantation. Basad et al[9] investigated this issue further with a randomized controlled trial comparing matrix-associated autologous chondrocyte implantation and microfracture, specifically for defects larger than 4 cm^2, and found significantly better results with autologous chondrocyte

Table 1
Treatment Algorithm for Cartilage Repair in the Tibiofemoral Compartment[a]

Small Defects (< 2 to 4 cm²)		Large Defects (> 2 to 4 cm²)	
Very Small (< 2 cm²) Osteochondral Autograft	Small Microfracture	Autologous Chondrocyte Implantation	Osteochondral Allograft
+ Mature hyaline cartilage + Primary bone healing + Quicker recovery and return to sports than after microfracture – Technically difficult (mini-open) – Donor-site morbidity with multiple plugs	+ No donor-site morbidity + Arthroscopic procedure – Complex rehabilitation (continuous passive motion and touch-down weight bearing for 6 to 8 weeks) – Prolonged delay before return to sports (6 to 9 months)	+ No size limitation + Hyaline-like cartilage + Autologous tissue – Arthrotomy required – High reoperation rate when using periosteum – Very complex rehabilitation (continuous passive motion and touch-down weight bearing for 6 to 8 weeks) – Prolonged delay before return to sports (12 to 18 months) – High cost	+ No size limitation + Mature hyaline cartilage + Simple rehabilitation – Arthrotomy required – Graft availability – Disease transmission – Graft failure occurs through bone, transforming a chondral into an osteochondral defect – Prolonged delay before return to sports (9 to 12 months) – High cost

[a]Plus signs indicate advantages, and minus signs indicate disadvantages

implantation. Another recent randomized controlled trial, by Saris et al,[10,11] demonstrated that the histologic and functional outcomes of autologous chondrocyte implantation were significantly better than those of microfracture even for smaller defects (average, 2.6 cm^2). Several other studies indicated that microfracture is not efficacious in large lesions.[12-15] Taken together, these studies suggest that treatment should be chosen on the basis of the size of the lesion, but whether to use 2, 3, or 4 cm^2 as the criterion for using a particular treatment approach is a subjective determination by the treating physician and should be individualized to the specific patient. For example, while a 3-cm^2 lesion represents only a portion of the weight-bearing area of the condyle in a 74-inch-tall (1.9-m) man, and could be considered small, a similar size lesion in a 62-inch (1.6-m) woman likely encompasses the entire weight-bearing area of the condyle and is comparatively large. Unfortunately, there are no data to help guide this individualized decision.

Small Lesions (< 2 to 4 cm^2) in the Femoral Condyle

Both microfracture and osteochondral autograft transfer for the treatment of lesions in this location and of this size consistently produce good and excellent results in 60% to 80% of patients.[12-18]

The decision regarding which of these two procedures to use is based on surgeon preference and familiarity with the techniques, the patient's functional demands, and associated bone loss. Although the issue of donor-site morbidity after osteochondral autograft transfer is controversial, the harvest of one to two grafts appears safe and provides sufficient material to fill a lesion 1 to 2 cm^2 in size. Athletes have been shown to return to sports activity more quickly after osteochondral autograft transfer than after microfracture treatment (percentage that return to sports, 93% versus 52%, respectively).[16] Osteochondral autograft transfer is recommended for smaller lesions, lesions in high-demand athletes, and lesions with associated bone loss, whereas microfracture is well suited for the treatment of medium-size defects with little or no bone loss in lower-demand patients.

More complex procedures, such as autologous chondrocyte implantation and the use of osteochondral allograft, can effectively treat lesions in this size range. However, increased morbidity and cost make them less attractive; therefore, these more complex procedures should be reserved for revision situations.

Large Lesions (> 2 to 4 cm^2) in the Femoral Condyle

The results of microfracture treatment of lesions of this size are less encouraging, and microfracture is not recommended for these larger lesions. Some have reported good results with osteochondral autograft transfer in these and even larger lesions, but donor-site morbidity is a concern and a limiting factor.[19]

Both autologous chondrocyte implantation and osteochondral allografts have produced good and excellent results in more than 70% of patients, but this chapter's authors are not aware of any randomized controlled trials comparing the two procedures.[7,19-28] Surgeon and patient preference are factors when deciding between osteochondral allografts and autologous chondrocyte implantation for this group of lesions. Bone loss associated with osteochondral defects can influence the decision. Defects deeper than 8 to 10 mm can be treated with autologous chondrocyte implantation, but bone grafting of the osseous defect needs to be done in a staged or concurrent fashion (sandwich autologous chondrocyte implantation).[29] When there are multiple lesions, especially associated lesions in the patellofemoral joint, autologous chondrocyte implantation is the more flexible treatment option.

Osteochondritis Dissecans Lesions in the Femoral Condyle

Symptomatic osteochondral defects, such as osteochondritis dissecans lesions, should be repaired whenever possible, although nonsurgical treatment of stable lesions can lead to healing in an adolescent with open physes. Stable, nondisplaced lesions can be treated with antegrade or retrograde drilling in an attempt to induce bone healing. Unstable or displaced defects are better treated with internal fixation with compressive screws.[30] Both metal and resorbable devices can be used, but they should be seated well under the articular surface. Metal implants ideally should be removed before full weight bearing.

Fragment removal alone without subsequent repair provides good short-term pain relief and therefore can be considered in specific circumstances—for example, for in-season athletes, very small defects, and patients unable or unwilling to follow the rehabilitation protocol associated with repair. Long-term follow-up studies,[31-33] however, have shown high rates of osteoarthritis as early as 9 years after fragment removal, especially when the lesion was larger than 2 cm^2. Overall, repair of osteochondritis dissecans lesions results in better outcomes than does fragment removal followed by secondary cartilage repair with osteochondral allograft transplantation.[34] A randomized controlled trial comparing osteochondral autograft transfer with microfracture for treatment of osteochondritis dissecans reported a better outcome with osteochondral autograft transfer (rate of excellent or good results, 83% versus 63%) at 4 years.[35] The success rate has been reported to be more than 80% with autologous chondrocyte implantation[36,37] and approximately 70% with osteochondral allograft transplantation.[23] Specific treatment recommendations follow the same size-based algorithm discussed previously.

Patellofemoral Compartment

The patellofemoral compartment is a difficult location for cartilage repair, and all techniques performed here are less successful than those done on the femoral condyles. The correction of adverse factors, such as abnormal tracking of the patella, is crucial for success.

Although microfracture, osteochondral autograft transfer, and osteochondral allograft transplantation have generally good outcomes in the femoral condyles, there is a growing consensus that they should be used cautiously in the patellofemoral compartment except in very specific cases. Kreuz et al[6] found only transient improvement after microfracture in the patellofemoral compartment, with worsening after 18 to 36 months. The use of osteochondral autograft transfer in the patellofemoral compartment has shown varying results. Hangody and Füles[17] reported that the results were only slightly worse than those in the femoral condyle, but Bentley et al[7] reported almost universal failure of osteochondral autograft transfer in the patella. Jamali et al[38] investigated the use of osteochondral allografts in the patellofemoral compartment and reported 60% good and excellent results.

The first study on autologous chondrocyte implantation demonstrated dismal results in the patellofemoral compartment, with only two of seven patients having a good or excellent outcome.[21] However, with increased understanding of patellofemoral joint biomechanics and more aggressive treatment of tracking abnormalities of the patella, results have improved dramatically. Recent studies have shown successful outcomes of autologous chondrocyte implantation in the patellofemoral compartment in more than 80% of patients.[39-42] Even though a defect in the patella is an off-label indication for autologous chondrocyte implantation, this treatment has emerged as the cartilage repair option of choice for all but the smallest defects in the patellofemoral compartment.

Patient Age and Defect Chronicity

The results of microfracture treatment in patients older than 30 years are not as good as the outcomes in younger patients.[8,16,43,44] In general, the same has been found with osteochondral autograft transfer and autologous chondrocyte implantation, although one study of autologous chondrocyte implantation demonstrated low failure rates in patients older than 45 years.[45] The patient's age does not substantially affect the results after use of an osteochondral allograft. The effect of defect chronicity on the outcomes of cartilage repair is not well established, although

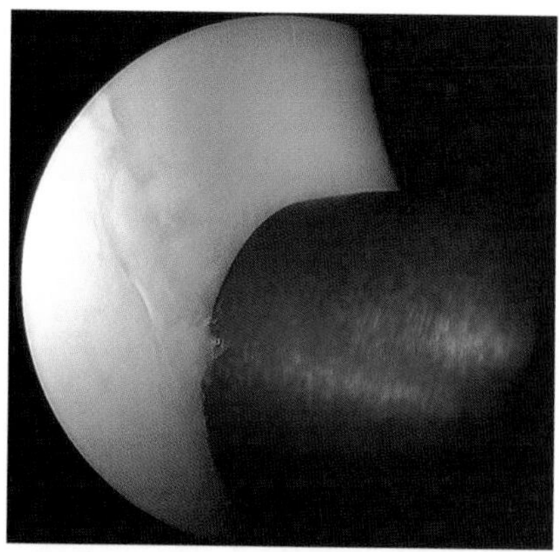

Figure 1 A sizing rod has been placed on the defect to measure the diameter of the required graft.

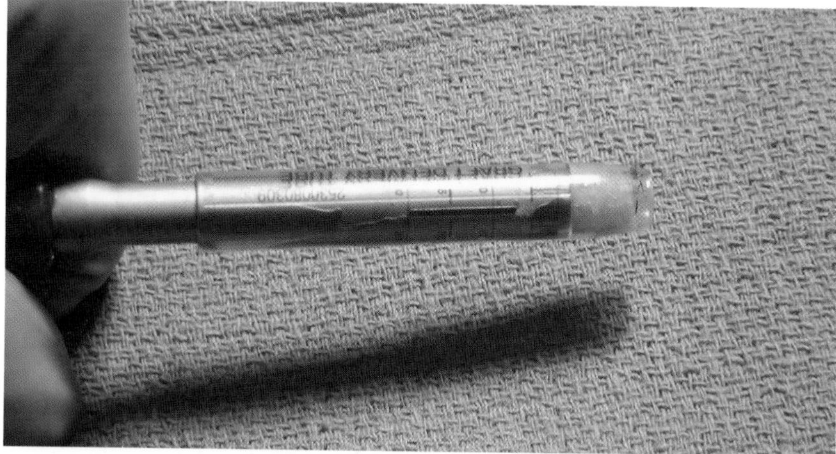

Figure 2 An osteochondral cylinder has been harvested and is ready for implantation.

repairs of acute injuries (sustained less than 1 year before treatment) tend to have better results.[12]

Surgical Procedures for the Treatment of Small and Medium-Size Cartilage Defects

Débridement and chondroplasty (removal of degenerated tissue and creation of mechanically stable cartilage with vertical shoulders), generally performed arthroscopically, can be the definitive treatment of cartilage lesions noted as an incidental finding or for the initial treatment of symptomatic defects before consideration of more invasive cartilage repair procedures. Patients recover quickly after a débridement and chondroplasty and can bear full weight. Knee pain and swelling should be absent before the patient returns to activities.

Osteochondral autograft transfer requires careful restoration of the curvature of the articular surface and may involve accessory arthroscopic portals or a mini-open approach. After the diagnostic portion of the arthroscopic procedure has been completed, accessory portals or incisions are created to allow orientation of the instruments perpendicular to the articular surfaces in both the harvest and the recipient location. If a transpatellar tendon approach is required, the tendon should be split in line with its fibers and repaired at the end of the procedure. Sizing rods are used to determine the size and number of required grafts (**Figure 1**). Then an appropriately sized harvester is selected, and an osteochondral plug, usually approximately 10 to 15 mm in length, is obtained, with the graft harvested perpendicular to the articular surface. There are several suitable donor sites for osteochondral plug harvest in the knee. These sites are located in areas of less weight bearing in the knee—for example, the medial and lateral trochlear ridge, the intercondylar notch, or the sulcus terminalis on the lateral femoral condyle, which is the transition zone between the tibiofemoral and patellofemoral weight-bearing areas.[46] The graft length and any angulation are noted. A defect harvester of slightly smaller diameter is used to create a recipient hole in the defect area that corresponds in length, diameter, and angulation to the donor plug. Depending on the specific system used, the graft is transferred to a different device or remains in its harvesting tube. The plug is advanced within the tube so that the end is just

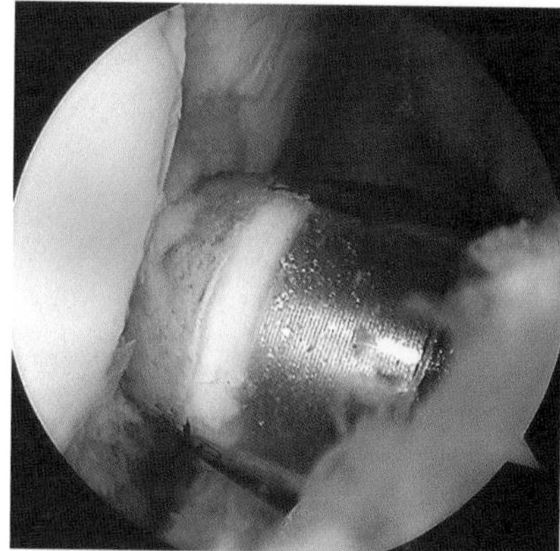

Figure 3 The graft is being introduced into the recipient slot.

visible (**Figure 2**). The harvester is introduced into the joint and placed over the recipient hole; the graft is then slowly introduced into the defect until it is almost seated (**Figure 3**). Subsequently, the harvester is removed, and the graft is seated flush with the surrounding articular surface by gentle pressure with an oversized tamp. Excessive force and the use of a mallet should be avoided because they cause chondrocyte death.[38,47,48] Overall, a slightly recessed graft is preferable to one that is proud, although recessing the graft by 2 mm or more also has deleterious effects on the cartilage.[49]

The process is then repeated until the defect is filled. Close contact with

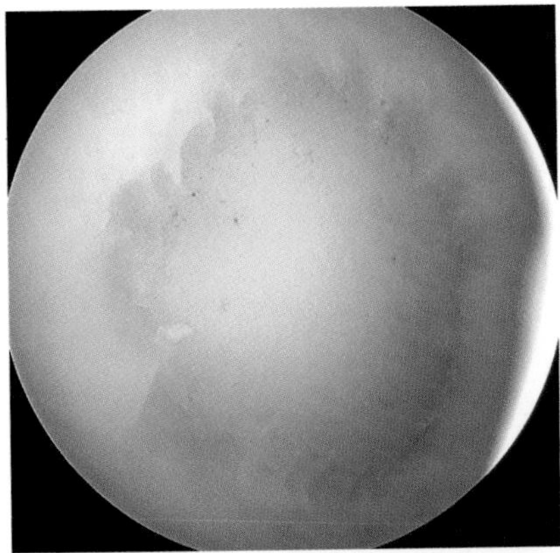

Figure 4 Arthroscopic view of a cartilage defect that has been prepared for microfracture. Any degenerated or loose tissue has been removed; the layer of calcified cartilage has been débrided; and stable, vertical shoulders have been created.

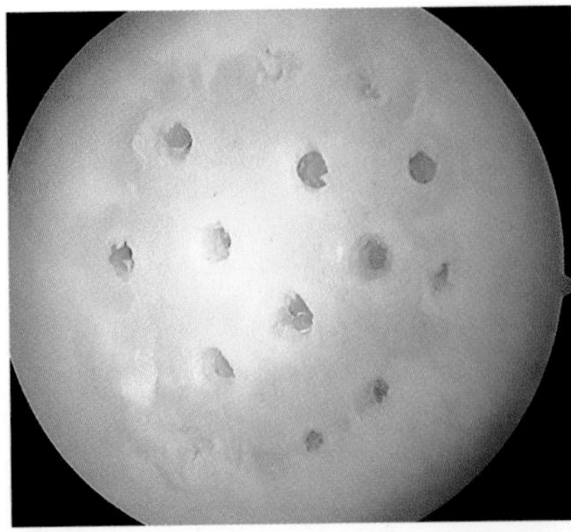

Figure 5 Final appearance after microfracture, before release of the tourniquet.

the surrounding host bone, which is difficult to obtain with multiple plugs surrounding a central plug, is important because, without close contact with the native cancellous bone, integration is compromised and plug resorption and necrosis may follow. The donor site(s) can be left vacant or be filled—for example, with synthetic back-fill plugs, which potentially decrease the risk of postoperative hematoma.

After surgery, the patient maintains touch-down weight bearing for a period ranging from 4 weeks when there is a small defect (one or two plugs surrounded by intact cartilage) to 8 weeks when the defect is larger. Continuous passive motion is optional, but if there are concerns about postoperative stiffness, it can be used for 2 to 3 weeks. Return to athletic activities is delayed for 4 to 6 months to allow restoration of quadriceps strength and proprioception.

Microfracture is also an arthroscopic procedure, with accessory portals sometimes used to improve access to the cartilage lesion. The initial blood from the treated site is believed to contain more marrow elements than the subsequent blood, so if multiple arthroscopic procedures are done, microfracture should be performed last.

With microfracture treatment, a curet is used to trim any soft and fissured cartilage along the defect rim to create vertical shoulders of mechanically stable cartilage (**Figure 4**). The layer of calcified cartilage is débrided to improve the volume of regenerative tissue, but the subchondral plate should not be violated.[50] After thorough débridement, multiple holes are created in the subchondral plate with a microfracture awl (**Figure 5**). The procedure starts at the rim, directly adjacent to the surrounding cartilage. Ideally, microfracture holes should be spaced approximately 3 to 4 mm apart so that they do not break into each other and destabilize the subchondral plate. The awl should be kept as perpendicular to the subchondral bone as possible, which may require accessory arthroscopic portals. After completing the procedure, the tourniquet is deflated, and the pump pressure is lowered; bleeding should be observed from all holes.

After surgery, the patient maintains touch-down weight bearing for a period ranging from 4 weeks when the defect is small (< 1 cm^2) and well contained to 8 weeks when it is larger and/or uncontained. Continuous passive motion for 6 weeks, 6 to 8 hours per day, is recommended. Return to athletic activities is delayed for 6 to 9 months to allow tissue maturation.

Advanced Surgical Procedures to Address Complex Defects (Large, Multiple, or Osteochondral Lesions)

Autologous chondrocyte implantation is a two-stage, cell-based cartilage repair technique indicated for the treatment of medium-to-large (more than 3 to 4 cm^2) full-thickness, focal cartilage defects of the femoral condyles and trochlea of the knee. Ideally, the lesion has a stable rim of intact cartilage (is contained) to support suturing of the cover membrane. Defects that are deeper than 8 to 10 mm in the subchondral bone require staged or concomitant bone grafting.

Arthroscopic Cartilage Biopsy

Initially, the defect should be evaluated arthroscopically, and the joint should be assessed for ligamentous instability, abnormality of patellar tracking, or meniscal deficiency. The number, size, and location of chondral defects should be noted. The opposite articular surface should be carefully evaluated for a bipolar (kissing) lesion. The quality and thickness of the surrounding articular cartilage are assessed to determine whether the lesion is contained or uncontained. If the defects are amenable to autologous chondrocyte implantation, full-thickness cartilage is harvested with a sharp gouge from the superolateral aspect of the intercondylar notch (**Figure 6**) or the medial aspect of the proximal part of the trochlea. The harvested cartilage should be approximately 5 mm wide and 10 mm long and weigh 200 to 300 mg. The cartilage is placed di-

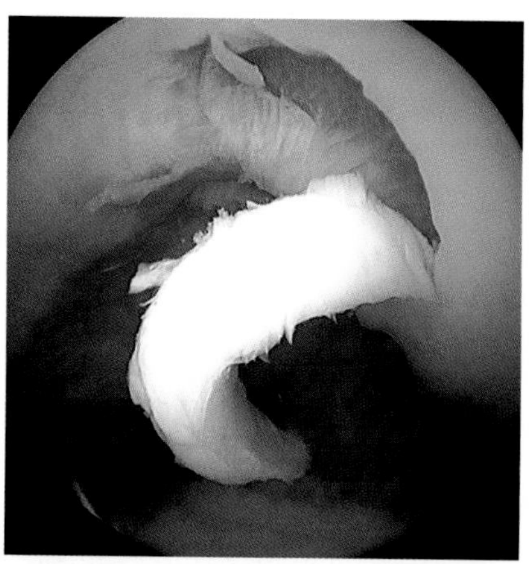

Figure 6 A cartilage biopsy specimen is being obtained from the superolateral aspect of the intercondylar notch.

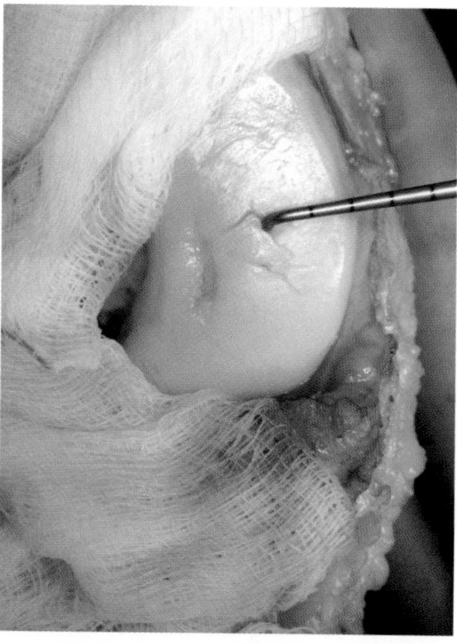

Figure 7 A cartilage defect of the medial femoral condyle with a large surrounding area of fissured and softened cartilage.

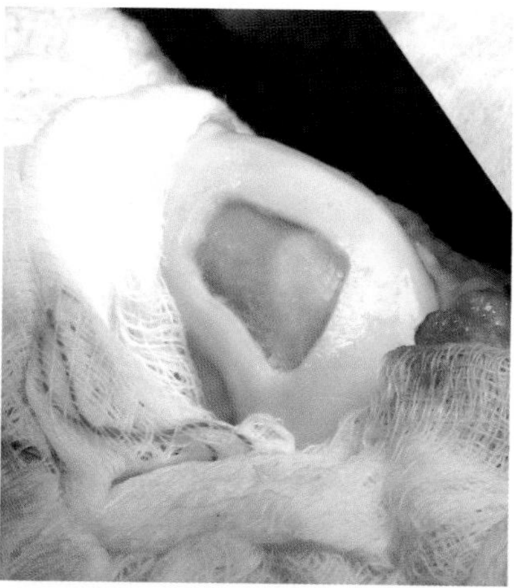

Figure 8 The defect after débridement of all degenerated tissue back to stable and healthy cartilage.

rectly in sterile transport medium and shipped for cell culturing. To obtain cultured cartilage cells, the cartilage is enzymatically digested, and the approximately 200,000 to 300,000 cells contained in the cartilage sample are amplified to approximately 12 million cells per 0.4 mL of culture medium. This takes approximately 6 weeks, but the process can be interrupted after 2 weeks by cryopreservation if necessary. Up to 1.2 mL (48 million cells) can be obtained through standard culture, but additional cells can be obtained with additional cell passage.

Autologous Chondrocyte Implantation

Adequate exposure is critical to allow proper defect preparation and suturing. A limited medial or lateral parapatellar arthrotomy is used for isolated lesions of the femoral condyles. Multiple and larger femoral lesions require a more extensile approach, and tibial plateau lesions frequently require detachment of the anterior meniscal horn insertion, with repair after grafting is complete. A bent Hohmann retractor placed in the intercondylar notch will displace the patella to the contralateral side to assist with exposure.

Defect Preparation

The defect must be cleaned of all degenerated tissue to achieve a stable rim of healthy cartilage with vertical shoulders (**Figure 7**). First, the defect is outlined with a fresh scalpel down to the subchondral plate. The degenerated cartilage is débrided with small curets, with removal of all unstable or undermined cartilage (**Figure 8**), unless this removal changes a contained lesion into an uncontained one. If that is about to happen, the surgeon should leave a small rim of degenerated cartilage to sew into, rather than using bone tunnels or suture anchors. The calcified cartilage should be débrided but not the intact subchondral plate so that bleeding is minimized. Bleeding from the subchondral bone allows a mixed stem cell population into the chondral defect, diluting the end-differentiated chondrocytes grown in vitro. Bleeding can also compromise the mechanical stability or even rupture the cover membrane or suture line. Minor punctate bleeding is frequently encountered but can usually be controlled with thrombin or epinephrine-soaked sponges, fibrin glue, or electrocautery. After débridement, the defect is templated with aluminum foil or glove packaging paper (**Figure 9**). If periosteum is used to cover the chondrocyte graft, the template should be oversized by 1 to 2 mm in all dimensions to accommodate for shrinkage of the periosteal flap after harvest.

Patch Cover

Two options are available to cover the defect. A periosteal patch is the only Food and Drug Administration (FDA)-approved method, but these patches have been abandoned in Europe because of their propensity to hypertrophy, with arthroscopic débridement of areas of periosteal hypertrophy required in 20% to 50% of patients.[45,50-52] Good outcomes and lower reoperation rates have been reported with the use of a collagen membrane.[51,53,54] Coverage of a cartilage defect with a collagen membrane is an off-label use of the membrane and must be discussed with the patient.[53]

The recommended site for procurement of periosteum is the proximal-medial aspect of the tibia, just distal to

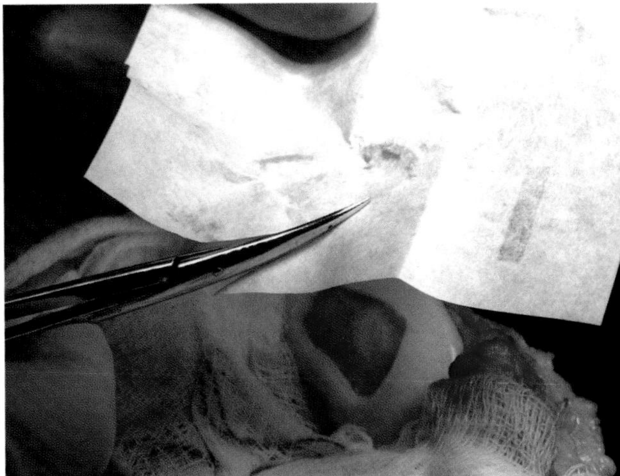

Figure 9 Templating of the defect with glove packaging paper.

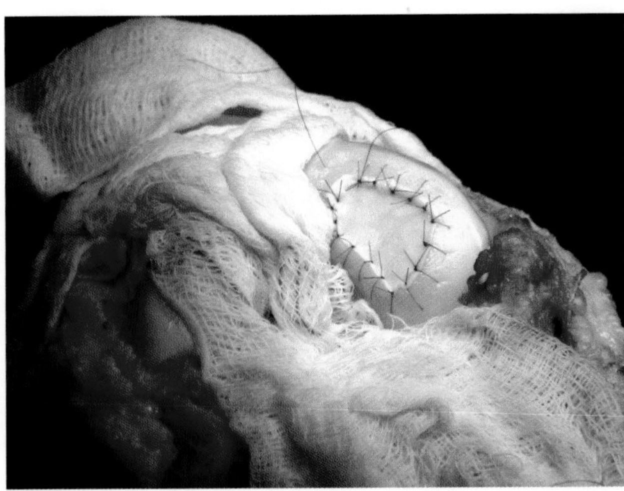

Figure 10 The membrane has been secured with multiple interrupted sutures.

the insertion of the pes anserinus. Fibers of the sartorius blend with the periosteum more proximally, potentially compromising graft quality. The periosteum is exposed, and a periosteal patch is outlined on the basis of the template. The superficial surface and orientation of the patch are marked with a pen. The periosteum is divided with a fresh scalpel blade and is then mobilized with a small, sharp periosteal elevator. After the patch has been harvested, it should be spread out on a moist sponge to avoid desiccation and shrinkage. If a tourniquet was used, it can be deflated at this point and for the remainder of the procedure.

The cartilage defect is dried, and the periosteal patch is placed over the defect with the cambium layer facing toward the defect bed. The patch is gently unfolded and is stretched with nontoothed forceps; it is then trimmed to fit the defect. The patch is sutured in place with 6-0 resorbable suture on a cutting needle that was immersed in sterile mineral oil or glycerin for better handling. The suture is placed first through the patch and then through the surrounding articular cartilage, exiting approximately 3 mm from the defect edge; the patch edge is everted slightly to provide a better seal against the defect wall. The knots are tied on the patch side, seated below the level of the adjacent cartilage (**Figure 10**). Interrupted sutures are placed on each side of the patch (at 3, 6, 9, and 12 o'clock), with the tension of the patch adjusted after each suture and the patch trimmed as needed so that it is neither loose enough to sag into the defect nor so tight that it cuts out of the sutures. Ideally, the patch should re-create the contour of the articular surface. The surgeon should leave an opening in the most superior aspect of the patch that is wide enough to accept an angiocatheter to inject the chondrocytes. The suture line is waterproofed with fibrin glue. The suture line is tested by slowly injecting saline solution into the covered defect with a tuberculin syringe and a plastic 18-gauge angiocatheter. Leakage is addressed by sealing with additional sutures or fibrin glue. The saline solution should be aspirated to prepare the defect for injection of the chondrocyte suspension.

Using a sterile technique, the chondrocytes are aspirated from the transport vials through a flexible, 2-inch (5-cm) plastic 18-gauge angiocatheter. The angiocatheter is placed into the defect through the residual opening, and, as the angiocatheter is slowly withdrawn, cells are injected until the defect is filled with the cell suspension (**Figure 11**). One or two additional sutures and fibrin glue are used to close the injection site.

Rehabilitation

There are three phases of rehabilitation after autologous chondrocyte implantation. These follow the progress of tissue maturation: proliferation, transition, and remodeling. Initially, the cell graft is soft and not strongly integrated with the surrounding cartilage and underlying bone. It is vulnerable to shear and compression forces, which need to be avoided while the graft is protected. Continuous passive motion is used for 6 to 8 hours per day for 6 weeks after the surgery, and the patient uses crutches with toe-touch weight bearing. The exact rehabilitation protocol depends on the defect location. Patients with condylar defects are allowed a full active range of motion, whereas those with patellofemoral defects are limited to passive extension and active flexion. Likewise, the range of the continuous passive motion is advanced as tolerated to 90° for patients with condylar lesions but is held at 40° for those with patellofemoral defects. To decrease the risk of arthrofibrosis, the patient dangles the leg over the side of the bed at least three times per day to achieve 90° of flexion by 3 weeks after surgery. During the second phase (beginning 7 weeks after surgery), the patient gradually transitions to full weight bearing and begins closed-chain strengthening exercises. The third phase (beginning at 12 weeks) starts a slow return to activities of daily living, with progression of strengthening and proprioceptive exercises. Patients are restricted from impact activities, such as running, for 12 to 18 months and from sports involving cutting motions for at least 18 months.

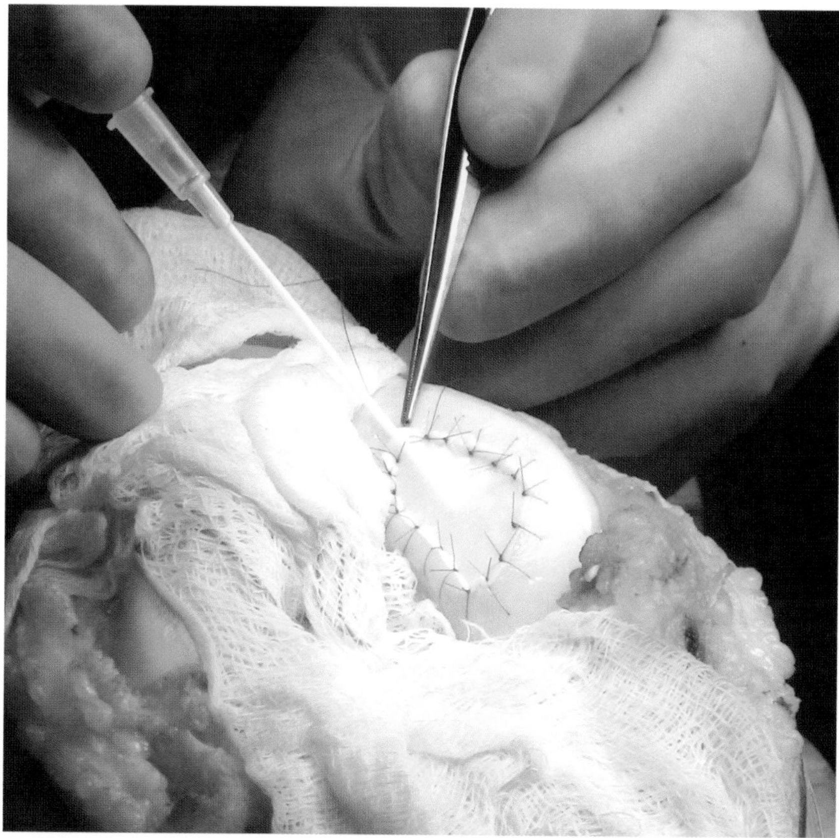

Figure 11 The chondrocyte suspension is being injected into the defect with an angiocatheter.

Osteochondral Allograft Transplantation

The use of osteochondral allografts dates to the early 20th century but was done sparingly before the last decade.[55-60] The purpose of osteochondral allograft transplantation is to implant fully developed tissue capable of withstanding normal load transmission. The hyaline cartilage already has a mature matrix, and the intact subchondral bone remains integrated at the cartilage-bone interface. The matrix and chondrocytes have been shown to survive in long-term recovery studies.[61-63] Furthermore, the allograft chondrocytes are immunoprivileged, in part as a result of protection by the avascular and dense cartilage matrix. Allograft failure does not appear to be a result of an immune reaction to the transplanted cartilage but rather seems to be caused by failure of the transplanted bone.[61,62,64] The allograft articular cartilage is fully developed at the time of implantation and does not need to heal. The allograft bone needs to heal and acts as a scaffold that incorporates over time by creeping substitution.[63] Successful integration into the host bone is critical for the graft's ultimate function and load transmission. However, the transplanted bone generates an immunologic reaction primarily from remaining donor blood elements. Patients with a positive result on antihuman leukocyte antigen antibody screening after osteochondral allograft transplantation have greater surrounding bone edema and more abnormal graft marrow than do those patients in whom screening results are negative.[65] For this reason, as little bone as necessary should be transplanted and as many donor marrow cells as possible should be removed through lavage before transplantation.[23,26]

The FDA began regulatory oversight of the use of cadaver tissue in 1993. Safety guidelines established by the American Association of Tissue Banks advocate extensive serologic, bacterial, and viral testing; donor screening; procurement and storage requirements; and graft quarantine until negative testing results are ensured.[66,67] The risk of HIV transmission is estimated to be approximately 1 in 1.6 million, and there have been no reported cases of this route of disease transmission since the late 1980s.[66] When tissue is obtained from tissue centers that follow the FDA's Current Good Tissue Practice rules and the guidelines of the American Association of Tissue Banks, the safety of allograft implants is maximized.

Typical indications for use of an osteochondral allograft are traumatic or degenerative chondral and osteochondral lesions of the femoral condyles of more than 2 cm^2, particularly when

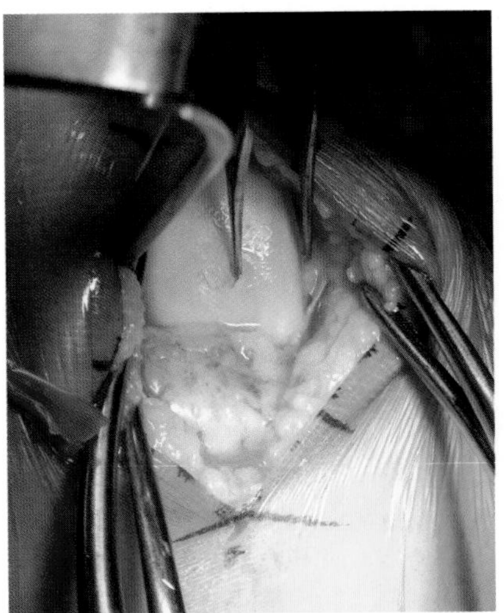

Figure 12 The defect has been exposed and sized.

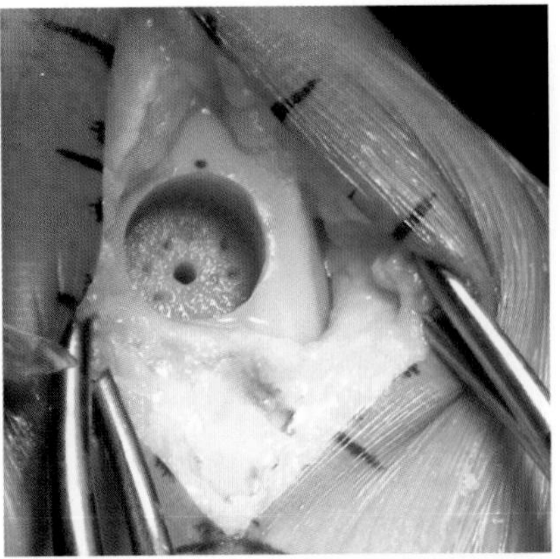

Figure 13 The defect has been reamed over the guidewire down to healthy-appearing bone.

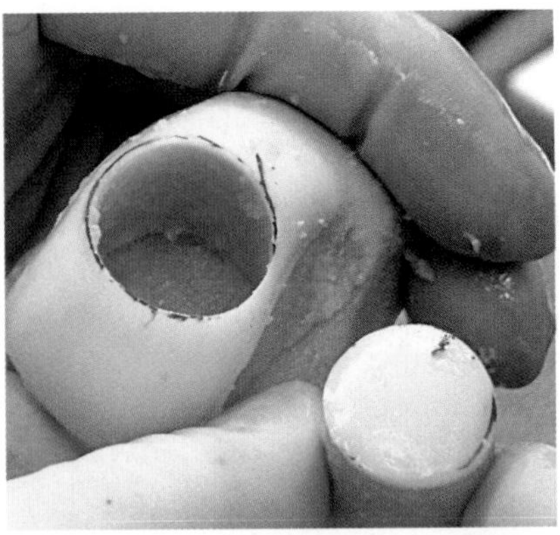

Figure 14 The donor graft has been obtained from the matched donor hemicondyle with use of a circular coring reamer.

the accompanying bone loss is more than 6 mm. Osteochondral allografts can be used to revise a prior failed cartilage repair. Use in the tibial plateau or the patellofemoral joint is best suited for younger patients without arthritic changes.[26,38]

Contraindications to osteochondral allograft transplantation are inflammatory arthritis (rheumatoid or any other systemic arthritis), advanced degenerative changes, diffuse corticosteroid-induced osteonecrosis, uncorrectable knee instability, or knee malalignment.[23,26-28,67]

Graft Viability

Fresh refrigerated allografts are the standard for osteochondral allograft transfers because frozen and freeze-dried cartilage has insufficient viable cartilage cells.[27,59,60,66] In fresh refrigerated allograft cartilage, up to 98% of the chondrocytes are viable for 7 days; this decreases to 70% by 28 days.[68,69] This decreased viability is accompanied by diminished cell density and decreased metabolic activity.[69,70] Safety testing takes 14 to 20 days, so the window for implantation is approximately 10 to 14 days from the time the tissue is released from quarantine. A delay in implantation affects chondrocyte viability and tissue metabolism but does not affect the hyaline matrix or biomechanical properties of the allograft bone; the effect of this delay on clinical outcome is unknown.[69-71]

Surgical Technique

A size-matched and side-matched allograft is preferred. Size is determined by using magnification markers on AP and lateral radiographs to measure femoral condylar and tibial width and height.[26-28]

The most common location requiring an osteochondral allograft is the weight-bearing surface of the medial or lateral femoral condyle. An arthrotomy with a medial or lateral capsular incision to displace the patella is usually sufficient for smaller defects, but larger defects may require subluxation of the patella during exposure to ensure perpendicular access to the defect.

Press-fit cylindrical osteochondral plugs are recommended for most defects.[26,56,72,73] A guidewire is placed in the center of the defect, and a reamer is used to remove any remaining tissue and subchondral bone down to healthy cancellous bone (**Figures 12** and **13**). As little as 3 to 5 mm of bone can be removed for purely chondral lesions, whereas deeper lesions or necrotic bone from osteochondritis dissecans or osteonecrosis can require up to 8 to 10 mm of bone removal. The remnants of healthy bone from reaming this area should be saved and used to fill the cavity to minimize the defect depth. The depth in all four quadrants is measured and recorded.

The osteochondral allograft is harvested from the corresponding location on the allograft hemicondyle. The graft location and orientation are marked. On a back table, a matching-size coring reamer is used to harvest the donor allograft cylinder (**Figure 14**). The cancellous allograft bone is trimmed to match the depth measurements from the defect. Pulsatile lavage is used on the osseous portion of the graft to remove any remaining marrow elements. The edges are beveled to facilitate insertion. The graft is pushed in place by hand; a tamp is not used because it will injure the superficial chondrocytes. The knee is placed through a range of motion to assist with seating of the allograft (**Figure 15**). Press-fit fixation alone is usually adequate, but supplemental fixation with pins or screws can be used if needed. Irregularly shaped lesions may

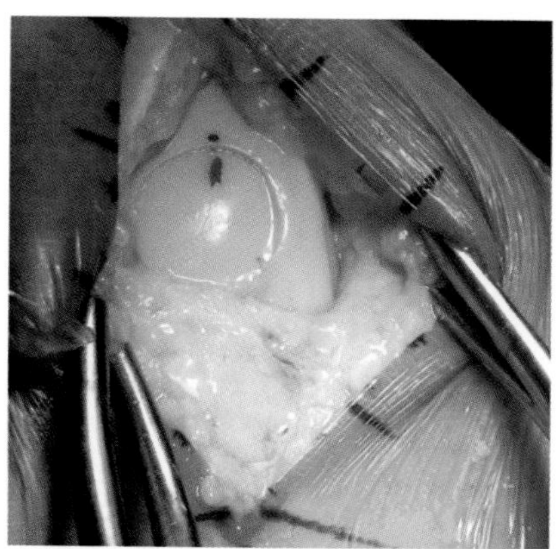

Figure 15 After matching of the depth of the graft to the donor site and use of pulsatile lavage on the osseous portion of the graft, the graft is press-fit flush with the articular surface.

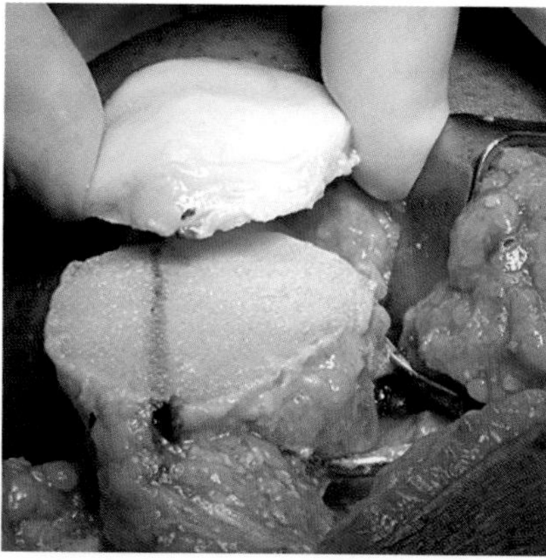

Figure 16 The allograft surface separated from the donor patella matches the depth of the resection performed in the patient. The line marking the host median ridge is used to orient the donor graft along the same axis.

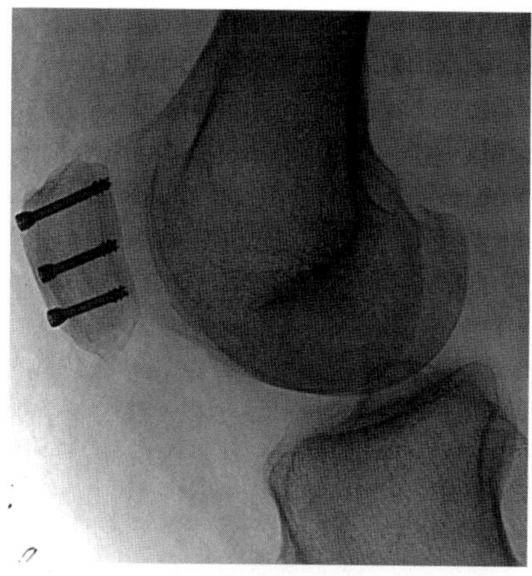

Figure 17 Lateral knee radiograph showing the final patellar resurfacing after insertion of double-pitched screws along the axis of the median ridge, providing rigid fixation and allowing early motion.

require a freehand technique, and these grafts frequently require supplemental fixation. The implants for fixation should be placed below the articular surface; ideally, screws should be placed either in the intercondylar notch or on the edge of the condyles away from the articular surface.[23,26]

Osteochondral allograft transplantation at the trochlea and patella presents special challenges because of the complex anatomy and topography. Peripheral lesions on the medial or lateral aspect of the trochlear groove may be amenable to cylindrical plugs, but it is difficult to match the central sulcus anatomy with plugs. For more extensive lesions of the trochlea, a shell allograft can be fashioned much like a patellofemoral arthroplasty, with a trochlear graft fashioned to match the anterior femoral resection and fixed with absorbable pins and/or peripheral screws.[23,26]

Press-fit cylindrical plugs should be used for isolated patellar facet lesions or lesions centered on the median ridge. Extensive patellar lesions can be treated with patellar allograft resurfacing.[38,55] The diffusely damaged patellar surface is resected in its entirety with an oscillating saw, much like the technique for arthroplasty. The surgeon should leave sufficient patellar bone (at least 12 to 14 mm) after the resection. The allograft patellar surface is harvested in a similar fashion, making the osteochondral portion of the allograft essentially the entire surface of the patella. The osteochondral graft is placed on the resected host bone (**Figure 16**), and fixation is obtained with the use of small double-pitched screws placed from anterior to posterior along the median ridge with threads in the subchondral bone in the allograft just below the articular surface (**Figure 17**). Any patellar tracking problems should be corrected during the same procedure.

The most common indication for an osteochondral tibial allograft is a tibial plateau fracture malunion or bone loss from trauma.[74] The technique allows restoration of up to 15 mm of lost bone. Typically, the allograft plateau and attached meniscus are transplanted together. The tibial plateau of the host is resected as is done for an onlay unicompartmental arthroplasty. The cuts on the allograft tibial plateau are matched, and fixation is performed with screws placed off the articular surface. Fluoroscopy assists with evaluation of the alignment. The compartment should not be overstuffed or understuffed, and an off-loading osteotomy should be done if necessary. The periphery of the transferred allograft meniscus is sewn to the meniscal synovial junction.

Rehabilitation

Rehabilitation after osteochondral allograft transplantation must prevent overloading of the graft-host interface until osseous union is achieved. Touch-down weight bearing for 6 to 12 weeks is recommended, with the duration depending on the location and size of the graft. Progressive range-of-motion exercises are encouraged early, although open-chain exercises are avoided by patients with a patellofemoral allograft. Pulsed ultrasound has been shown to improve graft healing.[75]

Osteochondral allograft failure usually results from unsuccessful osseous integration and subsequent subchondral collapse.[61,63] It may also be the re-

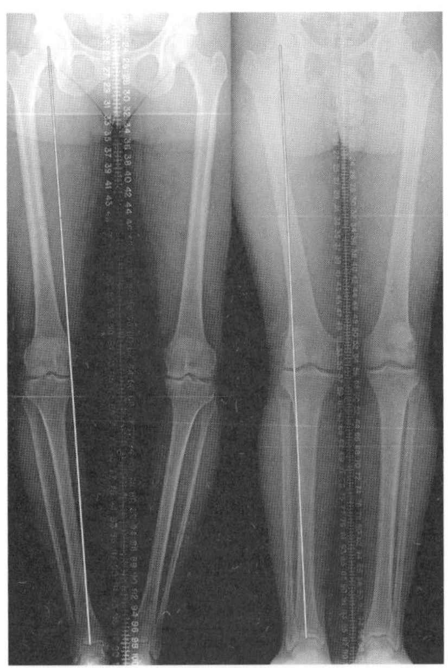

Figure 18 AP standing radiographs demonstrating varus malalignment with the mechanical axis shifted into the medial compartment (left) and valgus malalignment with the mechanical axis shifted into the lateral compartment (right).

sult of technical problems with achieving press-fit fixation or uncorrected coexisting joint pathology, such as malalignment or instability, which continues to overload the graft. Allografts of the tibial plateau and those used in compromised (osteonecrotic) bone have higher failure rates.[59] Graft failure with collapse or fragmentation requires revision with repeat allografting or unicompartmental or total joint arthroplasty.[26] As would be expected, patients with a unipolar lesion and a normal mechanical axis have the best outcomes, whereas patients who have transplants for patellofemoral disease, osteonecrosis, or arthrosis of both the femur and the tibia have less consistent results.

Articular Comorbidities

Malalignment

Malalignment of the knee frequently accompanies articular cartilage defects, and restoration of a neutral biomechanical environment is the single most important factor contributing to the success of any cartilage repair procedure. A medial opening-wedge high tibial osteotomy for varus malalignment and a lateral opening-wedge distal femoral osteotomy for valgus malalignment are the most common methods for correcting malalignment. Overcorrection with a proximal tibial osteotomy, although beneficial for advanced degenerative joint disease, is not well tolerated by younger patients, who typically have an isolated articular cartilage defect. Therefore, correction to neutral alignment with the mechanical axis falling centrally between the tibial spines is recommended. Overcorrection by shifting the axis more into the contralateral compartment is indicated only if there are arthritic changes in the joint. Generally, the necessary amount of correction is calculated on the basis of preoperative standing AP radiographs from the hip to the ankle, with lines drawn from the hip and ankle joints to the center of the tibial plateau (or to the contralateral tibial spine should mild overcorrection be desired). The angular difference between the two lines is the necessary angle of correction. This angle should be transformed into the amount of opening required during the osteotomy because angles are difficult to measure intraoperatively, whereas the opening of the osteotomy can be easily assessed with a ruler.

During opening-wedge osteotomies, there is a tendency to change sagittal alignment. The surgeon should take care that the surgical correction does not inadvertently increase posterior tibial slope.[76,77] The normal posterior slope of the tibia ranges from 3° to 10°; an increase in the posterior slope promotes anterior translation of the tibia on the femur and will worsen the effect of anterior cruciate ligament deficiency or, conversely, diminish posterior cruciate ligament deficiency.

Indications

Patients with a cartilage defect of the femoral condyle and a mechanical axis outside the neutral zone bordered by the tibial spines (**Figure 18**) should have an osteotomy as a part of the cartilage repair treatment.[78-80]

An osteotomy is contraindicated if there is articular cartilage degeneration in the contralateral or patellofemoral compartment, less than 90° of knee flexion, a knee flexion contracture of more than 20°, nonconcordant pain (knee pain outside the involved medial or lateral compartment), inflammatory arthritis, or ongoing infection.[80,81] Patients who have a body mass index greater than 30 to 35 kg/m^2, who continue to smoke, or who fail or are unable to comply with restricted weight-bearing precautions during the postoperative period have higher failure rates; these factors are relative contraindications to an osteotomy.[81-85]

Surgical Technique

Medial Opening-Wedge High Tibial Osteotomy

The posteromedial aspect of the tibia is exposed with subperiosteal dissection; a blunt retractor is placed behind the posterior cortex at the site of the osteotomy to protect the neurovascular structures, and another retractor is placed anteriorly to protect the patellar tendon. When a high tibial osteotomy is combined with open intra-articular procedures such as osteochondral allografting or autologous chondrocyte implantation, separate incisions can be used. The osteotomy incision is made directly in line with the posteromedial cortex of the tibia, and the longitudinal arthrotomy incision is made 5 to 7 cm anterior to it. Using two incisions decreases the length of an anterior single incision for the arthrotomy and allows its placement in the ideal location for all present and any future intra-articular procedures. Should osteotomy implants have to be removed at a later date, the posteromedial incision makes it possible to avoid opening the front of the knee.

An oblique osteotomy of the tibia is performed just proximal to the tibial tubercle, directed toward the superior tip of the fibular head (**Figure 19**). An oblique osteotomy does not substantially affect patellar height, whereas a transverse osteotomy is more likely to create mild-to-moderate patella baja.[86,87] The surgeon should leave at least 1.5 to 2 cm of lateral cortex below the joint line so that the lateral compartment is not violated and so that fixation on the lateral side is possible if the lateral cortex is inadvertently disrupted.[88,89] Aiming the osteotome at the fibular head minimizes the risk of the osteotomy inadvertently extending up into the lateral compartment. Disruption of the lateral cortex causes a 58% reduction in axial stiffness, a 68% reduction in torsional stiffness of the tibia, and micromotion at the osteotomy site,[89] all of which increase the chances of delayed union, nonunion, and loss of correction. However, the application of a staple or small periarticular plate to the disrupted lateral cortex restores the axial and torsional stiffness.[89] It is much easier to deal with this pitfall of medial opening-wedge high tibial osteotomy intraoperatively than to later revise the osteotomy because of loss of correction and/or nonunion.

To avoid increasing the posterior slope, lateral fluoroscopic views are used to place guidewires to align the cutting jig or platform parallel to the anatomic posterior slope. With use of a combination of an oscillating saw and osteotomes, the osteotomy is continued to between 75% and 80% of the way across the tibia. Thin and/or flexible osteotomes assist in ensuring that

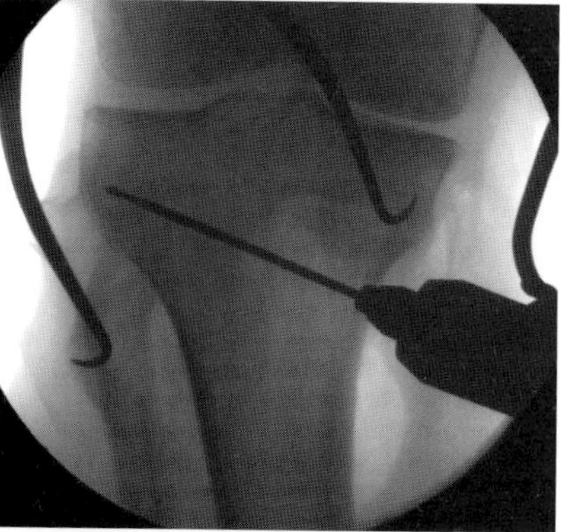

Figure 19 The aiming point for the high tibial osteotomy should never be more proximal than the tip of the fibular head. This allows for sufficient lateral tibial cortex below the joint line for fixation should the lateral cortex fracture and also reduces the risk of inadvertent propagation of the osteotomy into the lateral tibial plateau.

the cortex is completely cut anteriorly and posteriorly. A 3.5-mm drill bit is used to make two or three small drill holes in the lateral cortex to provide stress relief to the bone during opening. The medial side is gradually opened using wedged-shaped tamps, wedged osteotomes, or lamina spreaders put in place anteriorly and posteriorly. The lamina spreaders are used, allowing one or two clicks at a time, followed by a period allowing stress relaxation within the bone. When the approximate opening is obtained within the expected range of correction, long-limb alignment is checked. The leg is axially loaded in full extension, and the mechanical axis is determined with fluoroscopy by placing an alignment rod or the electrocautery cord at the center of the femoral head and the center of the ankle. Any bump or other buildup that had been placed under the patient's hip for positioning should be removed so that a true re-creation of weight bearing is obtained. Final correction is adjusted by further opening or closing the osteotomy to

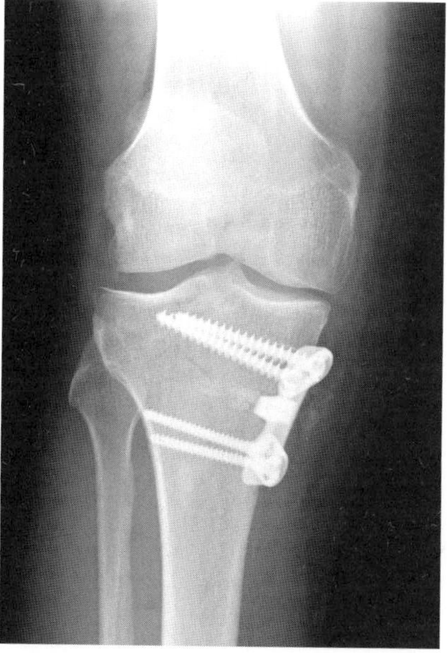

Figure 20 Final appearance after locking plate fixation.

create the degree of desired correction as determined by the mechanical axis through the knee. The preferred type of internal fixation is placed (**Figure 20**). Plate position should be as posterior on the tibia as possible to avoid increasing the tibial slope. It has been shown that anterior and central plate position as well as larger correction angles increase posterior tibial slope.[77,90] Strong plates and locking screws are recommended.[84,91,92] The gap is filled with bone graft. Allograft wedges and cancellous chips, hydroxyapatite, tricalcium phosphate, and tricortical iliac crest and cancellous plug autografts are all options that have been used successfully.[83,93-95] However, the fixation method may be more important than the specific type of bone graft.[91,94]

Lateral Opening-Wedge Distal Femoral Osteotomy

One of this chapter's authors' (SDG) preferred technique for distal femoral osteotomy is a modification of the technique described by Puddu et al.[96] This modification better controls sag-

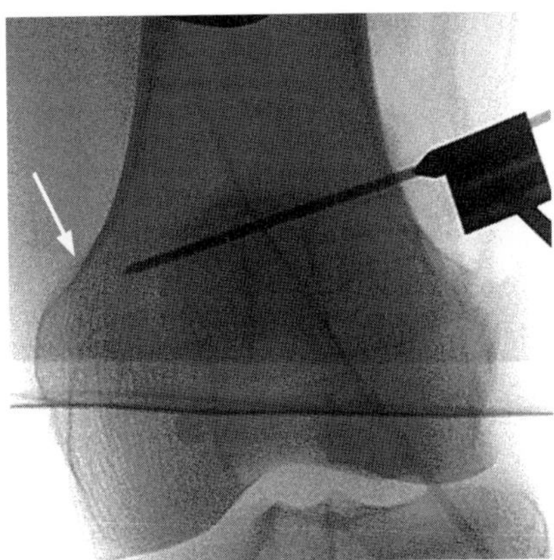

Figure 21 Placement of the guidewire for a distal femoral osteotomy; it is aimed just distal to where the medial cortex fades (arrow).

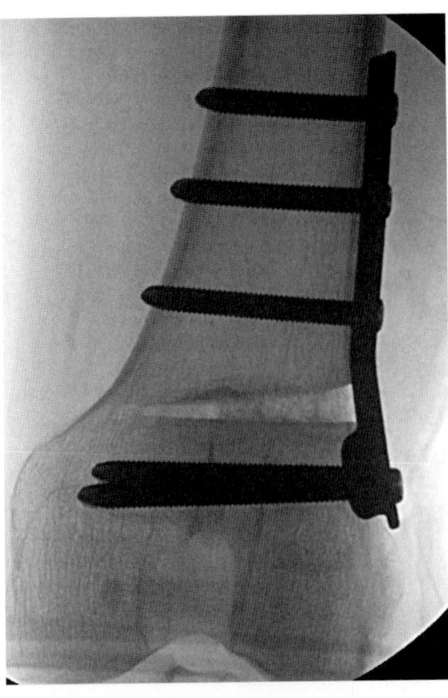

Figure 22 The sliding screw has been removed and replaced by locking screws providing rigid fixation. Bone graft fills the opening of the osteotomy.

ittal and rotational alignment during the distal femoral osteotomy. There are multiple variables that affect rotational and sagittal alignment in the distal part of the femur. One variable is the anatomic obliquity of the distal part of the femur. An osteotomy aimed at the distal medial cortex creates a medial hinge that is less stable than a flat cortical hinge. In addition, this unstable medial hinge is exposed to deforming forces of the quadriceps, gastrocnemius, hamstrings, iliotibial band, and adductors. To eliminate this unstable medial cortical hinge, a modified technique was developed that uses definitive distal fixation and provisional proximal fixation with a sliding screw technique, all before completion of the osteotomy and before correction of coronal alignment is attempted.

The sliding screw technique is performed with lateral exposure in line with the distal part of the femur, splitting the iliotibial band and retracting the vastus lateralis and distal quadriceps anteriorly, and placing a retractor posterior to and directly on bone to protect the neurovascular structures.

The planned trajectory in the coronal plane starts just proximal to the metaphyseal flare of the lateral femoral condyle and aims at the most distal aspect of the medial cortex. A fixation plate is temporarily approximated on the lateral aspect of the femur to get an idea of the plate fit and the starting point for the osteotomy. Aiming the osteotomy toward a more proximal end point on the medial side increases the risk of medial hinge disruption because the thicker cortical bone in this area is more susceptible to fracture. Conversely, a more distal medial hinge, located at the metaphyseal-diaphyseal junction, has thinner cortical bone that is more viscoelastic and therefore less likely to break when the osteotomy is wedged open. After the correct coronal trajectory for the oblique osteotomy is marked with a Kirschner wire (**Figure 21**), the lateral view is used to place another Kirschner wire through a flat surface cutting guide so that the osteotomy will be perpendicular to the shaft of the femur.

The osteotomy is started with an oscillating saw blade traversing about three-quarters of the way across the femur while the anterior and posterior soft tissues are protected. The osteotomy is not opened, and the femur therefore remains stable. A locking T-plate (Synthes, West Chester, PA) is then placed on the lateral aspect of the femur while ensuring appropriate placement with fluoroscopy. Distal fixation with two locked cancellous 6.5-mm screws keeps the plate in position. Provisional proximal fixation is then obtained with one unicortical 4.5-mm screw that is not fully tightened in the distal end of the sliding oblong hole of the plate. Two or three 3.2-mm-diameter drill holes in line with the osteotomy are made in the medial cortex to stress relieve the osseous hinge. Osteotomes and two lamina spreaders or wedges are then used anterior and posterior to the plate to gradually open the osteotomy without breaking the medial hinge. The sliding hole allows approximately 10 mm of opening before it has to be repositioned, should more opening be required. The mechanical axis is then checked. Once neutral alignment is achieved, fixation is completed with three or four locked bicortical screws proximally and two or three locked unicortical cancellous screws distally (**Figure 22**). When fixation is secured, bone graft or allograft wedges are used to fill any gap in the bone.

Rehabilitation

The fixation is strong enough to allow an unrestricted range of motion and weight bearing as tolerated.[96] The rehabilitation program is, therefore, determined by the type of concomitant cartilage repair that has been done.

Patellar Maltracking

Patellofemoral pain and/or instability are a subset cause of anterior knee pain, as are chondral lesions. The management of patients with patellofemoral pain is complicated and the subject of many excellent books and papers. Articular cartilage is aneural and pain can arise from other sources, so it is imperative that all sources of pain are identified and a comprehensive treatment plan is established before performing patellofemoral cartilage repair surgery. Initially, an extensive physical therapy program will be successful for most patients.[97] A smaller number of patients with patellofemoral pain will need surgery, and both autologous chondrocyte implantation and osteochondral allograft transplantation have been reported to provide good outcomes for patients with a monopolar cartilage lesion, but autologous chondrocyte implantation provides more positive outcomes than does allografting for patients with bipolar lesions.[24,37,39] The goal of patellofemoral surgery combined with cartilage restoration is to optimize the environment for the cartilage implant to heal. Patellofemoral pathology is typically multifactorial but can be divided into three primary areas of concern: (1) tibial tuberosity location, (2) medial soft tissues (specifically, the medial patellofemoral ligament), and (3) lateral soft tissues. Often it is best to make minor adjustments to each of these sites rather than to attempt to solve the problem by addressing only one issue.

Tibial Tuberosity Position

The tibial tuberosity is the distal attachment of the extensor mechanism of the knee and is key to alignment and patellar tracking. The lateral position of the tibial tuberosity relative to the trochlear groove (an average tibial tubercle-to-trochlear groove distance of approximately 13 mm) places a lateral force vector on the patella during knee motion that is balanced by medial soft-tissue restraints. An excessively lateral position of the tibial tuberosity (a tibial tubercle-to-trochlear groove distance of > 20 mm) results in high lateral force vectors that may lead to elevated stress in the patellofemoral compartment and/or contribute to the potential for lateral patellar instability. Restoration of patellofemoral cartilage without treating other patellofemoral abnormalities generally yields poor results, but using the same cartilage restoration technique with attention to patellofemoral stresses has improved outcomes.[37,40,41,97] The tibial tuberosity location may be normal; excessively lateral; or in the case of prior tuberosity surgery, excessively medial, posterior, and/or distal. In addition, even with a normal tuberosity position, the patella may be too distal because of prior trauma (patella baja) or may be congenitally too proximal (patella alta). The treatment goal is to optimize force and the contact area between the patella and the femur. The tuberosity may be moved medially, laterally, proximally, and/or distally to normalize the position of the patella relative to the trochlear groove. Moving the tibial tubercle incorrectly results in a poor outcome.[98-100] In addition to normalization of the tuberosity position, anterior displacement of the patella, which has been shown to decrease patellofemoral forces in both Fuji film and Tekscan studies, may be performed.[101] When the tuberosity position is excessively lateral, anterior displacement of the tibial tuberosity may be combined with medial displacement. If the tibial tubercle-to-trochlear groove distance is normal, straight anterior displacement may be performed to decrease patellofemoral stress; it should be noted that there is concomitant rotation of patellar contact areas proximally. Each surgical procedure for patellofemoral cartilage restoration must be carefully custom tailored to the patient's specific chondral pathology.

Medial Soft Tissues (Specifically, the Medial Patellofemoral Ligament)

Proximally, the main medial soft-tissue dynamic restraint is the vastus medialis muscle, and the static restraints are the medial patellofemoral ligament, the medial patellotibial ligament, the medial patellomeniscal ligament, and the medial joint capsule. Although in vitro studies vary in terms of the reported magnitude of restraint to lateral displacement forces by each of these tissues, all investigators have agreed that more than 50% is derived from the medial patellofemoral ligament, with lesser contributions from the medial patellomeniscal ligament and the medial patellotibial ligament.[102-105] Lateral patellar instability (patellar dislocation) results in injury to the medial soft-tissue restraints (the medial patellofemoral ligament) and is often associated with patellofemoral chondral injury.[98] The chondral injury is often distal and medial; therefore, the medial soft-tissue restraints need to be normalized so as to not overload the medial patellofemoral compartment, in addition to preventing pathologic lateral displacement. Historically, nonanatomic medial repairs have resulted in a high incidence of arthrosis,[99] and thus the current recommendation is to focus on the medial patellofemoral ligament. Elias and Cosgarea[100] showed that, regardless of the specific technique, it is important to properly reestablish the correct anatomic attachment sites, which allow the patella to be checkreined against lateral displacement forces. Under normal circumstances, there are low loads in the medial patellofemoral ligament and from approximately 30° of flexion to higher degrees of flexion the ligament should become progressively more lax.[106] **Table 2** shows techniques that have been used in various studies for addressing deficiencies of the medial patellofemoral ligament.[107-117]

Table 2
Techniques for Addressing Deficiency of the Medial Patellofemoral Ligament

Authors (Year)	Graft	Patellar Fixation	Femoral Fixation
Schöttle et al[107] (2009)	Double-arm gracilis autograft	Swivel lock anchors (Arthrex, Naples, FL)	Interference screw
Ahmad et al[108] (2009)	Double-arm semitendinosus autograft	Patellar docking technique	Biotenodesis (Arthrex)
Schöttle et al[109] (2007)	Free gracilis autograft	Suture anchor and bone trough	Interference screw
Noyes and Albright[110] (2006)	Autologous quadriceps tendon strip from native attachment		Soft-tissue fixation to medial retinaculum
Farr and Schepsis[111] (2006)	Double-arm semitendinosus autograft	Suture-anchor fixation	
Steiner et al[112] (2006)	Adductor tendon autograft	Bone tunnel, soft-tissue fixation	Bone tunnel, screw fixation
Nomura et al[113] (2005)	Repair augmented with medial retinaculum slip	Primary repair	Cancellous screw and spiked washer
Ellera Gomes et al[114] (2004)	Single-arm semitendinosus autograft	Patellar bone tunnel	Soft-tissue fixation tied over gracilis
Nomura and Inoue[115] (2003)	Single-arm medical retinaculum graft	Graft looped through a patellar tunnel	Staple fixation at femur
Deie et al[116] (2003)	Transferred semitendinosus tendon	Sutured through a bone tunnel	Looped under medial collateral ligament from native attachment
Drez et al[11] (2001)	Semitendinosus and gracilis autograft	Suture anchor	Sutured to periosteum

Lateral Soft Tissues

Proximally, the main lateral soft-tissue dynamic restraint is the vastus lateralis muscle, and the static restraints are the two layers of the lateral retinaculum: the superficial oblique layer confluent from the iliotibial band and the deep transverse capsular layer, which contains the lateral patellofemoral ligament. Patellofemoral cartilage restoration is commonly performed in patients with lateral patellar instability who have a chronic static lateral position (without current instability) of the patella relative to the trochlear groove (subluxation) and/or patellar lateral tilt, but not all of these patients benefit from a lateral release, especially in isolation. In fact, although somewhat counterintuitive, if the medial patellofemoral ligament is pathologically lax, the lateral retinaculum provides restraint to lateral displacement forces.[118,119] Thus, a lateral release may increase lateral patellar instability.[120] Furthermore, an overzealous lateral release may lead to the development of iatrogenic medial instability.[121] Although empirically it may appear that releasing the lateral retinaculum decreases patellofemoral stress, in vitro studies have failed to demonstrate this benefit.[122] When patellar tilt is seen on CT or MRI scans, a limited lateral release is appropriate to balance soft tissues. The lateral release extends only proximally to allow reversal of tilt and never into the vastus lateralis. An alternative to lateral release is lateral lengthening as described by Biedert.[123] By step-cutting the superficial and deep layers of the lateral retinaculum, it is possible to lengthen the retinaculum 1 to 2 cm while maintaining the lateral checkrein, thus avoiding medial subluxation. Additionally, this provides closure of the joint.

Meniscal Deficiency

Meniscal tears are the most commonly treated lesions of the knee; many patients with articular cartilage damage have meniscal tears. Although meniscal repair is possible in some cases, most meniscal tears are treated with partial meniscectomy. In those knees treated with a partial meniscectomy, the typical posterior horn pathology often results in segmental loss. To the untrained eye, this may seem to represent only one third of the meniscal volume. However, biomechanical studies have shown that disruption of the circumferential hoop bundles at any location results in biomechanical loss of that entire hoop.[124] For example, both the loss of a posterior 2-cm segment to a remnant rim of less than 3 mm and a radial posterior horn root tear to within 3 mm of the periphery have the same biomechanical effect as removal of an entire bucket-handle tear with a remnant of 3 mm. Sequential segmental removal of meniscal tissue in a laboratory setting resulted in a linear loss of articular cartilage contact area and a resultant increase in peak loads and stress in that compartment.[125] On the

Table 3
Outcomes of Meniscal Allograft Transplanations

Author(s) (Year)	No. of Patients	Mean or Range of Follow-up	Reported Outcomes
Milachowski et al[130] (1989)	22	14 months	86% of patients had improvement with surgery
Garrett[131] (1993)	43	2-7 years	81% arthroscopically visualized as successful or clinically "silent"
Noyes et al[132] (2004)	38	40 months	89% rated the knee condition as improved; 76% returned to light low-impact sports without problems
van Arkel and de Boer[133] (1995)	23	2-5 years	87% successful
Cameron and Saha[134] (1997)	63	31 months	87% good-to-excellent results
Goble et al[135] (1999)		4 years	94% of patients had improvement with surgery
Carter[136] (1999)		3 years	88% of patients had improvement with surgery
Rodeo[137] (2001)	33	2 years	67% moderate-to-good results after implantation without bone plugs; 88% moderate-to-good results after implantation with bone plugs
Stollsteimer et al[138] (2000)	23	1-5 years	100% with decreased symptoms
Rath et al[139] (2001)	23	2-8 years	64% improved; 36% became symptomatic, requiring subsequent meniscectomy
Ryu et al[140] (2002)	25	1-6 years	83% reported overall satisfaction
Verdonk et al[128] (2006)	42 (medial meniscal transplantation + high tibial osteotomy, n = 11)	10 years	90% satisfied with outcome; 18% failure rate
Sekiya et al[141] (2006)	25	2-6 years	96% with improved function and activity
Cole et al[142] (2006)	32	2 years	77.5% reported being completely or mostly satisfied
Hommen et al[143] (2007)	22	10 years	90% with improvement in Lysholm and pain scores

basis of this in vitro study, most cartilage restoration algorithms dictate treatment of the meniscal remnant as if it is functional if it is 5 mm or wider and as if it is biomechanically absent if it is less than 3 mm anywhere along the circumferential hoop fibers. The effect of meniscal tissue loss is evident sooner in the lateral compartment, but over time the medial compartment articular cartilage begins to break down in a large percentage of patients. These detrimental effects on native cartilage are also believed to be detrimental to cartilage restoration. Meniscal transplantation decreases the stresses in a compartment with meniscal loss.[126,127] The potentially positive protective effects of in situ meniscal transplantation on the results of articular cartilage repair are suggested by the long-term case study of humans by Verdonk et al[128] and by a study of a sheep model by Szomor et al.[129] The negative effect of meniscal loss and the potentially positive effects of meniscal transplantation are the basis for adding meniscal transplantation to articular cartilage restoration surgery when the meniscus is biomechanically absent. Separate prospective case-series studies by Farr et al[97] and Rue et al[120] demonstrated the safety, feasibility, and efficacy of performing the two techniques concomitantly.

Meniscal allograft transplantation was performed initially to treat patients with chronic rotational instability of the knee who had both ligamentous and meniscal deficiencies.[130] **Table 3** summarizes other studies supporting that approach.[128,130-143] Allograft size and position are critical, and a 10% mismatch in size has major negative consequences with regard to the contact area. The correctly sized meniscal allograft needs to be ordered. Standard AP and lateral radiographs are corrected for magnification, and then anteroposterior and mediolateral meniscal dimensions are calculated.[144] A typical meniscal anteroposterior distance is between 35 and 45 mm. A 10% "allowable mismatch" error range is, therefore, 3.5 to 4.5 mm. Currently, meniscal transplant availability allows rejection of graft-size approximations that differ from the calculated measurements by more than 2 to 3 mm. However, even a properly sized meniscus placed in a nonanatomic position will not reestablish proper contact areas within the compartment, as noted by authors of in vitro studies.[145,146] The meniscal transplant horns are positioned to the patient's native attachment sites, but this does not guarantee proper placement. Allowing the surgeon to "place the anterior horn to effect proper tension" will often not place the horn attachment in the original attachment site and should be discouraged. The decision to use a bone bridge with a slot technique or bone plugs with a socket technique is determined by surgeon preference, but in vitro biomechanical testing suggests that soft-tissue anchoring alone is inadequate.

Summary

Cartilage defects in the knee are common, but not all are symptomatic. If pain persists despite an appropriate nonsurgical treatment regimen, cartilage repair is indicated. Multiple procedures are available, which should be seen as complementary, rather than competitive, allowing treatment of the entire spectrum of lesions from small focal lesions on the femoral condyles to large bipolar or multiple lesions in the patellofemoral joint. Normalization of the biomechanical joint environment through osteotomy or meniscal transplantation is crucial to the success of any cartilage repair technique.

References

1. Heir S, Nerhus TK, Røtterud JH, et al: Focal cartilage defects in the knee impair quality of life as much as severe osteoarthritis: A comparison of knee injury and osteoarthritis outcome score in 4 patient categories scheduled for knee surgery. *Am J Sports Med* 2010;38(2):231-237.
2. Rosenberg TD, Paulos LE, Parker RD, Coward DB, Scott SM: The forty-five-degree posteroanterior flexion weight-bearing radiograph of the knee. *J Bone Joint Surg Am* 1988;70(10):1479-1483.
3. Potter HG, Chong R: Magnetic resonance imaging assessment of chondral lesions and repair. *J Bone Joint Surg Am* 2009;91(Suppl 1): 126-131.
4. Jaiswal PK, Macmull S, Bentley G, Carrington RW, Skinner JA, Briggs TW: Does smoking influence outcome after autologous chondrocyte implantation? A case-controlled study. *J Bone Joint Surg Br* 2009;91(12):1575-1578.
5. Curl WW, Krome J, Gordon ES, Rushing J, Smith BP, Poehling GG: Cartilage injuries: A review of 31,516 knee arthroscopies. *Arthroscopy* 1997;13(4): 456-460.
6. Kreuz PC, Steinwachs MR, Erggelet C, et al: Results after microfracture of full-thickness chondral defects in different compartments in the knee. *Osteoarthritis Cartilage* 2006;14(11):1119-1125.
7. Bentley G, Biant LC, Carrington RW, et al: A prospective, randomised comparison of autologous chondrocyte implantation versus mosaicplasty for osteochondral defects in the knee. *J Bone Joint Surg Br* 2003;85(2): 223-230.
8. Knutsen G, Engebretsen L, Ludvigsen TC, et al: Autologous chondrocyte implantation compared with microfracture in the knee: A randomized trial. *J Bone Joint Surg Am* 2004;86-A(3): 455-464.
9. Basad E, Ishaque B, Bachmann G, Stürz H, Steinmeyer J: Matrix-induced autologous chondrocyte implantation versus microfracture in the treatment of cartilage defects of the knee: A 2-year randomised study. *Knee Surg Sports Traumatol Arthrosc* 2010;18(4): 519-527.
10. Saris DB, Vanlauwe J, Victor J, et al; TIG/ACT/01/2000&EXT Study Group: Treatment of symptomatic cartilage defects of the knee: Characterized chondrocyte implantation results in better clinical outcome at 36 months in a randomized trial compared to microfracture. *Am J Sports Med* 2009;37(Suppl 1):10S-19S.
11. Saris DB, Vanlauwe J, Victor J, et al: Characterized chondrocyte implantation results in better structural repair when treating symptomatic cartilage defects of the knee in a randomized controlled trial versus microfracture. *Am J Sports Med* 2008;36(2): 235-246.
12. Mithoefer K, Williams RJ III, Warren RF, et al: The microfracture technique for the treatment of articular cartilage lesions in the knee: A prospective cohort study. *J Bone Joint Surg Am* 2005;87(9): 1911-1920.
13. Mithoefer K, Williams RJ III, Warren RF, Wickiewicz TL, Marx RG: High-impact athletics after knee articular cartilage repair: A prospective evaluation of the microfracture technique. *Am J Sports Med* 2006;34(9):1413-1418.
14. Kon E, Gobbi A, Filardo G, Delcogliano M, Zaffagnini S, Marcacci M: Arthroscopic second-generation autologous chondrocyte implantation compared with microfracture for chondral lesions of the knee: Prospective nonrandomized study at 5 years. *Am J Sports Med* 2009;37(1):33-41.
15. Steadman JR, Briggs KK, Rodrigo JJ, Kocher MS, Gill TJ, Rodkey WG: Outcomes of microfracture for traumatic chondral defects of the knee: Average 11-year follow-up. *Arthroscopy* 2003; 19(5):477-484.
16. Gudas R, Kalesinskas RJ, Kimtys V, et al: A prospective randomized clinical study of mosaic osteochondral autologous transplantation versus microfracture for the treatment of osteochondral defects in the knee joint in young athletes. *Arthroscopy* 2005;21(9): 1066-1075.
17. Hangody L, Füles P: Autologous osteochondral mosaicplasty for the treatment of full-thickness defects of weight-bearing joints: Ten years of experimental and clinical experience. *J Bone Joint Surg Am* 2003;85-A(Suppl 2): 25-32.

18. Hangody L, Kish G, Kárpáti Z, Szerb I, Udvarhelyi I: Arthroscopic autogenous osteochondral mosaicplasty for the treatment of femoral condylar articular defects: A preliminary report. *Knee Surg Sports Traumatol Arthrosc* 1997; 5(4):262-267.
19. Bartlett W, Skinner JA, Gooding CR, et al: Autologous chondrocyte implantation versus matrix-induced autologous chondrocyte implantation for osteochondral defects of the knee: A prospective, randomised study. *J Bone Joint Surg Br* 2005;87(5): 640-645.
20. Behrens P, Bitter T, Kurz B, Russlies M: Matrix-associated autologous chondrocyte transplantation/implantation (MACT/MACI): 5-year follow-up. *Knee* 2006; 13(3):194-202.
21. Brittberg M, Lindahl A, Nilsson A, Ohlsson C, Isaksson O, Peterson L: Treatment of deep cartilage defects in the knee with autologous chondrocyte transplantation. *N Engl J Med* 1994; 331(14):889-895.
22. Peterson L, Minas T, Brittberg M, Nilsson A, Sjögren-Jansson E, Lindahl A: Two- to 9-year outcome after autologous chondrocyte transplantation of the knee. *Clin Orthop Relat Res* 2000;374: 212-234.
23. Emmerson BC, Görtz S, Jamali AA, Chung C, Amiel D, Bugbee WD: Fresh osteochondral allografting in the treatment of osteochondritis dissecans of the femoral condyle. *Am J Sports Med* 2007;35(6):907-914.
24. Shasha N, Aubin PP, Cheah HK, Davis AM, Agnidis Z, Gross AE: Long-term clinical experience with fresh osteochondral allografts for articular knee defects in high demand patients. *Cell Tissue Bank* 2002;3(3):175-182.
25. Aubin PP, Cheah HK, Davis AM, Gross AE: Long-term followup of fresh femoral osteochondral allografts for posttraumatic knee defects. *Clin Orthop Relat Res* 2001;391(Suppl):S318-S327.
26. Görtz S, Bugbee WD: Allografts in articular cartilage repair. *J Bone Joint Surg Am* 2006;88(6):1374-1384.
27. LaPrade RF, Botker J, Herzog M, Agel J: Refrigerated osteoarticular allografts to treat articular cartilage defects of the femoral condyles: A prospective outcomes study. *J Bone Joint Surg Am* 2009; 91(4):805-811.
28. McCulloch PC, Kang RW, Sobhy MH, Hayden JK, Cole BJ: Prospective evaluation of prolonged fresh osteochondral allograft transplantation of the femoral condyle: Minimum 2-year follow-up. *Am J Sports Med* 2007; 35(3):411-420.
29. Bartlett W, Gooding CR, Carrington RW, Skinner JA, Briggs TW, Bentley G: Autologous chondrocyte implantation at the knee using a bilayer collagen membrane with bone graft: A preliminary report. *J Bone Joint Surg Br* 2005;87(3):330-332.
30. Gomoll AH, Flik KR, Hayden JK, Cole BJ, Bush-Joseph CA, Bach BR Jr: Internal fixation of unstable Cahill Type-2C osteochondritis dissecans lesions of the knee in adolescent patients. *Orthopedics* 2007;30(6):487-490.
31. Murray JR, Chitnavis J, Dixon P, et al: Osteochondritis dissecans of the knee: Long-term clinical outcome following arthroscopic debridement. *Knee* 2007;14(2): 94-98.
32. Aglietti P, Ciardullo A, Giron F, Ponteggia F: Results of arthroscopic excision of the fragment in the treatment of osteochondritis dissecans of the knee. *Arthroscopy* 2001;17(7):741-746.
33. Wright RW, McLean M, Matava MJ, Shively RA: Osteochondritis dissecans of the knee: Long-term results of excision of the fragment. *Clin Orthop Relat Res* 2004;424:239-243.
34. Pascual-Garrido C, Friel NA, Kirk SS, et al: Midterm results of surgical treatment for adult osteochondritis dissecans of the knee. *Am J Sports Med* 2009;37 (Suppl 1):125S-130S.
35. Gudas R, Simonaityte R, Cekanauskas E, Tamosiūnas R: A prospective, randomized clinical study of osteochondral autologous transplantation versus microfracture for the treatment of osteochondritis dissecans in the knee joint in children. *J Pediatr Orthop* 2009;29(7):741-748.
36. Krishnan SP, Skinner JA, Carrington RW, Flanagan AM, Briggs TW, Bentley G: Collagen-covered autologous chondrocyte implantation for osteochondritis dissecans of the knee: Two- to seven-year results. *J Bone Joint Surg Br* 2006;88(2):203-205.
37. Peterson L, Minas T, Brittberg M, Lindahl A: Treatment of osteochondritis dissecans of the knee with autologous chondrocyte transplantation: Results at two to ten years. *J Bone Joint Surg Am* 2003;85-A(Suppl 2):17-24.
38. Jamali AA, Emmerson BC, Chung C, Convery FR, Bugbee WD: Fresh osteochondral allografts: Results in the patellofemoral joint. *Clin Orthop Relat Res* 2005;437:176-185.
39. Farr J: Autologous chondrocyte implantation improves patellofemoral cartilage treatment outcomes. *Clin Orthop Relat Res* 2007;463:187-194.
40. Henderson IJ, Lavigne P: Periosteal autologous chondrocyte implantation for patellar chondral defect in patients with normal and abnormal patellar tracking. *Knee* 2006;13(4):274-279.
41. Minas T, Bryant T: The role of autologous chondrocyte implantation in the patellofemoral joint. *Clin Orthop Relat Res* 2005;436: 30-39.

42. Pascual-Garrido C, Slabaugh MA, L'Heureux DR, Friel NA, Cole BJ: Recommendations and treatment outcomes for patellofemoral articular cartilage defects with autologous chondrocyte implantation: Prospective evaluation at average 4-year follow-up. *Am J Sports Med* 2009; 37(Suppl 1):33S-41S.

43. Kreuz PC, Erggelet C, Steinwachs MR, et al: Is microfracture of chondral defects in the knee associated with different results in patients aged 40 years or younger? *Arthroscopy* 2006;22(11): 1180-1186.

44. Asik M, Ciftci F, Sen C, Erdil M, Atalar A: The microfracture technique for the treatment of full-thickness articular cartilage lesions of the knee: Midterm results. *Arthroscopy* 2008;24(11):1214-1220.

45. Rosenberger RE, Gomoll AH, Bryant T, Minas T: Repair of large chondral defects of the knee with autologous chondrocyte implantation in patients 45 years or older. *Am J Sports Med* 2008; 36(12):2336-2344.

46. Garretson RB III , Katolik LI, Verma N, Beck PR, Bach BR, Cole BJ: Contact pressure at osteochondral donor sites in the patellofemoral joint. *Am J Sports Med* 2004;32(4):967-974.

47. Pylawka TK, Wimmer M, Cole BJ, Virdi AS, Williams JM: Impaction affects cell viability in osteochondral tissues during transplantation. *J Knee Surg* 2007; 20(2):105-110.

48. Görtz S, Bugbee WD: Allografts in articular cartilage repair. *Instr Course Lect* 2007;56:469-480.

49. Huang FS, Simonian PT, Norman AG, Clark JM: Effects of small incongruities in a sheep model of osteochondral autografting. *Am J Sports Med* 2004;32(8): 1842-1848.

50. Zaslav K, Cole B, Brewster R, et al; STAR Study Principal Investigators: A prospective study of autologous chondrocyte implantation in patients with failed prior treatment for articular cartilage defect of the knee: Results of the Study of the Treatment of Articular Repair (STAR) clinical trial. *Am J Sports Med* 2009;37(1): 42-55.

51. Gooding CR, Bartlett W, Bentley G, Skinner JA, Carrington R, Flanagan A: A prospective, randomised study comparing two techniques of autologous chondrocyte implantation for osteochondral defects in the knee: Periosteum covered versus type I/III collagen covered. *Knee* 2006; 13(3):203-210.

52. Kreuz PC, Steinwachs M, Erggelet C, et al: Classification of graft hypertrophy after autologous chondrocyte implantation of full-thickness chondral defects in the knee. *Osteoarthritis Cartilage* 2007;15(12):1339-1347.

53. Gomoll AH, Probst C, Farr J, Cole BJ, Minas T: Use of a type I/III bilayer collagen membrane decreases reoperation rates for symptomatic hypertrophy after autologous chondrocyte implantation. *Am J Sports Med* 2009; 37(Suppl 1):20S-23S.

54. Haddo O, Mahroof S, Higgs D, et al: The use of chondrogide membrane in autologous chondrocyte implantation. *Knee* 2004; 11(1):51-55.

55. Chu CR, Convery FR, Akeson WH, Meyers M, Amiel D: Articular cartilage transplantation. Clinical results in the knee. *Clin Orthop Relat Res* 1999;360: 159-168.

56. Garrett JC: Fresh osteochondral allografts for treatment of articular defects in osteochondritis dissecans of the lateral femoral condyle in adults. *Clin Orthop Relat Res* 1994;303:33-37.

57. Ghazavi MT, Pritzker KP, Davis AM, Gross AE: Fresh osteochondral allografts for post-traumatic osteochondral defects of the knee. *J Bone Joint Surg Br* 1997;79(6):1008-1013.

58. Lexer E: Joint transplantations and arthroplasty. *Surg Gynecol Obstet* 1925;40:782-809.

59. McDermott AG, Langer F, Pritzker KP, Gross AE: Fresh small-fragment osteochondral allografts: Long-term follow-up study on first 100 cases. *Clin Orthop Relat Res* 1985;197:96-102.

60. Meyers MH, Akeson W, Convery FR: Resurfacing of the knee with fresh osteochondral allograft. *J Bone Joint Surg Am* 1989;71(5): 704-713.

61. Kandel RA, Gross AE, Ganel A, McDermott AG, Langer F, Pritzker KP: Histopathology of failed osteoarticular shell allografts. *Clin Orthop Relat Res* 1985;197: 103-110.

62. Williams SK, Amiel D, Ball ST, et al: Analysis of cartilage tissue on a cellular level in fresh osteochondral allograft retrievals. *Am J Sports Med* 2007;35(12):2022-2032.

63. Czitrom AA, Keating S, Gross AE: The viability of articular cartilage in fresh osteochondral allografts after clinical transplantation. *J Bone Joint Surg Am* 1990;72(4): 574-581.

64. Langer F, Gross AE: Immunogenicity of allograft articular cartilage. *J Bone Joint Surg Am* 1974; 56(2):297-304.

65. Sirlin CB, Brossmann J, Boutin RD, et al: Shell osteochondral allografts of the knee: Comparison of mr imaging findings and immunologic responses. *Radiology* 2001;219(1):35-43.

66. Mroz TE, Joyce MJ, Steinmetz MP, Lieberman IH, Wang JC: Musculoskeletal allograft risks and recalls in the United States. *J Am Acad Orthop Surg* 2008;16(10):559-565.

67. Shelton WR, Treacy SH, Dukes AD, Bomboy AL: Use of allografts in knee reconstruction:

II. Surgical considerations. *J Am Acad Orthop Surg* 1998;6(3): 169-175.

68. Pearsall AW IV, Tucker JA, Hester RB, Heitman RJ: Chondrocyte viability in refrigerated osteochondral allografts used for transplantation within the knee. *Am J Sports Med* 2004;32(1): 125-131.
69. Williams SK, Amiel D, Ball ST, et al: Prolonged storage effects on the articular cartilage of fresh human osteochondral allografts. *J Bone Joint Surg Am* 2003; 85-A(11):2111-2120.
70. Ball ST, Amiel D, Williams SK, et al: The effects of storage on fresh human osteochondral allografts. *Clin Orthop Relat Res* 2004;418:246-252.
71. Kwan MK, Wayne JS, Woo SL, Field FP, Hoover J, Meyers M: Histological and biomechanical assessment of articular cartilage from stored osteochondral shell allografts. *J Orthop Res* 1989;7(5): 637-644.
72. Bugbee WD: Fresh osteochondral allografts for the knee. *Tech Knee Surg* 2004;3:1-9.
73. Bugbee WD: Fresh osteochondral allografts. *J Knee Surg* 2002;15(3): 191-195.
74. Shasha N, Krywulak S, Backstein D, Pressman A, Gross AE: Long-term follow-up of fresh tibial osteochondral allografts for failed tibial plateau fractures. *J Bone Joint Surg Am* 2003; 85-A(Suppl 2):33-39.
75. Cook SD, Salkeld SL, Patron LP, Doughty ES, Jones DG: The effect of low-intensity pulsed ultrasound on autologous osteochondral plugs in a canine model. *Am J Sports Med* 2008;36(9):1733-1741.
76. Giffin JR, Vogrin TM, Zantop T, Woo SL, Harner CD: Effects of increasing tibial slope on the biomechanics of the knee. *Am J Sports Med* 2004;32(2):376-382.
77. Rubino LJ, Schoderbek RJ, Golish SR, Baumfeld J, Miller MD: The effect of plate position and size on tibial slope in high tibial osteotomy: A cadaveric study. *J Knee Surg* 2008;21(1):75-79.
78. Gillogly S: Autologous chondrocyte implantation: Complex defects and combined procedures. *Oper Tech Sports Med* 2002;10: 120-128.
79. Minas T: Nonarthroplasty management of knee arthritis in the young individual. *Curr Opin Orthop* 1998;9:46-52.
80. Wright JM, Crockett HC, Slawski DP, Madsen MW, Windsor RE: High tibial osteotomy. *J Am Acad Orthop Surg* 2005;13(4): 279-289.
81. Brinkman JM, Lobenhoffer P, Agneskirchner JD, Staubli AE, Wymenga AB, van Heerwaarden RJ: Osteotomies around the knee: Patient selection, stability of fixation and bone healing in high tibial osteotomies. *J Bone Joint Surg Br* 2008;90(12):1548-1557.
82. Miller BS, Downie B, McDonough EB, Wojtys EM: Complications after medial opening wedge high tibial osteotomy. *Arthroscopy* 2009;25(6):639-646.
83. Noyes FR, Mayfield W, Barber-Westin SD, Albright JC, Heckmann TP: Opening wedge high tibial osteotomy: An operative technique and rehabilitation program to decrease complications and promote early union and function. *Am J Sports Med* 2006; 34(8):1262-1273.
84. Spahn G: Complications in high tibial (medial opening wedge) osteotomy. *Arch Orthop Trauma Surg* 2004;124(10):649-653.
85. Spahn G, Kirschbaum S, Kahl E: Factors that influence high tibial osteotomy results in patients with medial gonarthritis: A score to predict the results. *Osteoarthritis Cartilage* 2006;14(2):190-195.
86. El-Azab H, Glabgly P, Paul J, Imhoff AB, Hinterwimmer S: Patellar height and posterior tibial slope after open- and closed-wedge high tibial osteotomy: A radiological study on 100 patients. *Am J Sports Med* 2010;38(2): 323-329.
87. Matar WY, Boscariol R, Dervin GF: Open wedge high tibial osteotomy: A roentgenographic comparison of a horizontal and an oblique osteotomy on patellar height and sagittal tibial slope. *Am J Sports Med* 2009;37(4):735-742.
88. Amendola A, Fowler PJ, Litchfield R, Kirkley S, Clatworthy M: Opening wedge high tibial osteotomy using a novel technique: Early results and complications. *J Knee Surg* 2004;17(3):164-169.
89. Miller BS, Dorsey WO, Bryant CR, Austin JC: The effect of lateral cortex disruption and repair on the stability of the medial opening wedge high tibial osteotomy. *Am J Sports Med* 2005; 33(10):1552-1557.
90. Rodner CM, Adams DJ, Diaz-Doran V, et al: Medial opening wedge tibial osteotomy and the sagittal plane: The effect of increasing tibial slope on tibiofemoral contact pressure. *Am J Sports Med* 2006;34(9):1431-1441.
91. Dorsey WO, Miller BS, Tadje JP, Bryant CR: The stability of three commercially available implants used in medial opening wedge high tibial osteotomy. *J Knee Surg* 2006;19(2):95-98.
92. Niemeyer P, Koestler W, Kaehny C, et al: Two-year results of open-wedge high tibial osteotomy with fixation by medial plate fixator for medial compartment arthritis with varus malalignment of the knee. *Arthroscopy* 2008;24(7):796-804.
93. Moyad TF, Minas T: Opening wedge high tibial osteotomy: A novel technique for harvesting autograft bone. *J Knee Surg* 2008; 21(1):80-84.
94. Takeuchi R, Ishikawa H, Aratake M, et al: Medial opening

wedge high tibial osteotomy with early full weight bearing. *Arthroscopy* 2009;25(1):46-53.

95. Yacobucci GN, Cocking MR: Union of medial opening-wedge high tibial osteotomy using a corticocancellous proximal tibial wedge allograft. *Am J Sports Med* 2008;36(4):713-719.

96. Puddu G, Cipolla M, Cerullo G, Franco V, Giannì E: Osteotomies: The surgical treatment of the valgus knee. *Sports Med Arthrosc* 2007;15(1):15-22.

97. Farr J, Rawal A, Marberry KM: Concomitant meniscal allograft transplantation and autologous chondrocyte implantation: Minimum 2-year follow-up. *Am J Sports Med* 2007;35(9):1459-1466.

98. Nomura E, Inoue M: Second-look arthroscopy of cartilage changes of the patellofemoral joint, especially the patella, following acute and recurrent patellar dislocation. *Osteoarthritis Cartilage* 2005;13(11):1029-1036.

99. Nomura E, Inoue M, Kobayashi S: Long-term follow-up and knee osteoarthritis change after medial patellofemoral ligament reconstruction for recurrent patellar dislocation. *Am J Sports Med* 2007;35(11):1851-1858.

100. Elias JJ, Cosgarea AJ: Technical errors during medial patellofemoral ligament reconstruction could overload medial patellofemoral cartilage: A computational analysis. *Am J Sports Med* 2006;34(9):1478-1485.

101. Cohen ZA, Henry JH, McCarthy DM, Mow VC, Ateshian GA: Computer simulations of patellofemoral joint surgery: Patient-specific models for tuberosity transfer. *Am J Sports Med* 2003;31(1):87-98.

102. Hughston JC, Walsh WM: Proximal and distal reconstruction of the extensor mechanism for patellar subluxation. *Clin Orthop Relat Res* 1979;144:36-42.

103. Warren LF, Marshall JL: The supporting structures and layers on the medial side of the knee: An anatomical analysis. *J Bone Joint Surg Am* 1979;61(1):56-62.

104. Conlan T, Garth WP Jr, Lemons JE: Evaluation of the medial soft-tissue restraints of the extensor mechanism of the knee. *J Bone Joint Surg Am* 1993;75(5):682-693.

105. Panagiotopoulos E, Strzelczyk P, Herrmann M, Scuderi G: Cadaveric study on static medial patellar stabilizers: The dynamizing role of the vastus medialis obliquus on medial patellofemoral ligament. *Knee Surg Sports Traumatol Arthrosc* 2006;14(1):7-12.

106. Amis AA, Firer P, Mountney J, Senavongse W, Thomas NP: Anatomy and biomechanics of the medial patellofemoral ligament. *Knee* 2003;10(3):215-220.

107. Schöttle P, Schmeling A, Romero J, Weiler A: Anatomical reconstruction of the medial patellofemoral ligament using a free gracilis autograft. *Arch Orthop Trauma Surg* 2009;129(3):305-309.

108. Ahmad CS, Brown GD, Stein BS: The docking technique for medial patellofemoral ligament reconstruction: Surgical technique and clinical outcome. *Am J Sports Med* 2009;37(10):2021-2027.

109. Schottle PB, Romero J, Schmeling A, Weiler A: Technical note: Anatomical reconstruction of the medial patellofemoral ligament using a free gracilis autograft. *Arch Orthop Trauma Surg* 2008;128(5):479-484.

110. Noyes FR, Albright JC: Reconstruction of the medial patellofemoral ligament with autologous quadriceps tendon. *Arthroscopy* 2006;22(8):904, e1-e7.

111. Farr J, Schepsis AA: Reconstruction of the medial patellofemoral ligament for recurrent patellar instability. *J Knee Surg* 2006;19(4):307-316.

112. Steiner TM, Torga-Spak R, Teitge RA: Medial patellofemoral ligament reconstruction in patients with lateral patellar instability and trochlear dysplasia. *Am J Sports Med* 2006;34(8):1254-1261.

113. Nomura E, Inoue M, Osada N: Augmented repair of avulsion-tear type medial patellofemoral ligament injury in acute patellar dislocation. *Knee Surg Sports Traumatol Arthrosc* 2005;13(5):346-351.

114. Ellera Gomes JL, Stigler Marczyk LR, César de César P, Jungblut CF: Medial patellofemoral ligament reconstruction with semitendinosus autograft for chronic patellar instability: A follow-up study. *Arthroscopy* 2004;20(2):147-151.

115. Nomura E, Inoue M: Surgical technique and rationale for medial patellofemoral ligament reconstruction for recurrent patellar dislocation. *Arthroscopy* 2003;19(5):E47.

116. Deie M, Ochi M, Sumen Y, Yasumoto M, Kobayashi K, Kimura H: Reconstruction of the medial patellofemoral ligament for the treatment of habitual or recurrent dislocation of the patella in children. *J Bone Joint Surg Br* 2003;85(6):887-890.

117. Drez D Jr, Edwards TB, Williams CS: Results of medial patellofemoral ligament reconstruction in the treatment of patellar dislocation. *Arthroscopy* 2001;17(3):298-306.

118. Desio SM, Burks RT, Bachus KN: Soft tissue restraints to lateral patellar translation in the human knee. *Am J Sports Med* 1998;26(1):59-65.

119. Christoforakis J, Bull AM, Strachan RK, Shymkiw R, Senavongse W, Amis AA: Effects of lateral retinacular release on the lateral stability of the patella. *Knee Surg Sports Traumatol Arthrosc* 2006;14(3):273-277.

120. Rue JP, Yanke AB, Busam ML, McNickle AG, Cole BJ: Prospective evaluation of concurrent meniscus transplantation and articular cartilage repair: Minimum 2-year follow-up. *Am J Sports Med* 2008;36(9):1770-1778.

121. Hughston JC, Deese M: Medial subluxation of the patella as a complication of lateral retinacular release. *Am J Sports Med* 1988; 16(4):383-388.

122. Ostermeier S, Holst M, Hurschler C, Windhagen H, Stukenborg-Colsman C: Dynamic measurement of patellofemoral kinematics and contact pressure after lateral retinacular release: An in vitro study. *Knee Surg Sports Traumatol Arthrosc* 2007;15(5):547-554.

123. Biedert R: Complicated case studies, in Sanchis-Alfonso V, ed: *Anterior Knee Pain and Patellar Instability.* London, England, Springer-Verlag, 2005, pp 323-336.

124. Jones RS, Keene GC, Learmonth DJ, et al: Direct measurement of hoop strains in the intact and torn human medial meniscus. *Clin Biomech (Bristol, Avon)* 1996; 11(5):295-300.

125. Lee SJ, Aadalen KJ, Malaviya P, et al: Tibiofemoral contact mechanics after serial medial meniscectomies in the human cadaveric knee. *Am J Sports Med* 2006; 34(8):1334-1344.

126. Paletta GA Jr, Manning T, Snell E, Parker R, Bergfeld J: The effect of allograft meniscal replacement on intraarticular contact area and pressures in the human knee: A biomechanical study. *Am J Sports Med* 1997;25(5):692-698.

127. Verma NN, Kolb E, Cole BJ, et al: The effects of medial meniscal transplantation techniques on intra-articular contact pressures. *J Knee Surg* 2008;21(1):20-26.

128. Verdonk PC, Verstraete KL, Almqvist KF, et al: Meniscal allograft transplantation: Long-term clinical results with radiological and magnetic resonance imaging correlations. *Knee Surg Sports Traumatol Arthrosc* 2006;14(8): 694-706.

129. Szomor ZL, Martin TE, Bonar F, Murrell GA: The protective effects of meniscal transplantation on cartilage: An experimental study in sheep. *J Bone Joint Surg Am* 2000;82(1):80-88.

130. Milachowski KA, Weismeier K, Wirth CJ: Homologous meniscus transplantation: Experimental and clinical results. *Int Orthop* 1989; 13(1):1-11.

131. Garrett J: Meniscal transplantation: A review of 43 cases with 2- to 7-year follow-up. *Sports Med Arthrosc Rev* 1993;1:164-167.

132. Noyes FR, Barber-Westin SD, Rankin M: Meniscal transplantation in symptomatic patients less than fifty years old. *J Bone Joint Surg Am* 2004;86-A(7):1392-1404.

133. van Arkel ER, de Boer HH: Human meniscal transplantation: Preliminary results at 2 to 5-year follow-up. *J Bone Joint Surg Br* 1995;77(4):589-595.

134. Cameron JC, Saha S: Meniscal allograft transplantation for unicompartmental arthritis of the knee. *Clin Orthop Relat Res* 1997; 337:164-171.

135. Goble EM, Kohn D, Verdonk R, Kane SM: Meniscal substitutes: Human experience. *Scand J Med Sci Sports* 1999;9(3):146-157.

136. Carter T: Meniscal allograft transplantation. *Sports Med Arthrosc Rev* 1999;7:51-62.

137. Rodeo SA: Meniscal allografts: Where do we stand? *Am J Sports Med* 2001;29(2):246-261.

138. Stollsteimer GT, Shelton WR, Dukes A, Bomboy AL: Meniscal allograft transplantation: A 1- to 5-year follow-up of 22 patients. *Arthroscopy* 2000;16(4):343-347.

139. Rath E, Richmond JC, Yassir W, Albright JD, Gundogan F: Meniscal allograft transplantation: Two- to eight-year results. *Am J Sports Med* 2001;29(4):410-414.

140. Ryu RK, Dunbar V WH, Morse GG: Meniscal allograft replacement: A 1-year to 6-year experience. *Arthroscopy* 2002; 18(9):989-994.

141. Sekiya JK, West RV, Groff YJ, Irrgang JJ, Fu FH, Harner CD: Clinical outcomes following isolated lateral meniscal allograft transplantation. *Arthroscopy* 2006; 22(7):771-780.

142. Cole BJ, Dennis MG, Lee SJ, et al: Prospective evaluation of allograft meniscus transplantation: A minimum 2-year follow-up. *Am J Sports Med* 2006;34(6):919-927.

143. Hommen JP, Applegate GR, Del Pizzo W: Meniscus allograft transplantation: Ten-year results of cryopreserved allografts. *Arthroscopy* 2007;23(4):388-393.

144. Pollard ME, Kang Q, Berg EE: Radiographic sizing for meniscal transplantation. *Arthroscopy* 1995; 11(6):684-687.

145. Kohn D, Moreno B: Meniscus insertion anatomy as a basis for meniscus replacement: A morphological cadaveric study. *Arthroscopy* 1995;11(1):96-103.

146. von Lewinski G, Kohn D, Wirth CJ, Lazovic D: The influence of nonanatomical insertion and incongruence of meniscal transplants on the articular cartilage in an ovine model. *Am J Sports Med* 2008;36(5):841-850.

Technical Aspects of Anterior Cruciate Ligament Reconstruction for the General Orthopaedic Surgeon

Matthew L. Busam, MD
John P. Fulkerson, MD
Trevor R. Gaskill, MD
Claude T. Moorman III, MD
Frank R. Noyes, MD
Marc T. Galloway, MD

Abstract

Anterior cruciate ligament reconstruction is the sixth most common procedure performed by orthopaedic surgeons. The goals of the procedure are to restore knee stability and patient function. These goals are dependent on proper graft positioning and incorporation. Anterior cruciate ligament reconstruction involves a technically complicated series of steps, all of which affect graft healing and clinical outcome. A wide variety of graft choices and surgical techniques are currently available for use. It is important for orthopaedic surgeons performing anterior cruciate ligament reconstructions to be aware of the indications for graft selection, techniques for correct graft placement, and the biologic implications related to these factors.

Instr Course Lect 2011;60:485-497.

It is estimated that more than 150,000 patients are treated with anterior cruciate ligament (ACL) reconstructions in the United States each year.[1,2] Many studies have reported consistently high success rates that are characterized by the restoration of knee function and the ability of patients to return to their desired level of activity.[1-3] Most of these reports arise from centers in which surgeons have significant experience with the procedure. The literature suggests that postoperative complications following total joint arthroplasty correlate with the number of procedures performed by the surgeon each year.[4] Records from the American Board of Orthopaedic Surgery indicate that most ACL reconstructions are done by surgeons who perform fewer than 10 such procedures per year.[5]

Reconstructing the ACL is a technically demanding procedure that involves a series of steps, all of which

Dr. Busam or an immediate family member has received research or institutional support from Arthrex and DJ Orthopaedics. Dr. Fulkerson or an immediate family member serves as a board member, owner, officer, or committee member of the Patellofemoral Foundation; the American Orthopaedic Society for Sports Medicine; the Arthroscopy Association of North America; and the International Society of Arthroscopy, Knee Surgery, and Orthopaedic Sports Medicine; has received royalties from Arthrex, DJ Orthopaedics, and Lippincott; serves as an unpaid consultant to DJ Orthopaedics, the Musculoskeletal Transplant Foundation, and Smith & Nephew; has received research or institutional support from Kinamed; has stock or stock options held in DJ Orthopaedics; and has received nonincome support (such as equipment or services), commercially derived honoraria, or other non–research-related funding (such as paid travel) from SLACK. Dr. Moorman or an immediate family member serves as a board member, owner, officer, or committee member of the Southern Orthopaedic Association; is a member of a speakers' bureau or has made paid presentations on behalf of Nutramax; has received research or institutional support from Histogenics, Stryker, Breg, and Mitek; and has stock or stock options held in Healthsport. Dr. Noyes or an immediate family member serves as a board member, owner, officer, or committee member of the Cincinnati Sports Medicine Research and Education Foundation Board of Directors; has received royalties from Smith & Nephew; has received research or institutional support from Arthrex, DePuy, DJ Orthopaedics, Genzyme, Mitek, Regeneration Technologies, Stryker, and AlloSource; and has received nonincome support (such as equipment or services), commercially derived honoraria, or other non–research-related funding (such as paid travel) from Saunders/Mosby-Elsevier. Dr. Galloway or an immediate family member has received research or institutional support from Arthrex and DJ Orthopaedics. Neither Dr. Gaskill nor any immediate family member has received anything of value from or owns stock in a commercial company or institution related directly or indirectly to the subject of this chapter.

impact graft incorporation, biologic function, and ultimately clinical outcome. There is no standard surgical technique that is applicable to every patient. Those surgeons performing the procedure less frequently may not have the opportunity to gain the necessary expertise for consistently good outcomes. A review of the various considerations and surgical techniques that impact outcomes following ACL reconstruction are discussed in this chapter.

Biologic Implications of Graft Selection

Perhaps the most important choice to consider when planning an ACL reconstruction is graft choice. A wide variety of tissues are available, including autogenous and allograft tendon. Autogenous choices can be divided into those including a tendon-bone composite, such as a bone-patellar tendon-bone graft, quadriceps tendon graft with a bone block, and all soft-tissue grafts (such as hamstrings and quadriceps tendon). Allograft choices include patellar tendon, Achilles tendon, tibialis anterior, and hamstring tendon grafts. The choice of graft should be based on considerations that are unique to each patient, including age, required activity level, the condition of the joint, and the ability of the patient to participate in a rehabilitation program. Understanding the biology of graft incorporation also helps to guide the decision-making process.

Scheffler et al[6] divided ACL healing into three phases, including an early graft healing phase; a proliferation phase; and a ligamentization phase, which is an ongoing process that can take up to 3 years. The early graft healing phase (0 to 4 weeks) is characterized by creeping necrosis of the graft, which is most markedly present centrally. It is important to note that autografts, unlike allografts, may never become totally necrotic during the incorporation process. The original cells are replaced between 2 to 4 weeks following the graft placement. During the early healing phase, the normal collagen structure and crimp pattern is well maintained. This correlates with no weakening of the graft during this time. Graft failure during this phase of graft healing typically occurs at the bone attachment site and is a function of the strength of fixation.

The proliferation phase lasts between 4 and 12 weeks and is a time of maximal cellular activity.[6] Mesenchymal stem cells have been described at the periphery of the graft, and growth factor release has been reported to peak between weeks 4 and 6 and is complete by 12 weeks following graft implantation. During this phase, there is maximal matrix alteration; consequently, a decrease in mechanical properties (strength) occurs. Because of these changes within the graft, the graft is weakest between 6 and 8 weeks following implantation. The ligamentization phase is an ongoing process during which more normal graft cellularity and vascularity is restored. However, complete matrix maturation may take up to 3 years, and the normal bimodal distribution of large and small diameter collagen fibrils is never completely restored.[6]

Bone-to-bone healing, such as is present with bone-patellar tendon-bone grafts, is complete by 8 weeks, whereas tendon-to-bone healing, such as occurs with hamstring grafts, may require between 8 and 12 weeks.[6] Because the tendons retain their initial biomechanical properties for several months following implantation, early rehabilitation is more a function of fixation strength than graft choice. Histologic and biochemical incorporation is slow and may take up to 2 years before there is complete incorporation of autograft tissue.

In a classic study, Jackson et al[7] described allograft versus autograft healing using a bone-patellar-tendon graft in a goat model. Animals were examined at 6 weeks and 6 months. At 6 months, the autograft group showed less anteroposterior displacement and had ultimate failure loads twice as great as those in the allograft group. In addition, the autograft group showed a larger cross-sectional area and more extensive remodeling. The authors concluded that "a more robust biologic response, improved stability, and increased strength to failure" is present in autograft tissue.[7] Scheffler et al[6] compared healing between allografts and autografts using semitendinosus tendon. The authors reported faster revascularization and remodeling in the autograft group, and the autografts appeared stronger at 1-year follow-up than the allografts.

Human studies examining graft incorporation following ACL reconstruction have consisted of serial MRI and biopsy studies. Muramatsu et al[8] performed serial MRIs on bone-patellar tendon-bone autografts and allografts. A slower onset and rate of revascularization was present in the allograft group. The autograft group had peak revascularization and incorporation activity between 4 to 6 months, whereas the allograft group showed continued remodeling for up to 2 years. Malinin et al[9] performed graft retrievals from patients between 20 days and 10 years following ACL reconstruction with allografts. Central areas of graft acellularity were present up to 2 years, with incomplete bony attachment being observed in this group. The authors concluded that remodeling could take up to 3 years following reconstructions with allografts. Understanding the differences in the rates and degree of healing between the grafts available for reconstructing the ACL allows the surgeon to better counsel patients concerning graft choices and the rehabilitation process following surgery.

Graft Placement and Implications

For most patients, a single-bundle ACL reconstruction can provide excellent knee stability. Studies show that a more oblique single-graft orientation in the sagittal and coronal plane achieved from a central anatomic femoral and tibial location provides rotational stability similar to a double-bundle ACL graft.[10-13] Insufficient experimental and clinical data are available to recommend the more complex double-bundle ACL graft technique over a central anatomic single graft in terms of restoring knee rotational stability.

The details of the recommended surgical technique and supporting experimental and clinical studies are described in detail in the literature[14,15] and in chapter 38. ACL graft placement varies between surgeons and is dependent on the surgical technique selected. For single grafts, an anatomic central ACL placement locates the femoral guide pin just above the midpoint of the proximal-to-distal length of the ACL attachment and 7 to 8 mm from the posterior articular cartilage edge. After the tunnel has been drilled, 3 to 4 mm of the posterior tunnel wall should remain. It is important to determine the graft length to ensure that a mismatch does not occur in terms of tunnel and intra-articular length and graft length.

A technique in which the femoral tunnel is drilled independently of the tibial tunnel provides the most accurate graft placement. Although a transtibial tunnel technique to drill the femoral tunnel is frequently used, this procedure has the potential to result in a more vertical graft orientation. Vertical graft placement must be avoided if this technique is used. It is advised that the femoral tunnel be drilled either through the anteromedial portal or with a two-incision technique. These two drilling options for femoral tunnel placement reliably achieve the desired femoral graft location. In the two-incision technique, the tunnel is drilled in either a retrograde or an antegrade procedure.[14] The tunnel is drilled to the appropriate diameter for a snug graft fit in the tunnel. In the anteromedial portal technique, the knee is placed at 120° flexion to avoid drill penetration into the posterior femoral articular cartilage. An alternative technique places a curved guide pin and flexible retractor through the anteromedial portal, which places the graft tunnel into the desired position, avoiding the hyperflexed knee position (and any associated decreased visualization with hyperflexion).

Reconstruction Using a Bone-Patellar Tendon-Bone Autograft

Graft Selection: Indications and Contraindications

Bone-patellar tendon-bone autogenous graft is indicated for knees with physiologically lax posterolateral structures, for knees with chronic superficial medial collateral ligament (MCL) insufficiency, and for knees requiring a revision ACL reconstruction with a grade 3 pivot-shift test.

A bone-patellar tendon-bone autograft is not recommended in patients with associated patellofemoral disorders and is not used in patients who are unable or unwilling to follow the more involved rehabilitation program or withstand the initial pain related to this graft. In knees with an associated complete rupture of the medial or posterolateral ligament structures that require surgical repair with the ACL reconstruction, a bone-patellar tendon-bone autograft harvest adds morbidity to the procedure and is used only in select athletic knees. Additional contraindications include skeletally immature patients with open growth plates and low performance knees in which a semitendinosus-gracilis graft is preferred.

Surgical Technique

A meticulous surgical technique for ACL reconstruction is necessary, including identifing the appropriate landmarks to achieve correct graft placement in the anatomic femoral and tibial footprint. This chapter's authors have a strong preference for autografts compared with allografts in both primary and revision ACL surgery for many reasons, including increased rates of success and lower failure rates.[3,16-18] Before surgery, the length of the patient's patellar tendon is determined on lateral radiographs. The normal patellar length based on the Linclau technique ranges from 35 to 45 mm.[5] It is important to determine the graft length to ensure that a mismatch does not occur in terms of tunnel and intra-articular length and graft length. The patient is positioned supine on the operating table, all extremities are well padded, and a tourniquet is placed on the middle to proximal thigh. All knee ligament tests are performed after the induction of anesthesia in both limbs. The amount of increased anterior and posterior tibial translation, lateral and medial joint opening, and external tibial rotation are documented. A thorough arthroscopic examination is conducted, noting articular cartilage surface abnormalities and the condition of the menisci. Appropriate débridement and meniscal repair or partial excision are performed as necessary.

Graft Harvest

To harvest the graft, a tourniquet is inflated to 275 mm of pressure. A 3- to

4-cm vertical medial incision is made just adjacent to the medial border of the patellar tendon, avoiding the tibial tubercle. The incision is located just medial to the inferior pole of the patella. A cosmetic approach is used, with the plane beneath the subcutaneous tissues dissected to allow a limited skin incision. The patellar retinaculum is carefully incised and reflected medially and laterally only for the width of the graft that is being removed. The retinaculum is protected to allow closure over the bone-grafted patellar defect. A similar procedure is used at the tibial tuberosity.

The patellar tendon is incised 9 to 10 mm in the midportion. A powered, handheld saw with a thin-width blade is marked with a thin adhesive strip 9 to 10 mm from the tip. A trapezoidal bone-block graft from the patella is removed by angling the saw 15° at each side of the cut. The bone cut extends to the inferior pole, and the insertion site of the patellar tendon is protected. A 4-mm osteotome is used to gently remove the patella bone block without wedging the side walls, which could induce a lateral fracture. A similar procedure is followed in harvesting the tibial bone block. The tourniquet is deflated, and a cotton sponge is placed in the wound.

The bone blocks are prepared in a manner that will allow easy passage through the tunnels. The diameters of the tunnels are configured 1 mm larger than that of the bone blocks. A 2-mm drill hole is placed one third of the distance from the end of each bone block for sutures. The tips of the bone block are fashioned into a bullet-tip configuration for tunnel passage. Two No. 2 nonabsorbable FiberWire (Arthrex, Naples, FL) sutures are passed into the bone blocks. The graft is wrapped in the blood-soaked sponge, which protects the graft, maintains a moist blood environment, and theoretically allows cells to survive in the graft remodeling process.

Placement of the Tibial Tunnel

The center of the ACL is located 16 to 20 mm anterior to the interspinous ridge. The guide pin is placed eccentric and 2 to 3 mm anterior and medial to the true ACL center. This eccentric tunnel will place most of the graft within the central tibial attachment. The tibial tunnel is placed in a coronal manner, at a 55° to 60° angle, allowing a tunnel length of 35 to 40 mm. The tunnel is begun just anterior and adjacent to the superficial MCL. It is usually 25 to 30 mm medial to the tibial tubercle and 10 mm distal to the most proximal point of the patellar tendon tibial tubercle insertion. The tunnel is drilled to the desired graft diameter, and the joint tunnel edges are chamfered to prevent graft abrasion.

Placement of the Femoral Tunnel

The surgeon may drill the femoral tunnel using either a retrograde or antegrade procedure, based on the necessity of adding additional suture after fixation at the femoral site. In the retrograde drilling procedure, a lateral incision 2 to 3 cm in length is made at the posterior third of the iliotibial band. The posterior third of the iliotibial band is incised 4 to 6 cm to allow exposure. The interval posterior to the vastus lateralis is entered, and the muscle is protected. An S retractor is placed beneath the vastus lateralis oblique to gently lift the muscle anteriorly. The proximal edge of the lateral femoral condyle is bluntly palpated with an instrument. The goal is to locate the tunnel entrance just anterior and not distal to this point. A 15-mm periosteal incision is made, and an elevator is used to remove soft tissues from the site for the tunnel proximal entrance.

In most chronic ACL-deficient knees, a notchplasty is required to remove overgrowth of cartilage and spur formation in the femoral notch to prevent ACL graft impingement. An anterior notchplasty of a few millimeters is usually required in acute ACL-injured knees because of the central placement of the tibial tunnel. A lateral notchplasty is performed, when required, if there is insufficient width between the posterior cruciate ligament and lateral femoral notch wall to accommodate the ACL graft.

The ACL femoral attachment is mapped based on the bony landmarks. The guidewire is placed within the central ACL attachment, which is midway between the lateral notch roof and distal articular cartilage edge, 8 mm from the posterior articular cartilage edge. With a central femoral tunnel, the posterior back wall is 3 to 4 mm thick, and the graft occupies approximately two thirds to three fourths of the ACL footprint. Once the center point is selected, the knee is flexed to the desired position. The tunnel is drilled to the appropriate diameter to allow the graft to fit snugly in the tunnel. The edges of the tunnel are chamfered to prevent graft abrasion.

Graft Tunnel Passage: Conditioning and Fixation

The graft is passed in a retrograde manner with a 20-gauge looped wire passed from the femur to the tibial tunnel. The graft is gently lifted up through the tibia and guided into the femoral tunnels with a nerve hook. The graft is marked at the bone-tendon junction to adjust its length in each tunnel and is then brought proximally until the bone is flush with the tibia. In most knees, the femoral portion of the graft is at or just proximal to the inside femoral tunnel. The femoral bone graft plug is fixed with a metallic or an absorbable-type interference screw. Graft conditioning is performed by placing approximately 44 N tension on the distal graft sutures and flexing the knee from 0° to 135° for 30 to 40 flexion-extension cycles. The arthroscope is placed to verify that the graft position is ideal and there is no impingement against the lateral femoral condyle or notch with full hyperextension. The knee is placed at 20° of flexion, and the tension on the graft is reduced to approximately 10 to 15 N to avoid overconstraining the tibial anteroposterior translation. A finger is placed on the anterior tibia to maintain the posterior gravity position of the tibia. An interference screw (usually absorbable) is placed. In cases in which the interference screw fixation is not ideal or the screw resistance on placement is not acceptable, the sutures are tied over a suture post. The arthroscope is placed into the joint, and a final graft inspection is performed. A Lachman test is then performed. There should be 3 mm of anteroposterior translation, indicating that the graft has not been overtightened. If the graft has a "bowstring," tight appearance with little to no anterior tibial translation on testing, the distal tensioning and fixation procedure is repeated with less tension placed on the graft.

Closure

The patellar tendon graft harvest site is loosely approximated with No. 2-0 absorbable sutures. A coring reamer used for the femoral and tibial tunnels is used to provide a large dowel of cancellous bone to completely fill the patellar and tibial defects. The bone-grafted sites are smoothed to remove any pressure points. Two horizontal mattress sutures are placed at the inferior pole of the patella and at the superior tendon attachment at the tibia to create a buttress or pocket to maintain the position of the bone graft at each site. This prevents the bone graft from displacing and becoming a source of future pain. The patella retinaculum is carefully closed to provide soft-tissue coverage over the patella defect. The retinaculum soft tissues are closed using No. 2-0 absorbable horizontal mattress sutures.

Postoperative Care

The first postoperative week represents a critical time period to control knee joint pain and swelling, regain adequate quadriceps muscle contraction, begin immediate knee motion exercises, and maintain limb elevation. Cryotherapy is begun in the recovery room. A bulky compression dressing is used for 48 hours and then converted to compression stockings, with an additional elastic bandage if necessary. Patients are encouraged to stay in bed and elevate the limb above the heart for the first 5 to 7 days, only rising to perform exercises and attend to personal hygiene needs. Prophylaxis against deep venous thrombosis includes one aspirin a day for 10 days, ambulation (with crutch support) six to eight times a day for short periods of time, ankle pumping every hour that the patient is awake, and close observation of the lower limb by the therapist and surgeon. Nonsteroidal anti-inflammatory drugs are administered for at least 5 days postoperatively. Appropriate pain medication is prescribed to provide relief and allow performance of the immediate exercise protocol. Electrogalvanic stimulation or high voltage electrical muscle stimulation is used to augment the ice, compression, and elevation program to control swelling and to facilitate an adequate quadriceps contraction.

Patients should perform passive and active range-of-motion knee exercises in a seated position for 10 minutes per session, approximately four to six times per day. The goal in the first postoperative week is to obtain 0° to 90° of knee motion and then advance to 135° by weeks 5 to 6. Partial weight bearing is permitted immediately postoperatively. Initially, bilateral crutches may be used with 50% of the body weight placed on the involved limb. The amount of weight the patient is allowed to place on the involved limb is progressed as tolerated to allow full weight bearing by the third to fourth postoperative week. Quadriceps isometrics and straight leg raises are initiated the day after surgery.

Reconstruction Using a Hamstring Graft

Graft Selection: Indications and Contraindications

After the decision is made to reconstruct the ACL, all graft types should be routinely discussed with the patient. This chapter's authors typically elect to use a quadrupled hamstring autograft for several reasons. First, it appears autograft tendons have virtually no risks of disease transmission and a lower risk of inflammatory reaction. Hamstring autografts tend to cause less postoperative knee discomfort and have a relatively smaller overall harvest morbidity profile. Because these grafts are biologic grafts, revascularization and stress relaxation can be expected. The quadrupled hamstring graft has a high ultimate tensile load and stiffness that should surpass the native ACL strength despite the typical loss of graft strength after incorporation. It should be noted that in some patients (such as those with generalized ligamentous laxity and some collision athletes), the bone-patellar tendon-bone graft may have advantages over the quadrupled hamstring autograft.

Surgical Technique

After general or regional anesthesia (preferably) has been administered, a

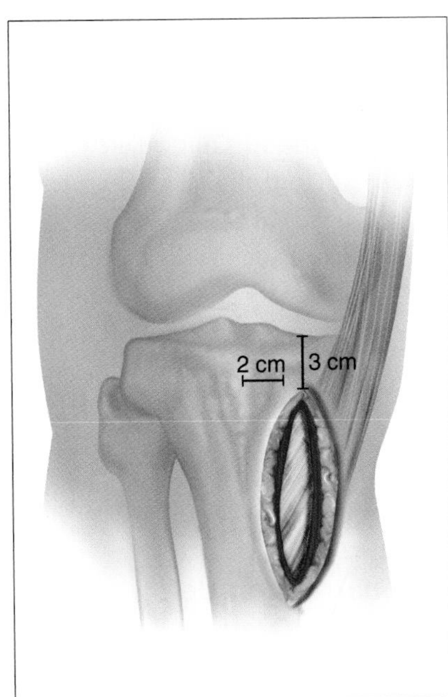

Figure 1 Illustration of the typical hamstring harvest approach with the hamstring insertion and overlying sartorius fascia. (Reproduced with permission from Noyes FR, Barber-Westin SD: Anterior cruciate ligament primary and revision reconstruction, in Noyes FR, ed: *Noyes' Knee Disorders: Surgery, Rehabilitation, Clinical Outcomes.* Philadelphia, PA, WB Saunders, 2009, pp 140-228.)

comprehensive physical examination of the injured extremity is performed to confirm the preoperative diagnosis. Pressure points are then carefully padded, and a nonsterile tourniquet is placed as proximally as possible on the operative extremity, although the tourniquet is not routinely inflated. Pneumatic compression stockings are used on the contralateral extremity. Standard prepping and draping techniques are used, and preoperative antibiotics are administered. When instability is confirmed by preoperative examination, the hamstring tendons are harvested before beginning the arthroscopic portion of the procedure. This allows ample time for an assistant to prepare the graft for use.

Graft Harvest

A 3- to 4-cm vertical incision is made beginning approximately 2 cm medial to the tibial tubercle and 3 cm distal to the joint line with the knee at 90° of flexion. The location of the incision can be modified based on patient size and palpation of the hamstring tendons (**Figure 1**). This incision is bluntly carried through the subcutaneous tissues in an effort to avoid damaging the saphenous nerve or its infrapatellar branch. The distal sartorius aponeurosis is identified, and the gracilis and semitendinosus tendons are located by palpation. A split is made in the overlying sartorius fascia in line with and between these tendons. This chapter's authors routinely use a quadrupled tendon graft, harvesting both the gracilis and semitendinosus tendons. After locating the hamstring insertion, a right angle clamp is used to deliver the gracilis tendon into the split created in the sartorius fascia. Prior to detachment from its tibial insertion, adhesions are carefully removed, and a Linvatec tendon harvester (Conmed Linvatec, Largo, FL) is used to release the tendon proximally from its muscle belly. Once the proximal end is delivered into the wound, the distal insertion is detached, freeing the tendon. A graft of 24 cm is preferable. Detaching the tibial attachment last and dissecting the investing fascia and periosteum off the tibia can afford an additional 1 to 2 cm of graft length if needed. The semitendinosus is then harvested in a similar fashion.

Graft Preparation

Each tendon is prepared by initially removing residual muscle from the aponeurosis using the backside of a No. 10 scalpel blade. The peripheral 20 mm of each tendon is tubularized and whipstitched using No. 2 Orthocord (DePuy Mitek, Raynham, MA). The grafts are doubled through a 15-mm fixed loop Endobutton (Smith & Nephew, Memphis, TN), creating a four-strand hamstring graft. It is then sized using sizing tubes (ACUFEX, Smith & Nephew). The graft is moistened using a damp sponge and kept in a Graft Preparation System (Arthrex, Raynham, MA).

Notchplasty

When performing notchplasty, an anterolateral portal is established, and the joint is insufflated. A medial working portal is established, and routine diagnostic arthroscopy is performed. Any meniscal or chondral work is completed before ACL reconstruction. The remnant ACL is removed from its tibial and femoral attachment using a mechanical shaver. The synovium and fat pad are débrided sufficiently to afford adequate visualization. Iatrogenic posterior cruciate ligament and meniscal injury must be avoided. A minimal superior and lateral notchplasty is performed from the anteromedial portal using a 4.5-mm arthroscopic burr. Only the amount of bone necessary to allow passage of the graft without impingement is removed.

Tunnel Placement

A tibial drill guide is used to fashion the tibial tunnel. The tip of the guide is placed intra-articularly through the anteromedial portal in the anatomic footprint of the native ACL. The base of the guide is rotated medially into the hamstring graft harvest incision and placed along the anterior fibers of the superficial MCL to ensure adequate coronal obliquity of the graft. On average, the guide is set at approximately 60°. A guide pin is placed through the guide under direct arthroscopic visualization. An appropriately sized tunnel is reamed (typically 8 to 9 mm) based on the size of the harvested graft. Placing the femoral tunnel at the intersection between the apex of the femoral condyle and the most posterior aspect of the posterior condylar articular surface is recommended. If the tibial tunnel is appropriately placed, a transtibial femoral tunnel can be used to reach this starting point, thus establishing appropriate coronal obliquity. If it is not possible to reach the starting point transtibially, the femoral tunnel is fashioned though an accessory medial portal. Femoral tunnel preparation is accomplished through the medial portal in 40% of cases and through a transtibial femoral tunnel in 60% of cases. A guide pin is placed, stopped just through the lateral femoral cortex, and measured using the guide pin. The femoral tunnel is reamed (based on size of the harvested graft) within 10 to 12 mm of the lateral wall to facilitate Endobutton deployment.

Graft Placement

To place the graft, a shuttle stitch is passed using the guide pin eyelet, and the Endobutton is shuttled with the graft through the tibial tunnel and out the lateral cortex. The Endobutton is deployed and checked. Aperture fixation is achieved by placing a 7- × 23-mm interference screw (MILAGRO, DePuy Mitek) into the femoral tunnel. Hand tension is applied, and the graft is cycled 10 times to remove graft creep. At 90° of flexion, the graft is tied over a 6.5-mm low-profile screw (Arthrex, Naples, FL) with a washer. An additional 7- × 23-mm interference screw is then placed to achieve aperture fixation (**Figure 2**).

This fixation provides excellent graft stiffness. The graft is examined through a full range of motion to ensure that it is free of impingement. The knee is then thoroughly irrigated to remove residual debris. Arthroscopic portals are closed with locking horizontal mattress stitches. The graft harvest incision is closed with 2-0 Vicryl (Ethicon, Somerville, NJ) for the subcutaneous tissue and a running 3-0 Prolene (Ethicon) subcuticular stitch for the skin. A bulky sterile dressing, hinged knee brace, and polar care are applied.

Reconstruction Using a Central Quadriceps Tendon Without Bone

Graft Selection: Indications and Contraindications

Marshall et al[19] and Blauth[20] originally used central quadriceps tendon with bone for successful ACL reconstructions. This technique proved highly effective because this robust graft has desirable mechanical properties.[21,22] With the advent of improved soft-tissue, tendon graft, and fixation methods for cruciate reconstruction, the central quadriceps as a free tendon graft was first introduced in 1999.[23] In 2005, Joseph et al[24] reported superior short-term recovery and a reduced need for analgesics in patients treated with ACL reconstruction with central quadriceps tendon without bone compared with comparable patient groups treated with bone-patellar tendon-bone autograft and hamstring autograft. DeAngelis and Fulkerson[25] and Geib et al[26] subsequently reported very favorable clinical results in using quadriceps tendon without bone for ACL reconstruction.

The central quadriceps tendon without bone graft yields stability results similar to those of bone-patellar tendon-bone, hamstring, and allograft ACL reconstructions, while avoiding some of the complications ascribed to the other graft types, such as difficulty kneeling (bone-patellar tendon-bone), patella fracture[27] (bone-patellar tendon-bone), patellofemoral pain,[28] loss of medial and posterior support of the knee (hamstrings), high cost, and the unknown effects of prions and other donor factors in allograft reconstructions. With a mean follow-up of 67 months (2-year minimum follow-up), DeAngelis and Fulkerson[25] reported that no patient had anterior knee pain as a result of central quadriceps free tendon ACL reconstruction. Geib et al[26] reported similar findings, with quadriceps tendon autograft showing significantly less morbidity than bone-patellar tendon-bone reconstructions. Single-leg hop testing was comparable (0.96) to the contralateral side at an average follow-up of 67 months, and two patients were able

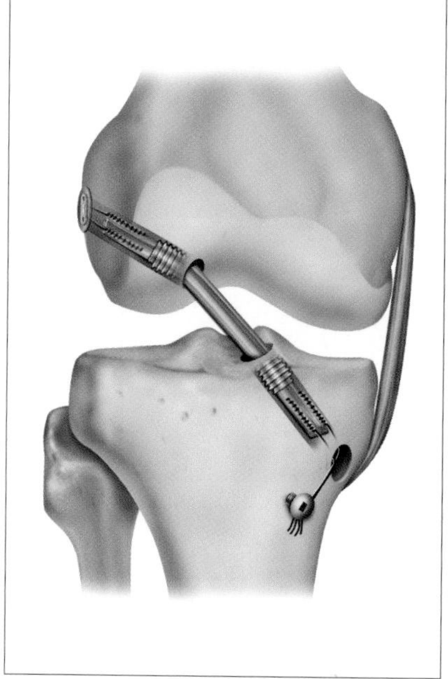

Figure 2 Illustration of the quadrupled hamstring construct using both aperture and backup fixation. Note that the tibial tunnel start point is just anterior to the MCL fibers, and the coronal obliquity of the femoral tunnel is critical. The femoral position, in this illustration, is meant to show the fixation technique, not placement. Refer to the section on anatomic graft placement for specific details on placement. (Reproduced with permission from Noyes FR, Barber-Westin SD: Anterior cruciate ligament primary and revision reconstruction, in Noyes FR, ed: *Noyes' Knee Disorders: Surgery, Rehabilitation, Clinical Outcomes.* Philadelphia, PA, WB Saunders, 2009, pp 140-228.)

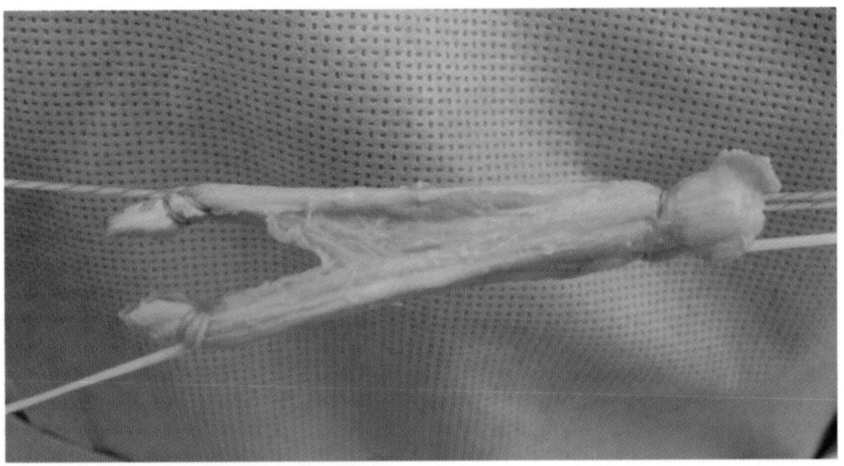

Figure 3 Photograph of a double-bundle construct fashioned by whipstitching the intermedius and rectus tendons separately. Quadriceps tendon may be placed for either single- or double-bundle reconstruction as desired.

to return to participation in Division 1 athletics (lacrosse and gymnastics).[25]

Based on the published studies to date, central quadriceps tendon without bone appears to be a very desirable autograft alternative for short-term rehabilitation, the reduction of short-term pain, and the probability of long-term success without pain following ACL reconstruction.

Graft Harvest

The quadriceps tendon graft without bone is harvested through a 1.5- to 2-inch incision starting at the proximal pole of the patella centrally and extending proximally. The entire anterior quadriceps tendon is exposed and examined. The autograft is harvested just medial to the most central aspect of the central quadriceps tendon because the tendon is thickest medially. The quadriceps tendon is 9 to 10 mm thick on average[29] compared with the patellar tendon, which averages 4.8 mm thick. Thus, a partial thickness quadriceps tendon graft can be harvested, leaving the posterior fibers of the intermedius intact so that the suprapatellar pouch is not entered. Two parallel longitudinal incisions are made in the quadriceps tendon approximately 10 mm apart using a No. 10 scalpel blade (with an approximate 7.5-mm width). The No. 10 scalpel blade may be buried in the tendon to provide a 7-mm depth of cut, leaving the posterior 2 mm of the quadriceps tendon intact. Suprapatellar incisions are extended proximally 8 to 9 cm from the proximal pole of the patella. A hemostat is used to spread the tendon graft at a 7-mm depth in the coronal plane to separate the anterior 7 mm of the central quadriceps tendon from the remaining 2 mm posteriorly. With experience, the graft may be routinely harvested without entering the joint. Once the graft is mobilized, it is released sharply with a No. 15 scalpel blade from the proximal pole of the patella and the distal end of the graft and grasped with a uterine T clamp. At this point, whipstitches[30] are placed in the distal quadriceps tendon graft with Orthocord, Durabraid (Smith & Nephew), FiberWire, No. 5 Ethibond (Ethicon), or similar strength nonabsorbable suture material. The graft is mobilized by blunt dissection, taking care to avoid entry into the suprapatellar pouch and keeping all fibers of the graft intact. The graft is then released proximally and sharply to yield a 7- to 8-cm long free tendon graft. The quadriceps tendon is stronger at load to failure after harvesting than the patellar tendon is before graft harvesting.[31] A minimum length of 7 cm is desirable.

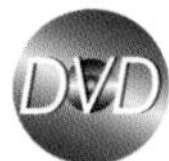

Video 37.1: ACL Reconstruction Using Quadriceps Free Tendon Autograft: Graft Harvest. John P. Fulkerson, MD (6 min)

Surgical Technique

To begin the ACL reconstruction, the residual fragments of the original ACL are resected, notchplasty is performed, and hemostasis is achieved using cautery. Because there are two distinct tendon components (rectus and intermedius) to the central quadriceps tendon, a double-bundle construct can be easily fashioned by whipstitching the intermedius and rectus tendons separately. The quadriceps tendon may be placed for either single- or double-bundle reconstruction as desired (**Figure 3**). After the whipstitches are placed, Endobuttons are tied through the central holes on the Endobutton to the exact length desired to allow a minimum of 2 cm of quadriceps tendon in each socket (**Figure 4**). The Endobutton may then be deployed into one or two femoral sockets as desired for single- or double-bundle reconstruction as the graft is drawn through the tibial tunnel by lead sutures. On the tibial side, one of this chapter's authors (JPF) prefers an absorbable interference screw, one size larger than the tunnel and recessed back from the intra-articular tunnel entry site by 5 to 8 mm. This fixation has been proven to be secure in laboratory testing by Nagarkatti et al.[32]

After the reconstruction has been tensioned appropriately and fixed se-

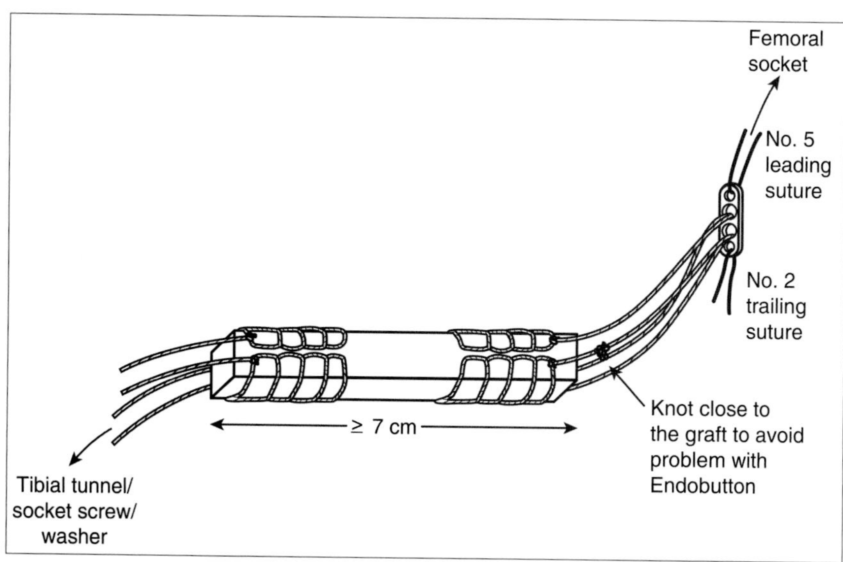

Figure 4 After the whipstitches are placed in quadriceps tendon ACL reconstruction, Endobuttons are tied through the central holes on the Endobutton to the exact length desired to allow a minimum of 2 cm of quadriceps tendon in each socket.

curely, the tourniquet is released, hemostasis is achieved, and the wounds are closed after irrigating. The defect in the central quadriceps tendon is left open so that it may reconstitute. In 15 years of experience using quadriceps tendon autograft, two of this chapter's authors (JPF and MTG) have never seen a quadriceps tendon rupture or a significant complication related to the graft harvest site.

Postoperative Care

In the postoperative period, the patient uses crutches with a knee immobilizer, is encouraged to bear partial weight, and is advised to remove the splint for motion several times a day. After 10 to 12 days, the immobilizer is discontinued, and the patient can participate in physical therapy for closed chain rehabilitation, full motion, and progressive weight bearing. Continuous passive motion and immediate physical therapy are not necessary, so patients can achieve some healing and comfort before entering formal rehabilitation. At the time of the first postoperative office visit, usually 10 to 12 days after surgery, many patients no longer need analgesics, have good quadriceps contraction, and often have achieved 90° flexion and full extension on their own. Most patients no longer need crutches by 3 weeks after surgery.

Primary Reconstruction Using an Allograft

Graft Selection: Indications and Contraindications

ACL reconstruction with allograft tissue is an attractive alternative when autograft reconstruction is not possible or otherwise contraindicated. Ideally, the graft chosen for the ACL reconstruction will have appropriate biomechanical properties and low morbidity, will incorporate quickly, will function well, and will meet the goals and needs of the patient and the surgeon.[33] Several randomized trials and systematic reviews have failed to show significant clinical differences when comparing allograft tissue to autograft tissue if irradiated and chemically processed grafts are excluded.[10-12,34] Many retrospective reviews have shown excellent clinical outcomes for allograft ACL reconstruction.[13,35-37] However, basic science and animal studies have shown longer graft incorporation times and delayed tendon remodeling when using allograft tissue.[8,38-41] In addition, several nonrandomized retrospective studies have shown higher than expected failure rates when using allogeneic tissue in patients with high levels of activity.[42,43]

Determining the proper graft for ACL reconstruction is a multifactorial issue and must take into account patient- and surgeon-specific factors. A recent survey indicated that the main factor influencing graft choice was the surgeon's recommendation.[44] That same report showed that most ACL reconstructions examined in that survey were performed with allograft tissue.[44] The potential advantages and disadvantages of allograft tissue must be considered in the decision-making process.

Although some surgeons routinely use allograft tissue for all reconstructions,[45] others use allograft only in select situations, such as older patients. The use of allograft tissue is indicated in less active patients, those with preexisting patellofemoral pathology, and in multiligament reconstructions. The basic tenet of any ACL reconstruction should be to replicate the form and function of the native ACL while minimizing potential adverse side effects. A biomechanically sufficient graft that is rigidly fixed in appropriately positioned tibial and femoral tunnels will generally result in a stable knee if the graft incorporates and complications are avoided.

Although allograft tissue has sufficient time zero strength, healing of the graft in the tunnel and ligamentization of the graft is delayed with allogeneic tissue.[33] This delay potentially places the patient at risk for recurrent instability and injury on return to participation in sports activities. Despite this information, clinical outcomes have not been shown to be worse for allografts. Allograft tissue also minimizes potential complications associated with autograft harvest, decreases the pain associated with surgery, and allows improved cosmesis because of smaller incisions. Although the patient typically experiences a more rapid early recovery, delayed healing and remodeling results in an effectively longer recovery period.

When counseling patients regarding graft selection, the surgeon's typical choice of autograft will often dictate which allograft will be offered to the patient. For example, if a surgeon typically uses a bone-patellar tendon-bone autograft, reconstruction with a bone-patellar tendon-bone allograft allows the surgeon to use the same instrumentation and technique. This also applies to soft-tissue grafts (hamstring as a primary graft and hamstring or tibialis tendon allograft). Achilles tendon allograft requires a hybrid technique with bone-to-bone fixation on one side and soft-tissue fixation on the other.

Regardless of the allograft chosen, proper preoperative patient counseling requires discussion of disease transmission risks. Allografts are very safe graft options if the tissue bank follows established guidelines for graft harvest and preparation. Although a full discussion of these guidelines is beyond the scope of this chapter, the patient should be counseled about the theoretic risk of disease transmission. Some sources have stated the risk of transmission of HIV and hepatitis to be approximately 1 in 1.6 million; however, the accuracy of this number is not known.[46] The American Association of Tissue Banks and the Food and Drug Administration have set standards for graft procurement and harvest; however, disease transmission has occurred. Gamma irradiation as an adjunct to terminally sterilize the graft has been proposed. A dose of 3 megarads is required to eliminate viral vectors,[47] but this dose of irradiation negatively impacts the biomechanical properties of the graft.[48] Therefore, using grafts irradiated to this level is not recommended.[49] Different tissue banks have a variety of proprietary methods to reduce the possibility of disease transmission while maintaining biomechanical properties. Awareness of the safety record of the tissue bank being used, its compliance with standards established by the American Association of Tissue Banks and the Food and Drug Administration, and understanding proper methods of graft preparation are essential for a surgeon treating patients with allograft tissue ACL reconstructions.

Surgical Technique

With soft-tissue or bone-patellar tendon-bone allograft reconstruction, a standard technique is usually possible. A problem often encountered with bone-patellar tendon-bone grafts and the single-incision endoscopic technique is graft-construct mismatch. A very long allograft used in a shorter patient can make distal fixation challenging. There are several options to address this problem. Recessing the femoral bone plug can shorten the graft, but the possibility of the screw wrapping the tendinous graft and lacerating it is a distinct possibility. After fixing the femoral side, rotating the graft up to 540° can shorten the graft by 5 to 6 mm.[50] If a more significant mismatch is noted, the distal bone plug can be sharply resected and fixed via a free bone-block technique.[51] This is a challenging procedure once the femoral side is fully fixed, but it does allow standard interference fixation.

Another excellent option for reconstruction is the two-incision technique. As the graft is fixed at the lateral femoral cortex proximally, the risk of graft laceration is quite low even if the graft is fully recessed into the tunnel. Just as important is the fact that the femoral tunnel is completely independent of the tibial tunnel, allowing anatomic tunnel placement, avoiding vertical and anteriorly placed femoral tunnels. Although some surgeons routinely use an anteromedial portal technique for femoral tunnel placement, the shorter tunnel created with this technique is not typically helpful if there is significant graft-construct mismatch. In the two-incision technique, placement of the femoral tunnel is guided via a rear-entry guide or via a guide placed in the lateral or central portal. Once the graft is placed, it can be recessed to any level to allow interference fixation on the femoral and tibial sides.

Postoperative Care

Postoperatively, after ACL allograft reconstruction, patients are routinely evaluated for therapy within 24 to 48 hours. The surgeon can assess the need for aspiration and change dressings at this evaluation. A large hemarthrosis can be aspirated to improve quadriceps control, decrease pain, and allow easier range of motion. Although many patients treated with allografts experience less pain initially than those treated with autografts, the surgeon and therapists must emphasize that full graft maturation takes longer with an allograft than with an autograft. For this reason, delaying full return to cutting and pivoting sporting activities for at least 6 months should be considered, provided that appropriate range of motion, strength, and stability has been achieved at that time.

Allograft reconstruction of the ACL has shown excellent clinical results and has a strong track record. Appropriate patient counseling, graft selection, surgical technique, and proper rehabilitation should allow return to work and participation in sport activities with a minimal risk of adverse events.

Summary

ACL reconstruction is a technically complicated procedure. Restoration of stability is dependent on surgical variables, including graft choice, tunnel placement, and secure graft fixation. The principles of proper graft placement must be understood and properly applied by the treating surgeon. Although the transtibial technique is appealing because of the ease and speed of the procedure, it is important to recognize that there will be times that an appropriately placed femoral tunnel cannot be obtained with this technique. Placing the tibial portal more posteriorly than intended to drill the femoral tunnel should be avoided. For this reason, the surgeon should be familiar with alternative methods of femoral placement, such as using a separate lateral incision or an anteromedial drilling portal. The choice of graft and the strength of the initial fixation influence the pace of rehabilitation and impact the timing and intensity of functional activities postoperatively. Autogenous tissue heals faster and more completely than allograft tissue and may be a better choice for patients attempting to return to more strenuous sports; however, the presence of associated conditions, such as a multiligament knee injury, prior surgery, and articular cartilage injury, are frequently best treated using allografts. Allografts are also frequently used in patients in whom less postoperative pain and a faster return to daily activity is a priority. Because healing following the use of an all soft-tissue autogenous graft may lag several weeks behind that of a bone-patellar tendon-bone autograft, this should be considered during the early rehabilitation of these patients. For surgeons performing fewer than 10 ACL reconstructions each year, it is advisable to take surgical skills courses available through organizations such as the American Academy of Orthopaedic Surgeons or other specialty societies and to use techniques with which they are most comfortable.

Acknowledgment

The authors wish to acknowledge Cassie Fleckenstein, MS, for her assistance in preparing this manuscript.

References

1. Gottlob CA, Baker CL Jr, Pellissier JM, Colvin L: Cost effectiveness of anterior cruciate ligament reconstruction in young adults. *Clin Orthop Relat Res* 1999;367: 272-282.
2. Spindler KP, Wright RW: Clinical practice: Anterior cruciate ligament tear. *N Engl J Med* 2008; 359(20):2135-2142.
3. Noyes FR, Barber-Westin SD: A comparison of results in acute and chronic anterior cruciate ligament ruptures of arthroscopically assisted autogenous patellar tendon reconstruction. *Am J Sports Med* 1997;25(4):460-471.
4. Manley M, Ong K, Lau E, Kurtz SM: Effect of volume on total hip arthroplasty revision rates in the United States Medicare population. *J Bone Joint Surg Am* 2008;90(11):2446-2451.
5. Garrett WE Jr, Swiontkowski MF, Weinstein JN, et al: American Board of Orthopaedic Surgery Practice of the Orthopaedic Surgeon: Part-II. Certification examination case mix. *J Bone Joint Surg Am* 2006;88(3):660-667.
6. Scheffler SU, Unterhauser FN, Weiler A: Graft remodeling and ligamentization after cruciate ligament reconstruction. *Knee Surg Sports Traumatol Arthrosc* 2008; 16(9):834-842.
7. Jackson DW, Grood ES, Wilcox P, Butler DL, Simon TM, Holden JP: The effects of processing techniques on the mechanical properties of bone-anterior cruciate ligament-bone allografts: An experimental study in goats. *Am J Sports Med* 1988;16(2):101-105.
8. Muramatsu K, Hachiya Y, Izawa H: Serial evaluation of human anterior cruciate ligament grafts by contrast-enhanced magnetic resonance imaging: Comparison of allografts and autografts. *Arthroscopy* 2008;24(9):1038-1044.
9. Malinin TI, Levitt RL, Bashore C, Temple HT, Mnaymneh W: A study of retrieved allografts used to replace anterior cruciate ligaments. *Arthroscopy* 2002;18(2): 163-170.
10. Edgar CM, Zimmer S, Kakar S, Jones H, Schepsis AA: Prospective comparison of auto and allograft hamstring tendon constructs for ACL reconstruction. *Clin Orthop Relat Res* 2008;466(9):2238-2246.
11. Sun K, Tian SQ, Zhang JH, Xia CS, Zhang CL, Yu TB: ACL reconstruction with BPTB autograft and irradiated fresh frozen allograft. *J Zhejiang Univ Sci B* 2009;10(4):306-316.
12. Sun K, Tian SQ, Zhang JH, Xia CS, Zhang CL, Yu TB: Anterior cruciate ligament reconstruction with bone-patellar tendon-bone autograft versus allograft. *Arthroscopy* 2009;25(7):750-759.
13. Poehling GG, Curl WW, Lee CA, et al: Analysis of outcomes of anterior cruciate ligament repair with 5-year follow-up: Allograft versus autograft. *Arthroscopy* 2005; 21(7):774-785.
14. Noyes FR, Barber-Westin SD: Anterior cruciate ligament primary and revision reconstruction: Diagnosis, operative techniques, and clinical outcomes, in Noyes FR, ed: *Noyes Knee Disorders: Surgery, Rehabilitation, Clinical Outcomes.* Philadelphia, PA, Saunders, 2009, pp 140-228.

15. Noyes FR: The function of the human anterior cruciate ligament and analysis of single- and double-bundle graft reconstructions. *Sports Health: A Multidisciplinary Approach* 2009:1:66-75.

16. Noyes FR, Barber-Westin SD, Roberts CS: Use of allografts after failed treatment of rupture of the anterior cruciate ligament. *J Bone Joint Surg Am* 1994;76(7):1019-1031.

17. Noyes FR, Barber-Westin SD: Revision anterior cruciate surgery with use of bone-patellar tendon-bone autogenous grafts. *J Bone Joint Surg Am* 2001;83-A(8):1131-1143.

18. Noyes FR, Barber-Westin SD: Anterior cruciate ligament revision reconstruction: Results using a quadriceps tendon-patellar bone autograft. *Am J Sports Med* 2006;34(4):553-564.

19. Marshall JL, Warren RF, Wickiewicz TL, Reider B: The anterior cruciate ligament: A technique of repair and reconstruction. *Clin Orthop Relat Res* 1979;143:97-106.

20. Blauth W: 2-strip substitution-plasty of the anterior cruciate ligament with the quadriceps tendon. *Unfallheilkunde* 1984;87(2):45-5.

21. Stäubli HU, Schatzmann L, Brunner P, Rincón L, Nolte LP: Quadriceps tendon and patellar ligament: Cryosectional anatomy and structural properties in young adults. *Knee Surg Sports Traumatol Arthrosc* 1996;4(2):100-110.

22. Stäubli HU, Schatzmann L, Brunner P, Rincón L, Nolte LP: Mechanical tensile properties of the quadriceps tendon and patellar ligament in young adults. *Am J Sports Med* 1999;27(1):27-34.

23. Fulkerson J: Central quadriceps free tendon for anterior cruciate ligament reconstruction. *Oper Tech Sports Med* 1999;7(4):195-200.

24. Joseph M, Fulkerson J, Nissen C, Sheehan TJ, Fulkerson J: Short-term recovery after anterior cruciate ligament reconstruction: A prospective comparison of three autografts. *Orthopedics* 2006;29(3):243-248.

25. DeAngelis JP, Fulkerson JP: Quadriceps tendon: A reliable alternative for reconstruction of the anterior cruciate ligament. *Clin Sports Med* 2007;26(4):587-596.

26. Geib TM, Shelton WR, Phelps RA, Clark L: Anterior cruciate ligament reconstruction using quadriceps tendon autograft: Intermediate-term results. *Arthroscopy* 2009;25(12):1408-1414.

27. Viola R, Vianello R: Three cases of patella fracture in 1,320 anterior cruciate ligament reconstructions with bone-patellar tendon-bone autograft. *Arthroscopy* 1999;15(1):93-97.

28. Sachs RA, Daniel DM, Stone ML, Garfein RF: Patellofemoral problems after anterior cruciate ligament reconstruction. *Am J Sports Med* 1989;17(6):760-765.

29. Fulkerson JP, Langeland R: An alternative cruciate reconstruction graft: The central quadriceps tendon. *Arthroscopy* 1995;11(2):252-254.

30. McKeon BP, Heming JF, Fulkerson J, Langeland R: The Krackow stitch: A biomechanical evaluation of changing the number of loops versus the number of sutures. *Arthroscopy* 2006;22(1):33-37.

31. Adams DJ, Mazzocca AD, Fulkerson JP: Residual strength of the quadriceps versus patellar tendon after harvesting a central free tendon graft. *Arthroscopy* 2006;22(1):76-79.

32. Nagarkatti DG, McKeon BP, Donahue BS, Fulkerson JP: Mechanical evaluation of a soft tissue interference screw in free tendon anterior cruciate ligament graft fixation. *Am J Sports Med* 2001;29(1):67-71.

33. Baer GS, Harner CD: Clinical outcomes of allograft versus autograft in anterior cruciate ligament reconstruction. *Clin Sports Med* 2007;26(4):661-681.

34. Krych AJ, Jackson JD, Hoskin TL, Dahm DL: A meta-analysis of patellar tendon autograft versus patellar tendon allograft in anterior cruciate ligament reconstruction. *Arthroscopy* 2008;24(3):292-298.

35. Indelli PF, Dillingham MF, Fanton GS, Schurman DJ: Anterior cruciate ligament reconstruction using cryopreserved allografts. *Clin Orthop Relat Res* 2004;420:268-275.

36. Bach BR Jr, Aadalen KJ, Dennis MG, et al: Primary anterior cruciate ligament reconstruction using fresh-frozen, nonirradiated patellar tendon allograft: Minimum 2-year follow-up. *Am J Sports Med* 2005;33(2):284-292.

37. Kuechle DK, Pearson SE, Beach WR, et al: Allograft anterior cruciate ligament reconstruction in patients over 40 years of age. *Arthroscopy* 2002;18(8):845-853.

38. Peterson RK, Shelton WR, Bomboy AL: Allograft versus autograft patellar tendon anterior cruciate ligament reconstruction: A 5-year follow-up. *Arthroscopy* 2001;17(1): 9-13.

39. Lomasney LM, Tonino PM, Coan MR: Evaluation of bone incorporation of patellar tendon autografts and allografts for ACL reconstruction using CT. *Orthopedics* 2007;30(2):152-157.

40. Lee CA, Meyer JV, Shilt JS, Poehling GG: Allograft maturation in anterior cruciate ligament reconstruction. *Arthroscopy* 2004;20(Suppl 2):46-49.

41. Scheffler SU, Schmidt T, Gangéy I, Dustmann M, Unterhauser F, Weiler A: Fresh-frozen free-

tendon allografts versus autografts in anterior cruciate ligament reconstruction: Delayed remodeling and inferior mechanical function during long-term healing in sheep. *Arthroscopy* 2008;24(4): 448-458.

42. Borchers JR, Pedroza A, Kaeding C: Activity level and graft type as risk factors for anterior cruciate ligament graft failure: A case-control study. *Am J Sports Med* 2009;37(12):2362-2367.

43. Singhal MC, Gardiner JR, Johnson DL: Failure of primary anterior cruciate ligament surgery using anterior tibialis allograft. *Arthroscopy* 2007;23(5):469-475.

44. Cohen SB, Yucha DT, Ciccotti MC, Goldstein DT, Ciccotti MA, Ciccotti MG: Factors affecting patient selection of graft type in anterior cruciate ligament reconstruction. *Arthroscopy* 2009; 25(9):1006-1010.

45. Clark JC, Rueff DE, Indelicato PA, Moser M: Primary ACL reconstruction using allograft tissue. *Clin Sports Med* 2009;28(2): 223-244.

46. Cohen SB, Sekiya JK: Allograft safety in anterior cruciate ligament reconstruction. *Clin Sports Med* 2007;26(4):597-605.

47. Fideler BM, Vangsness CT Jr, Moore T, Li Z, Rasheed S: Effects of gamma irradiation on the human immunodeficiency virus: A study in frozen human bone-patellar ligament-bone grafts obtained from infected cadavera. *J Bone Joint Surg Am* 1994;76(7): 1032-1035.

48. Gibbons MJ, Butler DL, Grood ES, Bylski-Austrow DI, Levy MS, Noyes FR: Effects of gamma irradiation on the initial mechanical and material properties of goat bone-patellar tendon-bone allografts. *J Orthop Res* 1991; 9(2):209-218.

49. Schwartz HE, Matava MJ, Proch FS, et al: The effect of gamma irradiation on anterior cruciate ligament allograft biomechanical and biochemical properties in the caprine model at time zero and at 6 months after surgery. *Am J Sports Med* 2006; 34(11):1747-1755.

50. Verma N, Noerdlinger MA, Hallab N, Bush-Joseph CA, Bach BR Jr : Effects of graft rotation on initial biomechanical failure characteristics of bone-patellar tendon-bone constructs. *Am J Sports Med* 2003;31(5):708-713.

51. Novak PJ, Wexler GM, Williams JS Jr , Bach BR Jr , Bush-Joseph CA: Comparison of screw post fixation and free bone block interference fixation for anterior cruciate ligament soft tissue grafts: Biomechanical considerations. *Arthroscopy* 1996;12(4):470-473.

Video Reference

37.1: Fulkerson JP: Video. Excerpt. ACL reconstruction using quadriceps free tendon autograft, in Fu FH, Howell SM, eds; *Masters Experience: Arthroscopic Surgical Techniques: Anterior Cruciate Ligament Reconstruction.* DVD. Rosemont, IL, Arthroscopy Association of North America and American Academy of Orthopaedic Surgeons, 2010.

Anterior Cruciate Ligament Graft Placement Recommendations and Bone-Patellar Tendon-Bone Graft Indications to Restore Knee Stability

Frank R. Noyes, MD
Sue D. Barber-Westin, BS

Abstract

The anterior cruciate ligament (ACL) resists the combined abnormal motions of anterior tibial translation and internal tibial rotation that occur in the pivot-shift phenomenon. The placement of a single ACL graft high and proximal at the femoral attachment and posterior at the tibial attachment results in a vertical graft orientation. This graft position has a limited ability to provide rotational stability. A more oblique ACL graft orientation in the sagittal and coronal planes achieved from a central anatomic femoral and tibial location provides an orientation that is better in resisting the pivot-shift phenomenon. Tibial and femoral tunnels are drilled independently; transtibial drilling of the femoral tunnel is not recommended. The meticulous surgical technique for ACL reconstruction includes identifying the appropriate landmarks to achieve correct graft placement. There are insufficient experimental and clinical data to recommend the more complex double-bundle ACL graft technique over a central anatomic single graft in terms of restoring knee rotational stability. Allografts are used only in select knees for which autograft tissue is not available. The postoperative rehabilitation program takes into account the condition of the menisci and articular cartilage and associated reconstructive procedures.

Instr Course Lect 2011;60:499-521.

Given the number of anterior cruciate ligament (ACL) reconstructions performed yearly (approximately 200,000), the average published failure rates of 5% to 10% potentially result in as many as 20,000 patients who may require ACL revision surgery with its well-known complications. Many factors can contribute to the outcome of ACL surgery, including making the correct diagnosis and treating all associated ligament structures and meniscus tears; selecting an appropriate preoperative rehabilitation protocol; technical issues related to surgery, graft selection, placement, and tensioning; biologic factors that affect graft healing and remodeling; and appropriate postoperative rehabilitation to achieve the return of muscle function, joint motion, and neuromuscular function.[1-13]

The surgical technique for ideally placing an ACL graft to resist abnormal anterior tibial translation and internal tibial rotation and the resultant anterior tibial subluxation in the pivot-shift phenomenon are discussed in this chapter. Indications and contraindications of the bone-patellar tendon-bone (BPTB) autograft are presented. Post-

Dr. Noyes or an immediate family member serves as a board member, owner, officer, or committee member of the Cincinnati Sports Medicine Research and Education Foundation Board of Directors; has received royalties from Smith & Nephew; has received research or institutional support from Arthrex, DePuy, DJ Orthopaedics, Genzyme, Mitek, Regeneration Technologies, Stryker, and AlloSource; and has received nonincome support (such as equipment or services), commercially derived honoraria, or other non–research-related funding (such as paid travel) from Saunders/Mosby-Elsevier. Neither Ms. Barber-Westin nor any immediate family member has received anything of value from or owns stock in a commercial company or institution related directly or indirectly to the subject of this chapter.

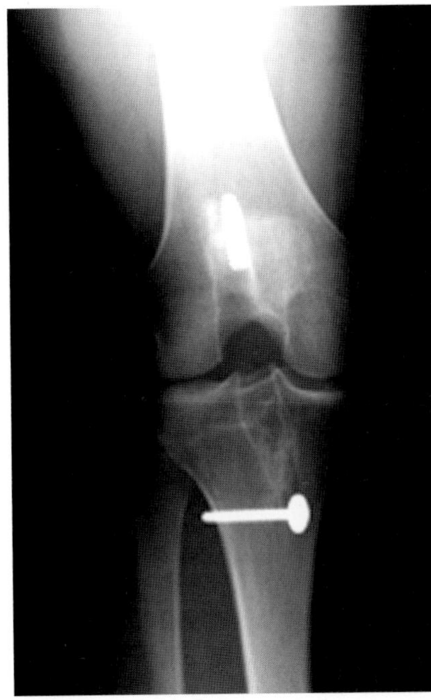

Figure 1 AP radiograph of a vertical coronal ACL graft orientation with most of the graft placed on the intercondylar roof outside the native ACL femoral attachment. Transtibial drilling of the femoral tunnel is the usual cause of a vertical graft. (Reproduced with permission from Noyes FR, Barber-Westin SD: ACL primary and revision reconstruction: Diagnosis, operative techniques, clinical outcomes, in Noyes FR, Barber-Westin SD, eds: *Noyes' Knee Disorders: Surgery, Rehabilitation, Clinical Outcomes.* Philadelphia, PA, WB Saunders, 2009, pp 140-228.)

Table 1
Indications for Bone-Patellar Tendon-Bone Autograft ACL Reconstruction

Competitive athlete
Physiologically lax posterolateral structures
Residual superficial medial collateral ligament insufficiency, increased medial tibiofemoral joint opening
ACL revision
Grade 3 pivot shift, gross anterior tibial subluxation (> 10 mm) indicating loss of secondary mediolateral restraints

operative rehabilitation programs are outlined according to the desired postoperative activity level and associated procedures. A summary of the previously published investigations is provided.[4,14,15]

One of the most common causes of a failed ACL reconstruction, regardless of the graft choice, is placing the graft in a tibial and femoral location that is vertical in a coronal or sagittal plane (or both) with limited ability to resist the pivot-shift phenomenon.[2,3,11,16] A vertical ACL graft orientation occurs when a graft is placed in a high proximal femoral attachment position and posterior tibial attachment location (**Figure 1**). The graft may be malpositioned and placed close to or on the femoral notch roof, outside the normal ACL femoral attachment, particularly when a transtibial drilling technique is used. A graft in this orientation may resist anterior tibial translation; however, abnormal midrange internal rotation still occurs with the symptomatic pivot-shift phenomenon experienced by the patient.[13,17,18]

The complications related to vertical ACL graft placement appear to have developed with the change in technique from a two-incision to a single-incision procedure using transtibial drilling of the femoral tunnel.[19] In the classic two-incision technique, the rear entry drill guide inserted through a limited lateral thigh incision placed the ACL graft femoral tunnel on the lateral femoral wall within the ACL attachment.[2,3,13,16,20,21] The tibial and femoral tunnels were placed in an independent manner and were not linked, parallel, or drilled together. Clinical studies of the two-incision ACL technique reported low failure rates.[7,20,22-24] ACL techniques that placed the ACL graft into the posterior tibial attachment became popular based on the belief that this portion of the native ligament could better resist the pivot-shift phenomenon; this belief has now been disproved.

Recently, authors have recommended a double-bundle ACL reconstruction to reduce the rate of failure (return of positive pivot shift).[25-29] There is disagreement among investigators regarding the advantages of this technique. This chapter's authors believe that a well-placed, central, anatomic, single graft restores knee stability and that the added complexity of a double-bundle ACL technique is not necessary. The rationale for anatomically placing a single ACL graft is summarized from recently published works of this chapter's authors.[4,14] Other studies have presented similar concepts.[30-34]

BPTB Autograft

There remains no standard graft choice for ACL reconstruction. Autograft tissue sources include BPTB, quadriceps tendon–patellar bone, and semitendinosus-gracilis tendons. This chapter's authors prefer using BPTB autogenous grafts in athletes (**Table 1**). This recommendation is supported by several long-term studies and by recent studies showing a higher rate of ACL primary reconstruction failure following treatment with allograft compared with autografts, especially in younger patients[35-40] (CC Kaeding et al, and KT Luber et al, Orlando, FL, unpublished data presented at the American Orthopaedic Society of Sports Medicine annual meeting, 2008). BPTB autograft is not recommended in patients with associated patellofemoral disorders (**Table 2**), those who are unable or unwilling to follow the more involved rehabilitation program, or patients who are unable to tolerate the initial pain related to BPTB grafting. In recreational athletes and more sedentary patients, a four-strand semitendinosus-gracilis autograft is recommended. Newer fixation methods have increased the success rate of this construct, and postoperative rehabilitation is less demanding for the patient. Allografts are reserved for multiligament reconstructions or patients who refuse to allow autograft harvest.[41] A BPTB allograft or an Achilles tendon-bone allograft is preferred over a posterior or anterior tibialis allograft.[42] At least one portion of the graft should have a bone plug for an increased rate of graft healing. All allografts must undergo secondary chemical sterilization; irradiation sterilization should be avoided.

Table 2
Contraindications for Bone-Patellar Tendon-Bone Autograft ACL Reconstruction

Patellofemoral disorders
Medial patellofemoral ligament deficiency, lateral patellar subluxation
Patellofemoral cartilage damage, symptomatic
Quadriceps atrophy
Prior surgery, difficulty regaining knee motion
Patellar tendon narrow, patella infera
Osgood-Schlatter disease
Multiligament reconstruction/dislocation
Lack of an experienced rehabilitation team
Lack of patient compliance, difficulty with rehabilitation
Low performance knee: semitendinosus gracilis graft would be effective
Open growth plates

In revision knee surgery, if the ipsilateral patellar tendon was previously harvested, the contralateral patellar tendon is a valid graft source. Reharvesting the patellar tendon is not recommended because of persistent MRI changes and graft morphology reported 7 to 10 years postoperatively.[43-47] A second option is a quadriceps tendon–patellar bone autograft taken from the same or opposite knee.[3] Any residual patellar bone defect is grafted. The quadriceps tendon has the greatest cross-sectional area (100 mm^2) and is ideal for use in revision knee surgery if the prior tunnels are in the desired anatomic ACL site but are slightly expanded. If autograft tissues are not available or the patient refuses harvest from the contralateral knee, a BPTB or Achilles tendon-bone allograft is recommended.

In knees with associated complete rupture of the medial or posterolateral ligament structures that require surgical repair with the ACL reconstruction, a BPTB autograft harvest adds morbidity to the procedure and is used in knees of only select athletes. Other graft options, such as a semitendinosus-gracilis autograft, have less morbidity, particularly in recreational athletes. In knees treated with multiligament reconstructions, the preferred graft for the ACL reconstruction is either a contralateral BPTB autograft or allograft as was previously discussed.

In knees with associated varus malalignment, the timing of the high tibial osteotomy (HTO) and ligament reconstructive procedures is based on the diagnosis of primary, double, or triple varus syndrome.[48] In knees with primary varus that do not show abnormal lateral tibiofemoral compartment opening or external tibial rotation, the HTO and ACL reconstruction may be done at the same setting. The preferred graft is a semitendinosus-gracilis autograft, which may be harvested from the involved limb with little morbidity. Most patients treated with HTO cannot return to strenuous activities; however, the semitendinosus-gracilis provides suitable stability for low-impact activities. BPTB autograft, harvested from the contralateral side, may be considered in knees with gross anterior tibial subluxation and a grade 3 pivot-shift test.

In double varus knees, lower limb varus malalignment results from two factors: (1) the tibiofemoral osseous and geometric alignment and (2) the separation of the lateral tibiofemoral compartment from deficient posterolateral structures. In these patients, the ACL reconstruction is staged after the HTO because the increase in lateral joint opening contraindicates a simultaneous ACL procedure. HTO is effective in decreasing abnormal loads in the lateral and posterolateral structures, allowing physiologic remodeling and shortening to occur. Posterolateral reconstruction or ACL reconstruction is often avoided.[49]

In triple varus knees, lower limb varus malalignment results from three factors: the tibiofemoral varus osseous malalignment, increased lateral tibiofemoral compartment separation caused by marked insufficiency of the posterolateral structures, and varus recurvatum in extension. In these patients, the ACL and posterolateral reconstructive procedures are performed after the HTO has healed. This chapter's authors believe that simultaneous HTO, ACL, and posterolateral reconstructions have a high morbidity rate, and ligamentous procedures should always be staged.

The repair of meniscal tears, including complex tears that extend into the avascular zone, has been advocated along with ACL reconstruction.[50-52] The deleterious effects of meniscectomy are well established, and the preservation of meniscal tissue is as important as a successful ACL reconstruction in these knees. Several long-term ACL reconstruction studies have recently reported a high rate of arthrosis in knees treated with functional ACL reconstructions in patients treated with prior meniscectomy.[53-55] Inside-out vertical divergent sutures are placed first on the superior surface to reduce the tear and then on the inferior surface to close the tear site. An accessory posteromedial or posterolateral limited incision and dissection is done.[56] The indications, contraindications, and technique have been described in detail elsewhere.[56] After meniscus repair, full knee motion is possible; however, weight bearing is limited for 4 weeks to protect the repair site.[57]

Clinical Evaluation

A thorough patient history is obtained, including a detailed account of all knee injuries and the surgical procedures performed. In revision knee procedures, prior surgical records are obtained to verify the surgical findings, the condition of the articular cartilage and menisci, and graft placement. A comprehensive physical examination is performed, including assessing knee flexion and extension, patellofemoral indices, tibiofemoral crepitus, tibiofemoral joint line pain, muscle strength, and gait abnormalities. All of the abnormal translations and rotations in the knee joint are determined with appropriate tests. The medial posterior tibiofemoral step-off on the posterior drawer test is done at 90° of flexion. The integrity of the ACL is determined with KT-2000 arthrometer testing at 20° of flexion (134 N force) to quantify total anteroposterior displacement. The pivot-shift test is recorded on a scale of 0 to 3, with a grade of 0 indicating no pivot shift; grade 1, a slip or glide; grade 2, a jerk with gross subluxation or clunk; and grade 3, gross subluxation with impingement of the posterior aspect of the lateral side of the tibial plateau against the femoral condyle.

Insufficiency of the posterolateral and medial ligament structures is determined by varus and valgus stress testing at 0° and 30° of knee flexion. The surgeon estimates the amount of joint opening (in mm) between the initial closed contact position of each tibiofemoral compartment, performed in a constrained manner avoiding internal or external tibial rotation, to the maximal opened position. The result is recorded according to the increase in the tibiofemoral compartment of the affected knee compared with that of the opposite normal knee. Abnormal medial or lateral joint openings may be measured with stress radiographs. The tibiofemoral rotation dial test at 30° and 90° detects increases in external tibial rotation with posterior subluxation of the lateral tibial plateau or anterior subluxation of the medial tibial plateau caused by medial ligament injury. It is important to recognize that it is possible to confuse increased external tibial rotation for a posterolateral injury and miss the medial-side ligament injury that requires correction.[58] The presence of a varus recurvatum in both the supine and standing positions should be carefully assessed. Gait analysis is performed to detect a varus, valgus, or hyperextension thrust. Patients can sometimes demonstrate knee instability while standing with a few degrees of knee flexion by producing an external femoral rotation that reproduces the pivot-shift phenomenon. The patient may also have an abnormal varus or valgus tibiofemoral joint opening.

Radiographs, including standing AP at 0°, lateral at 30° of knee flexion, weight-bearing PA at 45° of knee flexion, and patellofemoral axial views should be taken during the initial examination.[59] Double-stance standing radiographs of both lower extremities from the femoral heads to the ankle joints should be obtained in knees in which varus or valgus lower extremity alignment is detected on clinical examination. The mechanical axis and weight-bearing line should be measured.[48] MRI should be done to measure the length, width, and thickness of the patellar tendon.[60] In kness that have undergone revision, MRI is useful in providing additional details of tunnel placement and the condition of the articular cartilage and menisci. The tibial tunnel placement is visualized on sagittal views, and measurements are made to determine if the tunnel is too posterior, which requires a staged bone graft procedure. Fast spin-echo techniques are available to obtain superior quality articular cartilage images.[61]

At the Cincinnati SportsMedicine and Orthopaedic Center, patients complete questionnaires and are interviewed to assess symptoms, functional limitations, sports and occupational activity levels, and the patient's perception of his or her overall knee condition according to the Cincinnati Knee Rating System.[62]

ACL Graft Function Required to Resist the Pivot-Shift Phenomenon

Biomechanical studies show that the ACL is the primary restraint to anterior tibial translation, providing 87% of the total restraining force at 30° of knee flexion and 85% at 90° of flexion.[63] The iliotibial band, midmedial capsule, midlateral capsule, medial col-

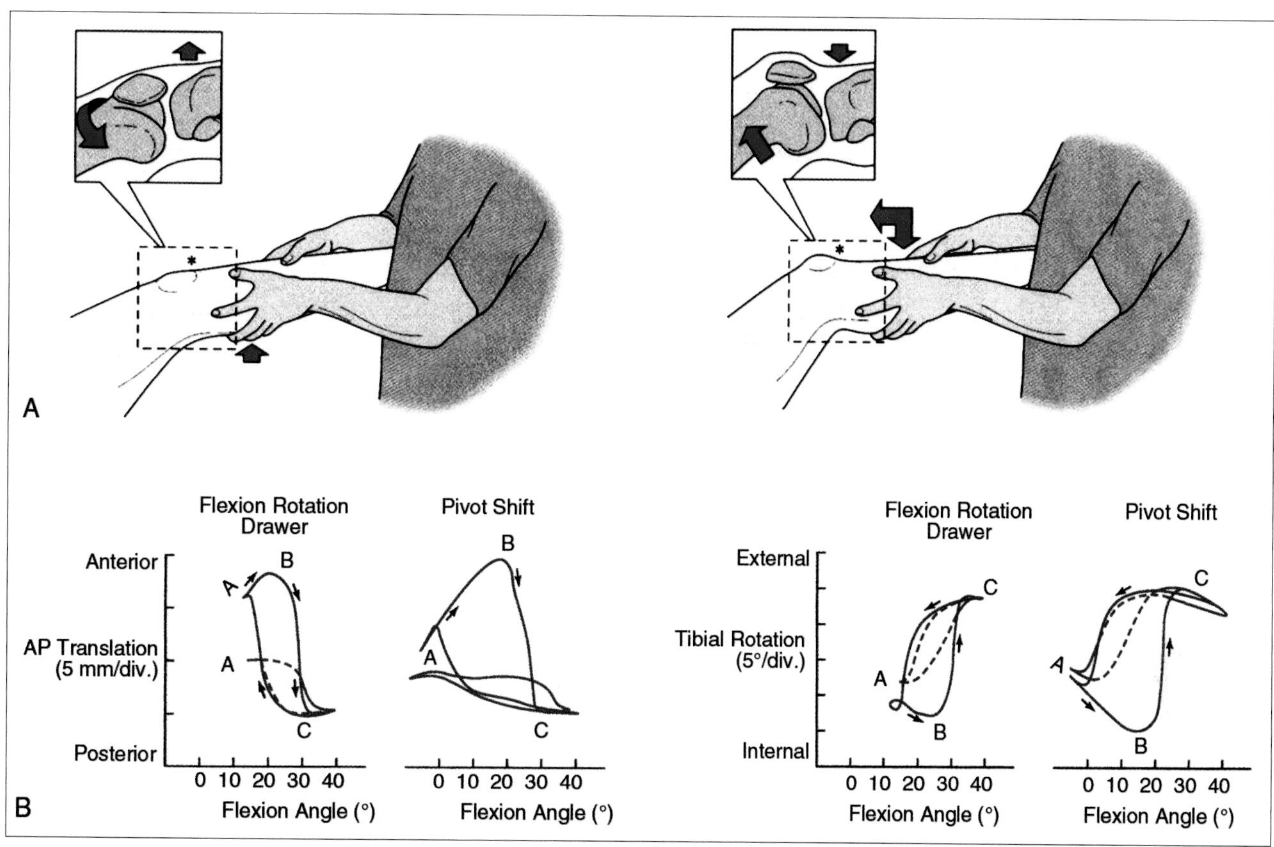

Figure 2 **A,** Illustrations showing the pivot-shift test. The leg is held with the knee at 15° to 20° of flexion. An anterior tibial load with internal tibial rotation produces anterior tibial subluxation (left). Gentle posterior loading, external tibial rotation, and valgus loading results in the reduced position (right). **B,** Grafts of knee motions during the pivot-shift test. "A" indicates the starting position; "B," the maximum subluxated position; and "C," the reduced position. The dashed figure represents the motions of the normal knee, and the solid figure is the condition after ACL sectioning. Note the major increases in both anterior translation and internal tibial rotation. (Reproduced with permission from Noyes FR, Barber-Westin SD: ACL primary and revision reconstruction: Diagnosis, operative techniques, clinical outcomes, in Noyes FR, Barber-Westin SD, eds: *Noyes' Knee Disorders: Surgery, Rehabilitation, Clinical Outcomes.* Philadelphia, PA, WB Saunders, 2009, pp 140-228.)

lateral ligament (MCL), and fibular collateral ligament all provide a secondary restraint to anterior tibial translation. The posteromedial and posterolateral capsules provide added resistance with knee extension. The secondary restraints (including the menisci) may be injured or become deficient with repeat injuries, resulting in major increases in anterior tibial subluxation and a grossly positive grade 3 pivot-shift test.[64,65]

Laboratory studies show that sectioning of the ACL produces only a small increase in the final limit of internal rotation.[65] Subsequent sectioning of the lateral structures produces sequentially larger increases in the final limit of internal tibial rotation. The final limit for internal tibial rotation is primarily resisted by the lateral extra-articular structures, which are tightened by internal tibial rotation and not by the ACL. This is an important concept because clinical and biomechanical studies frequently attempt to measure the increase in the final internal tibial rotation limits after ACL surgery to quantify ACL graft function.[66] Because the lateral structures resist the internal tibial rotation limit more than the ACL, this approach in measuring ACL function is not appropriate.

Sectioning the ACL results in large increases in both internal tibial rotation and anterior translation in the midportion of the motion envelopes (before the final limit of tibial rotation is reached). Therefore, during clinical testing, the Lachman and pivot-shift tests should be performed within the midportion of the tibial rotation envelope to avoid the constraining effect of medial or lateral restraints.[67]

The pivot-shift test[68,69] is illustrated in **Figure 2, A** and the increases in anterior translation and internal tibial rotation after ACL sectioning are shown in **Figure 2, B**. The function of the ACL is ideally described by its effect in limiting the combined motions of anterior tibial translation and internal tibial rotation and the resulting anterior subluxation of the lateral and medial tibiofemoral compartments (**Figure 3**). The effect of both the abnormally increased motions and the resulting tibial subluxation clinically represents the pivot-shift phenomenon.[64,67,70]

The abnormal increase in anterior translation and internal rotation results in anterior subluxation of the lateral and medial compartments[64] (**Figure 4**). The effect of sectioning the superficial MCL allows increased subluxation of both compartments and is associated with a grossly positive pivot-shift test.[64,70]

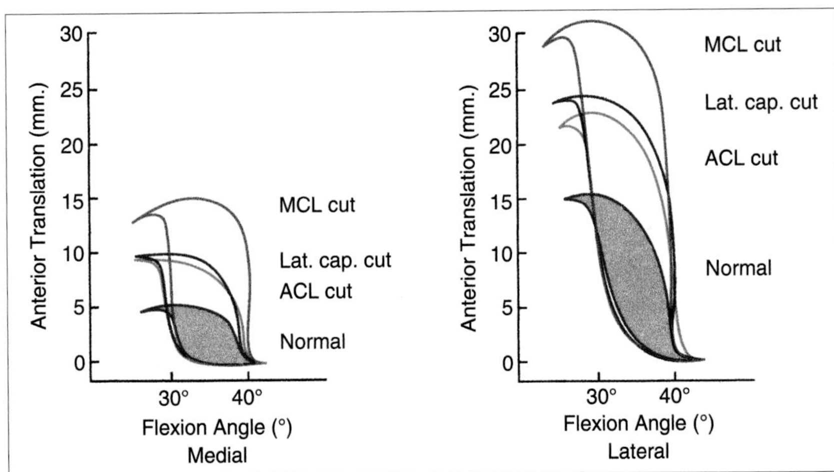

Figure 3 Graphs showing anterior tibial translation for the medial (left) and lateral (right) tibiofemoral compartments during the pivot-shift test in a normal knee and after ACL sectioning. The lateral compartment translation is greater than the medial compartment translation with the effect of additional ligament sectioning increasing the compartment subluxations. Lat cap = lateral capsule. (Adapted with permission from Noyes FR, Grood ES, Suntay WJ: Three-dimensional motion analysis of clinical stress tests for anterior knee subluxations. *Acta Orthopaedica Scand* 1989;60:308-319.)

Currently, no accurate clinical system is available to measure the abnormal motions and joint subluxation in the pivot-shift test. This is a prime area for future research. Measurements of the pivot-shift test by experienced knee surgeons using an instrumented cadaver knee joint with six degrees of freedom showed large variations in the techniques used and the resulting motions and joint subluxations induced during the test.[67] Some examiners applied a forcible internal tibial rotation that resulted in constraining the amount of anterior tibial translation. The flexion-rotation drawer test[68] is a modification of the pivot-shift test and avoids the sometimes painful thud or clunk sensation as the tibia reduces. The grading of the pivot-shift test is entirely qualitative. The variations in techniques between examiners administering the pivot-shift test and the loads applied prevent quantitative

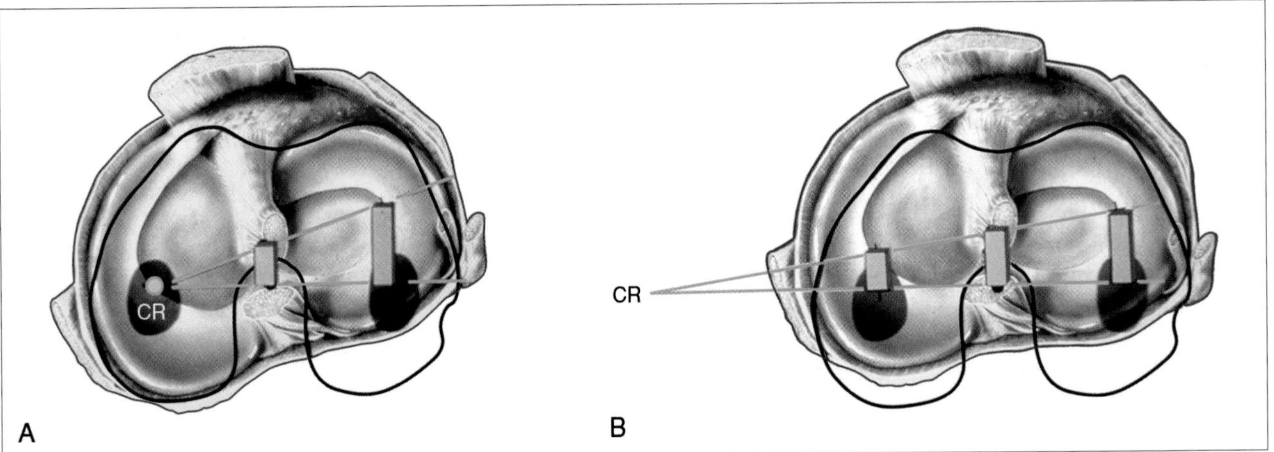

Figure 4 **A,** Illustration of an intact knee. **B,** Illustration showing the response to combined anterior tibial translation and internal rotation about a center of rotation (CR) resulting in anterior subluxation of the lateral and medial tibiofemoral compartments. (Reproduced with permission from Noyes FR: The function of the human anterior cruciate ligament and analysis of single- and double-bundle graft reconstruction. *Sports Health: A Multidisciplinary Approach* 2009; 1:66-75.)

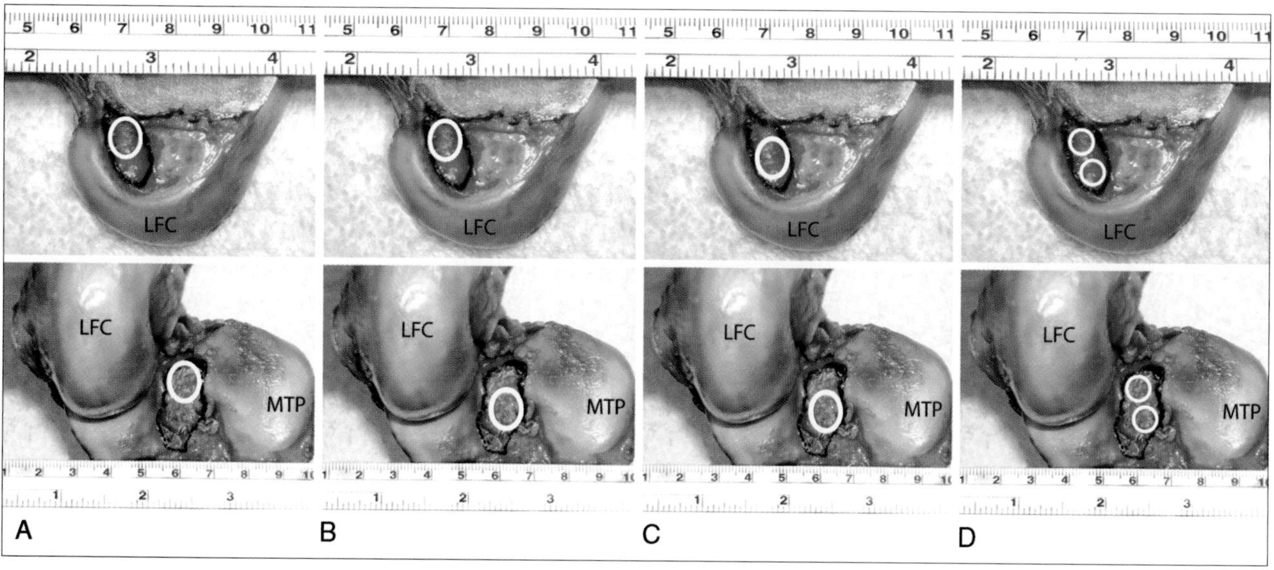

Figure 5 Summary of different femoral and tibial graft positions that are possible using anteromedial and posterolateral bundle terminology. **A,** Classic anteromedial femur to posterolateral tibia results in a vertical graft with a tibial tunnel placed too far posteriorly. **B,** A more central and anterior tibial tunnel is advantageous for controlling rotational stability; however, the femoral tunnel is still high and proximal. **C,** The ideal central femoral-tibial tunnel locations for a single graft reconstruction. **D,** The placement of a two-bundle ACL reconstruction. LFC = lateral femoral condyle, MTP = medial tibial plateau. (Reproduced with permission from Noyes FR, Barber-Westin SD: ACL primary and revision reconstruction: Diagnosis, operative techniques, clinical outcomes, in Noyes FR, Barber-Westin SD, eds: *Noyes' Knee Disorders: Surgery, Rehabilitation, Clinical Outcomes.* Philadelphia, PA, WB Saunders, 2009, pp 140-228.)

measurement for knee stability after ACL surgery. The KT-2000 arthrometer (Medmetric, San Diego, CA) underestimates the maximal lateral compartment translation because this device provides a quantitative assessment of the millimeters of translation at the center of the tibia. Even so, the quantitative data are important for published studies.

Ideal Femoral and Tibial ACL Graft Attachment Sites

Considerable variation exists between studies on the anatomic division of the ACL into two distinct fiber bundles, as well as attachment locations.[71] Some authors[28,72-75] report that an anatomic and functional division exists whereby the anteromedial bundle tightens with knee flexion,[72,76] and the posterolateral bundle is under tension with knee extension and relaxes with flexion. Other authors[71,77] express doubt that there is a true anatomic division, believing instead that the division is functional in nature. Under this condition, the ACL fibers participate in load sharing, with different percentages of load in fiber regions instead of reciprocal loading occurring between separate distinct fiber bundles.[78-80] This chapter's authors believe that the characterization of the ACL into two fiber bundles represents a gross oversimplification, which is not supported by biomechanical studies.[79,80]

The femoral and tibial graft attachment sites markedly affect the ability of the ACL graft to control the combined motions of anterior tibial translation and internal rotation (**Figure 5**). Given the variation in ACL anatomic shapes between specimens,[71,81] during surgery it is important (when possible) to outline the size and shape of the ACL attachment for each knee. This can be done in primary ACL reconstructions but is usually not possible in revision surgery. Because of the variation in ACL attachment shapes, it is also expected that the locations chosen for single- and double-bundle ACL graft locations vary among surgeons.

The length-tensile behavior of ACL fibers in resisting anterior tibial subluxation is greatly influenced by the femoral attachment in reference to the center of femoral flexion and extension rotation.[80] In **Figure 6**, the concept of a transition zone or a contour plot is shown for the ACL fibers at the femoral attachment.[80] A central zone is shown where the fiber separation distance (tibiofemoral attachment) undergoes a 2-mm change in length during knee flexion and extension. ACL fibers anterior to this zone have a tibiofemoral separation distance that lengthens with knee flexion, whereas the tibiofemoral separation distance of the posterior fibers lengthens with knee extension. ACL fibers in the posterior distal femoral attachment (posterolateral bundle) attach (in part) pos-

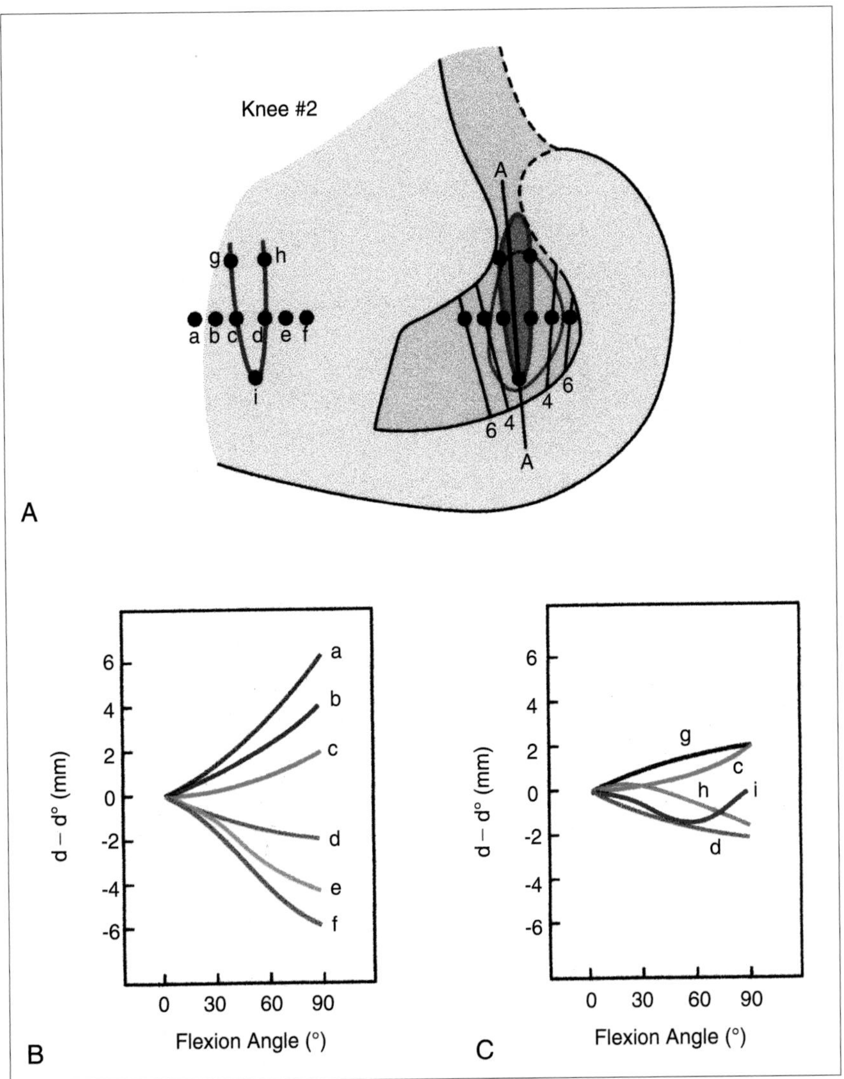

Figure 6 **A,** Typical contour plot for the ACL. This figure was determined for knee flexion from 0° to 90° while an anterior force of 100 N was applied to the tibia. The tibial attachment site used in the analysis was located in the geometric center of the tibial insertion of the ACL. **B,** The graph shows, for femoral attachments a through f, how the tibiofemoral distance (d) changes from its value at full extension. Points a, b, and c, located posterior to line A-A in the illustration (part **A** of this figure), all move away from the tibial attachment with flexion. Points d, e, and f, located posterior to line A-A, all move toward the tibial attachment. **C,** The graph shows separation distance curves for attachments located around the 2-mm contour line. Points g and c, located on the anterior branch of the 2-mm contour line, have separation distances that are longest at 90° of flexion. Points h and d, located on the posterior branch, have separation distances that are shortest at 90° of flexion. (Reproduced with permission from Hefzy MS, Grood ES, Noyes FR, et al: Factors affecting the region of most isometric femoral attachments: Part II. The anterior cruciate ligament. *Am J Sports Med* 1989;17:208-216.)

terior to the zone, explaining their increased function closer to full knee extension as the separation distance lengthens with knee extension. The central transition zone is not static and changes with knee flexion-extension.[80]

The ACL fiber separation distance data, although useful in understanding ACL fiber behaviors and graft placements, do not indicate the actual strain or tension developed in ACL fibers because the initial length of fibers and true fiber strain are not computed. The data provide information on the expected length-tension behaviors of a graft with parallel fibers of similar length.

An error in placing a graft in an anterior or posterior position has the greatest effect in producing deleterious lengthening and graft failure in comparison with the proximal or distal placement of a graft. For example, a graft placed anterior to the ACL femoral attachment (anterior to the "residents ridge") would undergo deleterious lengthening with knee flexion. A graft placed too posteriorly, with fibers in the most posterior aspect of the femoral tunnel, would undergo lengthening with knee extension and, when tensioned under large loads at surgery, may block knee extension. One qualification to the above data is important. The ACL femoral attachment of fibers has three-dimensional characteristics. Accordingly, fiber function described in a single plane does not truly represent fiber function in a three-dimensional plane; this is an important area for future research.[82]

Biomechanical Studies Supporting the Recommended Graft Placement

Several studies have reported that load sharing occurs between ACL fibers rather than as reciprocal loading between two distinct ACL bundles.[78,82,83] In a robotic cadaver study, Gabriel et al[78] reported that with anterior tibial loading, the anteromedial bundle was nearly equal in distributing in situ force to the posterolateral bundle at 15° of flexion; anteromedial forces increased with knee flexion. Under the rotational loads of valgus and internal tibial rotation, the forces in the anteromedial bundle were greater than those of the posteromedial bundle. In a cadaver robotic study, Mae et al[83] reported that the posterolateral bundle functioned best at distributing forces at low flexion angles and was equal to the anteromedial bundle at 10° of flexion. An increase in anteromedial bundle function was observed with increasing knee flexion. In an in vivo study of ACL kinematics during weight bearing, Li et al[82] reported no distinct separation of ACL function based on the bundle arrangement. The classic description of reciprocal loading between the posterolateral bundle (tight in extension) and the anteromedial bundle (tight in flexion) inadequately describes load sharing of ACL fibers and the theoretic basis for a double-bundle reconstruction.

Cadaver and robotic studies have typically analyzed single ACL grafts placed in the proximal femoral ACL attachment (1 o'clock position), with a posterior tibial ACL attachment, which produced a less than ideal vertical ACL graft construct.[72,74] Only a few studies compared a two-bundle graft construct with a single graft placed centrally in the femoral ACL footprint.[34,84] As a result, there are major differences in the functional properties between ACL single-graft reconstructions in cadaver studies based on the placement of the femoral and tibial grafts. Yamamoto et al[34] reported no statistical differences in the anterotibial translation or combined rotatory loading conditions between the intact ACL, single-graft, or double-bundle reconstructions except at high knee flexion. Markolf et al[33] reported that a single-bundle reconstruction restored mean tibial rotations and lateral plateau displacements to levels similar to those of the intact knee. The double-bundle reconstruction reduced combined rotations and displacements to levels less than those of the intact knee. The authors concluded that the overconstraint induced by the double-bundle reconstruction has unknown clinical consequences, and that the need for the added complexity of this procedure is questionable.

In a goat model, Ekdahl et al[85] showed that anatomic ACL graft placement (anteromedial-tibial to anteromedial-femoral) improved anterior tibial translation, in situ force, and ultimate failure load and resulted in less graft tunnel enlargement compared with two nonanatomic graft placements (posterolateral-tibial to anteromedial-femoral, and posterolateral-tibial to high anteromedial-femoral). The term anatomic was used in this context following a two-bundle ACL classification with the graft occupying the same bundle attachment at the tibial and femoral insertion. The effect of ACL graft position on knee rotatory stability was not studied.

Scanlan et al[86] reported that the walking mechanics of patients after ACL reconstruction was influenced by the ACL graft position. A more vertical coronal position produced a higher external knee flexion moment during walking (reduction in net quadriceps usage), which is a gait alteration similar to that found in ACL-deficient knees.

In a cadaver study on ACL graft placement, Steiner[87] reported that transtibial drilling of the femoral tunnel resulted in more vertical ACL graft placement, with the tibial tunnel more posterior and the femoral tunnel more superior in relationship to the native ACL attachment. Independent drilling of the tibial and femoral tunnels produced a more oblique coronal graft that was located more centrally in the ACL respective footprint, which better restored anterior and rotational knee stability. The author concluded that single-bundle ACL reconstruction results would be improved by independent tibial and femoral tunnel drilling to locate the ACL graft more precisely within the central tibial and femoral footprints; this recommendation has been described in other publications.[4,14]

Surgical Technique for Central Anatomic Tibial Graft Placement

The important anatomic landmarks for the ACL attachments have been well described.[21,71,81,88-97] The tibial attachments are easily visualized at surgery and include the medial tibial spine, posterior interspinous ridge of the proximal posterior cruciate ligament (PCL) fossa, and the attachment of the lateral meniscus (**Figure 7**). Because the PCL is a poor soft-tissue landmark for the posterior extent of the native ACL attachment, drill guides that use the PCL as a reference are not recommended.

A central, anatomic, ACL tibial attachment location directly adjacent and anterior to the posterior edge of the lateral meniscus anterior horn attachment is shown in **Figure 8**. The center of the ACL is usually 16 to 20 mm anterior to the posterior interspinous ridge. The most posterior extent of the ACL tibial attachment is 6 to 10 mm anterior to the retroeminence ridge or posterior interspinous ridge.[71,76,92] During surgery, the guide pin is placed eccentric and 2 to 3 mm anterior and medial to the true ACL center because the ACL graft displaces to the posterior and lateral aspect of the tibial tunnel.[98] The eccentric tunnel places most of the graft within the central and anterior aspect of the tibial attachment, adjacent and not behind the lateral meniscal attachment, which avoids a posterior ACL attachment location. To avoid a vertical graft

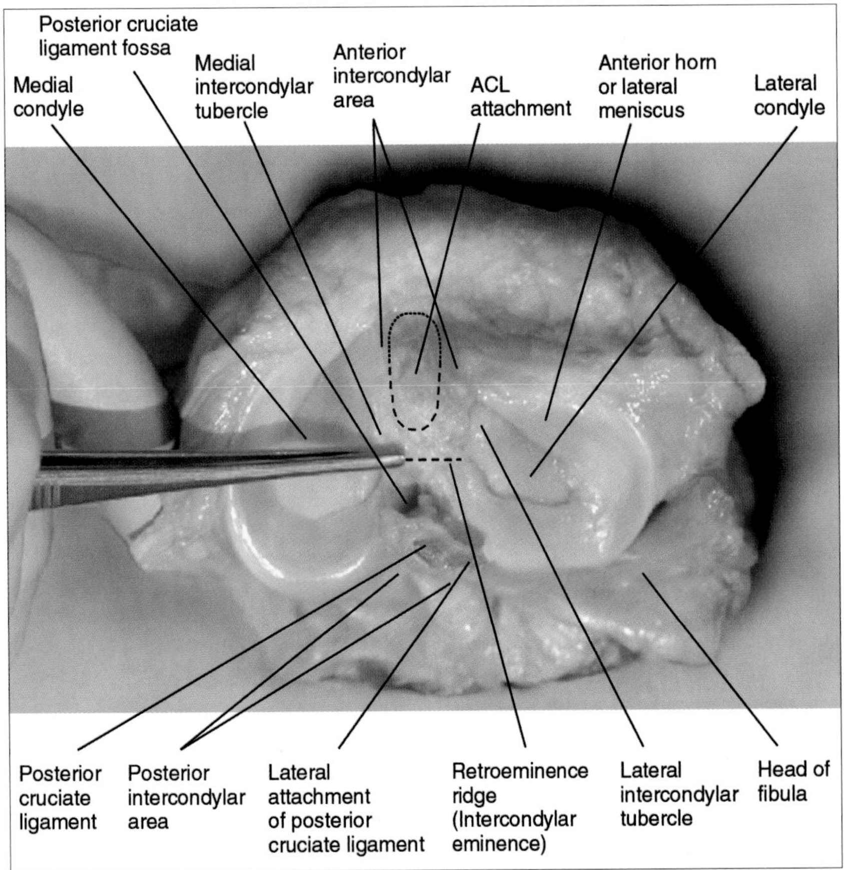

Figure 7 ACL tibial attachment anatomy. (Reproduced with permission from Noyes FR, Barber-Westin SD: ACL primary and revision reconstruction: Diagnosis, operative techniques, clinical outcomes, in Noyes FR, Barber-Westin SD, eds: *Noyes' Knee Disorders: Surgery, Rehabilitation, Clinical Outcomes.* Philadelphia, PA, WB Saunders, 2009, pp 140-228.)

orientation, the tibial drill must not inadvertently penetrate into or beyond the posterior one third of the ACL attachment and adjacent posterior interspinous ridge. It is important that graft impingement with knee extension does not occur. This is easily determined by direct viewing with the scope in the anteromedial portal and also with the scope placed within the tibial tunnel as the knee is brought into extension. The tibial central and anterior graft location frequently requires a limited anterior and medial femoral notchplasty, which this chapter's authors believe causes no morbidity.

The ideal tibial tunnel is placed in a coronal manner at a 55° to 60° angle, which allows a tunnel length of 35 to 40 mm. The tunnel is initiated just anterior and adjacent to the superficial MCL and is usually 25 mm medial to the tibial tubercle and 10 mm distal to the most proximal point of the tibial tubercle insertion into the patellar tendon. The tunnel is drilled to the desired graft diameter, and the joint tunnel edges are chamfered to prevent graft abrasion.

Surgical Technique for Central Anatomic Femoral Graft Placement

To anatomically place the femoral graft, the principle is to drill the femoral tunnel to the desired length and correct the central anatomic location independently of the femoral tunnel drilling. Important anatomic landmarks for the femoral ACL attachment are the posterior articular cartilage, the Blumensaat line, and the ACL attachment on the lateral femoral wall of the notch. It is important to emphasize that no native ACL fibers extend to the intercondylar roof; all the fibers are located on the lateral wall (**Figures 9** and **10**). The ACL femoral attachment is mapped based on the bony landmarks.

For single grafts, an anatomic central ACL placement locates the femoral guide pin just above the midpoint of the proximal-to-distal length of the ACL attachment and 7 to 8 mm from the posterior articular cartilage edge, leaving approximately 3 to 4 mm of a posterior tunnel wall (**Figure 11**). In this location, the graft will occupy approximately two thirds to three fourths of the ACL footprint. The ACL attachment is easily mapped at 30° of flexion with the arthroscope in the anteromedial portal. After the point of the ACL attachment and guide pin is marked, the knee can be placed in the final degrees of flexion based on the selected endoscopic technique. With knee flexion, the proximal-to-distal ACL attachment assumes a more horizontal appearance, which can be easily observed as the knee is taken into different knee flexion positions. It is more reliable to map the ACL femoral attachment at the 30° knee flexion position instead of a 90° position. The final 8- to 9-mm diameter femoral tunnel occupies the central ACL attachment, leaving the most proximal and distal few millimeters of the ACL attachment unoccupied by a graft.

Many techniques are available for drilling the femoral tunnel; the selected technique can be based on the surgeon's preference if the central anatomic graft position is achieved in a reliable and reproducible manner. The most common techniques include an

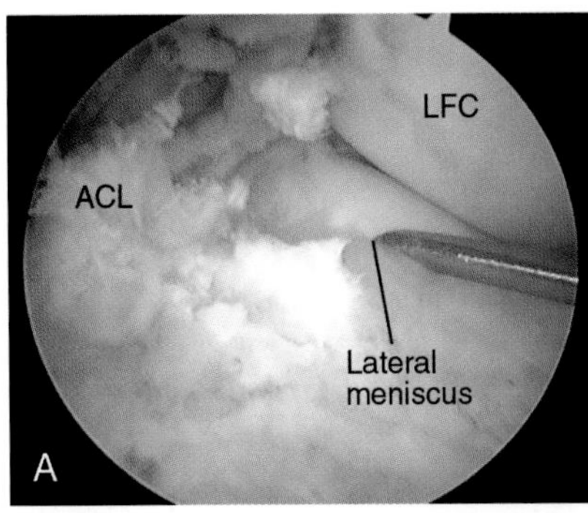

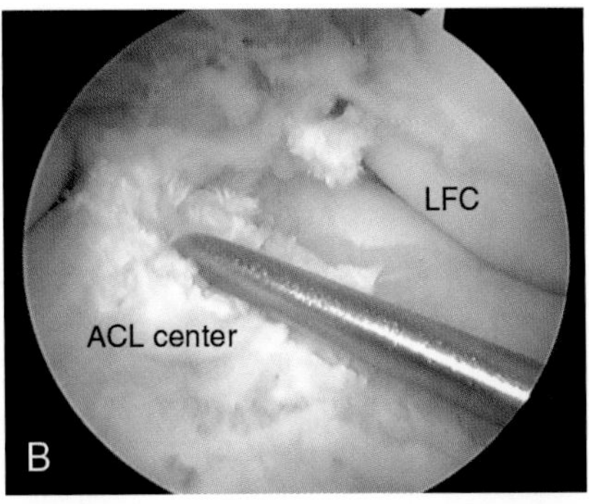

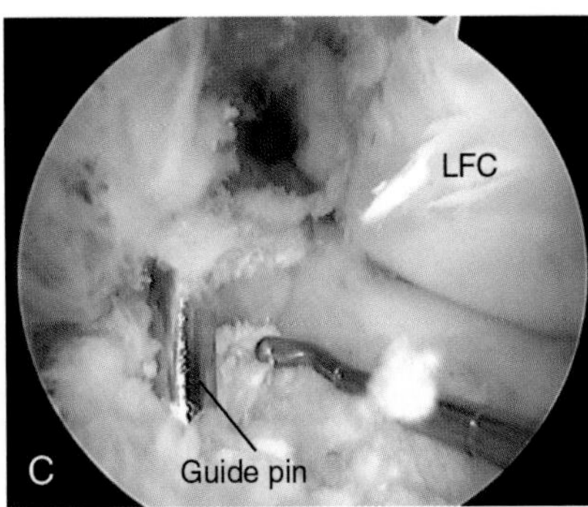

Figure 8 **A,** Arthroscopic image showing ACL tibial attachment anterior to the posterior edge of the lateral meniscus. **B,** The center of ACL tibial attachment is marked and is anterior to the lateral meniscus posterior edge. **C,** Placement of central guide pin for single tunnel ACL reconstruction. LFC = lateral femoral condyle. (Reproduced with permission from Noyes FR, Barber-Westin SD: ACL primary and revision reconstruction: Diagnosis, operative techniques, clinical outcomes, in Noyes FR, Barber-Westin SD, eds: *Noyes' Knee Disorders: Surgery, Rehabilitation, Clinical Outcomes.* Philadelphia, PA, WB Saunders, 2009, pp 140-228.)

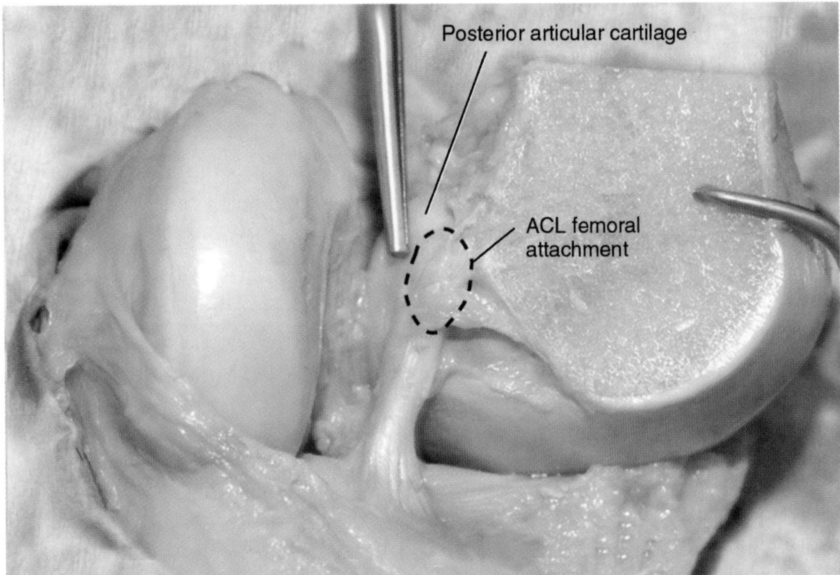

Figure 9 Image showing the entire ACL femoral attachment on the lateral wall of the notch. (Reproduced with permission from Noyes FR, Barber-Westin SD: ACL primary and revision reconstruction: Diagnosis, operative techniques, clinical outcomes, in Noyes FR, Barber-Westin SD, eds: *Noyes' Knee Disorders: Surgery, Rehabilitation, Clinical Outcomes.* Philadelphia, PA, WB Saunders, 2009, pp 140-228.)

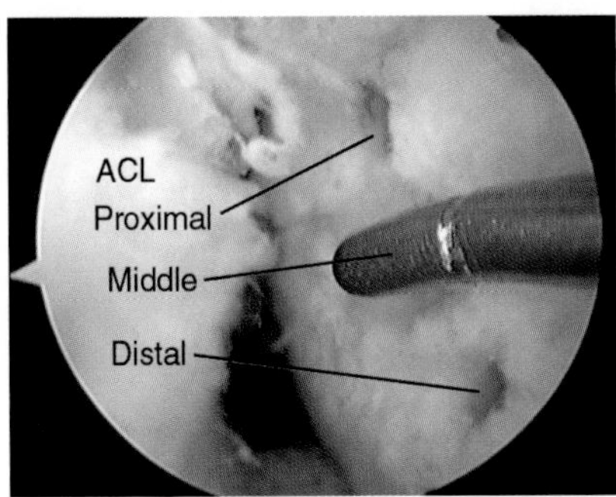

Figure 10 Three points are identified in the proximal, the middle, and the distal portions of the femoral ACL attachment viewed through the anteromedial portal at 30° of knee flexion. (Reproduced with permission from Noyes FR, Barber-Westin SD: ACL primary and revision reconstruction: Diagnosis, operative techniques, clinical outcomes, in Noyes FR, Barber-Westin SD, eds: *Noyes' Knee Disorders: Surgery, Rehabilitation, Clinical Outcomes.* Philadelphia, PA, WB Saunders, 2009, pp 140-228.)

all-endoscopic anteromedial portal technique with a hyperflexed knee position (≥ 120°) (**Figure 12**), and a two-incision technique (**Figure 13**). Flexible guides, guide pins, and drills are available, which some surgeons have found beneficial. Transtibial tunnel drilling of the femoral tunnel is not recommended by this chapter's authors because it may induce errors in the femoral tunnel location described by recent publications.[19,21,99-101] The tunnel is drilled to the appropriate diameter so that the graft fits snugly in the tunnel. The tunnel edges are chamfered to prevent graft abrasion.

The ACL femoral tunnel should not be placed too distally because this shortens the femoral socket and overall tibiofemoral graft length. This is particularly true when a BPTB graft is used, which may result in too much of the graft protruding outside the tibial tunnel. The location for a single-tunnel ACL reconstruction at the proximal one half or central one half of the femoral attachment will most

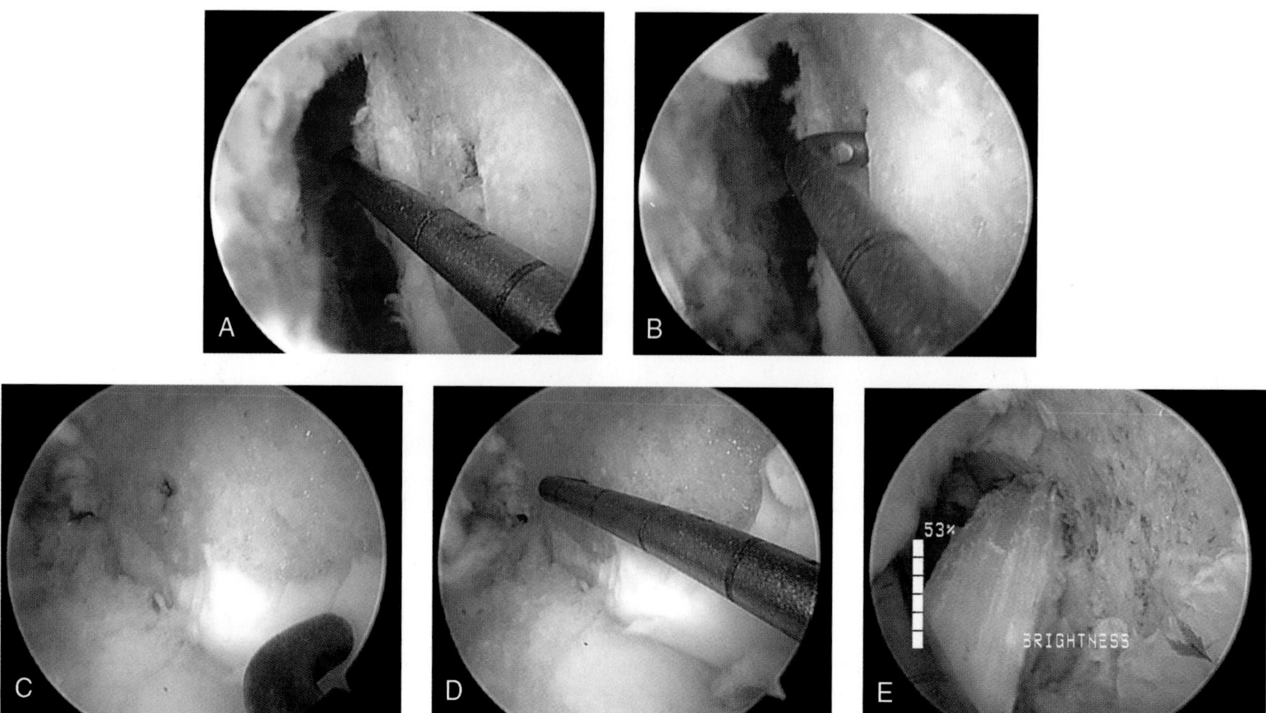

Figure 11 Arthroscopic images viewed through the anteromedial portal. The guide pin location on the lateral wall for the femoral tunnel is shown at 30° of knee flexion (**A** and **B**) and 90° of knee flexion (**C** and **D**). The anterolateral portal commonly provides insufficient visualization and is not recommended. **E,** Arthroscopic view of the final graft placement.

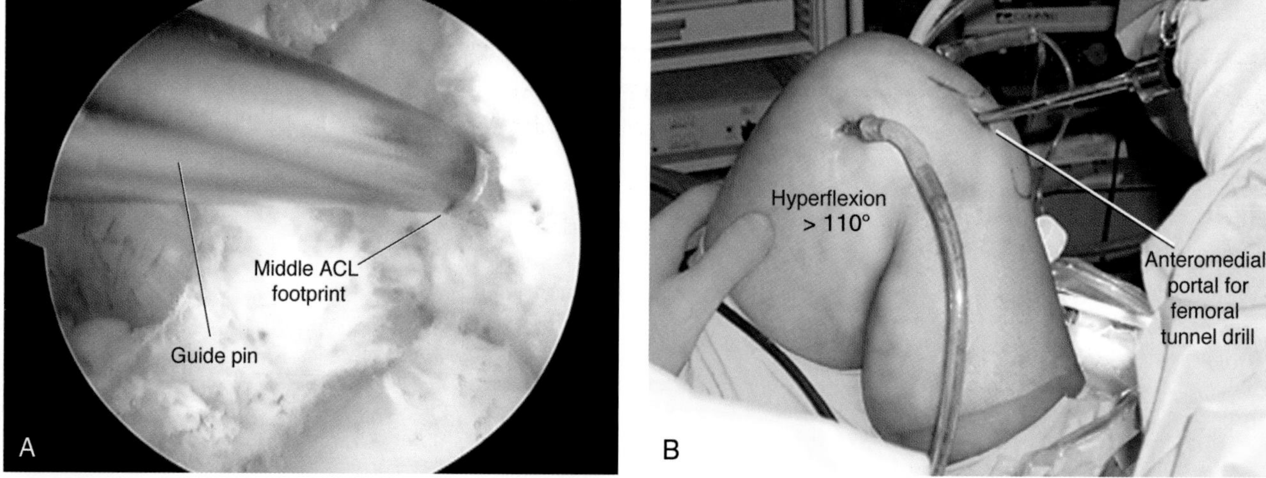

Figure 12 **A,** The ACL central point is reached with an endoscopic technique. **B,** The knee is hyperflexed 120°, and an anteromedial portal is used to drill the femoral tunnel. (Reproduced with permission from Noyes FR, Barber-Westin SD: ACL primary and revision reconstruction: Diagnosis, operative techniques, clinical outcomes, in Noyes FR, Barber-Westin SD, eds: *Noyes' Knee Disorders: Surgery, Rehabilitation, Clinical Outcomes.* Philadelphia, PA, WB Saunders, 2009, pp 140-228.)

likely have the same graft function and characteristics. The principle is to place the graft within the ACL femoral attachment, with no portion of the graft extending proximally onto the intercondylar roof. Equally important, as was previously discussed, is to avoid graft placement that is too anterior or posterior, which would produce abnormal graft displacement and tensioning in extension or flexion. This tensioning should be checked after

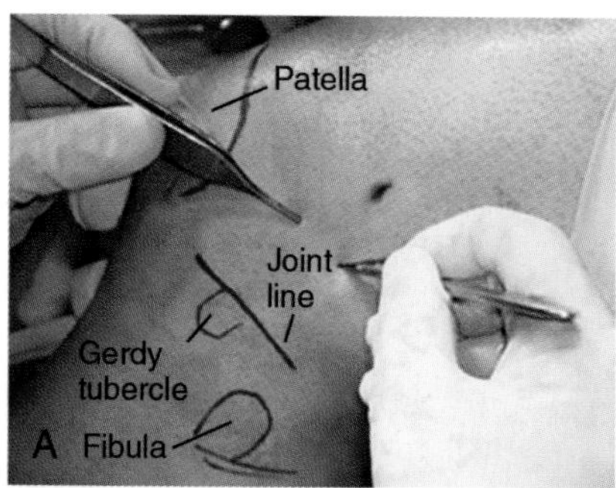

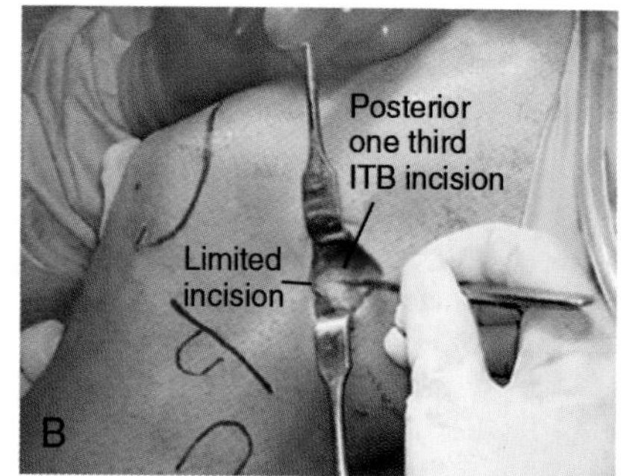

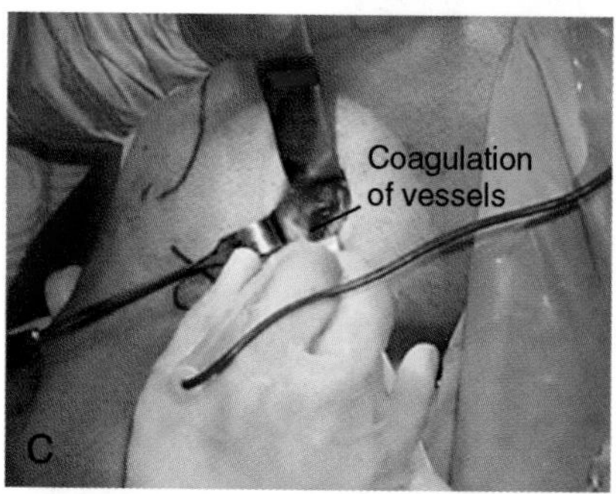

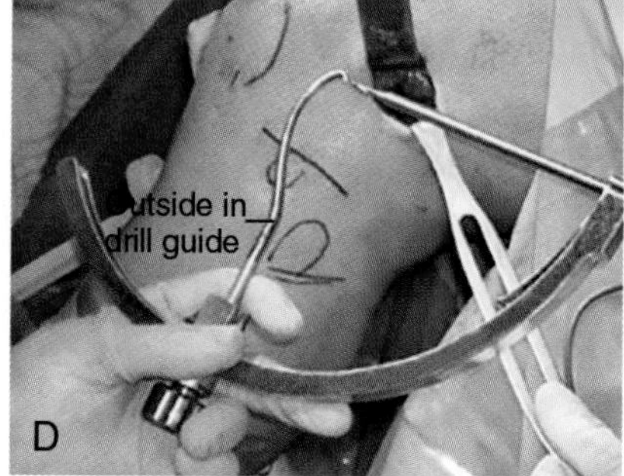

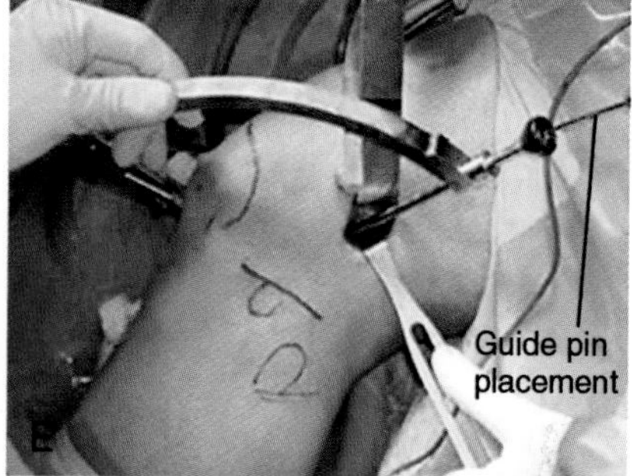

Figure 13 The ACL procedure with a two-incision technique for drilling the femoral tunnel. **A,** The anatomic landmarks are shown. The joint line, the tibial tubercle, and the fibula are marked. **B,** A 2-cm incision is made in the posterior one third of the iliotibial band (ITB) as described in the text. **C,** Electrocoagulation of vessels. **D,** A commercially available drill guide is used. **E,** The guide pin is placed. (Reproduced with permission from Noyes FR, Barber-Westin SD: ACL primary and revision reconstruction: Diagnosis, operative techniques, clinical outcomes, in Noyes FR, Barber-Westin SD, eds: *Noyes' Knee Disorders: Surgery, Rehabilitation, Clinical Outcomes.* Philadelphia, PA, WB Saunders, 2009, pp 140-228.)

graft placement and during the graft conditioning cycles before graft fixation.

Outcomes of Single- and Double-Bundle ACL Grafting

Several clinical studies have compared the outcomes of primary single- and double-bundle ACL reconstructions.[17,25-27,30-32,102-105] A critical review of these studies is beyond the scope of this chapter. Most of the authors used a vertically oriented ACL graft for the single-bundle construct (via a transtibial technique), which produced a greater number of patients with a positive pivot-shift test postoperatively compared with those treated with the double-bundle procedures.[17] However, not all the investigators reported a significant difference in postoperative knee stability; therefore, some authors did not support the use of the double-bundle procedure.[30-32,105] None of the studies reported clinical differences between the procedures because all subjective and functional scores were comparable. Meredick et al[106] conducted a meta-analysis of level I through III clinical studies comparing single- and double-bundle reconstructions and reported no clinically relevant difference in arthrometer (KT-2000) and pivot-shift test data. A mean difference of 0.5 mm was reported between the reconstructed and contralateral knee on knee arthrometer testing; the reconstruction method resulted in no difference in the odds of having a normal or nearly normal pivot-shift test result.

Discussion

In the past, authors have recommended that an ACL graft be placed in the proximal one third of the femoral attachment, believing this represented the most isometric zone. The adoption of the transtibial technique for drilling the femoral tunnel achieved this proximal graft placement; however, this technique required a posterior tibial tunnel. This resulted in a hybrid graft that was in a more vertical position in both the coronal and sagittal planes. Biomechanical studies have shown that this is not the ideal graft placement to resist the pivot-shift phenomenon.

Studies recommending double-bundle ACL reconstructions commonly compared this construct with a vertically oriented graft. Recent biomechanical studies of a more ideal single graft placed within the central femoral and tibial ACL insertion sites show the ability of the graft to resist the combined motions of anterior translation and internal tibial rotation

Table 3
Major Complications to Avoid in ACL Reconstruction

BPTB autograft reconstruction in the poorly motivated, recreational athlete with low pain tolerance who is unable to fully rehabilitate the knee
Failure to achieve adequate bone grafting of the patellar and tibial graft harvest sites: increased risk of patellar fracture; prevents kneeling
Posterior tibial tunnel leading to vertical ACL graft
Proximal and high femoral tunnel with portions of graft extending to roof, fails to control pivot-shift phenomenon
Failure to obtain 0° of extension and 90° of flexion with active quadriceps control by 2 to 3 weeks postoperatively
Failure to recognize an associated lateral/medial ligament insufficiency requiring reconstruction
Failure to recognize varus angulated knee with an abnormal lateral tibiofemoral joint opening
ACL revision: failure to bone graft prior tunnels, placing revision graft in previously malpositioned tibial and femoral tunnels.

ACL = anterior cruciate ligament, BPTB = bone-patellar tendon-bone

that occur in the pivot-shift phenomenon.

The rationale is to locate single-strand ACL grafts in the central region of their anatomic insertion with the graft occupying as much of the native ACL femoral and tibial footprint as possible. This requires independent drilling of the tibial and femoral tunnels.

The ACL is not an isometric structure, and the length-tension behavior of its fibers cannot be truly represented by a functional division into two fiber bundles. Rather than a reciprocal tensioning of the two bundles, there is load sharing between all ACL fibers with differing percentages of resistance based on the fiber attachment and the knee position. Native ACL function most likely cannot be replicated by either single- or double-bundle grafts.

Independent drilling of the femoral tunnel requires either an anteromedial portal antegrade drilling technique with the knee in hyperflexion or a two-incision retrograde technique. The use of the transtibial drilling technique for the femoral tunnel is recommended by some authors using a tibial tunnel entrance through the MCL fibers and beneath the medial plateau; however, the tibial tunnel is still in a less than ideal posterior tibial position.

The evolution of the double-bundle ACL technique has the theoretic advantage of locating grafts and collagen fibers throughout the entire ACL anatomic attachment sites. The concepts of ACL double-bundle grafts have prompted a worthwhile reevaluation of ACL anatomy and study of the ideal location for both single- and double-bundle grafts. The surgical complexity added by using a double-bundle graft may be found to be unnecessary when comparisons with a well-placed central ACL anatomic single strand graft are made in future clinical outcome studies.

ACL double-bundle techniques frequently use soft-tissue allografts to achieve the desired cross-sectional area of the two grafts. Allografts may pose the added problem of a higher failure rate because of delayed graft incorporation and healing compared with autografts, thereby possibly obviating the benefits of the double-bundle procedure.

Future clinical studies require objective clinical testing methods to measure the coupled motions of anterior tibial translation and internal tibial rotation and the resultant anterior tibial translation of the lateral and medial tibiofemoral compartments in the pivot-shift phenomenon. The lack of objective testing methods currently represents an unsolved problem that limits clinical comparisons of knee stability in ACL reconstruction studies.

Avoiding Complications

The major complications in ACL reconstruction are listed in **Table 3**. Complications may be related to improper diagnosis and treatment of associated ligament instabilities, poor patient selection, improper surgical techniques, and inadequate postoperative rehabilitation. The postoperative complication of arthrofibrosis, or a limitation of knee flexion and extension resulting from other factors such as a cyclops lesion, is frequently reported after ACL reconstruction. The causes, risk factors, preventive measures, and effective treatment strategies for knee motion complications are discussed in the literature.[107]

Postoperative Rehabilitation

The Cincinnati SportsMedicine and Orthopaedic Center rehabilitation program is summarized in **Tables 4** and **5**.[15] Each patient is taken through the appropriate rehabilitation program at a rate that considers sports and occupational goals; the condition of the articular surfaces, menisci, and other knee ligaments; concomitant surgical procedures performed with the ACL reconstruction; the type of graft used; postoperative healing and response to surgery; and biologic principles of graft healing and remodeling. The protocol shown in **Table 4** was designed to delay or diminish knee joint and graft loading for patients treated with ACL revision reconstruction, primary ACL allograft or semitendinosus-gracilis autograft reconstruction, BPTB autogenous reconstruction with

Table 4
Cincinnati SportsMedicine and Orthopaedic Center Rehabilitation Protocol for ACL Reconstruction: Revision Knees, Allografts, Complex Knees

	Postoperative Weeks					Postoperative Months			
	1-2	3-4	5-6	7-8	9-12	4	5	6	7-12
Brace: postoperative and functional	X	X	X	X	(X)			X	X
Range of motion minimum goals:									
0° to 90°	X	X							
0° to 120°			X						
0° to 135°				X					
Weight bearing:									
Toe touch	X								
1/4 to 1/2 body weight		X							
3/4 to full			X						
Patella mobilization	X	X	X						
Modalities:									
Electrical muscle stimulation	X	X	X	X					
Pain/edema management (cryotherapy)	X	X	X	X	X	X	X	X	X
Stretching:									
Hamstring, gastrocnemius-soleus complex, iliotibial band, quadriceps	X	X	X	X	X	X	X	X	X
Strengthening:									
Quadriceps isometrics, quadriceps-hamstring isometrics, co-contraction, straight leg raises, active knee extension	X	X	X	X	X				
Closed-chain: gait retraining, toe raises, wall sits, minisquats	X	X	X	X	X	X			
Knee flexion hamstring curls (90°)			X	X	X	X	X	X	X
Knee extension quadriceps (90° to 30°)			X	X	X	X	X	X	X
Hip abduction-adduction, multihip			X	X	X		X	X	X
Leg press (70° to 10°)			X	X	X	X	X	X	X
Balance/proprioceptive training:									
Weight-shifting, cup walking, BBS	X	X	X	X	X				
BBS, BAPS, perturbation training, balance board, minitrampoline					X	X	X	X	X
Conditioning:									
UBC		X	X	X					
Bike (stationary)			X	X	X	X	X	X	X
Aquatic program				X	X	X	X	X	X
Elliptical machine				X	X	X	X	X	X
Swimming (kicking)					X	X	X	X	X
Walking					X	X	X	X	X
Stair climbing machine					X	X	X	X	X
Ski machine					X	X	X	X	X
Running: straight								X	X
Cutting: lateral carioca, figure 8s									X
Plyometric training									X
Full sports									X

ACL = anterior cruciate ligament, BAPS = Biomechanical Ankle Platform System (Camp, Jackson, MI), BBS = Biodex Balance System (Biodex Medical Systems, Shirley, NY), UBC = upper body cycle (Biodex Medical Systems). (Adapted with permission from Heckmann TP, Noyes FR, Barber-Westin SD: Rehabilitation of primary and revision anterior cruciate ligament reconstructions, in Noyes FR, Barber-Westin SD, eds: *Noyes' Knee Disorders: Surgery, Rehabilitation, Clinical Outcomes*. Philadelphia, PA, WB Saunders, 2009, pp 306-336.)

major associated procedures such as a complex meniscus repair, or for significant articular cartilage lesions found during surgery. Delaying return to full weight bearing, initiating certain strengthening and conditioning exercises, beginning running and agility drills, and a return to full sports activities are incorporated into the protocol.

Table 5

Cincinnati SportsMedicine and Orthopaedic Center Rehabilitation Protocol for Primary ACL Reconstruction: Early Return to Strenuous Activities

	Postoperative Weeks					Postoperative Months			
	1-2	3-4	5-6	7-8	9-12	4	5	6	7-12
Brace: immobilizer for patient comfort	X	(X)							
Range of motion minimum goals:									
0° to 110°	X								
0° to 120°		X							
0° to 135°			X						
Weight bearing:									
1/2 body weight	X								
Full body weight		X							
Patella mobilization	X	X	X						
Modalities:									
Electrical muscle stimulation	X	X	X						
Pain/edema management (cryotherapy)	X	X	X	X	X	X	X	X	X
Stretching:									
Hamstring, gastrocnemius-soleus complex, iliotibial band, quadriceps	X	X	X	X	X	X	X	X	X
Strengthening:									
Quadriceps isometrics, straight leg raises, active knee extension	X	X	X	X					
Closed-chain: gait retraining, toe raises, wall sits, minisquats	X	X	X	X	X	X			
Knee flexion hamstring curls (90°)	X	X	X	X	X	X	X	X	X
Knee extension quadriceps (90° to 30°)	X	X	X	X	X	X	X	X	X
Hip abduction-adduction, multihip	X	X	X	X	X	X	X	X	X
Leg press (70° to 10°)	X	X	X	X	X	X	X	X	X
Balance/proprioceptive training:									
Weight-shifting, cup walking, BBS	X	X	X	X					
BBS, BAPS, perturbation training, balance board, minitrampoline				X	X	X	X	X	
Conditioning:									
UBC	X	X	X						
Bike (stationary)		X	X	X	X	X	X	X	X
Aquatic program		X	X	X	X	X	X	X	X
Swimming (kicking)				X	X	X	X	X	X
Walking				X	X	X	X	X	X
Stair climbing machine			X	X	X	X	X	X	X
Ski machine			X	X	X	X	X	X	X
Elliptical machine				X	X	X	X	X	X
Running: straight					X	X	X	X	X
Cutting: lateral carioca, figure-8s						X	X	X	X
Plyometric training						X	X	X	X
Full sports							X	X	X

ACL = anterior cruciate ligament, BAPS = Biomechanical Ankle Platform System (Camp, Jackson, MI), BBS = Biodex Balance System (Biodex Medical Systems, Shirley, NY), UBC = upper body cycle (Biodex Medical Systems). (Adapted with permission from Heckmann TP, Noyes FR, Barber-Westin SD: Rehabilitation of primary and revision anterior cruciate ligament reconstructions, in Noyes FR, Barber-Westin SD, eds: *Noyes' Knee Disorders: Surgery, Rehabilitation, Clinical Outcomes*. Philadelphia, PA, WB Saunders, 2009, pp 306-336.)

This protocol is designed to protect healing in concomitant meniscal or ligament repairs and allograft tissues, and to avoid exacerbating articular cartilage deterioration or symptoms.

The rehabilitation protocol shown in **Table 5** was designed for patients treated with primary BPTB autogenous reconstruction of the ACL who desire a return to strenuous sports or work activities as soon as possible after surgery. All patients are warned that the early postoperative return to strenuous activities carries a risk of reinjury to the ACL-reconstructed knee or a

Table 6
Summary of Conclusions From ACL Clinical Studies by This Chapter's Authors

Variable	Conclusion
Type of graft	BPTB autografts preferred whenever possible, decreased failure rate in chronic knees, and more rapid graft healing Autografts provide higher success rate in subjective, objective, and functional parameters Allografts reserved for multiligament surgery, knee dislocations, and special situations
Sex	No difference in outcomes between males and females No scientific basis to use sex as selection criterion for reconstruction
Chronicity of injury	No difference in objective stability after BPTB autograft reconstruction Significantly poorer results in chronic knees for symptoms, limitations with sports and daily activities, and patient rating of knee condition for chronic knees caused by loss of meniscal tissue and preexisting joint damage Reconstruct ACL early after injury in active patients
Concomitant surgical procedures	Meniscus repairs frequently needed; results may be improved by concomitant ACL reconstruction High success rates, even in complex tears extending into central one third region, regardless of patient age Posterolateral injuries frequently accompanied by ACL ruptures: reconstruct all ligamentous ruptures concurrently MCL injuries usually do not require surgical treatment
Preexisting joint arthrosis	Symptomatic unstable knees can be improved by ACL reconstruction; advise return to low-impact activities
Varus osseous malalignment	ACL reconstruction is usually staged after osteotomy in symptomatic unstable knees ACL reconstruction not required after osteotomy in knees that are asymptomatic; patient willing to modify activities
Rehabilitation program	Immediate motion and rehabilitation safe, not deleterious to healing graft, low incidence (< 1%) of arthrofibrosis Identify and immediately treat limitation of knee motion with overpressure program Full motion regained within weeks of surgery (with exception of PCL reconstructions where hyperflexion is delayed)
Insurance	No difference in outcome between workers' compensation and privately insured patients except days of lost employment Reconstruct ACL in workers' compensation patients earlier after injury
Revision ACL reconstruction	BPTB or quadriceps tendon–patellar bone autograft preferred over allografts; high success rates for restoration of stability

ACL = anterior cruciate ligament, BPTB = bone-patellar tendon-bone, MCL = medial collateral ligament (Adapted with permission from Noyes FR, Barber-Westin SD: Anterior cruciate ligament primary and revision reconstruction: Diagnosis, operative techniques, and clinical outcomes, in Noyes FR, Barber-Westin SD, eds: *Noyes' Knee Disorders: Surgery, Rehabilitation, Clinical Outcomes*. Philadelphia, PA, WB Saunders, 2009, pp 140-228.)

new injury to the contralateral knee. If postoperative complications (such as knee motion problems, chronic effusion, patellofemoral pain, or patellar tendinitis) develop, the patient should be advised to slow the rehabilitation progression rate until the complications are resolved.

In all patients, the first postoperative week represents a critical time period for controlling knee joint pain and swelling, showing adequate quadriceps muscle contraction, initiating immediate knee motion exercises, and maintaining adequate limb elevation. A bulky compression dressing is used for 48 hours and then converted to compression stockings with an additional elastic bandage, if necessary. Patients are encouraged to stay in bed and elevate the limb above the heart for 5 days postoperatively, rising only to perform exercises and attend to personal and bathing needs. Prophylaxis against deep venous thrombosis includes using full-limb compression stockings, one aspirin per day for 10 days, ambulation (with crutch support) six to eight times a day for short periods of time, ankle pumping every hour that the patient is awake, and close observation of the lower limb by the therapist and surgeon. Knee joint hemarthroses require aspiration. Nonsteroidal anti-inflammatory drugs are taken for at least 5 days postoperatively. Appropriate medication is prescribed to provide pain relief and allow participation in an immediate exercise protocol.

Clinical Studies

A series of clinical outcome studies have been published on BPTB autografts in ACL reconstruction that provide information regarding the effects of the following variables on clinical outcomes: sex,[108] chronicity of injury,[20] concomitant surgical procedures,[51,52] preexisting joint arthritis,[109] the rehabilitation program,[110-112] the type of insurance (workers' compensation versus private),[113] and revision reconstructions[2,3] (**Table 6**). A higher rate of ACL graft failure was noted in knees with chronic ACL ruptures treated with fresh-frozen or irradiated allografts (16% to 30%) compared with those treated with autografts (3% to 8%). Autogenous tissue is preferred whenever possible for all ACL reconstructions. In a prospective level II study of 94 patients, no difference was noted in outcomes between men and women.[108] It was concluded that equal consideration should be given to active patients for ACL reconstruction regardless of gender. When assessing the effect of the chronicity of the ACL rupture, patients surgically treated in the acute/subacute time period had less postoperative pain, fewer limitations with sports functions, and were able to return to more strenuous activities than those who had chronic deficiencies.[20] It was concluded that joint stabilization should be performed early in active patients before reinjuries and loss of meniscal tissue. Two studies found that ACL reconstruction was effective in reducing symptoms and functional limitations and increasing activity levels in approximately two thirds of patients with advanced articular cartilage damage.[109,114]

Studies on rehabilitation protocols showed that immediate knee motion following ACL reconstruction was effective in reducing the risk of arthrofibrosis and was not deleterious to the healing graft.[110-112] There was no association found between the initial onset of abnormal AP knee displacements (> 3 mm increased displacement on knee arthrometer testing) and either the amount of time after surgery or the rehabilitation program. The failure rate was an acceptable 5%.

In ACL revision reconstructions, it was reported that either a BPTB or a quadriceps tendon–patellar bone autograft had increased success rates in terms of restoring stability compared with allograft tissues;[2,3] however, the failure rates were greater than those in primary reconstructions. Most revision knees had one or more compounding morbidities, including articular cartilage damage, meniscectomy, varus malalignment, and additional ligamentous injuries, which affected the outcome.

Summary

The ACL resists the combined motions of anterior tibial translation and internal tibial rotation that occur in the pivot-shift phenomenon. An oblique graft orientation in the sagittal and coronal planes achieved from an anatomic femoral and tibial location is effective in resisting the pivot-shift test. Tibial and femoral tunnels are drilled independently with a two-incision technique. Insufficient clinical and experimental data exist to recommend the more complex double-bundle ACL graft technique. BPTB autografts are recommended for athletes, and semitendinosus-gracilis autografts are used for recreational athletes or more sedentary patients. The postoperative rehabilitation program takes multiple factors into account and is initiated the day following surgery. The outcomes from multiple clinical studies provide the basis of recommendations for treating ACL ruptures.

References

1. Noyes FR, Barber-Westin SD, Roberts CS: Use of allografts after failed treatment of rupture of the anterior cruciate ligament. *J Bone Joint Surg Am* 1994;76(7):1019-1031.
2. Noyes FR, Barber-Westin SD: Revision anterior cruciate surgery with use of bone-patellar tendon-bone autogenous grafts. *J Bone Joint Surg Am* 2001;83-A(8): 1131-1143.
3. Noyes FR, Barber-Westin SD: Anterior cruciate ligament revision reconstruction: Results using a quadriceps tendon-patellar bone autograft. *Am J Sports Med* 2006; 34(4):553-564.
4. Noyes FR, Barber-Westin SD: Anterior cruciate ligament primary and revision reconstruction: Diagnosis, operative techniques, and clinical outcomes, in Noyes FR, Barber-Westin SD, eds: *Noyes' Knee Disorders: Surgery, Rehabilitation, Clinical Outcomes.* Philadelphia, PA, WB Saunders, 2009, pp 140-228.
5. Jackson DW, Simon TM: Donor cell survival and repopulation after intraarticular transplantation of tendon and ligament allografts. *Microsc Res Tech* 2002;58(1): 25-33.
6. Beynnon BD, Johnson RJ, Abate JA, Fleming BC, Nichols CE: Treatment of anterior cruciate ligament injuries: Part I. *Am J Sports Med* 2005;33(10): 1579-1602.
7. Beynnon BD, Johnson RJ, Abate JA, Fleming BC, Nichols CE: Treatment of anterior cruciate ligament injuries: Part 2. *Am J Sports Med* 2005;33(11): 1751-1767.
8. Arnoczky SP, Bullough PG: Healing of knee ligaments and menisci, in Insall JN, Scott WN, eds: *Surgery of the Knee.* Philadelphia, PA, WB Saunders, 2001, pp 457-471.
9. Beynnon BD, Johnson RJ, Fleming BC: The science of anterior cruciate ligament rehabilitation. *Clin Orthop Relat Res* 2002;402: 9-20.
10. Howell SM, Taylor MA: Failure of reconstruction of the anterior

cruciate ligament due to impingement by the intercondylar roof. *J Bone Joint Surg Am* 1993;75(7): 1044-1055.

11. Carson EW, Anisko EM, Restrepo C, Panariello RA, O'Brien SJ, Warren RF: Revision anterior cruciate ligament reconstruction: Etiology of failures and clinical results. *J Knee Surg* 2004; 17(3):127-132.
12. Denti M, Lo Vetere D, Bait C, Schönhuber H, Melegati G, Volpi P: Revision anterior cruciate ligament reconstruction: Causes of failure, surgical technique, and clinical results. *Am J Sports Med* 2008;36(10):1896-1902.
13. George MS, Dunn WR, Spindler KP: Current concepts review: Revision anterior cruciate ligament reconstruction. *Am J Sports Med* 2006;34(12):2026-2037.
14. Noyes FR: The function of the human anterior cruciate ligament and analysis of single- and double-bundle graft reconstructions. *Sports Health: A Multidisciplinary Approach* 2009;1:66-75. http://sph.sagepub.com/content/1/1.toc. Accessed June 11, 2010.
15. Heckmann TP, Noyes FR, Barber-Westin SD: Rehabilitation of primary and revision anterior cruciate ligament reconstructions, in Noyes FR, Barber-Westin SD, eds: *Noyes' Knee Disorders: Surgery, Rehabilitation, Clinical Outcomes.* Philadelphia, PA, WB Saunders, 2009, pp 306-336.
16. Diamantopoulos AP, Lorbach O, Paessler HH: Anterior cruciate ligament revision reconstruction: Results in 107 patients. *Am J Sports Med* 2008;36(5):851-860.
17. Kondo E, Yasuda K, Azuma H, Tanabe Y, Yagi T: Prospective clinical comparisons of anatomic double-bundle versus single-bundle anterior cruciate ligament reconstruction procedures in 328 consecutive patients. *Am J Sports Med* 2008;36(9):1675-1687.
18. Busam ML, Provencher MT, Bach BR Jr: Complications of anterior cruciate ligament reconstruction with bone-patellar tendon-bone constructs: Care and prevention. *Am J Sports Med* 2008;36(2):379-394.
19. Rue JP, Ghodadra N, Bach BR Jr: Femoral tunnel placement in single-bundle anterior cruciate ligament reconstruction: A cadaveric study relating transtibial lateralized femoral tunnel position to the anteromedial and posterolateral bundle femoral origins of the anterior cruciate ligament. *Am J Sports Med* 2008;36(1):73-79.
20. Noyes FR, Barber-Westin SD: A comparison of results in acute and chronic anterior cruciate ligament ruptures of arthroscopically assisted autogenous patellar tendon reconstruction. *Am J Sports Med* 1997;25(4):460-471.
21. Heming JF, Rand J, Steiner ME: Anatomical limitations of transtibial drilling in anterior cruciate ligament reconstruction. *Am J Sports Med* 2007;35(10):1708-1715.
22. Brandsson S, Faxén E, Eriksson BI, Swärd L, Lundin O, Karlsson J: Reconstruction of the anterior cruciate ligament: Comparison of outside-in and all-inside techniques. *Br J Sports Med* 1999;33(1):42-45.
23. Hess T, Duchow J, Roland S, Kohn D: Single-versus two-incision technique in anterior cruciate ligament replacement: Influence on postoperative muscle function. *Am J Sports Med* 2002; 30(1):27-31.
24. Panni AS, Milano G, Tartarone M, Demontis A, Fabbriciani C: Clinical and radiographic results of ACL reconstruction: A 5- to 7-year follow-up study of outside-in versus inside-out reconstruction techniques. *Knee Surg Sports Traumatol Arthrosc* 2001; 9(2):77-85.
25. Aglietti P, Giron F, Cuomo P, Losco M, Mondanelli N: Single- and double-incision double-bundle ACL reconstruction. *Clin Orthop Relat Res* 2007;454: 108-113.
26. Järvelä T, Moisala AS, Sihvonen R, Järvelä S, Kannus P, Järvinen M: Double-bundle anterior cruciate ligament reconstruction using hamstring autografts and bioabsorbable interference screw fixation: Prospective, randomized, clinical study with 2-year results. *Am J Sports Med* 2008;36(2):290-297.
27. Siebold R, Dehler C, Ellert T: Prospective randomized comparison of double-bundle versus single-bundle anterior cruciate ligament reconstruction. *Arthroscopy* 2008;24(2):137-145.
28. Zelle BA, Vidal AF, Brucker PU, Fu FH: Double-bundle reconstruction of the anterior cruciate ligament: Anatomic and biomechanical rationale. *J Am Acad Orthop Surg* 2007;15(2):87-96.
29. Zhao J, Peng X, He Y, Wang J: Two-bundle anterior cruciate ligament reconstruction with eight-stranded hamstring tendons: Four-tunnel technique. *Knee* 2006;13(1):36-41.
30. Streich NA, Friedrich K, Gotterbarm T, Schmitt H: Reconstruction of the ACL with a semitendinosus tendon graft: A prospective randomized single blinded comparison of double-bundle versus single-bundle technique in male athletes. *Knee Surg Sports Traumatol Arthrosc* 2008;16(3):232-238.
31. Asagumo H, Kimura M, Kobayashi Y, Taki M, Takagishi K: Anatomic reconstruction of the anterior cruciate ligament using double-bundle hamstring tendons: Surgical techniques, clinical outcomes, and complications. *Arthroscopy* 2007;23(6):602-609.
32. Adachi N, Ochi M, Uchio Y, Iwasa J, Kuriwaka M, Ito Y: Reconstruction of the anterior cruci-

ate ligament: Single- versus double-bundle multistranded hamstring tendons. *J Bone Joint Surg Br* 2004;86(4):515-520.

33. Markolf KL, Park S, Jackson SR, McAllister DR: Simulated pivot-shift testing with single and double-bundle anterior cruciate ligament reconstructions. *J Bone Joint Surg Am* 2008;90(8):1681-1689.

34. Yamamoto Y, Hsu WH, Woo SL, Van Scyoc AH, Takakura Y, Debski RE: Knee stability and graft function after anterior cruciate ligament reconstruction: A comparison of a lateral and an anatomical femoral tunnel placement. *Am J Sports Med* 2004;32(8):1825-1832.

35. Drogset JO, Grøntvedt T, Robak OR, Mølster A, Viset AT, Engebretsen LA: A sixteen-year follow-up of three operative techniques for the treatment of acute ruptures of the anterior cruciate ligament. *J Bone Joint Surg Am* 2006;88(5):944-952.

36. Hart AJ, Buscombe J, Malone A, Dowd GS: Assessment of osteoarthritis after reconstruction of the anterior cruciate ligament: A study using single-photon emission computed tomography at ten years. *J Bone Joint Surg Br* 2005;87(11):1483-1487.

37. Hertel P, Behrend H, Cierpinski T, Musahl V, Widjaja G: ACL reconstruction using bone-patellar tendon-bone press-fit fixation: 10-year clinical results. *Knee Surg Sports Traumatol Arthrosc* 2005;13(4):248-255.

38. Lebel B, Hulet C, Galaud B, Burdin G, Locker B, Vielpeau C: Arthroscopic reconstruction of the anterior cruciate ligament using bone-patellar tendon-bone autograft: A minimum 10-year follow-up. *Am J Sports Med* 2008;36(7):1275-1282.

39. Wu WH, Hackett T, Richmond JC: Effects of meniscal and articular surface status on knee stability, function, and symptoms after anterior cruciate ligament reconstruction: A long-term prospective study. *Am J Sports Med* 2002;30(6):845-850.

40. Krych AJ, Jackson JD, Hoskin TL, Dahm DL: A meta-analysis of patellar tendon autograft versus patellar tendon allograft in anterior cruciate ligament reconstruction. *Arthroscopy* 2008;24(3):292-298.

41. Malinin TI, Levitt RL, Bashore C, Temple HT, Mnaymneh W: A study of retrieved allografts used to replace anterior cruciate ligaments. *Arthroscopy* 2002;18(2):163-170.

42. Singhal MC, Gardiner JR, Johnson DL: Failure of primary anterior cruciate ligament surgery using anterior tibialis allograft. *Arthroscopy* 2007;23(5):469-475.

43. Bernicker JP, Haddad JL, Lintner DM, DiLiberti TC, Bocell JR: Patellar tendon defect during the first year after anterior cruciate ligament reconstruction: Appearance on serial magnetic resonance imaging. *Arthroscopy* 1998;14(8):804-809.

44. Kartus J, Stener S, Lindahl S, Eriksson BI, Karlsson J: Ipsi- or contralateral patellar tendon graft in anterior cruciate ligament revision surgery: A comparison of two methods. *Am J Sports Med* 1998;26(4):499-504.

45. LaPrade RF, Hamilton CD, Montgomery RD, Wentorf F, Hawkins HD: The reharvested central third of the patellar tendon: A histologic and biomechanical analysis. *Am J Sports Med* 1997;25(6):779-785.

46. Lidén M, Ejerhed L, Sernert N, Bovaller A, Karlsson J, Kartus J: The course of the patellar tendon after reharvesting its central third for ACL revision surgery: A long-term clinical and radiographic study. *Knee Surg Sports Traumatol Arthrosc* 2006;14(11):1130-1138.

47. Lidén M, Movin T, Ejerhed L, et al: A histological and ultrastructural evaluation of the patellar tendon 10 years after reharvesting its central third. *Am J Sports Med* 2008;36(4):781-788.

48. Noyes FR, Barber-Westin SD: Primary, double, and triple varus knee syndromes: Diagnosis, osteotomy techniques, and clinical outcomes, in Noyes FR, Barber-Westin SD, eds: *Noyes' Knee Disorders: Surgery, Rehabilitation, Clinical Outcomes*. Philadelphia, PA, WB Saunders, 2009, pp 821-895.

49. Noyes FR, Barber SD, Simon R: High tibial osteotomy and ligament reconstruction in varus angulated, anterior cruciate ligament-deficient knees. A two- to seven-year follow-up study. *Am J Sports Med* 1993;21(1):2-12.

50. Rubman MH, Noyes FR, Barber-Westin SD: Arthroscopic repair of meniscal tears that extend into the avascular zone: A review of 198 single and complex tears. *Am J Sports Med* 1998;26(1):87-95.

51. Noyes FR, Barber-Westin SD: Arthroscopic repair of meniscus tears extending into the avascular zone with or without anterior cruciate ligament reconstruction in patients 40 years of age and older. *Arthroscopy* 2000;16(8):822-829.

52. Noyes FR, Barber-Westin SD: Arthroscopic repair of meniscal tears extending into the avascular zone in patients younger than twenty years of age. *Am J Sports Med* 2002;30(4):589-600.

53. Shelbourne KD, Gray T: Minimum 10-year results after anterior cruciate ligament reconstruction: How the loss of normal knee motion compounds other factors related to the development of osteoarthritis after surgery. *Am J Sports Med* 2009;37(3):471-480.

54. Nakata K, Shino K, Horibe S, et al: Arthroscopic anterior cruci-

ate ligament reconstruction using fresh-frozen bone plug-free allogeneic tendons: 10-year follow-up. *Arthroscopy* 2008;24(3):285-291.

55. Cohen M, Amaro JT, Ejnisman B, et al: Anterior cruciate ligament reconstruction after 10 to 15 years: Association between meniscectomy and osteoarthrosis. *Arthroscopy* 2007;23(6):629-634.
56. Noyes FR, Barber-Westin SD: Meniscus tears: Diagnosis, repair techniques, and clinical outcomes, in Noyes FR, Barber-Westin SD, eds: *Noyes' Knee Disorders: Surgery, Rehabilitation, Clinical Outcomes.* Philadelphia, PA, WB Saunders, 2009, pp 733-771.
57. Heckmann TP, Noyes FR, Barber-Westin SD: Rehabilitation of meniscus repair and transplantation procedures, in Noyes FR, Barber-Westin SD, eds: *Noyes' Knee Disorders: Surgery, Rehabilitation, Clinical Outcomes.* Philadelphia, PA, WB Saunders, 2009, pp 806-817.
58. Noyes FR, Cummings JF, Grood ES, Walz-Hasselfeld KA, Wroble RR: The diagnosis of knee motion limits, subluxations, and ligament injury. *Am J Sports Med* 1991;19(2):163-171.
59. Rosenberg TD, Paulos LE, Parker RD, Coward DB, Scott SM: The forty-five-degree posteroanterior flexion weight-bearing radiograph of the knee. *J Bone Joint Surg Am* 1988;70(10):1479-1483.
60. Chang CB, Seong SC, Kim TK: Preoperative magnetic resonance assessment of patellar tendon dimensions for graft selection in anterior cruciate ligament reconstruction. *Am J Sports Med* 2009; 37(2):376-382.
61. Potter HG, Foo LF: Magnetic resonance imaging of articular cartilage: Trauma, degeneration, and repair. *Am J Sports Med* 2006; 34(4):661-677.
62. Barber-Westin SD, Noyes FR, McCloskey JW: Rigorous statistical reliability, validity, and responsiveness testing of the Cincinnati knee rating system in 350 subjects with uninjured, injured, or anterior cruciate ligament-reconstructed knees. *Am J Sports Med* 1999;27(4):402-416.
63. Butler DL, Noyes FR, Grood ES: Ligamentous restraints to anterior-posterior drawer in the human knee: A biomechanical study. *J Bone Joint Surg Am* 1980; 62(2):259-270.
64. Noyes FR, Grood ES: Classification of ligament injuries: Why an anterolateral laxity or anteromedial laxity is not a diagnostic entity. *Instr Course Lect* 1987;36: 185-200.
65. Wroble RR, Grood ES, Cummings JS, Henderson JM, Noyes FR: The role of the lateral extraarticular restraints in the anterior cruciate ligament-deficient knee. *Am J Sports Med* 1993; 21(2):257-262, discussion 263.
66. Monaco E, Labianca L, Conteduca F, De Carli A, Ferretti A: Double bundle or single bundle plus extraarticular tenodesis in ACL reconstruction? A CAOS study. *Knee Surg Sports Traumatol Arthrosc* 2007;15(10):1168-1174.
67. Noyes FR, Grood ES, Cummings JF, Wroble RR: An analysis of the pivot shift phenomenon: The knee motions and subluxations induced by different examiners. *Am J Sports Med* 1991; 19(2):148-155.
68. Noyes FR, Bassett RW, Grood ES, Butler DL: Arthroscopy in acute traumatic hemarthrosis of the knee: Incidence of anterior cruciate tears and other injuries. *J Bone Joint Surg Am* 1980;62(5):687-695.
69. Noyes FR, Grood ES, Suntay WJ: Three-dimensional motion analysis of clinical stress tests for anterior knee subluxations. *Acta Orthop Scand* 1989;60(3):308-318.
70. Haimes JL, Wroble RR, Grood ES, Noyes FR: Role of the medial structures in the intact and anterior cruciate ligament-deficient knee: Limits of motion in the human knee. *Am J Sports Med* 1994;22(3):402-409.
71. Edwards A, Bull AM, Amis AA: The attachments of the anteromedial and posterolateral fibre bundles of the anterior cruciate ligament: Part 1. Tibial attachment. *Knee Surg Sports Traumatol Arthrosc* 2007;15(12):1414-1421.
72. Yagi M, Wong EK, Kanamori A, Debski RE, Fu FH, Woo SL: Biomechanical analysis of an anatomic anterior cruciate ligament reconstruction. *Am J Sports Med* 2002;30(5):660-666.
73. Zelle BA, Brucker PU, Feng MT, Fu FH: Anatomical double-bundle anterior cruciate ligament reconstruction. *Sports Med* 2006; 36(2):99-108.
74. Petersen W, Tretow H, Weimann A, et al: Biomechanical evaluation of two techniques for double-bundle anterior cruciate ligament reconstruction: One tibial tunnel versus two tibial tunnels. *Am J Sports Med* 2007;35(2): 228-234.
75. Zantop T, Wellmann M, Fu FH, Petersen W: Tunnel positioning of anteromedial and posterolateral bundles in anatomic anterior cruciate ligament reconstruction: Anatomic and radiographic findings. *Am J Sports Med* 2008;36(1): 65-72.
76. Amis AA, Dawkins GP: Functional anatomy of the anterior cruciate ligament: Fibre bundle actions related to ligament replacements and injuries. *J Bone Joint Surg Br* 1991;73(2): 260-267.
77. Edwards A, Bull AM, Amis AA: The attachments of the fiber bundles of the posterior cruciate ligament: An anatomic study. *Arthroscopy* 2007;23(3):284-290.

78. Gabriel MT, Wong EK, Woo SL, Yagi M, Debski RE: Distribution of in situ forces in the anterior cruciate ligament in response to rotatory loads. *J Orthop Res* 2004; 22(1):85-89.

79. Sidles JA, Larson RV, Garbini JL, Downey DJ, Matsen FA III: Ligament length relationships in the moving knee. *J Orthop Res* 1988; 6(4):593-610.

80. Hefzy MS, Grood ES, Noyes FR: Factors affecting the region of most isometric femoral attachments: Part II. The anterior cruciate ligament. *Am J Sports Med* 1989;17(2):208-216.

81. Edwards A, Bull AM, Amis AA: The attachments of the anteromedial and posterolateral fibre bundles of the anterior cruciate ligament: Part 2. femoral attachment. *Knee Surg Sports Traumatol Arthrosc* 2008;16(1):29-36.

82. Li G, Defrate LE, Rubash HE, Gill TJ: In vivo kinematics of the ACL during weight-bearing knee flexion. *J Orthop Res* 2005;23(2): 340-344.

83. Mae T, Shino K, Miyama T, et al: Single- versus two-femoral socket anterior cruciate ligament reconstruction technique: Biomechanical analysis using a robotic simulator. *Arthroscopy* 2001;17(7): 708-716.

84. Markolf KL, Park S, Jackson SR, McAllister DR: Contributions of the posterolateral bundle of the anterior cruciate ligament to anterior-posterior knee laxity and ligament forces. *Arthroscopy* 2008; 24(7):805-809.

85. Ekdahl M, Nozaki M, Ferretti M, Tsai A, Smolinski P, Fu FH: The effect of tunnel placement on bone-tendon healing in anterior cruciate ligament reconstruction in a goat model. *Am J Sports Med* 2009;37(8):1522-1530.

86. Scanlan SF, Blazek K, Chaudhari AM, Safran MR, Andriacchi TP: Graft orientation influences the knee flexion moment during walking in patients with anterior cruciate ligament reconstruction. *Am J Sports Med* 2009;37(11): 2173-2178.

87. Steiner ME: Independent drilling of tibial and femoral tunnels in anterior cruciate ligament reconstruction. *J Knee Surg* 2009;22(2): 171-176.

88. Hutchinson MR, Ash SA: Resident's ridge: Assessing the cortical thickness of the lateral wall and roof of the intercondylar notch. *Arthroscopy* 2003;19(9):931-935.

89. Harner CD, Baek GH, Vogrin TM, Carlin GJ, Kashiwaguchi S, Woo SL: Quantitative analysis of human cruciate ligament insertions. *Arthroscopy* 1999; 15(7):741-749.

90. Girgis FG, Marshall JL, Monajem AL: The cruciate ligaments of the knee joint: Anatomical, functional and experimental analysis. *Clin Orthop Relat Res* 1975;106:216-231.

91. Ferretti M, Ekdahl M, Shen W, Fu FH: Osseous landmarks of the femoral attachment of the anterior cruciate ligament: An anatomic study. *Arthroscopy* 2007;23(11): 1218-1225.

92. Colombet P, Robinson J, Christel P, et al: Morphology of anterior cruciate ligament attachments for anatomic reconstruction: A cadaveric dissection and radiographic study. *Arthroscopy* 2006; 22(9):984-992.

93. Petersen W, Zantop T: Anatomy of the anterior cruciate ligament with regard to its two bundles. *Clin Orthop Relat Res* 2007;454: 35-47.

94. Luites JW, Wymenga AB, Blankevoort L, Kooloos JG: Description of the attachment geometry of the anteromedial and posterolateral bundles of the ACL from arthroscopic perspective for anatomical tunnel placement. *Knee Surg Sports Traumatol Arthrosc* 2007;15(12):1422-1431.

95. Stäubli HU, Rauschning W: Tibial attachment area of the anterior cruciate ligament in the extended knee position. Anatomy and cryosections in vitro complemented by magnetic resonance arthrography in vivo. *Knee Surg Sports Traumatol Arthrosc* 1994; 2(3):138-146.

96. Siebold R, Ellert T, Metz S, Metz J: Tibial insertions of the anteromedial and posterolateral bundles of the anterior cruciate ligament: Morphometry, arthroscopic landmarks, and orientation model for bone tunnel placement. *Arthroscopy* 2008; 24(2):154-161.

97. Takahashi M, Matsubara T, Doi M, Suzuki D, Nagano A: Anatomical study of the femoral and tibial insertions of the anterolateral and posteromedial bundles of human posterior cruciate ligament. *Knee Surg Sports Traumatol Arthrosc* 2006;14(11):1055-1059.

98. Clancy WG Jr, Nelson DA, Reider B, Narechania RG: Anterior cruciate ligament reconstruction using one-third of the patellar ligament, augmented by extra-articular tendon transfers. *J Bone Joint Surg Am* 1982;64(3): 352-359.

99. Steiner ME, Murray MM, Rodeo SA: Strategies to improve anterior cruciate ligament healing and graft placement. *Am J Sports Med* 2008;36(1):176-189.

100. Arnold MP, Kooloos J, van Kampen A: Single-incision technique misses the anatomical femoral anterior cruciate ligament insertion: A cadaver study. *Knee Surg Sports Traumatol Arthrosc* 2001;9(4):194-199.

101. Simmons R, Howell SM, Hull ML: Effect of the angle of the femoral and tibial tunnels in the coronal plane and incremental excision of the posterior cruciate ligament on tension of an anterior

cruciate ligament graft: An in vitro study. *J Bone Joint Surg Am* 2003;85-A(6):1018-1029.

102. Muneta T, Koga H, Mochizuki T, et al: A prospective randomized study of 4-strand semitendinosus tendon anterior cruciate ligament reconstruction comparing single-bundle and double-bundle techniques. *Arthroscopy* 2007;23(6): 618-628.

103. Yasuda K, Kondo E, Ichiyama H, Tanabe Y, Tohyama H: Clinical evaluation of anatomic double-bundle anterior cruciate ligament reconstruction procedure using hamstring tendon grafts: Comparisons among 3 different procedures. *Arthroscopy* 2006;22(3): 240-251.

104. Yagi M, Kuroda R, Nagamune K, Yoshiya S, Kurosaka M: Double-bundle ACL reconstruction can improve rotational stability. *Clin Orthop Relat Res* 2007;454: 100-107.

105. Hamada M, Shino K, Horibe S, et al: Single- versus bi-socket anterior cruciate ligament reconstruction using autogenous multiple-stranded hamstring tendons with endoButton femoral fixation: A prospective study. *Arthroscopy* 2001;17(8):801-807.

106. Meredick RB, Vance KJ, Appleby D, Lubowitz JH: Outcome of single-bundle versus double-bundle reconstruction of the anterior cruciate ligament: A meta-analysis. *Am J Sports Med* 2008; 36(7):1414-1421.

107. Noyes FR, Barber-Westin SD: Prevention and treatment of knee arthrofibrosis, in Noyes FR, Barber-Westin SD, eds: *Noyes' Knee Disorders: Surgery, Rehabilitation, Clinical Outcomes*. Philadelphia, PA, WB Saunders, 2009, pp 1053-1095.

108. Barber-Westin SD, Noyes FR, Andrews M: A rigorous comparison between the sexes of results and complications after anterior cruciate ligament reconstruction. *Am J Sports Med* 1997;25(4): 514-526.

109. Noyes FR, Barber-Westin SD: Anterior cruciate ligament reconstruction with autogenous patellar tendon graft in patients with articular cartilage damage. *Am J Sports Med* 1997;25(5):626-634.

110. Barber-Westin SD, Noyes FR: The effect of rehabilitation and return to activity on anterior-posterior knee displacements after anterior cruciate ligament reconstruction. *Am J Sports Med* 1993; 21(2):264-270.

111. Barber-Westin SD, Noyes FR, Heckmann TP, Shaffer BL: The effect of exercise and rehabilitation on anterior-posterior knee displacements after anterior cruciate ligament autograft reconstruction. *Am J Sports Med* 1999;27(1): 84-93.

112. Noyes FR, Berrios-Torres S, Barber-Westin SD, Heckmann TP: Prevention of permanent arthrofibrosis after anterior cruciate ligament reconstruction alone or combined with associated procedures: A prospective study in 443 knees. *Knee Surg Sports Traumatol Arthrosc* 2000;8(4):196-206.

113. Noyes FR, Barber-Westin SD: A comparison of results of arthroscopic-assisted anterior cruciate ligament reconstruction between workers' compensation and noncompensation patients. *Arthroscopy* 1997;13(4):474-484.

114. Noyes FR, Barber-Westin SD: Arthroscopic-assisted allograft anterior cruciate ligament reconstruction in patients with symptomatic arthrosis. *Arthroscopy* 1997; 13(1):24-32.

Management of Complex Knee Ligament Injuries

Gregory C. Fanelli, MD
James P. Stannard, MD
Michael J. Stuart, MD
Peter B. MacDonald, MD, FRCS
Robert G. Marx, MD, FRCSC
Daniel B. Whelan, MD, FRCSC
Joel L. Boyd, MD
Bruce A. Levy, MD

Abstract

The ideal management of the dislocated knee remains controversial. These injuries often can be elusive; a significant number of dislocated knees spontaneously reduce and appear relatively benign on routine radiographs. A high index of suspicion, based on the mechanism of injury, soft-tissue assessment of the limb, and the level of knee instability should alert the physician to the possibility of a dislocated knee. Early recognition and appropriate neurovascular assessment is paramount to the successful treatment of these complex injuries.

Controversies exist regarding surgical versus nonsurgical management, early versus delayed surgery, the use of allograft versus autograft tissue, the decision to repair versus reconstruct torn ligamentous structures, and the type of reconstruction technique and postoperative rehabilitation program.

To achieve optimal patient care, it is important to be aware of the current evaluation and treatment strategies for complex knee ligament injuries, including modern anatomic reconstruction techniques. Current recommendations include measurement of the ankle-brachial indices in each patient, early surgical management, the use of autograft or allograft tissue, reconstruction as opposed to repair alone of the fibular collateral ligament/posterolateral corner structures, reconstruction of the anterior and posterior cruciate ligaments, and repair and/or reconstruction of the medial collateral ligament/posteromedial corner depending on the injury pattern and the quality of tissue.

Instr Course Lect 2011;60:523-535.

Initial Evaluation of Acute and Chronic Multiligament Knee Injuries

Initial evaluation of a knee with multiple ligament injuries begins with a thorough and complete neurovascular examination, an assessment of the soft tissue, and determination of the instability pattern. Failure to recognize a vascular injury can lead to catastrophic limb dysfunction and ultimately to amputation. Injury to the tibial and/or peroneal nerves can also have devastating consequences and is encountered in almost 25% of dislocated knees.[1] The modified Schenck classification, in which not only ligamentous structures but also neurovascular injury and the presence of periarticular fracture are taken into account, is widely used to describe these injuries.[2]

Vascular Assessment

There are several algorithms for the assessment of vascular injury of the lower limb. Vascular assessment may include physical examination alone, use of the ankle-brachial index, arterial ultrasound, and conventional and/or CT angiography. A palpable pulse may be present distal to a complete popliteal arterial occlusion because of the presence of collateral flow (**Figure 1**). When a patient presents with "hard signs" of ischemia, which include a cool, pulseless, obviously dysvascular limb, immediate vascular surgery consultation is warranted. When

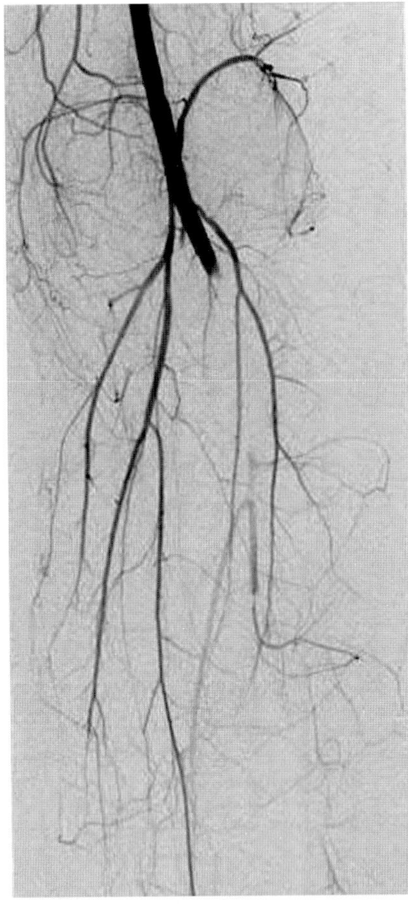

Figure 1 Conventional arteriogram showing collateral flow to the distal part of the lower extremity despite complete popliteal artery occlusion.

the level of the lesion (for example, the popliteal artery in the setting of a dislocated knee) is known, the vascular surgeon may opt for immediate surgical exploration or proceed with angiography. Typically, a saphenous vein bypass graft obtained from the contralateral side is used to reestablish arterial flow, and concomitant prophylactic four-compartment fasciotomies are

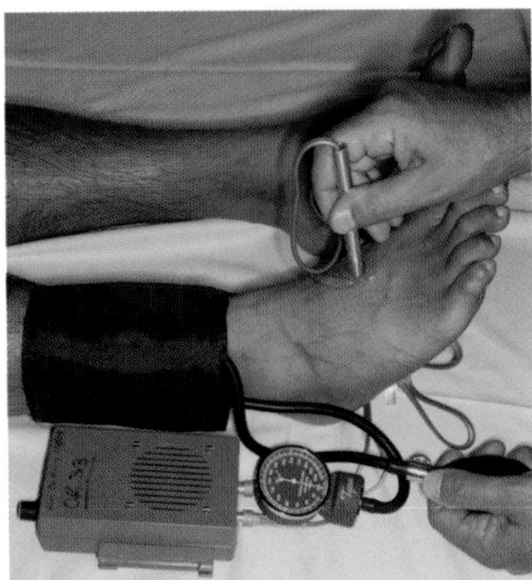

Figure 2 Measurement of the ankle-brachial index.

done. When a patient presents with "soft signs" of ischemia, including palpable but asymmetric pulses and asymmetric warmth and/or color of the limb, further assessment is needed.

The ankle-brachial index is determined by obtaining the systolic blood pressure of the affected limb at the level of the ankle and comparing it with the systolic blood pressure of the ipsilateral arm at the level of the brachial artery (**Figure 2**): ankle-brachial index = Doppler systolic arterial pressure in the injured limb (ankle) ÷ Doppler systolic arterial pressure in the uninjured limb (brachial).

Mills et al[3] showed that when the ankle-brachial index is 0.9 or greater, there is no risk of a major arterial injury, but because delayed thrombus is a risk, serial pulse examination should be done every 4 to 6 hours for a period of 24 hours. When the ankle-brachial index is less than 0.9, either arterial ultrasound or CT angiography should be done.[4] Duplex arterial ultrasound has excellent sensitivity and specificity; however, it is technician-dependent, and not all centers have around-the-clock access to an ultrasound technician. The advantage of CT angiography over conventional angiography is that there is fewer than one fourth the dose of radiation, access is obtained through the antecubital fossa as opposed to the groin, and CT angiography is 100% sensitive and specific.[5] Conventional angiography has a 5% to 7% false-positive rate.

Neurologic Assessment

Niall et al[1] reported the risk of peroneal nerve injury with dislocation of the knee to be approximately 25%. In their series, fewer than 50% of the patients had nerve recovery. Prompt placement of an ankle-foot orthosis in the early postinjury period is important to prevent equinus deformity from Achilles tendon contracture.

Treatment of a peroneal nerve palsy can include sural nerve grafting, direct repair, neurolysis, and tibial tendon transfer, but the success of treatment can vary widely. The direct transfer of tibial nerve motor branches to the peroneal nerve has promise, but the long-term results of this procedure are unknown.

Diagnostic Imaging

A substantial number of dislocated knees spontaneously reduce, and radiographic findings may be subtle, but standard AP and lateral radiographs of the knee are necessary following this injury. Joint asymmetry, mild tibio-

Dr. Stannard or an immediate family member serves as a board member, owner, officer, or committee member of the Orthopaedic Trauma Association; is a member of a speakers' bureau or has made paid presentations on behalf of Medtronic and Synthes; serves as a paid consultant to or is an employee of Medtronic and NovaLign; and has received research or institutional support from Kinetic Concepts, Medtronic, Smith & Nephew, and Synthes. Dr. Stuart or an immediate family member has received royalties from Fios; serves as a paid consultant to or is an employee of Arthrex and Fios; and has received research or institutional support from DePuy, Biotmet, Stryker, and Zimmer. Dr. MacDonald or an immediate family member is a member of a speakers' bureau or has made paid presentations on behalf of Linvatec; serves as an unpaid consultant to Linvatec; and has received research or institutional support from Linvatec and Ossur. Dr. Boyd or an immediate family member serves as a paid consultant to or is an employee of Zimmer and serves as an unpaid consultant to Regeneration Technologies. Dr. Levy or an immediate family member has received royalties from VOT Technologies; serves as a paid consultant to or is an employee of Arthrex; and has received research or institutional support from National Institutes of Health (NIAMS & NICHD). None of the following authors nor any immediate family member has received anything of value from or owns stock in a commercial company or institution related directly or indirectly to the subject of this chapter: Dr. Fanelli, Dr. Marx, and Dr. Whelan.

femoral subluxation, avulsion fractures, and rim fractures are clues to the extent of the injury. In the nonacute setting, bilateral comparison stress radiography (varus, valgus, and posterior) can help to determine the extent of ligamentous instability. LaPrade et al[6] reported that demonstration of a side-to-side difference of 2.7 mm on comparison of varus stress AP radiographs indicates a fibular collateral ligament injury, whereas a side-to-side difference of more than 4.0 mm indicates a fibular collateral ligament and posterolateral corner injury. In the acute setting, fluoroscopic stress examination under anesthesia helps to confirm clinical and/or MRI findings.

MRI is the diagnostic imaging modality of choice after radiographs have been obtained. MRI identifies the ligament injury and its specific location and extent, both of which are critical for surgical planning.

Indications for Emergency Surgical Treatment

The indications for emergency surgical treatment include an open knee dislocation, an irreducible knee dislocation, and a compartment syndrome. Open knee dislocations require aggressive irrigation and débridement and placement of antibiotic bead pouches and/or a wound vacuum-assisted closure device (VAC; Kinetic Concepts, San Antonio, TX) and may warrant plastic surgery for soft-tissue coverage. The irreducible knee dislocation is typically a posterolateral dislocation in which the medial femoral condyle buttonholes through the medial aspect of the capsule and/or the medial collateral ligament, causing a classic puckering of the medial skin. Prompt reduction is imperative to avoid skin necrosis and typically requires an open arthrotomy. In emergency cases such as these, definitive ligament repair or reconstruction is usually performed in a staged fashion, once all débridement and/or wound considerations have been addressed and the soft tissues have healed satisfactorily to allow additional surgery. Indications for the immediate placement of joint-spanning external fixation include vascular injury requiring repair, an open knee dislocation, and the inability to maintain tibiofemoral joint reduction by other means.[7,8]

Combined Posterior and Anterior Cruciate Ligament Reconstruction

The principles of reconstruction in a knee with multiple ligament injuries include identification and treatment of all torn ligaments with accurate tunnel placement, anatomic graft insertion sites, utilization of strong graft material, secure graft fixation, and an extensive postoperative rehabilitation program.[8-24]

An Achilles tendon allograft is the preferred graft of this chapter's authors for single-bundle posterior cruciate ligament reconstructions, and the Achilles tendon and tibialis anterior allografts are preferred for double-bundle posterior cruciate ligament reconstructions. Either a tibialis anterior or a patellar tendon allograft is preferred for anterior cruciate ligament reconstructions. The allograft tissue is prepared, and arthroscopic instruments are placed with the inflow in the superolateral portal, the arthroscope in the inferolateral patellar portal, and instruments in the inferomedial patellar portal. An accessory extracapsular extra-articular posteromedial safety incision is used to protect the neurovascular structures and to confirm the accuracy of tibial tunnel placement.

Notch preparation is performed first and consists of anterior cruciate and posterior cruciate ligament stump débridement, bone removal, and contouring of the medial and lateral walls and roof of the intercondylar notch. Specially designed 90° curets and rasps placed through the notch to the posterior aspect of the tibia are used to elevate the capsule and clearly identify the tibial footprint of the posterior cruciate ligament.

The arm of the posterior cruciate ligament–anterior cruciate ligament guide is inserted through the inferomedial patellar portal to begin creation of the tibial tunnel for the posterior cruciate ligament graft. The tip of the guide is positioned at the inferolateral aspect of the anatomic insertion site of the posterior cruciate ligament. The bullet portion of the guide contacts the anteromedial surface of the proximal part of the tibia at a point midway between the posteromedial border of the tibia and the anterior aspect of the tibial crest approximately 1 cm below the tibial tubercle. This will provide an angle of graft orientation such that the graft will turn two very smooth 45° angles on the posterior aspect of the tibia and will not have an acute 90°-angle turn, which may cause pressure necrosis of the graft. The tip of the guide in the posterior aspect of the tibia is confirmed with the surgeon's finger through the extracapsular extra-articular posteromedial safety incision. Intraoperative AP and lateral radiographs may also be used. The surgeon's finger confirms the position of the guidewire through the posteromedial safety incision, providing a double safety check. The appropriately sized standard cannulated reamer is used to create the tibial tunnel. The surgeon's finger through the extracapsular extra-articular posteromedial incision monitors the position of the guidewire. The drill is advanced until it comes to the posterior cortex of the tibia. The chuck is disengaged from the drill, and the tibial tunnel is completed by hand, which provides an additional margin of safety for completing the tibial tunnel.

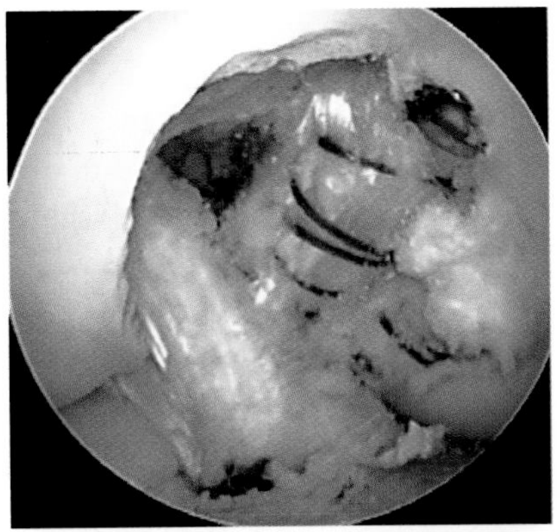

Figure 3 Double-bundle posterior cruciate ligament reconstruction with of an Achilles tendon allograft (anterolateral bundle) and a tibialis anterior allograft (posteromedial bundle) is shown, as well as anterior cruciate ligament reconstruction with an Achilles tendon allograft.

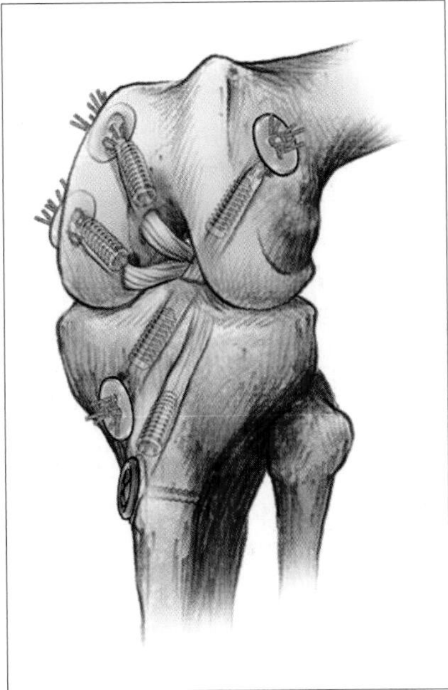

Figure 4 Illustration showing fixation, tunnel, and graft positioning in a combined reconstruction of the posterior and anterior cruciate ligaments. Note the primary aperture-opening fixation combined with cortical suspensory back-up fixation. (Reproduced with permission from Fanelli GC: *Rationale and Surgical Technique for PCL and Multiple Knee Ligament Reconstruction.* Warsaw, IN, Biomet Sports Medicine, 2008.)

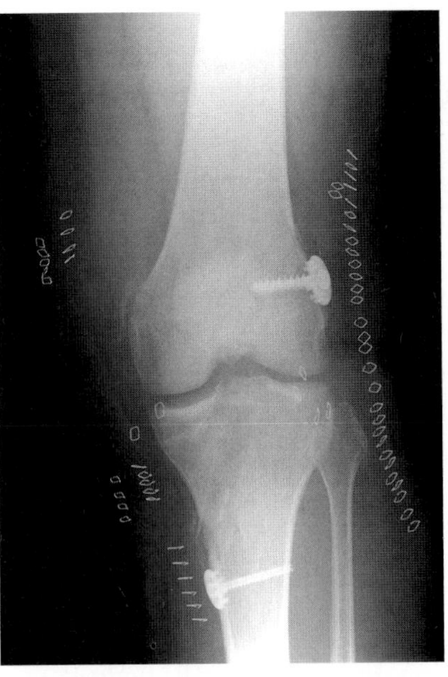

Figure 5 Postoperative radiograph made after reconstruction of the anterior cruciate ligament, posterior cruciate ligament, and posterolateral corner.

The femoral tunnels for single- or double-bundle reconstruction of the posterior cruciate ligament can be made from inside out. Inserting the appropriately sized double-bundle aimer through a low anterolateral patellar arthroscopic portal creates the femoral tunnel for the anterolateral bundle of the posterior cruciate ligament graft. The double-bundle aimer is positioned directly on the femoral footprint of the insertion site of the anterolateral bundle of the posterior cruciate ligament graft. The appropriately sized guidewire is drilled through the aimer, through the bone, and out a small skin incision. The double-bundle aimer is removed, and an acorn reamer is used to drill endoscopically from inside out the femoral tunnel for the anterolateral bundle of the posterior cruciate ligament graft. When the surgeon chooses to perform a double-bundle double-femoral-tunnel reconstruction of the posterior cruciate ligament, the same process is repeated for the posteromedial bundle of the posterior cruciate ligament graft. There should be at least 5 mm of bone between the two drill holes.

The tunnels for anterior cruciate ligament reconstruction are created with a single-incision technique. The tibial tunnel begins externally at a point 1 cm proximal to the tibial tubercle on the anteromedial surface of the proximal part of the tibia to emerge through the center of the stump of the anterior cruciate ligament tibial footprint. The femoral tunnel is positioned next to the over-the-top position on the medial wall of the lateral femoral condyle near the anatomic insertion site of the anterior cruciate ligament. The anterior cruciate ligament graft is positioned and is anchored on the femoral side; this is followed by tensioning and tibial fixation of the anterior cruciate ligament graft[25] (**Figures 3**, **4**, and **5**).

Lateral-Sided Reconstruction

The lateral side of the knee is commonly injured as part of a multiligament knee dislocation complex. The modified Schenck classification[2,26] of knee dislocations includes KD IIIL (injuries involving the anterior and posterior cruciate ligaments as well as the lateral complex). KD IV is less common and more severe because this injury involves both the medial and lateral sides as well as both cruciate ligaments. The mechanism of this injury includes a strong, high-energy, varus and external rotation force.[26] The lateral side of the knee is complex anatomically and therefore difficult to replicate with reconstructive techniques.

The lateral side consists of static and dynamic stabilizers. The static stabilizers include the fibular collateral ligament and the popliteofibular liga-

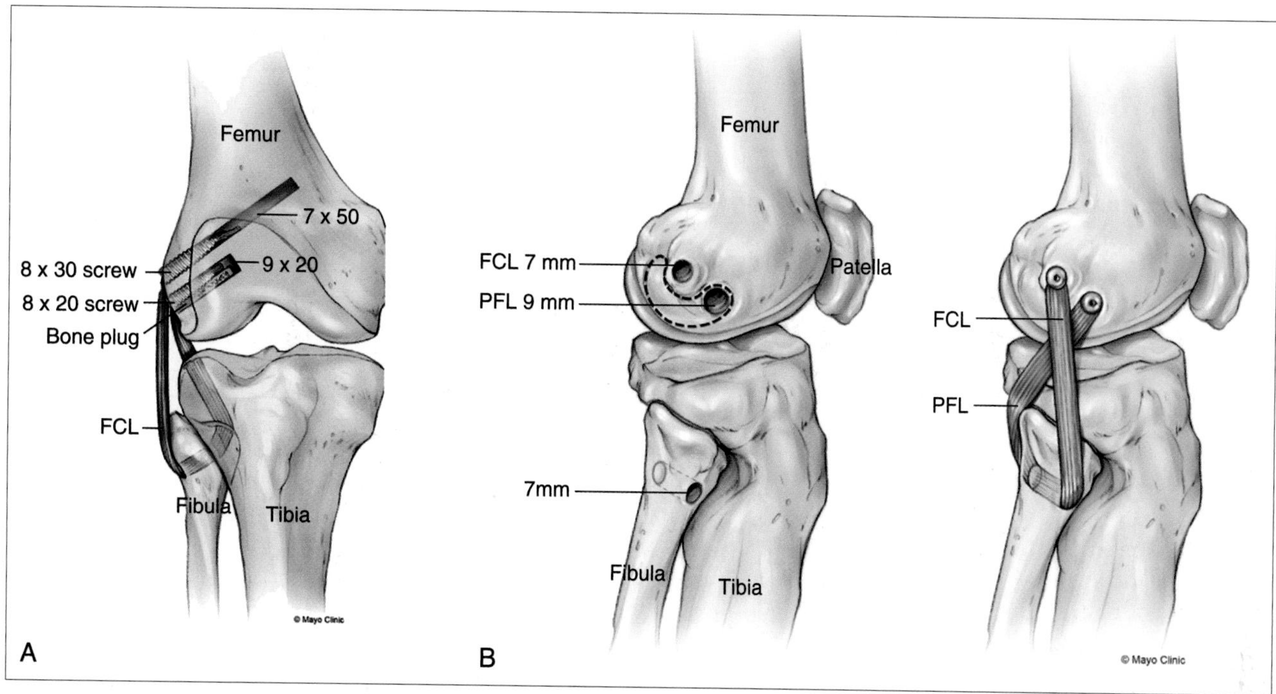

Figure 6 Anterior (**A**) and lateral (**B**) pictorial representations of fibular and femoral-based reconstructions of the fibular collateral ligament (FCL) and the posterolateral corner. PFL = popliteofibular ligament. (Reproduced with permission from the Mayo Foundation for Medical Education and Research, Rochester, MN.)

ment as well as the posterolateral aspect of the capsule. The popliteus muscle and tendon act as both a static and a dynamic stabilizer to control posterolateral rotation of the knee. The fibular collateral ligament acts as a primary restraint to varus stress and a secondary restraint to posterolateral rotation of the tibia on the femur. The popliteofibular ligament acts as a primary restraint to external rotation of the tibia on the femur at 30° of flexion, as does the popliteus muscle and tendon. The posterolateral aspect of the capsule acts in a secondary supportive role to resist external rotation, hyperextension, and varus moments.[27-29]

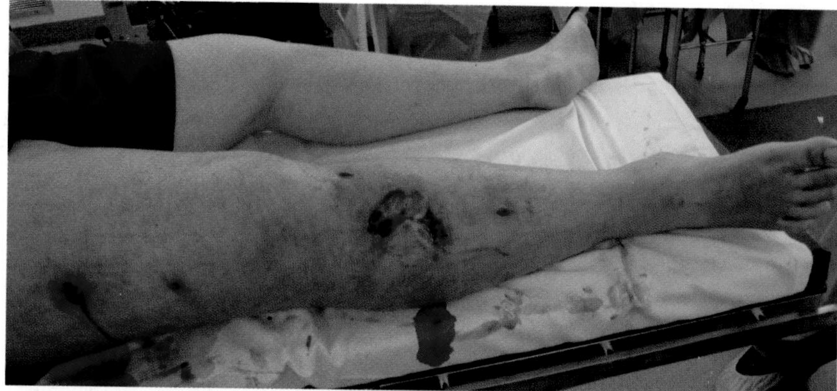

Figure 7 Clinical photograph of a knee dislocation requiring spanning external fixation with substantial soft-tissue injury.

The challenge of anatomic reconstructions is to re-create the posterolateral anatomy as closely as possible, usually with a combination of femoral, tibial, and fibular drill holes and allograft tissue. An alternative is to simplify the repair by performing a fibular and femoral-based reconstruction alone[14,21,30-32] (**Figure 6**). There are few studies comparing types of reconstructions in the literature, but, with other knee reconstructions, the more anatomic restorations tend to produce the best results. A reconstruction described by LaPrade et al[33] is often mentioned as the closest reproduction of normal anatomy and will be described later in this chapter.

The timing of surgery has been one of the most controversial aspects of knee dislocation management. Recent studies have indicated that earlier reconstruction may be better,[34] but the evidence is not strong. The benefits of early surgery must be balanced against the risks of arthrofibrosis and the risks of infection where open wounds persist from either external fixation pin sites or wounds from soft-tissue injury (**Figure 7**). The decision when to operate needs to be individualized.

Another controversial issue is whether to repair or reconstruct the posterolateral corner. Recent work by both Stannard et al[34] and Levy et al[35] indicates that reconstruction is probably better than repair. When surgery is performed within the first 3 weeks after the injury, a combination of repair and reconstruction can be done and should provide the best chance of producing a stable posterolateral corner. Stannard et al[34] recently reported a trial of repair versus reconstruction of the posterolateral corner in 57 knees. Forty-four of 57 patients (77%) had sustained multiple ligament injuries of the knee, and the minimum duration of follow-up was 24 months. The repair failure rate was 37%, compared with a reconstruction failure rate of 9%. Reconstruction was found to have a significant advantage over repair in terms of stability on clinical examination.

In a study by Levy et al,[35] patients with multiligament knee injuries treated by a single surgeon were identified in a prospective database. Between February 2004 and May 2005, patients underwent repair of medial- and lateral-sided injuries, followed by delayed cruciate ligament reconstructions. Between May 2005 and February 2007, patients underwent single-stage multiligament knee reconstruction. Forty-five knees (42 patients) with a minimum of 2 years of follow-up were identified. Four of 10 repairs of the fibular collateral ligament and posterolateral corner and 1 of 18 reconstructions of the fibular collateral ligament and posterolateral corner failed ($P = 0.04$). Although neither of these studies[34,35] was randomized, the findings of the two studies were quite similar, with both showing the rate of failure of repairs of the fibular collateral ligament and posterolateral corner to be significantly higher than the rate of failure of reconstructions of those structures.

Numerous surgical techniques to treat posterolateral corner injury have been described, with varying clinical outcomes.[14,36-38] Stannard et al[36] used a modified two-tailed technique that reconstructs the popliteofibular ligament and fibular collateral ligament through transtibial and transfibular bone tunnels and around a single screw on the lateral femoral condyle. Twenty-two knees were followed for a minimum of 2 years, and the mean range of motion at the time of follow-up was 133°. The mean Lysholm knee score was 90 points for the entire group, 92 points for the knees with multiligament injuries, and 88 points for those with an isolated posterolateral corner reconstruction. There were two failures (13%) in the group with multiligament knee injuries, compared with no failures in the group with an isolated posterolateral corner reconstruction.

Strobel et al[37] evaluated the clinical outcomes after single-stage anterior cruciate ligament, posterior cruciate ligament, and posterolateral corner reconstruction in 17 patients with chronic knee injuries and a minimum duration of follow-up of 24 months. The posterolateral corner was reconstructed with a graft passed through the proximal part of the fibula, with both graft limbs inserting at an isometric point on the femur. At the final evaluation, performed with the International Knee Documentation Committee (IKDC) score, the result was graded as nearly normal for 5 of the 17 patients, as abnormal for 10 patients, and as grossly abnormal for 2 patients. The mean postoperative subjective IKDC score was 71.8 ± 19.3 points.

The LaPrade technique has been popularized as a stable and anatomically complete reconstruction using a two-tailed graft (usually an Achilles tendon allograft) and reconstructing the fibular collateral ligament, the popliteofibular ligament, and the popliteus tendon.[33] This technique requires four tunnels: two in the femur (for the insertion of the fibular collateral ligament and the popliteus tendon), one in the fibula, and one in the proximal part of the tibia. The Achilles tendon can be split into two separate grafts and bone blocks. Both bone blocks are inset into the femoral tunnels and secured with interference screws, replicating the insertions of the fibular collateral ligament and popliteus tendon, respectively. The fibular collateral ligament graft then runs from anterior to posterior through the tunnel in the fibula and subsequently into the tibia. The popliteus portion then runs from the femur into the tibial tunnel to join the other graft. A large bioabsorbable screw is then placed from anterior to posterior with the two graft limbs under tension at 30° of flexion and slight internal rotation. Excessive internal rotation force can constrain the knee excessively. Although the procedure is technically challenging, the results of this reconstruction appear to be good.

When the posterolateral corner is torn, there are usually other knee ligament injuries. Therefore, when the posterolateral corner is being repaired, the lateral collateral ligament and the popliteofibular ligament complexes should be repaired as well. Allograft tissue is recommended for posterolateral corner reconstruction so that autogenous grafts can be used to repair the other ligaments and donor site morbidity is kept to a minimum. Numerous surgical techniques are available, but varus and posterolateral rotatory stability are best restored by the technique with which the surgeon is most familiar.

Reconstruction of the Medial Collateral Ligament and Posteromedial Corner

Combined injuries of the anterior cruciate ligament, posterior cruciate ligament, and medial collateral ligament/posteromedial corner are classified as type III according to the modified Schenck anatomic classification scheme. The anatomic structures on the medial side are arranged in three distinct layers. Layer 1 is the sartorius and sartorius fascia; layer 2 is the superficial medial collateral ligament, posterior oblique ligament, and semimembranosus; and layer 3 is the deep medial collateral ligament (the meniscofemoral and meniscotibial ligaments) and the posteromedial aspect of the capsule. The gracilis and semitendinosus tendons are found between layers 1 and 2. These layers are not always separate because layers 1 and 2 blend anteriorly, whereas layers 2 and 3 blend posteriorly.

LaPrade et al[39] described the clinically relevant medial knee anatomy. There are three osseous prominences on the medial aspect of the distal part of the femur: the medial epicondyle, the adductor tubercle, and the gastrocnemius tubercle. The femoral origin of the superficial medial collateral ligament is approximately 3 mm proximal and 5 mm posterior to the epicondyle, whereas the tibial insertion is approximately 6 cm distal to the joint line. The deep medial collateral ligament inserts along the tibial plateau margin, just distal to the articular cartilage. The femoral origin of the posterior oblique ligament is approximately 8 mm distal and 6 mm posterior to the adductor tubercle. These anatomic sites correspond to the radiographic landmarks described by Wijdicks et al.[40] The combination of recognition of osseous prominences and radiographic identification helps to guide the surgeon to the proper ligament origin and insertion sites during repair or reconstruction. In a study of cadaver knees, Stannard et al[41] reported that using radiographic landmarks, rather than palpating the osseous prominences, led to better reproduction of the isometry of the superficial medial collateral ligament.

More than 10 mm of medial joint opening with the knee in full extension is the hallmark finding in a knee with a combined injury involving the medial side and both cruciate ligaments. Stress examination, with the patient under anesthesia, with the use of fluoroscopy or radiography to compare the joint space opening of the injured knee with that of the contralateral knee, helps the surgeon to understand the extent of pathologic ligament laxity. MRI is a sensitive tool for identifying injured structures.

Once the soft tissues are satisfactory, acute surgery (performed 1 to 3 weeks after the injury) is indicated when there is extensive medial disruption, a displaced meniscal tear, or a so-called Stener lesion of the knee in which the distal medial collateral ligament is flipped over the pes anserinus tendons. Delayed surgical intervention (at more than 3 weeks after the injury) may be necessary to allow the swelling to resolve and knee motion to return. When the only medial damage is a femoral medial collateral ligament avulsion, healing may occur and only the cruciate ligaments need to be repaired. When the anterior cruciate ligament, posterior cruciate ligament, and medial side need to be repaired, a single-stage procedure with anterior and posterior cruciate ligament reconstructions along with repair or reconstruction of the medial collateral ligament and posteromedial corner, as indicated, is best.

In the acute setting, a femoral or tibial-sided avulsion of the medial collateral ligament with good ligament substance can be repaired to the anatomic origin with a suture post and ligament washer. **Figure 8** shows an example of a tibial-sided disruption of the medial collateral ligament. The intact ligament with excellent tissue substance allows a secure repair without the need for augmentation or reconstruction. The deep meniscotibial ligament can be reattached with suture anchors. The repair should be tensioned with the knee at 30° of flexion, a varus stress, and slight tibial external rotation. Injuries of the posterior oblique ligament and the posteromedial aspect of the capsule are also repaired anatomically with suture anchors and tensioning near full extension. It is important to avoid overtensioning in flexion, because this may prevent full knee extension.

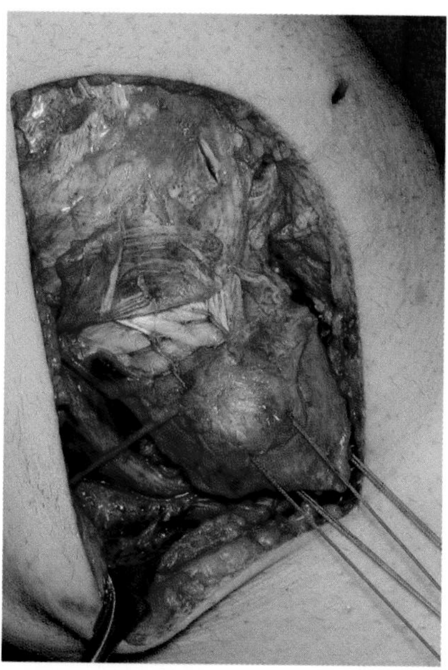

Figure 8 A tibial-sided disruption of the medial collateral ligament with excellent tissue substance that is amenable to direct repair is shown.

Numerous reconstruction techniques for treatment in the chronic setting have been described.[23,42-44] This chapter's authors prefer to use an Achilles tendon allograft with the bone plug fixed in a femoral socket with an interference screw and the tendon se-

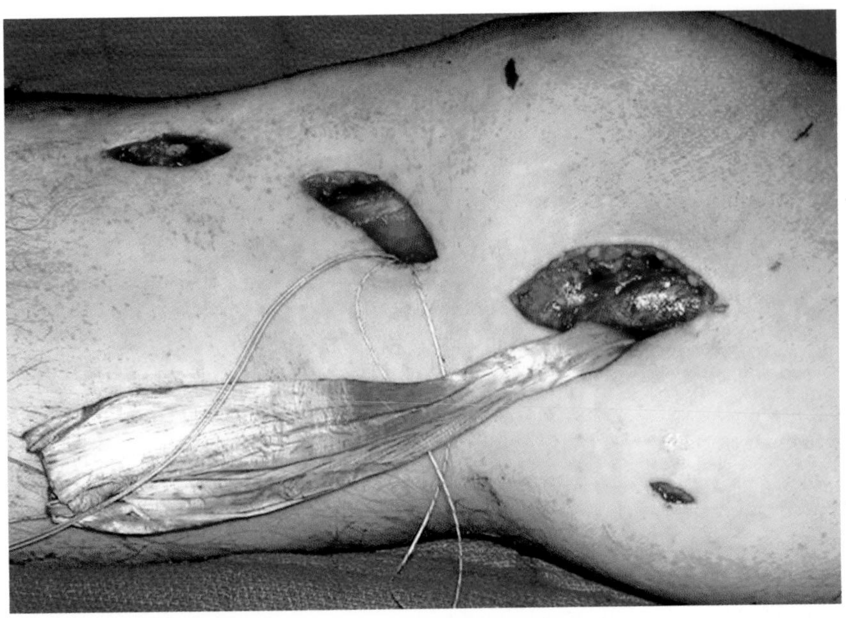

Figure 9 A reconstruction of the medial collateral ligament with an Achilles tendon allograft after fixation of the bone block in the femoral socket is shown.

cured to the tibia with a suture post/ligament washer construct. **Figure 9** shows the Achilles tendon allograft after fixation of the femoral attachment. The posterior oblique ligament and posteromedial aspect of the capsule are repaired if necessary.

A detailed search of the literature from 1978 through 2008 identified all studies with outcome data on repair or reconstruction of the medial collateral ligament in the setting of combined ligament injuries.[8] Only eight studies met the inclusion criteria: five were on medial collateral ligament repair, and three were on medial collateral ligament reconstruction. No prospective studies directly compared medial collateral ligament repair or reconstruction with nonsurgical treatment or compared medial collateral ligament reconstruction with repair. The collective results suggest that either repair or reconstruction in the knee with multiple ligament injuries yields satisfactory outcomes. Owens et al[45] reported on 11 knees with injuries to the anterior cruciate ligament, posterior cruciate ligament, and medial collateral ligament, with the medial collateral ligament repaired only if it was avulsed; all were stable to valgus stress at the time of final follow-up. In a 2005 study on nine knees with injuries to the anterior cruciate ligament, posterior cruciate ligament, and medial collateral ligament, all were stable to valgus stress, including seven that were treated surgically.[22] In a study by Hayashi et al[46] in which seven reconstructions of the anterior cruciate ligament, posterior cruciate ligament, and medial collateral ligament were performed with use of a semitendinosus autograft, the average Lysholm knee score was 95.1 points. Stannard et al[41] reported on 73 dislocated knees with posteromedial corner injuries. Forty-eight underwent autograft or allograft reconstruction of the medial collateral ligament, and 24 had a medial collateral ligament repair. On the basis of a 20% failure rate in the repair group compared with a 4% failure rate in the reconstruction group, Stannard et al[41] concluded that medial collateral ligament repair is inferior to reconstruction in a knee with multiple ligament injuries.

It is important to make an accurate anatomic diagnosis with the use of a physical examination, imaging studies, and bilateral comparison stress radiographs. The surgeon needs to determine the safe and appropriate timing of surgery and then proceed with reconstruction of the anterior and posterior cruciate ligaments along with repair or reconstruction of the medial collateral ligament, posterior oblique ligament, and posteromedial aspect of the capsule.

Postoperative Rehabilitation

The knee should be kept in full extension for a minimum of 3 weeks, and the patient should not bear weight for 6 weeks.[47] Progressive range-of-motion exercises start 3 weeks after surgery. The brace should be unlocked at the end of the third week, and the use of crutches is discontinued once the patient can bear full weight. Progressive closed kinetic-chain strength training and continued motion exercises are performed. Use of the brace should be discontinued after the 10th week. The patient can return to sports and strenuous labor after the ninth postoperative month as long as sufficient strength, proprioceptive skills, and motion have returned.[11,48] A loss of 10° to 15° of terminal flexion might be expected after these complex knee ligament reconstructions.

Fracture-Dislocations

Fracture-dislocations of the knee are severe injuries that have frequently been associated with poor outcomes.[49-54] The most common fracture around the knee associated with a multiligament knee injury is a tibial plateau fracture. It is difficult to treat patients who have instability of both the bone (a fracture) and ligaments of the knee. Reconstructing ligaments is a challenge when it is necessary to anchor a reconstruction in fractured bone. The risk of failure of early reconstruction of the posterolateral corner with use of the modified two-tailed technique is higher in patients with a tibial plateau fracture than it is in patients who do not have a fracture.[34,36]

Knee fracture-dislocations occur more frequently than generally believed and are particularly challenging to diagnose. It is difficult to determine the stability of the knee in a patient with a tibial plateau fracture. These patients also frequently have multiple injuries that divert the attention of treating teams away from the knee injury. As identified with MRI, the prevalence of concomitant ligament injuries with tibial plateau fractures has been reported to be as low as 33% and as high as 90%.[55-58] Although many of these injuries do not represent fracture-dislocations, in a series of 103 consecutive tibial plateau fractures, more than 50% of the patients had multiple ligament injuries, and 26% had a fracture-dislocation.[55] MRI is an important adjunct to an examination under anesthesia for the successful diagnosis of fracture-dislocations of the knee.

There are very few published studies dedicated to the topic of fracture-dislocation of the knee. The published results show a high prevalence of poor outcomes, with pain, instability, and arthrofibrosis being the most common complications.[49-54] Conservative treatment is associated with poor results, and most authors have recommended surgical treatment for patients with a fracture-dislocation. Delamarter et al[59] reported that 40% of their patients with a fracture-dislocation had a poor outcome after nonsurgical treatment compared with a 16% rate of poor results in those who were surgically treated. Stannard et al[60] developed a staged treatment protocol for fracture-dislocations, in which the treatment of the fracture is separated from that for the dislocation, and it has yielded good functional outcomes in most patients. Outcome scores after using this staged protocol have been encouraging in patients with these complex injuries.

The initial phase of treatment of a patient with a fracture-dislocation of the knee is on the day of injury. The mechanism of injury, radiographic findings, and examination of the skin lead to a suspicion of a fracture-dislocation. The fracture is gently reduced with traction, and a careful vascular examination is performed. If the knee remains reduced, the extremity should be immobilized with a splint or knee-immobilizer, and MRI should be performed. In most cases, the skin and soft-tissue injury are so severe that surgical treatment should be delayed for at least 3 to 7 days. Once the condition of the soft tissues around the knee is satisfactory, the second phase of treatment can begin.

Phase two is surgical stabilization of the fracture and any avulsions of major ligaments. Locked plates are frequently necessary to stabilize the complex fractures associated with fracture-dislocations. Preoperative planning is critical, both for successful treatment of the fracture and to ensure that the implants do not block future tunnels that will be necessary for reconstruction of the injured ligament. A knee immobilizer should be applied after stabilization of the fracture, and one must be certain that the knee stays reduced.

Phase three is the early reconstructive phase of the protocol. If the condition of the patient and the soft tissues allow it, this chapter's authors advance to this phase during week 3 or 4 following the injury. Allograft ligament reconstruction is the mainstay of this phase. There are no definitive data in the literature regarding the timing or staging of ligament reconstructions in patients following knee dislocations. On the basis of the findings in the series evaluated by Stannard et al,[34,36] reconstruction of the anterior cruciate ligament and posterolateral corner should be delayed for approximately 4 months to allow early healing of the tibial plateau before tunnels are drilled through the tibia. Those authors reported a failure rate of more than 30% when posterolateral corner reconstructions had been performed during phase three compared with a failure rate of 8% when the same posterolateral corner reconstruction technique had been performed in patients without a tibial plateau fracture.[34,36] A hinged external fixator is placed at the end of the surgery in phase three, providing a stable environment for early ligament healing. Gentle motion is initiated on postoperative day 1 if the condition of the soft tissue allows it.

Phase four is the late reconstructive phase. The patient should have at least 80° of knee flexion before starting phase four. The hinged external fixator is removed, and the anterior cruciate ligament and posterolateral corner are reconstructed if the knee remains unstable. Again, allograft tissue is normally used for the reconstructions. Early motion after surgery is used to minimize arthrofibrosis.

In series evaluated by Stannard et al,[60] good functional outcomes were achieved in patients in whom a fracture-dislocation had been treated with this staged protocol. In a series of 50 patients with a total of 54 fracture-dislocations, the final Lysholm knee score averaged 86 points (range, 50 to 100 points). According to the final objective IKDC scores, there were 32 normal or nearly normal knees and 17 abnormal knees. However, although good function was achieved, patients required an average of four surgical procedures to complete their treatments.

Complications

Complications are frequent after knee dislocations and fracture-dislocations. Complications include a wide variety of conditions, including wound healing and vascular and neurologic problems. The most common complications remain pain, arthrofibrosis, and ligament instability despite reconstruction. Pain is a difficult complication to quantify objectively, but many patients report chronic pain following these injuries. The prevalence of chronic pain has ranged from 25% to 68%.[61] Arthrofibrosis remains a substantial source of pain and disability following knee dislocations. The prevalence has ranged from 5% to 71% in the published literature, with a mean of 29% of patients having arthrofibrosis requiring surgical treatment.[61] The prevalence of persistent instability was 100% after nonsurgical treatment, and it ranged from 18% to 100% after surgical treatment, with a mean of 42% of patients having instability in at least one plane.[61]

Results of Treatment of Knee Dislocations

Outcomes after knee dislocation are difficult to quantify in large part because the injuries are heterogeneous.[62] A knee dislocation can range from a three-ligament noncontact injury that reduced spontaneously to one sustained in a high-speed motor vehicle crash and is associated with severe neurologic and vascular injuries. The data on the outcomes of these injuries are summarized below.

Levy et al[8] performed a systematic review of 413 articles on this topic. They evaluated studies that compared surgical treatment with nonsurgical treatment,[63-66] studies that compared repair with reconstruction,[34,67] and studies that compared early and late surgical treatment.[21,68-71]

Of the four studies that compared surgical and nonsurgical treatment,[63-66] one was a meta-analysis of investigations published before 2000.[63] In three studies in which the Lysholm knee score was used to record postoperative outcomes, surgical treatment resulted in higher mean scores,[63-65] with one of the differences being significant.[64] The surgical group also had higher IKDC scores.[64,66] Return to work and sports activities was also better overall in the surgically treated group.

Two studies that compared surgical repair with reconstruction were identified.[34,67] Direct repair of cruciate ligaments resulted in inferior motion, a higher rate of positive posterior sag signs, and a lower rate of return to the preinjury activity level.[67] The rate of failure after repair of the posterolateral corner was also found to be higher than that after reconstruction.[34]

In general, 3 weeks was the most consistent time point up to which surgery was described as "early." Overall, the patients who had early surgery had improved outcomes for several parameters.[21,68-71] However, there is potential for substantial bias with respect to the timing of surgery because the reason for early or late surgery may be related to prognosis (such as other injuries or the status of the soft tissues around the knee).

An excellent prospective cohort study with a minimum 2-year follow-up after reconstruction for treatment of knee dislocations was performed by Engebretsen et al.[72] Inclusion criteria were injury to both the anterior and the posterior cruciate ligaments as well as an injury to the medial and/or lateral side. Patients were treated with surgical reconstruction within 2 weeks after the injury, when that was not contraindicated by other injuries. The authors used both autograft and allograft tissue, with a trend toward using autograft later in the study enrollment period. Of 121 patients who were initially eligible, 85 patients had sufficient follow-up. Approximately 50% of the patients in this cohort sustained what was considered high-energy knee dislocations. The median Lysholm knee score for the patients who were followed was 83 points, and the median Tegner activity score was 5 points. The authors found that injuries resulting from high-energy trauma and those involving all four major ligaments resulted in worse outcomes than did those resulting from low-energy trauma and those involving three ligaments.

Despite some excellent case series as well as comparative studies and the prospective cohort study by Engebretsen et al,[72] this chapter's authors are not aware of any randomized controlled trials to assist with outcome assessment after knee dislocation. These injuries are complex and not easily amenable to randomized trials for many reasons.[62] Additional research is needed to identify prognostic factors and treatment algorithms to improve outcomes after these rare and devastating injuries.

Summary

Recent advances in surgical techniques, including anatomic reconstructions, for the management of knees with multiple ligament injuries have led to improved patient outcomes. Current recommendations include measurement of the ankle-brachial index in each patient, early surgical management (earlier than 3 weeks postinjury), the use of autograft or allograft tissue, reconstruction as opposed to repair alone of the fibular collateral ligament and posterolateral corner structures, reconstruction of the anterior and posterior cruciate ligaments, and repair and/or reconstruction of the medial collateral ligament and posteromedial corner, depending on the injury pattern and quality of tissue. Future research, including the establishment of multicenter working groups and the collection of prospective data, may hold the key to identifying optimal treatment protocols for these complex injuries.

References

1. Niall DM, Nutton RW, Keating JF: Palsy of the common peroneal nerve after traumatic dislocation of the knee. *J Bone Joint Surg Br* 2005;87(5):664-667.
2. Wascher DC: High-velocity knee dislocation with vascular injury: Treatment principles. *Clin Sports Med* 2000;19(3):457-477.
3. Mills WJ, Barei DP, McNair P: The value of the ankle-brachial index for diagnosing arterial injury after knee dislocation: A prospective study. *J Trauma* 2004; 56(6):1261-1265.
4. Levy BA, Zlowodzki MP, Graves M, Cole PA: Screening for extermity arterial injury with the arterial pressure index. *Am J Emerg Med* 2005;23(5):689-695.
5. Redmond JM, Levy BA, Dajani KA, Cass JR, Cole PA: Detecting vascular injury in lower-extremity orthopedic trauma: The role of CT angiography. *Orthopedics* 2008;31(8):761-767.
6. LaPrade RF, Heikes C, Bakker AJ, Jakobsen RB: The reproducibility and repeatability of varus stress radiographs in the assessment of isolated fibular collateral ligament and grade-III posterolateral knee injuries: An in vitro biomechanical study. *J Bone Joint Surg Am* 2008;90(10):2069-2076.
7. Levy BA, Krych AJ, Shah JP, Morgan JA, Stuart MJ: Staged protocol for initial management of the dislocated knee. *Knee Surg Sports Traumatol Arthrosc*, in press.
8. Levy BA, Dajani KA, Whelan DB, et al: Decision making in the multiligament-injured knee: An evidence-based systematic review. *Arthroscopy* 2009;25(4): 430-438.
9. Fanelli GC, ed: *The Multiple Ligament Injured Knee: A Practical Guide to Management.* New York, NY, Springer, 2004.
10. Fanelli GC, ed: *Posterior Cruciate Ligament Injuries: A Practical Guide to Management.* New York, NY, Springer, 2001.
11. Edson CJ: Postoperative rehabilitation of the multiligament-reconstructed knee. *Sports Med Arthrosc* 2001;9:247-254.
12. Fanelli GC: Double-bundle compared with single-bundle posterior cruciate ligament reconstruction. *Orthop Today* 2008;28:58.
13. Fanelli GC, Edson CJ: Arthroscopically assisted combined anterior and posterior cruciate ligament reconstruction in the multiple ligament injured knee: 2- to 10-year follow-up. *Arthroscopy* 2002;18(7):703-714.
14. Fanelli GC, Edson CJ: Combined posterior cruciate ligament-posterolateral reconstructions with Achilles tendon allograft and biceps femoris tendon tenodesis: 2- to 10-year follow-up. *Arthroscopy* 2004;20(4):339-345.
15. Fanelli GC, Edson CJ, Orcutt DR, Harris JD, Zijerdi D: Treatment of combined anterior cruciate-posterior cruciate ligament-medial-lateral side knee injuries. *J Knee Surg* 2005;18(3): 240-248.
16. Fanelli GC, Edson CJ, Reinheimer KN: Evaluation and treatment of the multiligament-injured knee. *Instr Course Lect* 2009;58: 389-395.
17. Fanelli GC, Edson CJ, Reinheimer KN: Posterior cruciate ligament reconstruction: Transtibial tunnel surgical technique. *Orthop Today* 2007;27(2):40-46.
18. Fanelli GC, Edson CJ, Reinheimer KN, Beck J: Arthroscopic single-bundle versus double-bundle posterior cruciate ligament reconstruction. *Arthroscopy* 2008; 24:e26.
19. Fanelli GC, Edson CJ, Reinheimer KN, Garofalo R: Posterior cruciate ligament and posterolateral corner reconstruction. *Sports Med Arthrosc* 2007;15(4): 168-175.
20. Fanelli GC, Feldmann DD: Management of combined anterior cruciate ligament/posterior cruciate ligament/posterolateral complex injuries of the knee. *Oper Tech Sports Med* 1999;7:143-149.
21. Fanelli GC, Giannotti BF, Edson CJ: Arthroscopically assisted combined anterior and posterior cruciate ligament reconstruction. *Arthroscopy* 1996;12(1):5-14.
22. Fanelli GC, Orcutt DR, Edson CJ: The multiple-ligament injured knee: Evaluation, treatment, and results. *Arthroscopy* 2005;21(4):471-486.
23. Fanelli GC, Tomaszewski DJ: Allograft use in the treatment of the multiple ligament injured knee. *Sports Med Arthrosc* 2007; 15(3):139-148.
24. Levy BA, Fanelli GC, Whelan DB, et al; Knee Dislocation Study Group: Controversies in the treatment of knee dislocations and multiligament reconstruction. *J Am Acad Orthop Surg* 2009; 17(4):197-206.
25. Fanelli GC: *Rationale and Surgical Technique for PCL and Multiple Knee Ligament Reconstruction: Surgical Technique Guide.* Warsaw, IN, Biomet Sports Medicine, 2008.
26. Schenck RC Jr, Kovach IS, Agarwal A, et al: Cruciate injury patterns in knee hyperextension: A cadaveric model. *Arthroscopy* 1999;15(5):489-495.
27. Baker CL Jr, Norwood LA, Hughston JC: Acute posterolateral

rotatory instability of the knee. *J Bone Joint Surg Am* 1983;65(5): 614-618.

28. LaPrade RF, Wentorf FA, Fritts H, Gundry C, Hightower CD: A prospective magnetic resonance imaging study of the incidence of posterolateral and multiple ligament injuries in acute knee injuries presenting with a hemarthrosis. *Arthroscopy* 2007;23(12): 1341-1347.
29. Sanchez AR II, Sugalski MT, LaPrade RF: Anatomy and biomechanics of the lateral side of the knee. *Sports Med Arthrosc* 2006; 14(1):2-11.
30. Nau T, Chevalier Y, Hagemeister N, Deguise JA, Duval N: Comparison of 2 surgical techniques of posterolateral corner reconstruction of the knee. *Am J Sports Med* 2005;33(12):1838-1845.
31. Schechinger SJ, Levy BA, Dajani KA, Shah JP, Herrera DA, Marx RG: Achilles tendon allograft reconstruction of the fibular collateral ligament and posterolateral corner. *Arthroscopy* 2009;25(3):232-242.
32. Sekiya JK, Kurtz CA: Posterolateral corner reconstruction of the knee: Surgical technique utilizing a bifid Achilles tendon allograft and a double femoral tunnel. *Arthroscopy* 2005;21(11):1400.
33. LaPrade RF, Johansen S, Wentorf FA, Engebretsen L, Esterberg JL, Tso A: An analysis of an anatomical posterolateral knee reconstruction: An in vitro biomechanical study and development of a surgical technique. *Am J Sports Med* 2004;32(6):1405-1414.
34. Stannard JP, Brown SL, Farris RC, McGwin G Jr , Volgas DA: The posterolateral corner of the knee: Repair versus reconstruction. *Am J Sports Med* 2005;33(6):881-888.
35. Levy BA, Dajani KA, Morgan JA, Shah JP, Dahm DL, Stuart MJ: Repair versus reconstruction of the fibular collateral ligament and posterolateral corner in the multiligament-injured knee. *Am J Sports Med* 2010;38(4):804-809.
36. Stannard JP, Brown SL, Robinson JT, McGwin G Jr, Volgas DA: Reconstruction of the posterolateral corner of the knee. *Arthroscopy* 2005;21(9):1051-1059.
37. Strobel MJ, Schulz MS, Petersen WJ, Eichhorn HJ: Combined anterior cruciate ligament, posterior cruciate ligament, and posterolateral corner reconstruction with autogenous hamstring grafts in chronic instabilities. *Arthroscopy* 2006;22(2):182-192.
38. Yoon KH, Bae DK, Ha JH, Park SW: Anatomic reconstructive surgery for posterolateral instability of the knee. *Arthroscopy* 2006; 22(2):159-165.
39. LaPrade RF, Engebretsen AH, Ly TV, Johansen S, Wentorf FA, Engebretsen L: The anatomy of the medial part of the knee. *J Bone Joint Surg Am* 2007;89(9):2000-2010.
40. Wijdicks CA, Griffith CJ, LaPrade RF, et al: Radiographic identification of the primary medial knee structures. *J Bone Joint Surg Am* 2009;91(3):521-529.
41. Stannard JP, Volgas DA, Azbell CH: Posteromedial corner injury in knee dislocations. *AOSSM 2009 Annual Meeting Final Program.* Rosemont, IL, American Orthopaedic Society for Sports Medicine, 2009, p 385.
42. Borden PS, Kantaras AT, Caborn DN: Medial collateral ligament reconstruction with allograft using a double-bundle technique. *Arthroscopy* 2002;18(4):E19.
43. Kim SJ, Lee DH, Kim TE, Choi NH: Concomitant reconstruction of the medial collateral and posterior oblique ligaments for medial instability of the knee. *J Bone Joint Surg Br* 2008;90(10): 1323-1327.
44. Lind M, Jakobsen BW, Lund B, Hansen MS, Abdallah O, Christiansen SE: Anatomical reconstruction of the medial collateral ligament and posteromedial corner of the knee in patients with chronic medial collateral ligament instability. *Am J Sports Med* 2009; 37(6):1116-1122.
45. Owens BD, Neault M, Benson E, Busconi BD: Primary repair of knee dislocations: Results in 25 patients (28 knees) at a mean follow-up of four years. *J Orthop Trauma* 2007;21(2):92-96.
46. Hayashi R, Kitamura N, Kondo E, Anaguchi Y, Tohyama H, Yasuda K: Simultaneous anterior and posterior cruciate ligament reconstruction in chronic knee instabilities: Surgical concepts and clinical outcome. *Knee Surg Sports Traumatol Arthrosc* 2008;16(8):763-769.
47. Higgins L, Clatworthy M, Harner CD: Multiligament injuries of the knee, in Garrett WE Jr, Speer KP, Kirkendall DT, eds: *Principles and Practice of Orthopedic Sports Medicine.* Philadelphia, PA, Lippincott Williams & Wilkins, 2000, pp 805-817.
48. Fanelli GC: Posterior cruciate ligament rehabilitation: How slow should we go? *Arthroscopy* 2008; 24(2):234-235.
49. Berg EE: Comminuted tibial eminence anterior cruciate ligament avulsion fractures: Failure of arthroscopic treatment. *Arthroscopy* 1993;9(4):446-450.
50. Dendrinos GK, Kontos S, Katsenis D, Dalas A: Treatment of high-energy tibial plateau fractures by the Ilizarov circular fixator. *J Bone Joint Surg Br* 1996; 78(5):710-717.
51. Hohl M: Tibial condylar fractures. *J Bone Joint Surg Am* 1967; 49(7):1455-1467.

52. Mills WJ, Nork SE: Open reduction and internal fixation of high-energy tibial plateau fractures. *Orthop Clin North Am* 2002; 33(1):177-198, ix.

53. Moore TM: Fracture-dislocation of the knee. *Clin Orthop Relat Res* 1981;156:128-140.

54. Stokel EA, Sadasivan KK: Tibial plateau fractures: Standardized evaluation of operative results. *Orthopedics* 1991;14(3):263-270.

55. Stannard JP, Schmidt AH, Kregor PJ, eds: *Surgical Treatment of Orthopaedic Trauma.* New York, NY, Thieme, 2007.

56. Gardner MJ, Yacoubian S, Geller D, et al: The incidence of soft tissue injury in operative tibial plateau fractures: A magnetic resonance imaging analysis of 103 patients. *J Orthop Trauma* 2005;19(2):79-84.

57. Holt MD, Williams LA, Dent CM: MRI in the management of tibial plateau fractures. *Injury* 1995;26(9):595-599.

58. Shepherd L, Abdollahi K, Lee J, Vangsness CT Jr: The prevalence of soft tissue injuries in nonoperative tibial plateau fractures as determined by magnetic resonance imaging. *J Orthop Trauma* 2002; 16(9):628-631.

59. Delamarter RB, Hohl M, Hopp E Jr: Ligament injuries associated with tibial plateau fractures. *Clin Orthop Relat Res* 1990; 250(250):226-233.

60. Stannard J, Bankston L, Volgas DA, McGwin G Jr: Fracture dislocation of the knee: Clinical outcomes with a treatment protocol using a hinged external fixator. *AOSSM 2005 Annual Meeting Final Program.* Rosemont, IL, American Orthopaedic Society for Sports Medicine, 2005, p 89.

61. Stannard J, Schenck RC Jr, Fanelli G: Knee dislocations and fracture-dislocations, in Bucholz RW, Heckman JD, Court-Brown CM, Tornetta P III, eds: *Rockwood and Green's Fractures in Adults,* ed 7. Philadelphia, PA, Lippincott Williams & Wilkins, 2009, pp 1832-1866.

62. Levy BA, Marx RG: Outcome after knee dislocation. *Knee Surg Sports Traumatol Arthrosc* 2009; 17(9):1011-1012.

63. Dedmond BT, Almekinders LC: Operative versus nonoperative treatment of knee dislocations: A meta-analysis. *Am J Knee Surg* 2001;14(1):33-38.

64. Richter M, Bosch U, Wippermann B, Hofmann A, Krettek C: Comparison of surgical repair or reconstruction of the cruciate ligaments versus nonsurgical treatment in patients with traumatic knee dislocations. *Am J Sports Med* 2002;30(5):718-727.

65. Ríos A, Villa A, Fahandezh H, de José C, Vaquero J: Results after treatment of traumatic knee dislocations: A report of 26 cases. *J Trauma* 2003;55(3):489-494.

66. Wong CH, Tan JL, Chang HC, Khin LW, Low CO: Knee dislocations: A retrospective study comparing operative versus closed immobilization treatment outcomes. *Knee Surg Sports Traumatol Arthrosc* 2004;12(6):540-544.

67. Mariani PP, Santoriello P, Iannone S, Condello V, Adriani E: Comparison of surgical treatments for knee dislocation. *Am J Knee Surg* 1999;12(4):214-221.

68. Harner CD, Irrgang JJ, Paul J, Dearwater S, Fu FH: Loss of motion after anterior cruciate ligament reconstruction. *Am J Sports Med* 1992;20(5):499-506.

69. Liow RY, McNicholas MJ, Keating JF, Nutton RW: Ligament repair and reconstruction in traumatic dislocation of the knee. *J Bone Joint Surg Br* 2003;85(6): 845-851.

70. Tzurbakis M, Diamantopoulos A, Xenakis T, Georgoulis A: Surgical treatment of multiple knee ligament injuries in 44 patients: 2-8 years follow-up results. *Knee Surg Sports Traumatol Arthrosc* 2006;14(8):739-749.

71. Wascher DC, Becker JR, Dexter JG, Blevins FT: Reconstruction of the anterior and posterior cruciate ligaments after knee dislocation: Results using fresh-frozen nonirradiated allografts. *Am J Sports Med* 1999;27(2):189-196.

72. Engebretsen L, Risberg MA, Robertson B, Ludvigsen TC, Johansen S: Outcome after knee dislocations: A 2-9 years follow-up of 85 consecutive patients. *Knee Surg Sports Traumatol Arthrosc* 2009; 17(9):1013-1026.

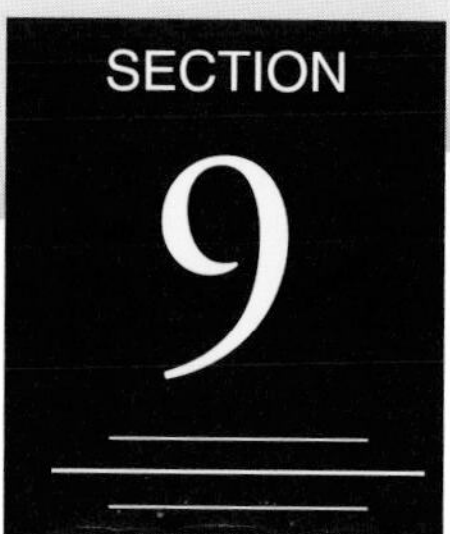

SECTION 9

Orthopaedic Medicine

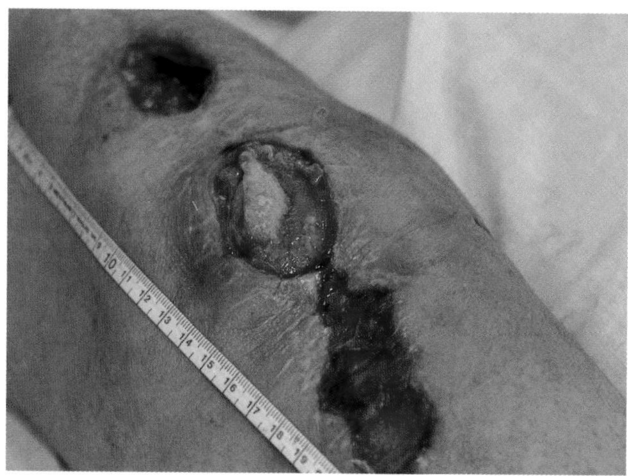

Surgical Site Infection Prevention and Control: An Emerging Paradigm

Richard P. Evans, MD
Terry A. Clyburn, MD
Calin S. Moucha, MD
Laura Prokuski, MD
The American Academy of Orthopaedic Surgeons Patient Safety Committee

Abstract

Examining the current state of infection in orthopaedic surgery provides tools and techniques to reduce the risks of nosocomial infections and prevent and treat infections from drug-resistant organisms. It is important for surgeons to recognize modifiable surgical risk factors and be aware of the importance of preoperative patient screening in reducing surgical site infections. The latest evidence-based data from scientific exhibits, instructional course lectures, and the Orthopaedic Knowledge Online continuing medical education module gathered during the past 5 years by the American Academy of Orthopaedic Surgeons Patient Safety Committee are useful in understanding and controlling the increasing and vital problem of surgical site infection.

Instr Course Lect 2011;60:539-543.

This chapter, along with chapters 41, 42, and 43, reviews nosocomial infections, drug-resistant organisms, modifiable surgical risk factors, preoperative screening, and the tools and techniques shown to affect orthopaedic surgical site infections (SSIs). These infection-control techniques are provided using an outside-to-inside methodology, incorporating the latest evidence-based data gathered by the American Academy of Orthopaedic Surgeons (AAOS) Patient Safety Committee over the past 5 years from scientific exhibits; instructional course lectures; and the continuing education module developed for Orthopaedic Knowledge Online, which is available at the AAOS Website. A commentary on the importance of SSI prevention is that completion of the AAOS Orthopaedic Knowledge Online SSI prevention continuing medical education module is required by 11 states and 3 insurance companies for malpractice insurance premium discounts. Additionally, the American Board of Orthopaedic Surgeons has incorporated this module into its maintenance of certification requirement.

Scope of the Problem

SSIs are not just an orthopaedic problem. The increasing incidence and enormous cost of SSIs and the epidemic of methicillin-resistant organisms are affecting public health policy (**Figure 1**). The Centers for Disease Control and Prevention (CDC) estimates that 22% of all health care-associated infections are SSIs. In 2001, the CDC estimated that approximately 290,000 SSIs occur annually in the United States, resulting in $1 billion to $10 billion in direct and

Dr. Evans or an immediate family member is a member of a speakers' bureau or has made paid presentations on behalf of Cubist; serves as a paid consultant to or is an employee of DePuy and Smith & Nephew; and has received research or institutional support from Cubist. Dr. Clyburn or an immediate family member has received royalties from Nimbic Systems and is a member of a speakers' bureau or has made paid presentations on behalf of Conformis. Dr. Moucha or an immediate family member serves as a board member, owner, officer, or committee member of the American Academy of Orthopaedic Surgeons. Neither Dr. Prokuski nor any immediate family member has received anything of value from or owns stock in a commercial company or institution related directly or indirectly to the subject of this chapter.

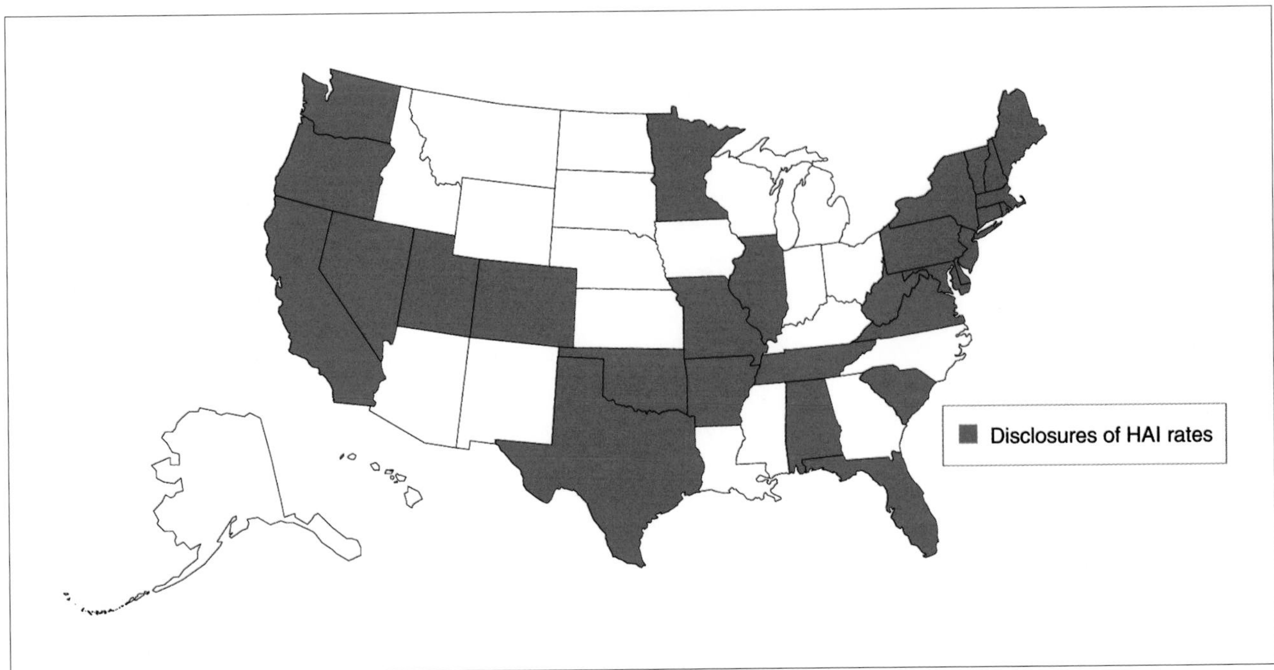

Figure 1 Map showing state initiatives for the public reporting of health care-associated infections. (Reproduced with permission from the Centers for Disease Control and Prevention, Atlanta, GA.)

indirect medical costs.[1] Approximately 8,000 patient deaths are associated with these infections. *Staphylococcus* species, including *Staphylococcus aureus*, are the leading nosocomial pathogens in hospitals throughout the world and made up approximately 30% of the pathogenic isolates of health care-associated infections reported to the National Healthcare Safety Network from January 2006 to October 2007.[1]

More recent data document that the largely solvable problem of hospital-acquired infections (HAIs) now occur in 1 of 20 patients (5%) and result in an estimated 1.7 million HAIs annually, leading to approximately 100,000 deaths each year and costing $26 to $33 billion in health care costs. The most common types of infection are urinary tract, surgical site, and bloodstream infections.[2]

Organisms resistant to multiple drugs include methicillin-resistant *S aureus* (MRSA) and vancomycin-resistant enterococci, which colonize the skin and are spread by contact. The CDC estimates that 94,360 invasive MRSA infections occurred in the United States in 2005. Of these infections, approximately 86% were health care-associated and 14% were community-associated.[3] The death rate from MRSA is 2.5 times greater than from nonresistant *S aureus*. More than 18,650 MRSA deaths were recorded in 2005. More than 30% of the population is colonized with *S aureus*, and an increasing proportion of these bacteria are MRSA. As many as 4% of health care workers may be colonized with MRSA, with up to 5% having a clinical infection.[4]

These bacteria contribute to two types of infection: surgical and so-called nonsurgical MRSA infections. Additionally, there are two types of MRSA. Both community-acquired MRSA and hospital-associated MRSA have resulted in an increase in the incidence of all types of nonsurgical infections. Because of the increasing incidence, severity, and extent of disease caused by multiple drug-resistant organisms, the prevention and treatment of these infections have become a national priority.

Health Care Organizations and Initiatives

The Healthcare Infection Control Practices Advisory Committee is a federal advisory committee composed of 14 external infection control experts who provide advice and guidance to the CDC and the Secretary of the Department of Health and Human Services regarding the practice of health care infection control and strategies for the surveillance, prevention, and control of health care-associated infections in US health care facilities. The CDC established the National Nosocomial Infections Surveillance System in 1970. Selected US hospitals routinely report nosocomial infection surveillance data for aggregation into a national database. In 1999, the CDC published a guideline presenting evidence-based recommendations for the prevention of SSIs and providing a

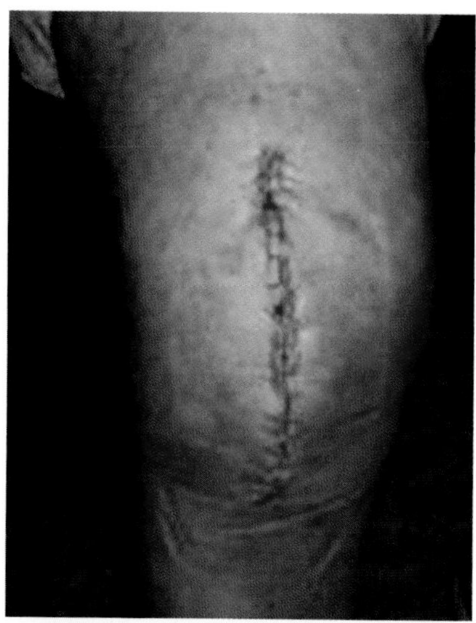

Figure 2 Photograph of the knee of a patient colonized with MRSA who was screened and treated with mupirocin with prophylactic vancomycin before total knee replacement surgery. The outcome was successful.

Table 1
SCIP Milestones for Infection Prevention Pertaining to Orthopaedic Procedures

Measure	Performance Measure
SCIP Infection 1	Prophylactic antibiotic received within 1 hour before surgical incision
SCIP Infection 2	Prophylactic antibiotic selection for surgical patients
SCIP Infection 3	Prophylactic antibiotics discontinued within 24 hours after surgery end time
SCIP Infection 5	Postoperative SSI diagnosed during index hospitalization
SCIP Infection 6	Surgery patients with appropriate hair removal

SCIP = Surgical Care Improvement Project; SSI = surgical site infection

detailed discussion of the preoperative, intraoperative, and postoperative issues relevant to the genesis of SSIs.[5]

The Centers for Medicare and Medicaid Services (CMS)-CDC Surgical Infection Prevention Project was implemented in 2002 by the CMS in collaboration with the CDC. The goal of the project is to decrease the morbidity and mortality associated with postoperative SSI by promoting appropriate selection and timing when administering prophylactic antimicrobials. The project was based on the experience that the CDC had gained from implementation of the National Nosocomial Infection Surveillance System and on efforts by the CMS to improve health care quality through its Medicare Quality Improvement Organization program. Effective July 1, 2006, the Joint Commission (formerly the Joint Commission on the Accreditation of Healthcare Organizations) transitioned the Surgical Infection Prevention Project to the Surgical Care Improvement Project (SCIP).

SCIP is a national partnership of government organizations committed to improving the safety of surgical care through the reduction of postoperative complications. Initiated in 2003 by the CMS and the CDC, the SCIP partnership is coordinated through a steering committee of 10 national organizations. More than 20 organizations provide expertise to the steering committee through a panel of technical experts. The goal of SCIP is to reduce the incidence of surgical complications nationally by 25% by the year 2010. Some SCIP milestones for infection prevention[6,7] are shown in **Table 1**.

Surveillance

Surveillance is the ongoing and systematic collection, analysis, interpretation, and dissemination of data regarding a health-related event for use in public health actions to reduce morbidity and mortality and improve health. Surveillance is becoming increasingly common in three major areas. The first area is a surgeon's own local surveillance of patients, which is accomplished by tracking postoperative infections as well as screening patients preoperatively for MRSA. The second area is national surveillance of infection rates and resistance, which is predominately provided by government agencies. The third area is public surveillance of hospitals for infection rates by consumer advocate organizations. Each of these surveillance methods increases awareness and enables proactive improvements in infection prevention.

Surveillance performed on a provider level includes postoperative surveillance for determining the rate and resistance of SSI organisms, including preoperative surveillance for methicillin resistance. Approximately 32% (89.4 million individuals) and 0.8% (2.3 million individuals) of the US population is colonized with *S aureus* and MRSA, respectively.[8] A standardized method of screening and decolonization for MRSA carriers has not been established, although there are reports of successful implementation of MRSA screening methods. Decolonization protocols and vancomycin prophylaxis for patients colonized with MRSA can improve the likelihood of an expected surgical outcome (**Figure 2**) and reduce the likelihood of the development of a MRSA infection[9,10] (**Figure 3**). Numerous governmental agencies, such as the Veterans Health Administration, have mandated MRSA screening programs. States, including California, Washington, Illinois, New Jersey, and Pennsylvania, also are mandating similar MRSA screening tests.

In 2008, the National Healthcare Safety Network Surveillance System,

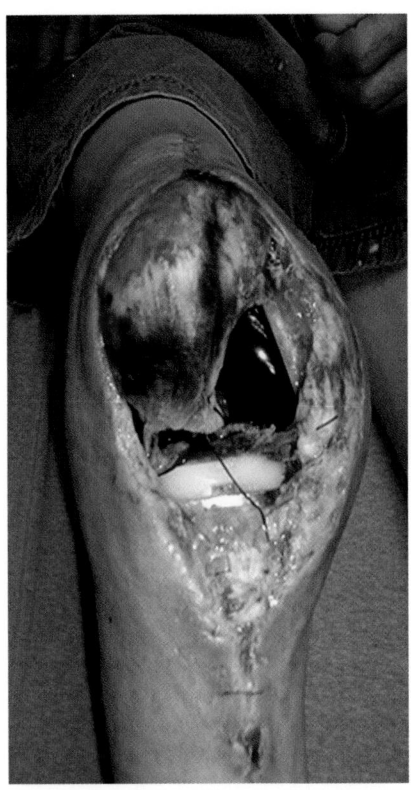

Figure 3 Photograph of an unsuccessful total knee replacement in a patient colonized with MRSA who was given cefazolin preoperatively.

which is supported by the Division of Healthcare Quality Promotion and the CDC, reported that approximately 2% of all surgical procedures result in infection, with orthopaedic procedures responsible for 18% of the SSIs. Coagulase-negative staphylococci and *S aureus* were the most prevalent pathogens causing SSI. Overall, most orthopaedic isolates were coagulase-negative staphylococci (15%), *S aureus* (49%), *Enterococcus* species (9%), *Candida* species (11%), *Escherichia coli* (3%), *Pseudomonas aeruginosa* (3%), and *Enterobacter* species (3%).[1]

Although there have been general improvements in the SCIP measures for preoperative antibiotic administration with 1 hour of surgery and discontinuance within 24 hours of surgery, the number of infections acquired in hospitals continued to rise in 2009. Warnings of government sanctions and efforts by some hospitals to combat the problem have not achieved a decrease in HAI rates.[11] The Secretary of Health and Human Services believes that a new reform law (effective in 2015) will help decrease the HAI rate by imposing a 1% pay-for-performance Medicare penalty for hospitals with high infection rates.

Recent progress has been made in raising awareness, improving event reporting systems, and establishing national standards for data collection. The Patient Safety and Quality Improvement Act of 2005 provides for the voluntary formation of patient safety organizations. Under this legislation, these entities can receive and analyze patient safety data and work with providers to improve care without fear of legal discovery. Currently, 69 organizations have been listed by the Department of Health and Human Services as patient safety organizations.

Public reporting of HAIs has become common.[12] Mandatory reporting of HAIs will provide consumers and stakeholders with additional information for making informed health care choices. However, these reported HAIs are not risk adjusted and may penalize the highest quality tertiary caregivers and institutions. Reports from private systems suggest that participation in an organized ongoing system for monitoring and reporting of HAIs may reduce HAI rates.[13,14] Web available report cards on individual hospitals have become readily accessible.[15,16]

Summary

There are few complications that can compromise a patient's outcome as severely as a nosocomial infection. This complication can range from mild and annoying cellulitis to severe and life-threatening SSIs and sepsis. Although the threat of SSIs remains ever present, an emerging paradigm of SSI infection prevention and control has matured.

It is likely that SSIs are underreported because they may become evident after patients are discharged from the hospital, and patients may not return to the original treating faculty for subsequent treatment. Prioritization of SSI surveillance efforts and advances in information technology should lead to improved participation in surveillance efforts by hospitals. The evolution of the National Nosocomial Infection Surveillance System into the Web-based National Healthcare Safety Network at the CDC should address the need for SSI data collection at the local level and allow prevention efforts to be more sharply focused.

References

1. Hidron AI, Edwards JR, Patel J, et al: NHSN annual update: Antimicrobial-resistant pathogens associated with healthcare-associated infections. Annual summary of data reported to the National Healthcare Safety Network at the Centers for Disease Control and Prevention, 2006-2007. *Infect Control Hosp Epidemiol* 2008; 29(11):996-1011.
2. The Centers for Disease Control and Prevention (CDC): Public Health Grand Rounds: Office of the Director. *Toward the Elimination of Healthcare-Associated Infections. October 15,* 2009. CDC website. http://www.cdc. gov/about/grand-rounds/archives/2009/download/GR-101509.pdf. Accessed August 31, 2010.
3. Klevens RM, Morrison MA, Nadle J, et al: Invasive methicillin-resistant Staphylococcus aureus infections in the United States. *JAMA* 2007; 298(15):1763-1771.
4. Albrich WC, Harbarth S: Health-care workers: Source, vector, or victim of MRSA? *Lancet Infect Dis* 2008;8(5):289-301.

5. Mangram AJ, Horan TC, Pearson ML, Silver LC, Jarvis WR; Hospital Infection Control Practices Advisory Committee: Guideline for prevention of surgical site infection, 1999. *Infect Control Hosp Epidemiol* 1999;20(4):250-280.
6. Fry DE: Surgical site infections and the Surgical Care Improvement Project (SCIP): Evolution of national quality measures. *Surg Infect (Larchmt)* 2008;9(6):579-584.
7. Fact Sheet SC: Specifications Manual: Discharges 04/1/2008 to 09/30/2008. QualityNet Website. http://www.qualitynet.org/dcs/ContentServer?cid=1192804535739&pagename=QnetPublic%2FPage%2FQnetTier3&c=Page. Accessed August 31, 2010.
8. Kuehnert MJ, Kruszon-Moran D, Hill HA, et al: Prevalence of Staphylococcus aureus nasal colonization in the United States, 2001-2002. *J Infect Dis* 2006; 193(2):172-179.
9. Kotilainen P, Routamaa M, Peltonen R, et al: Elimination of epidemic methicillin-resistant Staphylococcus aureus from a university hospital and district institutions: Finland. *Emerg Infect Dis* 2003;9(2):169-175.
10. Bode LG, Kluytmans JA, Wertheim HF, et al: Preventing surgical-site infections in nasal carriers of Staphylococcus aureus. *N Engl J Med* 2010;362(1):9-17.
11. US Department of Health & Human Services: 2009 National Healthcare Quality Report. AHRQ Publication No. 10-0003. March 2010. USHHS website. http://www.ahrq.gov/qual/qrdr09.htm. Accessed August 31, 2010.
12. McKibben L, Horan T, Tokars JI, et al: Guidance on public reporting of healthcare-associated infections: Recommendations of the Healthcare Infection Control Practices Advisory Committee. *Am J Infect Control* 2005;33(4): 217-226.
13. McCall JL, Macchiaroli S, Brown RB, et al: A method to track surgical site infections. *Qual Manag Health Care* 1998;6(3):52-62.
14. Centers for Disease Control and Prevention (CDC): Monitoring hospital-acquired infections to promote patient safety: United States, 1990-1999. *MMWR Morb Mortal Wkly Rep* 2000;49(8): 149-153.
15. Doctors and hospitals: Deadly infections. Hospitals can lower the risk, but many fail to act. March 2010. Consumer Reports Health .org Website. http://www.consumerreports.org/health/doctors-hospitals/hospital-infection/deadly-infections-hospitals-can-lower-the-danger/overview/deadly-infections-hospitals-can-lower-the-danger.htm. Accessed August 31, 2010.
16. Consumers Union: Safe Patient Project: Topics. Consumers Union Website. http://www.safepatient project.org/topics.html. Accessed August 31, 2010.

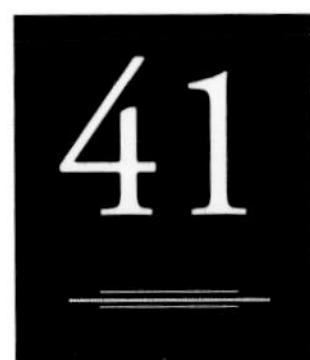

Prophylactic Antibiotics in Orthopaedic Surgery

Laura Prokuski, MD
Terry A. Clyburn, MD
Richard P. Evans, MD
Calin S. Moucha, MD

Abstract

The use of prophylactic antibiotics in orthopaedic surgery has been proven effective in reducing surgical site infections after hip and knee arthroplasty, spine procedures, and open reduction and internal fixation of fractures. To maximize the beneficial effect of prophylactic antibiotics, while minimizing any adverse effects, the correct antimicrobial agent must be selected, the drug must be administered just before incision, and the duration of administration should not exceed 24 hours.

Instr Course Lect 2011;60:545-555.

Approximately 27 million surgical procedures are performed in the United States each year.[1] Surgical site infections (SSIs) are a major source of postoperative illness. The Centers for Disease Control and Prevention (CDC) estimate that approximately 500,000 SSIs occur annually in the United States.[2] The National Nosocomial Infections Surveillance System (NNIS), established in 1970, monitors reported trends in nosocomial infections in US acute-care hospitals.[3]

Despite advances in infection control practices, SSIs remain a substantial cause of morbidity and mortality among hospitalized patients. Among surgical patients, SSIs were the most common nosocomial infection. Patients in whom an SSI developed were five times more likely to be readmitted to the hospital, 60% more likely to spend time in an intensive care unit, and twice as likely to die compared with patients without an SSI.[4] In surgical patients with an SSI who died, 89% of the deaths were attributable to the infection.[5]

Criteria for Defining SSI

The NNIS has developed standardized surveillance criteria for defining SSIs. These definitions have been applied consistently by surveillance personnel and are currently a national standard. SSIs are classified as superficial if they involve only skin and subcutaneous tissue and deep if the infection is within the fascia or muscle. Organ/space SSIs involve any part of the anatomy, other than incised body wall layers, which were opened or manipulated during surgery. Osteomyelitis, epidural abscess, diskitis, septic bursitis, and septic arthritis are considered organ/space SSIs. These criteria also specify that a superficial wound infection occurs within 30 days after surgery, but a deep wound infection occurs up to 1 year from the time of surgery if an implant is in place.[3]

Pathogenesis

Bacteria contaminate every surgical wound. The most common source is the endogenous flora of the skin, which is usually composed primarily of aerobic gram-positive cocci. The

Dr. Clyburn or an immediate family member has received royalties from Nimbic Systems and is a member of a speakers' bureau or has made paid presentations on behalf of Conformis. Dr. Evans or an immediate family member is a member of a speakers' bureau or has made paid presentations on behalf of Cubist; serves as a paid consultant to or is an employee of DePuy and Smith & Nephew; and has received research or institutional support from Cubist. Dr. Moucha or an immediate family member serves as a board member, owner, officer, or committee member of the American Academy of Orthopaedic Surgeons. Neither Dr. Prokuski nor any immediate family member has received anything of value from or owns stock in a commercial company or institution related directly or indirectly to the subject of this chapter.

This chapter adapted from Prokuski L: Prophylactic antibiotics in orthopaedic surgery. J Amer Acad Orthop Surg *2008;16(5):283-293.*

skin may also harbor fecal organisms, including gram-negative rods and anaerobes. SSI occurs when the bacterial load in the wound cannot be managed by the host defenses. The amount of bacteria required to cause infection is variable and depends on the virulence of the organisms, the condition of the wound (such as the quantity of necrotic tissue), the presence of nonbiologic substances (such as metallic implants), and host immune competence. Bacteria may enter the surgical wound through hematogenous dissemination or from the exogenous environment. Bacteria may have adaptive strategies to increase their virulence. Of particular importance to orthopaedic surgeons are the surface compounds that some bacteria produce; these compounds inhibit phagocytosis and facilitate adherence to implants, shielding them from immune defenses.[3,6]

The NNIS has reported that the distribution of pathogens isolated from SSIs did not change markedly from 1986 to 1996.[7] *Staphylococcus aureus*, coagulase-negative staphylococci, *Enterococcus* species, and *Escherichia coli* were the most frequently isolated pathogens. Recent data have shown that an increasing proportion of SSIs are caused by antimicrobial-resistant pathogens, such as methicillin-resistant *Staphylococcus aureus* (MRSA).[3] The changing spectrum of organisms associated with orthopaedic SSIs will be an important factor in directing future recommendations for surgical antibiotic prophylaxis. Existing recommendations are based on current knowledge.

Antimicrobial Prophylaxis in General Orthopaedic Surgery

Surgical antimicrobial prophylaxis is not administered to sterilize the tissues but as an adjunct to modulate intraoperative contamination of the surgical wound to a level that will not overwhelm the defenses of the host.[3] Optimal prophylaxis ensures that an adequate concentration of an antimicrobial agent is present in the serum and tissue during the entire time the surgical wound is open. The antibiotic should be active against bacteria that are likely to contaminate the wound and should be both safe and inexpensive. The antibiotic prophylaxis should have the smallest impact possible on the normal bacterial flora of the patient and should take into account the biogram (the common infecting organisms in a particular community) of the community.[8]

Choice of Antimicrobial Agent

Cephalosporins

In clean orthopaedic surgery, bacteria found on the skin, primarily aerobic gram-positive cocci, are a cause for concern. A first-generation cephalosporin, such as cefazolin, provides adequate coverage against most staphylococci and other gram-positive bacteria that may contaminate the wound. Second-generation cephalosporins, such as cefuroxime, have a slightly broader spectrum, covering some gram-negative bacteria while remaining effective against gram-positive organisms. Cephalosporins also rapidly achieve optimal tissue concentrations in subcutaneous tissue, muscle, and bone. First- and second-generation cephalosporins have a long enough half-life to provide adequate tissue concentrations during the entire time the wound is open in most orthopaedic procedures. The cost of these agents is relatively low. Adverse effects are rare but include a spectrum of allergic reactions.[9]

Drug Allergies

Although many patients have drug allergies documented in their medical records, efforts should be made to determine if a true allergy (such as urticaria, pruritus, bronchospasm, hypotension) or a serious risk for an adverse drug reaction (such as drug fever or drug-induced hypersensitivity reaction) really exists. The incidence of adverse reactions to cephalosporins among patients with reported penicillin allergy is rare. Patients with a history of penicillin allergy and negative penicillin skin test results are not at an increased risk of an adverse reaction to cephalosporins.[9] Alternative antimicrobial agents should be considered for patients who have a high likelihood of serious adverse reaction or allergy based on their history and/or skin testing. Vancomycin or clindamycin may be used for patients with a true β-lactam allergy.[3,9,10] Penicillin allergy skin testing can decrease prophylactic vancomycin use in patients treated with elective orthopaedic surgery.[11]

Vancomycin and MRSA

The routine use of vancomycin for surgical prophylaxis in orthopaedic surgery has been discouraged. Increased exposure to vancomycin provides evolutionary pressure for organisms to develop vancomycin resistance and is a risk factor for the development of a vancomycin-resistant enterococcus infection.[12] Vancomycin has been traditionally reserved for the treatment of serious infections with β-lactam resistant organisms.

MRSA has become more prevalent in the community, with MRSA colonization reported in 3% to 20% of patients.[13] Price et al[14] reported an increase from 0% in 2003 to 4% in 2005 in MRSA nasal colonization identified by preoperative screening in patients undergoing outpatient orthopaedic surgery.

MRSA is now subclassified into community-associated and health care-associated MRSA. Each type differs in its pathogenic capacity, virulence, and antibiotic resistance profile and in the patient population affected.[15] Groups at risk for community-associated MRSA include athletes in contact sports, children at day care centers, homeless people, intravenous drug users, men who have sex with men, military personnel, certain ethnic groups, and prison inmates. Other risk factors include antibiotic use within the preceding year, crowded living conditions, and chronic wounds.[15-17]

Individuals at risk for health care-associated MRSA are those who have been hospitalized, had surgery or dialysis, or had residency in a long-term care facility in the past year. Also at risk are patients with a permanent indwelling catheter or percutaneous medical device, those with previous MRSA infection and/or colonization, patients receiving recent antimicrobial therapy, and those in proximity to or contact with a patient colonized or infected with MRSA.[17]

Knowledge of patient risk factors can help the physician determine if vancomycin is an appropriate prophylactic agent. Current or previous infection with MRSA, known MRSA colonization, and the presence of MRSA risk factors are indications to choose vancomycin for surgical prophylaxis. Sanderson[18] states that MRSA infection or colonization should label the patient colonized for life because subsequent negative screening swabs may not be accurate.

Vancomycin may also be an appropriate prophylactic agent in facilities with recent MRSA outbreaks. Some physicians believe that vancomycin is the correct prophylactic agent in institutions with a "high" prevalence of MRSA. Unfortunately, no threshold exists as to what constitutes a "high" enough prevalence rate to use vancomycin for routine surgical prophylaxis. There is no evidence that routine use of vancomycin instead of cephalosporins for prophylaxis in institutions with perceived high rates of MRSA infection will result in fewer SSIs.[9] In an institution with a perceived high rate of MRSA infection, Finkelstein et al[19] randomized 885 cardiac surgery patients to prophylaxis with cefazolin or vancomycin. There was no difference in the SSI rates between the two groups. Patients who received cefazolin and later developed an SSI were more likely to be infected with MRSA. Patients in whom an SSI developed after vancomycin prophylaxis were more likely to be infected with methicillin-sensitive *S aureus*. The choice of antimicrobial used for prophylaxis changed the infecting organism but did not alter the infection rate.

Preoperative Screening and Decolonization

Nasal colonization with *S aureus* increases the risk of SSI with *S aureus*. Preoperative nasal swabbing can detect 80% to 90% of carriers and may be a helpful screening test for elective surgery.[18] Mupirocin is a topical antimicrobial agent that is effective against *S aureus*, and it can be used in the perioperative period to reduce nasal colonization. It is applied inside the nose for 3 to 5 days, has few adverse side effects (similar to placebo), and is relatively inexpensive. Mupirocin resistance does not appear to be a problem with short-term use.[20] Agents used to reduce *S aureus* on skin include soaps containing triclosan or chlorhexidine.

There is support for preoperative decolonization in patients. Kalmeijer et al[21] studied patients undergoing orthopaedic surgery with prosthetic implants. Nasal carriage of *S aureus* was the most important independent risk factor for the development of an SSI. It is believed that the elimination of nasal carriage of *S aureus* will decrease SSI rates. Gernaat-van der Sluis et al[22] reported that the overall rate of SSI and the rate of *S aureus* SSI was significantly lower in a group that received mupirocin versus a group of historic control subjects. Kalmeijer et al[23] randomized patients to receive either placebo or mupirocin nasal ointment before knee arthroplasty, hip arthroplasty, or spinal surgery. Eradication of *S aureus* nasal carriage was significantly more effective in patients who received mupirocin; however, the overall SSI rates and the *S aureus* SSI rates were comparable in the two groups. A recent, randomized, double-blind, placebo-controlled, multicenter trial found that the preoperative use of mupirocin and chlorhexidine soap in patients with nasal colonization of *S aureus* resulted in a deep surgical wound infection rate of 0.9% compared with 4.4% in a group that did not receive the decolonization treatment.[24]

The effect of prophylactic mupirocin specifically on MRSA SSIs in orthopaedic surgery has also been examined. Wilcox et al[25] reported on a consecutive series of patients undergoing orthopaedic surgery involving the insertion of metal prostheses or internal fracture fixation. The treatment group received perioperative prophylaxis with nasal mupirocin and triclosan soap. A group of patients undergoing similar procedures served as the control group. There was a marked decrease in the incidence of MRSA nasal carriage in the mupirocin/triclosan group. After introduction of the mupirocin/triclosan protocol, MRSA SSIs decreased from 23 per 1,000 to 3.3 to 4 per 1,000. Of the 11 MRSA SSIs that occurred in the mupirocin/triclosan group, only one patient received the intervention correctly. The number of SSIs caused by other pathogens was not affected by the intervention. The relative contributions of mupirocin and triclosan could not be determined. Nevertheless, the authors stated their results justify empirical, as opposed to targeted, usage of mupirocin prophylaxis because current health care practices make it almost impossible to preoperatively assess MRSA carriage and subsequently treat all patients undergoing orthopaedic surgery. It is concerning that Rotger et al[26] found that 27% of MRSA isolates causing hip or knee prosthetic joint infections were resistant to mupirocin.

Timing of Administration

In a 1961 study using guinea pigs, Burke[27] investigated the effects of parenteral antibiotics on inflammation of surgical incisions contaminated with *S aureus*. Antibiotics were administered at different times in relationship to the inoculation of the wound with bacteria. When antibiotics were given 1 hour before the inoculation, there was no inflammatory response. These wounds did not differ either clinically or microscopically from incisions inoculated with dead bacteria. When antibiotics were given 1 hour after inoculation, a greater inflammatory response was observed. When antibiotics were administered 3 hours or longer after inoculation, the inflammatory response was no different than that observed in animals that had received no antibiotics. Burke concluded the susceptibility of bacteria was greatest when the antimicrobial agent was in the tissue when the bacteria arrived, and the effective period of antibiotic action was restricted to the initial few hours after inoculation.

The lowest rate of SSI has been observed with antibiotics given shortly before incision. Classen et al[28] prospectively studied patients undergoing a variety of clean or clean-contaminated surgical procedures. The patients who received antibiotic prophylaxis during the 2 hours prior to incision had the lowest rates of SSI. Relative risk for SSI increased with antibiotic administration during the 3 hours after incision (2.4), 3 to 24 hours after incision (5.8), and 2 to 24 hours before incision (6.7).

Infusion of cephalosporins and clindamycin should begin within 60 minutes of incision and be completed at the time of incision. Administration of vancomycin should begin 1 to 2 hours before incision to accommodate the extended infusion time. Administration of the antimicrobial agent at the time of anesthesia induction is safe and results in adequate tissue drug levels at the time of incision.[9,29] The concentration of cephalosporins in serum, bone, synovial fluid, and wound drainage during knee and hip arthroplasty was measured by Schurman et al.[30] The antibiotics were administered with the induction of anesthesia, and high concentrations of antibiotics were found in all samples. Cefazolin administered immediately preoperatively has resulted in the bone cefazolin concentration to be 60 times the minimum inhibitory concentration for penicillin-resistant *S aureus*.[29]

Tourniquet use is a specific consideration when considering the timing of prophylactic antibiotic administration in extremity surgery. The concentrations of cephalosporin in serum and bone are high immediately after administration and were reported to be adequate even with the use of a tourniquet.[30] Johnson[31] investigated the concentration of cefuroxime in bone and subcutaneous fat during knee arthroplasty. Patients were randomized to receive 1.5 g of cefuroxime 5, 10, 15, and 20 minutes before tourniquet inflation. All patient groups had antibiotic levels greater than the minimal bactericidal concentration for *S aureus* in bone. In the subcutaneous fat, 86% of the group treated at 5 minutes had antibiotic concentrations lower than the minimal bactericidal concentration for *S aureus*; however, the levels were adequate in the other groups. The authors concluded that 10 minutes would be an appropriate amount of time between administration and tourniquet inflation to achieve adequate tissue levels of cefuroxime. Deacon et al[32] reported that adequate tissue concentrations of cephalosporins can be achieved in the foot after tourniquet inflation. Cefazolin concentrations in the medial eminence of the first metatarsal reached adequate levels when administration was 30 to 60 minutes before surgery and a pneumatic ankle tourniquet was used during the bunion surgery.

Dosing

Cefazolin dosing is 1 to 2 g, with 2 g recommended if the patient weighs more than 80 kg.[3,9] The dose of cefuroxime is 1.5 g. The optimal dose of vancomycin and clindamycin is related to the patient's body mass. Pediatric dosing is based on the patient's mass. The optimal dose may also change with specific conditions or diseases that affect the metabolism of the drug. If there is a question regarding the appropriate dose, consultation with a pharmacist may be helpful.

Additional doses of antibiotic are warranted if the duration of the procedure exceeds one to two times the half-life of the antibiotic,[19,33,34] or if there is significant blood loss during the procedure.[12,32,35] In a study of 40 patients undergoing major surgery with significant blood loss and intraoperative blood salvage, the minimal inhibitory concentration for several cephalosporins in tissue was barely adequate after 4 hours, indicating that redosing could be beneficial.[36]

Duration

The shortest effective duration of antimicrobial administration for preventing postoperative infection is not known.[9,11] Most published evidence shows that antimicrobial prophylaxis after wound closure does not provide additional protection against SSI. Studies comparing single-dose prophylaxis with multiple-dose prophylaxis have shown no reduction in the SSI rate with the additional doses.[9,34] Continuing antibiotic prophylaxis longer than 24 hours after wound closure has not proven to be beneficial and may contribute to the development of antimicrobial resistance.[9,11] Continuing prophylactic antibiotics for the duration of time that drains and catheters are in place has not been shown to reduce SSI rates.[9,37]

Prophylactic Antibiotics in Orthopaedic Surgical Subspecialties

The practice of orthopaedic surgery is becoming increasingly subspecialized. A summary of information related to the use of surgical antimicrobial prophylaxis in orthopaedic subspecialties follows.

Hip and Knee Arthroplasty

Although the infection rate is fairly low after hip and knee arthroplasty, the consequences of a prosthetic infection are severe. Prophylactic antibiotics have been shown to reduce the incidence of infection after primary joint arthroplasty. Early studies show antibiotic prophylaxis is more effective than placebo in the prevention of postoperative wound infections in patients treated with total joint arthroplasty.[38] In 1973, Ericson et al[39] compared infection rates in patients receiving either placebo or cloxacillin before major surgery of the hip. In the first 6 months after the procedure, 12 of 88 patients in the placebo group had an infection compared with none of the 83 patients in the cloxacillin group. Carlsson et al[40] followed this group for 7 years and reported the infection rate without prophylaxis was 15.4% compared with 2% with prophylaxis. Subsequent investigations have shown the efficacy of prophylactic antibiotics in reducing SSI after hip or knee arthroplasty.[28,41]

The preferred antimicrobial agents for prophylaxis in patients undergoing hip or knee arthroplasty are cefazolin and cefuroxime.[9,10,12,33,34,42-44] The rise in the incidence of MRSA infections prompted Ritter et al[45] to examine an alternative prophylactic antibiotic regimen. A series of 201 consecutive patients treated with total joint arthroplasty received a single dose of 1 g vancomycin and 80 g of gentamycin. Trough levels of vancomycin up to 24 hours later exceeded the minimum inhibitory concentration for all sensitive organisms. No postoperative infections were reported. The authors concluded this was a safe and effective method of prophylaxis for joint arthroplasty. Gram-negative organisms are reported to account for 20% to 30% of SSIs reported to the NNIS for cardiac surgery and total joint arthroplasty.[46] Therefore, antibiotic prophylaxis for joint arthroplasty may evolve to include antimicrobial agents active against gram-negative organisms.

The optimal duration of antimicrobial prophylaxis is not known. No further benefit has been shown with extending antibiotic prophylaxis beyond 24 hours in arthroplasty patients.[47-50] It has not been proved that continuing antibiotic prophylaxis until removal of drains and catheters reduces the incidence of SSIs.[10]

The data supporting prophylactic antibiotics in hip and knee arthroplasty are sufficiently strong that national organizations have published recommendations for their use. The Surgical Care Improvement Committee Project has issued recommendations on the use of intravenous antibiotic prophylaxis in primary total joint arthroplasty that are similar to those previously described.[9] The American Academy of Orthopaedic Surgeons (AAOS) has issued recommendations on the use of intravenous prophylactic antibiotics in primary total joint arthroplasty[33] (**Table 1**).

Spine Surgery

Early retrospective studies generally supported the use of prophylactic antibiotics for spine surgery.[38,51-53] Later randomized underpowered trials did not overwhelmingly prove the efficacy of prophylactic antimicrobial agents in reducing SSIs in spine surgery.[54-58] Barker[59] performed a meta-analysis of antibiotic prophylaxis in spine surgery that include 843 patients from 6 randomized controlled trials. The meta-analysis provided statistically significant ($P < 0.01$) evidence that prophylactic antibiotic use is effective in reducing SSI rates in spine surgery.

The timing of administration of prophylactic antimicrobial agents has been shown to be critical in reducing SSIs in spine surgery. Antibiotics administered more than 2 hours before incision or after completion of the procedure produced higher rates of SSI.[53,58]

Redosing antimicrobial agents intraoperatively to maintain adequate tissue levels has been found to be important in spine surgery. Swoboda et al[35] examined patients undergoing elective spinal instrumentation. Blood loss correlated with the change in tissue antibiotic concentrations of cefazolin. Based on measured pharmacokinetic values, the authors recommended that additional doses of cefazolin should be administered when the operation approaches 4 hours or blood loss is greater than 1,500 mL.

There is support for the use of prophylactic antibiotics in spine surgery. Special emphasis exists in the data on the importance of timing the administration and intraoperative redosing of antibiotics to maximize efficacy.

Table 1

AAOS Recommendations for the Use of Intravenous Antibiotic Prophylaxis in Primary Total Joint Arthroplasty

Recommendation 1: The antibiotic used for prophylaxis should be carefully selected, consistent with current recommendations in the literature, taking into account the issues of resistance and patient allergies.

Currently, cefazolin and cefuroxime are the preferred antibiotics for patients undergoing orthopaedic procedures. Clindamycin or vancomycin may be used for patients with a confirmed β-lactam allergy. Vancomycin may be used in patients with known colonization with methicillin-resistant *Staphylococcus aureus* (MRSA) or in facilities with recent MRSA outbreaks. In multiple studies, exposure to vancomycin is reported as a risk factor in the development of vancomycin-resistant enterococcus (VRE) colonization and infection. Therefore, vancomycin should be reserved for the treatment of serious infection with β-lactam-resistant organisms or for the treatment of infection in patients with life-threatening allergy to β-lactam antimicrobial agents.

Recommendation 2: Timing and dosage of antibiotic administration should optimize the efficacy of the therapy.

Prophylactic antibiotics should be administered within 1 hour before skin incision. Due to an extended infusion time, vancomycin should be started within 2 hours before incision. When a proximal tourniquet is used, the antibiotic must be completely infused before inflation of the tourniquet. Dose amount should be proportional to patient weight; for patients more than 80 kg, the doses of cefazolin should be doubled. Additional intraoperative doses of antibiotic are advised when the duration of the procedure exceeds one to two times the antibiotic's half-life or when there is significant blood loss during the procedure.

The general guidelines for frequency of intraoperative antibiotic administration are as follows: cefazolin every 2-5 hours, cefuroxime every 3-4 hours, clindamycin every 3-6 hours, vancomycin every 6-12 hours.

Recommendation 3: Duration of prophylactic antibiotic administration should not exceed the 24-hour postoperative period.

Prophylactic antibiotics should be discontinued within 24 hours of the end of surgery. The medical literature does not support the continuation of antibiotics until all drains or catheters are removed and provides no evidence of benefit when they are continued past 24 hours.

Arthroscopy

The incidence of infection after arthroscopic surgery has been reported to be extremely low (approximately 0.2%).[60,61] D'Angelo and Ogilvie-Harris[62] retrospectively reviewed patients who had infections after knee and shoulder arthroscopic procedures performed without prophylactic antibiotics and reported a septic arthritis rate of 0.23%. After comparing the cost of treating the infections and the cost of administering prophylactic antibiotics universally, the authors concluded that it may be cost-effective to use antibiotic prophylaxis to reduce hospital costs and patient morbidity when performing arthroscopic surgery. However, this would need to be proven in a better designed study. A prospective, randomized, double-blind study of 437 patients undergoing arthroscopic procedures on the knee, shoulder, ankle, elbow, and wrist was performed by Wieck et al.[61] Procedures included subacromial decompression, lateral release, meniscal repair, and synovectomy. No implants or grafts were inserted. Patients either received cefazolin or placebo preoperatively. No deep infections occurred in either group; one superficial infection occurred in a patient who received placebo. The authors concluded that the routine use of prophylactic antibiotics is not indicated for patients treated with arthroscopic surgery.

Kurzweil[63] expressed concerns regarding antibiotic prophylaxis in contemporary arthroscopic procedures. Many procedures are not performed exclusively arthroscopically and involve making incisions. Other procedures can require prolonged surgical times. More complex arthroscopic procedures may involve the use of implants. All these conditions present additional risk factors for the development of an SSI. No study has truly examined the effect of prophylactic antibiotics along the spectrum of contemporary arthroscopic procedures. Kurzweil[63] recommended that routine antibiotic prophylaxis should be provided for patients who undergo arthroscopic surgery.

The few available studies are not sufficiently designed or powered to provide meaningful conclusions about the efficacy of prophylactic antibiotics in the full spectrum of arthroscopic surgery.

Pediatric Orthopaedics

Pediatric patients are subject to many of the same procedures performed on adults, but pediatric-specific antibiotic prophylaxis data are sparse. A case-control study to identify risk factors for SSIs after spinal fusion in children found that antibiotic prophylaxis was more frequently suboptimal in patients in whom an SSI developed.[64] Of the 13 cases of infection, one patient did not receive antibiotic prophylaxis. Ten of the remaining 12 cases received appropriate doses of cefazolin, but timing was optimal in only 3 cases.

No well-controlled studies have evaluated the efficacy of antimicrobial prophylaxis in pediatric patients undergoing clean orthopaedic procedures. In most instances, pediatric recommendations have been extrapolated from studies performed on adults.[11]

Foot and Ankle

Few studies have examined the effect of prophylactic antibiotics on SSI rates exclusively in foot and ankle surgery. Zgonis et al[65] performed a retrospective review of 555 patients treated with elective foot and ankle surgery for nontraumatic conditions; no revision procedures were included. The wound infection rate was 1.6% with prophylactic antibiotics and 1.4% without. The authors concluded that prophylactic antibiotic use in routine elective foot and ankle surgery is not warranted. Paiement et al[66] performed a double-blind randomized prospective study in 122 patients treated with open reduction and internal fixation of isolated closed ankle fractures. No statistical difference in the rates of infections with or without prophylactic antibiotics was found. The authors, however, recognized that the study may have been underpowered.

No recommendations exist for the use of prophylactic antibiotics in patients with diabetes mellitus who are undergoing clean elective foot surgery. Diabetic patients are at a higher risk for postoperative infection, and their infections are typically polymicrobial. Extrapolation of recommendations from other studies may not be accurate.[11]

Few studies are available and are not sufficiently designed or powered to provide meaningful conclusions about the efficacy of prophylactic antibiotics in foot and ankle surgery.

Hand Surgery

Few studies address the use of antibiotic prophylaxis in patients treated with clean elective hand surgery. Kleinert et al[67] prospectively studied 2,337 patients treated with elective upper extremity surgery. Perioperative antibiotics were given unpredictably and never before incision. Infection developed in 2.6% of patients who received systemic antibiotics and in 1.2% who did not. The statistical analysis determined that systemic administration of antibiotics was not a predictor of infection.

Hanssen et al[68] reported a retrospective 0.447% infection rate after carpal tunnel release; most patients did not receive perioperative antibiotics. Platt and Page[69] prospectively analyzed 112 patients treated with elective hand surgery. The decision to use antibiotics was made by the operating surgeon, and several different antibiotic regimens were used. No difference in the postoperative infection rate was reported among the 48 patients who received antibiotics and the 64 patients who received no antibiotics. Limitations in the study were a failure to randomize the patients and the small numbers of patients.

A multicenter, retrospective review of carpal tunnel release procedures showed that antibiotic use did not decrease the risk of infection in the study population, including patients with diabetes.[70] The authors concluded that routine antibiotic prophylaxis for carpal tunnel release is not indicated.

No randomized controlled studies exist on the efficacy of prophylactic antibiotics in metacarpophalangeal, wrist, or elbow arthroplasty. Many authors recommend prophylactic antibiotics in upper extremity arthroplasty, extrapolating from studies of hip and knee arthroplasty or justifying their use by emphasizing the seriousness of an arthroplasty infection.[69,71]

Prophylactic antibiotics have not been proven efficacious in clean elective hand procedures. Properly designed and powered studies do not exist to definitively answer this question. In a review article, Hoffman and Adams[71] state that it would be reasonable to use prophylactic antibiotics in reconstructive procedures involving large flaps, procedures of prolonged duration, and arthroplasty.

Closed Fracture Fixation

Preoperative prophylactic antibiotics are beneficial in reducing SSIs after surgical treatment of hip fractures. Boyd et al[72] studied 280 patients with hip fractures randomized to receive either nafcillin or a placebo. The infection rate in the nafcillin group was 0.8%, and the infection rate in the placebo group was 4.8%. Similar benefits of prophylactic antibiotics have been shown by other investigators.[73,74] A meta-analysis showed that antibiotic prophylaxis significantly reduced the rate of wound infections after hip fracture surgery when compared with placebo. One preoperative dose of intravenous antibiotics was as effective as multiple doses.[75]

Prophylactic antibiotics also have been shown to be effective in reducing SSIs with internal fixation of other closed fractures.[76] The Dutch Trauma Trial was a prospective, randomized, double-blind, placebo-controlled study of antibiotic prophylaxis in the primary surgical treatment of 2,195 closed fractures.[77] Hip, femur, patella, tibia, fibula, ankle, foot, humerus, forearm, and hand fractures were included. Patients received preoperative ceftriaxone or placebo. The infection rate was 3.6% in the ceftriaxone group and 8.3% in the placebo group. A meta-analysis by Gillespie and Walenkamp[78] examined the effects of preoperative antibiotics on 8,307 patients in 22 studies treated with fracture surgery. In those treated using closed fracture fixation, single-dose antibiotic prophylaxis significantly reduced the number of deep wound, superficial wound, urinary tract, and respiratory tract infections. Multiple-dose prophylaxis was not superior to single-dose prophylaxis in reducing the rate of SSI.

Prophylactic Antibiotics in Irrigation Solution

The use of prophylactic intravenous antibiotics has been shown to reduce the infection rate in elective clean orthopaedic surgeries and open fractures. The addition of antibiotics to the irrigation solution has become common in an attempt to further decrease the rate of postoperative infections. However, the efficacy of using antibiotics in irrigation fluid has not been proved.

Two early clinical studies examined the efficacy of antibiotic irrigation in orthopaedic surgery. One study found that topical antibiotics reduced the subsequent rate of infection,[79] and the other did not.[80]

Information on antibiotic irrigation during spine surgery exists in the neurosurgical literature. Savitz et al[81] examined antibiotic irrigation in elective clean spinal surgery. Intravenous antibiotic prophylaxis was also used. No wound infections occurred. The authors stated the lack of laboratory methodology and statistical analysis precluded an exact explanation for the success in eliminating postoperative sepsis. Haines[82] concluded that the existing published evidence did not support the use of antibiotic irrigation for clean neurosurgical procedures for which postoperative infection rates were less than 5%. Brown et al[83] discouraged the inclusion of antibiotics in the irrigation fluid because their antibacterial actions are unpredictable and the effectiveness of this practice has not been proved.

Kleinert et al[67] studied postoperative infection after elective outpatient procedures on the upper extremity. The authors reported variable use of parenteral antibiotics and antibiotics in irrigation fluid. The wound infection rate was 2.2% in 179 wounds irrigated with antibiotic solution and 1.2% in 1,385 wounds that had been irrigated with a solution that did not contain antibiotics; this was not a significant difference.

Anglen[84] studied open fracture wounds of the lower extremity, randomizing patients to receive either bacitracin or castile soap added to irrigation fluid. There was no significant difference in the infection rate between the two groups. Wound healing complications occurred in 9.5% of the bacitracin irrigation group and in 4% of the castile soap irrigation group. The author concluded that irrigation of open fracture wounds with antibiotic solution offered no advantage over the soap solution, and it may increase the risk of wound healing complications.

Several concerns exist with regard to antibiotic irrigation.[85] Adverse reactions to topically applied antibiotics occur. Anaphylaxis after irrigation with bacitracin solution has been reported.[86,87] Neomycin has prominent neuromuscular blocking actions and may contribute to prolonged unconsciousness and respiratory depression/apnea, bradycardia, and hypotension. Neomycin has caused postoperative deafness and renal failure.[87,88] The cost of using antibiotics in irrigation adds to the total cost of patient care. The routine use of antibiotic irrigation may contribute to the development of antibiotic resistance.[85]

Summary

Knowledge concerning SSIs is changing rapidly. Recommendations are based on current knowledge but may change over time. The use of prophylactic antibiotics in orthopaedic surgery has been proven effective in reducing SSI rates in studies of hip and knee arthroplasty, spine surgery, and open reduction and internal fixation of fractures. To maximize the beneficial effect of prophylactic antibiotics while minimizing adverse effects, the correct antimicrobial agents must be selected, the drug must be administered just before incision, and the duration of administration should not exceed 24 hours.

References

1. Centers for Disease Control and Prevention, National Center for Health Statistics: *Vital and Health Statistics, Detailed Diagnoses and Procedures, National Hospital Discharge Survey, 1994.* Hyattsville, MD, Department of Health and Human Services, 1997, vol 127.
2. Wong ES: Surgical site infections, in Mayhall DG, ed: *Hospital Epidemiology and Infection Control,* ed 2. Philadelphia, PA, Lippincott, Williams & Wilkins, 1999, pp 189-210.
3. Mangram AJ, Horan TC, Pearson ML, Silver LC, Jarvis WR; Hospital Infection Control Practices Advisory Committee: Guideline for prevention of surgical site infection, 1999. *Infect Control Hosp Epidemiol* 1999;20(4): 250-280.
4. Kirkland KB, Briggs JP, Trivette SL, Wilkinson WE, Sexton DJ: The impact of surgical-site infections in the 1990s: Attributable mortality, excess length of hospitalization, and extra costs. *Infect Control Hosp Epidemiol* 1999;20(11):725-730.
5. Horan TC, Culver DH, Gaynes RP, et al: Nosocomial infections in surgical patients in the United States, January 1986-June 1992. *Infect Control Hosp Epidemiol* 1993;14(2):73-80.
6. Rimoldi RL, Haye W: The use of antibiotics for wound prophylaxis in spinal surgery. *Orthop Clin North Am* 1996;27(1):47-52.
7. Centers for Disease Control and Prevention: National Nosocomial Infections Surveillance (NNIS) report, data summary from October 1986-April 1996, issued May 1996: A report from the National Nosocomial Infections Surveillance (NNIS) System. *Am J Infect Control* 1996;24(5):380-388.
8. Raymond DP, Kuehnert MJ, Sawyer RG: Preventing antimicrobial-resistant bacterial infections in surgical patients. *Surg Infect (Larchmt)* 2002;3(4): 375-385.

9. Bratzler DW, Houck PM, et al; Surgical Infection Prevention Guidelines Writers Workgroup: Antimicrobial prophylaxis for surgery: An advisory statement from the National Surgical Infection Prevention Project. *Clin Infect Dis* 2004;38(12):1706-1715.

10. American Society of Health-System Pharmacists: ASHP therapeutic guidelines on antimicrobial prophylaxis in surgery. *Am J Health Syst Pharm* 1999;56(18): 1839-1888.

11. Li JT, Markus PJ, Osmon DR, Estes L, Gosselin VA, Hanssen AD: Reduction of vancomycin use in orthopedic patients with a history of antibiotic allergy. *Mayo Clin Proc* 2000;75(9):902-906.

12. Medical Letter: Antimicrobial prophylaxis in surgery. *Med Lett Drugs Ther* 2001;43(1116-1117): 92-97.

13. Lucet JC, Chevret S, Durand-Zaleski I, Chastang C, Régnier B, Multicenter Study Group: Prevalence and risk factors for carriage of methicillin-resistant Staphylococcus aureus at admission to the intensive care unit: Results of a multicenter study. *Arch Intern Med* 2003;163(2):181-188.

14. Price CS, Williams A, Philips G, Dayton M, Smith W, Morgan S: Staphylococcus aureus nasal colonization in preoperative orthopaedic outpatients. *Clin Orthop Relat Res* 2008;466(11):2842-2847.

15. Patel A, Calfee RP, Plante M, Fischer SA, Arcand N, Born C: Methicillin-resistant Staphylococcus aureus in orthopaedic surgery. *J Bone Joint Surg Br* 2008;90(11): 1401-1406.

16. Muto CA, Jernigan JA, Ostrowsky BE, et al: SHEA guideline for preventing nosocomial transmission of multidrug-resistant strains of Staphylococcus aureus and enterococcus. *Infect Control Hosp Epidemiol* 2003;24(5):362-386.

17. Marcotte AL, Trzeciak MA: Community-acquired methicillin-resistant Staphylococcus aureus: An emerging pathogen in orthopaedics. *J Am Acad Orthop Surg* 2008;16(2):98-106.

18. Sanderson PJ: The role of methicillin-resistant Staphylococcus aureus in orthopaedic implant surgery. *J Chemother* 2001; 13(Spec No 1):89-95.

19. Finkelstein R, Rabino G, Mashiah T, et al: Vancomycin versus cefazolin prophylaxis for cardiac surgery in the setting of a high prevalence of methicillin-resistant staphylococcal infections. *J Thorac Cardiovasc Surg* 2002;123(2): 326-332.

20. Kallen AJ, Wilson CT, Larson RJ: Perioperative intranasal mupirocin for the prevention of surgical-site infections: Systematic review of the literature and meta-analysis. *Infect Control Hosp Epidemiol* 2005;26(12):916-922.

21. Kalmeijer MD, van Nieuwland-Bollen E, Bogaers-Hofman D, de Baere GA: Nasal carriage of Staphylococcus aureus is a major risk factor for surgical-site infections in orthopedic surgery. *Infect Control Hosp Epidemiol* 2000; 21(5):319-323.

22. Gernaat-van der Sluis AJ, Hoogenboom-Verdegaal AM, Edixhoven PJ, Spies-van Rooijen NH: Prophylactic mupirocin could reduce orthopedic wound infections: 1,044 patients treated with mupirocin compared with 1,260 historical controls. *Acta Orthop Scand* 1988;69(4): 412-414.

23. Kalmeijer MD, Coertjens H, van Nieuwland-Bollen PM, et al: Surgical site infections in orthopedic surgery: The effect of mupirocin nasal ointment in a double-blind, randomized, placebo-controlled study. *Clin Infect Dis* 2002;35(4): 353-358.

24. Bode LG, Kluytmans JA, Wertheim HF, et al: Preventing surgical-site infections in nasal carriers of Staphylococcus aureus. *N Engl J Med* 2010;362(1):9-17.

25. Wilcox MH, Hall J, Pike H, et al: Use of perioperative mupirocin to prevent methicillin-resistant Staphylococcus aureus (MRSA) orthopaedic surgical site infections. *J Hosp Infect* 2003;54(3): 196-201.

26. Rotger M, Trampuz A, Piper KE, Steckelberg JM, Patel R: Phenotypic and genotypic mupirocin resistance among Staphylococci causing prosthetic joint infection. *J Clin Microbiol* 2005;43(8): 4266-4268.

27. Burke JF: The effective period of preventive antibiotic action in experimental incisions and dermal lesions. *Surgery* 1961;50:161-168.

28. Classen DC, Evans RS, Pestotnik SL, Horn SD, Menlove RL, Burke JP: The timing of prophylactic administration of antibiotics and the risk of surgical-wound infection. *N Engl J Med* 1992; 326(5):281-286.

29. Cunha BA, Gossling HR, Pasternak HS, Nightingale CH, Quintiliani R: The penetration characteristics of cefazolin, cephalothin, and cephradine into bone in patients undergoing total hip replacement. *J Bone Joint Surg Am* 1977;59(7):856-859.

30. Schurman DJ, Hirshman HP, Burton DS: Cephalothin and cefamandole penetration into bone, synovial fluid, and wound drainage fluid. *J Bone Joint Surg Am* 1980;62(6):981-985.

31. Johnson DP: Antibiotic prophylaxis with cefuroxime in arthroplasty of the knee. *J Bone Joint Surg Br* 1987;69(5):787-789.

32. Deacon JS, Wertheimer SJ, Washington JA: Antibiotic prophylaxis and tourniquet application in podiatric surgery. *J Foot Ankle Surg* 1996;35(4):344-349.

33. American Academy of Orthopaedic Surgeons Infections Commit-

tee: American Academy of Orthopaedic Surgeons Advisory Statement: Recommendations for the use of intravenous antibiotic prophylaxis in primary total joint arthroplasty. http://www.aaos.org/about/papers/advistmt/1027.asp. Accessed September 2, 2010.

34. Dellinger EP, Gross PA, Barrett TL, et al: Quality standard for antimicrobial prophylaxis in surgical procedures. *Clin Infect Dis* 1994;18(3):422-427.

35. Swoboda SM, Merz C, Kostuik J, Trentler B, Lipsett PA: Does intraoperative blood loss affect antibiotic serum and tissue concentrations? *Arch Surg* 1996;131(11): 1165-1172.

36. Dehne MG, Mühling J, Sablotzki A, Nopens H, Hempelmann G: Pharmacokinetics of antibiotic prophylaxis in major orthopedic surgery and blood-saving techniques. *Orthopedics* 2001;24(7):665-669.

37. Oishi CS, Carrion WV, Hoaglund FT: Use of parenteral prophylactic antibiotics in clean orthopedic surgery: A review of the literature. *Clin Orthop Relat Res* 1993;296:249-255.

38. Fogelberg EV, Zitzmann EK, Stinchfield FE: Prophylactic penicillin in orthopaedic surgery. *J Bone Joint Surg Am* 1970;52(1): 95-98.

39. Ericson C, Lidgren L, Lindberg L: Cloxacillin in the prophylaxis of postoperative infections of the hip. *J Bone Joint Surg Am* 1973; 55(4):808-813, 843.

40. Carlsson AK, Lidgren L, Lindberg L: Prophylactic antibiotics against early and late deep infections after total hip replacements. *Acta Orthop Scand* 1977;48(4): 405-410.

41. Hill C, Flamant R, Mazas F, Evrard J: Prophylactic cefazolin versus placebo in total hip replacement: Report of a multicentre double-blind randomised trial. *Lancet* 1981;1(8224):795-796.

42. Bratzler DW, Houck PM, Richards C, et al: Use of antimicrobial prophylaxis for major surgery: Baseline results from the National Surgical Infection Prevention Project. *Arch Surg* 2005;140(2): 174-182.

43. Williams DN, Gustilo RB: The use of preventive antibiotics in orthopaedic surgery. *Clin Orthop Relat Res* 1984;190:83-88.

44. Page CP, Bohnen JM, Fletcher JR, McManus AT, Solomkin JS, Wittmann DH: Antimicrobial prophylaxis for surgical wounds: Guidelines for clinical care. *Arch Surg* 1993;128(1): 79-88.

45. Ritter MA, Barzilauskas CD, Faris PM, Keating EM: Vancomycin prophylaxis and elective total joint arthroplasty. *Orthopedics* 1989;12(10):1333-1336.

46. Bratzler DW, Hunt DR: The surgical infection prevention and surgical care improvement projects: National initiatives to improve outcomes for patients having surgery. *Clin Infect Dis* 2006; 43(3):322-330.

47. Pollard JP, Hughes SP, Scott JE, Evans MJ, Benson MK: Antibiotic prophylaxis in total hip replacement. *Br Med J* 1979;1(6165): 707-709.

48. Nelson CL, Green TG, Porter RA, Warren RD: One day versus seven days of preventive antibiotic therapy in orthopedic surgery. *Clin Orthop Relat Res* 1983;176: 258-263.

49. Heydemann JS, Nelson CL: Short-term preventive antibiotics. *Clin Orthop Relat Res* 1986;205: 184-187.

50. Mauerhan DR, Nelson CL, Smith DL, et al: Prophylaxis against infection in total joint arthroplasty: One day of cefuroxime compared with three days of cefazolin. *J Bone Joint Surg Am* 1994;76(1):39-45.

51. Keller RB, Pappas AM: Infection after spinal fusion using internal fixation instrumentation. *Orthop Clin North Am* 1972;3(1):99-111.

52. Lonstein J, Winter R, Moe J, Gaines D: Wound infection with Harrington instrumentation and spine fusion for scoliosis. *Clin Orthop Relat Res* 1973;96: 222-233.

53. Horwitz NH, Curtin JA: Prophylactic antibiotics and wound infections following laminectomy for lumber disc herniation. *J Neurosurg* 1975;43(6):727-731.

54. Geraghty J, Feely M: Antibiotic prophylaxis in neurosurgery: A randomized controlled trial. *J Neurosurg* 1984;60(4):724-726.

55. Young RF, Lawner PM: Perioperative antibiotic prophylaxis for prevention of postoperative neurosurgical infections: A randomized clinical trial. *J Neurosurg* 1987;66(5):701-705.

56. Bullock R, van Dellen JR, Ketelbey W, Reinach SG: A double-blind placebo-controlled trial of perioperative prophylactic antibiotics for elective neurosurgery. *J Neurosurg* 1988;69(5):687-691.

57. Rubinstein E, Findler G, Amit P, Shaked I: Perioperative prophylactic cephazolin in spinal surgery: A double-blind placebo-controlled trial. *J Bone Joint Surg Br* 1994; 76(1):99-102.

58. Wimmer C, Nogler M, Frischhut B: Influence of antibiotics on infection in spinal surgery: A prospective study of 110 patients. *J Spinal Disord* 1998;11(6): 498-500.

59. Barker FG II: Efficacy of prophylactic antibiotic therapy in spinal surgery: A meta-analysis. *Neurosurgery* 2002;51(2):391-401.

60. Luer MS, Hatton J: Appropriateness of antibiotic selection and use in laminectomy and microdiskectomy. *Am J Hosp Pharm* 1993; 50(4):667-670.

61. Wieck JA, Jackson JK, O'Brien TJ, Lurate RB, Russell JM, Dorchak JD: Efficacy of prophylactic antibiotics in arthroscopic surgery. *Orthopedics* 1997;20(2):133-134.

62. D'Angelo GL, Ogilvie-Harris DJ: Septic arthritis following arthroscopy, with cost/benefit analysis of antibiotic prophylaxis. *Arthroscopy* 1988;4(1):10-14.

63. Kurzweil PR: Antibiotic prophylaxis for arthroscopic surgery. *Arthroscopy* 2006;22(4):452-454.

64. Labbé AC, Demers AM, Rodrigues R, Arlet V, Tanguay K, Moore DL: Surgical-site infection following spinal fusion: A case-control study in a children's hospital. *Infect Control Hosp Epidemiol* 2003;24(8):591-595.

65. Zgonis T, Jolly GP, Garbalosa JC: The efficacy of prophylactic intravenous antibiotics in elective foot and ankle surgery. *J Foot Ankle Surg* 2004;43(2):97-103.

66. Paiement GD, Renaud E, Dagenais G, Gosselin RA: Double-blind randomized prospective study of the efficacy of antibiotic prophylaxis for open reduction and internal fixation of closed ankle fractures. *J Orthop Trauma* 1994;8(1):64-66.

67. Kleinert JM, Hoffmann J, Miller Crain G, Larsen CF, Goldsmith LJ, Firrell JC: Postoperative infection in a double-occupancy operating room: A prospective study of two thousand four hundred and fifty-eight procedures on the extremities. *J Bone Joint Surg Am* 1997;79(4):503-513.

68. Hanssen AD, Amadio PC, DeSilva SP, Ilstrup DM: Deep postoperative wound infection after carpal tunnel release. *J Hand Surg Am* 1989;14(5):869-873.

69. Platt AJ, Page RE: Post-operative infection following hand surgery: Guidelines for antibiotic use. *J Hand Surg Br* 1995;20(5):685-690.

70. Harness NG, Inacio MC, Pfeil FF, Paxton LW: Rate of infection after carpal tunnel release surgery and effect of antibiotic prophylaxis. *J Hand Surg Am* 2010;35(2):189-196.

71. Hoffman RD, Adams BD: The role of antibiotics in the management of elective and post-traumatic hand surgery. *Hand Clin* 1998;14(4):657-666.

72. Boyd RJ, Burke JF, Colton T: A double-blind clinical trial of prophylactic antibiotics in hip fractures. *J Bone Joint Surg Am* 1973;55(6):1251-1258.

73. Burnett JW, Gustilo RB, Williams DN, Kind AC: Prophylactic antibiotics in hip fractures: A double-blind, prospective study. *J Bone Joint Surg Am* 1980;62(3):457-462.

74. Tengve B, Kjellander J: Antibiotic prophylaxis in operations on trochanteric femoral fractures. *J Bone Joint Surg Am* 1978;60(1):97-99.

75. Southwell-Keely JP, Russo RR, March L, Cumming R, Cameron I, Brnabic AJ: Antibiotic prophylaxis in hip fracture surgery: A metaanalysis. *Clin Orthop Relat Res* 2004;419:179-184.

76. Gatell JM, Garcia S, Lozano L, Soriano E, Ramon R, SanMiguel JG: Perioperative cefamandole prophylaxis against infections. *J Bone Joint Surg Am* 1987;69(8):1189-1193.

77. Boxma H, Broekhuizen T, Patka P, Oosting H: Randomised controlled trial of single-dose antibiotic prophylaxis in surgical treatment of closed fractures: The Dutch Trauma Trial. *Lancet* 1996;347(9009):1133-1137.

78. Gillespie WJ, Walenkamp G: Antibiotic prophylaxis for surgery for proximal femoral and other closed long bone fractures. *Cochrane Database Syst Rev* 2001;1:CD000244.

79. Maguire WB: The use of antibiotics, locally and systemically, in orthopaedic surgery. *Med J Aust* 1964;2:412-414.

80. Nachamie BA, Siffert RS, Bryer MS: A study of neomycin instillation into orthopedic surgical wounds. *JAMA* 1968;204:687-689.

81. Savitz SI, Savitz MH, Goldstein HB, Mouracade CT, Malangone S: Topical irrigation with polymyxin and bacitracin for spinal surgery. *Surg Neurol* 1998;50(3):208-212.

82. Haines SJ: Topical antibiotic prophylaxis in neurosurgery. *Neurosurgery* 1982;11(2):250-253.

83. Brown EM, Pople IK, de Louvois J, et al: Spine update: Prevention of postoperative infection in patients undergoing spinal surgery. *Spine (Phila Pa 1976)* 2004;29(8):938-945.

84. Anglen JO: Comparison of soap and antibiotic solutions for irrigation of lower-limb open fracture wounds: A prospective, randomized study. *J Bone Joint Surg Am* 2005;87(7):1415-1422.

85. Anglen JO: Wound irrigation in musculoskeletal injury. *J Am Acad Orthop Surg* 2001;9(4):219-226.

86. Dirschl DR, Wilson FC: Topical antibiotic irrigation in the prophylaxis of operative wound infections in orthopedic surgery. *Orthop Clin North Am* 1991;22(3):419-426.

87. Golightly LK, Branigan T: Surgical antibiotic irrigations. *Hosp Pharm* 1989;24(2):116-119.

88. Gelman ML, Frazier CH, Chandler HP: Acute renal failure after total hip replacement. *J Bone Joint Surg Am* 1979;61(5):657-660.

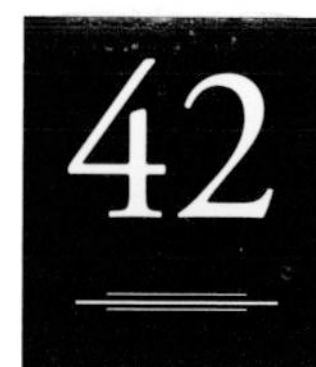

Modifiable Risk Factors for Surgical Site Infection

Calin S. Moucha, MD
Terry A. Clyburn, MD
Richard P. Evans, MD
Laura Prokuski, MD

Abstract

Multiple risk factors for orthopaedic surgical site infection have been identified. Some of these factors directly affect the wound-healing process, whereas others can lead to blood-borne sepsis or relative immunosuppression. Modifying a patient's medications; screening for comorbidities, such as HIV or diabetes mellitus; and advising the patient on options to diminish or eliminate adverse behaviors, such as smoking, should lower the risk for surgical site infections.

Instr Course Lect 2011;60:557-564.

Multiple risk factors for orthopaedic surgical site infection, including a wide variety of demographic, comorbid, surgical, and postoperative variables, have been identified.[1] The patient as a host is an important risk factor for infection, and many (if not most) patients are in suboptimal health. Optimizing the patient's medical condition before surgery and eliminating or even diminishing modifiable risk factors for infection should lower the risk of surgical site infection (**Figure 1**). Direct scientific evidence showing that modifying these risk factors will lead to a decrease in surgical site infections is not readily available, and much work in this field remains to be done. It is imperative that surgeons have an extensive knowledge of modifiable risk factors affecting the wound-healing process and subsequent wound complications.

Modifiable Risk Factors and Possible Preoperative Interventions

Rheumatoid Arthritis

Patients with rheumatoid arthritis have an increased risk of infection following orthopaedic procedures. Patients with rheumatoid arthritis treated with total joint arthroplasty have a two to three times greater risk of acquiring a postoperative surgical site infection than do patients with osteoarthritis.[2-4] Patients with rheumatoid arthritis are often treated with complex drug regimens that include nonsteroidal anti-inflammatory drugs, corticosteroids, methotrexate, and biologics, all of which have an effect on wound healing and the risk of infection. There are insufficient data from patients who have undergone orthopaedic procedures to make evidence-based recommendations about most of these medications. A good working relationship with the patient's rheumatologist is critical to making decisions about these medications; however, it is helpful to be familiar with possible effects on surgical infections, which have been suggested by a synthesis of the available data.

Nonsteroidal Anti-inflammatory Drugs

Although the use of nonsteroidal anti-inflammatory drugs does not seem to increase transfusion requirements, morbidity, and mortality directly, they

Dr. Moucha or an immediate family member serves as a board member, owner, officer, or committee member of the American Academy of Orthopaedic Surgeons. Dr. Clyburn or an immediate family member has received royalties from Nimbic Systems and is a member of a speakers' bureau or has made paid presentations on behalf of Conformis. Dr. Evans or an immediate family member is a member of a speakers' bureau or has made paid presentations on behalf of Cubist; serves as a paid consultant to or is an employee of DePuy and Smith & Nephew; and has received research or institutional support from Cubist. Neither Dr. Prokuski nor any immediate family member has received anything of value from or owns stock in a commercial company or institution related directly or indirectly to the subject of this chapter.

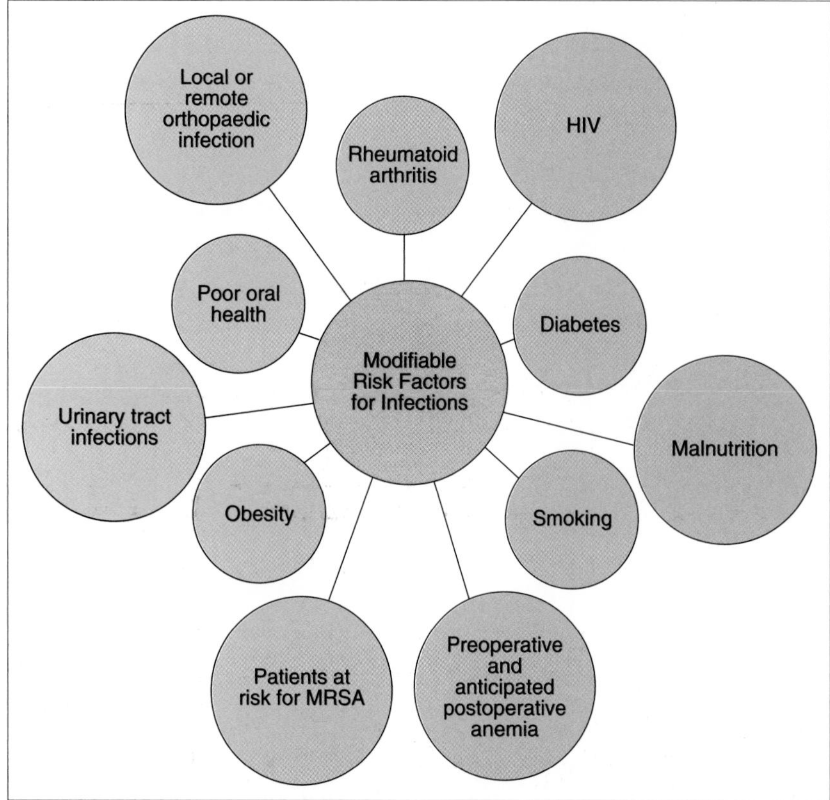

Figure 1 Diagram showing modifiable risk factors for infection. Many patients have risk factors that make them more susceptible to the development of infections. Some infections may be preventable through the identification and treatment of modifiable risk factors. MRSA = methicillin-resistant *Staphylococcus aureus*. (Reprinted with permission from The American Academy of Orthopaedic Surgeons Patient Safety Committee, Evans RP: Surgical site infection prevention and control: An emerging paradigm. *J Bone Joint Surg Am* 2009;91 [Suppl 6]:2-9.)

may increase intraoperative and postoperative bleeding. Increased bleeding may lead to a postoperative infection, especially in already compromised hosts.[5,6] Medications with short half-lives (ibuprofen and indomethacin) should be discontinued 1 to 2 days before surgery. Drugs with longer half-lives (naproxen) should be discontinued 3 days before surgery. Aspirin should be discontinued 7 to 10 days before surgery to allow regeneration of unaffected platelets. Although cyclooxygenase-2-specific nonsteroidal anti-inflammatory drugs may not be associated with as much bleeding as non–cyclooxygenase-2-specific nonsteroidal anti-inflammatory drugs, bone healing may be affected by the latter. As such, the data are controversial with regard to the best way to use these newer drugs.

Corticosteroids

Inadequate doses of corticosteroids lead to disease flares and, in rare instances, adrenal insufficiency. Corticosteroids have been shown to increase infection rates and affect wound healing.[7] In general, all patients being treated with chronic corticosteroid therapy should receive their regular dose of corticosteroids perioperatively.

The use of stress dose steroids remains controversial, and guidelines are difficult to establish. Stress dose steroids should probably not be routinely prescribed but should be individualized on the basis of the length of time for which steroid treatment has been used, the anticipated stress level of the surgery, and the presence of other risk factors for infection.[5,6]

Methotrexate

Most studies on the perioperative use of methotrexate have not shown an increased risk of infection. The dose of methotrexate in many of these studies, however, was lower than the doses that are often used currently. In general, methotrexate should not be discontinued perioperatively. Patients with renal insufficiency (preoperatively or postoperatively), poorly controlled diabetes, lung or liver disease, or a history of alcohol abuse should discontinue preoperative use of methotrexate.[5,6] This recommendation is especially important for patients undergoing high-stress procedures such as arthroplasty or tumor resection.

Other Disease-Modifying Antirheumatic Drugs

Few data are available on which to base recommendations about medications such as hydroxychloroquine, azathioprine, leflunomide, or sulfasalazine. Hydroxychloroquine has few immunosuppressive properties, and it appears safe for perioperative use. The other medications have immunosuppressive properties, and some interfere with warfarin dosing.[5,6] Preoperative consultation with a rheumatologist is highly recommended.

Biologics: Tumor Necrosis Factor and Interleukin-1 Antagonists

Medications such as etanercept, adalimumab, and infliximab are tumor necrosis factor antagonists. Serious infection is a known complication of tumor necrosis factor inhibitor therapy.[8] However, perioperative use of such therapy has been shown to be safe in foot and ankle surgery.[9] Anakinra is an interleukin-1 antagonist. There are minimal data and experience on which to base strict recommendations about either of these classes of drugs. At this time, a conservative approach should be taken. For patients treated with intensive procedures in particular, these medications should be withheld preoperatively for at least one dosing cycle and postoperatively until adequate wound healing is observed.

Human Immunodeficiency Virus

The increased life expectancy of HIV-positive patients has created a new subset of potential candidates for total joint arthroplasties and other orthopaedic procedures.[10] Several retrospective reports, most involving a small numbers of patients, have provided mixed results. Whereas some studies showed an alarming rate of postoperative infection in patients with HIV, other studies did not.[11-15] Prospective randomized studies on this topic are lacking.

Studies from outside orthopaedics, however, suggest that specific risk factors influencing surgical morbidity, especially infections related to wound healing, include an absolute CD4 cell count of less than 200 cells/mm^3 or a viral load of more than 10,000 copies/mL.[16] As such, every attempt should be made to coordinate care with infectious disease specialists to optimize the immune systems of these patients. It is imperative to try to diminish and/or eliminate other modifiable risk factors (injection drug use, smoking, serum glucose level, and obesity) and optimize psychosocial issues before elective surgical treatment.[14]

Diabetes Mellitus and Hyperglycemia

Diabetes has been associated with an increased risk of surgical site infection in several areas of orthopaedics.[4,17] Although this "diabetic disadvantage" may be caused, in part, by the impact of the pathologic changes resulting from diabetes, it is more likely that the acute effects of perioperative hyperglycemia are even more detrimental.[18]

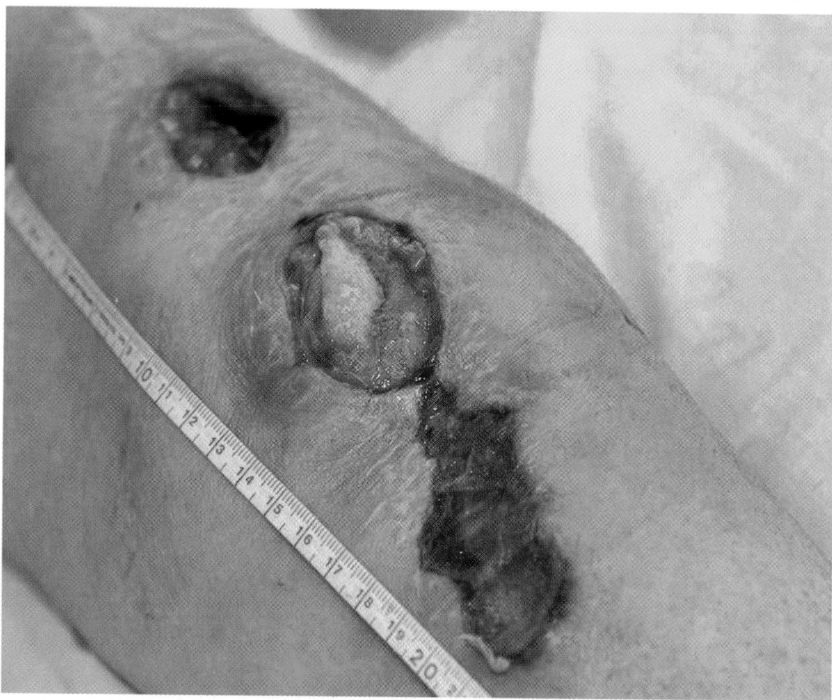

Figure 2 Infected wound dehiscence in a 63-year-old woman with poorly controlled type I diabetes treated with a total knee replacement.

The increased risk of infection in diabetic patients undergoing orthopaedic surgery is often associated with complications related to wound healing (**Figure 2**). To achieve appropriate wound healing, the nutritional status and insulin regimen of a diabetic patient must be optimized before any surgical procedure. The primary goal of these efforts is to obtain close perioperative glucose control, not necessarily an improvement in the hemoglobin A1C level, as the latter is a marker of long-term glucose control and may take too much time to improve. A recent study evaluating surgical site infections following orthopaedic spinal surgery identified hyperglycemia in patients not previously diagnosed with diabetes as a potential risk factor.[17] Further research is needed to evaluate whether patients who are scheduled for elective orthopaedic surgery should have routine screening for diabetes and hyperglycemia, as has been done for patients who are to have cardiothoracic surgery.[19]

Malnutrition

Malnutrition is a known risk factor for deep infection after a variety of orthopaedic surgical procedures. Optimizing nutrition is important to ensure proper immune function and postoperative wound healing. Nutritional status should be checked preoperatively in patients at risk for malnutrition, such as elderly patients and those who have gastrointestinal diseases, renal failure, alcoholism, cancer, or any chronic disease.[20-22] A total lymphocyte count of less than 1,500/mm^3 (1.5×10^9/L), a serum albumin level of less than 3.5 g/dL, or a transferrin level of less than 226 mg/dL has been associated with an increased rate of wound complications.[21] Other markers of malnutrition that need further study include prealbumin and retinol-binding protein. Specific recommendations about nutrition should be individualized to each patient on the basis of age, nutritional status, and other comorbid conditions. Preoperative nutritional supplementation may benefit all patients with abnormal nutritional markers.[23] Patients should obtain sufficient protein intake and specific daily vitamin and mineral supplementation (vitamins A and C, zinc, and copper).[24,25]

Smoking

Smoking is a well-known risk factor for the development of a variety of postoperative complications, including infection.[26] Tobacco products, including cigarettes, cause microvascular vasoconstriction because of nicotine and the activation of the sympathetic nervous system. Carbon monoxide found in cigarette smoke also contributes to tissue hypoxia by binding to hemoglobin to form carboxyhemoglobin.[27-29] Carboxyhemoglobin has a high affinity for oxygen and decreases the delivery of oxygen to tissues.[30]

Smoking intervention programs have been studied extensively in several surgical disciplines, including orthopaedics. It appears that such programs decrease the risk of postoperative complications, especially wound healing, even when they are instituted 4 to 6 weeks before elective surgery.[31-35]

Obesity

Several studies have shown that a body mass index of 30 kg/m^2 or greater, the definition of obesity, increases the risk of postoperative complications, including surgical site infection.[17,36-38] One study reported that the risk of an infection was 6.7 times higher in obese patients treated with total knee replacement and 4.2 times higher in obese patients treated with total hip replacement.[39]

Several factors explain this relationship. Surgical time is often longer for obese patients.[36] The extent of surgical dissection can be greater and lead to hematoma and/or seroma formation and subsequent prolonged drainage.[40] The subcutaneous fat layer is poorly vascularized. The diets of many obese patients, although high in calories, are often devoid of essential nutrients, vitamins, and minerals. The dose of prophylactic antibiotics is often not adjusted to weight, and antibiotic serum levels are inadequate in many of these patients.[41] Obese patients undergoing surgery have significantly lower subcutaneous oxygen tensions and, compared with nonobese patients, require a significantly greater fraction of inspired oxygen (FiO_2) to reach an arterial oxygen tension of 150 mm Hg.[42] Type 2 diabetes mellitus and obesity share a pathogenic relationship, and both have rapidly increased in prevalence over the past decade.[43]

Obese patients should be counseled well in advance of elective orthopaedic procedures about methods of weight loss, including bariatric surgery when appropriate.[44] Improvement in the quality of their nutritional intake is also important. These patients should be screened for hyperglycemia and referred to their physician for improvement of perioperative glycemic control as needed. It is not advisable to recommend that patients lose weight in a short period of time before a surgical procedure because this leads to a catabolic state that could lead to wound-healing and infectious complications. It also is recommended that surgeons collaborate with the anesthesia team preoperatively in an effort to provide an adequate dose of prophylactic antibiotics based on the patient's weight.

Colonization With *Staphylococcus aureus*

One of the most common organisms found in orthopaedic surgical site infections is *Staphylococcus aureus.* There is a strong association between nasal carriage of *S aureus* and the development of *S aureus* surgical site infections. Carriers are two to nine times more likely to acquire *S aureus* surgical site infections than are noncarriers.[45] In patients who acquire *S aureus* surgical site infections, paired *S aureus* isolates from the wound match those from the nares 80% to 85% of the time.[46]

A preoperative screening and topical decolonization protocol that has been proposed and studied at length includes administering mupirocin ointment to the nares twice daily.[47] Some investigators include the use of a chlorhexidine bath once daily for 5 days before surgery.

Studies on this topic vary in terms of randomization, sample size, type of surgery, and the method of intervention. Interpretation of the literature from a variety of disciplines suggests that a preoperative decolonization protocol may decrease the risk of surgical site infections in colonized patients.[48,49] Whether screening and treating all surgical patients will lead to a decrease in overall *S aureus* surgical site infections warrants additional studies.[50]

Until more information is obtained from such studies, it is recommended that patients at risk for *Staphylococcus* colonization be screened and treated preoperatively with a decolonization regimen. Risk factors for such colonization include previous methicillin-resistant *S aureus* (MRSA) infection; being a health care worker, nursing home patient, or prisoner; and contact with a patient who has MRSA colonization. In patients who are found preoperatively to be carriers of MRSA, the use of antibiotics such as vancomycin in place of (or possibly in addition to) cefazolin as a prophylactic antibiotic just before the surgical incision may be beneficial, although strict guidelines cannot be established. Similar prophylactic decisions on the choice of an antibiotic should be considered in hospitals with antibiogram data that indicate a high percentage of *Staphylococcus* resistance.[51]

Poor Oral Health

It is well known that bacteremia after dental procedures can cause hematogenous seeding of bacteria onto joint implants, both in the early postoperative period and for many years following implantation.[52-55] Prophylactic antibiotic prophylaxis before dental intervention may be beneficial in certain patients who have previously been treated with total joint arthroplasty, although debate over this topic continues.[56,57]

An equally rational approach to diminishing the risk of surgical site infections may be to finish any anticipated dental treatment before elective orthopaedic surgery.[58,59] Decayed teeth, untreated dental abscesses, advanced gingivitis, and periodontitis can all progress to become potential sources of infection. Inadequate patient education, financial constraints, and dental phobias often cause patients to ignore their dental health. Although this chapter's authors are not aware of any scientific studies directly showing the benefits of preoperative dental screening, this low-risk, common-sense approach, previously advocated by cardiac surgeons for their patients, may prove beneficial.

Urinary Tract Infections

Urinary tract infections are generally classified into upper and lower tract infections. Lower tract infections, particularly cystitis, are more common than upper tract infections in patients being evaluated for elective orthopaedic surgery. Postoperative urinary tract infection has been identified as a risk factor for periprosthetic joint infection in several but not all studies.[60] Deep infection in the involved joint after hip or knee arthroplasty may be the result of hematogenous seeding from the urinary tract. It is unclear whether there is an association between preoperative bladder infections and deep infection at the site of an arthroplasty implant; however, patients should be asked preoperatively about urinary tract symptoms.

A synthesis of the literature allows some recommendations.[61,62] If symptoms are present, a urinalysis and a urine culture should be considered. If symptoms are not present, a urinalysis and a urine culture should be considered for patients with other risk factors for postoperative surgical site infection. Elderly patients often do not have classic symptoms of urinary tract infection, such as dysuria, urgency, and/or frequency.

The surgery can proceed when bacteriuria is present without symptoms of urinary irritation or obstruction. Patients with urine colony counts of more than 10^3/mL should be treated with a postoperative course of an appropriate oral antibiotic. The surgeon also can proceed with surgery if bacteriuria is present with irritative symptoms in combination with a bacterial count of less than 10^3/mL or if urinalysis does not suggest infection.

The surgeon should consider postponing surgery, especially in high-risk patients, when the preoperative evaluation shows symptoms related to obstruction of the urinary pathway or the patient has dysuria and urinary frequency symptoms in combination with a bacterial count greater than 10^3/mL on urine culture.

Preoperative Anemia

Some reports have indicated that postoperative anemia treated with allogenic blood transfusion is a risk factor for surgical site infections.[60,63] Several studies have shown that, when preoperative anemia is corrected, the risk of postoperative allogenic blood transfusions is diminished.[64] Several blood conservation regimens are available, and the literature is not clear about the best method for decreasing the risk of postoperative allogenic blood transfusion.

Screening for preoperative anemia and correcting the condition with recombinant human erythropoietin (epoetin alfa) therapy has been studied in orthopaedic patients and has proven to be beneficial in some but not all instances.[65,66] Epoetin alfa directly increases preoperative red blood cell mass, hemoglobin concentration, and hematocrit levels. Even when a patient has chosen to donate autologous blood preoperatively, erythropoietin may be used as an adjunct to further diminish the risk of postoperative allogenic blood transfusion.[67] Because iron deficiency has been shown to be a common reason for erythropoietin treatment failure, iron levels should be supplemented while the patient is being treated with recombinant erythropoietin.[68,69]

Local or Remote Orthopaedic Infections

Prior surgery increases the rate of deep infection after revision arthroplasty procedures. A history of an infection following the primary arthroplasty procedure increases the risk of an infection after the revision arthroplasty. Infection is one cause of nonunion requiring revision surgery after fracture surgery.[70] In joint arthroplasty surgery, but probably in all types of orthopaedic surgery, serum studies should be obtained for any patient scheduled for revision surgery for any reason. An elevated leukocyte count with differential, erythrocyte sedimentation rate, and C-reactive protein level should raise suspicion of an underlying infection. If one of these values is elevated in a patient scheduled for joint arthroplasty, additional preoperative testing (aspiration and bone marrow and/or white blood cell scan) or intraoperative testing (cell counts and frozen-section sampling) should be done.[71,72] Evaluations for infection after other types of procedures involve similar principles but may vary in some respects. Elective surgery should be postponed until the elimination of all possible orthopaedic sources of infection in the patient.

Summary

Risk factors for infection have been identified for multiple orthopaedic procedures. Some of these risk factors can be eliminated or modified preoperatively. The strategy of diminishing the rate of surgical site infection is logical and should be broadly adopted.

References

1. American Academy of Orthopaedic Surgeons Patient Safety Committee; Evans RP: Surgical site infection prevention and control: An emerging paradigm. *J Bone Joint Surg Am* 2009; 91(Suppl 6): 2-9.
2. Poss R, Thornhill TS, Ewald FC, Thomas WH, Batte NJ, Sledge CB: Factors influencing the incidence and outcome of infection following total joint arthroplasty. *Clin Orthop Relat Res* 1984;182:117-126.
3. Wilson MG, Kelley K, Thornhill TS: Infection as a complication of total knee-replacement arthroplasty: Risk factors and treatment in sixty-seven cases. *J Bone Joint Surg Am* 1990;72(6): 878-883.
4. Luessenhop CP, Higgins LD, Brause BD, Ranawat CS: Multiple prosthetic infections after total joint arthroplasty: Risk factor analysis. *J Arthroplasty* 1996; 11(7):862-868.
5. Howe CR, Gardner GC, Kadel NJ: Perioperative medication management for the patient with rheumatoid arthritis. *J Am Acad Orthop Surg* 2006;14(9):544-551.
6. Scanzello CR, Figgie MP, Nestor BJ, Goodman SM: Perioperative management of medications used in the treatment of rheumatoid arthritis. *HSS J* 2006;2(2): 141-147.
7. Wicke C, Halliday B, Allen D, et al: Effects of steroids and retinoids on wound healing. *Arch Surg* 2000;135(11):1265-1270.
8. Giles JT, Bartlett SJ, Gelber AC, et al: Tumor necrosis factor inhibitor therapy and risk of serious postoperative orthopedic infection in rheumatoid arthritis. *Arthritis Rheum* 2006;55(2):333-337.
9. Bibbo C, Goldberg JW: Infectious and healing complications after elective orthopaedic foot and ankle surgery during tumor necrosis factor-alpha inhibition therapy. *Foot Ankle Int* 2004;25(5): 331-335.
10. Govender S, Harrison WJ, Lukhele M: Impact of HIV on bone and joint surgery. *Best Pract Res Clin Rheumatol* 2008;22(4): 605-619.
11. Parvizi J, Sullivan TA, Pagnano MW, Trousdale RT, Bolander ME: Total joint arthroplasty in human immunodeficiency virus-positive patients: An alarming rate of early failure. *J Arthroplasty* 2003;18(3):259-264.
12. Harrison WJ, Lavy CB, Lewis CP: One-year follow-up of orthopaedic implants in HIV-positive patients. *Int Orthop* 2004;28(6): 329-332.
13. Mahoney CR, Glesby MJ, DiCarlo EF, Peterson MG, Bostrom MP: Total hip arthroplasty in patients with human immunodeficiency virus infection: Pathologic findings and surgical outcomes. *Acta Orthop* 2005;76(2): 198-203.
14. Habermann B, Eberhardt C, Kurth AA: Total joint replacement in HIV positive patients. *J Infect* 2008;57(1):41-46.
15. Young WF, Axelrod P, Jallo J: Elective spinal surgery in asymptomatic HIV-seropositive persons: Perioperative complications and outcomes. *Spine (Phila Pa 1976)* 2005;30(2):256-259.
16. Davison SP, Reisman NR, Pellegrino ED, Larson EE, Dermody M, Hutchison PJ: Perioperative guidelines for elective surgery in the human immunodeficiency virus-positive patient. *Plast Reconstr Surg* 2008;121(5): 1831-1840.
17. Olsen MA, Nepple JJ, Riew KD, et al: Risk factors for surgical site infection following orthopaedic spinal operations. *J Bone Joint Surg Am* 2008;90(1):62-69.
18. Furnary AP, Wu Y: Eliminating the diabetic disadvantage: The Portland Diabetic Project. *Semin Thorac Cardiovasc Surg* 2006; 18(4):302-308.
19. Latham R, Lancaster AD, Covington JF, Pirolo JS, Thomas CS: The association of diabetes and glucose control with surgical-site infections among cardiothoracic surgery patients. *Infect Control Hosp Epidemiol* 2001;22(10): 607-612.
20. Dreblow DM, Anderson CF, Moxness K: Nutritional assessment of orthopedic patients. *Mayo Clin Proc* 1981;56(1): 51-54.
21. Greene KA, Wilde AH, Stulberg BN: Preoperative nutritional status of total joint patients: Relationship to postoperative wound complications. *J Arthroplasty* 1991;6(4):321-325.

22. Jensen JE, Jensen TG, Smith TK, Johnston DA, Dudrick SJ: Nutrition in orthopaedic surgery. *J Bone Joint Surg Am* 1982;64(9):1263-1272.

23. Smith TK: Prevention of complications in orthopedic surgery secondary to nutritional depletion. *Clin Orthop Relat Res* 1987;222: 91-97.

24. Fairfield KM, Fletcher RH: Vitamins for chronic disease prevention in adults: Scientific review. *JAMA* 2002;287(23):3116-3126.

25. Fletcher RH, Fairfield KM: Vitamins for chronic disease prevention in adults: Clinical applications. *JAMA* 2002;287(23): 3127-3129.

26. Møller AM, Pedersen T, Villebro N, Munksgaard A: Effect of smoking on early complications after elective orthopaedic surgery. *J Bone Joint Surg Br* 2003;85(2): 178-181.

27. Benowitz NL: Clinical pharmacology of nicotine. *Annu Rev Med* 1986;37:21-32.

28. Forrest CR, Pang CY, Lindsay WK: Pathogenesis of ischemic necrosis in random-pattern skin flaps induced by long-term low-dose nicotine treatment in the rat. *Plast Reconstr Surg* 1991;87(3): 518-528.

29. Sørensen LT, Jørgensen S, Petersen LJ, et al: Acute effects of nicotine and smoking on blood flow, tissue oxygen, and aerobe metabolism of the skin and subcutis. *J Surg Res* 2009;152(2): 224-230.

30. Heliövaara M, Karvonen MJ, Vilhunen R, Punsar S: Smoking, carbon monoxide, and atherosclerotic diseases. *Br Med J* 1978; 1(6108):268-270.

31. Lindström D, Sadr Azodi O, Wladis A, et al: Effects of a perioperative smoking cessation intervention on postoperative complications: A randomized trial. *Ann Surg* 2008;248(5):739-745.

32. Livingston EH, Arterburn D, Schifftner TL, Henderson WG, DePalma RG: National Surgical Quality Improvement Program analysis of bariatric operations: Modifiable risk factors contribute to bariatric surgical adverse outcomes. *J Am Coll Surg* 2006; 203(5):625-633.

33. Møller A, Villebro N: Interventions for preoperative smoking cessation. *Cochrane Database Syst Rev* 2005;3(3):CD002294.

34. Møller AM, Villebro N, Pedersen T, Tønnesen H: Effect of preoperative smoking intervention on postoperative complications: A randomised clinical trial. *Lancet* 2002;359(9301):114-117.

35. Sørensen LT, Jørgensen T: Short-term pre-operative smoking cessation intervention does not affect postoperative complications in colorectal surgery: A randomized clinical trial. *Colorectal Dis* 2003; 5(4):347-352.

36. Porter SE, Graves ML, Qin Z, Russell GV: Operative experience of pelvic fractures in the obese. *Obes Surg* 2008;18(6):702-708.

37. Lübbeke A, Moons KG, Garavaglia G, Hoffmeyer P: Outcomes of obese and nonobese patients undergoing revision total hip arthroplasty. *Arthritis Rheum* 2008; 59(5):738-745.

38. Dowsey MM, Choong PF: Early outcomes and complications following joint arthroplasty in obese patients: A review of the published reports. *ANZ J Surg* 2008; 78(6):439-444.

39. Namba RS, Paxton L, Fithian DC, Stone ML: Obesity and perioperative morbidity in total hip and total knee arthroplasty patients. *J Arthroplasty* 2005;20 (7, suppl 3)46-50.

40. Patel VP, Walsh M, Sehgal B, Preston C, DeWal H, Di Cesare PE: Factors associated with prolonged wound drainage after primary total hip and knee arthroplasty. *J Bone Joint Surg Am* 2007; 89(1):33-38.

41. Freeman JT, Anderson DJ, Hartwig MG, Sexton DJ: Surgical site infections following bariatric surgery in community hospitals: A weighty concern? *Obes Surg* 2010; 20. http://www.springerlink.com/content/h3238k2630h11666/. Accessed December 3, 2010.

42. Fleischmann E, Kurz A, Niedermayr M, et al: Tissue oxygenation in obese and non-obese patients during laparoscopy. *Obes Surg* 2005;15(6):813-819.

43. Anaya DA, Dellinger EP: The obese surgical patient: A susceptible host for infection. *Surg Infect (Larchmt)* 2006;7(5):473-480.

44. Parvizi J, Trousdale RT, Sarr MG: Total joint arthroplasty in patients surgically treated for morbid obesity. *J Arthroplasty* 2000;15(8): 1003-1008.

45. Wenzel RP, Perl TM: The significance of nasal carriage of Staphylococcus aureus and the incidence of postoperative wound infection. *J Hosp Infect* 1995;31(1):13-24.

46. Perl TM, Cullen JJ, Wenzel RP, et al: Intranasal mupirocin to prevent postoperative Staphylococcus aureus infections. *N Engl J Med* 2002;346(24):1871-1877.

47. Rao N, Cannella B, Crossett LS, Yates AJ Jr, McGough R III: A preoperative decolonization protocol for staphylococcus aureus prevents orthopaedic infections. *Clin Orthop Relat Res* 2008;466(6): 1343-1348.

48. van Rijen M, Bonten M, Wenzel R, Kluytmans J: Mupirocin ointment for preventing Staphylococcus aureus infections in nasal carriers. *Cochrane Database Syst Rev* 2008;4(4):CD006216.

49. van Rijen MM, Kluytmans JA: New approaches to prevention of staphylococcal infection in surgery. *Curr Opin Infect Dis* 2008; 21(4):380-384.

50. Trautmann M, Stecher J, Hemmer W, Luz K, Panknin HT: Intranasal mupirocin prophylaxis in elective surgery: A review of published studies. *Chemotherapy* 2008;54(1):9-16.
51. Meehan J, Jamali AA, Nguyen H: Prophylactic antibiotics in hip and knee arthroplasty. *J Bone Joint Surg Am* 2009;91(10):2480-2490.
52. Kaar TK, Bogoch ER, Devlin HR: Acute metastatic infection of a revision total hip arthroplasty with oral bacteria after noninvasive dental treatment. *J Arthroplasty* 2000;15(5):675-678.
53. LaPorte DM, Waldman BJ, Mont MA, Hungerford DS: Infections associated with dental procedures in total hip arthroplasty. *J Bone Joint Surg Br* 1999; 81(1):56-59.
54. Waldman BJ, Mont MA, Hungerford DS: Total knee arthroplasty infections associated with dental procedures. *Clin Orthop Relat Res* 1997;343:164-172.
55. Lindqvist C, Slätis P: Dental bacteremia: A neglected cause of arthroplasty infections? Three hip cases. *Acta Orthop Scand* 1985; 56(6):506-508.
56. Kuong EE, Ng FY, Yan CH, Fang CX, Chiu PK: Antibiotic prophylaxis after total joint replacements. *Hong Kong Med J* 2009;15(6):458-462.
57. Berbari EF, Osmon DR, Carr A, et al: Dental procedures as risk factors for prosthetic hip or knee infection: A hospital-based prospective case-control study. *Clin Infect Dis* 2010;50(1):8-16.
58. Yasny JS, White J: Dental considerations for cardiac surgery. *J Card Surg* 2009;24(1):64-68.
59. Harms KA, Bronny AT: Cardiac transplantation: Dental considerations. *J Am Dent Assoc* 1986; 112(5):677-681.
60. Pulido L, Ghanem E, Joshi A, Purtill JJ, Parvizi J: Periprosthetic joint infection: The incidence, timing, and predisposing factors. *Clin Orthop Relat Res* 2008; 466(7):1710-1715.
61. David TS, Vrahas MS: Perioperative lower urinary tract infections and deep sepsis in patients undergoing total joint arthroplasty. *J Am Acad Orthop Surg* 2000;8(1): 66-74.
62. Rajamanickam A, Noor S, Usmani A: Should an asymptomatic patient with an abnormal urinalysis (bacteriuria or pyuria) be treated with antibiotics prior to major joint replacement surgery? *Cleve Clin J Med* 2007; 74(Suppl 1):S17-S18.
63. Innerhofer P, Klingler A, Klimmer C, Fries D, Nussbaumer W: Risk for postoperative infection after transfusion of white blood cell-filtered allogeneic or autologous blood components in orthopedic patients undergoing primary arthroplasty. *Transfusion* 2005; 45(1):103-110.
64. Keating EM, Ritter MA: Transfusion options in total joint arthroplasty. *J Arthroplasty* 2002;17(4, Suppl 1):125-128.
65. Faris PM, Ritter MA, Abels RI; The American Erythropoietin Study Group: The effects of recombinant human erythropoietin on perioperative transfusion requirements in patients having a major orthopaedic operation. *J Bone Joint Surg Am* 1996;78(1): 62-72.
66. Vitale MG, Privitera DM, Matsumoto H, et al: Efficacy of preoperative erythropoietin administration in pediatric neuromuscular scoliosis patients. *Spine (Phila Pa 1976)* 2007;32(24):2662-2667.
67. Shapiro GS, Boachie-Adjei O, Dhawlikar SH, Maier LS: The use of Epoetin alfa in complex spine deformity surgery. *Spine (Phila Pa 1976)* 2002;27(18):2067-2071.
68. Auerbach M, Goodnough LT, Picard D, Maniatis A: The role of intravenous iron in anemia management and transfusion avoidance. *Transfusion* 2008;48(5): 988-1000.
69. Cuenca J, García-Erce JA, Martínez AA, Solano VM, Molina J, Muñoz M: Role of parenteral iron in the management of anaemia in the elderly patient undergoing displaced subcapital hip fracture repair: Preliminary data. *Arch Orthop Trauma Surg* 2005;125(5): 342-347.
70. Lynch JR, Taitsman LA, Barei DP, Nork SE: Femoral nonunion: Risk factors and treatment options. *J Am Acad Orthop Surg* 2008;16(2):88-97.
71. Della Valle CJ, Sporer SM, Jacobs JJ, Berger RA, Rosenberg AG, Paprosky WG: Preoperative testing for sepsis before revision total knee arthroplasty. *J Arthroplasty* 2007;22(6, Suppl 2):90-93.
72. Schinsky MF, Della Valle CJ, Sporer SM, Paprosky WG: Perioperative testing for joint infection in patients undergoing revision total hip arthroplasty. *J Bone Joint Surg Am* 2008;90(9):1869-1875.

Surgical Site Infection Prevention: The Operating Room Environment

Terry A. Clyburn, MD
Richard P. Evans, MD
Calin S. Moucha, MD
Laura Prokuski, MD

Abstract

Surgical site infections can complicate orthopaedic procedures and contribute to morbidity, mortality, and health care costs. Extensive literature has been published on this topic; however, the quality of data using standards of evidence-based medicine is variable with a lack of well-controlled studies. A review of the literature concerning measures to prevent surgical site infections in the operating room environment may be helpful in preventing such infections.

Instr Course Lect 2011;60:565-574.

Surgical site infections (SSIs) are a major worldwide problem, contributing to patient morbidity and mortality and adding significant costs to the health care system. The problem is staggering, with at least 27 to 30 million surgical procedures performed annually in the United States, and a SSI rate of 2% to 5% (up to 20% in some studies) coupled with estimated direct costs of treatment of at least $50,000 per case.[1-6] The frequency of SSI is increasing. Over the past 20 years, hospital-acquired infections have increased 36%, with direct and indirect costs estimated to be as much as $10 billion annually in the United States.[7-9]

Preoperative and postoperative measures, especially antibiotic prophylaxis, have been shown to be effective in reducing SSI rates. In this chapter, the critically important variables in the operating room environment, which can be controlled by the surgeon, are discussed.

Dr. Clyburn or an immediate family member has received royalties from Nimbic Systems and is a member of a speakers' bureau or has made paid presentations on behalf of Conformis. Dr. Evans or an immediate family member is a member of a speakers' bureau or has made paid presentations on behalf of Cubist; serves as a paid consultant to or is an employee of DePuy and Smith & Nephew; and has received research or institutional support from Cubist. Dr. Moucha or an immediate family member serves as a board member, owner, officer, or committee member of the American Academy of Orthopaedic Surgeons. Neither Dr. Prokuski nor any immediate family member has received anything of value from or owns stock in a commercial company or institution related directly or indirectly to the subject of this chapter.

Operating Room Air Handling

Clean Air

If it is assumed that the quantity of particulate matter and colony-forming units (CFUs) in the operating room air are related to the rate of SSI, then producing "clean air" in the operating room should be effective in reducing infection rates. Studies have shown a correlation between airborne bacterial contamination and postoperative joint sepsis in joint arthroplasty surgery.[10-12]

Other studies have evaluated the potential for airborne bacteria to cause bacterial deposition in surgical wounds.[13-17] The literature regarding the relationship between airborne particulates and airborne microbes is unclear. Landrin et al[18] reported no correlation between particle and bacteria counts in operating rooms, whereas Seal and Clark[19] found a correlation. The study by Landrin et al[18] was conducted in an empty operating room, which does not represent the movements of equipment, operating room staff, and the patient, which are typical during orthopaedic surgery. The data in the Seal and Clark[19] study were collected from only two surgical procedures, which makes the generalizability of their results questionable.

Particulate matter in the operating room comes primarily from people.[20] Reports in the current literature that used modern devices for measuring the density of particulate matter and CFUs in the operating room air and in the air immediately adjacent to the wound have shown increased particle and CFU counts with the increasing duration of surgery and the number of people in the room.[21-26]

All people shed large amounts of particulate matter from their bodies, but certain individuals (referred to as shedders) produce many times the average amount of particulate matter, There is evidence that the presence of a shedder in the operating room is associated with an increased risk of infection.[27,28] Using bacterial fingerprinting, one study traced the actual infectious organism in postoperative wound infections to specific members of the surgical team.[29] Ritter[25] reported a statistically significant increase in the bacterial count in the operating room when the door remained open and five people were added to the room.

Elevated ambient air pressure in the operating room will theoretically prevent contaminated air from the outer corridors from entering the room. The Centers for Disease Control and Prevention (CDC) recommend at least a 0.03-inch water-gauge positive pressure difference between the operating room and adjoining areas.[30]

There is good support in the literature for limiting the number of personnel in the operating room and the movement of these individuals.[31] Presumably, particulate matter in the operating room air and in the areas by the surgical instruments and the wound affect the amount of CFUs and may affect the rate of infection. Means are available to control the concentrations of these particulates and CFUs in the operating room air; some of these control methods have been in use for many years.

Laminar Airflow and Body Exhaust Suits

The design of the operating room, including the room's size, shape, and air handling devices, may affect the rate of SSI. It may be assumed that larger rooms would be favorable, but there are no scientific data to support this assumption. Air handling has received much attention, but definitive data are lacking regarding its effect on SSI. One method to reduce the amount of particulate matter in the air is the use of laminar airflow systems. Several studies have shown a reduced infection rate in orthopaedic implant surgeries performed in ultraclean air facilities with surgical teams wearing body exhaust (evacuation) suits.[32-36] Laminar airflow results in a statistically significant reduction in airborne bacterial CFUs,[35] but a statistically significant decrease in infection rates has not been definitively shown. These studies have numerous uncontrolled variables, including horizontal versus vertical laminar airflow, variation in the use of body exhaust suits, and great variations in the use of prophylactic antibiotics. The CDC also confirms that variables during multiple evaluations of laminar airflow may have "confounded the associations." Based on this information, some authors have disputed the results of studies showing the efficacy of laminar airflow in reducing SSI.[37,38]

Laurence[39] showed that body exhaust suits were effective in reducing bacterial counts in the air, but data did not prove a reduction in SSI. It is doubtful that a definitive study of laminar airflow will be undertaken because, with an infection rate of approximately 1% in joint arthroplasty surgeries, a very large series of homologous surgical cases would be needed to show statistically significant results. The CDC advises that the surgeon should "consider performing orthopedic implant operations in operating rooms with ultraclean air and body exhaust suits."[22] The cost of building operating rooms with laminar airflow systems is significant. Organizations such as the American College of Healthcare Architecture recommend maintaining positive pressure in the conventional operating room and providing greater than 15 operating room air volume exchanges per hour through high-efficiency particulate air (HEPA) filters (**Figure 1**).

The use of body exhaust suits in conjunction with laminar airflow provides patients with additional protection from bacterial shedding from the hair, exposed skin, and mucus membranes of operating room personnel.[40,41] Body exhaust suits may also prevent the patient from contaminating operating room personnel, although this reverse isolation protection is still unstudied. Although widely used and accepted, it has not been proven that body exhaust suits alone are effective in reducing SSI.

The Mask

It is assumed that by covering the oral cavity, indigenous bacteria and particulate matter are isolated from the operating room air; however, several studies have not definitively shown that CFUs are reduced with surgical masks.[42-44] One study reported effectiveness if the mask was worn under a hood, theoretically directing the airflow back under the cap.[45]

This chapter's authors believe it is reasonable to assume that clean scrub attire and the proper use of a hat and mask (such that the mouth, nose, and all hair are covered) are appropriate precautions to limit the risk of SSI. More importantly, the surgeon should set the standard for the operating room personnel and should expect adherence to this standard.

The Surgical Team

Hand Scrubbing

The ritual of the surgeon "scrubbing up" at the sink is indigenous to the surgical culture. Clocks and timers have been installed and used to mandate the traditional 10-minute scrub with the use of a nail cleaner and a scrub brush.[7] The current recommendations require an antimicrobial soap to scrub the hands and forearms for the length of time recommended by the manufacturer, which can range from 2 to 6 minutes. When using an alcohol-based surgical hand-scrub product with persistent activity, it is important to follow the manufacturer's instructions. Before applying the alcohol solution, the hands and forearms should be prewashed with a nonantimicrobial soap and completely dried. After applying the alcohol-based product as recommended, the hands and forearms should be allowed to dry thoroughly before donning gloves and gown.

Alcohol-based agents immediately reduce resident flora by 95%, with a 99% reduction with repeated applications.[46] Chlorhexidine can be left on the hands and will continue to lower bacterial counts during the procedure.[47] Again, it is important for the surgeon to set the example for the surgical team.

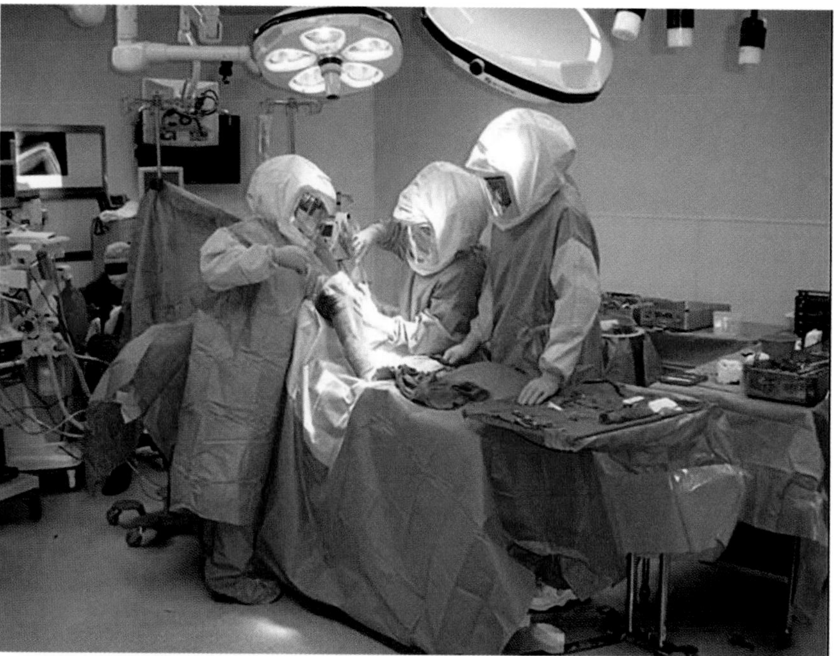

Figure 1 Photograph of a large, modern, operating room with high-efficiency particulate air filtered with a high rate of turnover. Most operating rooms do not have laminar airflow systems. Body exhaust suits are commonly used during total joint arthroplasty surgery.

Gloves and Gown

Double gloving in orthopaedic surgery is a common practice, but an evidence basis for this practice is not clear. Some studies have shown a similar incidence of wound contamination when single and double gloving were compared.[48] Sanders et al[49] showed that a cloth glove over a latex glove resulted in fewer punctures of the inner glove; however, even with double gloving, the puncture rate increased in procedures with surgical times of more than 3 hours compared with shorter surgical times. Although the evidence is soft, double gloving and changing gloves during prolonged procedures is recommended. It is generally recommended that surgical gowns and drapes should be nonwoven or tightly woven and water repellent; staff should minimize handling of the material.[50] There are good data to support more occlusive clothing because bacterial contamination is significantly lower.[51]

The Surgical Site

Shaving

Shaving the hair about the surgical area is another procedure steeped in tradition. In the past, it was not unusual for the entire leg to be shaved the evening before a knee arthrotomy. However, shaving with a safety razor more than 24 hours preoperatively carries a 20% infection rate.[52] Shaving with a safety razor immediately before surgery carries a 3.1% risk of infection. Using a depilatory agent or no hair removal has the lowest SSI rate of 0.6%.[53] It is recommended that when shaving is necessary, an electric razor should be used.

Surgical Preparation

The surgical "scrub" of the patient is another step steeped in ritual. It has been shown that preparing the patient with a traditional povidone-iodine scrub and paint is quite effective, but the bacterial killing potential ceases upon completion of the scrubbing process, and drape adhesion may be compromised. The one-step, water-insoluble, iodophor-in-alcohol solution fulfills the requirements for surgical site skin preparation and significantly improves drape adhesion;[54] however, available data give conflicting reports of its effectiveness.[55] Recent studies have compared

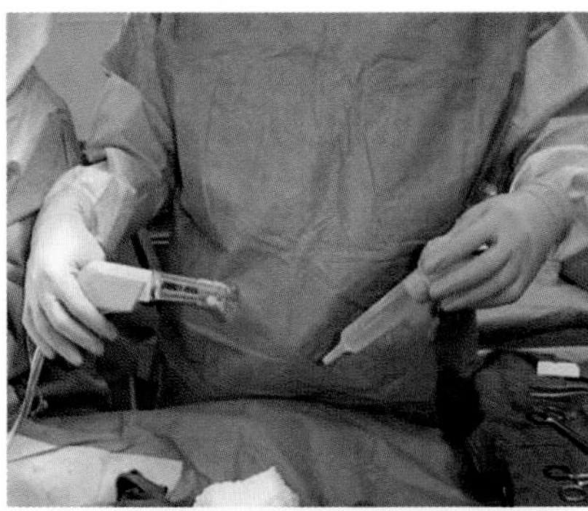

Figure 2 Modern pulse lavage systems (left) have been shown to be superior to a bulb syringe (right) for irrigation.

chlorhexidine-alcohol to povidone-iodine.[56] In 849 surgeries performed at six Veterans Administration hospitals, the overall infection rate was 9.5% in the chlorhexidine-alcohol group compared with 16.1% in the povidone-iodine group (P = 0.004). The deep incisional infection rate was 1% and 3%, respectively.

In another study, three different preparation protocols were used for 6 consecutive months and compared, with SSI as the measured outcome.[57] In the first period, the povidone-iodine scrub, isopropyl alcohol, and then povidone-alcohol paint were used; the overall infection rate was 6.4%. In the second period, 2% chlorhexidine and 70% isopropyl alcohol were used; the infection rate was 7.1%. In the third period, iodine povacrylex in isopropyl alcohol was used. This protocol resulted in a statistically significantly lower rate of infection of 3.9% (P = 0.002). Although each protocol is effective, the literature does not clearly support the superiority of a given technique for surgical site preparation.

Adhesive Drapes

Surgical adhesive drapes have been the topic of several studies. French et al[58] concluded that the drape prevents bacterial penetration and multiplication and precludes bacterial migration beneath the drape. In a study by Fairclough et al,[59] the authors reported that bacterial sampling of the wound at the end of the procedure (using a iodophor-impregnated adhesive drape) showed that wound contamination was reduced from 15% to 1.6%. However, in a report based on a study of 123 surgical patients, 68 with a drape and 55 without, there was a 54.5% infection rate without the drape and 44.1% with the drape, which was not statistically different.[60] Overall, there is significant support for using the adhesive drape, but the drape must adhere to the skin throughout the procedure to be effective.

Antibiotic Irrigation

Empirically, most surgeons believe that dilution offers a solution to controlling polluting agents, but disagreement continues with regard to what solutions are best, what delivery method is optimal, and how much diluting fluid is required. One study compared 208 spinal surgery patients treated with wound irrigation with povidone-iodine and 206 with no povidone-iodine irrigation. The infection rates were 0.5% and 2.9%, respectively, which was significantly different (P = 0.0146).[61] Antibiotic irrigation has been used for many years, but evidence of efficacy is lacking. Roth et al[62] concluded there is no evidence that antibiotic irrigation is effective in prophylaxis of infection in orthopaedic procedures. Detergents and castile soaps also have been used for many years but have never been highly accepted, although there is literature to support their efficacy. Burd et al[63] reported a statistically significant difference between groups (control versus detergent irrigation) for the total number of culture positive sites (P < 0.0001), culture positive animals (P = 0.02), and quantitative cultures (P < 0.02). The authors found lower bacterial counts in polymicrobial wounds treated with surfactant irrigation. An in vitro animal wound model showed that surfactant irrigation was superior to saline or antibiotic solution in removing adherent bacteria from metallic surfaces, bone, and bovine muscle.[64] It can be concluded that antibiotic solutions are not effective, and povidone-iodine solution as well as surfactants may be effective in lowering bacterial counts.

It has not been clearly determined how much irrigating solution is optimal. Empirically, in open fractures the use of 10 L is generally taught. One study sequentially measured cement debris in the suction canister during irrigation in cemented total knee arthroplasties and found that 4 L of irrigating solution was necessary to remove all debris.[65]

There is some literature comparing pulse lavage to bulb syringe irrigation (**Figure 2**). In one study, the pulse lavage group had a significantly lower total infection rate and, specifically, a decreased joint-space or deep infection rate compared with the group treated with jug or syringe irrigation.[66] Too much irrigation pressure, however, may be detrimental. A study by Hassinger et al[67] reported that high-pressure pulsatile lavage caused deeper bacterial penetration and resulted in greater bacterial retention in soft tissues when compared with low pressure lavage. Povidone-iodine, surfactants, and castile soap have been shown to be superior irrigating solutions compared with antibiotic solutions, and pulsatile lavage is superior to bulb syringe irrigation. Based on the best available information, the use of at least 4 L of irrigating solution may be appropriate.

Tools and Instruments

Studies have shown that large volumes of air pass through the suction tip, and airborne bacteria that collect on the suction tip can be transferred to the wound.[68-70] A Scandinavian study reported that after an average of 100 minutes of surgical time, 12 of 22 suction tips (55%) were contaminated with bacteria.[70] Greenough[68] reported 11 of 30 suction tips (37%) were contaminated at the end of a hip arthroplasty compared with only 1 of 31 (3%) when the tip had been exchanged before preparation of the femoral canal. Intermittently changing the suction tip and turning the suction system on only before its actual use may help to minimize this source of bacterial contamination.

The splash basin has been referred to as the "bacterial dip." The practice of placing used instruments into a basin of saline prevents blood and debris from drying on the instruments, thus making them easier to clean. However, the instruments are often used again during the surgical procedure even though normal saline with blood and tissue represents an excellent culture media for bacteria. In one study, 58 of 78 splash basins (74%) were culture positive at the end of the orthopaedic procedure.[71] Thirty-four of 58 positive cultures (59%) yielded multiple organisms. The most common organism was coagulase-negative *Staphylococcus,* which is the organism most frequently associated with deep periprosthetic infections. Instruments placed into the splash basin should never be returned for use on the operative wound.

With time, the instruments on the back table are exposed to the operating room environment and contamination; this is believed to be a factor for infection risk, although definitive correlation has not been established.[72] Cleaning and sterilizing instruments should follow the manufacturer's recommendations. Definitive data are not available, but reports indicate that when flash sterilization is not used, hospital infection rates are reduced.[73]

Wound Drainage

The debate concerning the use of a drain evokes passionate disagreement among orthopaedic surgeons. A study by Drinkwater and Neil[74] found no clear benefit in using a drain, raised the concern over track drainage and a potential passageway for infection, and showed an increased infection rate if the drain remained in place for more than 24 hours. However, the argument for using a drain in a wound with a high risk of hematoma formation and the relationship of hematoma to infection risk is also recognized. In another study in which a drain was used on only one side in bilateral knee surgery, no difference in swelling, quadriceps function, drainage, or infection was reported.[75] A meta-analysis showed that drains increase the need for transfusion in postoperative total hip and knee arthroplasty patients and provide no major benefit.[76] The literature does not support the routine use of drains in total joint arthroplasty except when hematoma is a significant risk; if used, attempts should be made to remove the drain within 24 hours.

Wound Closure

There has been recent mention in the lay press regarding the risk of infection associated with certain suture materials (**Figure 3**); however, the medical literature is very limited on this topic. In a study of skin closure in dogs comparing Monocryl (Ethicon, New Brunswick, NJ) to Vicryl (Ethicon), less early inflammation was reported with Monocryl, but no late differences were reported.[77] In another study of 81 patients treated with breast reduction surgery, there was less inflammation and the formation of fewer keloids with Monocryl compared with Vicryl.[78] In a study comparing abdominal wound closure with Vicryl and Vicryl Plus (coated with triclosan), the Vicryl group had a 10.8% infection rate, and the Vicryl Plus group had a 4.9% infection rate.[79] Although these reported infection rates are higher than comparable studies, the differences are statistically significant.

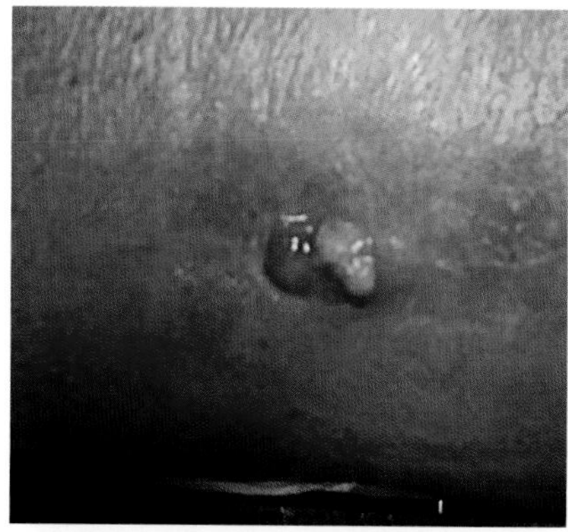

Figure 3 Clinical photograph of an abscess that formed around a retained suture.

The Patient Factor

Patient factors, such as age, general health, and body weight, are risk factors for infection that cannot be controlled by the surgeon. The Surgical Care Improvement Project (SCIP) recommends maintaining normothermia, normoglycemia, and adequate oxygen levels in the operating room.[80] Individually, these measures lack strong literature-based evidence, but there is good support in the literature for the effectiveness of SCIP measures in total.[81] Pushback on the incorporation of SCIP measures has resulted in specific studies to evaluate the value of some measures. Moretti et al[82] hypothesized that the use of warm airflow systems over the patient may induce greater particulate counts at the wound site. The hypothesis was found to be false. Meyhoff et al[83] showed administering oxygen at 80% as opposed to 30% did not affect SSI; however, a meta-analysis of five randomized, controlled studies including 3,001 subjects reported an overall reduction in SSI from 12% to 9% in the hyperoxic group ($P = 0.006$).[84] Although the data are not compelling, it is reasonable to conclude that these measures are rational.

Local Antibiotic Delivery at the Wound

Direct Antibiotic Placement

There are few data in the literature with regard to placing antibiotics directly within a wound, although the practice is common. One recent study using an animal model compared systemic cephalosporin with local injection of gentamicin and found that the gentamicin was more effective than parenteral cephalosporin but not as effective as the combination of parenteral cephalosporin and locally administered gentamicin.[85] Although animal studies are encouraging, the local administration of antibiotic into the wound at closure is not approved by the Food and Drug Administration (FDA). Direct application of high levels of antibiotics into blast injuries and coverage with a plastic dressing, thus creating an antibiotic bead pouch, has been shown to be effective.[86]

Antibiotic-Loaded Bone Cement

For many years, antibiotics have been added to polymethylmethacrylate bone cement.[87] Antibiotic-loaded cement has also been commercially available outside the United States for many years. It has been shown that commercially produced antibiotic-loaded bone cement has superior mechanical properties compared with surgeon-mixed preparations.[88] The FDA has recently approved the sale of commercially produced antibiotic-loaded cement in the United States but only for use in second-stage revision surgeries. The commercially available compounds in the United States contain either 1.2 g of tobramycin, 1.0 g of gentamycin, or 1.0 g of vancomycin per 40 g of cement. This dose is adequate for prophylaxis but not for treating infection. Commercially available prosthesis antibiotic-loaded acrylic cement contains only low-dose antibiotics and is not adequate for treating infection. The most significant data with regard to the prophylactic use of antibiotic-loaded cement comes from European Registry data. The revision rates in 56,275 cemented and uncemented primary total hip arthroplasties were followed for 0 to 16 years.[89] It was noted that the risk of revision because of infection was equal for prostheses implanted with antibiotic cement and uncemented implants. These findings can be explained by the reduced resistance to infection caused by the cement, which appears to be neutralized by adding antibiotic to the cement. Prostheses implanted with antibiotic cement were superior to cemented arthroplasties without antibiotic cement. Prostheses implanted with antibiotic cement were superior to cemented arthroplasties without antibiotic cement. Antibiotic bone cement with systemic antibiotics was found to be more effective in preventing deep infection than using systemic antibiotics alone or antibiotic bone cement alone ($P < 0.001$).

Common concerns with antibiotic-loaded bone cement are the potential for the development of allergic reaction and the promotion of resistant strains. However, in the Norwegian registry of more than 100,000 patients, there have been no reports of an allergic reaction and no evidence of the development of resistance.[89] A 2002 study by Chiu et al[90] compared 178 knees treated with cefuroxime-impregnated cement versus 162 without added cement. Two superficial infections occurred in both groups, but the antibiotic cement group had no deep infections, whereas the control group had five.

In a study using up to 3 g of vancomycin per 60 g of cement, no degradation of the mechanical properties of the cement was reported, and the antibiotic was undetectable in urine by day 10.[91] Antibiotic drainage levels were well below toxic levels, and bone levels were well above effective levels. The authors expressed concerns about the development of resistant strains and allergic reactions to antibiotics.

At this time, US orthopaedic surgeons should strongly consider using one of the commercially available antibiotic-loaded cement preparations when reimplanting a previously infected total joint arthroplasty. Antibiotic cement is not FDA approved in the United States for primary arthroplasties but may be considered if a risk stratification approach indicates its usefulness.

Antibiotic Coating of Implants

New biodegradable drug delivery systems are being developed with the goal of providing local prophylaxis and for treating osteomyelitis.[92] Polylactic acid has shown promise as a delivery device, producing a predictable release of antibiotic, leaving no residual carrier material, and having no adverse effect on bone healing.[93-95] In a study in which trabecular metal implants were inserted into the forelimb of rabbits and inoculated with *Staphylococcus aureus*, there was a statistically significant reduction in the occurrence of infection when the implant was protected with antibiotic microspheres (CG Ambrose, MD, and TA Clyburn, MD, unpublished data, Houston, TX, 2005). In another animal study, spinal implant infections were significantly reduced with the use of gentamicin microspheres.[96] Local antibiotic protection of implants promises better wound protection and lowered risks of the systemic ill effects of antibiotics, but reports are limited to in vitro and animal studies.

Silver coatings have been used with some success in applications such as fixation pins and megaprostheses.[97]

Summary

There is extensive literature available that is relative to SSI reduction. Within the operating room environment, there are many variables that the orthopaedic surgeon can control. Many established protocols and methods are considered "good practices." Evaluation using standards of evidence-based medicine support the use of laminar flow with body exhaust suits; data also support the effectiveness of several surgical skin preparations. Particulate matter in the operating room is related to the density of CFUs and correlates with the number of people in the room. Attention to detail and protocol in the operating room is strongly recommended, but many specific measures may not meet the requirements to be considered evidence-based standards.

References

1. Delgado-Rodríguez M, Sillero-Arenas M, Medina-Cuadros M, Martínez-Gallego G: Nosocomial infections in surgical patients: Comparison of two measures of intrinsic patient risk. *Infect Control Hosp Epidemiol* 1997;18(1):19-23.
2. Horan TC, Culver DH, Gaynes RP, et al: Nosocomial infections in surgical patients in the United States, January 1986-June 1992. *Infect Control Hosp Epidemiol* 1993;14(2):73-80.
3. Wallace WC, Cinat M, Gornick WB, Lekawa ME, Wilson SE: Nosocomial infections in the surgical intensive care unit: A difference between trauma and surgical patients. *Am Surg* 1999;65(10):987-990.
4. National Nosocomial Infections Surveillance (NNIS) report, data summary from October 1986-April 1996, issued May 1996: A report from the National Nosocomial Infections Surveillance (NNIS) System. *Am J Infect Control* 1996;24(5):380-388.
5. Auerbach AD: Prevention of surgical site infections, in Shojania KG, Duncan BW, McDonald KM, Wachter RM, Markowitz AJ, eds: *Making Health Care Safer: A Critical Analysis of Patient Safety Practices. Evidence Report/Technology Assessment 43, publication 01-E058.* Rockville, MD, Agency for Healthcare Research and Quality, 2001, pp 221-244.
6. Maderazo EG, Judson S, Pasternak H: Late infections of total joint prostheses: A review and recommendations for prevention. *Clin Orthop Relat Res* 1988;229:131-142.
7. Gilbert P, McBain AJ: Literature-based evaluation of the potential risks associated with impregnation of medical devices and irrigation with triclosan. *Surg Infect (Larchmt)* 2002;3(Suppl 1):S55-S63.
8. Fry DE: The economic costs of surgical site infection. *Surg Infect (Larchmt)* 2002;3(Suppl 1):S37-S48.
9. Urban JA: Cost analysis of surgical site infections. *Surg Infect (Larchmt)* 2006;7(Suppl 1):S19-S22.
10. Gosden PE, MacGowan AP, Bannister GC: Importance of air quality and related factors in the prevention of infection in orthopaedic implant surgery. *J Hosp Infect* 1998;39(3):173-180.
11. Lidwell OM, Lowbury EJ, Whyte W, Blowers R, Stanley SJ, Lowe D: Airborne contamination of wounds in joint replacement operations: The relationship to sepsis rates. *J Hosp Infect* 1983;4(2):111-131.
12. Lidwell OM, Elson RA, Lowbury EJ, et al: Ultraclean air and antibiotics for prevention of postoperative infection: A multicenter study of 8,052 joint replacement operations. *Acta Orthop Scand* 1987;58(1):4-13.
13. Friberg B, Friberg S, Burman LG: Inconsistent correlation between aerobic bacterial surface and air counts in operating rooms with ultra clean laminar air flows: Proposal of a new bacteriological standard for surface contamination. *J Hosp Infect* 1999;42(4):287-293.
14. Friberg B, Friberg S, Ostensson R, Burman LG: Surgical area contamination: Comparable bacterial counts using disposable head and mask and helmet aspirator system, but dramatic increase upon omission of head-gear. An experimental study in horizontal laminar air-flow. *J Hosp Infect* 2001;47(2):110-115.
15. Friberg B, Friberg S, Burman LG: Correlation between surface and air counts of particles carrying aerobic bacteria in operating rooms with turbulent ventilation: An experimental study. *J Hosp Infect* 1999;42(1):61-68.
16. Knobben BA, van Horn JR, van der Mei HC, Busscher HJ: Evaluation of measures to decrease intra-operative bacterial contamination in orthopaedic implant surgery. *J Hosp Infect* 2006;62(2):174-180.
17. Whyte W, Hodgson R, Tinkler J: The importance of airborne bacterial contamination of wounds. *J Hosp Infect* 1982;3(2):123-135.
18. Landrin A, Bissery A, Kac G: Monitoring air sampling in operating theatres: Can particle counting replace microbiological sampling? *J Hosp Infect* 2005;61(1):27-29.
19. Seal DV, Clark RP: Electronic particle counting for evaluating the quality of air in operating theatres: A potential basis for stan-

dards? *J Appl Bacteriol* 1990; 68(3):225-230.

20. Lidwell OM, Lowbury EJ, Whyte W, Blowers R, Stanley SJ, Lowe D: Effect of ultraclean air in operating rooms on deep sepsis in the joint after total hip or knee replacement: A randomised study. *Br Med J (Clin Res Ed)* 1982; 285(6334):10-14.
21. Stocks GW, Self SD, Thompson B, Adame XA, O'Connor DP: Predicting bacterial populations based on airborne particulates: A study performed in nonlaminar flow operating rooms during joint arthroplasty surgery. *Am J Infect Control* 2010;38(3):199-204.
22. Mangram AJ, Horan TC, Pearson ML, Silver LC, Jarvis WR; Hospital Infection Control Practices Advisory Committee: Guideline for prevention of surgical site infection, 1999. *Infect Control Hosp Epidemiol* 1999;20(4): 250-280.
23. Whyte W, Hambraeus A, Laurell G, Hoborn J: The relative importance of the routes and sources of wound contamination during general surgery: II. Airborne. *J Hosp Infect* 1992;22(1): 41-54.
24. Clarke MT, Lee PT, Roberts CP, Gray J, Keene GS, Rushton N: Contamination of primary total hip replacements in standard and ultra-clean operating theaters detected by the polymerase chain reaction. *Acta Orthop Scand* 2004; 75(5):544-548.
25. Ritter MA: Surgical wound environment. *Clin Orthop Relat Res* 1984;190:11-13.
26. Howard JL, Hanssen AD: Principles of a clean operating room environment. *J Arthroplasty* 2007; 22(7, Suppl 3):6-11.
27. Davies RR, Noble WC: Dispersal of bacteria on desquamated skin. *Lancet* 1962;2(7269):1295-1297.
28. Walter CW, Kundsin RB: The airborne component of wound contamination and infection. *Arch Surg* 1973;107(4):588-595.
29. Edmiston CE Jr, Seabrook GR, Cambria RA, et al: Molecular epidemiology of microbial contamination in the operating room environment: Is there a risk for infection? *Surgery* 2005;138(4): 573-582.
30. Sehulster L, Chinn RY; CDC, HICPAC: Guidelines for environmental infection control in health-care facilities: Recommendations of CDC and the Healthcare Infection Control Practices Advisory Committee (HICPAC). *MMWR Recomm Rep* 2003; 52(RR-10):1-42.
31. Nelson CL: Prevention of sepsis. *Clin Orthop Relat Res* 1987;222: 66-72.
32. Charnley J: Postoperative infection after total hip replacement with special reference to air contamination in the operating room. *Clin Orthop Relat Res* 1972;87: 167-187.
33. Lidwell OM: Clean air at operation and subsequent sepsis in the joint. *Clin Orthop Relat Res* 1986; 211:91-102.
34. Nelson CL: Environmental bacteriology in the unidirectional (horizontal) operating room. *Arch Surg* 1979;114(7):778-882.
35. Nelson JP, Glassburn AR Jr , Talbott RD, McElhinney JP: The effect of previous surgery, operating room environment, and preventive antibiotics on postoperative infection following total hip arthroplasty. *Clin Orthop Relat Res* 1980;147:167-169.
36. Salvati EA, Robinson RP, Zeno SM, Koslin BL, Brause BD, Wilson PD Jr: Infection rates after 3175 total hip and total knee replacements performed with and without a horizontal unidirectional filtered air-flow system. *J Bone Joint Surg Am* 1982;64(4): 525-535.
37. Franco JA, Baer H, Enneking WF: Airborne contamination in orthopedic surgery: Evaluation of laminar air flow system and aspiration suit. *Clin Orthop Relat Res* 1977;122:231-243.
38. Laufman H: Airflow effects in surgery. *Arch Surg* 1979;114(7): 826-830.
39. Laurence M: Ultra-clean air. *J Bone Joint Surg Br* 1983;65(4): 375-377.
40. Dharan S, Pittet D: Environmental controls in operating theatres. *J Hosp Infect* 2002;51(2):79-84.
41. Owers KL, James E, Bannister GC: Source of bacterial shedding in laminar flow theatres. *J Hosp Infect* 2004;58(3):230-232.
42. Mitchell NJ, Hunt S: Surgical face masks in modern operating rooms: A costly and unnecessary ritual? *J Hosp Infect* 1991;18(3): 239-242.
43. Ritter MA, Eitzen H, French ML, Hart JB: The operating room environment as affected by people and the surgical face mask. *Clin Orthop Relat Res* 1975;111: 147-150.
44. Tunevall TG: Postoperative wound infections and surgical face masks: A controlled study. *World J Surg* 1991;15(3):383-388.
45. Letts RM, Doermer E: Conversation in the operating theater as a cause of airborne bacterial contamination. *J Bone Joint Surg Am* 1983;65(3):357-362.
46. Ayliffe GA: Surgical scrub and skin disinfection. *Infect Control* 1984;5(1):23-27.
47. Dahl J, Wheeler B, Mukherjee D: Effect of chlorhexidine scrub on postoperative bacterial counts. *Am J Surg* 1990;159(5):486-488.
48. Ritter MA, French ML, Eitzen H: Evaluation of microbial contamination of surgical gloves during actual use. *Clin Orthop Relat Res* 1976;117:303-306.

49. Sanders R, Fortin P, Ross E, Helfet D: Outer gloves in orthopaedic procedures: Cloth compared with latex. *J Bone Joint Surg Am* 1990;72(6):914-917.

50. Bergman BR, Hoborn J, Nachemson AL: Patient draping and staff clothing in the operating theatre: A microbiological study. *Scand J Infect Dis* 1985;17(4):421-426.

51. Whythe W, Bailey PV, Hamblen DL, Fisher WD, Kelly IG: A bacteriologically occlusive clothing system for use in the operating room. *J Bone Joint Surg Br* 1983; 65(4):502-506.

52. Cruse PJ, Foord R: The epidemiology of wound infection: A 10-year prospective study of 62,939 wounds. *Surg Clin North Am* 1980;60(1):27-40.

53. Seropian R, Reynolds BM: Wound infections after preoperative depilatory versus razor preparation. *Am J Surg* 1971;121(3): 251-254.

54. Gilliam DL, Nelson CL: Comparison of a one-step iodophor skin preparation versus traditional preparation in total joint surgery. *Clin Orthop Relat Res* 1990;250: 258-260.

55. Ritter MA, French ML, Eitzen HE, Gioe TJ: The antimicrobial effectiveness of operative-site preparative agents: A microbiological and clinical study. *J Bone Joint Surg Am* 1980;62(5):826-828.

56. Darouiche RO, Wall MJ Jr, Itani KM, et al: Chlorhexidine-alcohol versus povidone-iodine for surgical-site antisepsis. *N Engl J Med* 2010;362(1):18-26.

57. Swenson BR, Hedrick TL, Metzger R, Bonatti H, Pruett TL, Sawyer RG: Effects of preoperative skin preparation on postoperative wound infection rates: A prospective study of 3 skin preparation protocols. *Infect Control Hosp Epidemiol* 2009;30(10): 964-971.

58. French ML, Eitzen HE, Ritter MA: The plastic surgical adhesive drape: An evaluation of its efficacy as a microbial barrier. *Ann Surg* 1976;184(1):46-50.

59. Fairclough JA, Johnson D, Mackie I: The prevention of wound contamination by skin organisms by the pre-operative application of an iodophor impregnated plastic adhesive drape. *J Int Med Res* 1986;14(2): 105-109.

60. Breitner S, Ruckdeschel G: Bacteriologic studies of the use of incision drapes in orthopedic operations. *Unfallchirurgie* 1986;12(6): 301-304.

61. Cheng MT, Chang MC, Wang ST, Yu WK, Liu CL, Chen TH: Efficacy of dilute betadine solution irrigation in the prevention of postoperative infection of spinal surgery. *Spine (Phila Pa 1976)* 2005;30(15): 1689-1693.

62. Roth RM, Gleckman RA, Gantz NM, Kelly N: Antibiotic irrigations: A plea for controlled clinical trials. *Pharmacotherapy* 1985;5(4):222-227.

63. Burd T, Christensen GD, Anglen JO, Gainor BJ, Conroy BP, Simpson WA: Sequential irrigation with common detergents: A promising new method for decontaminating orthopedic wounds. *Am J Orthop (Belle Mead NJ)* 1999;28(3):156-160.

64. Anglen JO, Gainor BJ, Simpson WA, Christensen G: The use of detergent irrigation for musculoskeletal wounds. *Int Orthop* 2003;27(1):40-46.

65. Niki Y, Matsumoto H, Otani T, Tomatsu T, Toyama Y: How much sterile saline should be used for efficient lavage during total knee arthroplasty? Effects of pulse lavage irrigation on removal of bone and cement debris. *J Arthroplasty* 2007;22(1):95-99.

66. Hargrove R, Ridgeway S, Russell R, Norris M, Packham I, Levy B: Does pulse lavage reduce hip hemiarthroplasty infection rates? *J Hosp Infect* 2006;62(4): 446-449.

67. Hassinger SM, Harding G, Wongworawat MD: High-pressure pulsatile lavage propagates bacteria into soft tissue. *Clin Orthop Relat Res* 2005;439:27-31.

68. Greenough CG: An investigation into contamination of operative suction. *J Bone Joint Surg Br* 1986;68(1):151-153.

69. Moeckel B, Huo MH, Salvati EA, Pellicci PM: Total hip arthroplasty in patients with diabetes mellitus. *J Arthroplasty* 1993;8(3):279-284.

70. Strange-Vognsen HH, Klareskov B: Bacteriologic contamination of suction tips during hip arthroplasty. *Acta Orthop Scand* 1988; 59(4):410-411.

71. Baird RA, Nickel FR, Thrupp LD, Rucker S, Hawkins B: Splash basin contamination in orthopaedic surgery. *Clin Orthop Relat Res* 1984;187:129-133.

72. Fitzgerald RH Jr, Washington JA II: Contamination of the operative wound. *Orthop Clin North Am* 1975;6(4):1105-1114.

73. Nimmo L: Meeting standards, following guidelines: Hospital eliminates routine flash sterilization, reduces infection risk. Interview by Alan Joch. *Mater Manag Health Care* 2009;18(3):9-11.

74. Drinkwater CJ, Neil MJ: Optimal timing of wound drain removal following total joint arthroplasty. *J Arthroplasty* 1995;10(2): 185-189.

75. Beer KJ, Lombardi AV Jr, Mallory TH, Vaughn BK: The efficacy of suction drains after routine total joint arthroplasty. *J Bone Joint Surg Am* 1991;73(4): 584-587.

76. Parker MJ, Roberts CP, Hay D: Closed suction drainage for hip and knee arthroplasty: A meta-

analysis. *J Bone Joint Surg Am* 2004;86-A(6):1146-1152.

77. Kirpensteijn J, Maarschalkerweerd RJ, Koeman JP, Kooistra HS, van Sluijs FJ: Comparison of two suture materials for intradermal skin closure in dogs. *Vet Q* 1997;19(1):20-22.

78. Niessen FB, Spauwen PH, Kon M: The role of suture material in hypertrophic scar formation: Monocryl vs. Vicryl-rapide. *Ann Plast Surg* 1997;39(3):254-260.

79. Justinger C, Moussavian MR, Schlueter C, Kopp B, Kollmar O, Schilling MK: Antibacterial [corrected] coating of abdominal closure sutures and wound infection. *Surgery* 2009;145(3):330-334.

80. Fry DE: Surgical site infections and the surgical care improvement project (SCIP): Evolution of national quality measures. *Surg Infect (Larchmt)* 2008;9(6):579-584.

81. Liau KH, Aung KT, Chua N, et al: Outcome of a strategy to reduce surgical site infection in a tertiary-care hospital. *Surg Infect (Larchmt)* 2010;11(2):151-159.

82. Moretti B, Larocca AM, Napoli C, et al: Active warming systems to maintain perioperative normothermia in hip replacement surgery: A therapeutic aid or a vector of infection? *J Hosp Infec* 2009;73(1):58-63.

83. Meyhoff CS, Wetterslev J, Jorgensen LN, et al: Effect of high perioperative oxygen fraction on surgical site infection and pulmonary complications after abdominal surgery: The PROXI randomized clinical trial. *JAMA* 2009;302(14):1543-1550.

84. Qadan M, Akça O, Mahid SS, Hornung CA, Polk HC Jr: Perioperative supplemental oxygen therapy and surgical site infection: A meta-analysis of randomized controlled trials. *Arch Surg* 2009;144(4):359-367.

85. Cavanaugh DL, Berry J, Yarboro SR, Dahners LE: Better prophylaxis against surgical site infection with local as well as systemic antibiotics: An in vivo study. *J Bone Joint Surg Am* 2009;91(8):1907-1912.

86. Henry SL, Ostermann PA, Seligson D: The antibiotic bead pouch technique: The management of severe compound fractures. *Clin Orthop Relat Res* 1993;295:54-62.

87. Buchholz HW: Proceedings: Deep infections as a result of hip-joint replacement (author's transl). *Langenbecks Arch Chir* 1973;334:547-553.

88. Postak PD, Greenwald AS: The influence of antibiotics on the fatigue life of acrylic bone cement. *J Bone Joint Surg Am* 2006;88(Suppl 4):148-155.

89. Engesaeter LB, Espehaug B, Lie SA, Furnes O, Havelin LI: Does cement increase the risk of infection in primary total hip arthroplasty? Revision rates in 56,275 cemented and uncemented primary THAs followed for 0-16 years in the Norwegian Arthroplasty Register. *Acta Orthop* 2006;77(3):351-358.

90. Chiu FY, Chen CM, Lin CF, Lo WH: Cefuroxime-impregnated cement in primary total knee arthroplasty: A prospective, randomized study of three hundred and forty knees. *J Bone Joint Surg Am* 2002;84-A(5):759-762.

91. Chohfi M, Langlais F, Fourastier J, Minet J, Thomazeau H, Cormier M: Pharmacokinetics, uses, and limitations of vancomycin-loaded bone cement. *Int Orthop* 1998;22(3):171-177.

92. Kent ME, Rapp RP, Smith KM: Antibiotic beads and osteomyelitis: Here today, what's coming tomorrow? *Orthopedics* 2006;29(7):599-603.

93. Calhoun JH, Mader JT: Treatment of osteomyelitis with a biodegradable antibiotic implant. *Clin Orthop Relat Res* 1997;341:206-214.

94. Ambrose CG, Clyburn TA, Louden K, et al: Effective treatment of osteomyelitis with biodegradable microspheres in a rabbit model. *Clin Orthop Relat Res* 2004;421:293-299.

95. Ambrose CG, Gogola GR, Clyburn TA, Raymond AK, Peng AS, Mikos AG: Antibiotic microspheres: Preliminary testing for potential treatment of osteomyelitis. *Clin Orthop Relat Res* 2003;415:279-285.

96. Stall AC, Becker E, Ludwig SC, Gelb D, Poelstra KA: Reduction of postoperative spinal implant infection using gentamicin microspheres. *Spine (Phila Pa 1976)* 2009;34(5):479-483.

97. Hardes J, von Eiff C, Streitbuerger A, et al: Reduction of periprosthetic infection with silver-coated megaprostheses in patients with bone sarcoma. *J Surg Oncol* 2010;101(5):389-395.

Principles of Biomechanics and Biomaterials in Orthopaedic Surgery

S. Raymond Golish, MD, PhD
William M. Mihalko, MD, PhD

Abstract

There are few surgical procedures within the field of orthopaedic surgery that do not entail the basis or need for understanding basic biomechanical principles. Every subspecialty field requires some aspect of biomechanics to properly understand and perform surgical procedures, patient examinations, and clinical treatment. A proper review of these principles will allow surgeons to better approach all treatment modalities used for patient care.

Instr Course Lect 2011;60:575-581.

Advances in orthopaedic surgery have been based on biomechanical principles for years. Engineering advances in metallurgy, polymer science, ceramic technology, and manufacturing processes lead to improvements in the devices that orthopaedic surgeons use and thus to better performance in the fields of orthopaedics, especially arthroplasty, spine surgery, trauma, and arthroscopy.

Biomechanics and biomaterials as broad topics may seem overwhelming, but they are manageable when approached by reviewing applications directly related to clinical practice. This chapter reviews the basic aspects of biomaterials relevant to clinical practice, including their mechanical properties and uses for implants, and outlines the clinically relevant aspects, principles, and facts that are germane to many surgical decisions.

Basic Mechanics

The surgeon's understanding of orthopaedic implant technology is enhanced by a basic knowledge of mechanics. Understanding how mechanical properties of materials are determined provides a better appreciation of why certain materials are used in orthopaedics.

The first concept to emphasize is the stress-strain diagram, a useful graphic tool for illustrating the static behavior of systems that are elastic, viscoelastic, and plastic. The full meaning of these terms is clarified in the following sections.

Stress and Strain

Stress is defined as the applied force per unit cross-sectional area of the test piece (newtons per millimeter^2 [N/mm^2]). Strain is defined as the increase in length (in millimeters) as a fraction of the original length (in millimeters).[1] A servohydraulic materials testing machine allows for either load or displacement control to test the mechanical integrity of a specimen or device. A standard materials test piece uses a small volume with a constant cross-sectional area loaded to failure according to protocols that are standardized by ASTM International and the International Organization for Standardization (ISO). With these testing protocols, the stress-strain curve can be plotted, and multiple material properties of the specimen can be calculated.

Dr. Golish or an immediate family member serves as a board member, owner, officer, or committee member of the American Academy of Orthopaedic Surgeons Biomedical Engineering Committee; serves as a paid consultant to or is an employee of Cytonics; and owns stock or stock options in Cytonics. Dr. Mihalko or an immediate family member has received royalties from Aesculap/B. Braun; is a member of a speakers' bureau or has made paid presentations on behalf of Aesculap/B. Braun; serves as a paid consultant to or is an employee of Aesculap/B. Braun; has received research or institutional support from Aesculap/B. Braun, Smith & Nephew, Stryker, and Corin U.S.A.; and has received nonincome support (such as equipment or services), commercially derived honoraria, or other non–research-related funding (such as paid travel) from Aesculap/B. Braun.

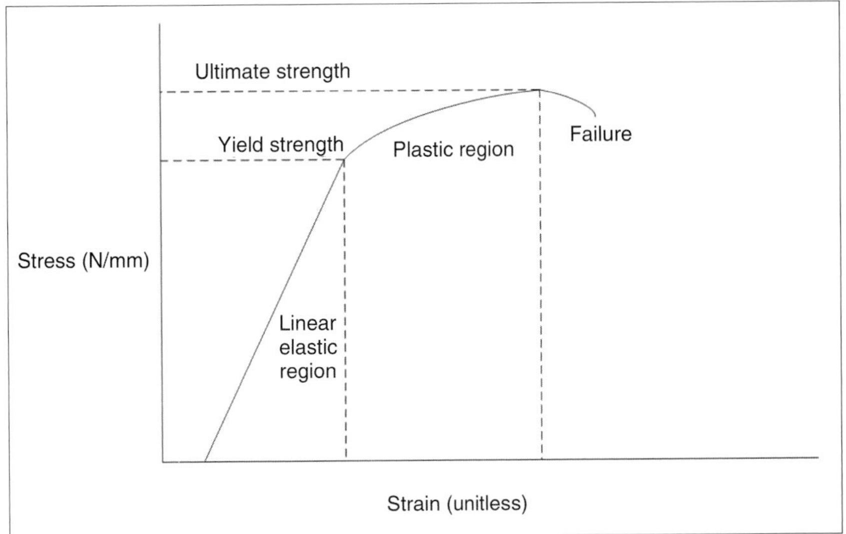

Figure 1 A representative stress-strain diagram (for a ductile material).

A representative stress-strain diagram is shown in **Figure 1**.

Several features of the stress-strain diagram in **Figure 1** are important and define the mechanical properties of the material or device being tested. These features are the linear elastic region, yield point, plastic region, ultimate strength, and failure. As a convention, the properties of materials are most often illustrated with use of a longitudinal force and measurement of the material's tensile strength. A similar curve can be constructed for materials subjected to other forces, such as compression or shear.

Linear Elastic Region

In the linear region of the stress-strain diagram, the test piece behaves as a simple spring. When the stress is increased, the strain increases proportionally.[2] If the same amount of stress is let off, the strain decreases to the previous length. No permanent deformation of the test piece occurs. The strain may be altered any number of times with the same results. The slope of the linear region equals the modulus of elasticity (or the Young modulus) of the material. On the stress-strain curve, stiffer materials have greater slope on the linear portion of the curve.

Yield Point

The yield point is the stress at which there is a change from elastic to plastic deformation. Graphically, on the stress-strain curve, the yield point occurs at the transition of a straight line with constant slope to a curved line of variable slope. On the stress-strain diagram, the yield point is not always visually apparent as it is in **Figure 1**. Consequently, a stress resulting in a 0.2% change in strain is conventionally chosen as the numerical definition of the yield point.

Plastic Region

In the plastic region, when the stress is increased, the strain increases in a more complex way than it does in the elastic region. The stress-strain curve may decrease for a small interval or it may continue to increase but at a lower or more variable rate relative to that in the linear elastic region.

The essential feature of plastic deformation is that it is not completely reversible. If the stress is let off, the test piece will not return to its original length. The molecular mechanisms that mediate plastic deformation are complex. Plastic deformation may result in a phenomenon known as work hardening or strain hardening.

Ultimate Strength

The ultimate strength is the maximum stress that a material can withstand before impending failure. The ultimate strength is not as important for orthopaedic implants as it is in other settings. For orthopaedic implants, fatigue strength is more important and is not necessarily related to ultimate strength.

Failure

Failure occurs when the test piece or material fractures. Numerous modes of failure are possible.[3] Ductile materials have a process of impending failure that occurs immediately after the stress surpasses the material's ultimate strength. Brittle materials are the opposite of ductile materials. Very brittle materials, such as some ceramics, fail in the linear elastic region or after a very small amount of plastic deformation. Brittle materials have a simple stress-strain diagram, and their yield strength, ultimate strength, and failure strength are the same.

Mechanical Properties

Modulus of Elasticity

The modulus of elasticity is the stress per unit strain in the linear elastic portion of the stress-strain curve. The Young modulus is the modulus of elasticity for tensile strength (measured with use of a longitudinal force). As a rule, the stress-strain diagram is for tensile testing (demonstrating the Young modulus) unless stated otherwise. The units for the Young modulus are megapascals (MPa).[2]

Strength

The yield strength is the stress in megapascals at the yield point on the stress-strain curve. This is the strength at the end of linear elastic behavior and at the onset of plastic deformation.[4] The ultimate strength is the stress at the apex of the stress-strain curve. This is the strength at the end of the plastic deformation portion of the curve if it is higher than the yield point. This strength denotes the end of work hardening and the beginning of necking, which precedes fracture (**Figure 1**).

Failure strength is defined as the point of fracture, beyond the linear elastic region and after plastic deformation. In principle, the strength at the failure or fracture point can be measured. In practice, there is rarely a distinction between the ultimate strength and the strength at failure. Since necking has begun, the failure of the test piece is impending with further strain after the ultimate strength. Therefore, the ultimate strength is often reported as the final strength measurement of a material.

Fatigue Strength

Fatigue strength is defined as the maximum stress at which a material can withstand 10 million cyclic loading cycles without failure. (The number 10 million is arbitrary but widely used.) In the stress-strain diagram, the test piece is subjected to a static load instead of a repetitive load. Incremental increases in loading result in elastic deformation, followed by plastic deformation and eventual failure. In fatigue failure, repetitive cyclic loading below the yield strength produces failure after numerous cycles.

Hardness

The most common measure of the hardness of orthopaedic implants involves indentation of the material by a small indenter made of a very hard material (such as diamond).[2] The Rockwell C scale is based on a test using a small diamond indenter with nearly 1,500 N of force. The scratch resistance of materials is a distinct but related concept of hardness that is important for articulating total joint components, although it is less commonly reported as a materials property.

Toughness

Toughness is defined as the amount of energy (per unit volume) that a material can absorb up to the failure strength. Intuitively, toughness is a measure of the fracture resistance of a material when it is subjected to stress. The units are joules per cubic meter (J/m^3).

Roughness

Roughness is a measurement of the surface finish of a test piece. As such, it is not a property of the material alone; it is also a property of the manufacturing processes used to create the surface finish. Ra is the average deviation of the peaks and valleys on a microscopic level (in micrometers or microinches). Ra is the most common roughness measure used for orthopaedic implant surfaces.[5] Roughness may impact the ultimate and fatigue strength material properties of an implant. The greater the roughness of the material's surface, the higher the stress concentrations at the valleys of the surface. Crack initiation and propagation in a device can originate in the valleys of the surface, and roughness has an impact on the longevity of a device that is loaded for millions of cycles during its lifetime.

Static Versus Dynamic Analysis

Stress-strain diagrams are usually an illustration of static analysis, but materials also can be studied with dynamic analysis. Static analysis reveals the properties of materials independent of time. For example, a material in the linear region of a stress-strain diagram is held at an initial stress, with some deformation (strain). If the stress is increased a small amount and then held steady, a new strain is measured without taking into account what occurs during the time period when the testing machine is adjusting the applied stress. When measurements are made during changes that are applied very slowly, or when a substantial time period elapses between changes and remeasurement, the behavior of the test piece and material appears static.

In reality, no practical situation is truly independent of time (static). The alternative to static analysis is dynamic analysis, in which the time-dependent behavior at all time points is considered. If measurements are made when large changes in stress are applied, when changes are made very quickly, or when very little time has elapsed between changes and remeasurement, the behavior of the test piece and material will appear time dependent. A dynamic system that reaches steady-state equilibrium with respect to applied changes appears static if measurements are made only after equilibration.

Linear Elastic Behavior

The assessment of linear elasticity is the simplest type of static analysis and is useful for materials in the linear elastic region of the stress-strain diagram undergoing slow changes in stress, especially metals and alloys under static loading.[2] In a linear elastic system, the measured strain is directly proportional to the applied stress at the jig. The constant of proportionality, or the slope of the stress-strain diagram, is called the Young modulus for tensile testing. There are several synonymous terms for linear elasticity, such as the Hooke law and the simple spring.

The input-output diagrams for a linear elastic system are illustrated in **Figure 2**. When the input load changes instantaneously in the testing of these kinds of materials, the output also changes instantaneously. This is an

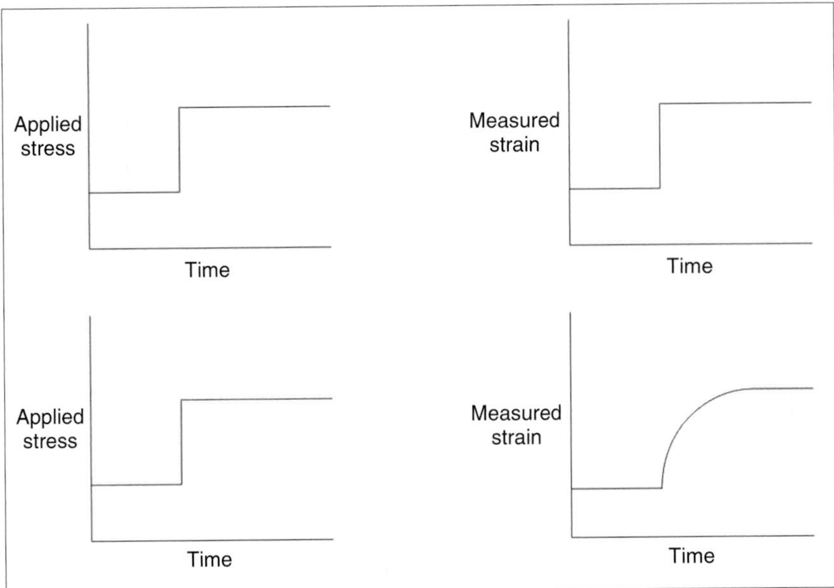

Figure 2 Time course of changes in measured strain for an instantaneous change in applied stress for both linear elastic (top) and linear viscoelastic (bottom) behavior. Because of its simplicity, linear elastic behavior may be viewed as time independent (static), whereas the more complex linear viscoelastic behavior is time dependent (dynamic). However, both models are abstractions. A system may appear to be static versus dynamic depending on the time scale of measurements and the size of changes of applied stresses.

idealization because the change only appears instantaneous at an appropriately coarse time scale. If the time scale is finer, the system may appear dynamic and viscoelastic.

Linear Viscoelastic Behavior

Linear viscoelasticity is another relatively simple type of dynamic analysis. It is useful for materials in the linear elastic region of the stress-strain diagram undergoing rapid changes in stress,[6] especially amorphous polymers under dynamic loading. In a linear viscoelastic system, the measured strain is directly proportional to the applied stress at the jig at final equilibrium but approaches the new steady state exponentially.

Time-dynamic behavior of viscoelastic systems can be described by the terms stress relaxation and creep. **Figure 2** illustrates creep, in which deformation takes some time to reach a final value after application of a new load. A complementary view of the same phenomenon is stress relaxation, in which the measured stress gradually approaches some new final value when the test piece is suddenly adjusted to a new length.

Other Behavior

An important exception to viscoelastic behavior is plastic behavior beyond the yield point, the point of transition from elastic to plastic deformation, in the stress-strain diagram. In plastic deformation, changes in length are not reversible with changes in load. The test piece is permanently deformed, and neither static nor dynamic elastic models describe the behavior beyond the yield point. Many biologic tissues exhibit nonlinear viscoelastic behavior that can be extremely complex.[6] Nonlinear viscoelasticity is dynamic behavior that is not described by linear time-invariant differential equations. Cartilage has complex nonlinear viscoelastic behavior. When a new load is applied slowly, such as with slow walking, the modulus of elasticity is lower, the deformation is increased, and the time to final deformation is increased. When a new load is applied quickly with a sudden weight-bearing impact, the modulus of elasticity is higher, the deformation is decreased, and the time to final deformation is decreased. Although important for biologic tissues and some polymers, nonlinear viscoelasticity does not need to be taken into account for most engineering purposes involving materials.

Continuum Mechanics

Continuum mechanics is used in the study of elastic, viscoelastic, and plastic behaviors of structures containing a variety of materials with different properties, often with complex geometry. Although the principles of complex systems are the same as those of simple test geometries of a single material, the practical situation is much more complex. Computers are used to solve large systems of equations to simulate the mechanics of complex designs (for example, finite element analysis).[2]

Some features of continuum mechanics are important clinically. For example, stress shielding can result when a mismatch in the elastic modulus occurs between two adjacent materials, such as a relatively stiff femoral stem and the cortical/cancellous bone in the proximal part of the femur. The proximal femoral region experiences a relative decrease in stress because of the stiff implant carrying stress to the cortical bone of the femoral diaphysis. This may result in relative osteopenia of the stress-shielded bone visible on a radiograph.[7]

Corrosion

The corrosion resistance of an implant has several components. The material and surface finish combine with the geometry of the test piece interacting with the biologic environment. Corrosion varies widely among orthopaedic implants, with some polymer implants, such as bioabsorbable implants, being designed to degrade completely and other implants being designed to resist corrosion as completely as possible.[8]

Chemical Corrosion

Chemical corrosion is a process by which there is a chemical reaction of a material with the biologic environment. The chemical reaction results in new compounds at the surface of the implant, which can change the mechanical properties. Metals often undergo oxidation, which may be catalyzed by other chemicals in the biologic milieu, especially halide ions such as chloride. Polymers undergo a variety of corrosive and degradative processes, including hydrolysis of the polymer bonds into shorter-chain polymers by thermal and enzymatic processes. The process of chemical corrosion can be altered by alterations in the chemistry of the biologic environment, such as the decrease in pH that may be present with bacterial infection.

Crevice and Pitting Corrosion

Crevice and pitting corrosion are two distinct but related processes that occur when local chemistry established in a small feature of the test piece causes increased corrosion in a small area. Crevice corrosion occurs when a small machined feature on the surface traps the local chemical environment and results in increased corrosion. Pitting corrosion is caused by a small pit, which can exist even on a smooth surface, with an altered chemical environment caused by an impurity resulting from statistical variation. This local pit sets up a catalytic process that leads to a larger pit with even more altered chemistry. Even a tiny pit can ultimately lead to catastrophic failure.

Galvanic Corrosion

Galvanic corrosion is caused by differences in electrochemical potential between two distinct metals in an electrolyte solution, creating an electric current between the two metals. This battery effect results in physical migration of metal ions. There is concern that galvanic corrosion in mixed-metal implants (especially cobalt-chromium and stainless-steel combinations) can change the geometry of the implant and weaken it over time. There is only limited evidence that this phenomenon represents a clinically relevant problem with commonly used metal.[9] Nevertheless, informed decisions that include an understanding of galvanic and other corrosion modes should be made regarding the use of mixed-metal implants.

Fretting

Fretting is a chemical and mechanical process in which corrosion occurs between two mating surfaces in micromotion. It includes both the chemical corrosion of freshly exposed surfaces and wear caused by the mechanical friction of corrosion products. Fretting is an important issue with articulating components of total joint arthroplasties, such as tibial trays articulating with polyethylene inserts in total knee arthroplasty, which can produce polyethylene debris affecting the tibial side.[10]

Corrosion and Biocompatibility

Titanium-aluminum-vanadium alloy (Ti-6Al-4V) is highly resistant to corrosion in biologic environments. Commercially pure titanium has a high affinity for oxygen; however, Ti-6Al-4V forms a stable, adherent oxide layer in aqueous environments in a process termed self-passivation. The resultant film stabilizes the alloy to resist further oxidation and chemical corrosion, including that caused by halide ions such as chloride. Passivation is a key to the corrosion resistance of Ti-6Al-4V.[8] Materials that resist corrosion by passivation are subject to pitting corrosion and crevice corrosion, in which an altered local chemistry in small pits or crevices inhibits the passivation layer, leading to progressive corrosion. This can be influenced by small scratches, pits, or design features and contributes to notch sensitivity induced by intraoperative handling and metal-metal interfaces.

Ti-6Al-4V is regarded as a highly biocompatible alloy. There is virtually no nickel in this alloy, so it is useful in patients with documented nickel sensitivity.[11] Corrosion modes, resistance, and biocompatibility are distinct for all orthopaedic metals and biomaterials, including 316L stainless steel, cobalt-chromium-molybdenum (Co-Cr-Mo) alloy, highly cross-linked ultra-high molecular weight polyethylene, poly-L-lactic acid polymer, and other commonly used materials. However, the considerations listed here for titanium alloys are representative of the considerations and reasoning for all materials.[11]

Alloys in Use

ASTM International is an international standards organization responsible for the standardization of materials in industrial use. Previously known as the American Society for Testing and Materials, the organization now has a global scope and charter. The existence of standards allows for trade of materials with known engineering performance among international vendors.[12] The society for medical devices is designated F-04, and the breadth and number of standards applicable to the

Table 1
Mechanical Properties of Commonly Used Alloys

Property	Porous Tantalum	Ti-6Al-4V	Co-Cr-Mo	316L Stainless Steel
Modulus of elasticity (GPa)	2.5-3.9	106-115	210	230
Yield strength (MPa)	35-51	860	825	170-690
Ultimate strength (MPa)	50-110	780-1050	430-1028	515-860
Hardness (on Rockwell C scale)	N/A	36	42	60
Fatigue strength (MPa at 10^7 cycles)	18-20	480-590	310	180-300
Mass density (g/cm^3)	N/A	4.4	8.3	8.0

Ti-6Al-4V = titanium-aluminum-vanadium alloy; Co-Cr-Mo = cobalt-chromium-molybdenum alloy.

field of orthopaedic surgery are astounding. The following are a few examples of standards for titanium alloys in current use in orthopaedic surgery.

ASTM F-136

This alloy is Ti-6Al-4V and is used in many orthopaedic applications in North America.[13]

ASTM F-67

This alloy is commercially pure titanium and is used for spinal rods, plasma-spray coatings on Ti-6Al-4V implants, and some other applications.

ASTM F-1295

This alloy contains titanium, aluminum, and niobium and has been used for applications similar to ASTM F-136 in the European and North American markets.

ASTM F-2063

This alloy is commonly called nitinol and contains nickel and titanium in nearly equal ratios. It has the peculiar property of being a shape memory alloy, in which heating after deformation restores the material to its prior shape. It has found wide application for intraluminal stents and arthroscopic suture passers but only scant application for orthopaedic implants.

Mechanical Properties of Common Materials in Orthopaedics

With an understanding of how mechanical properties of materials are determined, the reasons certain materials in orthopaedics are used over others can be better appreciated. Comparing these properties to bone allows a better comparison of the material's properties and use in orthopaedics (**Table 1**). The more similar a material's mechanical properties are to bone, the less stress shielding is created. For example, if the properties of a femoral component in a total hip replacement are more similar to bone, there will be less stress shielding of proximal femoral bone and a lower stress riser at the tip of the femoral stem, thereby decreasing the risk of periprosthetic fracture. This is just one of multiple examples of how a better understanding of biomechanics and material properties enhances a surgeon's ability to make an educated decision concerning the products used in the treatment of his or her patients.

Summary

The terminology and principles involved in mechanics, materials, and engineering for orthopaedic surgery are manageable. The availability of sources that provide a better understanding of applications to orthopaedic surgery is paramount to enable surgeons to better treat their patients and comprehend the rationale behind many surgical procedures. It is hoped that this chapter will serve as a resource to aid orthopaedic surgeons in obtaining this goal.

References

1. Stress and strain, in Özkaya N, Nordin M, eds: *Fundamentals of Biomechanics: Equilibrium, Motion, and Deformation*, ed 2. New York, NY, Springer, 1999, pp 125-152.
2. Properties of materials, in Ratner B, Hoffman AS, Schoen FI, Lemons JE, eds: *Biomaterials Science: An Introduction to Materials in Medicine*, ed 2. San Diego, CA, Elsevier Academic Press, 2004, pp 23-66.
3. Implants, devices, and biomaterials: Issues unique to this field, in Ratner B, Hoffman AS, Schoen FI, Lemons JE, eds: *Biomaterials Science: An Introduction to Materials in Medicine*, ed 2. San Diego, CA, Elsevier Academic Press, 2004, pp; 753-782.
4. Multiaxial deformations and stress analyses, in Özkaya N, Nordin M, eds: *Fundamentals of Biomechanics: Equilibrium, Motion, and Deformation*, ed 2. New York, NY, Springer, 1999, pp 153-194.

5. Forbes A, Tomlins P, Gurdak E, Illsely M, James S, James E: Methodologies for assessing local surface texture features that are relevant to cell attachment. *J Mater Sci Mater Med* 2010;21(8):2463-2477.
6. Mechanical properties of biological tissues, in Özkaya N, Nordin M, eds: *Fundamentals of Biomechanics: Equilibrium, Motion, and Deformation*, ed 2. New York, NY, Springer, 1999, pp 195-218.
7. Glassman AH, Bobyn JD, Tanzer M: New femoral designs: Do they influence stress shielding? *Clin Orthop Relat Res* 2006; 453:64-74.
8. Degradation of materials in the biological environment, in Ratner B, Hoffman AS, Schoen FI, Lemons JE, eds: *Biomaterials Science: An Introduction to Materials in Medicine*, ed 2. San Diego, CA, Elsevier Academic Press, 2004, pp 411-454.
9. Virtanen S, Milosev I, Gomez-Barrena E, Trebse R, Salo J, Konttinen YT: Special modes of corrosion under physiological and simulated physiological conditions. *Acta Biomater* 2008;4(3): 468-476.
10. Engh GA, Ammeen DJ: Epidemiology of osteolysis: Backside implant wear. *Instr Course Lect* 2004; 53:243-249.
11. Host reactions to biomaterials and their evaluation, in Ratner B, Hoffman AS, Schoen FI, Lemons JE, eds: *Biomaterials Science: An Introduction to Materials in Medicine*, ed 2. San Diego, CA, Elsevier Academic Press, 2004, pp 293-354.
12. New products and standards, in Ratner B, Hoffman AS, Schoen FI, Lemons JE, eds: *Biomaterials Science: An Introduction to Materials in Medicine*, ed 2. San Diego, CA, Elsevier Academic Press, 2004, pp 783-804.
13. Healy WL, Tilzey JF, Iorio R, Specht LM, Sharma S: Prospective, randomized comparison of cobalt-chrome and titanium trilock femoral stems. *J Arthroplasty* 2009;24(6):831-836.

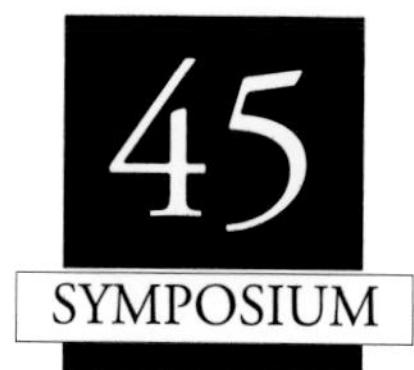

Applied Biomechanics in Articular Injuries: Perspectives in the Basic Investigation of Articular Injuries and Clinical Application

Steven A. Olson, MD, FACS
Thomas D. Brown, PhD
Kyriacos A. Athanasiou, PhD, PE
Roman M. Natoli, MD, PhD
Douglas R. Dirschl, MD

Abstract

Joint injury is an important cause of arthritis. Although the treatment of injury, in general, has been widely studied, the contribution of injury to the development of posttraumatic arthritis is still a relatively understudied area. One of the most perplexing aspects of investigating articular injuries is the complex nature of the injury itself and the multiple facets of the injury mechanism that can potentially lead to the development of arthritis.

A symposium by the Orthopaedic Research Society and the American Academy of Orthopaedic Surgeons was designed to examine the spectrum of basic science to clinical investigation in the role of biomechanics in the study of joint injury and subsequent posttraumatic arthritis. Four perspectives in the clinical aspects of managing articular injuries were investigated, including the clinical applications of basic science findings, the challenges and advancements in measuring and modeling articular fractures, the relationship of articular cartilage mechanical injuries and osteoarthritis, and the controlled creation of an intra-articular fracture to permit observations of the natural history of posttraumatic arthritis.

Instr Course Lect 2011;60:583-594.

Dr. Olson or an immediate family member serves as a board member, owner, officer, or committee member of the SouthEastern Fracture Consortium Foundation; is a member of a speakers' bureau or has made paid presentations on behalf of Synthes; and has received research or institutional support from Synthes. Dr. Brown or an immediate family member serves as a paid consultant to or is an employee of Smith & Nephew. Dr. Athanasiou or an immediate family member serves as a paid consultant to or is an employee of Arthrex; has received research or institutional support from Springer; and owns stock or stock options in VidaCare Diabetica Solutions. Dr. Dirschl or an immediate family member serves as a board member, owner, officer, or committee member of the American Orthopaedic Association and has received royalties from Biomet. Neither Dr. Natoli nor any immediate family member has received anything of value from or owns stock in a commercial company or institution related directly or indirectly to the subject of this chapter.

The overall effect of the condition of the musculoskeletal system on health in the United States is increasing. Recently, a working group of the Bone and Joint Decade initiative has attempted to quantify the burden of musculoskeletal disease in the United States.[1] Two of the major contributors to this burden of disease include arthritis and injuries. In adults, arthritis is the most common cause of disability in the United States and is among the leading conditions causing work limitations.[1] From 2003 to 2005, arthritis was diagnosed in approximately 21% or slightly more than 46 million patients in the United States. By the year 2030, it is projected that 25% of the US adult population will have physician-diagnosed arthritis. Injuries to the musculoskeletal system account for another large portion of overall disease in the United States. In 2004, approximately 57 million musculoskeletal injury episodes were treated in physician offices, emergency departments, clinics, and other medical institutions. More than 33% of all injuries were reported as strains and sprains. Fractures represented nearly 25% of all reported musculoskeletal injuries.[1]

The subgroup of patients with injuries to the musculoskeletal system (particularly major joint injuries) in whom arthritis develops is less well defined. This population of patients with posttraumatic arthritis is a distinct group of patients contributing to the overall burden of musculoskeletal disease.[2] As a disease entity, posttraumatic arthritis is relatively unstudied. Although arthritis can develop after any injury to a major joint, it most predictably and rapidly develops after intra-articular fractures.[3] The traditional view of the development of arthritis after an articular fracture has been one of focal stress elevation related to articular malreduction following surgical or nonsurgical treatment of the injury.[4] More recent studies suggest that elements of posttraumatic arthritis serve as components of the overall mechanism of disease and may alter chondrocyte viability, incite an acute inflammatory response, and contribute to altered mechanical wear.[5,6]

Many factors contribute to the relative lack of knowledge concerning posttraumatic arthritis.[3] From a research perspective, posttraumatic arthritis is a difficult topic to study. The overall spectrum of disease that can lead to clinical arthritis after injury is extensive, ranging from articular fractures to injuries with ligamentous disruption to joint contusion without fracture.[7,8] Articular fractures are examples of worst-case scenarios, with physical disruption of the articular surface, blunt impaction of the articular surface, and local hemarthrosis; these fractures are often associated with a systemic inflammatory response. Each of these aspects of injury represents a unique physiologic and biomechanical mechanism that can contribute to the overall outcome of the patient. Traditional investigative techniques that study isolated mechanisms of disease have been applied to these mechanisms.[5,7,9,10] Although these investigations provide new information, they do not replicate the complex conditions of an articular fracture, making clinical translation less certain.

Perhaps one of the most perplexing aspects of investigating articular fractures is the complex nature of the injury and the effects of the treatments designed to restore the displaced articular surface. Clinicians have inadequate tools to accurately and reliably assess the effects of the various aspects of injury on the ultimate clinical outcome.[11] The physical disruption of the joint, the physiologic response to injury, and impaction of the articular surface are all inseparably related. For example, how can posttraumatic arthritis be prevented in a patient with a comminuted articular fracture? Should prevention efforts be focused on restoring articular reduction, mitigating the effects of impaction injury to the cartilage, enhancing a combination of local and systemic physiologic response to the injury, or should all of these areas be addressed? To improve patient functioning following a displaced articular injury, it is critical to develop research strategies to investigate the role of injury mechanisms that will allow the development of new therapies to limit or prevent posttraumatic osteoarthritis (OA).

The material presented in this chapter is based on a combined Orthopaedic Research Society and American Academy of Orthopaedic Surgeons (AAOS) symposium designed to examine the spectrum of basic science to clinical investigation in the role of biomechanics in the study of joint injury and subsequent posttraumatic arthritis.

Clinical Applications of Basic Science Findings

Like much of orthopaedic practice, fracture surgery is ruled by tenets. Common sense, the desire to serve patients, and the substantial influence of the AO group and its educational network have resulted in ideas that have become "fracture dogma." Two of the most closely and passionately guarded tenets in managing articular fractures are as follows: the objective of treatment is precise reconstruction of the articular surface, and patient outcomes will vary based on the accuracy of articular reduction.

A review of the published literature shows that the necessary precision recommended for articular reconstruction has changed over time. In the tibial plateau, for example, the "necessary" threshold for articular congruity has decreased over the past 20 years from 8 mm to 2 mm.[12-16] Outcomes following care, however, appear to be largely unchanged.[12-16] It appears that the threshold for acceptable reduction has more closely followed improvements in the technical abilities of surgeons rather than improvements in outcomes. Another important factor is that a surgeon's ability to reliably measure articular incongruity (even at a flat surface like the tibial plateau) is rather poor, with a 95% confidence interval of ±12 mm for quantifying articular step-off.[11]

In numerous instances, a perfect reduction in a simple, low-energy fracture will result in significant pain and extremely poor function. In contrast, there are other cases in which a poor reduction in a highly comminuted fracture results in little pain and good function. Despite the desire to follow established fracture tenets and principles, observations indicate that the relationship between articular reduction and outcome is neither as direct nor as simple as it appears.

The simple but nonintuitive truth is that articular congruity is not the only factor that influences outcomes after fracture. An array of confounding variables, many of which are poorly understood, have a profound impact on the patient's outcome following an articular injury. Some of these factors include the magnitude and type of articular injury, the magnitude of the soft-tissue injury, the patient's response to the injury, morphologic and mechanical differences between joints, subtle but pronounced effects of joint kinematics and dynamic instability, cartilage biology and its response to injury, the patient's age and its effect on injury response, and the effects of load distribution that is not restored with the restoration of articular congruity.

Current research is helping clinicians understand these factors. Appreciating the value of this new research and incorporating it into clinical practice requires that clinicians challenge their traditional thinking about articular fractures. For example, articular congruity; injury to the articular cartilage; and other factors such as limb alignment, joint stability, and kinematics can independently and in combination have an impact on patient outcomes. Most orthopaedic fracture surgeons focus on the primacy of articular reduction in improving outcomes. This approach is overly simplistic and does not take into account other factors that have a profound impact on outcomes. To overcome this bias, it is important to recognize several truths. (1) All of the factors affecting outcomes are inextricably linked; there is no rational or realistic way to separate the effects of one from the others. (2) There is much evidence (new and old) in the literature to indicate that articular reduction may not be the most important factor in determining outcomes. (3) The appropriate weight of various factors is not yet known. If these truths are accepted, the clinician can acknowledge factors other than articular reduction as critically important to patient outcomes and can begin to incorporate these factors in the clinical care of patients with fractures.

In science, only what can be measured can be known. As medical scientists, orthopaedic fracture surgeons should embrace work that tries to improve methods to measurably characterize articular injury; the body's response to it; and the mechanical, kinematic, and biologic effects of treatment. Research currently in progress includes finite element modeling of injured and reconstructed joints,[17] methods for quantifying injury severity,[17] methods for measuring cartilage health and response to injury,[6,18] methods for measuring dynamic mechanical stresses,[19-21] methods for correlating measurements with outcomes,[2,17] and methods for predicting outcomes and guiding treatment. The goals of these and other research studies should be to better determine the relationships between articular cartilage injury, articular reduction, other mechanical factors, and patient outcomes. The support of orthopaedic clinicians is needed to continue this type of research.

In daily interactions with colleagues, staff, and patients, surgeons should indicate that they understand that factors other than articular alignment are important to patient outcomes. Surgeons should be willing to recommend treatment other than open reduction and internal fixation when it is not clear that articular reduction will change the patient's outcome. Cartilage biology, joint and limb mechanics, and articular congruity should be considered when making treatment decisions and counseling patients.

Challenges and Advancements in Measuring and Modeling Articular Fractures

Despite the need to objectively characterize articular injury, quantify injury response at the tissue and whole-joint level, and measure the mechanical and biologic effects of treatment, there are few appropriate techniques to achieve these goals. Developing or refining assessment tools to yield reliable mechanical data on joint injuries poses substantial biomechanical technical challenges. Although joint injuries are "global" events, the resulting pathophysiology originates locally at the tissue and cell level; the efficacy of therapeutic interventions (surgical and nonsurgical) depends on achieving favorable local effects.

One of the classic challenges has been to measure chronic cartilage insult caused by residual incongruities following imprecise reduction of intra-articular fractures.[22] Empirical clinical experience has shown that different joints and different specific fractures of these joints produce different tolerance levels for articular incongruity. Trying to reach agreement on specific acceptable tolerance levels has often resulted in controversy among leading surgeons. Corresponding aberrations of cartilage stress, either quasi-static stress concentrations locally near sites of surface irregularity or abrupt transients of cartilage stress associated with joint instability events, probably constitute much of the unifying explanation of why different joints behave or respond so differently.

Two distinct measurement methodologies using Fuji film (Sensor Products, Madison, NJ) or Tekscan pressure mapping (Tekscan, South Boston, MA) have been developed for measuring cartilage contact stress. The Fuji film method involves a mechanochemical transduction process based on pressure-dependent rupture of populations of microcapsules (containing a photoreactive liquid) deposited on the surface of paperlike acetate sheets. The sheets can be easily cut by hand to fit the articular anatomy of interest. The higher the contact pressure, the greater the fraction of microcapsules that rupture and the more intense the resulting (red) stain.[23] The intensity of the Fuji staining is normally quantified using laser scanning and digital image analysis. Accuracies in the range of 10% to 15% are the generally accepted norm. Because of the size scale of the microcapsules, for practical purposes the resulting stain patterns are essentially continuous, thus providing excellent spatial resolution for assessing local details of pressure aberrations into the submillimeter range. The primary limitation of this method is that the data captures are necessarily static, reflecting the high-water mark of pressure experienced at any given site on the film. Despite this limitation, the Fuji film method has been useful in answering many pragmatic surgical questions concerning alternative fracture reconstruction techniques and dose-response relationships between incongruity and the resulting pressure abnormality at various anatomic sites.[24,25]

The Tekscan transduction modality uses an entirely different methodology. It involves pressure-dependent changes in the electrical resistance between large numbers of intersection sites between rows and columns of conductors, separated by a thin layer of piezoresistive elastomer. This system enables transient recordings, although the spatial resolution of such recordings is limited by the row-column density of the conductor grid. Because trimming the sensors would destroy the electrical circuitry, the Tekscan system lacks the versatility of Fuji film to be easily cut to fit the anatomy of interest. Past biomechanical applications have usually involved general purpose sensor geometries designed for industrial purposes; therefore, this system may provide suboptimal coverage of an anatomic joint surface, or it may be difficult to accommodate the necessary (fragile) connecting cables. Recently, there have been several varieties of custom biomechanical sensors developed for specific anatomic locations (the knee, the ankle, and the hip), providing for well-conforming articular surface coverage and anatomically cognizant cable protection.[26] Currently, maximum data capture rates exceed 100 frames per second, and available spatial resolutions are on the order of 0.5 mm^2 per sampling site. A major advantage of transient data collection is that a loaded joint can be studied throughout its range of motion, thereby providing information about habitual cartilage loading, rather than just snapshot information at specific instants that may not be representative of the duty cycle and may not identify worst-case situations. Recent Tekscan measurements focusing on tibial plafond fractures have identified incongruity-dependent abnormalities of local contact stress magnitude and contact stress rates of change, shifts of global load transmission patterns, and the occurrence of seemingly dramatically deleterious fluctuations of loading under conditions of joint instability.[20,21]

Computational advancements in articular joint contact mechanics have greatly reduced the need for dependence on physical experimentation. Finite element techniques have spearheaded those developments. Previous limitations, which have recently been overcome, are the ability to simulate cartilage contact under physiologically realistic joint-loading magnitudes and the rates of change of joint-loading magnitudes in the presence of local incongruities.[27] Another important development has been the use of numerical techniques to study the interaction of solid and fluid components of cartilage matrix for situations involving articular surface contact. This is an important consideration in evaluating local incongruities because of the heightened ease for fluid egress from ruptured cartilage surfaces. Another class of developments has been the ability to realistically simulate cartilage impaction events, both for impulsive loadings between native joint surfaces and for laboratory impaction events involving platen loading of exposed joint surfaces or of specialty osteochondral explant preparations. Probably the most important current improvement in articular contact finite element analysis has been the development of novel meshing techniques to accommodate arbitrary derangements of joint surface geometry.[26,28] These improvements have allowed the study of actual clinically occurring fractures rather than geometrically idealized situations, such as straight-edged step-offs. These meshing techniques can be applied to prospective clinical studies to quantify risk factors for degenerative change.[29]

Assessing injury severity has been another fertile area for computational innovation. It was intuitively accepted that joint fractures resulting from high-energy mechanisms had a greater risk for posttraumatic OA than low-energy fractures; however, a method to directly quantify the involved energy did not exist. A fundamental tenet of engineering fracture mechanics of brittle solids holds that the kinetic energy absorbed during the fracture event is transformed into free-surface energy of the resulting fragment fracture surfaces. In human clinical fractures, information on fragment free-surface energy is available postfacto from CT images of the fracture bed and is based on segmentation (edge delineation) of all individual fragments, a process that is well suited to automated computational analysis. This has allowed "backing out" a measurement of the mechanical energy absorbed in bone fracture events. A series of laboratory computational/experimental studies has documented the quantitative accuracy of the essential concept.[30,31] After several computational developments to streamline and expedite the analysis, it has now been applied to human prospective studies,[17] allowing objective identification of the relative risk of posttraumatic OA to individual patients.

Another new area of computational development is the identification of anatomically correct reconstructions of displaced comminuted articular fractures. Surgical reduction of such fractures must be done piece by piece, with limited visibility, and with no way of knowing in advance if the reassembled fragments will result in gaps (especially periarticularly) because of missing or compacted fragments. An analogous process of three-dimensional puzzle solving performed computationally provides advanced information about appropriate geometric reassembly of individual fragments and identifies any region(s) of void that will necessarily result.[32] To implement this process, the puzzle-solving algorithm begins with automated segmentations of the bony fragments, with their respective surface facets identified as being native periosteal surface, native subchondral plate, or de novo fracture surface. Native fragment surface facets are computationally matched to geometrically corresponding sectors on a surface template that is defined by mirror imaging of the intact contralateral limb. Successive fragment facets are then computationally "locked into place" using an iterative closest point algorithm in a manner that minimizes their topographic disparity with corresponding sectors on the template surface. Homogeneous surrogates with biofidelity, which were fractured under controlled laboratory conditions, were initially used to tune the puzzle solver to achieve fragment reassembly accuracy in the range of a few tenths of 1 mm. After porting this computational procedure (with appropriate modifications) to cadaver material, submillimeter accuracies in fitting the template surfaces were maintained. Facilitated by new computational procedures to expedite fragment segmentation and an advanced surgeon-friendly graphic interface to manipulate fragments, the procedure has been applied to "puzzle-solve" a clinical case series of comminuted tibial plafond fractures, to compare geometrically ideal versus surgically obtained reconstructions, and to help understand the practical difficulties in obtaining fully anatomic reconstructions (especially of the articular surface) on a case-by-case basis.

A large-animal survival model of intra-articular fracture that allows orthopaedic interventions analogous to those for human clinical cases is also being developed. This model complements the capabilities of a recently developed mouse model, whose primary strengths were the ability to understand the pathophysiology and natural history of intra-articular fractures, especially in concert with genetic-level assessments and interventions. The large-animal model involves evaluating the hock joint of the adult Yucatan minipig after fractures with controlled morphology (for example, replicable fracture line location on the articular surface) are achieved by a specially developed offset impaction technique. The investigator has knowledge and control of the delivery energy and impaction force. At the whole-joint level, the fracture patterns closely resemble those of human tibial pilon fractures. At the cellular and tissue levels, the patterns of matrix damage and cell death (and its temporal and spatial progression after impaction) closely resemble those seen for impaction fractures of fully viable normal human ankle specimens obtained from above-knee tumor amputation patients. Minipigs are clinically tolerant of both plate and screw internal fixation and spanning external fixation of the hock joint; the pigs shortly resume non–weight-bearing protected limb usage. This model offers exciting promise for evaluating the efficacy of novel therapeutic interventions screened in vitro and in small-animal (nonreconstructible) fracture models and is a key laboratory testing step before translation to human clinical trials.

Articular Cartilage Mechanical Injuries and OA

Mechanical injuries of articular cartilage can result from events such as motor vehicle crashes, falls, and sports injuries. Such injuries can lead to posttraumatic OA, although the pathophysiologic processes are not fully understood.[3,7,33] Articular cartilage responds to injury by two separate processes that are linked to each other through mechanotransduction.[34,35] During the injurious event, the tissue responds mechanically by deforming according to the applied load. Subsequently, the biologic response starts when the mechanical forces applied to the tissue activate intracellular signaling.

OA can be thought of as a condition that develops as a result of the overloading of healthy tissue (acute trauma) or from normal loading of abnormal tissue. Overloading of healthy cartilage can immediately cause surface fissuring, cell death, and damage to the extracellular matrix from which the tissue cannot recover. Alternatively, overloading of normal cartilage may cause subcritical damage that leads to less robust tissue. Subsequent loading of this abnormal cartilage, even at physiologic levels, can result in chronic injury and damage accumulation that eventually manifest as OA. Articular cartilage does not heal well.[36] Attempted self-repair results in the formation of mechanically inferior fibrocartilage-like tissue, which has more collagen type I and contains less glycosaminoglycan than normal articular cartilage.[37,38] These biochemical changes lead to changes in the tissue's mechanical properties, preventing normal function.[39,40]

Changes in the physical properties of articular cartilage contribute significantly to the development of OA. Because of damage and loss of extracellular matrix, the compressive and tensile stiffness decreases and permeability increases.[41] Cartilage from osteoarthritic joints is thinner and more hydrated than healthy tissue. For example, a review by Knecht et al[42] reported that the compressive stiffness of articular cartilage decreases by 20% in early stages of the disease, a change that probably would be undetected by current clinical assessment methods. The decrease in compressive stiffness correlates with increased scores on the Mankin histologic scoring system for articular cartilage, increased tissue hydration, and decreased sulfated glycosaminoglycan content. The fact that changes in tissue occur so early suggests that timely intervention is needed to alter the course of OA.

Mechanical Considerations for In Vitro Studies of Cartilage Injury

Because the first response of articular cartilage to injury is mechanical, it is essential to understand the intrinsic mechanical characteristics of the tissue and the mechanical features of the external system causing injury. The mechanical properties of articular cartilage are the macroscopic result of its underlying organization and biochemical content. The collagen network of the tissue governs tensile behavior, whereas proteoglycans are necessary for resisting compression.[43] The tensile stiffness of articular cartilage positively correlates tissue collagen content and collagen cross-linking. Within cartilage, collagen is arranged in a depth-dependent manner. Collagen is parallel to the articular surface in the superficial zone, oriented randomly in the middle zone, and is perpendicular in the deep zone as it anchors into the calcified cartilage layer. In the superficial zone, collagen also follows preferred directions known as split lines. The tissue is stiffer when pulled in the direction of split lines when compared with off-axis pulling. The proteoglycan content of the tissue gives articular cartilage its ability to resist compressive loads because of the electrostatic repulsion of the negatively charged glycosaminoglycans when forced into close proximity.[44] Injuries to articular cartilage that affect collagen or proteoglycans alter the biomechanical behavior of the tissue.

The mechanical features of the external system used for in vitro study of cartilage mechanical injury are also important because the type of loading, boundary conditions, and preinjury tissue processing all affect experimental outcome. Loading regimens have varied and include injurious compression, single impacts, and cyclical loads.[45-57] Different load magnitudes and rates have been used with each of these regimens. Experimental setup (boundary conditions) must also be considered. Different setups with respect to the presence or absence of underlying bone and loading methods have been used.[53,58-63] The loading methods include confined compression, unconfined compression, and indentation. Each method radially constrains surrounding tissue differently. Some studies have included preinjury tissue processing steps, including the use of full-thickness cartilage versus cartilage with the superficial zone removed,[46] and equilibrating tissue in a culture medium before loading.[64] These factors must be considered when comparing studies.

Early Postinjury Biology and Treatment

Following the mechanical response of cartilage to injury, a biologic response occurs. Within the tissue, mechanical loading generates streaming potentials, stress-strain fields, and hydrostatic pressure. The biologic response starts when chondrocytes experience the mechanical forces applied to the tissue and intracellular signaling cascades are activated through stretch activated channels and integrins located in the cell membrane.[34,35,65] Following this mechanotransduction, the biologic response to injury evolves over time. Time-points for investigation after an in vitro mechanical injury have ranged from 3 hours to 2 weeks. Several cell matrix adhesion molecules have shown decreased expression as early as 3 hours after injury.[66] With the exception of *SOX9*, a transcription factor promoting collagen type II, there is generally upregulation of gene expression from 4 to 24 hours after injury.[67-69] Examples of upregulated genes include matrix metalloproteinases (MMPs), aggrecanases, and inhibitors of MMPs. These enzymes break down type II collagen and aggrecan. Further study has suggested these changes in gene expression normalize by 2 weeks after injury, and MMP-3 expression switches from increased to decreased expression,[70] suggesting that MMP-3 could be a marker for time after injury.

Articular cartilage degradation is mediated by several factors, such as cell death, matrix degrading enzymes, and inflammation. In attempts to mitigate some of these changes, the poloxamer P188 has been used to decrease cell death. P188 is an 8.4 kDa nonionic surfactant triblock copolymer of polyoxyethylene and polyoxypropylene that inserts into lipid membranes.[71] Postinjury, promising results have been reported with P188 in both in vitro and in vivo rabbit models.[72-75] In a study by Phillips and Haut,[72] P188 (8 mg/mL) was delivered in the culture medium following a 25-MPa load to cartilage explants. With P188 treatment, there were more viable cells in the superficial zone at 1 hour and in all zones at 24 hours but only if the explants were manually compressed. Compression presumably aided P188 entry into the tissue. In a 4-day in vivo study, a one-time intra-articular injection of P188 was effective at reducing cell death in impacted retropatellar cartilage.[64] A more recent study reported that P188 reduced cell death in tibiofemoral cartilage 6 weeks after injury.[75] Natoli and Athanasiou[76] evaluated P188 (8 mg/mL) following two levels of impact loading (1.1 and 2.8 J) using continuous treatment. They reported a 75% decrease in cell death at 1 week following the 1.1 J impact. In contrast to the study by Phillips and Haut,[72] no compression protocol was needed to achieve this benefit, perhaps because of the adoption of a continuous treatment regimen compared with a one-time treatment. A recent 2009 study showed that P188 treatment was more effective at decreasing cell death in human ankle cartilage after impact than inhibition of caspase 3 or 9 (two enzymes that drive apoptosis).[77] Future research should investigate combining treatments for apoptotic and necrotic cell death to further chondrocyte preservation after injury.

Osteoarthritic chondrocytes do not behave like native, healthy chondrocytes.[78] Because traumatic injury may shift the phenotype of chondrocytes remaining in the tissue toward catabolic processes, the previously described studies of treatment to decrease cell death should be interpreted cautiously. The catabolic nature of these cells (for example, the production of matrix-degrading enzymes and inflammatory signals) is evident based on the continued degradation of articular cartilage after the inciting event.[69] Although chondrocyte survival postinjury is necessary for tissue healing, it may not be sufficient. Future research must also address the behavior of viable chondrocytes after injury and should include measurements of tissue mechanical properties to assess tissue functionality. Researchers should also seek interventions that promote a healing response. In addition to preventing cell death, research has been directed at decreasing extracellular matrix degradation and inflammation after mechanical injury with methods such as pharmaceutical therapy.[79]

Controlled Creation of an Intra-Articular Fracture: Observations on the Natural History of Posttraumatic Arthritis

The mechanisms leading to the progression of posttraumatic arthritis following articular fracture are not well understood. After injury, several factors may affect the development of posttraumatic arthritis, including disruption of the articular surface, variable amounts of impaction of the articular cartilage, residual displacement of the articular surfaces, and exposure of blood and marrow products to the articular surface and synovium.[3] Because these predisposing factors are inseparably clinically linked with the injury, investigations of traumatic joint injury that focus on a single aspect of the acute injury, such as blunt trauma to the articular surface, are too limited. Traditional models of investigating a single aspect of injury trade simplicity for the complexity of a more realistic injury model system.

To gain a broader perspective on the effects of intra-articular fracture, it is necessary to understand the natural history of the development, over time, of posttraumatic arthritis in a displaced articular injury. A model was developed to create a closed joint injury in a relatively reproducible fashion that was usable in a survival animal model. Furman et al[80] described work to prove the concept that established the ability to create a closed fracture of the tibial plateau with varying degrees of severity. A single hind limb fracture was created in strain C57/BL6 mice. The fracture was allowed to heal without attempts at fracture reduction or fixation, thus allowing the natural history of posttraumatic arthritis to be studied; the contralateral limb served as an internal control. Faxitron imaging, micro-CT at the time of limb harvest, and histologic analysis were used to assess the joints of both extremities from each specimen. In the C57/BL6 mice, this injury reliably resulted in the development of a tricompartmental arthritis at 4 and 8 weeks after injury, with complete loss of articular cartilage by 50 weeks after injury.[80]

Application of this method to the MRL/MpJ strain of mice proved enlightening. Clark et al[81] was the first to describe the unique healing characteristics of MRL/MpJ mice. Because these mice were able to spontaneously regenerate tissue in ear punch holes without scarring, the strain was called the "super-healer." The creation of similar types of closed tibial plateau fractures in the MRl/MpJ mice did not result in the development of articular degeneration, despite articular fracture and displacement.[82] The observation that a displaced fracture results in ar-

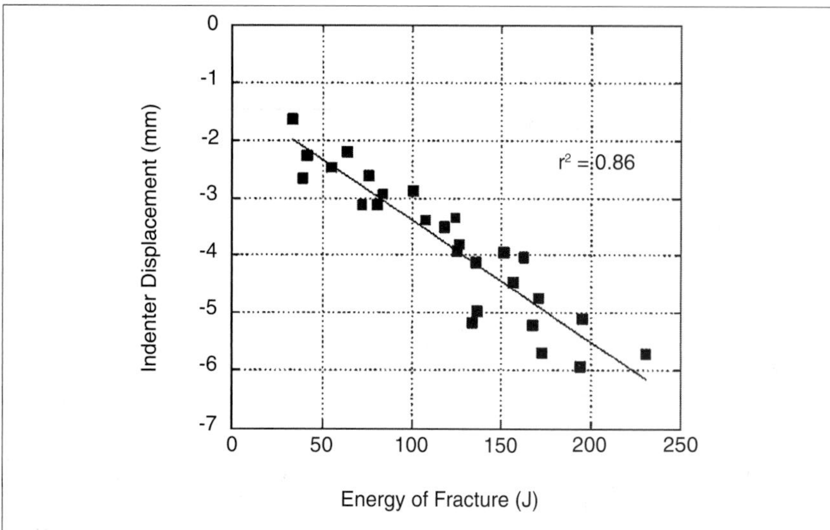

Figure 1 Graph illustrating the relationship between applied load (as represented by indenter displacement) and energy of fracture in the creation of a closed articular fracture in a murine model. (Reproduced with permission from Furman BD, Strand J, Hembree WC, Ward BD, Guilak F, Olson SA: Joint degeneration following closed intraarticular fracture in the mouse knee: A model of posttraumatic arthritis. *J Orthop Res* 2007;25(5):578-592.)

thritis in one strain but not in the other suggests altering physiologic response to injury is a potential intervention strategy.

Assessing the severity of injury is challenging. Three methods of injury severity assessment were applied in this model. (1) A modification of the AO/OTA classification for clinical fractures was applied to data from faxitron imaging and microCT.[80] The basis for a classification system is, in part, to stratify discrete events into varying categories of severity. (2) The applied energy and the energy of injury at time of fracture are both known.[80] A plot showing the relationship between applied energy and the energy of fracture is shown in **Figure 1**. This relationship allows the energy of fracture to be controlled. (3) Micro-CT from both control and experimental limbs were used to determine the liberated fracture surface as a third severity measure. Authors have described the assessment of liberated fracture as a means of assessing injury severity.[17,83] In the murine model of tibial plateau fracture, the energy of fracture has an excellent correlation with the liberated fracture area.[84]

Interest in the physiologic response following articular fracture in the C57/BL6 and the MRL/MpJ mice strains stimulated the development of novel techniques of assessing the response. Standard serum analysis of cytokines and biomarkers is a valuable technique. However, serum levels alone reflect incomplete information about physiologic response to injury. A novel technique was developed for quantitatively assessing cytokines and biomarkers in synovial fluid of the knee of mice following injury. Using small amounts of a calcium sodium alginate compound to absorb synovial fluid with controlled lyase digestion allows a quantitative analysis.[85] Gene activation following injury can be assessed from synovial tissue.[86] The small amount of synovial tissue available from this technique in mice typically requires pooling of specimens to obtain adequate amounts of DNA to generate reliable data. Histologic analysis allows assessment of proteoglycan staining of cartilage and synovial cellular response to fracture.[87] Determining the cellular viability and immunohistochemistry of the joints allows assessment of the variation of response, over time, following articular fracture.

The initial focus of research has been on understanding the initial events in the development of tricompartmental arthritis after fracture in the C57/BL6 mouse strain. Early effects of injury in the C57/BL6 strain show that the loss of cellular viability of chondrocytes parallels the structural damage of the articular surface as determined by the modified Mankin histologic scoring system for articular cartilage.[80] Additionally, changes in the synovium with increasing cellularity are proportional to the increasing energy of fracture.

Preliminary results of comparisons of early events following articular fracture in the C57/BL6 and MRL/MpJ strains indicate important differences. The severity of injury and the basic fracture characteristics are similar between mice strains, as is the initial increase in the cellularity of the synovial layer; however, local gene activation, synovial fluid levels, and serum levels of cytokines differ between strains.[88] In the C57/BL6 strain there is a significantly more robust inflammatory response to injury compared with the MRL/MpJ strain. One example of the effect of this response is a markedly increased presence of activated macrophages in the synovial lining of the C57/BL6 mice that persists weeks after injury, whereas a transient blush of activated macrophages occurs initially in the synovium and then returns to levels of the control limb in the MRL/MpJ mice.[88]

This simple observation provides the basis for new hypotheses regarding mechanisms beyond the traditional view of residual displacement of the articular surface as the cause of arthritis following fracture. Recent work in immunology suggests that, in the presence of necrotic material, macrophages become activated or primed to produce more inflammatory cytokines.[89,90] Disruption of the articular surface inherently produces necrotic chondrocytes and other cell types. Is this a signal that can result in activation of synovial macrophages? The question suggests a shift in perspective from posttraumatic arthritis as a consequence of injury to the articular surface to that of an organ-level response to injury in which there is physiologic signaling between articular cartilage and other tissues within the joint. New methods of investigating the effects of injury that consider the organ level response of the joint may offer new insights into this important area.

Summary

Injury to the articular surface contributes to the development of the clinical condition recognized as posttraumatic arthritis in a large number of patients each year. The basic mechanisms by which articular injury contributes to the development of joint degeneration remain incompletely characterized. Currently, the clinical treatment of the fracture itself is the primary form of intervention in attempting to prevent the development of posttraumatic arthritis. There are no pharmacologic interventions or other therapies available that can prevent or delay the onset of posttraumatic arthritis. Several lines of ongoing research discussed in this chapter have the potential to add to the knowledge of posttraumatic arthritis, with the potential to identify future targets for intervention.

Although patients with articular injury generally have an increased risk for the development of joint degeneration, an improved ability to predict what injury patterns and patient characteristics are at a true high risk for joint degeneration is needed to study interventions as they become available. The need for prospective registries with longitudinal follow-up is important to identify these at-risk patient populations. Approaching posttraumatic arthritis from these varied perspectives will contribute to a better understanding of how articular injury contributes to this condition and will improve patient care.

Acknowledgments

The authors wish to acknowledge the contributions of Farshid Guilak, PhD, and Bridgette Furman, BA, to this chapter.

References

1. Jacobs JJ: *The Burden of Musculoskeletal Diseases in the United States.* Rosemont, IL, American Academy of Orthopaedic Surgeons, 2008.
2. Brown TD, Johnston RC, Saltzman CL, Marsh JL, Buckwalter JA: Posttraumatic osteoarthritis: A first estimate of incidence, prevalence, and burden of disease. *J Orthop Trauma* 2006;20(10):739-744.
3. Olson SA, Guilak F: From articular fracture to posttraumatic arthritis: A black box that needs to be opened. *J Orthop Trauma* 2006;20(10):661-662.
4. Marsh JL, Buckwalter J, Gelberman R, et al: Articular fractures: Does an anatomic reduction really change the result? *J Bone Joint Surg Am* 2002;84-A(7):1259-1271.
5. Borrelli J Jr: Chondrocyte apoptosis and posttraumatic arthrosis. *J Orthop Trauma* 2006;20(10):726-731.
6. Martin JA, McCabe D, Walter M, Buckwalter JA, McKinley TO: N-acetylcysteine inhibits post-impact chondrocyte death in osteochondral explants. *J Bone Joint Surg Am* 2009;91(8):1890-1897.
7. Borrelli J Jr, Ricci WM: Acute effects of cartilage impact. *Clin Orthop Relat Res* 2004;423:33-39.
8. McKinley TO, Rudert MJ, Koos DC, Brown TD: Incongruity versus instability in the etiology of posttraumatic arthritis. *Clin Orthop Relat Res* 2004;423:44-51.
9. Llinas A, McKellop HA, Marshall GJ, Sharpe F, Kirchen M, Sarmiento A: Healing and remodeling of articular incongruities in a rabbit fracture model. *J Bone Joint Surg Am* 1993;75(10):1508-1523.
10. Bálint L, Park SH, Bellyei A, Luck JV Jr, Sarmiento A, Lovász G: Repair of steps and gaps in articular fracture models. *Clin Orthop Relat Res* 2005;430:208-218.
11. Martin J, Marsh JL, Nepola JV, Dirschl DR, Hurwitz S, DeCoster TA: Radiographic fracture assessments: Which ones can we reliably make? *J Orthop Trauma* 2000;14(6):379-385.
12. Lucht U, Pilgaard S: Fractures of the tibial condyles. *Acta Orthop Scand* 1971;42(4):366-376.
13. Rasmussen PS: Tibial condylar fractures: Impairment of knee joint stability as an indication for surgical treatment. *J Bone Joint Surg Am* 1973;55(7):1331-1350.
14. Lansinger O, Bergman B, Körner L, Andersson GB: Tibial condylar fractures: A twenty-year follow-up. *J Bone Joint Surg Am* 1986;68(1):13-19.
15. Koval KJ, Sanders R, Borrelli J, Helfet D, DiPasquale T, Mast JW: Indirect reduction and percutaneous screw fixation of displaced tibial plateau fractures. *J Orthop Trauma* 1992;6(3):340-346.

16. Honkonen SE: Indications for surgical treatment of tibial condyle fractures. *Clin Orthop Relat Res* 1994;302:199-205.
17. Anderson DD, Mosqueda T, Thomas T, Hermanson EL, Brown TD, Marsh JL: Quantifying tibial plafond fracture severity: Absorbed energy and fragment displacement agree with clinical rank ordering. *J Orthop Res* 2008; 26(8):1046-1052.
18. Hembree WC, Ward BD, Furman BD, et al: Viability and apoptosis of human chondrocytes in osteochondral fragments following joint trauma. *J Bone Joint Surg Br* 2007;89(10):1388-1395.
19. Anderson DD, Goldsworthy JK, Shivanna K, et al: Intra-articular contact stress distributions at the ankle throughout stance phase-patient-specific finite element analysis as a metric of degeneration propensity. *Biomech Model Mechanobiol* 2006;5(2-3):82-89.
20. McKinley TO, Tochigi Y, Rudert MJ, Brown TD: The effect of incongruity and instability on contact stress directional gradients in human cadaveric ankles. *Osteoarthritis Cartilage* 2008;16(11): 1363-1369.
21. McKinley TO, Tochigi Y, Rudert MJ, Brown TD: Instability-associated changes in contact stress and contact stress rates near a step-off incongruity. *J Bone Joint Surg Am* 2008;90(2):375-383.
22. Brown TD, Anderson DD, Nepola JV, Singerman RJ, Pedersen DR, Brand RA: Contact stress aberrations following imprecise reduction of simple tibial plateau fractures. *J Orthop Res* 1988;6(6): 851-862.
23. Huberti HH, Hayes WC: Patellofemoral contact pressures: The influence of q-angle and tendofemoral contact. *J Bone Joint Surg Am* 1984;66(5):715-724.
24. Malkani AL, Voor MJ, Rennirt G, Helfet D, Pedersen D, Brown T: Increased peak contact stress after incongruent reduction of transverse acetabular fractures: A cadaveric model. *J Trauma* 2001; 51(4):704-709.
25. Moed BR, Ede DE, Brown TD: Fractures of the olecranon: An in vitro study of elbow joint stresses after tension-band wire fixation versus proximal fracture fragment excision. *J Trauma* 2002;53(6):1088-1093.
26. Brown TD, Rudert MJ, Grosland NM: New methods for assessing cartilage contact stress after articular fracture. *Clin Orthop Relat Res* 2004;423:52-58.
27. Goreham-Voss CM, McKinley TO, Brown TD: A finite element exploration of cartilage stress near an articular incongruity during unstable motion. *J Biomech* 2007;40(15):3438-3447.
28. Anderson DD, Goldsworthy JK, Li W, James Rudert M, Tochigi Y, Brown TD: Physical validation of a patient-specific contact finite element model of the ankle. *J Biomech* 2007;40(8):1662-1669.
29. Li W, Anderson DD, Goldsworthy JK, Marsh JL, Brown TD: Patient-specific finite element analysis of chronic contact stress exposure after intraarticular fracture of the tibial plafond. *J Orthop Res* 2008;26(8):1039-1045.
30. Beardsley CL, Heiner AD, Brandser EA, Marsh JL, Brown TD: High density polyetherurethane foam as a fragmentation and radiographic surrogate for cortical bone. *Iowa Orthop J* 2000;20: 24-30.
31. Beardsley CL, Bertsch CR, Marsh JL, Brown TD: Interfragmentary surface area as an index of comminution energy: Proof of concept in a bone fracture surrogate. *J Biomech* 2002;35(3): 331-338.
32. Willis AR, Anderson DD, Thomas TP, Brown TD, Marsh JL: 3D reconstruction of highly fragmented bone fractures. *SPIE Medical Imaging* 2007;6512: 6512(1P1)-6512(1P10).
33. Chrisman OD, Ladenbauer-Bellis IM, Panjabi M, Goeltz S: The relationship of mechanical trauma and the early biochemical reactions of osteoarthritic cartilage. *Clin Orthop Relat Res* 1981;161: 275-284.
34. Wang JH, Thampatty BP: An introductory review of cell mechanobiology. *Biomech Model Mechanobiol* 2006;5(1):1-16.
35. Knobloch TJ, Madhavan S, Nam J, Agarwal S Jr, Agarwal S: Regulation of chondrocytic gene expression by biomechanical signals. *Crit Rev Eukaryot Gene Expr* 2008;18(2):139-150.
36. Hunziker EB: Articular cartilage repair: are the intrinsic biological constraints undermining this process insuperable? *Osteoarthritis Cartilage* 1999;7(1):15-28.
37. Campbell CJ: The healing of cartilage defects. *Clin Orthop Relat Res* 1969;64:45-63.
38. Gerber BE, Robinson D, Nevo Z, et al: Mechanical resistance of biological repair cartilage: Comparative in vivo tests of different surgical repair procedures. *Int J Artif Organs* 2002;25(11):1109-1115.
39. Silver FH, Bradica G, Tria A: Relationship among biomechanical, biochemical, and cellular changes associated with osteoarthritis. *Crit Rev Biomed Eng* 2001;29(4): 373-391.
40. Boschetti F, Peretti GM: Tensile and compressive properties of healthy and osteoarthritic human articular cartilage. *Biorheology* 2008;45(3-4):337-344.
41. Hasler EM, Herzog W, Wu JZ, Müller W, Wyss U: Articular cartilage biomechanics: Theoretical models, material properties, and biosynthetic response. *Crit Rev Biomed Eng* 1999;27(6):415-488.

42. Knecht S, Vanwanseele B, Stüssi E: A review on the mechanical quality of articular cartilage: Implications for the diagnosis of osteoarthritis. *Clin Biomech (Bristol, Avon)* 2006;21(10):999-1012.
43. Responte DJ, Natoli RM, Athanasiou KA: Collagens of articular cartilage: Structure, function, and importance in tissue engineering. *Crit Rev Biomed Eng* 2007;35(5): 363-411.
44. Mow VC, Ratcliffe A, Poole AR: Cartilage and diarthrodial joints as paradigms for hierarchical materials and structures. *Biomaterials* 1992;13(2):67-97.
45. Duda GN, Eilers M, Loh L, Hoffman JE, Kääb M, Schaser K: Chondrocyte death precedes structural damage in blunt impact trauma. *Clin Orthop Relat Res* 2001;393:302-309.
46. Kurz B, Jin M, Patwari P, Cheng DM, Lark MW, Grodzinsky AJ: Biosynthetic response and mechanical properties of articular cartilage after injurious compression. *J Orthop Res* 2001;19(6): 1140-1146.
47. Quinn TM, Allen RG, Schalet BJ, Perumbuli P, Hunziker EB: Matrix and cell injury due to subimpact loading of adult bovine articular cartilage explants: Effects of strain rate and peak stress. *J Orthop Res* 2001;19(2):242-249.
48. Morel V, Quinn TM: Cartilage injury by ramp compression near the gel diffusion rate. *J Orthop Res* 2004;22(1):145-151.
49. Aspden RM, Jeffrey JE, Burgin LV: Impact loading of articular cartilage. *Osteoarthritis Cartilage* 2002;10(7):588-590.
50. Finlay JB, Repo RU: Instrumentation and procedure for the controlled impact of articular cartilage. *IEEE Trans Biomed Eng* 1978;25(1):34-39.
51. Jeffrey JE, Gregory DW, Aspden RM: Matrix damage and chondrocyte viability following a single impact load on articular cartilage. *Arch Biochem Biophys* 1995;322(1):87-96.
52. Huser CA, Davies ME: Validation of an in vitro single-impact load model of the initiation of osteoarthritis-like changes in articular cartilage. *J Orthop Res* 2006;24(4):725-732.
53. Scott CC, Athanasiou KA: Design, validation, and utilization of an articular cartilage impact instrument. *Proc Inst Mech Eng H* 2006;220(8):845-855.
54. Quinn TM, Grodzinsky AJ, Hunziker EB, Sandy JD: Effects of injurious compression on matrix turnover around individual cells in calf articular cartilage explants. *J Orthop Res* 1998;16(4):490-499.
55. Clements KM, Burton-Wurster N, Lust G: The spread of cell death from impact damaged cartilage: Lack of evidence for the role of nitric oxide and caspases. *Osteoarthritis Cartilage* 2004; 12(7):577-585.
56. Borazjani BH, Chen AC, Bae WC, et al: Effect of impact on chondrocyte viability during insertion of human osteochondral grafts. *J Bone Joint Surg Am* 2006; 88(9):1934-1943.
57. Pylawka TK, Wimmer M, Cole BJ, Virdi AS, Williams JM: Impaction affects cell viability in osteochondral tissues during transplantation. *J Knee Surg* 2007; 20(2):105-110.
58. Radin EL, Paul IL: Importance of bone in sparing articular cartilage from impact. *Clin Orthop Relat Res* 1971;78:342-344.
59. Krueger JA, Thisse P, Ewers BJ, Dvoracek-Driksna D, Orth MW, Haut RC: The extent and distribution of cell death and matrix damage in impacted chondral explants varies with the presence of underlying bone. *J Biomech Eng* 2003;125(1):114-119.
60. Torzilli PA, Grigiene R, Borrelli J Jr, Helfet DL: Effect of impact load on articular cartilage: Cell metabolism and viability, and matrix water content. *J Biomech Eng* 1999;121(5):433-441.
61. Ewers BJ, Dvoracek-Driksna D, Orth MW, Haut RC: The extent of matrix damage and chondrocyte death in mechanically traumatized articular cartilage explants depends on rate of loading. *J Orthop Res* 2001;19(5):779-784.
62. Lewis JL, Deloria LB, Oyen-Tiesma M, Thompson RC Jr, Ericson M, Oegema TR Jr: Cell death after cartilage impact occurs around matrix cracks. *J Orthop Res* 2003;21(5):881-887.
63. Milentijevic D, Torzilli PA: Influence of stress rate on water loss, matrix deformation and chondrocyte viability in impacted articular cartilage. *J Biomech* 2005;38(3): 493-502.
64. Rundell SA, Haut RC: Exposure to a standard culture medium alters the response of cartilage explants to injurious unconfined compression. *J Biomech* 2006; 39(10):1933-1938.
65. Wilkins RJ, Browning JA, Urban JP: Chondrocyte regulation by mechanical load. *Biorheology* 2000;37(1-2):67-74.
66. Chan PS, Schlueter AE, Coussens PM, Rosa GJ, Haut RC, Orth MW: Gene expression profile of mechanically impacted bovine articular cartilage explants. *J Orthop Res* 2005;23(5): 1146-1151.
67. Burton-Wurster N, Mateescu RG, Todhunter RJ, et al: Genes in canine articular cartilage that respond to mechanical injury: Gene expression studies with Affymetrix canine GeneChip. *J Hered* 2005; 96(7):821-828.
68. Lee JH, Fitzgerald JB, Dimicco MA, Grodzinsky AJ: Mechanical injury of cartilage explants causes specific time-dependent changes in chondrocyte gene expression. *Arthritis Rheum* 2005;52(8):2386-2395.

69. Natoli RM, Scott CC, Athanasiou KA: Temporal effects of impact on articular cartilage cell death, gene expression, matrix biochemistry, and biomechanics. *Ann Biomed Eng* 2008;36(5): 780-792.
70. Ashwell MS, O'Nan AT, Gonda MG, Mente PL: Gene expression profiling of chondrocytes from a porcine impact injury model. *Osteoarthritis Cartilage* 2008;16(8):936-946.
71. Maskarinec SA, Hannig J, Lee RC, Lee KY: Direct observation of poloxamer 188 insertion into lipid monolayers. *Biophys J* 2002;82(3):1453-1459.
72. Phillips DM, Haut RC: The use of a non-ionic surfactant (P188) to save chondrocytes from necrosis following impact loading of chondral explants. *J Orthop Res* 2004;22(5):1135-1142.
73. Baars DC, Rundell SA, Haut RC: Treatment with the non-ionic surfactant poloxamer P188 reduces DNA fragmentation in cells from bovine chondral explants exposed to injurious unconfined compression. *Biomech Model Mechanobiol* 2006;5(2-3): 133-139.
74. Rundell SA, Baars DC, Phillips DM, Haut RC: The limitation of acute necrosis in retropatellar cartilage after a severe blunt impact to the in vivo rabbit patello-femoral joint. *J Orthop Res* 2005;23(6):1363-1369.
75. Isaac DI, Golenberg N, Haut RC: Acute repair of chondrocytes in the rabbit tibiofemoral joint following blunt impact using P188 surfactant and a preliminary investigation of its long-term efficacy. *J Orthop Res* 2010;28(4): 553-558.
76. Natoli RM, Athanasiou KA: P188 reduces cell death and IGF-I reduces GAG release following single-impact loading of articular cartilage. *J Biomech Eng* 2008; 130(4):041012.
77. Pascual Garrido C, Hakimiyan AA, Rappoport L, Oegema TR, Wimmer MA, Chubinskaya S: Anti-apoptotic treatments prevent cartilage degradation after acute trauma to human ankle cartilage. *Osteoarthritis Cartilage* 2009;17(9):1244-1251.
78. Yagi R, McBurney D, Laverty D, Weiner S, Horton WE Jr: Intrajoint comparisons of gene expression patterns in human osteoarthritis suggest a change in chondrocyte phenotype. *J Orthop Res* 2005;23(5):1128-1138.
79. Natoli RM, Athanasiou KA: Traumatic loading of articular cartilage: Mechanical and biological responses and post-injury treatment. *Biorheology* 2009;46(6): 451-485.
80. Furman BD, Strand J, Hembree WC, Ward BD, Guilak F, Olson SA: Joint degeneration following closed intraarticular fracture in the mouse knee: A model of posttraumatic arthritis. *J Orthop Res* 2007;25(5):578-592.
81. Clark LD, Clark RK, Heber-Katz E: A new murine model for mammalian wound repair and regeneration. *Clin Immunol Immunopathol* 1998;88(1):35-45.
82. Ward BD, Furman BD, Huebner JL, Kraus VB, Guilak F, Olson SA: Absence of posttraumatic arthritis following intraarticular fracture in the MRL/MpJ mouse. *Arthritis Rheum* 2008; 58(3):744-753.
83. Beardsley CL, Anderson DD, Marsh JL, Brown TD: Interfragmentary surface area as an index of comminution severity in cortical bone impact. *J Orthop Res* 2005;23(3):686-690.
84. Hembree W, Furman BD, Guilak F, Olson SA: *Early Effects of Intra-Articular Fracture in the C57/BL6 Mouse.* Durham, NC, Duke University Medical Center, 2010.
85. Seifer DR, Furman BD, Guilak F, Olson SA, Brooks SC III, Kraus VB: Novel synovial fluid recovery method allows for quantification of a marker of arthritis in mice. *Osteoarthritis Cartilage* 2008;16(12):1532-1538.
86. Buma P, Groenenberg M, Rijken PF, van den Berg WB, Joosten L, Peters H: Quantitation of the changes in vascularity during arthritis in the knee joint of a mouse with a digital image analysis system. *Anat Rec* 2001;262(4): 420-428.
87. Krenn V, Morawietz L, Burmester GR, et al: Synovitis score: Discrimination between chronic low-grade and high-grade synovitis. *Histopathology* 2006;49(4): 358-364.
88. Lewis J, Furman BD, Guilak F, Olson SA: *Comparison of Early Effects of Intra-Articular Fracture in the C57/BL6 and MRL/MpJ Strains.* Durham, NC, Duke University Medical Center, 2010.
89. Scaffidi P, Misteli T, Bianchi ME: Release of chromatin protein HMGB1 by necrotic cells triggers inflammation. *Nature* 2002; 418(6894):191-195.
90. Wermeling F, Karlsson MC, McGaha TL: An anatomical view on macrophages in tolerance. *Autoimmun Rev* 2009;9(1):49-52.

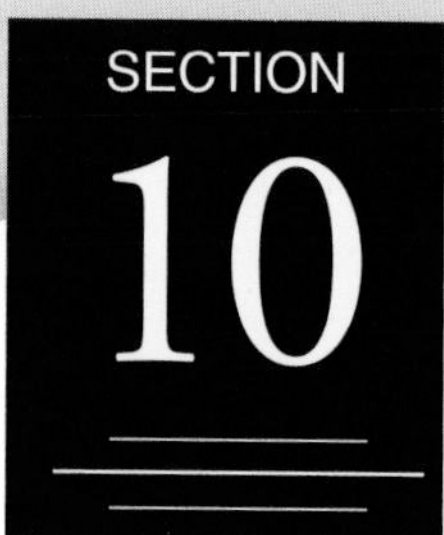

The Practice of Orthopaedics

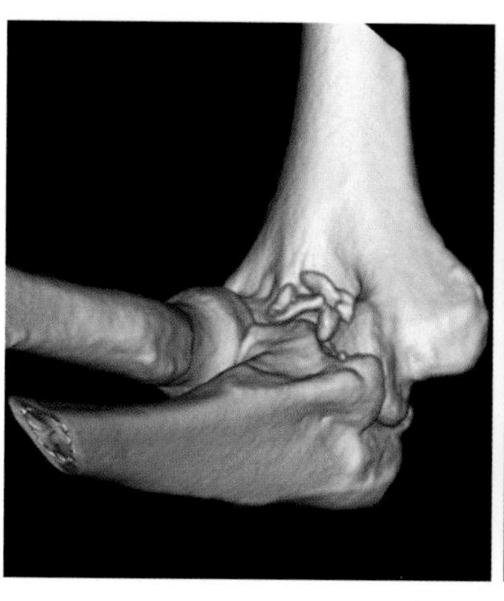

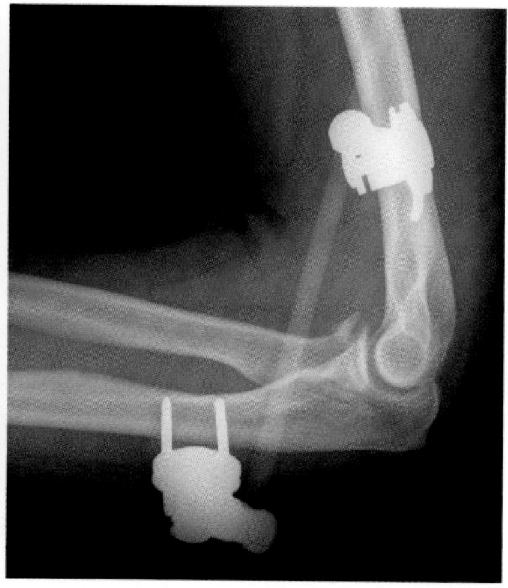

Orthopaedic Expert Opinion, Testimony, and the Physician as a Defendant

Charles Carroll IV, MD
David S. Wellman, MD

Abstract

Medicolegal issues continue to challenge orthopaedic surgeons. Although health reform legislation has passed Congress, the first phase has not incorporated any significant changes regarding liability reform for practicing orthopaedic surgeons. Medical malpractice, personal injury, and workers' compensation litigation remains an issue for patients and physicians.

Although orthopaedic surgeons can be defendants, it is more likely that they will be retained as treating physicians or experts as part of the litigation process. The involvement of a qualified physician as an expert witness is essential to the outcome of any litigation involving medical issues. As triers of the facts, the judge and jury members rely on quality medical testimony.

Expert witness testimony can be a time-consuming process. A physician who assumes the role must be able to spend the time necessary to do a good job. A prepared expert witness can have a profound effect on litigation. A poorly prepared physician expert witness can be harmful to a case and risks the loss of prestige, honor among colleagues, and future work. Sanctions may be imposed by professional organizations. Most importantly, a physician working within the legal system must remain honest and tell nothing but the truth.

Instr Course Lect 2011;60:597-605.

The current medicolegal environment demands that an orthopaedic surgeon thoroughly understand the legal context in which he or she practices. Although medical education in the United States provides physicians with the tools to be effective healers, it does not teach them how to effectively interface with the law. After completing their residency training, many physicians think of the law only in the context of medical malpractice. However, in the current legal system, the physician is much more likely to be asked to provide expert opinion than be called as a defendant. Understanding the various roles of an orthopaedic expert will help a practicing orthopaedic surgeon navigate the legal system and understand his or her role as a defendant in the event of a medical malpractice lawsuit.

An orthopaedic surgeon can expect, on average, to serve as a defendant in two lawsuits over the course of his or her career.[1] In 2005, the total cost of medical malpractice litigation reached $29.4 billion. Orthopaedic surgeons can anticipate that medical malpractice insurance costs will continue to increase; there is currently an 11.5% annual increase.[2] In medical malpractice, personal injury, and workers' compensation cases, orthopaedic surgeons may offer expert opinions regarding permanent damages and causality. Both the plaintiff and the defense may solicit expert opinions; in both instances, the orthopaedic surgeon may function as an expert. The physician serving as an expert witness is an essential aspect of a medical malpractice case because both sides assess damages, determine the standard of care, and participate in the process of finding of fact.

Dr. Carroll IV or an immediate family member serves as a board member, owner, officer, or committee member of the American Society for Surgery of the Hand and the American Academy of Orthopaedic Surgeons. Neither Dr. Wellman nor any immediate family member has received anything of value from or owns stock in a commercial company or institution related directly or indirectly to the subject of this chapter.

Expert testimony is required from physicians in many types of cases. Medical malpractice, personal injury, and workers' compensation cases all typically involve civil (not criminal) issues related to a contract.[3] In each scenario, the job of the orthopaedic expert is to offer opinions based on sound evidence and experience in practice. Both the plaintiff and defense may solicit opinions; these opinions not only constitute a critical component of both sides of the case but also are essential for the functioning of the medicolegal system in the United States.

In addition to serving as a defendant or a treating physician, the surgeon may also be asked to play the role of a controlled expert witness. In this situation, the plaintiff or defense team asks the orthopaedic surgeon to evaluate a patient or review records in a personal injury or workers' compensation case. A controlled expert witness may also act as a reviewer to help third parties determine the allotment of care and payment in particular cases.

For a variety of medically related lawsuits, an orthopaedic surgeon may be asked to serve in the critical role as an expert. This chapter provides a road map for navigating various roles, not only when participating in medical malpractice lawsuits but also in the countless legal depositions that may be provided as a treating physician or an expert in nonmedical malpractice cases, such as personal injury or workers' compensation matters.

The Physician as a Defendant

The role of defendant is one of the most stressful situations an orthopaedic surgeon can face. Lawsuits against orthopaedic surgeons are usually based on negligence, improper informed consent, or physician abandonment.

Negligence

Not practicing according to the standard of care is the most common claim faced by an orthopaedic surgeon. In a claim of negligence, an allegedly injured patient, represented by counsel (the plaintiff), attempts to prove that the physician breached the standard of care, generally defined as the skill, knowledge, expertise, and experience that another physician would possess and display in a similar situation and location.[3] State law dictates the specific definition of standard of care, and each state has subtle differences in interpretation. Successfully argued cases must prove that (1) the physician owed the patient a duty, (2) the physician breached the duty, (3) the breach led directly to the patient's injury, and (4) the injury caused legally recognizable damages.[1]

Improper Informed Consent

To obtain legal informed consent, a discussion must occur between the physician and patient regarding the potential risks and benefits of the proposed procedure, alternative treatments available, and the risks of refusing treatment.[1] The physician must provide a thorough list of all complications that a reasonable person in a similar situation would consider important.[1] An exhaustive list is not necessary. If proper informed consent is obtained, a physician will not generally be held liable in court if the procedure was performed according to the classic description and a recognized complication arises.[1]

To obtain proper informed consent, a patient must be allowed to make a decision voluntarily, be capable of decision making, and be able to understand the information presented.[4] Capacity to consent is a legal standard; ability to consent is determined by the physician. Consulting a second physician for a second opinion is advised when the patient's competence to consent is not clear.[4] The process of obtaining informed consent from a patient who is determined to be incompetent depends on state law and should be referenced before going forward with a procedure. Obtaining informed consent does not absolve the orthopaedic surgeon of possible negligence related to a procedure or medical intervention.

The risk of generating malpractice claims for lack of informed consent has been reviewed recently in the orthopaedic literature. Bhattacharyya et al[5] found that the risk of a malpractice claim significantly increased if the informed consent was obtained on the wards or in the preoperative holding suite. This risk significantly decreased if consent was obtained in the office and documented in the patient's chart.[5]

Physician Abandonment

Abandonment claims arise when a physician terminates care without notifying the patient or providing assistance in finding a new physician. In 1935, Utah courts advised physicians to "give the patient sufficient notice so the patient can procure other medical attention if he desires."[6] Physician abandonment claims in orthopaedic surgery often arise from a failure to provide proper follow-up, improper discharge instructions, or premature discharge from the hospital.[4,7] An orthopaedic surgeon's defense against abandonment claims hinges on proper documentation of follow-up instructions, transfer of care, and termination of services.

How to Avoid Being Named as a Defendant

Understanding the legal system is important for an orthopaedic surgeon's self-protection. Medical malpractice lawsuits are stressful to a practicing physician and his or her family. These lawsuits involve a major time commitment, might be perceived as an insult to professional integrity, and potentially may result in financial loss. Because an orthopaedic surgeon can expect to be named as a defendant in at least two medical malpractice cases during his or her career, it is prudent to be aware of proven strategies of self-protection to avoid litigation, and, in the unfortunate event of a malpractice lawsuit, to ease anxiety.

Personal Interaction

The prevalence of medical malpractice claims is related to the quality of the physician-patient relationship.[1] Certain communication strategies can reduce the risks and avoid patient complaints regarding personal interaction time with his or her orthopaedic surgeon. Medical malpractice attorneys recommend returning telephone calls personally, as well as reviewing test results and specific treatment recommendations directly with patients.[8] Office appointments should not be overbooked, and patients should not be made to sit in the waiting room for prolonged periods of time.

Effective communication is the foundation of the physician-patient relationship and an invaluable risk-management tool. An effective communicator is an active listener who asks open-ended questions in a pleasant and nonjudgmental manner, thereby developing a connection with each patient. Through listening and teaching, the orthopaedic surgeon is best prepared to assess the role of the disease process in the whole patient and treat the patient accordingly. Effective orthopaedic surgeons strive to work as a team with each patient and take a genuine interest in the patient's problems. A patient who believes that his or her physician is interested, competent, and personable is less likely to sue that physician.

Addressing Errors

The time spent formally addressing patients regarding mistakes is minuscule when compared with the time needed to prepare as a defendant in a medical malpractice court case.[1] Early in practice, orthopaedic surgeons should develop a plan to address mistakes and medical errors and discuss these with the affected patient. Prompt, honest disclosure to the patient is a tool that may reduce medical malpractice claims and should be used by all physicians.[1]

Complete Documentation

Complete and timely office documentation is one of the best methods of defense against litigation. All notes should be legible and include pertinent details. All interactions, including phone calls, should be recorded on the patient's chart. Timing is key; notes recorded months after the interaction or procedure occurred suggest that key details of the interaction may have been omitted or forgotten.[1] Corrections and changes to charts should always be made so that the original is still legible. Specifically, corrections should never be made after a lawsuit is filed. Attorneys for plaintiffs search for these occurrences and use them effectively to discredit defense arguments.[1] Reactionary revisions to documentation can be avoided by establishing a thorough system for initially recording information.

Preparing for the Role of Defendant

All orthopaedic surgeons should familiarize themselves with the statutes of their home state because they will likely be involved in a lawsuit during their careers. State laws dictate most aspects of providing medical opinions, and the physician will be expected to adhere to the particular state's regulations. Preparing to be a defendant in a medical malpractice action involves close communication with the participating attorneys and an understanding of state law.

If an orthopaedic surgeon is named as a defendant in a medical malpractice action, he or she should conduct a thorough review of the patient's chart, hospital records, and all other applicable information. A review of the pertinent medical literature is also essential. The newly named defendant-orthopaedic surgeon should attempt to recall any staff members present during the time of the alleged injury because their testimony could be beneficial. Depositions can be long, and trial testimony may be very stressful, so orthopaedic surgeons should expect to allocate significant time for review and preparation. Effective communication with attorneys will further help the defense team anticipate likely questions.

The orthopaedic surgeon-defendant's personal mental health is of critical importance during the stressful event of a lawsuit. The surgeon should depend on loved ones for mental support, keeping in mind that it is necessary to maintain the patient's privacy and also understanding that his or her family is also feeling stress because of the litigation. If the orthopaedic surgeon places the interests of the patient first during the litigation process, he or she can and should move on mentally after the lawsuit concludes, although this is sometimes challenging. The litigation process should be considered part of the price of being a physician and should not be taken as a personal affront.

An orthopaedic surgeon-defendant is also an expert witness for his or her own defense. The knowledge, expertise, and training of the orthopaedic surgeon-defendant will be called on in the trial. As a defendant, the orthopaedic surgeon can offer testimony concerning the medical care and the reasonable nature of that care. Similar to other expert witnesses in the trial, a prudent defense attorney will ask the orthopaedic surgeon-defendant to offer opinions about the care provided and whether it met the standard of care.

The Physician as an Expert Witness

Medical malpractice, personal injury, and workers' compensation court cases are often based on medical information that is beyond the understanding of a layperson; these cases require the expert opinion or testimony of a medical professional.[3] The jury must become knowledgeable about the standard of care in each case because they will ultimately determine liability. Thus, physicians are invited to act as expert witnesses to offer informed opinions to help determine the standard of care in each case. These physician-experts analyze data from the case, the pertinent literature, and provide practice experience to offer an opinion. A physician's professional interpretation is essential in determining the standard of care. Both plaintiffs and defendants are encouraged, expected, and may be required to provide expert witnesses.

States differ in standards for whom can provide expert opinions or testimony. Most states require the individual providing the opinion to be a licensed practitioner experienced with the issues in question.[3] Testimony is typically allowed if the medical facts of the case are within the proposed physician's area of expertise and the jury needs expert help to reach a decision.[3] Many states require the expert witness to practice within or be familiar with the community in which the defendant practices; this is called a locality rule. For example, in 2001 a Louisiana appellate court did not allow testimony from a physician who could not demonstrate having practiced in Louisiana or a similar demographic as the defendant in the case.[9] The trial judge makes the ultimate determination on whether an expert witness is allowed to testify.

A physician's area of expertise is not always clearly defined by his or her training. When a physician offers an opinion on an area of medicine outside his or her specialized training, it is called crossover testimony. The Idaho court system addressed this issue in 1988 by stating, "It is the scope of the witness' knowledge and not the artificial classification by title that should govern the threshold question of admissibility."[10] The final decision to allow an expert to give crossover testimony depends on the trial judge's interpretation of that state's law.

In the courtroom, a physician who provides expert opinion may face personal and professional judgment from the defendant, the jury, and the medical community in which he or she practices. In one survey of judges, 79% of respondents questioned the impartiality of expert witnesses, and 57% considered expert witnesses to be "hired guns."[11] This perception creates a "conspiracy of silence" environment in which qualified physicians actively avoid the role of an expert witness.[3] This is unfortunate because it is essential for physicians to offer appropriate and complete expert opinions as a critical part of the medicolegal process. As is evidenced in the Standards of Professionalism on Orthopaedic Expert Opinion and Testimony adopted by the fellowship of the American Academy of Orthopaedic Surgeons (AAOS), an orthopaedic surgeon does not compromise ethics or violate the community of physicians by providing qualified, informed, expert testimony.[12]

Definition of an Expert Witness

Rule 702 in the Federal Rules of Evidence defines the proper role of the expert witness in federal litigation; similar rules apply in every state. According to Rule 702, "If scientific, technical, or other specialized knowledge will assist the trier of fact to understand the evidence or to determine a fact in issue, a witness qualified as an expert by knowledge, skill, experience, training, or education, may testify thereto in the form of opinion or otherwise, if the testimony is based upon sufficient facts or data, the testimony is the product of reliable principles and methods, and the witness has applied the principles and methods reliably to the facts of the case."[13]

Physicians offering expert opinions have an exception to the requirement to testify to the facts rather than opinions because they are expected to draw inferences and opinions from the facts and present them to jury members who lack professional experience, which limits their analytic ability.

Types of Expert Witnesses

An orthopaedic surgeon can function in several roles when serving as an expert. Regardless of the role, the orthopaedic expert must first establish that a claim has merit. The doctor-patient relationship establishes the duty that the treating physician owes the patient. The duty has to have been breached by an action considered a violation of a standard of care. There has to be a causation of the action as it relates to the issues involved in the claim. The causation can be factual ("but for") or a substantial factor ("proximate cause"). The orthopaedic expert also may need to establish the damages to the plaintiff in the form of economic and noneconomic damages.

A physician can serve as an expert in the legal system as a nondisclosed consulting expert, an expert for the plaintiff, an expert for the defense, an expert for himself or herself (the physician as a defendant), or as a court-appointed expert. Each of these roles plays a critical part in the litigation process. As a nondisclosed consulting expert, the physician may advise an attorney, an insurance company, or a patient on the nature of the claim and the presence or absence of merit in a medical malpractice action. As a treating physician who works as a nondisclosed expert, an orthopaedic surgeon must be aware of his or her fiduciary duties to the patient and must not disclose information that can violate the doctor-patient privileged relationship or the Health Information Portability and Accountability Act (HIPAA) of 1996. The individual or organization seeking the opinion pays the professional fee for this service.

The expert for the plaintiff advises and testifies on the behalf of the plaintiff to establish the merit and causality of the actions in question. This expert must establish the violation of the standard of care and the presence of damage to the plaintiff. The plaintiff's legal team pays the professional fees for this service.

The expert for the defense testifies on the behalf of the physician, hospital, or party that has been named in the suit or claim. This expert attempts to refute merit, causality, violation of the standard of care, or the presence of damages. The defense pays all professional fees. An examination of the plaintiff may be required.

The physician as a defendant also can also act as his or her own expert. Although the physician-defendant is named in the lawsuit, he or she can still be qualified to act as an expert in addition to the outside expert retained or the controlled witnesses. The physician-defendant has treated the patient and is in a unique position to assist the jury in the finding of fact. This role can be critical in the defense of a medical malpractice claim and should not be ignored.

A court-appointed expert may be retained to educate and assist the jury in the finding of fact. This expert has not been retained by either party and must be impartial. An orthopaedic surgeon in this role functions as an educator and does not offer opinions at the request of the plaintiff or the defense. This expert may appear without compensation or may be compensated at a rate determined in discussion with the court.

Who Is Qualified?

Orthopaedic surgeons must be qualified before they can function as experts. It is necessary to use the knowledge obtained in medical school, residency, and fellowship along with the experience of practice and continuing medical education. Teaching at an academic medical center can enhance an orthopaedic surgeon's qualifications as an expert but is not required. Published material on the subject of interest also can be helpful; however, the expert must be sure that his or her opinions match those in the published material. If an opinion is contradictory, the orthopaedic surgeon should have new data available to explain the contradiction with his or her published article.

The medical details of the case should center on issues relevant to the expert's practice in orthopaedic surgery. The orthopaedic surgeon should be prepared to face issues involving subspecialties, such as pediatric, hand, spine, tumor, or foot and ankle surgery. Experts must be ready to answer questions about their qualifications as they apply to orthopaedic surgery or one of the subspecialties. A case involving other medical fields can be considered, but orthopaedic surgeons should be careful to adhere to the precedents of crossover testimony and not offer opinions outside their field of expertise.

Other personal issues also should be considered. The orthopaedic surgeon should have sufficient time in his or her practice to dedicate to the role of an expert. It is necessary to be prepared to deal with the pressures of testimony and speak in a clear and concise manner. Most importantly, the expert must be prepared to tell the truth, the whole truth, and nothing but the truth and adhere to the AAOS Standard of Professionalism on Orthopaedic Expert Opinion and Testimony.

The Role of the Treating Physician

The most likely role that most orthopaedic surgeons will play in litigation is that of a treating physician. In that context, the surgeon is functioning as a healer, not as a defendant. The established doctor-patient relationship must be kept in mind. The testimony will be based on direct observation of the patient, the care provided, and the outcome of the care. Much of the testimony will be a presentation of factual information that should be contained in the patient's medical chart. As part of that process, the treating orthopaedic surgeon has a fiduciary responsibility to the patient and must represent the interests of the patient. Because opinions may be solicited beyond the scope of the factual information, orthopaedic surgeons should be ready to state that they do not have an opinion in such instances.

All opinions should be based on scientific precedent and fact. Opinions should not be based only on speculative beliefs. As the field of evidence-based medicine continues to grow, a treating physician's opinions should have a basis in sound scientific literature.

The rules of discovery and HIPAA must be respected by the treating physician. The attorney for the patient may have unrestricted access to the treating physician under the law, but the other attorneys may not. Orthopaedic surgeons and their staff should be aware of the local rules of discovery deposition to prevent the inappropriate release of information, whether verbally or in writing. The attorneys may be required to subpoena all records. The legal teams are often able to speak with the treating physician at the time of a discovery or subsequent evidence deposition, and the treating physician should be prepared for these meetings.

The treating physician should be aware of external pressures. A patient may place subtle or obvious pressure on the treating orthopaedic surgeon to support the opinions of the patient or the patient's legal team. Any expressed opinion should be carefully considered. The orthopaedic surgeon should refrain from expressing an off-the-cuff opinion or comment that can present a problem at a later date. For example, a patient may ask at an office visit about the nature or quality of care provided by a previous physician. The answer should be carefully considered because a negative comment may become the basis of a subsequent legal action against the previous physician or the comment may be questioned during a deposition. A treating physician should consider having legal counsel at a discovery deposition, evidence deposition, or a trial to represent his or her personal interests.

Rules of Testimony as a Testifying Expert

As the trier of fact, the jury may need assistance in understanding pertinent medical issues. The expert physician functions as an educator and does not function as an attorney, judge, or jury. The expert physician must not act as an advocate and should be aware of any personal bias or conflict of interest relative to the matter at hand that could alter the expressed opinions.

Opinions must have a factual and scientific foundation. Treatment observations or a solicited medical examination can provide substantial information. The medical records and deposition testimony are also key sources of data. A physician's education, training, and experience can be used along with pertinent literature to formulate informed opinions. When a published paper or other material is cited, the expert should thoroughly review the literature and expect questions about less relevant material to test his or her understanding in cross-examination. It is important to be aware of conflicting literature. A source must be carefully chosen because the deposition record from a previous case may be presented if a different opinion was previously offered on the same issue. The testimony should never be based solely on the personal opinion of the physician because that can be speculative in nature; speculating is anathema in court cases.

Two cases have set precedent relating to the admissibility of an opinion in court or in deposition testimony. In *Frye v United States*,[14] it was established that opinions had to be generally accepted within the relevant scientific community to be admitted into evidence. An innovative procedure had to be published in a peer-reviewed journal. These rules apply in many state and local jurisdictions. In *Daubert v Merrell Dow Pharmaceuticals*,[15] the precedent was set that the trial judge must assess validity, reasoning, and methodology when considering the admissibility of a specific opinion. Judges require the separation of junk science from evidence-based medical testimony. This case dates to 1993 and is the standard in US Federal Court. A Daubert challenge to an expert physician's testimony will require the physician to produce the medical literature that is relevant to the opinion and 4 years of records relative to the physician's experience in the role as an expert witness. These principles are applied in the courts of many states and should be considered whenever preparing and presenting testimony.

Preparation for Testimony

The key concept in expert witness testimony is preparation. A thorough review of the patient's chart must be completed. The orthopaedic expert should formulate a timeline of events, procedures, testing, and outcomes of the medical care. All aspects of the patient's care should be reviewed because it may be pertinent to the final disposition of the patient and play a role in assessing damages. An orthopaedic surgeon should also review opinions of other experts involved in the case.

The orthopaedic expert must keep in mind that any notes prepared during the review process are subject to discovery. Discussions and letters written above and beyond a medical report are also subject to discovery. As a defendant, the rules are slightly different; a physician's verbal discussion with his or her personal attorney(s) may be subject to attorney-client privilege. Unless the attorney is representing a testifying expert in the matter of the discovery deposition, it should be assumed that any communications are subject to discovery.

An examination of the patient may be necessary and should be requested as needed by the expert. Any report generated will be discussed at the time of the discovery deposition, evidence deposition, and trial.

Prior to any deposition testimony of the expert, opinions must be formulated and communicated to all parties, with appropriate time to prepare for direct- or cross-examination. Opinions are prepared with the attorneys, and the orthopaedic expert should be comfortable with the wording of those opinions. Importantly, the opinions must be presented before the end of the time set aside for discovery by the trial court. Opinions not presented in the time frame ordered by the court may be declared inadmissible by the judge.

Appropriate time should be allowed to comprehensively review and prepare for testimony. A knowledge deficit can be exploited in a well-prepared cross-examination by an opposing attorney. The orthopaedic expert should be very familiar with the bases of his or her opinions, which will be probed during the discovery deposition. As part of proper preparation, the testifying expert should be aware of deadlines for discovery and trial. Any conflicts must be identified and discussed early in the process to prevent problems and possible applicable sanctions.

Deposition Testimony

There are two forms of deposition testimony: discovery deposition and evidence deposition. The discovery deposition is the initial opportunity for an expert witness to testify in a court-controlled environment. Direct-examination begins and is followed by cross-examination. A redirected examination can follow, clarifying the information in the cross-examination. The scope of the redirected examination deals only with material presented immediately before in the cross-examination; thus, the scope of the questioning remains focused. The physician expert must listen to the questions carefully and ask for clarification as needed. If a question is not understandable, this should be made known to ensure that the answer given reflects appropriate understanding. Compound questions should be broken up as needed. Answers should be given in a clear and succinct fashion, and an answer should be embellished only when necessary. As a retained expert, the physician should consult with the retaining attorney to ascertain which questions to expound on and which to answer succinctly. Questions must be answered in an honest and sincere fashion, and the retained expert should attempt to maintain a pleasant demeanor throughout. The length of the deposition may be 2 hours or more.

This deposition segues into an evidence deposition or trial testimony. If an expert is unable to be present, a verbal recording or videotaped deposition may be requested and played to the jury with editing.

It is essential to be prepared for a discovery deposition because the trial testimony or evidence deposition is determined by the information presented in the discovery deposition. All parties have the right to know an expert's opinions and bases for the opinions before the trial. It would be unusual for an expert not to be deposed in discovery by opposing counsel. Opinions expressed at an evidence deposition or trial must be consistent with the discovery deposition or may be inadmissible. New opinions cannot be presented at an evidence deposition or trial without proper discovery.

Trial Testimony

A trial can be a fascinating and taxing experience. An orthopaedic expert must be thoroughly prepared to discuss his or her opinions in front of all parties, a judge, and potentially a jury. The expert should dress neatly and remain polite to all parties; the courtroom belongs to the presiding judge, and that should never be forgotten. Appropriate time should be taken to prepare and confer with the expert's retaining attorneys. Opinions and scientific evidence must be known and rehearsed. Any opinions expressed should be consistent with those expressed in the discovery phase of the lawsuit. An argumentative, intentionally comical, and unresponsive expert may not be helpful and may be detrimental to a case.

Closure of a Case

An orthopaedic expert should attempt to end the testimony on a positive note. The expert should exit the courtroom quietly and with a pleasant demeanor. The retained expert should converse with the retaining attorney to discuss the testimony and accept praise or criticism as indicated. A bill should be submitted with realistic fees. Reimbursement for work as an expert witness can be subject to examination in a deposition or trial.

Qualities of a Good Defense Expert

A good defense expert will be well prepared and willing to spend the time and energy to work with the defense team. The time requirements can be significant; a good expert should be available to provide appropriate time for review, opinion formulation, deposition, and potentially trial testimony. All these activities can disrupt a busy medical practice; if time is not available, the physician should not serve as an expert witness.

The role of an expert witness requires affability. The experience will be stressful, and maintaining equanimity is essential. There is no purpose served in being rude or flippant while working as an expert. The court is under the purview of a judge who may not appreciate or allow poor behavior.

The ability to navigate the medicolegal system is central to the role of an orthopaedic expert. Speaking with clarity in an uncontrolled setting is an essential attribute. Critical and comprehensive analyses of large amounts of data are necessary. An expert must prepare a set of opinions that deal with relevant and recent medical data and present those opinions in a legal setting, which is quite different from an office or a clinical setting. Conviction and panache are important attributes that convey a sense of authority and influence.

Working in an academic practice can be helpful but is not necessary. Knowledge of both medical practice and the pertinent literature is essential. An expert should be aware of the nuances of health care in different regions. The standard of care can be open to interpretation based on the locale. A large urban area with many subspecialists may have a different set of parameters, which may be a different standard of care than in a rural setting.

A good defense expert will be prepared for the rigors of the case and the testimony. All experts must be ready to speak the truth and be fully prepared concerning the facts and outcomes of the issues presented.

Qualities of a Good Plaintiff's Expert

Testifying for a plaintiff can be rewarding because it may be helpful to an injured patient; however, the scrutiny from the defending physician can make the role difficult. A physician-defendant may possibly harbor negative sentiment toward the testifying physician. Complaints among peers and with professional societies can be lodged for testimony that is not perceived as being honest. The stress involved may be significant. In spite of that, fair and honest testimony is of paramount importance to the plaintiff and the plaintiff's legal team. It is necessary to control a strong bias. As with the defense expert, preparation is essential. A poorly prepared expert will not be helpful to a plaintiff. At deposition, poor preparation can be exposed with a good cross-examination. An effective plaintiff's expert should support the thesis of the allegedly injured party but should not be an advocate; that is the role of the attorney.

Penalties for Poor Testimony

Poorly prepared or executed expert witness testimony hinders all parties in the legal process. A poorly prepared expert must live with his or her conscience if the testimony is not based on appropriate medical facts and also can lose prestige among his or her colleagues. Poor testimony can lead to a sanction from a professional society and, in extreme cases, possible loss of membership. Future opportunities to testify may also be lost because attorneys will not be inclined to retain a poorly prepared expert. Failure to adequately prepare for a case hinders the legal process, and failure to tell the truth is unethical and potentially may damage the physician's career.

Rights and Responsibilities of an Expert Witness

Any expert witness should be treated with respect, as should the judge, jury, and participants in a case. An expert witness should be given the opportunity to understand the questions asked and should be addressed in an appropriate manner and tone. An expert witness is not required to tolerate inappropriate questions or be berated by a party to the lawsuit. A physician expert can complain to a local bar society about inappropriate behavior, which can then sanction or punish the offending attorney.

An expert has the right to be paid a fair wage for his or her time. The amount of compensation cannot be tied to the reward from a case. An expert may be asked to justify his or her fee to a law firm and perhaps to the court if the fee is perceived as being inappropriate for the jurisdiction. Unless the expert agrees to work pro bono, a fair and timely payment can be expected. These issues should be investigated, discussed, and agreed on before testimony is given. Communication can become more difficult after the lawsuit is resolved. The expert should produce a reasonable time log of hours spent preparing for the case for fee payment. Acceptable hourly rates for case preparation often vary among jurisdictions.

A plaintiff's expert must be honest, fair, and tell the truth because testimony is given under oath. Experts are providing opinions to assist and teach; they are not patient advocates.

Summary

A good orthopaedic expert will be honest and prepared. He or she should be available, affable, and able to speak and work under pressure. Mistakes in testimony are often caused by poor preparation and offering opinions that are not appropriate to the circumstances. Questions should be answered knowledgeably and have a scientific basis. Poor testimony can be harmful to the retaining party and may open the expert to legal and professional sanctions. Orthopaedic surgeons should be prepared to interface with the legal system numerous times during their careers, appreciate the different roles they may play in the legal system, and understand the laws dictating their involvement.

References

1. Hoffman PJ, Plump JD, Courtney MA: The defense counsel's perspective. *Clin Orthop Relat Res* 2005;433:15-25.
2. *2006 Update on U.S. Tort Cost Trends*. http://www.towersperrin.com/tp/getwebcachedoc?webc=TILL/USA/2006/200611/Tort_2006_FINAL.pdf. Accessed June 8, 2010.

3. Jerrold L: The role of the expert witness. *Surg Clin North Am* 2007;87(4):889-901, vii-viii.
4. Suk M, Udale AM, Helfet DL: Orthopaedics and the law. *J Am Acad Orthop Surg* 2005;13(6): 397-406.
5. Bhattacharyya T, Yeon H, Harris MB: The medical-legal aspects of informed consent in orthopaedic surgery. *J Bone Joint Surg Am* 2005;87(11):2395-2400.
6. *Ricks v Budge*, 64 P.2d 208, 211-212 (Utah 1937).
7. Gould MT, Langworthy MJ, Santore R, Provencher MT: An analysis of orthopaedic liability in the acute care setting. *Clin Orthop Relat Res* 2003;407:59-66.
8. Nichols JD: Lawyer's advice on physician conduct with malpractice cases. *Clin Orthop Relat Res* 2003;407:14-18.
9. *Roberts v Warren*, 782 So.2d 717 (Louisiana 2001).
10. *Clark v Prenger*, 760 P.2d 1182 (Idaho 1988).
11. Shuman DW, Whitaker E, Champagne A: An empirical examination of the use of expert witnesses in the courts: II. A three-city study. *Jurimetrics* 1994; 34:193-208.
12. American Academy of Orthopaedic Surgeons. *Standards of Professionalism: Orthopaedic Expert Opinion and Testimony.* http://www3.aaos.org/member/expwit/expertwitness.cfm. Accessed August 18, 2010.
13. Federal Rules of Evidence, 702 (2000).
14. *Frye v United States*, 293 F. 1013 (D.C. Cir. 1923).
15. *Daubert v Merrell Dow Pharmaceuticals*, 509 U.S. 579 (1993).

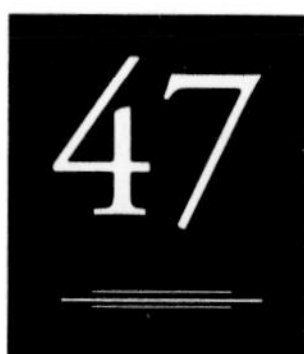

Using PubMed Effectively to Access the Orthopaedic Literature

J.F. Myles Clough, MD, DPhil, FRCSC
Kristin Hitchcock, MSI
David L. Nelson, MD

Abstract

PubMed is the free public Internet interface to the US National Library of Medicine's MEDLINE database of citations to medical scientific articles. Many orthopaedic surgeons use PubMed on a regular basis, but most orthopaedic surgeons have received little or no training in how to use PubMed effectively and express frustration with the experience. Typical problems encountered are data overload with very large numbers of returns to look through, failure to find a specific article, and a concern that a search has missed important papers. It is helpful to understand the system used to enter journal articles into the database and the classification of the common types of searches and to review suggestions for the best ways to use the PubMed interface and find sources for search teaching and assistance.

Instr Course Lect 2011;60:607-618.

The volume of new articles published in the orthopaedic literature is so large that "keeping up" is no longer an option.[1] "Just-in-time" updating of one's knowledge of current evidence and research on a particular subject is more appropriate; however, this requires the new skill of finding the relevant literature. Ten years ago, most literature searches were complicated, slow, and required the help of a medical librarian. Electronic searches have vastly sped up the process; the Internet has enabled everyone to conduct online searches. These changes, however, have introduced new problems, notably search failure through overload, a lack of specificity, and a lack of access.[2] To improve searches and reduce frustration, it is important to distinguish between these three forms of search failure.

MEDLINE is a biomedical and health literature database maintained by the National Library of Medicine (NLM) under the National Institutes of Health. PubMed,[3] introduced in 1996, is the free public online search engine interfacing with MEDLINE.[4] Although the names PubMed and MEDLINE are sometimes used interchangeably, it is important to make this distinction: MEDLINE is the database, and PubMed is the access facility. In addition to PubMed, several companies provide access to the MEDLINE database through proprietary, subscription-based search interfaces (including Ovid MEDLINE [Wolters Kluwer Health–Ovid, New York, NY]).[5] PubMed is an excellent choice because it is free; new records appear as soon as the NLM receives them from journal publishers. Other search systems require periodic data uploads.

Dr. Clough or an immediate family member serves as a board member, owner, officer, or committee member of Kamloops Surgical Center; serves as a paid consultant to or is an employee of eOrthopod Patient Information Collection and Medical Multimedia; and has stock or stock options held in Orthopaedic Web Links. Dr. Nelson or an immediate family member serves as a board member, owner, officer, or committee member of the American Society for Surgery of the Hand; has received royalties from Orthofix, Stryker, Synthes, and Smith & Nephew; is a member of a speakers' bureau or has made paid presentations on behalf of Pfizer, Synthes, and Orthofix; serves as a paid consultant to or is an employee of Orthofix; serves as an unpaid consultant to Orthofix; has stock or stock options held in Orthofix; and has received nonincome support (such as equipment or services), commercially derived honoraria, or other nonresearch-related funding (such as paid travel) from Springer, Biomet, DePuy, EBI, Hand Innovations, KMI, Orthofix, Stryker, Synthes, Trimed, Wright Medical Technology, and Zimmer. Neither Ms. Hitchcock nor any immediate family member has received anything of value from or owns stock in a commercial company or institution related directly or indirectly to the subject of this chapter.

Table 1
Types of Searches

Type/Category	Goal	Technique
1. Specific	A particular resource	Use known information (subject, author(s), journal, dates) in the search
2. Subject—Level 1: Just-in-time	Review of current clinical thinking	Rapid search (see technique below)
3. Subject—Level 2: Educational	Reading list for rounds or a presentation	MeSH-based search
4. Subject—Level 3: Research/meta-analysis	Comprehensive list of all publications on the subject	Elaborate search strategy in multiple databases with assistance from medical librarians

MeSH - medical subject heading

Most orthopaedic surgeons are aware of PubMed and use it on a regular basis to identify relevant literature; however, most surgeons receive little or no training in how to use PubMed effectively, and there have been few reviews of PubMed searching in the orthopaedic literature.[1,6-9] The PubMed site presents the user with a simple search box, like any other search engine, but its powerful capabilities can be confusing. Technical advice on framing search strings and the use of Boolean operators, search field tags, and medical subject heading (MeSH) terms has been offered[6,7,9] but only in the context of a comprehensive search of the literature. Inclusive strategies, such as using multiple databases, elaborate searching techniques, and obtaining the assistance of a librarian, have been emphasized. However, users have a range of information needs.[10] Most literature searches by orthopaedic surgeons do not have these comprehensive goals and require simpler techniques to obtain satisfying results.

It was recognized quite early that literature searches were either specific (in which a partially remembered resource is sought) or subject oriented (seeking literature to fill an information gap).[10] This chapter's authors propose a further categorization of the common types of searches into four types because each type requires a different search strategy (**Table 1**).

Information professionals can assist with all types of searches, from simple to complex; however, some orthopaedic surgeons may not have access to a librarian, prefer to be self-reliant, or require immediate results. Searches can be performed by any clinician who is prepared to learn a few basic PubMed features. Type 4 searches are covered by some of the articles already cited;[1,6,7] this chapter will focus on type 1, 2, and 3 searches—the simple searches that orthopaedic surgeons most regularly undertake. The goal is to provide background on the process and structure of PubMed and supply techniques and tips to help orthopaedic surgeons become more efficient (and less frustrated) PubMed users.

What PubMed Is and Is Not

Definitions

MEDLINE is the database containing information about journal articles that have been collected by the NLM. PubMed is the search engine for free public access to MEDLINE. Among many powerful search aids, it automatically translates the search terms supplied into MeSH terms. MeSH is the NLM-controlled vocabulary used for indexing articles for MEDLINE/PubMed.[11] MeSH terminology provides a consistent way to retrieve information that may use different words for the same concepts. With electronic searching, this standard set of terms is helpful because of the many synonyms, eponyms, and acronyms used in medicine.

MEDLINE, which contains more than 16 million article citations, is one of the largest biomedical literature databases. More than 5,200 journals are indexed, including more than 150 orthopaedic journals. Each record in the MEDLINE database stores core citation information: author name(s), title of the article, journal title, date, volume/issue, and pages. Abstracts are included (if available) along with the unique identifier, the PubMed identifier (PMID) of the article, and MeSH terms assigned to each article by the indexers. Although MEDLINE is a huge database, it is important to know that it does not contain citations from every biomedical journal published. The overlap with the European Excerpta Medica Database (EMBASE)[12] is approximately 50%. An NLM advisory board considers new journals for indexing.[13] Occasionally, a title is removed from the list of journals indexed by MEDLINE, usually because of a drastic change in the scope or the quality of the publication.

Not a Garden-Variety Search Engine

The PubMed interface continues to evolve with new features. The NLM released the current interface in fall 2009. The simple search screen that greets the user is reminiscent of other search engines, such as Google or Bing, and numerous new features provide more context-rich information for both novice and expert searchers. Although PubMed undergoes periodic revisions, the MEDLINE database it searches changes minimally other than yearly data maintenance. In many ways, PubMed provides an increasingly sophisticated point of access to what is essentially a legacy system. The computerized version of MEDLINE dates from 1971,[14] but print indexes to the medical literature existed before this time. PubMed searchers can now find citations dating back to 1948. Knowing that this system has evolved over time from an original print index helps to explain some of the quirks of PubMed searching.

Table 2
Steps in the Process of Adding New Journal Articles to MEDLINE

Steps to Adding Citations to MEDLINE	Status in PubMed
1. Publisher electronically submits article citations/abstracts to NLM.	[PubMed—as supplied by publisher]
2. Publisher either sends a print or electronic copy of the journal to NLM. Staff verifies the citation and begins indexing process.	[PubMed—in process]
3. NLM indexer reads article and assigns MeSH terms. Some MeSH terms are designated major topics. Some MeSH terms are assigned subheadings, which show relationships between concepts (such as "radius/surgery" or "infection/drug therapy).	[PubMed—indexed for MEDLINE]

NLM = National Library of Medicine, MeSH = medical subject heading.

Not an Online Library

Infrequent or new PubMed searchers may be disappointed in their attempts to locate free full-text articles identified in their search. PubMed is a search system, not a library; it provides direct access only to citations and abstracts, not to full-text articles. Viewing the article may require a subscription or pay-per-view fee; the NLM and PubMed are not involved in the transaction. Approximately 10% of recent journal articles are posted free of charge on the Internet either on the journal sites[15] or on PubMedCentral (PMC),[16] which is the NLM repository of open access articles.

Not Totally Automated

PubMed does not rely on robots to identify new content. Indexers provide a human touch to maintaining the underlying MEDLINE database. Approximately 2,000 to 4,000 citations are added to MEDLINE each business day.[14] Citations from many journals are added to PubMed as soon as, if not before, the journal issue is available in print. **Table 2** shows the stages in the process of adding new citations to PubMed. Search results in PubMed will show the status of a citation as it is added to the database and indexed for MEDLINE; "in process" or "provided by publisher" records appear at the top of the results list and may not have all the associated information and links described in this chapter.

The role of the NLM indexer (step 3 of **Table 2**) is extremely important. Indexers are not orthopaedic surgeons, but they have a science background and are carefully trained by the NLM in the principles of indexing. They also have many tools available to assist in the indexing process. Indexers decide which MeSH terms are covered in the article. For the PubMed analytic and translation system to work effectively, this assignment must be accurate and consistent. Details about MeSH terms are provided later in this chapter.

Each year, the NLM staff reviews and makes changes to the MeSH vocabulary to accommodate the evolving biomedical literature. NLM indexers note new terminology and concepts when the existing MeSH vocabulary is lacking; sometimes subject experts are consulted. Members of the public can also make suggestions online.[17]

By default, the list of citations displayed following a PubMed search is headed by the most recently added papers. It may be noted that the first few citations displayed have the status "PubMed—as supplied by publisher" or "PubMed—in process." These articles are in the earlier stages of indexing, so subject headings have not yet been assigned. In some cases they do not have a "Related articles" link.

Effective Use

This discussion of the ways to use PubMed will be more useful and easier to understand if the site is accessed (http://pubmed.gov) and the suggested actions are undertaken. Few ordinary features of the site involving display, sorting, selection, and storage will be discussed in this chapter. The focus will be on the issues most critical to successful searching, framing the search question, using the appropriate technique, and regrouping when necessary.

Framing the Search Question

In any inquiry, the answer is only as good as the question asked. The key skill is to define what is being looked for, visualizing the target resources. This requires orthopaedic knowledge and an understanding of the information gap that needs to be filled. The process cannot be delegated to anyone else, although a discussion with a colleague or a medical librarian may help

Table 3
The Patient-Intervention-Comparison-Outcome (PICO) System for Defining a Search Question

PICO	Heading	Examples
P	Patient specific	Diagnostic category, age category, general category (for example, multiple-trauma patient)
I	Intervention	Treatment modality, test, surgical procedure, drug regime
C	Comparison	Alternative intervention or patient category to compare with
O	Outcome	Treatment success or complication

to clarify the information that is sought.

Evidence-based medical literature offers the patient-intervention-comparison-outcome (PICO) format[18] as a valuable way of defining or refining the search question.[9,19] The value of this system (**Table 3**) is that it encourages the searcher to specify the question in at least four areas. Using this format will make the creation of a good search string almost automatic.

Creating a Good Search String

The search string presented to the PubMed search engine is usually a terse version of the search question. Words such as "and," "or," and "the" are called "stopwords" and should be eliminated from the search string because they are ignored by the search engine. A highly specific search string can be valuable at the start, making adjustments as needed. It is important to balance specificity against sensitivity. The more terms used in the search string, the greater the specificity. As the results pool gets smaller, it is easier to browse; however, the risk of not finding important articles becomes higher as well (reduced sensitivity). Searching is an iterative process. The desirable features of the search string are one or more terms for each of the PICO components, specific jargon terms, and terms that must be in the target article.

As an example of the transformation from a search question to a search string, consider a search related to outcomes after a hip fracture. Suppose the question to be answered is whether patients return to mobility quicker or more reliably after intertrochanteric fractures treated with a dynamic hip screw (DHS) sliding nail or an intramedullary fixation device. This question has covered the PICO categories but not in order. *P*atient: hip fracture; *I*ntervention: DHS; *C*omparison group: intramedullary device; *O*utcome: ambulatory status. By clarifying each element of the search question, the search string becomes: *hip fracture DHS intramedullary ambulation*. In accordance with the guidelines previously outlined, this string is quite long, does not have any stopwords, and includes two specific jargon terms (DHS and intramedullary).

Just-in-Time Searching: A Rapid PubMed Search

Commonly, the orthopaedic surgeon needs a quick review of current thinking to help with a case at hand. For this just-in-time searching, the process is quite straightforward: enter the search string, find a suitable up-to-date article on the subject to use as a "seed" article for a better list, and then use the "Related articles" link from the seed article to produce a more definitive list. If the indexers have been accurate, this list will start with articles on very similar subjects.

Step 1: Enter the Search String

After the search question and the initial search string have been formulated, the searcher should go to the PubMed site. The uniform resource locator (URL) should be bookmarked if that has not already been done. The search string is entered (for example, *hip fracture DHS intramedullary ambulation*) and "search" is clicked. **Figure 1** shows the page that would be returned with this search string.

This results page has several features. The search string is shown in the search box at the top of the page. The default list of citations is in summary format; each citation shows the title, author(s), reference, PMID number, PubMed status, and "Related articles" link. The title in each citation is a link to a page specific to that resource displaying the abstract (if there is one) and several other features (**Figure 2**). At the top right of the screen (**Figure 1**), there is a control to "Filter your results." This allows the searcher to change the nature of the articles listed, limiting the list either to review articles or to those available as free full-text articles. The number in brackets beside the filter shows how many articles will be shown. Once selected, a filter will remain in effect for all future searches; if the searcher wishes to see all articles in the database that match his or her search string, the filter setting should be restored to show "All."

A series of "discovery" panels appears on the right side of the PubMed results screen. The panels that appear will depend on what is displayed in the main screen. Features here include "Find related data," "Search details," and "Recent activity." The first option allows the search to be repeated in other NLM databases, such as "Books." "Recent activity" shows re-

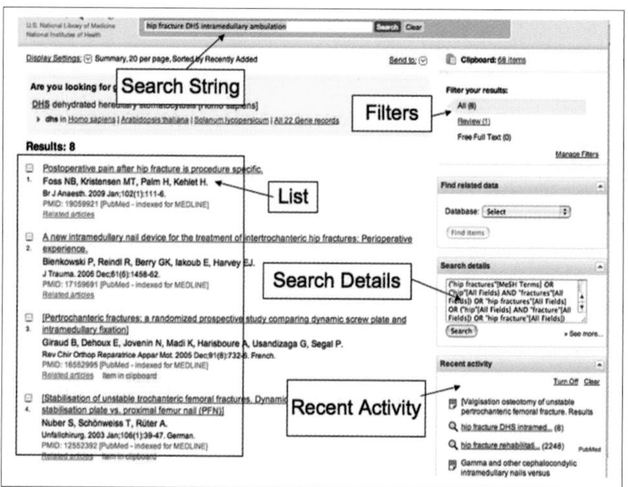

Figure 1 The results of a PubMed search. (National Center for Biotechnology Information, US National Library of Medicine, Bethesda, MD. http://www.ncbi.nlm.nih.gov/pubmed/.)

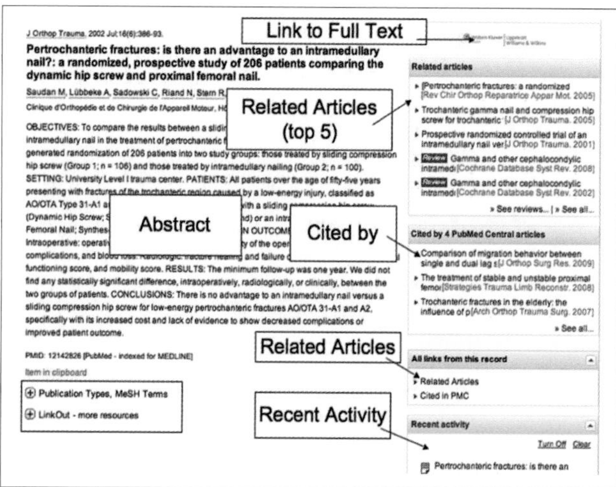

Figure 2 PubMed display of an abstract. (National Center for Biotechnology Information, US National Library of Medicine, Bethesda, MD. http://www.ncbi.nlm.nih.gov/pubmed/.)

cent searches and allows the searcher to return to those results without reentry. "Search details" shows the search translation and is discussed later in this chapter.

Step 2: Select a Suitable "Seed" Article

The list provided by the original search should be scanned to find a "seed" article. An ideal seed article would be one that is on the subject and recent. If a seed article cannot be found, then the search string must be modified and the search repeated (iteration).

Having found a suitable article, the searcher will click on the title link to see a display of the abstract (**Figure 2**) with additional useful information. To the left of the display, the reference (journal/title/author[s]) and text of the abstract are presented. Below the abstract, click on "Publication Types, MeSH Terms" to see the metadata assigned to the article by the NLM indexers—subject heading terms and the publication type (such as review, controlled clinical trial, comparative study). At the top right of the display, there is usually a link to the journal publisher's Website to view or purchase the article. The "LinkOut" control at the foot of the abstract gives other options for accessing full-text articles.

The top five related articles are displayed in a panel to the right of the abstract. The calculation of "related" is complex,[20] taking into account the subject headings (MeSH terms) assigned by the indexers and the words in the title and text of the abstract. In the absence of indexing, the article can be related to other articles based on the title and text words alone. If most of the articles in the top five "Related articles" box are on the proper subject, then the seed article is appropriate. If one or more of the related articles seems to be closer to an ideal paper on the subject, it may be better to select that article as the seed.

Below the panel of "Related articles" is one showing how many articles in PMC that have cited this article (**Figure 2**). Below this information, at the lower right of the screen, a box may be present with "All links from this record." This box is designed to provide contextual links to related material in any NLM online database. It may include a complete list of related articles in PubMed, a list of the articles in PMC that cite the current article, links to free full-text articles in PMC, and even links to free books and genetic information from the NLM. **Table 4** summarizes the use of some of the features of the abstract display.

Step 3: Generate a "Related Articles" List

Having selected a suitable seed article, a new list should be generated using the related articles function. This is done from the main search results list by using the "Related articles" link below a reference; it can also be done from the abstract display of the seed article using either the "See all" link in the "Related articles" panel or the "Related Articles" link in the "All links from this record" panel.

The related articles list will have approximately 100 articles. The first few should be on very similar subjects to the seed article. If they are not, or if the list is otherwise unsatisfactory, choose

Table 4
Using Some Features of the Abstract Display

Feature	Description	Use	Note
Abstract	Copy of the text of the abstract as it appears in the full article	Read this to make sure the article is on-subject	
Publication types: MeSH terms	Control to display this further information	Use to review the indexing of the article	Will not be present if the indexing is incomplete
Link to full text	Link to publisher's site and/or to PubMed Central if the article is archived there	Follow the link to see full text. Subscription or pay-per-view may be required for the publisher's site	Not always present
Top five related articles	Titles (and links to abstract display) of the five most closely related articles	Review to make sure the seed article is generating useful related articles; option to select a new seed article	Will be present whether or not the article is indexed but should be "better" when the indexing is complete.
Related articles links	Generate new list of articles in order of "relatedness" to the seed article	Use this to improve the specificity of the list of articles	"See all" in the "Related articles" box is one link; "Related Articles" in the "All links from this record" box is another

another seed article and repeat the process. Repetition (iteration) is a normal part of searching. If the aim of the search is to have a short reading list about the subject, the new list should be adequate, although not necessarily comprehensive.

Table 5
The Results of Using an Author's Name in a PubMed Search

Iteration	Search String	Number Found	Comment
1	Neer	881	Includes papers referring to Neer classification or hemiarthroplasty
2	Neer Classification	131	Target article is 130th on this list
3	Neer[AU]	377	Includes many other authors with last name Neer or van Neer
4	Neer CS[AU]	60[a]	Neer CS[author], "Neer CS"[au] and neer cs[au] all produce the same result
5	Neer CS 2nd[AU]	54	The 6 missing papers were also authored by him
6	Neer CS[AU] classification	6[b]	

[a]A reprint of the target article was at top of this list (January 2010).
[b]The original version of the target article [24] was fourth on this list.

Searching for a Specific Paper

Having a vague recollection of a paper and needing to locate the exact reference is a common experience. If only the subject is remembered, a rapid search may be the most useful approach, provided that the searcher can recognize the article in a list of possibilities. More often, there are other clues to help locate the paper: the author's name, the journal, or the approximate date of publication.

Rapid Search for an Author's Name

Table 5 shows using the author's name in a search for the original article describing the Neer classification of proximal humeral fractures.[21] Note that more than 50% of the papers found in the first iteration referred to Neer hemiarthroplasty or to the Neer classification and were not authored by him. The author [AU] tag specifies that the adjacent word should be searched for only in the author field of the database. The author's initials add to the specificity (iterations 3 and 4 in **Table 5**). One or two initials should be placed after the last name of the author. Do not add a period or space between the initials. Either uppercase or lowercase letters may be used. Suffixes such as "2nd" or "Jr" are allowed but are not always used by the journals and so may be unhelpful (search iteration 5 in **Table 5**).

The advance search function of PubMed also can be used to search for a specific author; however, searching for an author using the [AU] tag in the main PubMed search box allows quick editing of the search string to include additional search terms as needed. Often an author's name alone is not enough to identify a paper. In the example described, the addition of a term defining the subject (classification; iteration 6) was helpful, but the search term "Neer Classification" (iteration 2) was not helpful in finding the target article. In a search for papers that refer to the Neer classification but are not necessarily authored by him, the tag [TIAB] should be used for the title and abstract. This specifies that the term must appear in either the title or the abstract of the article.

Using Advanced Search

The advanced search function can be used to specify a journal and/or date as well as an author. (Prior to the fall 2009 PubMed update, these features were found using the "Limits" feature). Click on the "Advanced search" link above and to the right of the main PubMed search box. The first section of this page is the "History" feature that shows recent searches and allows a combination of previous searches without reentering them. Below that is a function to limit the search by author, journal, publication date, and other factors. When typing is started in one of these boxes, the system will provide suggestions for the query (**Figure 3**).

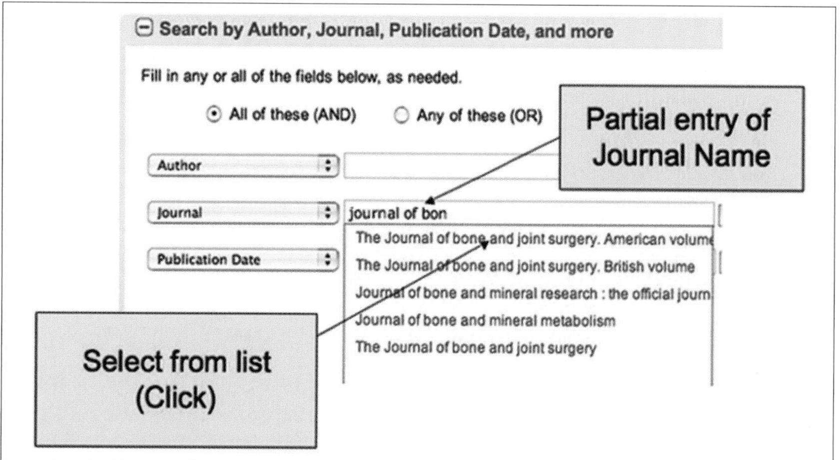

Figure 3 The "Advanced search" function for selecting the author, journal, or publication date. (PubMed, US National Library of Medicine, Bethesda, MD. http:// www.ncbi.nlm.nih.gov/pubmed/.)

As an example, an article is sought that was believed to have been published in the *Journal of Bone and Joint Surgery* in the late 1990s about weight bearing after intramedullary nailing of a fractured femur. A search for *intramedullary weight-bearing* yielded 553 search results, which was too many to browse to identify one article. Using the "Advanced search" function, a date range (1995-2000) and the journal title (*Journal of Bone and Joint Surgery American volume*) can be added to the search. After these additional limits were added, the target article[22] was located. By looking in "Search details," the complicated search string that PubMed actually created based on the entries can be seen: ("The Journal of bone and joint surgery. American volume"[Journal] AND ("1995"[PDAT]: "2000" [PDAT])) AND (intramedullary [All Fields] AND ("weight-bearing" [MeSH Terms] OR "weight-bearing" [All Fields] OR ("weight" [All Fields] AND "bearing" [All Fields]) OR "weight bearing"[All Fields])).

This search string could be assembled in the main PubMed search box if the searcher knew the syntax demanded by the PubMed search engine and was very accurate with quotes and opening and closing brackets. However, using the "Advanced search" function to compile such searches is much easier.

There are several other features of the advanced search function that should be explored as one learns more about PubMed. It is also possible to limit the search by language, sex, age groups, and other subsets or select only those citations that contain abstracts or links to full-text articles.

Educational Searches: Building a Reading List

Article-specific and just-in-time searches may be the most frequent types, but type 3 searches to create a more comprehensive reading list are also common, especially in an educational setting. A reasonably comprehensive collection of the relevant literature is obtainable using PubMed, but it usually requires using Boolean operators to combine terms and the conscious use of MeSH terms. In the context of type 3 searches, "failure to use the MeSH indexing ... is an important reason for failure."[6] Using MeSH terms will result in a list of citations that is more comprehensive, more concise, and more specific.

What Are MeSH Terms? How Are MeSH Terms Used?

NLM indexers describe the subjects of each article using a standard vocabulary. A MeSH term has the syntax "Standard Term"[MeSH terms], where the quotes and square brackets are required. If a MeSH term is used in a PubMed search, it is necessary to insert the term in the search string using the exact syntax. The use of MeSH terms helps define the content and assesses the similarity of articles for the PubMed searcher. Searching using MeSH terms will return all the articles that were indexed as being about that subject, regardless of the various synonyms that may actually have been used by authors. Retrieval depends not on the words in the title and text but on whether the indexers were consistent and accurate with their choice of MeSH terms to describe the content. There are three main methods to find MeSH terms.

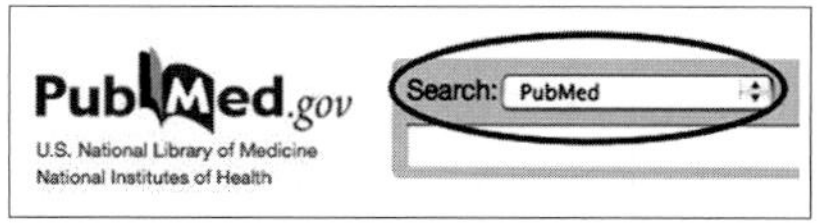

Figure 4 The location of the control to change the database being searched. (PubMed, US National Library of Medicine, Bethesda, MD. http://www.ncbi.nlm.nih.gov/pubmed/.)

Option 1: Find MeSH Terms Using the MeSH Database

At the top of any PubMed page, the searcher can change the database from PubMed to MeSH using the drop-down menu (**Figure 4**). After a search term is entered, the database will provide possible matches from the MeSH vocabulary. **Figure 5** is a display of the MeSH term "weight-bearing." The display includes a definition, subcategories, and entry terms. The entry terms are words or phrases that are automatically translated (mapped) into the MeSH term "weight-bearing" if they occur in a search. At the bottom of the display appear trees showing the relationship of this MeSH term with broader or narrower terms in the vocabulary.

To create a search string using a MeSH term or to add a MeSH term to an existing search string, use the drop-down "Send to" menu. To start with or to expand a search, select the option to send to "Search box with OR." If a new term will be used to narrow a search, use the option to send to "Search Box with AND." The contents of the search box can also be edited directly. After all the relevant terms have been combined in the search box, click on the "Search PubMed" button.

Option 2: Select MeSH Terms From a PubMed Abstract

MeSH terms may also be found on the abstract display of an article. Click on the "MeSH terms" control below the abstract to see the terms assigned by the indexers. Any terms believed suitable can be copied and then pasted to the search box.

Option 3: Locate MeSH Terms in the Search Details

Locating the MeSH terms in the search details may at first seem so complicated that it would seem unlikely that it would ever be used by an orthopaedic surgeon running an ordinary search. Regardless of the searcher's preferences, PubMed automatically translates many ordinary searches into search strings with multiple MeSH terms. By looking at the "Search details" function of the search (**Figure 1**), the searcher may find that a MeSH

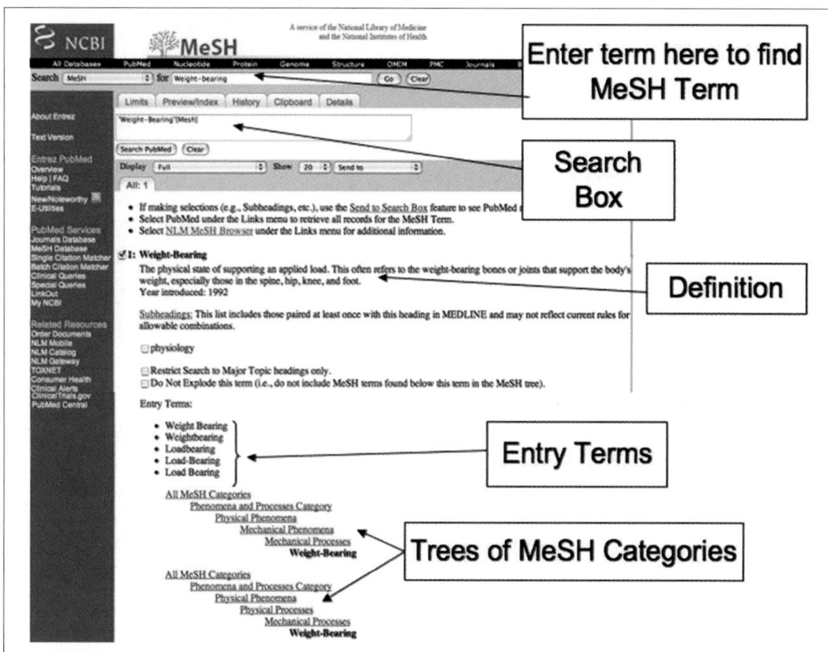

Figure 5 The MeSH database entry for weight-bearing. (http://www.ncbi.nlm.nih.gov/mesh.)

Operator		Translation
OR	A B — A OR B	Either/or; as well as
AND	A B — A AND B	Overlap with
NOT	A B — A NOT B	Excluding

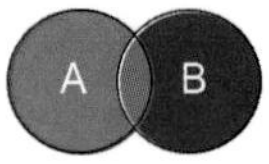

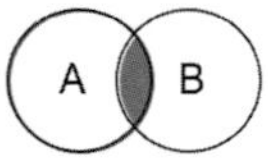

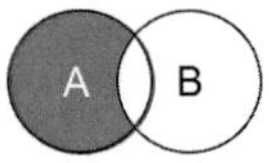

Figure 6 Logical (Boolean) operators.

term or an entry term mapped to a MeSH term was used.

The search system can usually accomplish what the user needs, but sometimes it is necessary to override the automatic process. It is important to understand the underlying process to be able to control it.

Boolean Operators, Quotes, and Brackets

Many of the examples discussed in this chapter use quotation marks, brackets, and logical operators such as "AND." To use PubMed effectively, it is necessary to understand how the search system interprets syntax.

Boolean Operators

Boolean (logical) operators are used to connect different words in a search string. The commonly used operators are OR, AND, and NOT (**Figure 6**). Operators must be in capital letters. Lowercase "and," "or," and "not" are ignored as stopwords. Although this subject may seem to be too complex for everyday use, it should not be dismissed outright. If more than one word is in the search string, the system inserts Boolean operators automatically. PubMed will automatically insert an AND into each gap (unless the searcher has already used quotes or another Boolean operator). To PubMed, "pelvis fracture" is equivalent to "pelvis AND fracture." It is better to use the operator consciously rather than get unexpected results. If the searcher intends to broaden the search, the operator "OR" must be entered. The word "NOT" should be used to exclude certain subjects (for example, "femur fracture NOT hip"). These two operators cannot be assumed and must be entered in capital letters. PubMed often uses a complex series of operators when translating the search. The operators used can be seen by looking at the "Search details."

Searching for a Phrase With Quotes

Quotation marks are used to designate a phrase or assign a string of words to a label. Most commonly, quotes are used when the searcher wishes to search for words placed together in a specific order, such as "Neer classification," and avoid off-subject articles in which the words Neer and classification are present but not together (for example, *Neer hemiarthroplasty—a classification of complications*). If it is necessary to assign a label, such as [MeSH terms] or [TIAB], to a phrase, it may also be necessary to use quotes so that PubMed recognizes the intended phrase in its entirety.

The way PubMed searches for these phrases is not as sophisticated as in some other databases. PubMed is not able to perform true phrase or proximity searching. It will not search through all records to find the word "Neer" next or near to the word "classification." Instead, NLM maintains a phrase index, a master list of some commonly encountered concepts that appear as multiword phrases. If like the phrase "Neer classification," the phrase placed in quotes appears on that master list, PubMed will return records that contain that phrase. If the phrase does not appear in the phrase index, the searcher will get an error message: "quoted phrase not found." This does not necessarily mean that the phrase does not appear in any PubMed records, only that it is not included in the phrase index; therefore, PubMed cannot locate it. In that case, PubMed reverts to applying its usual search algorithm, the results of which can be seen using the "Search details" feature.

Why Are Round Brackets Used?

Round brackets help to establish complex logic and relationships between search terms. Square brackets [like this] are used to designate field qualifiers such as [TI] or [AU]. Round brackets should be used liberally in searches. Care should be taken to close all round brackets—match each opening bracket with a closing bracket so that the search will have the intended results.

If unexpected search results are produced, it may be because PubMed is processing the search in an unintended way. This may occur if two words for the same concept are used in the search string with different spellings. For example, if the search string *scaphoid nonunion OR non-union* is entered, the searcher will get 2,062 citations. This may be more articles than would be expected on this topic; furthermore, many articles are off-subject. This unexpected result is because the PubMed search system does not recognize the implied relationships. It groups the first two words together (*scaphoid nonunion*) and the last one (*non-union*) on its own. The search retrieves articles on nonunion of the scaphoid, as well as (OR) non-union of any bone. Using round brackets forces PubMed to consider the correct terms together: *scaphoid AND (nonunion OR non-union).* This bracketed search results in 500 articles with better specificity.

Field Qualifiers

PubMed can be directed to look for a search string in a specific part of the citation, as was discussed in the search for a known paper. Common fields that nonlibrarians may use are listed in **Table 6**. The complete list of field qualifiers (or descriptions) is available in the PubMed "Help" section.[23] It is not necessary to use uppercase letters for these qualifiers but they must be enclosed in square brackets.

Failed Searches: It Is in the Details

The failure of a search is more common than success, even for expert searchers.

Table 6
Search Field Tags

Field Tag	Description	How the Search Functions
[ALL]	All fields	The search looks for the term in author, title, abstract, and journal fields
[AU]	Author	The search is restricted to the author fields
[TA]	Journal title	The search returns will all be from that journal if the specific NLM approved abbreviation for the journal (for example, J Bone Joint Surg Am) is supplied and qualified with [ta]
[MAJR]	MeSH term as a major topic	All the articles returned will have the topic as a major subject if the correct MeSH term is supplied and qualified with [MAJR].
[MH]	MeSH	If the correct MeSH term is supplied and qualified with [MH] or [MesH], all articles returned will have that topic as one of the subjects of the article (but not necessarily the major topic)
[TW]	Text words	Term found in the text
[TI]	Title	The search looks only in the title
[TIAB]	Title or abstract	The search looks in the title and abstract but not elsewhere

NLM = National Library of Medicine, MeSH = medical subject heading

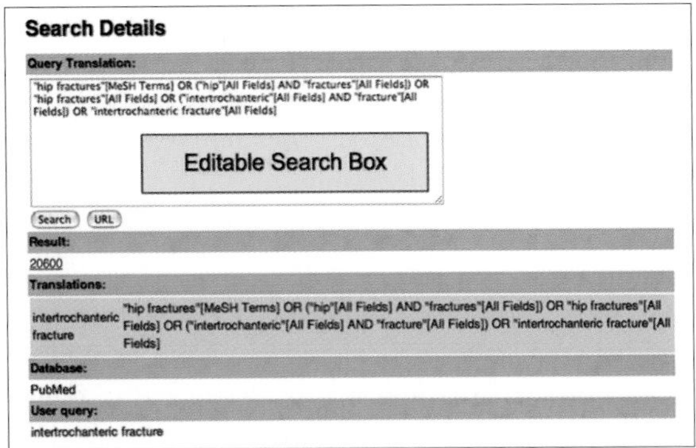

Figure 7 Search details for a PubMed search for intertrochanteric fracture. (US National Library of Medicine, Bethesda, MD. http://www.ncbi.nlm.nih.gov/mesh.)

Table 7
Internet Sources for Search Assistance

Workshop on using PubMed effectively to access the orthopaedic literature:
http://www.orthopaedia.com/display/Main/Informatics

NLM PubMed tutorial:
http://www.nlm.nih.gov/bsd/disted/pubmedtutorial/

PubMed help files:
http://www.ncbi.nlm.nih.gov/bookshelf/br.fcgi?book=helppubmed

National Network of Library of Medicine: membership directory:
http://nnlm.gov/members

AAOS ORACLE: assistance locating research information:
http://www.aaos.org/research/library/oracle.asp

The search results list frequently seems too long and irrelevant. The search string needs to be revised, but it may not be clear which part of the search string is causing trouble. A useful response is to use the "Search details" function to examine PubMed's automatic translation of the search string entered. PubMed often interprets the search in an unexpected way. To find the search details, the searcher should look at the "Search details" panel on the right side of the search results list (**Figure 1**). If the full display of details is needed, the searcher should click on the "See more" link in the "Search details" panel. The search details can also be found from the "Advanced search" page link at the top of the PubMed screen.

Normally, the query translation process is helpful, expanding the search to include MeSH terms that will make the search more comprehensive. **Figure 7** shows how the system can cause frustration. The search string in this example is *intertrochanteric fracture*. This term is automatically translated into "hip fractures," which seems reasonable. However, the MeSH term "hip fractures" encompasses all types of hip fractures, not just intertrochanteric fractures. There is no specific MeSH term for intertrochanteric fracture. Many articles on subjects such as osteoporosis and preventing falls have generic hip fracture as an outcome. The indexers see this outcome and assign "hip fractures" as a MeSH term. As a result, the translated *intertrochanteric fracture* search has more than 20,000 results. Many of the retrieved articles are about femoral neck fractures, periprosthetic hip fractures, or osteoporosis but not about the intertrochanteric fractures of original interest.

The search box in the "Search details" function can be edited. Currently it reads: "hip fractures"[MeSH Terms]

OR ("hip"[All Fields] AND "fractures"[All Fields]) OR "hip fractures"[All Fields] OR ("intertrochanteric"[All Fields] AND "fracture"[All Fields]) OR "intertrochanteric fracture"[All Fields]. It should be edited to eliminate all other references to hip fractures: ("intertrochanteric"[All Fields] AND "fracture"[All Fields]) OR "intertrochanteric fracture"[All Fields].

The edited search string can then be sent to the search system. It will still retrieve more than 900 articles, but at least all the articles will include the words *intertrochanteric* and *fracture* somewhere in the title, the abstract, or another part of the database record.

If the search string is edited in the "Search details" translation box, PubMed will not do any further translations. This is one way to force the system to perform the exact search that is desired. As more familiarity is gained with the search system, it is a good idea to frequently refer to the "Search details" box.

Search Assistance

Orthopaedic surgeons are not alone as they attempt to identify relevant literature. Building search skills is a process, and there are online tutorials that can help (**Table 7**). An online workshop demonstrating some of the procedures described in this chapter is posted in the Informatics section of Orthopaedia, the open source orthopaedic site.[24] Universities and many hospitals have information professionals who can help orthopaedic surgeons with their searches. Some medical libraries within the National Network of Library of Medicine provide services even for health professionals who are not affiliated with the library's own institution. The American Academy of Orthopaedic Surgeons (AAOS) Research and Scientific Affairs Department also provides ORACLE,[25] a free service to support the orthopaedic information needs of AAOS members. This service includes literature search assistance from the medical librarian at the AAOS and assistance in locating AAOS clinical practice guidelines and other data on orthopaedic practice in the United States. Because of copyright restrictions, the AAOS is unable to send copies of book chapters or articles to members, but it can refer members to a local medical library or document delivery service.

Summary

Using PubMed to search the orthopaedic literature is popular but can be frustrating without some training. Understanding the way PubMed conducts searches and reviewing practical suggestions for searching effectively will aid the orthopaedic surgeon in performing successful searches in a variety of common circumstances.

References

1. Gillespie LD, Gillespie WJ: Finding current evidence: Search strategies and common databases. *Clin Orthop Relat Res* 2003;413: 133-145.
2. Clough JF, Veillette CJ: Orthopaedic Web Links (OWL) and the Orthogate Classification of Subject Headings (OCOSH). *Clin Orthop Relat Res* 2010, in press.
3. PubMed Website. http://www.ncbi. nlm.nih.gov/pubmed/. Accessed January 4, 2010.
4. Canese K: PubMed celebrates its 10th anniversary! *NLM Tech Bull* 2006;352:e5. http://www.nlm.nih.gov/pubs/techbull/so06/so06_pm_10.html. Accessed January 4, 2010.
5. De Groote SL: PubMed, Internet Grateful Med, and Ovid: A comparison of three MEDLINE Internet interfaces. *Med Ref Serv Q* 2000;19(4):1-13.
6. Smith CG, Herzka AS, Wenz JF Sr: Searching the medical literature. *Clin Orthop Relat Res* 2004;421:43-49.
7. Zlowodzki M, Zelle BA, Keel M, Cole PA, Kregor PJ: Evidence-based resources and search strategies for orthopaedic surgeons. *Injury* 2006;37(4):307-311.
8. Biermann JS, Golladay GJ, Clough JF, Schelkun SR, Alexander AH: Orthopaedic information: How to find it fast on the Internet. *Instr Course Lect* 2007; 56:483-489.
9. Poolman RW, Kerkhoffs GM, Struijs PA, Bhandari M; International Evidence-Based Orthopedic Surgery Working Group: Don't be misled by the orthopedic literature: Tips for critical appraisal. *Acta Orthop* 2007;78(2):162-171.
10. Smith RS: Searching the medical literature. *Postgrad Med J* 1953; 29(332):313-315.
11. National Library of Medicine, National Institutes of Health: MeSH. http://www.nlm.nih.gov/mesh/meshhome.html. Accessed January 4, 2010.
12. Elsevier: Excerpta Medica Database (EMBASE). http://www.embase.com. Accessed January 4, 2010.
13. National Library of Medicine, National Institutes of Health: FAQ: Journal Selection for MEDLINE Indexing at NLM. http://www.nlm.nih.gov/pubs/factsheets/j_sel_faq.html. Accessed January 4, 2010.
14. National Library of Medicine, National Institutes of Health: Fact Sheet: MEDLINE. http://www.nlm.nih.gov/pubs/factsheets/medline.html. Accessed January 4, 2010.
15. Electronic journals: Orthopaedic web links. http://www.orthopaedicweblinks.com/Publications/Electronic_Journals/index.html. Accessed January 4, 2010.

16. PubMed Central Website. http://www.ncbi.nlm.nih.gov/pmc/. Accessed January 4, 2010.
17. National Library of Medicine, National Institutes of Health: Suggestions for medical subject heading changes. http://www.nlm.nih.gov/mesh/meshsugg.html. Accessed January 4, 2010.
18. Richardson WS, Wilson MC, Nishikawa J, Hayward RS: The well-built clinical question: A key to evidence-based decisions. *ACP J Club* 1995;123(3):A12-A13.
19. Schardt C, Adams MB, Owens T, Keitz S, Fontelo P: Utilization of the PICO framework to improve searching PubMed for clinical questions. *BMC Med Inform Decis Mak* 2007;7:16.
20. Computation of related articles. http://www.ncbi.nlm.nih.gov/bookshelf/br.fcgi?book=helppubmed&part=pubmedhelp#pubmedhelp.computation_of_relat. Accessed January 4, 2010.
21. Neer CS II: Displaced proximal humeral fractures: I. Classification and evaluation. *J Bone Joint Surg Am* 1970;52(6):1077-1089.
22. Brumback RJ, Toal TR Jr , Murphy-Zane MS, Novak VP, Belkoff SM: Immediate weight-bearing after treatment of a comminuted fracture of the femoral shaft with a statically locked intramedullary nail. *J Bone Joint Surg Am* 1999;81(11):1538-1544.
23. National Center of Biotechnology Information, National Library of Medicine: Search field descriptions: *PubMed Help*. Updated October 15, 2010. http://www.ncbi.nlm.nih.gov/books/bv.fcgi?rid=helppubmed.section.pubmedhelp.Search_Field_Descrip. Accessed November 23, 2010.
24. Informatics. *Orthopaedia, Collaborative Orthopaedic Knowledgebase.* http://www.orthopaedia.com/display/main/informatics. Accessed January 4, 2010.
25. American Academy of Orthopaedic Surgeons: Orthopaedic Research Assistance Center for Learning and Education (ORACLE). http://www.aaos.org/research/library/oracle.asp. Accessed January 4, 2010.

Resiliency and Medicine: How to Create a Positive Energy Balance

John D. Kelly, MD

Abstract

A career in orthopaedics is a race—a marathon. Many outside forces converge to increase stressors to high levels. Resiliency, or the ability to bounce back from difficulty, can be learned and nurtured. The management of energy, rather than time, holds the key to avoiding burnout. Orthopaedic surgeons must minimize "energy drain" by first recognizing their ability to become proactive and control their lives. Surgeons must learn how to say "no" and delegate work and responsibilities. A positive energy balance can be attained when relationships, not things, are given priority. A focus on passions and inspiration helps to maintain energy, while a connection to a "source" and living a morally just, service-oriented life will yield endless energy.

Instr Course Lect 2011;60:619-625.

A career in orthopaedic surgery is a race—a marathon. Burnout or erosion of the soul[1] is very common in medicine, with up to 38% of surgeons acknowledging this condition.[2] Symptoms include loss of emotional reserves, cynicism, perceived clinical ineffectiveness, and a sense of depersonalization in relationships with associates and/or patients.[3] A Canadian study reported that more than 50% of physicians admitted that their career choice interfered with their family and personal lives.[4] Physicians in leadership or academic roles and females may be especially vulnerable.[2,5,6] Resiliency, or the ability to "bounce back" from difficulty, can be achieved even in the most trying of times. Resiliency is not related as closely to the number of hours worked or hardships encountered as it is to the ability to manage one's energy. The flow of energy is very dependent on chosen values. Some values lead to a life of fear, insecurity, and continual energy depletion, whereas other values lead to a fulfilling life, peace, and energy renewal (**Figure 1**). We are free to choose the values that influence our decisions. The decisions we make on a daily basis will ultimately drain us or sustain us (**Figure 2**).

The real path to resiliency lies in minimizing energy drains and maximizing the things that replenishes us. To manage energy, the mind must be managed because distorted, negative thinking will sap our "life force." Resiliency can be learned because the brain is a rather "plastic" organ. Maladaptive thinking and behaviors can be replaced with healthy sustaining thoughts and actions so that the brain will be "hard wired" to more readily perform positive, energizing behaviors and avoid negative thinking and self-destructive actions. Regardless of your background, genetics, or station in life, you have the power to choose the life you want. Each of us has the power to choose "high octane values" and manage our minds.

Resilient people value seven characteristics: (1) Proactivity, which is the recognition that they are the creator of their life stories and have the power to choose their values. The choice of values will predict one's happiness and "energy index." (2) A connection to their "source" and a life based on morally sound and loving actions. Stress-resistant individuals live an honest, integrated life based on service and working for a common good. They love others and themselves and manage their ego by being "other centered." The extent that ego is devaluated will determine an individual's peacefulness and energy balance. (3) Mind management and living in the moment. Resilient individuals are not enslaved by an overactive mind but have a mind at their disposal. They do not allow their minds to be cluttered with racing thoughts, worry, or guilt. (4) The pursuit of excellence but not perfection. High-energy performers do not let the scourge of perfectionism sap their energy. (5) Relationships

Neither Dr. Kelly nor any immediate family member has received anything of value from or owns stock in a commercial or institution related directly or indirectly to the subject of this chapter.

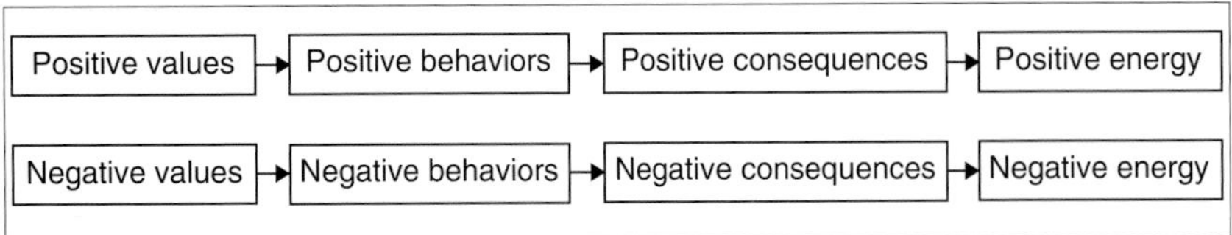

Figure 1 The effect of values on energy.

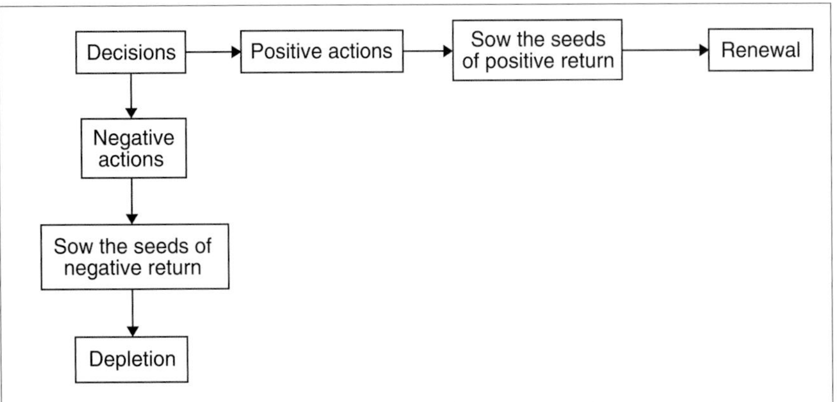

Figure 2 The power of decision.

(especially with one's spouse) are valued because resilient individuals recognize that the quality of their relationships will determine the quality of their lives. (6) Passion and inspiration, which are positive motivational guides, rather than fear and guilt. (7) Outside interests and hobbies. The resilient orthopaedic surgeon will seek continual renewal though the arts, hobbies, and fine literature.

The Value of Proactivity: We Can Create Our Life Story

In Steven Covey's masterpiece, *The Seven Habits of Highly Effective People*,[7] proactivity is described as the ability to base behaviors on decisions rather than conditions. The proactive person can subordinate feelings to a value. For example, proactive orthopaedic surgeons who value the responsible delivery of health care will decide to provide proper treatment for their patients despite the oppressive conditions created by insurers or other third parties. A feeling such as frustration will be subordinated to the value of responsible health care delivery. By being proactive, we gain control. The feeling that control has been lost is one of the strongest predictors of physician burnout.[1,8] Controlling our actions yields predictable consequences. In essence, when we decide to live our lives in accordance with "higher values," we predictably receive more energy and are at peace with ourselves and others because, as Covey states, "principles govern." In other words, principles of human existence predict that if life is lived in the right way, principles or natural law will predict positive consequences.

A principle is a timeless and self-evident natural law. For example, a commonly accepted principle is that consuming excess calories will lead to weight gain. This principle is changeless and timeless. Similarly, the principle of intimacy dictates that relationships must be constantly nurtured and repaired to flourish. Time must be shared between people to achieve intimacy. Every sustaining faith is based on enduring moral principles.

Two important principles pertaining to energy balance are as follows: adhering to morally sound, loving values yields high energy, and adopting self-centered values ultimately depletes energy. Choosing altruistic or egocentric/selfish motives will predict an individual's long-term energy balance.

Living our lives the right way can maintain long-term happiness and joy. Living in accordance with "high octane values" keeps our "tank full" and makes us more resistant to burnout.

The High-Octane Values

Honesty and integrity are essential to energy balance. Both virtues are very energy efficient. Honesty is "saying what I do," and integrity is "doing what I say." With honesty and integrity there are no coverups, no need to remember what I said, no protection of a pseudoself or someone you pretend to be. One must be true to oneself and not pose as someone else. Honest, integrated orthopaedic surgeons practice humility and stay within their honest abilities. If a surgeon is not a traumatologist, he or she will not try to treat a complex acetabular fracture. Poor choices made to protect a huge ego will deplete inner strength because energy must be expended to preserve an egocentric pseudoself.

When integrity is valued, promises to ourselves and others are kept. We demonstrate to others (and ourselves) that our word is our bond. Covey emphasizes that keeping promises is the very essence of proactivity. Keeping a promise is an affirmation that our lives are a product of our decisions rather than conditions. We are in control if we keep our word. We are deciding our life's direction, despite the current conditions. For example, if we make the proactive choice to value marriage, we will decide to spend time with our spouse—we keep our promise to have dinner Saturday night. We are true to our word, our spouse, and ourselves. Our decision is more important than our conditions or our mood (such as fatigue, other things to do, pressing agendas). As we become more proactive, we will experience more control over our lives. Being more in charge give us more hope, optimism, and energy. Embracing a posture of integrity and morally correct principles provides a sense of peace and self-respect that is otherwise unattainable. We will be respected (not necessarily liked) by others and will feel good about ourselves.

There are several reasons why operating from a principled core value system generates good feelings. Humans are hardwired for altruism, becoming more peaceful when we extend ourselves to others. We literally "get out of ourselves" when we become "other centered." As our problems receive less attention, we become more relaxed and more at ease. We reap what we sow. When we extend kind gestures to others, we will receive goodness in return. As one of my patients taught me, "If you want a smile, you give a smile." We recognize that something bigger than us may be at work. Some call it God, a higher power, or the universe. I use the term source, which describes the ultimate energy repository. When we align ourselves with our source, or the loving power of the universe, good will result, and we "plug into" our direct energy supply (**Figure 3**).

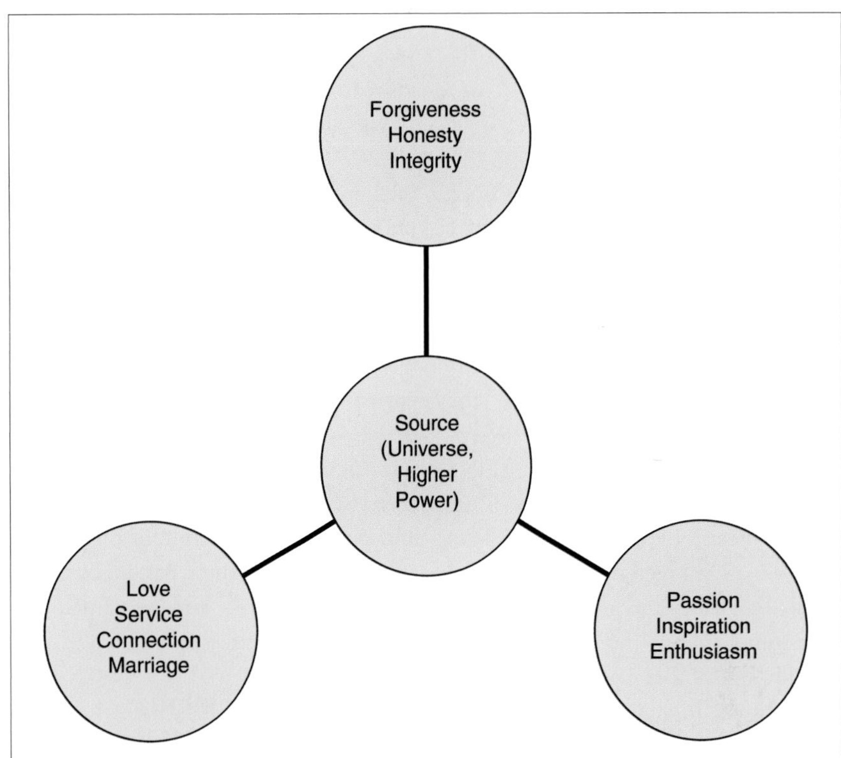

Figure 3 Aligning with an energy source.

If acting from a moral or principle-based system sustains us, why do we act otherwise? Ego, the constellation of our selfish motives, takes control. Ego is created by our minds to ease pain, but it separates rather than joins us to our source and others. Our ego is our fearful, insatiable self that wants more power, fame, and glory. It is possessed with agendas and focuses on "what's in it for me." It is never satisfied; the more it asserts itself, the more unhappy or unfulfilled it becomes. Individuals with large egos tend to have many accomplishments; however, the quality of their work is usually deficient because they operate from a posture of fear rather than abundance. They are removed from their source and the intrinsic energy supplies of inspiration and passion. The more things that ego drives one to accomplish, the more unfulfilled and unhappy one becomes. Childhood wounds and emotional pain feed the ego in the form of compulsive traits, such as doubt, guilty feelings, and an exaggerated sense of responsibility,[9] which are common characteristics in physicians. This compulsive triad of traits is the mechanism created by the ego to ease deep feelings of inadequacy.

Those who seek the greater good and a connection to others experience peace and a positive energy flow. They accomplish great things because they are creating from a source of abundance; the quality of their work reflects creativity and genuineness. Their energy is renewable because they are buoyed by the good feelings that a life of contribution generates. Those who drift away to their egocentric self will ultimately experience depletion.

We defend our ego by criticizing, complaining, comparing, and judging others and by justifying our actions and seeking perfection. We stay close to our source when we practice love, self-nurturance, forgiveness, and acceptance and offer compliments and gratitude. Forgiveness is absolutely essential to resiliency. When we do not extend forgiveness and hold onto hurt, we are merely defending our egocentric need to be right. Huge energy reserves can result when we realize it is more important to be at peace with our neighbor, our colleague, or our spouse rather than to be right. The daily practice of forgiveness allows us to start each day anew, fresh, and without "baggage."

The Value of Love

The value of love must apply to one's self first and foremost. To survive daily demands, the value of self-nurturance must be cultivated, and it must be remembered that principles govern well-being. To determine your self-nurturance value quotient, the following questions should be asked. (1) Do I get adequate sleep? (2) Do I have time to exercise? (3) Do I eat healthy meals? (4) Do I engage in a hobby? (5) Do I feed my soul with fine music, literature, and art? (6) Do I feel close to my friends and loved ones, especially my spouse? (7) Do I regularly connect to a "higher power"?

If the answer to any of these questions is no, basic needs are being neglected, and the soul in not being adequately fueled. More than a century ago, Sir William Osler wrote of the perils of ignoring self-nurturance, "Engrossed late and soon in professional cares . . . you may so lay waste that you may find, too late, with hearts given way, that there is no place in your habit-stricken souls for those gentler influences which make life worth living."[10]

Principles apply to sleep. A lack of sleep will hurt you.[11] Millions of years of evolution have determined that human beings need sleep. We cannot train ourselves to sleep less. Lack of sleep, over time, will lead to an increased risk of hypertension, diabetes, dementia, and harm to the immune system. Similarly, exercise and its effects are also based on principles. Exercise predictably leads to a positive mood, weight loss, disease reduction, and increased productivity. A 30-minute lunchtime workout can immeasurably boost afternoon productivity. Healthy meals are essential; we really are what we eat. Processed, sugar-laden foods do not lead to sustained energy but result in mood swings, fatigue, and periods of sleepiness. When the soul is fed with hobbies, music, and literature, we are adhering to the principles that you cannot give what you do not have, and a well-rested and happy physician will be more productive.[12] Self-nurturance by an orthopaedic surgeon promotes patient safety and reduces the incidence of medical errors.[13,14] When our "tank is full," we can extend the love and care that our families, friends, and patients need. Content physicians are perceived by their patients as rendering better care[15] and are named less often in malpractice suits.[16]

Managing Our Minds: The Value of Mindfulness

Depression and anxiety will sap energy and motivation. A return to mindfulness, or living in the moment, will restore us to healthy thinking and help us manage anxiety and depression.[17-19] Anxiety is merely worry about the future. Depression is largely based on guilt from the past. When we can return to the present moment, worry and guilt dissipate, and we can be energized by the wonders of the present world. When we can learn to live in the moment, we will not be at the mercy of our minds; rather, our minds will be at our disposal.

Thoughts of anxiety and depression are distortions; they are thinking that is controlled by the ego or the pseudo-self. The discipline of cognitive behavioral therapy[20] is predicated on the truth that dysfunctional thinking is not real. Negative thoughts about self-worth should be examined from a distance; then one should return to the present where ego can be suppressed and where we can act on our values and inspirations. Psychologists teach us that when we try to resist dysfunctional thinking, it grows and becomes more powerful. Negative thinking should be accepted but should not be believed or acted on.

If depression is deep, help may be needed. Self-nurturance is a sign of strength. Problems need to be addressed. Orthopaedic surgeons may feel that admitting depression is a sign of weakness. Admitting a problem and seeking help is a sign of real strength and character. More information on the importance of mindfulness can be found in chapter 49.

Value Excellence Rather Than Perfection

The field of medicine attracts perfectionists who are accustomed to harshly criticizing themselves and creating unrealistic expectations. Trying to attain perfection will result in a feeling of being continually disappointed and drained. Perfectionism usually has its roots in painful childhood experiences, such as being deprived of love from a parent or a caregiver. There is also evidence that some inherited genetic predisposition for obsessive traits may play a role in the need to strive for perfection. Perfectionists are unhappy individuals who live with a negative energy balance. They are always "missing the mark" and feel frustrated. Their dissatisfaction drives them to do more and more to prove their worth, only to feel more and more dissatisfied. Perfectionists tend to procrastinate, waiting for the perfect time to complete a task. This leaves them continually on edge as deadlines mount and psychic energy is consumed. Perfectionists are essentially defending the needs of their ego. The ego's need to be perfect will never be satiated. Perfection is an illusion. No person or thing is absolutely perfect. The antidote to this dysfunctional thinking is to recognize that perfection is an illusion and leads only to frustration and wounded self-esteem. To overcome perfectionism and return to a positive energy balance, it is necessary to accept and label the "voice of perfectionism" and practice detachment from it. The gentle movements of the spirit are in sharp contrast to the impulses of a perfectionist. For example, when the impulse to trim the meniscus to absolute perfection arises, take a deep breath, examine the impulse from a distance, return to the present moment, and be guided by inspiration rather than compulsion. The pursuit of excellence is noble; complacency is not advocated. When we strive for excellence, we are attempting to become our best selves and develop our talents to the best of our abilities. When we attain excellence in a given discipline, we experience feelings of accomplishment and the satisfaction that we are using our gifts to the highest degree. We must aim high for goals that stretch us, but we should also recognize the voice of ego, which tells us that we are not good enough and must achieve more to be considered worthy. We must return to the present and allow the gentle voices of fulfillment and satisfaction to inspire us to continue to strive for excellence rather than the unattainable perfection.

Relationships

The degree to which relationships are valued is proportional to life satisfaction. Career accomplishments pale in comparison with the life fulfillment achieved from positive relationships with families and friends. There are countless tales of aged workaholics lamenting the loss of intimacy with loved ones during their productive years. The proactive choice to value relationships is a decision to live a life of connection, support, and endless energy replenishment. Relationships are the true "tail winds" in life and must be kept in constant repair.

Marriage

Marriage is the most important relationship we establish and produces the most potential for energy replenishment. Marriage vows are the greatest promise we make; the quality of one's life will be in direct proportion to the quality of one's marriage.[21] Marital discord is the primary cause of adult depression in the United States and contributes to an estimated divorce rate of at least 50%.[22] Your marriage partner offers the greatest affirmation; investment in marriage yields great happiness.[23] Many physicians who devalue their marriages subsequently undermine their own happiness. In an effort to meet the needs of their egos by striving for extraordinary achievement and recognition, many physicians damage their families by their absence. In an effort to "build the practice," the spouse becomes an obstacle rather than a source of support, love, and protection from burnout.[2,24] When spouses are not growing closer, they are growing apart. In an effort to recapture happiness, many divorcees seek another partner, only to find the same issues and ego needs. Hendrix, in his enlightening book, *Getting the Love You Want*,[25] conveys the concept that when we make the proactive choice to love our spouses unconditionally, we are healing ourselves and our subconscious selves of old hurts. Hendrix's statement, "the trauma of childhood becomes the drama of adulthood" awakens us to the truth that we all have unfinished business as adults. In making the decision to honor our vows and "stay the course" with our spouses, we are working to recover from old wounds. Absolute commitment, for better or worse, holds great potential for growth. When we are not fully committed to marriage, we begin to see our spouses differently. It is important to focus on the positive aspects of marriage because commitment is vital to all relationships.

Spouses can teach us about ourselves if we are willing to manage our egos and accept the opportunity for real feedback and healing. Because the needs of our egos are projected on those closest to us, the characteristics that we dislike in our spouses hold clues to our own discomforting characteristics. Negative feelings elicited from a spouse are often linked to old childhood hurts. The security of commitment is needed to allow us to truly embrace the needs of our ego and begin the real work of healing.

Deciding to value one's marriage above everything else will provide a partner who will give lifelong support and sustenance. Higher quality work will arise from a place of abundance, not of fear or excessive ambition. It is important to work on marriage and persevere. Two thirds of unhappily married couples, when questioned 5 years later, report that they are happy.[26]

Mirror Neurons

Humans are hardwired to respond predictably to love and affirmation. Positive actions reap positive responses. When we form relationships, we must realize that what we give will be what we receive. When we choose to look for the good in others, we receive positive energy, and our mood is boosted. Consequently, when we affirm goodness in others, they will be inclined to respond in kind. Mirror neurons, located in the cerebral cortices, emit positive signals if positive energy is received, whereas the reception of negative impulses causes the cells to emit negative impulses.[27] For example, those who must associate with an individual who chronically complains are likely to begin complaining as well.

When relationships are valued, it behooves us to make the proactive choice to be an inspiration rather than a critic. As Wayne and Mary Sotile have elegantly stated in their writings on physician stress, resiliency is not about the absence of hassles; it is about the presence of "uplifts."[28] Wayne Sotile has coined the phrase, "emotions are contagious." We can decide what seeds to sow at work and at home. When we choose to offer a compliment, we flex our proactive muscles and gain more mastery of our lives.

Patients, Families, and Friends

Happiness is important for physicians because happiness increases productivity, allows better patient care, inspires patient compliance, and encourages the perception of competency. Likewise, investment in one's family generates peacefulness and resistance to stress. When we choose to value our families, they will value us in return. In Albom' s *Tuesdays with Morrie*,[29] Morrie Schwartz says his family is "what I call your spiritual security, knowing that your family will be there watching out for you. Nothing else will give you that. Not money. Not fame."

We enter this world and leave it with our families. No amount of material success will ever surpass the joy of a rich family life. It is important to prioritize our family life and carve out time daily to affirm and sow intimacy with our loved ones. Many orthopaedic surgeons work long hours to provide material goods for their families when the families most want only attention and time. The feeling that you matter in the lives of each of your children will buoy you through difficult events and in dealing with the most disgruntled patients.

Friendships outside the family are also crucial to attaining the emotional connections needed to remain resilient. Friends outside medicine are particularly helpful in seeing the world differently and experiencing life in ways unknown to medical families.

Passion and Inspiration

Interests and passions provide a renewable source of energy. When we gravitate to our interests and couple this with the value of service, we will be doubly energized. Giving back and trying to change the world for the better will lead to quantum energy. Causes or crusades to better the world are truly motivational, but the basic needs of living, loving, and learning should not be ignored. The author of *The Radical Leap*[30] lists the following energy generators in addition to love: great ideas, noble principles, leaping goals (goals that leap over your self-imposed limits), interesting work, and exciting challenges.

Inspiration, derived from the words breathed upon, indicates energy from a higher place. Following ideas that inspire us allows us to connect to our source and be sustained. If orthopaedic surgeons are inspired to change their practice venues or organizations, serious attention should be given to the matter. Enthusiasm, derived from the Greek word en theos meaning "having a God within," also is a means of connecting to a higher power. To better serve your patients and yourself, it is wise to determine your sources of enthusiasm and follow your passions.

Hobbies or Interests Outside Medicine as Energy Generators

Our souls need to be fed with activities that are done just for fun. The need to continually produce will ultimately lead to a loss of all energy. Resiliency blooms from indulging in regular hobbies that rest the nervous system and allow us to experience pleasure. Regularly engaging in a pleasant hobby will increase productivity. Every successful surgeon whom I know, who has enjoyed long-term productivity, has a passionate hobby. A continual preoccupation with only medical issues stunts personal growth, hampers relationships, and hinders physicians from achieving a realistic view of the world. Sporting events, art exhibits, concerts, plays, and events outside of medicine all help shift attention from draining wounds or litigious patients. Hobbies and interests help us to experience all that life has to offer and gain perspective. An appreciation of beauty in all its forms and acknowledging the concept of creativity help orthopaedic surgeons view the world differently.

Summary

For lasting energy and resiliency, it is necessary to choose high-octane values that sustain us rather than drain us. These values are in accordance with a moral center, with something bigger than us. Only by aligning ourselves with our source, or ultimate energy repository, will we retain a positive energy balance. True long-term fulfillment and happiness can only be attained when we live our lives the right way and reflect on the greater good—the higher calling. A loving, forgiving, and service-oriented spirit will enable an orthopaedic surgeon to accomplish more good works than ever could be imagined.

References

1. Maslach C, Leither MP: *The Truth About Burnout.* San Fransisco, CA, Jossey-Bass Publishers, 1997, pp 13-15.
2. Balch CM, Freischlag JA, Shanafelt TD: Stress and burnout among surgeons: Understanding and managing the syndrome and avoiding the adverse consequences. *Arch Surg* 2009;144(4): 371-376.
3. Spickard A Jr, Gabbe SG, Christensen JF: Mid-career burnout in generalist and specialist physicians. *JAMA* 2002;288(12): 1447-1450.

4. Sullivan P, Buske L: Results from CMA's huge 1998 physician survey point to a dispirited profession. *CMAJ* 1998;159(5):525-528.
5. McMurray JE, Linzer M, Konrad TR, et al: The work lives of women physicians results from the physician work life study. *J Gen Intern Med* 2000;15(6):372-380.
6. Saleh KJ, Quick JC, Conaway M, et al: The prevalence and severity of burnout among academic orthopaedic departmental leaders. *J Bone Joint Surg Am* 2007;89(4): 896-903.
7. Covey SR: *Seven Habits of Highly Effective People.* New York, NY, Free Press, 1989, p 71.
8. Freeborn DK: Satisfaction, commitment, and psychological well-being among HMO physicians. *West J Med* 2001;174(1):13-18.
9. Gabbard GO: The role of compulsiveness in the normal physician. *JAMA* 1985;254(20):2926-2929.
10. Osler W: Address to students of the Albany Medical College, February 1, 1899. *Albany Med Ann* 1899;20:307-309.
11. Sargent MC, Sotile W, Sotile MO, Rubash H, Barrack RL: Quality of life during orthopaedic training and academic practice: Part 1. Orthopaedic surgery residents and faculty. *J Bone Joint Surg Am* 2009;91(10):2395-2405.
12. Baruch-Feldman C, Brondolo E, Ben-Dayan D, Schwartz J: Sources of social support and burnout, job satisfaction, and productivity. *J Occup Health Psychol* 2000;7(1):84-93.
13. Shanafelt TD, Bradley KA, Wipf JE, Back AL: Burnout and self-reported patient care in an internal medicine residency program. *Ann Intern Med* 2002; 136(5): 358-367.
14. Firth-Cozens J, Greenhalgh J: Doctors' perceptions of the links between stress and lowered clinical care. *Soc Sci Med* 1997;44(7): 1017-1022.
15. Haas JS, Cook EF, Puopolo AL, Burstin HR, Cleary PD, Brennan TA: Is the professional satisfaction of general internists associated with patient satisfaction? *J Gen Intern Med* 2000;15(2): 122-128.
16. Crane M: Why burned-out doctors get sued more often. *Med Econ* 1998;75(10):210-218.
17. Christensen JB: Spirituality in everyday life. *West J Med* 2001; 174(1):75-76.
18. Epstein RM: Mindful practice. *JAMA* 1999;282(9):833-839.
19. Epstein RM: Just being. *West J Med* 2001;174(1):63-65.
20. Burns D: *The Feeling Good Handbook.* New York, NY, Plume Publishers, 1999.
21. Stack S, Eshleman JR: Marital status and happiness: A 17-nation study. *J Marriage Fam* 1998; 60(2):527-536.
22. Martin TC, Bumpass LL: Recent trends in marital disruption. *Demography* 1989;26(1):37-51.
23. Markman HJ, Stanley SM, Blumberg SL: *Fighting for Your Marriage: Positive Steps for Preventing Divorce and Preserving a Lasting Love.* Hoboken, NJ, Jossey-Bass, 2001.
24. Warde CM, Moonesinghe K, Allen W, Gelberg L: Marital and parental satisfaction of married physicians with children. *J Gen Intern Med* 1999;14(3):157-165.
25. Hendrix H: *Getting the Love You Want: A Guide for Couples,* ed 20. New York, NY, Henry Holt, 2007.
26. Waite LJ, Gallagher M: *The Case for Marriage.* New York, NY, Broadway Books, 2000.
27. Ramachandran VS: Mirror neurons and imitation learning as the driving force behind "the great leap forward" in human evolution. *Edge* Website. http://www.edge.org/3rd_culture/ramachandran/ramachandran_p1.html. Accessed May 19, 2010.
28. Sotile WM, Sotile MD: *The Resilient Physician: Effective Emotional Management for Doctors and Their Medical Organizations.* Chicago, IL, American Medical Association Press, 2001.
29. Albom M: *Tuesdays with Morrie.* New York, NY, Random House, 1997.
30. Farber S: *The Radical Leap.* Chicago, IL, Dearborn Trade Publishing, 2004.

Stress Management and Balance for the Orthopaedic Surgeon: Mindfulness

James C. Esch, MD

Abstract

Orthopaedic surgeons work in an environment in which decisions must be made in the moment, day-to-day, often with insufficient information and sometimes with immense uncertainty. Surgeons must discern patterns within the unfolding events of patient interviews or in the course of surgery. These patterns must be related to past experience, intuition, weighing the odds, and weighing the benefits and risks. To make these judgment calls, orthopaedic surgeons need ever-present awareness and integrity; they need the ability to embrace mindfulness, or to live in the moment. By tending to the moments of their lives, surgeons can be "in" the moment rather than carelessly letting it drift by. The practice of mindfulness dramatically reduces stress, worry, and regret and replaces these negative reactions with a vibrant awareness, joy, and enthusiasm, which are medicinal and spiritual.

Instr Course Lect 2011:60:627-631.

Taking a Fresh Look at Life to Attain Peaceful Living

In 1968 and 1969, I was a Mobile Army Surgical Hospital (MASH) surgeon in Da Nang, Vietnam. I had just finished my orthopaedic residency training when I was drafted in the doctor draft. With dizzying swiftness, I left my home and three children and found myself in downtown Da Nang. The foreign acrid smell, the depressing scene, and the fear and loneliness that swept over me with the realization that I would not see my family for a year are as vivid and unsettling today as they were then. But over the course of time, I learned to cope with the situation. I lived in a hooch with three other orthopaedic surgeons, and we became good friends. For 365 days, I cleaned wounds, watched as body bags were removed from helicopters, read books, quit smoking, wrote home, and even worked on my suntan. I learned to jog.

One day while jogging, I had a realization and jogged back to share my reflection with my friends. In a surprising moment for the four of us, we realized that our lives were not as bad as we had believed. All we really required was food, shelter, and a few friends—basic needs. From that moment on, we accepted our situation. We did not like it, but we were not suffering. Doing what was at hand? Could it actually be that simple?

Living in the Moment

Mindfulness is "living in the moment." It is about remaining calm, cool, and collected—whether one is sprawled out by a slowly flowing stream or in the throes of performing complex surgery. The very existence of orthopaedic surgeons is beset with endless distractions and tough decisions. We are inundated with phone calls to return, patients and operating rooms to schedule, partners to appease, and insurance companies to placate; and just when it seems we can finally go home to a reheated supper, we are called to the emergency department. Orthopaedic surgeons may sometimes feel frustrated by the lack of value that others assign to the time and energy that must be dedicated to education and work.

Multitasking Is Stressful

Orthopaedic surgeons become accustomed to multitasking but may neglect

Dr. Esch or an immediate family member has received royalties from Breg; is a member of a speakers' bureau or has made paid presentations on behalf of Smith & Nephew; serves as an unpaid consultant to Smith & Nephew and KFX Medical; and has stock or stock options held in KFX Medical.

to consider the stress such divided attention can place on their daily activities and equilibrium. A handy litmus test for just how much we divide our interests is to ask ourselves a few questions. Do I find myself listening to a patient while thinking of someone or something else? Am I rushing through my office or surgery schedule to make it to my next appointment? Am I constantly checking my smartphone for messages and answering e-mails? Do I use Twitter often? Do I find myself during the day thinking about what I am going to do after work? Do I often struggle to remain focused on the job at hand?

The answer to these questions is usually yes. The antidote begins with the ability to focus. The ability to focus may not come naturally to curious human creatures, although a youngster's fascination with a butterfly or an inchworm making its way through the grass might indicate otherwise. As we grow older and our distractions grow in number and seeming importance, focus is more likely a skill (or an art) that is acquired through intention and practice.

Ways to Maintain Focus

I find it easier to encourage and maintain focus if I do these things: (1) Read books on life, spirituality, success, and stress. (2) Control my office and the surgery environment so that I have time to see patients. This may require extending my office hours so that fewer patients are scheduled each hour. (3) Pursue friendships. As St Thomas Aquinas said, "Friendship is the source of the greatest pleasures, and without friends even the most agreeable pursuits become tedious."[1] (4) Reserve time every day to walk and exercise. (5) Meditate or write in my journal 10 to 20 minutes each day on some spiritual concept, a current stressor, or a thought or quote that enables me to get through the day. It takes a conscious decision and daily discipline to meditate or write in a journal until the day that meditating or writing becomes a working part of daily life. (6) Pursue some sort of spiritual group that meets regularly. This may vary from joining a book study group to attending regular spiritual meetings to going on retreats. The quiet that can be found on a retreat is the reason why spiritually minded men and women and mystics retreat to the mountains or to the desert to practice listening and awareness. It can be difficult not to talk, and listening requires an even greater effort for some people; thus, an environment that encourages such practices is helpful.

Befriend the Present Moment

The goal is to befriend the present moment and remain loyal to it. Just what does that mean and how is it done? First, it must be remembered that all we really have is the present—the moment at hand. Everything else is a summary or judgment on what has already occurred or a conjecture on what might be. It behooves us to truly live in the moment and to do so with excitement and joy.

This concept is complicated. Life is both sturdy and fragile. People we love die. Some do not have idyllic childhoods. As bittersweet as it can be, however, it is our perception of what has happened or is happening that colors our days rather than the facts. If I can be grateful for all the people I have loved and lost or for the many lessons learned the hard way, I can truly make the present moment my friend; by so doing, I can create room for joy and enthusiasm to sway the day.

For example, many orthopaedic surgeons both love and bemoan the game of golf. We crave the morning dew on the fairways, the jostling, the camaraderie, and that little white ball disappearing into the cup. But if one stays in the moment and allows excitement and joy to be their caddies, it is a good round—no matter the outcome. This holds true in everything I do, whether meditating, writing in my journal, reading a book, spending time with my children, performing surgery, or seeing patients in the office.

The present—this moment—is all that we have. It is best to make the moment our friend and ally. If we always fight off the present with thoughts of what is ahead or what just happened, we miss living. To be in a perpetually mindful state is to be alert, attentive, careful, and aware.

Mindful Awareness

Mindful awareness is the moment-by-moment process of actively and openly observing our mental, physical, and emotional experiences. These experiences must be "observed," without a constant stream of internal comment or judgment. This moment-by-moment process of actively observing our experiences is a form of meditation that bears fruit: a sense of well-being, lower blood pressure, and a growing sense of peace and wellness in life.

In his book on the healing power of meditation, Weiss[2] states that if we are mindful of the present moment, we develop concentration and focus. We gain insight and wisdom. This is the key to happiness—for us and for others. Thich Nhat Hanh,[3] a Vietnamese Buddhist monk, says, "The most precious gift we can offer others is our presence. When mindfulness embraces those we love, they will bloom like flowers." This inspiring image is true. At times, all physicians have experienced it when tending to patients. We are 100% in the moment with our patients, and they trust our reassurance implicitly. They do, in fact, seem to "bloom" right before our eyes.

When we learn to bring mindfulness into every moment of our lives, special things happen. Sports broadcasters speak of mindfulness as "being in the zone." So many times, in an interview, perhaps after a great game, a basketball player describes the hoop as looking as large as a bushel basket, or the quarterback says the receiver looked as if nobody was around him as he completed pass after pass.

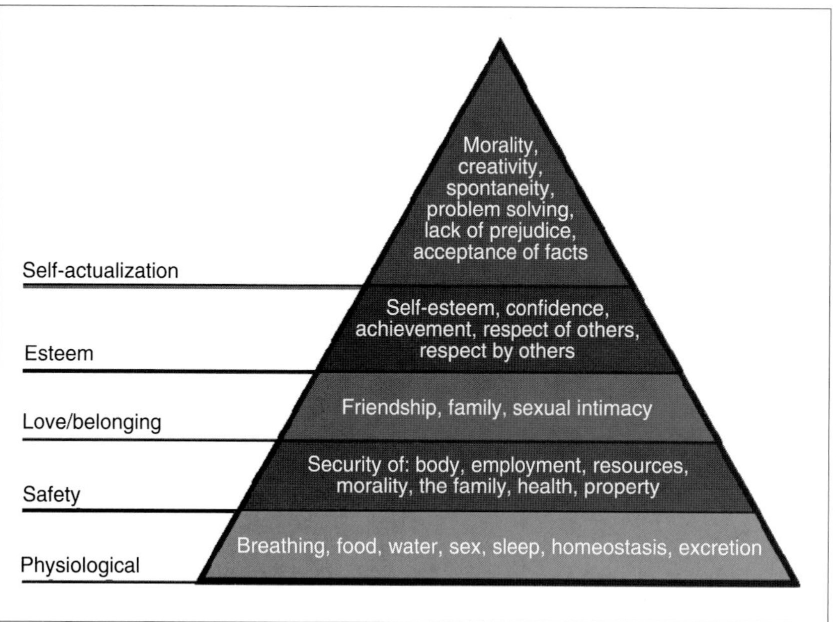

Figure 1 Maslow's hierarchy of needs. (Reproduced with permission from Wikipedia, http://en.wikipedia.org.)

Seeking Balance

Living in the moment is easier when living a balanced life, which can be difficult to achieve. Thinking of our days as residents will remind us of how seemingly impossible it can be to achieve balance. However, balance is possible with intention. Balance not only involves managing the use of time and energy at the office but also balancing time with family, travel, financial management, and living within one's means. Much of an orthopaedic surgeon's stress in these times of decreasing reimbursement may be related to being unable or unwilling to reduce expenses.

I do not believe we necessarily need to be in balance at all times. We just need to seek balance. In the *Book of Understanding*, the philosopher Osho[4] states: "Balance cannot be cultivated. Balance is something that comes out of experiencing all the dimensions of life. Balance is something that happens. It is not something that can be brought about by your efforts."

Maslow's Pyramid

Most physicians are familiar with Maslow's pyramid showing the hierarchy of human needs[5] (**Figure 1**). The base of the pyramid consists of basic needs, including shelter, sleep, and sex. Higher levels include safety and security, then love, belonging, and self-esteem. At the pinnacle of the pyramid is self-actualization, which is an elegant, essential blend of vitality, self-sufficiency, playfulness, and meaningfulness. We have all experienced or witnessed that without a secure base, we find ourselves in an unstable situation. I felt this instability when I first went to Da Nang, at other times when worry predominated, or when I momentarily lost sight of being grateful for my many responsibilities. In such times, we need a friend or the wisdom of a mentor.

Mentors

In his classic text, *Essay on Man*, Pope writes, "Thou wert my guide, philosopher and friend."[6] We need not travel alone. Much that I have gleaned in this life and included in this chapter has come by way of friends, authors, teachers, and advisors—those I have chosen to be my mentors. Some of these relationships grew from admiration and from my fervent wish to follow examples of good doctoring, office management, citizenship, success on the green, and the pursuit of a spiritual life. When you observe someone who is calm in crises or has skills you crave to possess, it is wise to ask, "How do you do that?" Asking such a question can yield lifelong guidance and friendship.

Mentoring gives away what has been given. My mentors include those brave souls who write books that speak to my heart and aspirations. Like others, I have sought answers to life's big questions in the work of Eckhart Tolle, a contemporary spiritual teacher who is not aligned with any particular religion or tradition. He has written several popular books, including *The Power of Now: A Guide to Spiritual Enlightenment* and *A New Earth: Awakening to Your Life's Purpose.* Many quotations from Tolle are quite helpful for daily living. Tolle tells us, "You are not your personal history, you are not your story."[7] If I am not an orthopaedic surgeon, not a member of the American Academy of Orthopaedic Surgeons, not the father of my children, not a golfer, then who am I? Tolle says not to define yourself by the things you do or who you think you are. This brings up basic philosophic questions. "Who am I? Where do I fit in the overall scheme of time and the universe? Another quotation from Tolle says, "No matter what has happened to you in the past, it has brought you to this moment now."[7] In this light, I am not where I was yesterday or this morning. I am here now, writing this. In time, reading these words, this is where you are. Both of these quotations ask that we decide if we are going to focus on our past stories or compose new stories in our lives; whether we (right now) are going to be grateful and enthusiastic—or not.

Breathing Is Helpful

Tolle offers this suggestion, "Being aware of your breathing takes away from thinking and creates space. It is one way of generating consciousness."[7] Breathing distracts you from your ego, which may be telling that you are a great surgeon who takes good care of your patients or reminds you of the multitude of obligations you must fulfill before settling down for a peaceful evening.

What Is Your Retirement Dollar Number?

To be truly in the moment, I cannot look to the hours ahead for peace, or next week, or even when I retire. If I do, peace will never find me. Thinking of tomorrow or the past keeps me from living in the present. In *The Number: A Completely Different Way to Think About the Rest of Your Life,*[8] Eisenberg speaks about interviewing people who are retired. I initially believed that this was a book about financial planning for retirement, about people "making their number." It turns out there really is no number. Everyone has his or her own dollar number that will permit retirement; however, almost everyone interviewed in the book was seeking fulfillment that lies beyond the financial realm.

Ego

Our ego causes us to seek attention and demand recognition. Ego is talking about our problems, telling stories about our illness, making a scene, providing an opinion when our advice is not sought, showing off our possessions. Ego makes us perpetually more concerned with how others see us, rather than being concerned with them.

The Essence

The essence of mindfulness is to befriend the present moment. Take deep breaths and enjoy the spaces between your deep breaths. Become aware of the space, the precious moments, between surgeries, golf shots, each step when walking, or whatever is being done. Try to find the inner peace in what is being done. This will not turn you into a procrastinator. You can still be a person of action planning a shoulder assessment, composing a book chapter, or preparing for a golf shot.

Learning to focus the mind can be a helpful antidote to the stresses and strains of our on-the-go lives. Mindfulness is the ability to pay attention to what you are experiencing moment to moment without drifting into thoughts of the past or concerns of the future or getting caught up in the opinions about what is going on. In an everyday sense, mindfulness means striving to bring a focused, nonjudgmental awareness to usual routines. Many people believe that the practice of meditation enhances everyday mindfulness.

Mindfulness Is Healthy

A questionnaire was developed by University of Rochester psychologists and administered to 1,500 people. Results showed that higher scorers on the Mindfulness Attention Awareness Scale were correlated with the established measurements of well-being, including better mood, optimism, openness to new experiences, and greater satisfaction with life.[9]

Much research on mindfulness also has been performed by the mindfulness-based Stress Reduction Clinic of the Massachusetts Medical School.[10] This program incorporated training in meditation to increase mindfulness during daily activities and discussions with other participants. Focusing attention on what you are experiencing from moment to moment is a daunting challenge in a hectic world, but science has begun to establish that it is a worthwhile habit to cultivate.

Summary

Mindfulness is bringing alertness or awareness to every moment during the day. Mindfulness will make life in the office, in the operating room, and at home more fruitful, more productive, and happier. The following poem by an anonymous author sums up the importance of mindfulness.

First I was dying to finish my high school and start college.
And then I was dying to marry and have children.
And then I was dying for my children to grow old enough so I could go back to work.
But then I was dying to retire.
And now I am dying.
And suddenly I realized,
I forgot to live.

References

1. Durepos J: *The Grandeur of God: Selections From Two Thousand Years of Catholic Spiritual Writing.* Chicago, IL, Loyola Press, p 36.
2. Weiss G: *The Healing Power of Meditation: Your Prescription for Getting Well and Staying Well With Meditation.* Laguna Beach, CA, Basic Health Publications, 2008.

3. Thich Nhat Hanh quotes. Think Exist Website. http://www.thinkexist.com/English/Author/x/Author_4223_2.htm. Accessed April 10, 2010.
4. Osho: *The Book of Understanding*. New York, NY, Harmony Books, 2006.
5. Maslow AH: *Toward a Psychology of Being*, ed 3. Hoboken, NJ, Wiley, 1998.
6. Pope A: *Essay on Man*. Epistle IV, line 390.
7. Tolle E: *A New Earth: Awakening to Your Life's Purpose*. London, England, Plume, 2006.
8. Eisenberg L: *The Number: A Completely Different Way to Think About the Rest of Your Life*. New York, NY, Free Press, 2006.
9. Brown KW, Ryan RM: The benefits of being present: Mindfulness and its role in psychological well-being. *J Pers Soc Psychol* 2003; 84(4):822-848.
10. Kabat-Zinn J: *Coming to Our Senses: Healing Ourselves and the World Through Mindfulness*. New York, NY, Hyperion Books, 2005.

Index

Page numbers with *f* indicate figures
Page numbers with *t* indicate tables

B

C

D

E

F

H

I

J

K

N

O

Q

R

S

T

W

Y

Z